Laser Therapy in Veterinary Medicine

Laser Therapy in Veterinary Medicine

Photobiomodulation

Second Edition

Edited by Christopher J. Winkler and Lisa A. Miller

WILEY

Published by John Wiley & Sons, Inc., Hoboken, New Jersey.
Published simultaneously in Canada.

Library of Congress Cataloging-in-Publication Data:
Names: Winkler, Christopher J., 1973– editor. | Miller, Lisa A. DVM, editor.
Title: Laser therapy in veterinary medicine : photobiomodulation / edited by Christopher J. Winkler and Lisa A. Miller.
Description: Second edition. | Hoboken, New Jersey : Wiley-Blackwell, [2025] | Includes bibliographical references and index.
Identifiers: LCCN 2024031882 (print) | LCCN 2024031883 (ebook) | ISBN 9781394205325 (hardback) | ISBN 9781394205332 (adobe pdf) | ISBN 9781394205349 (epub)
Subjects: MESH: Laser Therapy–veterinary | Low-Level Light Therapy–veterinary
Classification: LCC SF745 (print) | LCC SF745 (ebook) | NLM SF 745 | DDC 636.089/7058–dc23/eng/20240909
LC record available at https://lccn.loc.gov/2024031882
LC ebook record available at https://lccn.loc.gov/2024031883

Cover image: Courtesy of Kaitlan Hovis
Cover design: Wiley

Set in 9.5/12.5pt STIXTwoText by Straive, Pondicherry, India

Printed in Singapore
M008879280426

Dedication and Acknowledgments

This book is dedicated with deep appreciation to Ronald J. Riegel and John C. Godbold Jr. for all their previous hard work and efforts, the groundwork they have laid, their contributions to this work and to the field of veterinary medicine, and especially for the inspiration they so willingly and freely share with others.

We would like to thank the extraordinary efforts of our authors, experts, and their staffs for their distinct contributions to the subject of veterinary photobiomodulation. This past year has been a wonderfully illuminating education in each of your fields, and we are very proud and grateful for the privilege of presenting your brilliant work to our readers. It has been the greatest of pleasures collaborating with you. A heartfelt Thank You to you all.

To our editors, Vallikkannu Narayanan, Erica Judish, and Susan Engelken, for all your advice and assistance.

To my co-editor, Lisa Miller. I could not have done this without you. Words cannot express how much I admire your talent, your dedication, or my great appreciation for how synergistically we were able to complete this work together. May it not be our last.

To my family, friends, and colleagues for their support, especially to my parents, Nancy and Joseph, who taught me the value of a well-written word, and taught compassion and love by example. To my children, John and Kevin, who will forever remain my greatest endeavor, and to Nicole, my beloved wife and companion in this our adventure together. I love you all very much.

For Jack.

—Christopher

To my family, friends, and colleagues, thank you for your support and understanding for all the weekends of turned-down plans and late nights of working on this book. To my co-editor, Chris Winkler who is one of the most knowledgeable and kindest human beings I have met, and who kept the train on the tracks. To Dr. Juanita Anders, for being a pioneer and queen in the photobiomodulation world and for mentoring and guiding many of us. Lastly, to my colleagues who continue to inspire me daily with their innovation, passion, and dedication to the field of veterinary medicine; I thank you all.

Ad Astra Per Aspera.

—Lisa

Contents

Biography

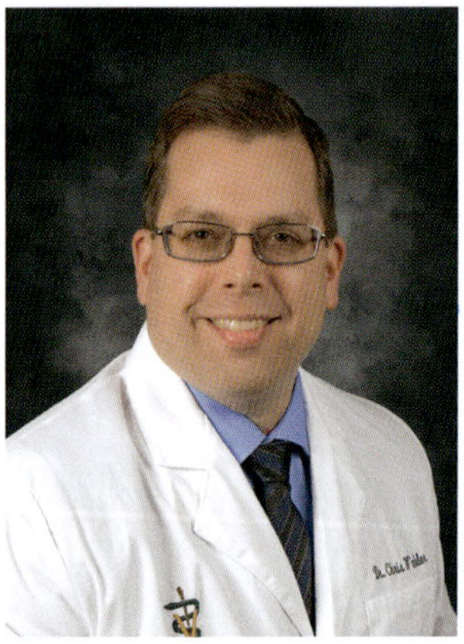

Christopher J. Winkler, DVM graduated from Ross University School of Veterinary Medicine in 2001, and worked on Long Island, New York, as an emergency room veterinarian and associate general practitioner before purchasing Suffolk Veterinary Group in 2006. Incorporating surgical and therapy lasers into his practice in 2010, he began formal training a short time later, earning certifications in Veterinary Laser Medicine and Surgery from the American Board of Laser Surgery (ABLS) in 2015, and Veterinary Medical Laser Safety Officer from the American Institute of Medical Laser Applications (AIMLA) in 2016.

Dr. Winkler has spoken on laser surgery and laser therapy and served as an associate laser surgery wet-lab instructor for a number of national veterinary conferences, including the NAVC, AVMA, the WVC, the Great Smokies Veterinary Conference, and the Colonial Veterinary Conference. He has also conducted webinars on laser therapy and laser safety for veterinary technicians and Ross University students, and published articles on laser surgery for Veterinary Practice News. He is a member of the American Society for Laser Medicine and Surgery (ASLMS), and is a Fellow and Faculty member of both the American Laser Medicine College and Board (ALMCB) and the American Laser Study Club (ALSC), for which he also sits on the editorial board of its journal. Dr. Winkler is editor and coauthor of the textbook *Laser Surgery in Veterinary Medicine* (Wiley-Blackwell, 2019), and he is the recipient of the 2021 Kumar C. Patel prize for outstanding contributions to veterinary laser surgery education. He receives referrals from and trains veterinarians locally and nationally on laser surgery and laser therapy procedures, continues to advise educating bodies on veterinary laser curricula, and offers his services as a laser consultant to veterinarians and equipment manufacturers.

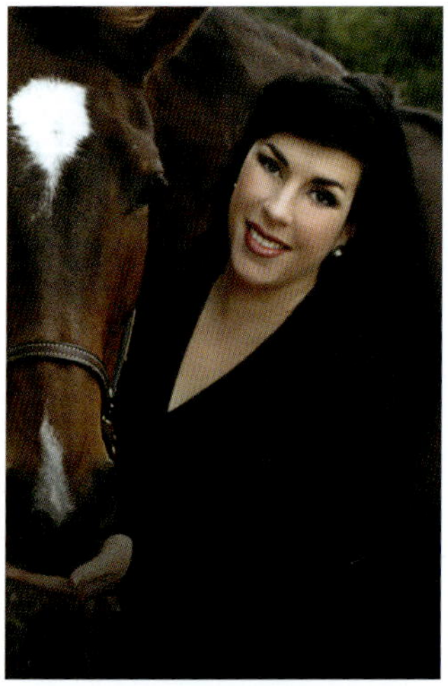

Dr. Lisa A. Miller is the vice president of Clinical Veterinary Medicine for Companion Animal Health and is a graduate of the University of Tennessee, College of Veterinary Medicine. After graduation, Dr. Miller completed an internship in internal medicine and then became certified in canine rehabilitation therapy. Working in a large referral hospital, she practiced rehabilitation, sports medicine, and acupuncture for several years before returning to general practice and later, joining the animal health industry.

Dr. Miller has been working with laser therapy/photobiomodulation (PBM) since 2006. She has lectured worldwide and led workshops on laser therapy and rehabilitation-related topics, including lectures at Western Veterinary Conference, VMX, the London Vet Show, Southern European Veterinary Conference, American Society of Laser Medicine & Surgery Conference, and Laser Florence. She has authored numerous research papers, articles, and chapters on PBM in veterinary practice. Her publications have appeared in *Photobiomodulation, Photomedicine, and Laser Surgery*, *Journal of Nanotechnology*

Research, Frontiers in Veterinary Science, Clinician's Brief, Integrative Veterinary Care, Today's Veterinary Practice, and the first edition of the textbook *Laser Therapy in Veterinary* Medicine. In her current role, she coordinates all veterinary and advanced PBM research involving Companion Animal Health technologies and is a consultant and reviewer for PBM research worldwide. Dr. Miller is a member of the American Veterinary Medical Association (AVMA), the American Association of Rehabilitation Veterinarians (AARV), the American Society of Laser Medicine & Surgery (ASLMS), and the World Association of Laser Therapy (WALT).

Contributing Author List

Steve Adair, MS, DVM, DACVS, DACVSMR
Department of Large Animal Clinical Science
University of Tennessee
College of Veterinary Medicine
Knoxville, TN, USA

João C. Alves, DVM, PhD, DECVSMR
Clinica Veterinária de Cães, Guarda Nacional Republicana
Lisbon, Portugal

Juanita J. Anders, PhD
Edward Hebert School of Medicine
Uniformed Services University of the Health Sciences
Bethesda, MD, USA

David S. Bradley, DVM, FASLMS
Veterinary Medical Director
Summus Medical Laser
Franklin, TN, USA

Micah C. Brodsky, VMD
Pono Scientific
Kaneohe, Hawaii, USA

Matthew W. Brunke, DVM, DACVSMR, CCAT, Fellow IAVRPT
Veterinary Referral Associates (VRAVet.com)
Gaithersburg, MD, USA

Liza Dadone, VMD
Giraffe Veterinary Services
Colorado Springs, CO, USA

Richard L. Godine, DVM
North American Association for Light Therapy
Ruckersville Animal Hospital and Veterinary
Laser Therapy Center
Ruckersville, VA, USA

Tara Harrison, DVM, MPVM, DACZM, DACVPM, DECZM (Zoo Health Management), CVA
North Carolina State College of Veterinary Medicine
Raleigh, NC, USA

Renaud "Ren" Houyoux, CVT, LVT, CVDT, VNA, VMLSO
Heartland Veterinary Partners
Chicago, IL, USA

Michael H. Jaffe, DVM, MS, CCRP, DACVS
Department of Small Animal Surgery
Mississippi State University
College of Veterinary Medicine
Mississippi State, MS, USA

Ann K. Ketz, PhD, RN
Recovery Sciences, Enovis
Lewisville, TX, USA

Ronald B. Koh, DVM, MS, DACVSMR, CVA, CCRV, CCRP, CVMMP, CVCH, CVFT
School of Veterinary Medicine
University of California, Davis, CA, USA

David Levine, PT, PhD, DPT, MPH, CCRP, FAPTA
Department of Physical Therapy
The University of Tennessee at Chattanooga
Chattanooga, TN, USA

Jörg Mayer, DVM, MS, DABVP (ECM), DECZM (Small Mammal)
Department of Small Animal Medicine and Surgery
University of Georgia
Athens, GA, USA

Diane J. Miller, MBA
The Animal Athlete
Newark, DE, USA

Lisa A. Miller, DVM, CCRT, CVA
Companion Animal Health
New Castle, DE, USA

Robert D. Ness, DVM
Ness Exotic Wellness Center
Lilse, IL, USA

Erin O'Leary, DVM
HEAL Mobile Laser Therapy
Cary, NC, USA

Michael C. Petty, DVM
Dogtor Consulting
Plymouth, MI, USA

Ronald J. Riegel, DVM
American Institute of Medical Laser Applications
Marysville, OH, USA

Julie Gard Schnuelle, DVM, PhD, DACT, BS
Professor Emeritus
Auburn University College of Veterinary Medicine
Auburn, AL, USA

Bryan J. Stephens, PhD
Multi Radiance Medical
Thompsons Station, TN, USA

Ashton B. Thompson, DVM, CCRP, cVMA
Companion Animal Health
New Castle, DE, USA

Deborah Gross Torraca, DPT, MSPT, DABPTS, CCRP, Fellow IAVRPT
Wizard of Paws Rehabilitation for Animals
Colchester, CT, USA

Chelsea Tripp, DVM, MS, DACVIM (O)
Bridge Animal Referral Center
Edmonds, WA, USA

Christopher J. Winkler, DVM, DABLS, VMLSO, FALSC, FASLMS
Suffolk Veterinary Group Animal Wellness and Laser Surgery Center
Selden, NY, USA

Foreword

In mid-2015, we took deep breaths and committed to coediting the pioneering textbook about the clinical use of photobiomodulation in veterinary medicine. Despite our prior experience in writing and publishing, neither of us had any idea of the scope of the task ahead. We did not realize the effort needed to gather 37 contributing authors from academia, clinical practice, and industry, nor did we anticipate the 18-month journey of editing 43 chapters covering nearly 500 pages. Regardless, the contributions of those chapter authors became the award-winning textbook *Laser Therapy in Veterinary Medicine: Photobiomodulation*.

The chapters on the history, theory, and science of photobiomodulation helped establish the credibility of therapeutic laser use. The chapters on clinical applications made the book a practical clinical reference across the full spectrum of veterinary practice. For the first time, a reliable, comprehensive, and evidence-based resource had been developed to provide practical insights into clinical veterinary photobiomodulation.

Even prior to the release of that first edition, we anticipated the rapid advancements in technology and the emergence of new research and clinical applications that would necessitate a second edition. Since its initial publication in 2017, the landscape of veterinary photobiomodulation therapy has evolved significantly, underscored by the publication of over 150 peer-reviewed articles. These developments have enriched our understanding of the conditions amenable to photobiomodulation therapy and refined our approach to its delivery.

With the aim of bringing new insight, energy, and perspective to *Laser Therapy in Veterinary Medicine: Photobiomodulation,* we engaged two gifted colleagues to coedit the second edition, Dr. Chris Winkler, and Dr. Lisa Miller. As coeditors, Chris and Lisa have again marshaled dozens of gifted contributing authors, authored chapters themselves, and overseen bringing veterinary medicine a new, up-to-date, and valuable resource for clinical photobiomodulation therapy.

Drs. Winkler and Miller have over 30 years of combined experience with therapeutic lasers. Both have general and specialty practice experience, as well as years of contributing to photobiomodulation therapy continuing education, research, and publication about the technology. Currently, Chris remains in general practice and Lisa is the vice president of Clinical Veterinary Medicine for Companion Animal Health. Their backgrounds and experiences, and their roles as leading experts on veterinary photobiomodulation, combine to bring the profession this valuable second edition.

While updating previous information in this book, Chris and Lisa continued to focus solely on photobiomodulation and the diagnostic technologies that support it. More complete and up-to-date information regarding dosing and treatment parameters is included. They make this edition usable by readers in a diversity of clinical settings since the information presented is not confined to specific techniques or equipment. Treatment procedures and protocols are provided in generic, noncommercially specific ways.

The editors include new chapters addressing urinary conditions, oncological applications, photobiomodulation in the critical care setting, and use for working dogs. Additionally, there is a new chapter on the use of thermal imaging to target photobiomodulation treatment areas and monitor response to therapy.

This second edition is now the definitive resource for veterinary students, general practitioners, specialists, and those involved in the continued development of new veterinary therapeutic laser devices. We thank the chapter authors, Chris and Lisa, for significantly improving our first edition. We are confident this text will prove to be an invaluable addition to readers' libraries, facilitating continued growth and excellence in the field of veterinary photobiomodulation therapy. It will be a well-used addition to our own libraries.

John C. Godbold, Jr., D.V.M.
Jackson, Tennessee

Ronald J. Riegel., D.V.M.
Marysville, Ohio

Preface

The United Nations fortuitously proclaimed 2015 as the International Year of Light and Light-Based Technologies. This seemed most apropos to me at the time, for it would also be the year I would begin to meet and work with many of the luminaries of veterinary laser medicine and surgery.

Having just finished a year of study and certification on the subject, I was then looking forward to my first conference of the American Society for Laser Medicine and Surgery. While there, I attended lectures on laser therapy delivered by Dr. Juanita Anders and Dr. Praveen Arany. It was at these that I first heard the word "photobiomodulation," and as I listened, I had the distinct sense of being present at an important milestone in science and medicine, the introduction of a new term and definition to our lexicon.

Another of those luminaries lecturing that week was Dr. Ron Riegel, one of several veterinarians speaking about laser applications in veterinary medicine. It was the first of many such lectures I have since heard from Dr. Riegel, and after bearing witness numerous times to his extensive expertise, his infectious exuberance, and his appreciable passion for this field, it came as absolutely no surprise to me that he would later go on with my first and most notable laser teacher, Dr. John C. Godbold Jr., to create the first edition of *Laser Therapy in Veterinary Medicine*.

The surprise came later when they both asked me to create the second edition.

Seeking assistance, I welcomed Dr. Godbold's recommendation of Dr. Lisa Miller. I had heard Dr. Miller speak at an American Institute of Medical Laser Applications function on the use of laser therapy for osteoarthritis, and from Dr. Godbold's confident description of her expertise, I knew she would be exactly what this project needed.

Our ideas for a second edition text were congruent from the beginning. We wanted to see the first edition text respected while also being updated with as much new information as possible. Indeed, the reader will note hundreds of new references, the majority of which are dated after the first edition's publication. We sought in this update to focus solely on photobiomodulation and the diagnostic technology that supports it, make it approachable and clinically usable by readers globally without specifically being beholden to singular techniques or equipment, and continue to provide more complete dose and parameter recommendations than previously available.

We wished to continue to push the envelope and offer better patient care as well as encourage both laser researchers and laser manufacturers to move forward with studies that challenge previous thoughts and technology innovations. We also wanted to add new content (particularly regarding veterinary oncology) while prompting our veterinary colleagues to continue to think outside the box, to consider treating new patients or conditions they may not have previously considered treating, and to utilize that same "veterinary ingenuity" that first interested them in this modality to begin with – something that John C. Godbold Jr. would always value and emphasize in his lectures. Colloquially (for now, anyway), while the first edition might say, "Never shine it in their eyes," this second edition would now say, "Don't shine it in their eyes – not yet."

The history of photobiomodulation research and clinical application is rather unfortunately marked by a plethora of underdosed and poorly or incorrectly reported parameters. It is for this reason that we further wish to encourage those desiring to perform research within the veterinary community to reach out to colleagues in the photobiomodulation world and learn more about how to optimally execute and report parameters with this exciting and effective modality, so that we can all continue to improve our knowledge base and optimize outcomes for our patients without repeating research and reporting mistakes of the past.

We certainly look forward with anticipation to exploring and discussing tomorrow's discoveries, innovations, and collaborations in future editions to come. Until then, we sincerely hope this new edition serves you well.

April 29, 2024

Christopher J. Winkler, DVM
Lisa A. Miller, DVM

Disclaimer

Please read the statements and the therapeutic protocols within this text carefully before utilizing any of this information. The information and recommendations are based on previously published scientific information and years of practice, clinical, and research experience by the contributing authors.

Knowledge about photobiomodulation (PBMT) is constantly changing through ongoing research, clinical trials, and day-to-day clinical experience. The information within this text is presented for educational purposes only and is designed to be a reference to complement formal training about laser therapy.

This text contains neither complete nor comprehensive information about any of the conditions addressed, and each condition should be evaluated on an individual basis in each patient prior to surgery. This text is not a substitute for professional advice, care, diagnosis, or treatment. It is the sole responsibility of the veterinarian, veterinary technician, veterinary assistant, and veterinary therapist to gain the knowledge and comply with all federal, national, provincial, state, and local laws regarding the use of therapeutic and surgical lasers for any condition. Dr. Christopher Winkler, Dr. Lisa Miller, all of the contributing authors of this text, and anyone involved with the publication of this text expressly disclaim any and all responsibility and legal liability for any kind of loss or risk, personal or otherwise, which is the result of the direct or indirect use or application of any of the material within this text.

Part I

The History of Laser Therapy

1

A Brief History of Laser Therapy

Christopher J. Winkler

Suffolk Veterinary Group Animal Wellness and Laser Surgery Center, Selden, NY, USA

1st Edition Contributor:

Ronald J. Riegel

American Institute of Medical Laser Applications, Marysville, OH, USA

Treatment with Light

Heliotherapy. Phototherapy. Light therapy. Cultures around the world have attributed many names to this remedy as they have practiced it in various forms over the past several millennia. Healers in Egypt and India used sunlight to treat leucoderma 3500 years ago (Hönigsmann, 2013). Physicians in Ancient Greece and Rome – including renowned Greek historian Herodotus in the sixth century BCE, and Hippocrates, the father of medicine – also realized the benefits of such therapy (Ellinger, 1957). Likewise, the Inca and Assyrian cultures worshiped the sun with the belief that it would bring them health. There are records in the Buddhist literature from around 200 CE and Chinese documentation from the tenth century recording similar therapeutic effects from light.

Niels Ryberg Finsen, a Faroese physician and scientist of Icelandic descent, is widely regarded as the original proponent of phototherapy. In 1903, he was awarded the Nobel Prize in Medicine and Physiology for the successful treatment of diseases using phototherapy, specifically lupus vulgaris, a skin infection caused by *Mycobacterium tuberculosis* (Nobel Prize, 2014b). He also famously utilized ultraviolet light to treat smallpox lesions (Nobel Lectures, 1967).

A Closer Look

In the seventeenth century, Sir Isaac Newton discovered that prisms could disassemble or separate white light into seven different visible colors, a phenomenon he described in his book *Opticks* (Newton, 1704). Newton first used the word *spectrum* (Latin for "appearance" or "apparition") while describing refracted light in 1671. Today we also use another word to describe these and other colors of light: *wavelengths.*

In 1916, Albert Einstein made several hypotheses to support his theory of relativity. Einstein proposed that an excited atom in isolation can return to a lower energy state while emitting photons, a process he termed "spontaneous emission." Other atoms will absorb such photons of the correct wavelength; causing those atoms to enter a higher-energy state and setting the stage for further spontaneous emission.

Einstein then predicted that as light passes through a substance, it stimulates the emission of more light (Hilborn, 1982). Einstein's theory hypothesized that a large collection of atoms already containing a great deal of excess energy will be ready to emit photons – photons that prefer to travel together in the same state. If one such stray photon of the correct wavelength passes by an atom already in an excited state, its presence will stimulate that atom to release its own photons early. The new photons will then travel together in the same direction as the original stray photon, with identical frequency and phase. A cascading effect could thus ensue: As the identical photons move through other atoms, ever more identical photons are emitted (Pais, 1982). Einstein termed this phenomenon "stimulated emission," postulating the theory of laser light 43 years prior to its realization.

A Momentous Device

On May 16, 1960, Theodore Maiman produced the first laser device at the Hughes Aircraft Research Laboratory in Malibu, California, using a simple flashlamp to stimulate

Laser Therapy in Veterinary Medicine: Photobiomodulation, Second Edition. Edited by Christopher J. Winkler and Lisa A. Miller.

a solid medium (a ruby rod) to emit collimated photons of coherent light. At a press conference to announce his invention, he predicted that such a light would be useful in medicine and surgery (Hecht, 2005). Maiman based his invention on Albert Einstein's explanation of stimulated emission of radiation, coupled with Charles Townes's and Arthur Schawlow's work with optical masers (Schawlow and Townes, 1958; Itzkan and Drake, 1997). The acronym LASER (Light Amplification by Stimulated Emission of Radiation) itself was first coined and recorded by Townes's graduate student Gordon Gould. Gould's subsequent struggles for recognition for his work with lasers would result in one of the most lengthy, controversial, and important patent battles in US history (Taylor, 2000). Meanwhile, advancements in the development of laser media and devices within other industries would indeed lead to new applications of lasers in medicine and surgery over the following decades.

Subsequent studies revealed that particular wavelengths of laser light could be produced by stimulating particular laser mediums. The first diode laser, utilizing coherent light emission from a gallium arsenide (GaAs) semiconductor diode, was revealed in 1962 by two groups: Robert N. Hall at the General Electric Research Center (Hall *et al.*, 1962) and Marshall Nathan at the IBM T.J. Watson Research Center (Nathan *et al.*, 1962).

In 1962, other teams at the MIT Lincoln Laboratory, Texas Instruments, and RCA Laboratories also demonstrated the emission of light and lasing in semiconductor diodes. Early in 1963, a team led by Nikolay Basov in the Soviet Union utilized GaAs lasers to achieve emission of light (Nobel Prize, 2014a).

In 1970, the first laser diode to achieve continuous-wave (CW) emission was revealed simultaneously by Zhores Alferov and his collaborators in the Soviet Union, and by Morton Panish and Izuo Hayashi in the United States (Ghatak, 2009). However, it is widely accepted that Alferov and his team reached the milestone first, and they were consequently awarded the Nobel Prize in Physics in 2000.

While many types of therapeutic lasers were in use around the world, it was not until 2002 that Class IIIb lasers gained Food and Drug Administration (FDA) approval for therapeutic purposes in the United States. These lasers are colloquially referred to as "cold lasers" or "low-level laser therapy" (LLLT) devices. They are limited to 500 mW and are considered effective in the treatment of superficial conditions. The term "cold lasers" refers to the lack of a heating effect on tissue cultures in early experiments, while the term "LLLT" helped to differentiate low-power therapeutic lasers from surgical lasers.

Class IV therapy lasers, operating in excess of 500 mW, were approved by the FDA in 2006. This was the dawn of "high-power laser therapy" (HPLT). Delivery systems and precise dosage software have evolved (over the past several decades) to allow the safe and effective delivery of 500 mW–60 W to target tissues.

An Innovative Therapy

Just a few years after the invention of the laser, Dr. Endre Mester became the first to experimentally document its healing effects. Because he used mice as his experimental model, this is also the first documented use of lasers to accelerate healing in veterinary medicine (Mester *et al.*, 1967). Considered the founding father of laser therapy for his pioneering work, Dr. Mester's experiments would also later prove that the acceleration of healing was actually a systemic event rather than merely a localized one (Perera, 1987). Mester observed a cascading effect of the healing process, motivating other researchers in Western and Eastern Europe to recognize the value of laser therapy and initiate studies of their own.

Early in the 1970s, the use of laser therapy was documented in Eastern Europe, China, and the Soviet Union; much of the early research emanates from these geographical regions. Over the next decade, the use of laser therapy spread to Western Europe and became accepted as an effective physical therapy modality (Goodson and Hunt, 1979).

Yo Cheng Zhou, an oral surgeon in China, was the first to stimulate an acupuncture point with a laser. He used laser stimulation instead of standard local anesthetic protocols during routine dental extractions. A beam from a 2.8–6.0 mW helium-neon laser apparatus (Model CW-12, Chengdu Thermometer Factory) was applied for 5 minutes before the removal of a tooth (Zhou, 1984).

From the mid-1970s to the early 1980s, laser therapy became an accepted physical therapy modality throughout Western European and several Asian countries. It finally appeared in the United States around 1977, but there were only a small number of therapists who understood its potential. Laser equipment in the United States during this time frame was limited to the 1–5 mW range, and acceptance by the medical and veterinary professions was very limited due to inconsistent clinical results. Extensive *in vitro* studies of the effects of various wavelengths of light on cell cultures was conducted throughout the 1980s and 1990s by researchers such as Dr. Tiina Karu, leading to a closer study of photoacceptors and the mechanisms of action of laser therapy (Karu, 1987). Laser therapy's association with cytochrome c oxidase and nitric oxide continues to be studied in innovative ways (Wong-Riley *et al.*, 2005).

The first Independent Institutional Review Board for Laser Acupuncture Research was established in 1993, based on research compiled by Margaret Naeser, Ph.D.,

Lic.Ac. through the Robert Wood Johnson Foundation of Princeton, New Jersey. This initiated the effort and motivation of several colleagues to compile enough current information and research to be in compliance with US FDA regulations. Dr. Naeser has since published papers on utilizing laser therapy in stroke cases (Naeser and Hamblin, 2011).

A New Name

The history of laser therapy and the development of laser therapy devices have produced confusing terminology. Multiple terms initially and rapidly sprang up to describe both this technology and its utilization, each of them often lacking adequate scope of the therapy they attempted to relate. Many such terms were more representative of the devices being used than of the therapy itself being provided.

Several associations have formed over the years to encourage scientists and practitioners to exchange knowledge and information on laser therapy. The American Society for Laser Medicine and Surgery (ASLMS), formed in 1981, was the first. It was the dream of its founders that this organization be unique and include physicians, clinicians, and outstanding researchers in the areas of biophysics, biochemistry, biomedical engineering, laser biology, and laser safety. In 1994, the World Association for Laser Therapy (WALT) was formed by combining the International Laser Therapy Association (ILTA) and the International Society for Medical Laser Applications (ISLA). The North American Association for Laser Therapy (NAALT) was established in 1998. It included the regions of Mexico, Canada, and the United States of America. In 2015, the association changed its name to the North American Association for Photobiomodulation Therapy, retaining the same acronym, NAALT. These organizations share the same common goals: improving the understanding of photobiological mechanisms, promoting research, establishing treatment and regulatory guidelines, and providing education, clinical applications, and new clinical techniques.

Recognizing that an accurate, clear, and unambiguous name was needed, 15 international participants joined in a nomenclature consensus meeting at the joint conference of NAALT and WALT in September 2014 (Anders *et al.*, 2015). Respected authorities Dr. Jan Bjordal and Dr. Juanita Anders co-chaired the meeting. The term "photobiomodulation therapy" (PBMT) was recognized as being most descriptive of a science that involves complex mechanisms, some that are stimulatory, some inhibitory. Since that meeting, the National Library of Medicine (United States) has added the term "photobiomodulation therapy" to the MeSH database (MeSH, 2016).

The committee defined the term photobiomodulation therapy as

> *"A form of light therapy that utilizes non-ionizing forms of light sources, including lasers, LEDs, and broadband light, in the visible and infrared spectrum. It is a nonthermal process involving endogenous chromophores eliciting photophysical (i.e., linear and nonlinear) and photochemical events at various biological scales. This process results in beneficial therapeutic outcomes including but not limited to the alleviation of pain or inflammation, immunomodulation, and promotion of wound healing and tissue regeneration."* (Anders et al., 2015)

Older terminology continues to be used even as photobiomodulation therapy becomes more commonplace in publications and practical applications. In this text, the terms "laser therapy" and "photobiomodulation therapy" (or simply "photobiomodulation," PBM) will be used interchangeably.

A Better Tomorrow

As thousands of veterinary practitioners around the world continue to adopt laser therapy into their practices and a wealth of evidence regarding the use and efficacy of laser therapy continues to be published, we as veterinarians should continue to be at the forefront of this scientifically and clinically proven modality. Continued collaboration and sharing of information between us is essential to the future development of this advanced medical technology. We invite you to be a part of both this distinguished history of laser therapy and the new developments within this burgeoning field, which tomorrow's veterinarians will continue to quote in the future.

References

Anders, J. *et al.* (2015). Low-level light/laser therapy versus photobiomodulation therapy. *Photomed Laser Surg.* 33(4):183–184.

Ellinger, F. (1957). *Medical Radiation Biology*. Literary Licensing, Springfield, IL.

Ghatak, A. (2009). *Optics*. Tata McGraw-Hill, New Delhi.

Goodson, W. and Hunt, T. (1979). Wound healing and the diabetic patient. *Surg Gynecol Obstet.* 149(4):600–608.

Hall, R.N. *et al.* (1962). Coherent light emission from GaAs junctions. *Phys Rev Lett.* 9(9):366–368.

Hecht, J. (2005). *Beam: The Race to Make the Laser.* Chapters 15 and 16, pp. 169–194. Oxford, University Press, New York.

Hilborn, R.C. (1982). Einstein coefficients, cross sections, f values, dipole moments, and all that. *Am J Phys.* 50(11):982.

Hönigsmann, H. (2013). History of phototherapy in dermatology. *Photochem Photobiol Sci.* 12(1):16–21. doi:10.1039/c2pp25120e PMID: 22739720.

Itzkan, I. and Drake, E. (1997). History of laser in medicine. In: *Lasers in Cutaneous and Aesthetic Surgery.* (eds. K. Arndt *et al.*), pp. 3–10. Lippincott-Raven, Philadelphia, PA.

Karu, T. (1987). Photobiological fundamentals of low-power laser therapy. *IEEE J Quantum Electron.* 23(10):1703–1717. doi:10.1109/JQE. 1987.1073236.

MeSH. (2016). Photobiomodulation. http://www.ncbi.nlm.nih.gov/mesh/?term=photobiomodulation (accessed November 30, 2016).

Mester, E. *et al.* (1967). Effect of laser on hair growth of mice. *Kiserl Orvostud.* 19:628–631.

Naeser, M. and Hamblin, M. (2011). Potential for transcranial laser or LED therapy to treat stroke, traumatic brain injury, and neurodegenerative disease. *Photomed Laser Surg.* 29(7):443–446.

Nathan, M.I. *et al.* (1962). Stimulated emission of radiation from GaAs p-n junctions. *Appl Phys Lett.* 1(3):62.

Newton, I. (1704). Opticks or, A Treatise of the Reflexions, Refractions, Inflexions and Colours of Light; also Two Treatises of the Species and Magnitude of Curvilinear Figures. Octavo, Palo Alto, CA

Nobel Lectures (1967). *Physiology or Medicine 1901–1921.* Elsevier, Amsterdam.

Nobel Prize. (2014a). Nicolay G. Basov – facts. Nobel Media AB. http://www.nobelprize.org/nobel_prizes/physics/laureates/1964/basov-facts.html (accessed November 30, 2016).

Nobel Prize. (2014b). Niels Ryberg Finsen – facts. Nobel Media AB. http://www.nobelprize.org/nobel_prizes/medicine/laureates/1903/finsen-facts.html (accessed November 30, 2016).

Pais, A. (1982). *Subtle Is the Lord: The Science and the Life of Albert Einstein.* Oxford University Press, New York.

Perera, J. (1987). The "healing laser" comes into the limelight. *New Scientist.* March 19.

Schawlow, A.L. and Townes, C.H. (1958). Principles of the optical laser. *Phys Rev Lett.* 1(1):1940–1949.

Taylor, N. (2000). *Laser (The Inventor, the Nobel Laureate, and the Thirty-Year Patent War).* Nick Taylor, Originally published by Simon and Shuster.

Wong-Riley. *et al.* (2005). Photobiomodulation directly benefits primary neurons functionally inactivated by toxins: role of cytochrome C oxidase. *J Biol Chem.* 280(6):4761–4771.

Zhou, Y. (1984). Innovations. An advanced clinical trial with laser acupuncture anesthesia for minor operations in the oro-maxillofacial region. *Lasers Surg Med.* 4(3):297–303.

Part II

The Theory and Science of Laser Therapy

2

Laser Physics in Veterinary Medicine

Bryan J. Stephens

Multi Radiance Medical, Thompsons Station, TN, USA

Introduction

Crucial to you getting the most out of the rest of this book is your understanding of some very basic properties of light. The more you understand about the complete set of characteristics of the magic that comes out of your therapy laser, the better equipped you will be to tailor your treatment protocols and enhance the clinical efficacy of your therapy. You are going to read chapters that tell you about *in vitro* experiments that demonstrate the enhancement of cellular mechanisms, followed by even more real-world data that show a broad range of clinical usefulness based on these mechanisms. Within this stockpile of evidence, there will be some basic recommendations on dose prescriptions, power settings, pulse frequency characteristics, and treatment periodicity. These will be necessarily broad, to account for patient and condition variations, but also because the parameters used throughout both the anecdotal reports and the well-controlled experiments are quite mixed. My goal in this chapter is to have an informal conversation (rather than an encyclopedic lookup) that identifies what can be tweaked, explains its significance, and gives you a glimpse of its clinical implications.

Why Use Light?

Simply put, we use light because it can penetrate into the body and then cause a physiological change once it gets inside. An eighth-grader may not agree with that, since he cannot see through his own hand, and when he shines a flashlight on his arm he does not start to grow another. However, you are not so naïve. You have seen x-rays that have allowed you to peer inside the body. And you can read these pages, so you accept the idea (however unconsciously) that light gets absorbed by the cones in your eyes, which causes chemical reactions that lead to electrical signals that affect your chemistry and even your mood, your behavior, and your health.

Yes, ducking when you see a baseball coming toward your head is a health-altering effect of light's interaction with your biological self. However, visible light does not penetrate very well into our bodies, and your eyes cannot see x-rays. So what is the difference between these and the other flavors of light you are here to read about?

Flavors of Light

Despite the wide range of interactions and applications of light, there is literally only one fundamental difference between any two types: wavelength. To understand what this means, we first need to know what light *is* – an oscillating electric and magnetic field that travels in a straight line and at a constant speed (the speed of light). This is why the technical term for light is "electromagnetic radiation." That is all that light is; what it *does* is much more complex, and we will dive into some of that in this chapter. So, since light always travels at the same speed, the structure of its oscillation can be described equivalently either by the distance between its peaks and valleys, or by how many peaks or valleys it has in a given time. We call these values the "wavelength" and "frequency," respectively. This is not to be confused with pulse frequency or repetition rate. That has to do with turning light on and off periodically. We will get to that later.

Going forward, I will refer to the different types of light by either of these characteristics, but you will know that they refer to the same thing, and that is this one-dimensional scale of the oscillating electromagnetic wave we call light.

Laser Therapy in Veterinary Medicine: Photobiomodulation, Second Edition. Edited by Christopher J. Winkler and Lisa A. Miller.

Growing up, my favorite A.M. sports radio station broadcasted using light at a frequency of 660 kHz; I heated up my tea in the microwave this morning with light at a frequency of 2.45 GHz, but my favorite color is 450 nm (the wavelength of blue light). Indeed, these are all just different colors of light; the human eye only evolved to contain cones that can detect wavelengths from about 390 to 700 nm, which is what we call the visible part of the spectrum. The near-infrared spectrum spans from about 700 to 1100 nm.

If you were clever, you would have hesitated when I said "one-dimensional scale," since you know we experience three dimensions. In one classical way to visualize light, it is made up of oscillating electric and magnetic fields; each of these fields oscillate in a plane perpendicular (90°) to each other, both of which are perpendicular (90°) from direction of propagation (see the top of Figure 2.1). So there are the other dimensions for you, three in total. This brings us to two characteristics of light you may have heard referenced: polarization, which simply means the alignment of the electric (or magnetic) fields of light, and coherence, which means that the peaks and valleys of two different pieces of light are lined up. However, these values (and these other two dimensions) only matter when whatever you are shining the light on is structured enough to make a difference. Biological matter generally is not; but we are jumping ahead a little. First, we have to define the interactions, and then things will clear up a bit.

One more fundamental property of light: It turns out that the energy of light is directly proportional to its frequency (and therefore inversely proportional to its wavelength). The amount of energy any "piece" of light carries is discrete or "quantized." Therefore, in a sense, light is made up of individual packets of light, called "photons." No reason to explore the wave–particle duality of light here, but it was important to mention, since it will affect how we talk about light a little later. Figure 2.1 illustrates the fundamental structure of an electromagnetic wave and the relationship between wavelength, frequency, and energy.

So, how does this one fundamental property of light (frequency or wavelength or energy, however you want to refer to it) lead to such different effects in the different regions of the spectrum? In other words, why do different colors of light interact differently with matter?

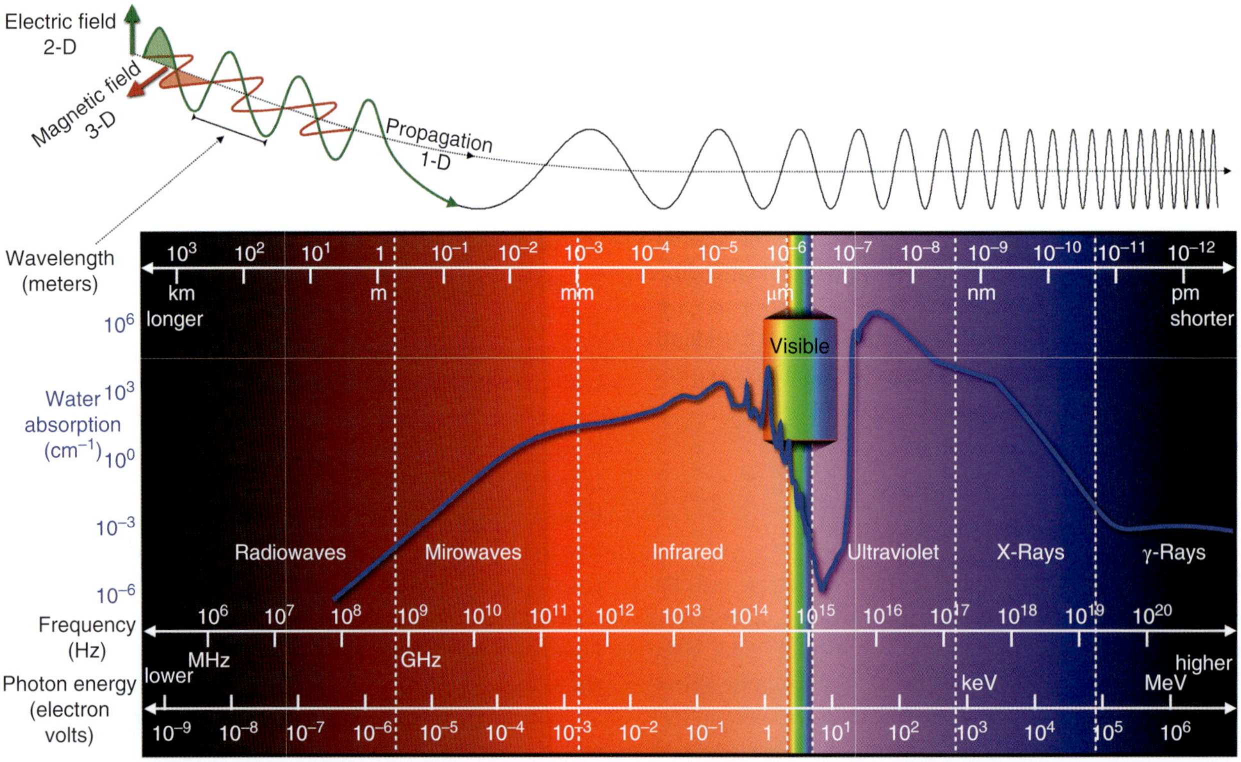

Figure 2.1 Electromagnetic structure and spectrum. The electric and magnetic fields of light are perpendicular to each other and to the direction of propagation. The name and effect of the radiation vary by wavelength (top axis), and equivalently by frequency and energy (bottom axes). The blue curve represents the absorption of water throughout the spectrum (Hale and Querry, 1973; Segelstein, 1981; Zolotarev *et al.*, 1969).

Interactions

In the region of the electromagnetic spectrum that concerns this book (the visible and near-infrared), there are two basic interactions: absorption and scatter. But before we get to these, we have to understand what we are shining the light on: biological matter. The body seems rigid enough, and it is at the scale of a baseball. However, when you are using light, you must see things at the scale of light, which we see is on the order of hundreds of nanometers (Figure 2.1). When you zoom in that closely, you will see that we are made up of molecules. If you zoomed in further, you would see atoms, but that would fall in the realm of x-rays (with wavelengths below 10 nm); visible and near-infrared light do not interact very strongly with objects that small.

Intra- and intermolecular bonds, however, are just the right size, and so they interact very well in this region. These bonds are nothing more than shared electron clouds (moving, charged particles), but they effectively act as springs between the constituent atoms. When charged particles are subject to an electric and magnetic field (like when you shine light on them), they experience forces, and since the field is oscillating, so do the bonds; and like strings on a guitar, they each have their own natural frequency.

Absorption

Absorption happens when the frequency of light is close to this natural frequency. Just like pushing someone on a swing or a mass on a spring, if you push in rhythm with the natural rhythm, you can transfer the most energy of your push to the system. In the visible and near-infrared region of the spectrum, photons of light either impart all their energy to the biological tissue they strike, or they bounce off; they are either completely absorbed or they scatter. So, in effect, light is absorbed by bonds that have just the right frequency, which makes it clear to see why absorption is wavelength- and tissue-dependent. Different tissues have different constituents, made up of bonds with different frequencies.

When these bonds absorb the light, they do what any excited spring does: bend, twist, expand, contract, and any combination of these. What this does, in effect, is change the shape of the molecule or chain of molecules. This is chemistry at its very core. You have to understand, the main way chemistry works (i.e., the way that two molecules combine) is a very sensitive, physical lock-and-key mechanism. Things that fit together nicely (both spatially and electrically) tend to bond together. If they do not fit, they do not bond. By changing the shape of one part of a molecule, even slightly and even on a very short time scale, you can cause the molecule to shed parts of itself or grab on to new things. What fascinating biochemical effects come from these absorption events is the topic of later chapters.

For those of you who have experience with surgical lasers (or kitchen microwaves, for that matter), you will realize that if you use enough light in a wavelength (or frequency) range that coincides with bonds that are prevalent in the tissue, these vibrations will reinforce themselves, create a lot of heat, and eventually shake molecules apart. Most of the time, the target molecules are water, and this boiling of water in the tissue either heats your food in a general way (if diffuse) or ablates the tissue in a very efficient, localized way (if focused).

In either case, absorption allows the targeting of molecules by light with the "right" frequency. However, statistically speaking, the majority of light bounces off something before it is absorbed.

Scatter

In the visible and near-infrared, virtually all of the scatter is elastic. In other words, photons retain their energy and simply bounce off particles in their path that do not have the "right" frequency to be absorbed (and even when they do, there is always a nonzero probability of each interaction). Which direction the photon travels after the bounce depends on what it bounced off of: mostly the size of the particle. Scattering of light by particles smaller than about 1/10th the wavelength of light is referred to as "Rayleigh scattering." Scattering by particles larger than that is referred to as "Mie scattering." The result of Rayleigh scattering is isotropic; the scattered light has equal intensity in all directions (except for at around 90°). Mie scattering, on the other hand, is very much forward-pointing, and the extent to which it points forward is represented by a number called the "anisotropy factor" (usually assigned the variable g) that can have values from +1 to −1. There are two ways to visualize this important concept: one with an individual photon in mind, and the other with a "beam" in mind. The technical way to define the anisotropy factor is the average cosine of the scattering angle of incoming light, which probably does not mean much to you as its written, but let us use some numbers. Anisotropy values for the near-infrared on biological tissue are in the 0.75–0.90 range, so let's take 0.85. This means that the average incoming photon is deflected by 31° ($\cos(31°) = 0.85$). If the incoming light was headed north, then after scattering it would be headed somewhere in the NNW/NNE direction. The other way to interpret this is to say that it is the average percentage of the beam that remains going forward: A value of 1 means 100% keeps going (no scattering at all); a value of −1 means full back-scattering (like a super-efficient mirror), and 0 means that the same amount of the beam goes forward and backward (and left and right and all around). So at g = 0.85, about 85% of the beam remains going in the same direction after scattering. You can see why I said that near-infrared scattering within the body is predominantly "forward-pointing."

How Much of Each

We do not talk about absorption and scattering on an individual basis, simply because there are more of these events in the first millimeter of skin than all of humanity could count in a lifetime. Instead, we talk about macroscopic quantities like absorption coefficients, μ_a, and reduced-scattering coefficients, μ_s', both of which have units of 1/length. These give you the average amount of absorption or scattering along the path of light and yield the shape of an exponential decay curve that describes the attenuation of light intensity (the percentage of the original beam) with depth. Inversely (i.e., if you take one divided by these quantities), you are left with what is called the "mean free path," which tells you the average distance between absorption and scattering events. Each of these quantities depends on both wavelength and tissue: for absorption, it is all about matching the frequency of light with the frequency of bonds, and for scatter, the story is dictated by how the wavelength of light relates to the size and number of the scattering particles (i.e., tissue composition and density).

Absorption coefficients are easy to understand, because a photon is either absorbed or it is not. Therefore, we use absorption coefficients along with depth from the surface to understand total absorption (and therefore the total relative intensity that is left in the beam). The blue curve in the background of Figure 2.1 shows the absorption coefficient of water throughout nearly the entire spectrum for reference.

Scattering is a bit trickier, because the direction the light bounces depends on what it bounced off of, and particularly its size. In addition, the path length of the light is never the same as the depth (and is usually a lot more), because of all the little bounces in different directions. Still, we do not track each bounce, but rather treat this directionality on average. This is why I referred to the *reduced* scattering coefficient, which incorporates the anisotropy into its calculation. Basically, the reduced scattering coefficient gives you a directionally corrected scattering coefficient that makes calculations simpler and lets you use the depth (which you know, or at least want to know) rather than individual path length of every light ray (which you do not know nor care about). The inverse, or reduced mean free path, thus gives you the average depth between scattering events.

These two quantities combine to form an effective attenuation coefficient, which is a generalized way of describing the loss of original beam intensity. With this, we can now understand how much light gets to what depth relative to how much we started with. Figure 2.2 illustrates the idea of attenuation in each of its mechanisms. Again, intensity is an exponentially decaying quantity, meaning that the deeper you go, the less light remains than in the original beam. That sounds simple enough. Just give me μ_a and μ_s' of a tissue, and I will tell how much light gets to that joint in the patient you are trying to treat.

Not so fast! In any target treatment area, there are many different amounts and types of tissue, which are not sliced and stacked neatly on top of on one another like deli meat in its packaging. So tracking the amount of absorption, type of scattering, and direction of scattering along the wide variety of interactions as light bounces around inside the body becomes a complicated mess. We can make some generalizations to help, though.

First, once inside the body, scattering is by far the dominant interaction in biological tissue, with its effect being strongest at shorter wavelengths. As some perspective, this means that the average depth of a scattering event is at most every half-millimeter (and usually less). At the skin, absorption and scattering play about equal roles, and there are a lot of both. Though the skin is not the ironclad barrier to the outside world as it is for, say, water, it is an obstacle for light. But since the anisotropy factor of visible and near-infrared light incident on biological tissue is very close to 1, on average these scattering events point the light even deeper into the patient.

Second, even though absorption is smaller in magnitude inside the body (a factor of 200–5000 times smaller than scattering coefficients), with absorption events taking place along the windy path, the light ends up bouncing along inside the body, and virtually all of the light that gets in is absorbed somewhere inside (Jacques, 2013). You do not see the animal glowing with near-infrared light as you treat them, even with an infrared camera. If you had a very sensitive detector, you would definitely find some light coming out, but the majority is absorbed by the body. In addition, a small fraction of absorption of a lot of photons still gives a lot of total absorption. How much are we talking about?

Units of Which You Have (Hopefully) Heard

We measure the energy of an individual photon in a unit called an electron volt (eV), with the energy of a photon

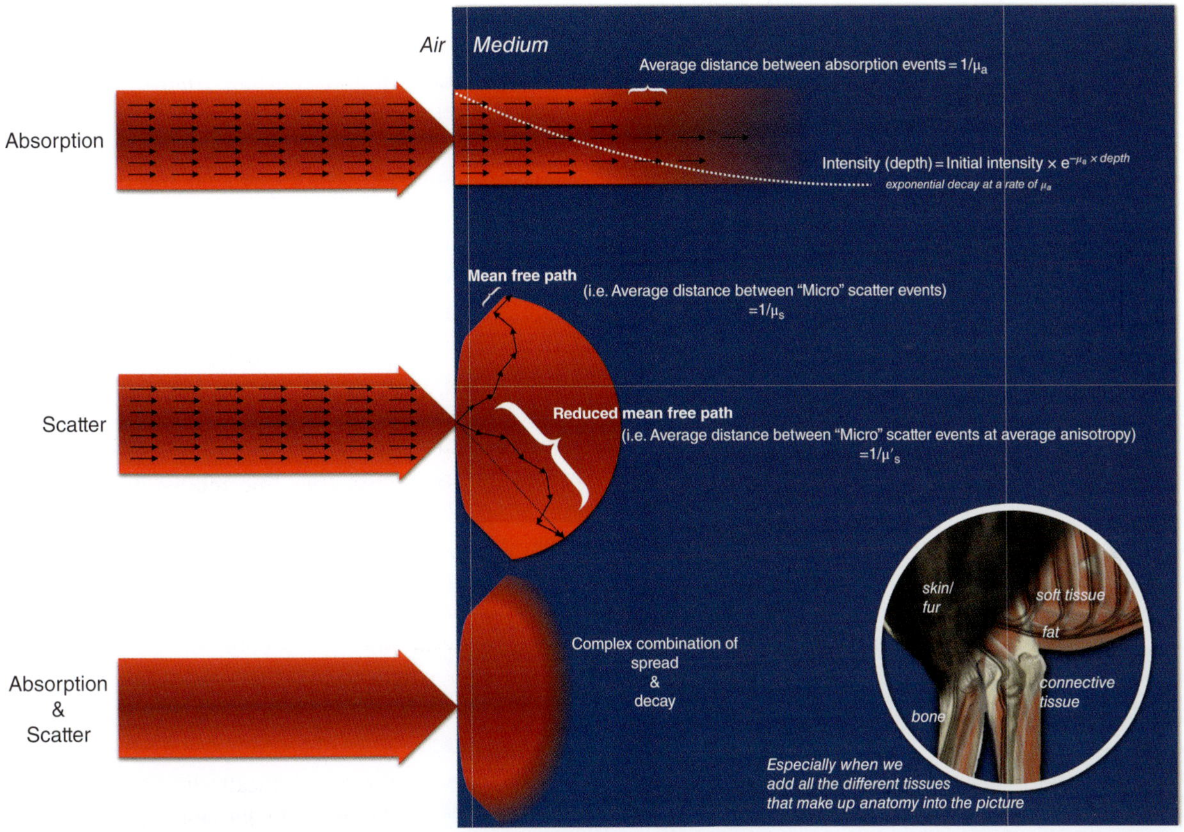

Figure 2.2 Attenuation mechanisms. Absorption is an exponential decay in intensity along any given path at a rate of μ_a. Many "micro" scattering events are often characterized by their average distance and angle, i.e., "macro" information, which is combined in the reduced scattering coefficient μ_s. Combined, these processes lead to a general "mushrooming" of the beam, i.e., a decay in intensity and spread of the beam with depth inside the patient.

equal to 1240 divided by the wavelength in nanometers. Therefore, a photon of red light at 620 nm carries 2 eV of energy. However, we measure the energy of a beam of light in a unit called joules (J). For reference, 1 J of energy is equal to 6 242 000 000 000 000 000 eV. So, 1 J of red light consists of 3 121 000 000 000 000 000 photons. Now you see what I meant when I said a small fraction of a big number is still a big number.

For another reference, 1 J of energy is how much it takes to lift a baseball 28 in. up off the ground. At the same time, when you drop a baseball from 28 in., it hits the ground with 1 J of energy. So why does your patient not feel like they are being bombarded with baseballs when you shine light at them? The reason is the flexibility of the molecular bonds in the body that we have been talking about. The body is not rigid when it comes to light, like it is with incoming baseballs. The energy absorbed (and we determined that the majority of the light you shine on the patient *is* absorbed by them) is transferred to the three-dimensional configuration of the billions of molecules and bonds in the treatment area on an individual basis and at varying depths within the tissue. Most of the absorbed vibrations turn into heat, which dissipates as the bonds come back to rest in their equilibrium states. We will return to the topic of heat later.

However, to say that you delivered 1 J of energy is meaningless. Did you expose the entire body to that energy, or just one part? Did you deliver that energy over the span of an hour or in a fraction of a second? Remember that photons move at the speed of light. Their absorption events are thus virtually instantaneous, so the time scale is very important.

For this reason, we prefer to use the quantity called "power," defined as the amount of energy delivered per time, and is usually measured in units of watts (W; 1 W = 1 J/sec). This gives a more accurate picture of the scale of interaction, because while we will see that the accumulation of light–tissue interactions is important, the body is living and moving, and so the amount of light delivered on any given time scale is important. As a clinician, you are not naïve enough to think that if you were to give 1 J of light to a patient once per day, by the time you had given them 100 J of energy their tissue or symptoms or overall condition would still be the same as when you started. If you delivered that same energy in 1 minute, it is very reasonable to assume that not much would have changed. However, we still have not answered the question relating to the size of the treatment area. Again, you know better than to think that 100 J across the whole animal would give the same clinical impact as if you only exposed the paw.

Therefore, while total energy and power are easy to calculate, they do not tell the whole story. This is important and dangerous, because without context, these quantities can be warped and used to manipulate the truth. The two quantities that give a more complete picture are *energy density* and *power density*, and they are simply the total energy and power per unit area, respectively.

As you deliver light to a patient and accumulate energy in a treatment area, you are forcing more light–tissue interactions in that area. Decades of research have shed the tiniest bit of light (pun definitely intended) on what biological, physiological, and clinical implications these interactions can initiate and sustain. Equally important has been the study of the time scale of these effects. So, while energy density, which we also call *dose* or *fluence* (energy per area, usually given in units of J/cm^2) and power density, which we also call *irradiance* (power per unit area, in W/cm^2) are better descriptors, one without the other still falls short of being explanatory because of the element of time. Dose is a description of deposition (how much), while irradiance describes exposure (how quickly). Dose and irradiance are exceedingly important when combined, and are dangerously hollow when discussed independent of one another. We will discuss this idea of reciprocity more later.

Deciding Dose

There is only one way to determine how much dose is best for a given treatment: precise science (trial and error). However, there are two places to start, both of which are important and independently necessary. First, you can start with the individual cells. Much of the research in the past two decades falls into this category, where people expose cells in a very controlled environment to different amounts of light and measure the magnitude of cellular effects, which can range from mitochondrial activity to adhesion to glass, luminescence, DNA replication rates, and much more. These studies have the benefit of being controlled, in that virtually all parameters other than the one you wish to change can be held fixed, and so individual mechanisms and their dose dependencies can be tracked. They are at the same time limited by their weak relation to real-world situations, where cell signaling and the transport of nutrients, wastes, and heat in the three-dimensional matrix of the cells that make up tissue are vastly different than in a monolayer of cells living on glass.

Nonetheless, for the determination of optimal dose, this is the cleanest method. Once you find the peak in the response curve, you then need to estimate the percentage of the light that reaches the cells that are at the heart of the condition you are treating. After reading the sections on absorption and scatter, you should be well-convinced that there is an enormous difference between what you expose to the surface and what actually reaches an internal structure. Penetration studies have been sprinkled within the literature (too sparsely, if you ask me) and lend some assistance in estimating this exposure-to-delivery ratio (Ash *et al.*, 2017; Chaki *et al.*, 2023). This is fundamentally the best strategy for an accurate dose prescription model.

However, we really care about the clinical efficacy, and so if the results do not follow from this prescription, we are forced to use the second starting point: the clinical version of trial and error, where we vary the parameters over a sample of patients and see what works best. This can be very scientific or anecdotal; in the coming chapters, you will see results of both versions. The obvious issue with this approach is the sheer size of "parameter space" (the impractically large number of combinations of all the relevant parameters you'd need to find an "optimal" result). The right path is to get your starting point from the fundamental calculations, then follow the translational research that progresses our understanding, down the path of simulations → ex-vivo studies → animal studies. From there you can learn to tweak protocols based on what we as a community have learned.

So, what else can you tweak, and which are the intelligent ways to do so?

Knobs to Turn

There are four knobs that virtually every laser has, whether they are physical knobs or not: wavelength, spot size, power, and time. Combined, these knobs determine the dose and irradiance of treatment. They are interdependent to some degree, however. Doubling the time and halving the power keeps the dose unchanged. Doubling the power and doubling the treatment area keeps the irradiance unchanged, which, given the same time, keeps the dose the same.

Advice about which to change for a given treatment should come from clinicians, and will in later chapters, but the meaningful limits of each are more fundamental than that, and mostly have to do with irradiance. Use a too-low irradiance and you might as well prescribe walks in the park for the animal, because the sun exposes your patient to about 33 mW/cm^2 of near-infrared light (ASTM, 2008). Use a too-high irradiance and heat will be deposited in the patient faster than its body can dissipate it, and so will accumulate, causing first pain and eventually irreversible tissue damage, which depends on both the temperature and the time exposed and varies per tissue type (more on this later). The threshold for pain is very much patient-dependent (and tissue- and wavelength-dependent, since different combinations absorb at different strengths), but a ballpark figure is that 1–2 W/cm^2 of near-infrared light will begin to hurt after a few seconds, and more than that will begin to hurt immediately. The body has a built in safety net, though: pain comes well before any serious damage can be done (unless you are working well above this irradiance). As long as you are not treating while the patient is writhing in pain, odds are you have not done any serious damage. Nevertheless, within this window of usefulness and comfort, there are knobs to turn.

Wavelength

Wavelength (per tissue) is the primary determiner of the absorption and scattering properties of that tissue, meaning it affects the spread of light through the tissue (both with depth and laterally). In recent years, laser manufacturers have created devices and protocols that not only mix wavelengths (multiple wavelengths per protocol, an industry standard by now), but also change that mixture, sometimes from protocol-to-protocol, sometimes from phase-to-phase within the same protocol.

Spot Size

Spot size is limited by the optical engineering of the light source and delivery apparatus. An instance where a small spot size (on the order of millimeters in diameter) is useful is in the practice of laser acupuncture, where the light can be used to stimulate qi meridians (see Chapter 31). Conditions such as otitis, where the infection stems from deep within the ear canal, are much easier and more effectively treated with a smaller spot size from a treatment head that can reach those types of areas. But while it may sound intuitive that if you have a more concentrated beam of light, your penetration will be higher, the opposite turns out to be true with beams less than about 10 mm in diameter (Ash *et al.,* 2017). From a clinical standpoint, it is difficult to cover a clinically significant area in a uniform manner with too small of an application. Also, as you decrease the spot size and keep other parameters constant, the irradiance increases, and without some software safeguards, you could produce too much heat and cause thermal damage to your patient.

The upper limit of spot size is determined by the optical coupling of the light source to the patient. We spoke about microscopic scatter earlier; macroscopically, scatter is very much angle-dependent. Administering light perpendicular to the surface minimizes scatter from the surface, with the amount of scatter increasing super-linearly with angle (the bigger the angle, the less light gets inside the patient). Therefore, the upper limit of the spot size is about the size of the handpiece from which the light originates; any larger than that, and the light on the edges of the treatment area will no longer be perpendicular to the surface, and the amount of light delivered inside the patient will be substantially diminished.

A quick aside on types of light sources. Lasers and light-emitting diodes (LEDs) are among the most popular light sources in the therapeutic world, and they have two fundamental differences, one that matters and one that likely does not: divergence and coherence. While technically both light sources produce somewhat divergent light, in general light from lasers is inherently much more collimated (all light rays within the beam are parallel to each other). This is not to say that the light emitted from either cannot pass through some focusing optics to produce similar beams of light. If it did, then their only difference would be that the light from the laser would be coherent (the peaks and valleys of all the constituent light would be aligned), but as discussed earlier, this only really matters when the light is shone on something that is structured enough to resolve it: usually crystalline lattices and metals. While LEDs can now be engineered to have relatively narrow emission angles, they are still inherently more divergent than lasers, and without any spherical or parabolic mirrors to reflect and focus the emitted light, they do not expose the patient to the total amount of light they produce; a nontrivial percentage of the light points in opposite or peripheral directions.

Power

Combined with spot size (and, obviously, wavelength), power dictates the real-time state of the laser. We just identified the upper and lower limits of irradiance, and since the spot size of your laser is usually fixed (or at least, fixed for any given treatment), the window of useful power output is set for you. The two principle reasons for changing power are to decrease your treatment time and to increase your effective treatment depth during a set treatment time.

"Whoa, whoa, whoa. Hold on. I thought wavelength determines the penetration?" Correct. Mostly. We talked about how both absorption and scattering lead to exponentially decaying intensities of light with depth inside the patient. And yes, the shape of these curves (how quickly the intensity drops) is dependent on the combination of wavelength and tissue type. If you start with more light, then you are left with more light at each depth. In fact, any percentage increase of power will lead to the same percentage decrease in treatment time required to deliver the same dose to the same depth. Refer to Figure 2.3. Suppose the goal is to deliver 20 J of energy to a depth A. We can see from the curve that only 50% of the beam's surface intensity remains at this depth. Thus, the 2 W laser would have to treat for 20 seconds to build up the desired dose, while the 8 W laser could deliver the exact same dose to the exact same depth in only 5 seconds (a quarter of the time, since the laser is four times as powerful).

To think of it from another perspective, one that really gets to the heart of this power-versus-penetration issue, let us consider the example of treating for a fixed amount of time and calculate the depth to which each laser will deliver the same dose. As before, treating for 20 seconds with a 2 W laser will deliver 20 J of energy to A. Now, even though the transmission percentage is four times lower at depth B (12.5%), since we start off with four times more photons with the higher-powered laser, the same 20 J of energy can be delivered to this deeper target (B vs. A) in the same treatment time. Again, the lower-powered laser can eventually accumulate the same amount of dose, but only with longer treatment time. It is important to note that the depth scale of Figure 2.3 is exaggerated to illustrate this point, so the distance between A and B might be quite small in highly attenuating tissue. So, yes, while the increase in penetration of an "effective dose" is *linear* with irradiance (more power means more penetration), it varies *exponentially* with wavelength and tissue type, so pairing the right wavelength with the appropriate tissue is much more effective.

An important disclosure of the "all else equal" assumptions in this analysis: In this discussion, we are assuming that none of the optical properties of the tissue are changing over time. As promised, we will dive deeper into the topic of heat a little later, but it is worth noting here that both the scatter and absorption coefficients of tissue can in fact increase (marginally, but not negligibly) with an increase in temperature (Iorizzo *et al.*, 2021) and you will see later that prolonged exposure to light can lead to an increase in heat.

Time

Where does the optimal treatment time come from? Realistically and unfortunately, the main factor is clinical feasibility. Nobody has time to treat each patient for an hour. In fact, any more than a few minutes begins to strain the animal's and the laser administrator's attention span. Most laser manufacturers develop protocols that fit into a given clinic's schedule. Also, the body does not heal in a matter of seconds-to-minutes; it takes time, and also depends on the acute vs. chronic nature of the injury. This is why most recommendations are for several treatments over a few weeks, as you will see throughout this book. Simply

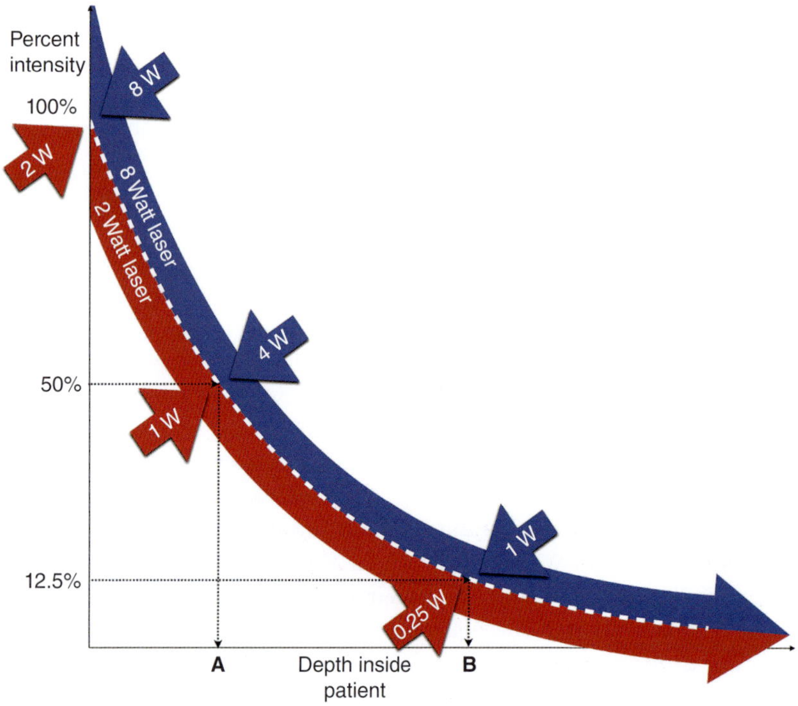

Figure 2.3 Comparison of penetration between lasers of different power output. To a given depth, a higher-powered laser delivers a dose in less time. In a given time, a higher-powered laser delivers the same dose to a greater depth.

blasting the body with light one time for a few seconds is not going to have a lasting effect. But you still have to perform these treatments within reasonable time frames over the course of the treatment period. That said, the industry now has lasers that can be sent home with the pet owner who, at the convenience of their couch and their own schedule, can deliver longer treatments over several days or weeks. Again, I will leave the treatment frequency (or "dosage") recommendations to the clinicians.

From a scientific perspective, though, the better way to calculate "how much time" starts with dose. We know how much dose we want at the target, back-calculate how much dose we need at the surface, and then set the power to whatever it needs to be to deliver that many joules in what we determine to be a "feasible treatment time."

More than Just Dose

In general, reciprocity is a serious question. Is the accumulation of dose, irrespective of the delivery method and light parameters, a sufficient predictor of clinical effect? In particular, on both the intra- and intertreatment timescales, should a treatment that aims to deliver 2 J/cm^2 of light take 2 minutes, 20 minutes, or 2 hours? Should those treatments be repeated every hour, every day, or every week? Or does it matter at all? Will all of these situations produce the same clinical effect as long as they deliver the same total dose?

These are ultimately clinical questions, but the literature suggests that while reciprocity does not seem to hold across the board (Karu *et al.*, 1996; Hashmi *et al.*, 2010), there are certain windows within the broad treatment spectrum where you can be reasonably confident that slight tweaks (such as when a pet owner could not get to the clinic that morning, or because you have the chance to deliver a second treatment while the animal is being boarded overnight) will not severely impact your standard expectation of therapeutic outcome.

A quick, but related aside having to do with this same idea of dose accumulation is the determination of treatment axis. We have covered enough about scatter to convince you that in the near-infrared spectrum and in biological tissue, the treatment beam does not look like a beam once it enters the body. Instead, the beam sort of "mushrooms" once it passes the skin and spreads out, principally inside the body. The clinicians again will have much to say about what joints and along which nerve routes and lymphatic paths to point the laser, but one thing to keep in mind is that dose is a cumulative quantity in the short term (on the order of seconds to minutes). There are many joints in the body that are more or less equidistant from two surfaces. It is often very useful to treat along different axes, always pointing at the same internal structure, in order to accumulate more dose at the intersection of axes than is delivered along any individual path. In radiation oncology with x-rays that encounter much less scatter, this technique is used in virtually every radiation treatment plan to spare benign tissues unnecessary dose while building up a toxic amount within the planned treatment volume. Granted, much more scatter is involved in the infrared, but in smaller geometries like the shoulders, hips, and more distal sites in the extremities, treating from under a leg or an arm can be a good adjunct, especially since the hair and fur (strong scatterers) are much less dense there.

Still, most of the advice you seek about the time scale of treatments will come from the clinicians in later chapters. But what about on a shorter time scale, like milliseconds?

Heat (Finally)

The topic of heat is interwoven throughout the story of light in the body, which is why you've seen it brought up in several sections of this chapter already. Fundamentally, almost every photon that enters the body is eventually absorbed, and that absorption event concludes in conversion to heat. Some of that heat conversion in the various chromophores leads to interesting and beneficial chemistry (a morphology change in hemoglobin that releases an oxygen molecule from the blood, or the redox of cytochrome c oxidase that leads to the creation of adenosine triphosphate, ATP), but at its core, photon in → heat out (Karu *et al.*, 2008). So light and heat *deposition* are linked; when and where you have a lot of light absorbed, you have a lot of heat created. But the *transport* of light and heat are very different. They travel at different speeds, by different mechanisms. When you turn off the light, the light is gone, instantly. That's not the case with heat. So we need to track the two separately. But first, let's recap why we care about heat.

Heat represents a threefold barrier in laser therapy: (i) patient comfort, (ii) clinical effect, and (iii) changes in optical properties of tissue. Because we must operate below the pain threshold, we cannot just use all the light we want to at the surface. On one hand, it has been shown that a modest increase of tissue temperature leads to an analgesic effect. In fact, the majority of therapy lasers in the human market have piggy-backed on the same general FDA clearance as an "infrared lamp" intended...

> *To emit energy in the infrared spectrum to provide* ***topical heating*** *for the purpose of elevating tissue temperature for the* ***temporary relief of minor***

muscle and joint pain and stiffness, or muscle spasm; the ***temporary increase in local blood circulation****; and/ or the temporary relaxation of muscle.*

And certain chemical processes in the body (i.e., endothermic and some anabolic reactions) are triggered, enabled, and/or enhanced by absorbing energy in the form of heat from the surroundings. But "too much" heat can in some cases saturate the body's biochemistry, at other levels inhibit it, and in extreme cases cause damage to tissue itself. There was a historically accepted threshold of 45 °C between hyperthermia and irreversible tissue damage. Much work has been done over the last decade on this subject (mostly related to targeting cancer while sparing healthy tissue around it) and now the literature talks about thermal damage to tissue in terms of Cumulative Equivalent Minutes (CEM) at 43 °C, with various models on different tissue types (Yarmolenko *et al.*, 2011, Assi *et al.*, 2022). I will not go into details here, but suffice to say that you do not want to be heating tissue into mid-to high 40s (above ~110 °F) for very long.

A quick note on barrier #3, namely the change in optical properties of tissue with temperature. Earlier I mentioned that both the scatter and absorption coefficients of tissue can in fact increase with temperature (Iorizzo *et al.*, 2021). Now we can put some numbers to those increases. In that paper, the authors measured (among other things) the absorption coefficient and reduced scattering coefficients of tissue at both 36 °C and 60 °C. The maximum change of either of those coefficients in the wavelength region of 600–1000 nm was less than 10% between 36 °C and 60 °C. So, when you treat below the thresholds of pain and irreversible tissue damage (always, I hope), this effect is minor.

What kind of parameters would get you close to these temperature limits, and how does that temperature profile look over time? Let us take opposite ends of the "therapeutic window" of wavelengths: 635 and 980 nm. Wavelengths below that are almost completely absorbed by the skin; we have evolved to grow hair and skin to protect us from the shorter wavelengths (UV) of sunlight, and if the majority of visible light went through us, we'd be walking translucent holograms. Wavelengths above that aren't absorbed much at all by biological tissue beyond the water inside us. Within this window, however, these two wavelengths represent relatively high and low absorption respectively, and so for a given irradiance represent relatively high and low temperature profiles. Figure 2.4 shows the spatial profile of the irradiance (A, B, and C) and temperature (D, E, and F) distribution on a model of tissue for these two different wavelengths in the form of a three-dimensional color map (COMSOL, n.d.). Imagine a light source incident from the top, and these plots have been cut in "quadrants" so you can see "inside" the tissue, both within and around the incident beam. Tissue parameters are listed in Table 2.1.

To begin, let's concentrate on the first two columns of plots. The initial irradiance in A, B, D, and E are the same: 0.5 W/cm^2. The only difference is the wavelength: 635 nm in A and D, and 980 nm in B and E. This is meant to illustrate the difference between a higher-skin-absorption scenario (635 nm) and a lower-skin-absorption scenario (980 nm).

Notice first that the light (irradiance) spreads wider and deeper than the temperature in all cases. This is a very good thing from a clinical and therapeutic standpoint. When we irradiate tissue, we get lots of beneficial "spread" of our beam. The 980 nm beam keeps its intensity (red-into-orange in the irradiance plot) intact through the epidermis because it has lower absorption in that tissue type. In fact, the irradiance of the 980 nm beam is higher through the first three layers of the model (epidermis, skin, subcutaneous fat). With 635 nm, however, it is a tale of only two tissues. Those first three layers absorb 635 nm (visible, red) light at much higher rates, illustrated as the plot shows a quicker change in color from red to light-blue. But within the muscle, 635 nm is actually absorbed *less* than 980 nm, so the little light that is left after the skin and fat actually permeates deeper. The problem is, very little is left. This is one of the big dilemmas in laser therapy. Red light has been shown to have really great photochemical benefits once absorbed in tissue and it can travel a relatively long distance within muscles; but it is *very* difficult to get it inside the body without burning a hole on its way down.

Speaking of the devil (aka high temperatures), notice that three things are "bigger" when it comes to 635 nm (the higher absorption scenario) vs. the 980 nm beam:

1) Maximum temperature of the tissue (46 °C vs. 39 °C);
2) Lateral spread of the heat (~8 mm vs ~4 mm, or 100% farther from the central axis until temperature reduced back to 38 °C);
3) Depth of the heat (~9.5 mm vs ~7.5 mm, or ~27% deeper from the surface along the central axis until temperature reduced back to 38 °C).

This helps us understand the effect of wavelength (and therefore absorption, scatter, and penetration) on temperature, but what of irradiance? That is where plots C and F come into play, showing that same 980 nm profile (irradiance and temperature), but an irradiance of 1.75 W/cm^2, which is 3.5 times higher than the first two scenarios. I chose this value because it is the point at which the maximum temperature of the 980 nm beam is the same as the equivalent exposure of the 635 nm beam.

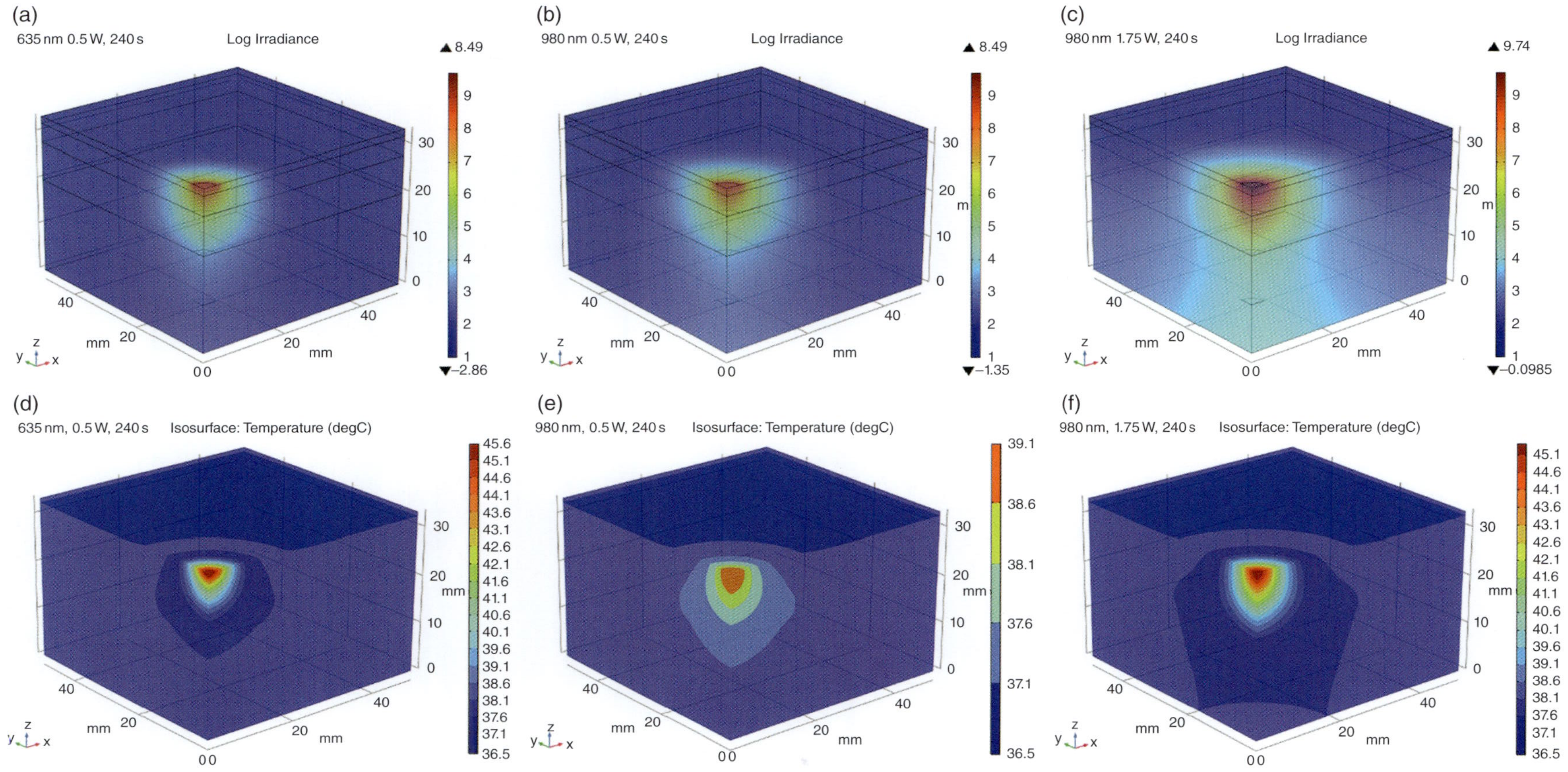

Figure 2.4 A 3-D irradiance (a, b, and c) and temperature (d, e, and f) profile with the following tissue and incident light parameters. Tissue layers detailed in Table 2.1. Light parameters: Power: 0.5 W (a, b, d, and e) and 1.75 W (c and f), Area: 1 cm^2, exposure time: 240 s.

Table 2.1 Tissue scattering – modeled parameters/tissue layer properties.

	635 nm		808 nm		980 nm		
Tissue layer	μ_a, cm^{-1}	μ_s', cm^{-1}	μ_a, cm^{-1}	μ_s', cm^{-1}	μ_a, cm^{-1}	μ_s', cm^{-1}	**Thickness- mm**
Epidermis	2.77	47.8	1.63	36.5	0.51	31.2	1
Dermis	1.55	29.8	1.18	22.5	0.81	18.9	4
Subcutaneous fat	1.52	25.4	1.06	20.0	0.90	17.8	10
Muscle	0.3	10	0.21	7.5	0.60	6.1	50[1]

Note: Tissue dimensions, optical absorption (μ_a), and reduced scattering (μ_s') for Caucasian skin (Adapted from Chaki *et al.*, 2023).

The take-home message here is the significance of wavelength in both depth of penetration and deposition of heat. In fact, you can use 350% more light at the surface to deliver nearly 550% more light to the fat/muscle barrier (a depth of 15 mm from the surface) with the *same* thermal impact on the skin by using one wavelength vs. the other (given the tissue conditions simulated here).

The last important aspect of the *heat* story is exposure time. Figure 2.4 showed the final results of a continuous exposure over 240 seconds. But let us take a look at more real-time models to illustrate what the tissue sees during an exposure. Figure 2.5 shows the maximum temperature profile over time along the central axis of the beam for three different wavelengths (635 nm, 808 nm, and 980 nm), given the same irradiance. First look at the left of the plot, which is continuous exposure for that same 240 seconds. All three curves follow a similar profile of increasing temperature, with 635 nm having the steepest slope (quickest to accumulate heat) and highest maximum temperature. At time = 240 seconds, the light sources were turned off to illustrate the natural thermal relaxation of tissue. Remember, this is simulation data, and does not account for any heat dissipation from bloodflow or pores in the skin that might aid in moving heat away from the treatment spot. Still, this shows the general behavior of tissue's thermal response under exposure to this range of wavelengths

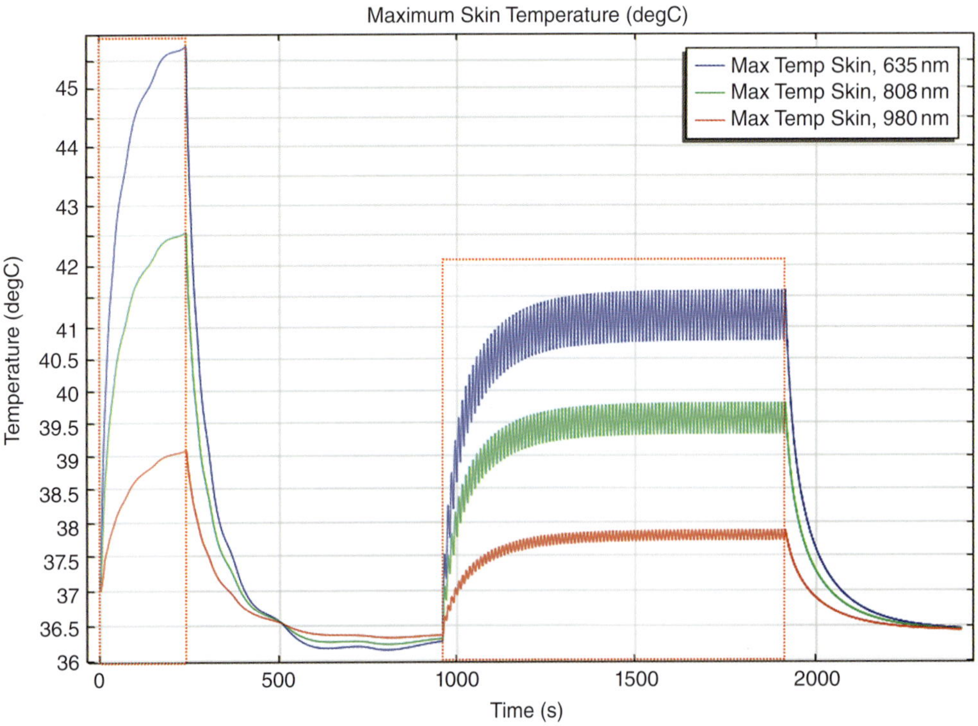

Figure 2.5 Maximum temperature over time along the central axis of the beam for three different wavelengths with the same tissue parameters as Figure 2.4. From time = 0–240 s there is continuous exposure. From 240 s > time > 1000 s there is no exposure. From 1000 s > time > 2000 s the beams are pulsed at a frequency of 5 s on and 5 s off.

and irradiances. Notice that it takes about half as much time for the tissue to return to baseline temperature (37 °C) as it took to get to its maximum temperature.

But at time = 1000s, I did something tricky: for the next 1000 seconds, the beam is "pulsed" on for 5 seconds and off for 5 seconds. Notice two BIG results: (i) the profile of the temperature rise is not as steep as continuous exposure, and (ii) the maximum temperature (even for the highest absorption scenario) is significantly lower than continuous exposure, never reaching the "danger zone." In fact, in all three cases, the temperature "levels off" at a lower maximum temperature and remains fairly constant.

This has two major macroscopic and microscopic implications. Macroscopically, what does this 5-second "pulse" structure mean? It means that if you expose an area for (on the order of) 5 seconds, then "move away" for about the same amount of time, then "come back," you can mitigate some serious thermal accumulation. Does that treatment technique sound familiar? This is the essence of the "scanning" treatment method that many (especially high-powered) laser manufacturers recommend, much of which you'll see in the coming chapters. Microscopically, however, while bulk tissue takes seconds to dissipate joules of energy, that translates to individual cells dissipating microjoules of energy (small fractions of the total beam) in microseconds. Therefore, if you can turn the beam on and off in around the same time it takes cells to return to equilibrium, you can mitigate the heat. If we can pulse the light source (turn it on and off periodically) at a frequency that coincides with the thermal dissipation rates of individual cells, then perhaps we can make the most out of the absorption events. If we pulse too quickly (or do not pulse at all) and we deliver more energy per time than the cells can dissipate, then we may actually be wasting a lot of the cellular energy and diminishing our clinical effect. If we pulse too slowly, then we are not taking full advantage of the cell's potential.

By this logic, it is reasonable to assume that since different types of cell have different densities (mostly due to differences in water content), each will have different average thermal dissipation rates and therefore respond optimally to different pulse frequencies.

There is much at play here, but suffice it to say that pulsing the light in your therapy can elicit some effects that continuous exposure cannot. Unfortunately, the clinical attempts to determine which are the appropriate parameters for which applications have been widely inconsistent, often due to bad reporting of data (Hashmi *et al.*, 2010), but more generally because clinicians simply do not have access to the large sample sizes needed to really isolate any optimizations. Scientists who have dug into the fundamentals, however, and who use biology laboratories with virtually limitless sample sizes, have uncovered several effects (by way of several isolated mechanisms) that are elicited from pulsed light and not from continuous-wave (CW) irradiation (Karu *et al.*, 1996, 1997).

With that comes some more nomenclature. *Frequency* tells you how many times the beam is on and then off per second, but an important quantity that people often overlook is the *duty cycle*. This is the percentage of time the *beam* is on versus off. By definition, then, continuous wave irradiation refers to 100% duty cycle. Two different pulse structures can lead to the same or very different average powers (the total amount of energy delivered per second). Figure 2.6 illustrates this idea.

With respect to pulsing, it is clear that the rule of reciprocity (that total exposure or dose determines clinical effect) does not hold across the board. The beneficial nature of pulsing relies on a specific timing of pulses, either in the time the light is on during a pulse or in the time the light is off between pulses. Therefore, it is clear that if you modified the pulse structure (e.g., by decreasing the peak power but increasing the pulse width proportionally), you could expect a very different intratissue effect, even though the total energy per pulse, and therefore delivered dose, would be identical. The point is, the pulse structure has at least some impact on the biological effect; if not, why are we pulsing at all? We still have much to learn here, but again, the goal is to bridge the gap between what scientists continue to uncover in cell cultures and what advantages clinicians might be able to exploit in the treatment of their patients.

Conclusion

I have told you a story that is made up of lots of little stories that do not tell the whole story. Why, to confuse you more than the last sentence did? No. I just think that understanding a little about all of the factors involved makes you better prepared to prescribe and administer an appropriate therapy. You are going to read a lot in the coming chapters about treating all sorts of injuries with a variety of clinical presentations, each with a variety of treatment prescriptions. The good news is that what follows is based on the fact that laser therapy works, to some degree or another. My goal for this chapter was to arm you with a more technical vocabulary so that you can more intelligently select the most appropriate laser(s) for your use and contribute to protocol development so we can all learn more. You should now have some idea of how these protocols have emerged and, more importantly, how you might modify them based on fundamental ideas in order to enhance your own treatments and the efficacy they induce.

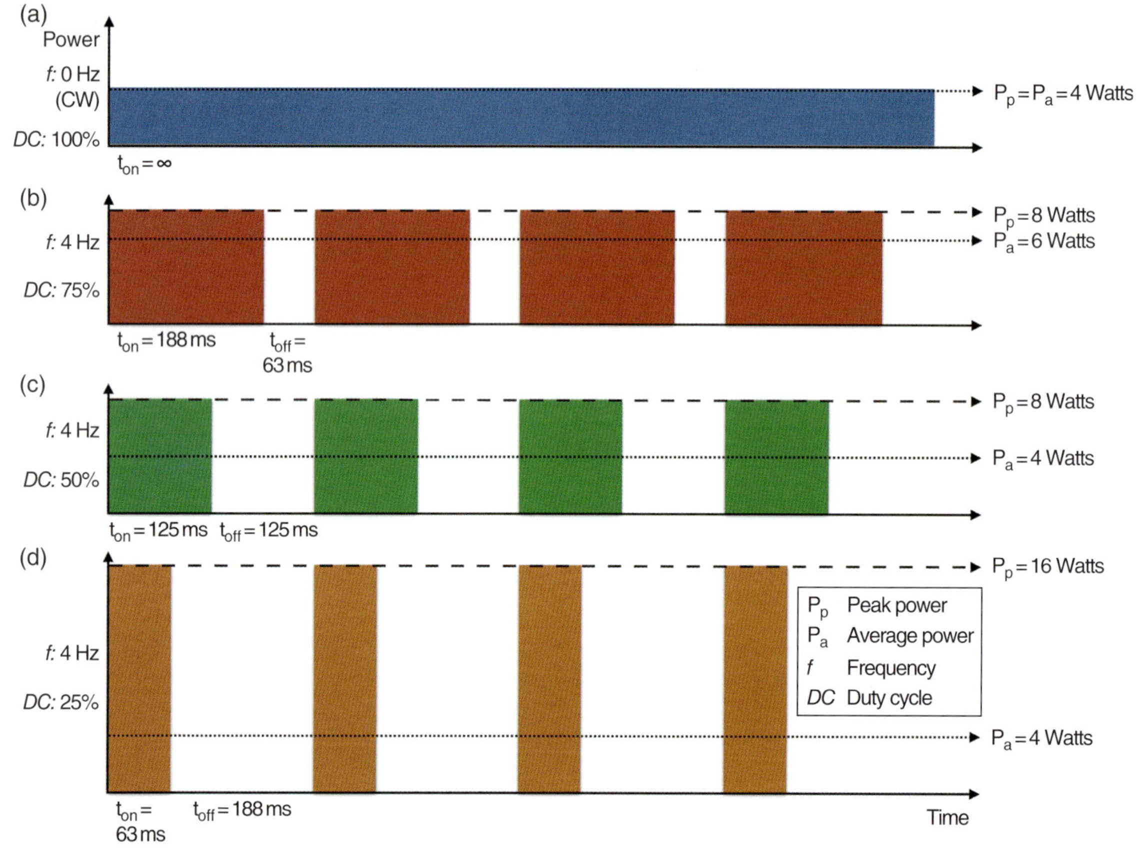

Figure 2.6 Pulse structure and its effect on average power. Pulse width (t_{on}) and dark period (t_{off}) combine to yield more common parameters – frequency and duty cycle – which, combined with peak power (P_p), can be used to calculate average power (P_a). Careful, though: these parameters alone can be misleading, as different combinations can lead to the same (a, c, and d) or different (b and c or d) average outputs.

Acknowledgment

A very special thanks to Luis De Taboada for his help on the second edition of this chapter. I only knew of Luis from our collective years in this industry (his trump mine, by a lot) and heard his name in reverent whispers as "the guy who knows." I've come to know him as a friend and colleague, and now I understand first-hand the esteem he deserves. We've spend many hours discussing this modality (and this chapter) and his insight and perspective have been invaluable to furthering the depth of my understanding. This chapter has benefited from his review, comments, suggestions, and most explicitly all the simulation work that generated the plots in Figures 2.4 and 2.5, not to mention the analysis surrounding them. This second edition is more robust than the first due to his impact more than any other reason. Thanks, Luis.

References

Ash, C. *et al.* (2017). Effect of wavelength and beam width on penetration in light-tissue interaction using computational models. *Lasers Med Sci.* 32:1909–1918.

Assi, H.T.I. *et al.* (2022). A new thermal dose model based on Vogel-Tammann-Fulcher behaviour in thermal damage processes. *Int J Hyperth.* 39(1):697–705.

ASTM (2008). Standard tables for reference solar spectral irradiances: direct normal and hemispherical on tilted surface. In: *ASTM Standard G173-03*. ASTM International, West Conshohocken.

Chaki, C. *et al.* (2023). Three-dimensional irradiance and temperature distributions resulting from transdermal application of laser light to the human knee – a numerical approach. *J Biophotonics*. 16(9):e202200283. doi:10.1002/jbio.202200283.

COMSOL (n.d.). Multiphysics® v. 6.2. www.comsol.com. COMSOL AB, Stockholm, Sweden.

Hale, G.M. and Querry, M.R. (1973). Optical constants of water in the 200 nm to 200 μm wavelength region. *Appl Opt*. 12(3):555–563.

Hashmi, J. *et al.* (2010). Effect of pulsing in low-level light therapy. *Lasers Surg Med*. 42(6):450–466.

Iorizzo, T.W. *et al.* (2021). Temperature induced changes in the optical properties of skin in vivo. *Nature Res*. 11:754.

Jacques, S. (2013). Optical properties of biological tissues: a review. *Phys Med Biol*. 58(11):R37–R61.

Karu, T.I. *et al.* (1996). Different sensitivity of cells from tumor-bearing organisms to continuous-wave and pulsed laser light (632.8 nm) evaluated by chemiluminescence test. *Lasers Life Sci*. 7(3):141–156.

Karu, T.I. *et al.* (1997). Nonmonotonic behavior of the dose dependence of the radiation effect on cells in vitro exposed to pulsed laser radiation at 820 nm. *Lasers Surg Med*. 21(5):485–492.

Karu, T.I. *et al.* (2008). Absorption measurements of cell monolayers relevant to mechanisms of laser phototherapy: reduction or oxidation of cytochrome c oxidase under laser radiation at 632.8 nm. *Photomed Laser Surg*. 26(6):593–599.

Segelstein, D.J. (1981). The complex refractive index of water. M.S. thesis. Department of Physics, University of Missouri–Kansas City.

Yarmolenko, P.S. *et al.* (2011). Thresholds for thermal damage to normal tissues: an update. *Int J Hyperth*. 27(4):320–343.

Zolotarev, V.M. *et al.* (1969). Dispersion and absorption of liquid water in the infrared and radio regions of the spectrum. *Opt Spectrosc*. 27:430–432.

3

Basic Principles of Photobiomodulation and Its Effects at the Cellular, Tissue, and System Levels

Juanita J. Anders[1] *and Ann K. Ketz*[2]

[1] *Edward Hébert School of Medicine, Uniformed Services University of the Health Sciences, Bethesda, MD, USA*
[2] *Recovery Sciences, Enovis, Lewisville, TX, USA*

Photobiomodulation: Nomenclature History

Dr. Theodore Maiman developed the first working laser at Hughes Research Laboratory, and published his paper describing its operation in *Nature* in 1960 (Maiman 1960). By 1963, pioneering experiments were being done on surgical applications of the laser (Mcguff *et al.,* 1964). Dr. Endre Mester is believed to have been the fourth physician to use lasers in medical applications, and he was the first to publish results suggesting that low-power lasers could have a stimulating effect on cells (Mester *et al.,* 1968a; Mester *et al.,* 1968c).

Surgical applications of lasers were (and still are) widely accepted due to a number of factors. The mechanisms behind how they work were identified, easily understood, and accepted. It was believed that the surgical use of lasers represented an improvement over the traditional scalpel by providing accurate cutting, coagulation, decontamination, and faster healing. Furthermore, the terminology used to describe the surgical applications of lasers was consistent and unified. In contrast, the use of low-powered lasers to alter cellular and tissue function was met with skepticism, for several reasons. The beneficial effects were subtle and difficult to study and measure, and the mechanistic basis for how photons could interact with cells to cause a positive therapeutic outcome was not known (Mick 2014).

Another factor adding to the confusion surrounding this emerging field was inconsistent terminology. In Mester's 1968 publication, he used the phrase "low power laser rays" (Mester *et al.,* 1968a), and he introduced the term "biostimulation" in 1985 (Mester *et al.,* 1985). A number of other terms were also introduced, such as "cool laser," "cold laser," "cold low-level laser therapy," "soft laser," and "low-power laser therapy." These terms were primarily industry-driven, in an attempt to distinguish these lasers from surgical lasers (Calderhead 1991). As pointed out by Calderhead (1991), all these terms were "hardware-related," and ignored the effect of the lasers on the tissue. Many were not accurate, since a high-powered surgical laser such as a carbon dioxide (CO_2) laser could be used as a low-power device if the beam were spread to a large spot size (Calderhead 1991).

The most important factor in selecting a term for this scientific and therapeutic field is the interaction of light with the target tissue, leading to a cascade of photon-driven cellular effects. A number of terms have been introduced to describe this light–tissue interaction, including "light therapy" or "phototherapy," "low reactive-level laser treatment," and "low level-laser therapy" (LLLT). It is interesting to note that it is now commonly thought that LLLT refers to the power of the laser. However, when this term was introduced by Calderhead (1991), it referred to the level of tissue reaction to the dose of light delivered. Thus, LLLT was defined as a dose of light that is below the level of the damage threshold and causes cellular photoactivation (Figure 3.1) (Calderhead 1991).

Mester reviewed his 20 years of clinical and experimental use of lasers in 1985 (Mester *et al.,* 1985). Though he notes in his abstract that "Low-energy laser radiation was found to have a stimulating effect on cells, and high-energy radiation had an inhibiting effect," the tremendous amount of data demonstrating stimulatory effects led him to propose the term "biostimulation."

Around the time (1988–89) that the first edition of the journal *Laser Therapy* was published, Calderhead recalls debating the use of the terms "photobiostimulation," "photobiomodulation," and "photobioactivation." The journal rejected the use of "photobiostimulation" because of the inhibitory effects observed with LLLT (e.g., decrease in collagen III synthesis in the prevention or remodeling of hypertrophic scars). "Photobioactivation" was chosen over "photobiomodulation" "because we felt it conveyed more

Laser Therapy in Veterinary Medicine: Photobiomodulation, Second Edition. Edited by Christopher J. Winkler and Lisa A. Miller.

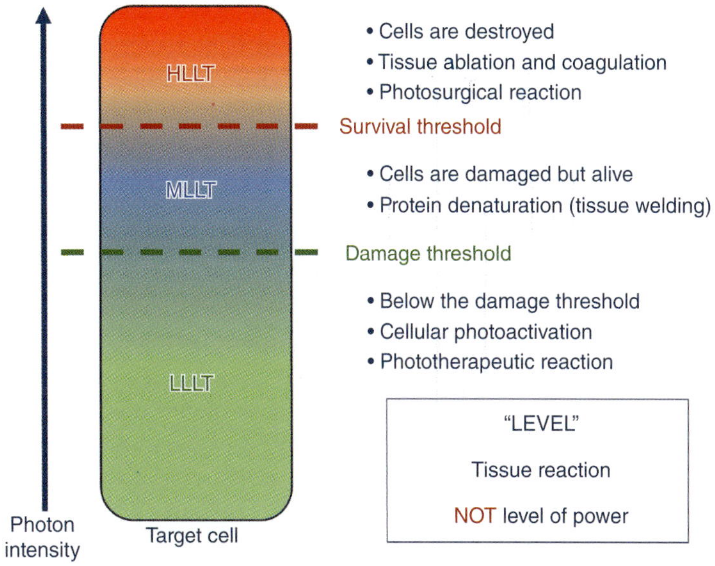

Figure 3.1 Tissue reaction to light, related to the parameters used. "High-level laser therapy" (HLLT) refers to the response of tissue to treatment parameters that are above the survival threshold, such as in surgical applications. "Medium-level laser therapy" (MLLT) is the response of tissue to laser parameters that are above the damage threshold but below the survival threshold. "Low-level laser therapy" (LLLT) is the modulation of functions of cells and tissues to parameters that are below the damage threshold. Adapted from Calderhead (1991).

accurately the overall effect on a target organism and its components" (Calderhead, pers. comm.). The term "photobioactivation" appeared in the subheading on the front cover and in the editorial of the pilot issue of *Laser Therapy* (Ohshiro 1989). In 1991, Calderhead expanded on the concept that light can cause stimulation or inhibition in relation to its dose, as well as on the selection of the term "photobioactivation" (Calderhead 1991).

With the recent advancement of laser technology producing higher-power devices (>0.5 W), another term, "high-intensity laser therapy (HILT)," has entered the literature. HILT can create warmth on the surface of the skin during treatment, but the main mechanism of action, as with the lower power lasers, is biochemical effects from light rather than heat.

The first formal reported use of "photobiomodulation" in the PubMed literature dates back to 1997 (Yu *et al.*, 1997a), though it had been used colloquially for several preceding years. In 2002, in conjunction with the Defense Advanced Research Projects Agency (DARPA) program titled "Persistence in Combat," which focused on the use of light to accelerate wound healing, a meeting was held at Uniformed Services University of the Health Sciences in Bethesda, Maryland, which included Drs. Tiina Karu, Ronald Waynant, Ilko Ilev, Kurt Henry, and Juanita Anders. At this meeting, it was decided that the term "photobiomodulation" should be used exclusively for this discipline. In 2003, Dr. Anders formally requested that the American Society for Laser Medicine & Surgery (ASLMS) change the name of their biostimulation abstract session to "Photobiomodulation." A major effort was made by many leaders in the field to use this term and to encourage others to do the same.

A nomenclature consensus meeting was organized under the auspices of the joint conference of the North American Association for Light Therapy and the World Association for Laser Therapy in 2014. It was attended by 15 international participants and co-chaired by Drs. Jan Bjordal and Juanita Anders. "Photobiomodulation" was considered by the majority of the participants to be the term of choice to describe the mechanistic and scientific basis for this photonic specialty, and "photobiomodulation therapy" the term for its therapeutic application. However, a major limitation to the adoption of this term was that "photobiomodulation therapy" was not a MeSH term of the National Library of Medicine (NLM)'s controlled vocabulary thesaurus. A request was submitted to the MeSH Section at the NLM, thanks to the efforts of Dr. Praveen Arany, and "photobiomodulation therapy" was added to the MeSH database's 2016 version as an entry term for the existing record of "laser therapy, low-level."

With the recent advancement of laser technology producing higher power devices (>0.5 W), another term, "high-intensity laser therapy (HILT)," has entered the literature in an attempt to differentiate from LLLT. HILT can create warmth on the surface of the skin during treatment but the main mechanism of action, like with the lower power lasers, is biochemical effects from light rather than heat therefore is also accurately describes as photobiomodulation therapy.

In summary, "photobiomodulation therapy" is an accurate and specific term for this effective and important therapeutic application of light. Universal use of "photobiomodulation" (PBM) and "photobiomodulation therapy" (PBMT) will eliminate confusion in the field and in the scientific, clinical, and lay literature. A suggested definition for PBMT was published in an editorial: "A form of light therapy that utilizes nonionizing forms of light sources including lasers, LEDs, and broadband light, in the visible and infrared spectrum. It is a nonthermal process involving endogenous chromophores eliciting photophysical, and photochemical events at various biological scales" (Anders *et al.*, 2015).

Making Sense of Commonly Used Device and Treatment Parameter Terminology

Besides the confusion that surrounded the name for this photonic science and therapy, a brief review of the PBM and PBMT literature will convince you of the nonstandardized and often confusing use of device parameters and treatment terms. Table 3.1 is a summary of terms commonly used to report device and treatment parameters, their definitions and abbreviations, and their synonyms.

Another problem plaguing the PBM and PBMT community is the lack of a complete description of the device and treatment parameters used in a laboratory or in clinical studies (Jenkins and Carroll 2011). A comprehensive list of device and treatment parameters to report was published in 2011 (Jenkins and Carroll). Not every parameter described in this report may be relevant to a specific experiment or treatment. For example, if an *in vivo* PBM treatment is targeting deep tissue with the handpiece in contact with the skin, then beam spot size and area irradiated at the depth of the target may be unknown. However, every parameter that can be measured should be included in the report.

Another error in describing treatment parameters that many scientists and clinicians still make is to report only the total joules (J) delivered. This parameter is useless on its own. The output power of the device, time of treatment, and spot size or treatment area are essential in order for the total joules delivered to be useful, repeatable data. Based on research from our laboratory, 65 J delivered transcutaneously to the transected peroneal nerve in a white New Zealand rabbit injury model either inhibited nerve regeneration or significantly increased the rate of regeneration, depending on the output power and treatment time (Anders *et al.*, 2014). The parameters used in this study were: control group (received no laser treatment), 2 W group (980 nm wavelength; continuous wave [CW]; output power: 2.0 W; treatment time: 32 seconds; 8 cm^2 area; 65 J), and 4 W group (output power: 4.0 W; treatment time: 16 seconds; 8 cm^2 area; 65 J) (Anders *et al.*, 2014). The fact that total joules reported on its own is a useless parameter was discussed by Calderhead (1991).

PBM Device and Treatment Parameters Based on Location of Target Tissue

Mester *et al.* (1971) reported that a dose of 1 J/cm^2 from a ruby laser caused significant stimulation of healing of cutaneous wounds and burns in a mouse model. In his *in vitro* and animal experiments, Mester tested the effects of fluences ranging from 0.05 to 4.0 J/cm^2 (Mester *et al.*, 1968b; Mester *et al.*, 1968a; Mester *et al.*, 1968c; Mester *et al.*, 1985; Mester *et al.*, 1971). These reported fluences had a significant impact on *in vitro* and preclinical animal studies. Indeed, a review of the literature on PBM effects on the proliferation of cultured cells concluded that a fluence of 0.5–4.0 J/cm^2 and a visible spectrum ranging from 600 to 700 nm enhanced the proliferation rate of various cell lines (Alghamdi *et al.*, 2012). Similarly, a review of the literature on *in vivo* rat and mouse animal studies of wound healing identified that use of red

Table 3.1 Summary of terms commonly used to report device and treatment parameters.

Term	Definition	Abbreviation (SI unit)	Formula	Synonym
Watt	Unit of power (Jenkins and Carroll 2011).	W	W = J/time(t)	Radiant power
Joule	Unit of work and energy (Jenkins and Carroll 2011).	J	J = W × t	Radiant energy
Fluence	The radiant energy received by a surface per unit area (Jenkins and Carroll 2011).	J/m^2, J/cm^2	J/cm^2	Radiant exposure; radiant fluence; energy density
Irradiance	The power received by or crossing a surface per unit area.	W/m^2, W/cm^2	W/cm^2	Intensity; power density
Fluence rate	W/m^2 seen by an absorber inside a medium (Anders *et al.*, 2014). It is only equal to irradiance when the beam is orthogonal to the surface (Mester *et al.*, 1971).	W/cm^2	W/cm^2	

or near-infrared wavelengths at a range of fluences with a median of 4.2 J/cm^2 resulted in significant improvement in wound healing (Peplow *et al.,* 2010b).

Therefore, many experiments supported the validity of Mester's original parameters for superficial applications. However, when clinicians began to use PBM to treat structures that were located deeper in the body, they persisted in using these parameters, with negative results. This led to the publication of a number of negative studies and the conclusion that there was inadequate evidence to recommend PBM for clinical use (Basford 1993; Basford 1995; Basford *et al.,* 1998). It is now obvious that the negative studies were the result of incorrect device and treatment parameters (Tuner and Hode 1998). Recently, two important advances have been made in PBMT: a broadening of the clinical application of this therapy to transcutaneous treatment of tissues and organs within the body, and the recognition that optimization of the therapeutic parameters should be based on the photonic dose reaching the target tissue (Anders *et al.,* 2014; Weersink *et al.,* 2007).

The wavelength of light used governs its depth of penetration into a tissue. Both absorption and scattering coefficients of living tissues are higher at shorter wavelengths, meaning near-infrared light penetrates more deeply than red light (Craig and Welch 2001). In 2005, we examined transcutaneous light penetration to the level of the spinal cord in adult, anesthetized Sprague–Dawley rats (Byrnes *et al.*). An incoherent broadband white light was applied to the surface of the skin over the thoracic vertebrae. A tissue-activated optical fiberprobe was inserted sequentially into the skin, subcutaneous connective tissue layer, deep connective tissue layer, dorsal muscle mass, and spinal cord within the vertebral column. At each of these layers, a transmission spectrum in the range of 500–1200 nm was collected. Analysis of the transmission spectra revealed the range of penetration was highest through all tissue layers overlying the spinal cord and through blood between the 770 and 850 nm wavelengths, with a peak at 810 nm. The 810 nm wavelength was minimally absorbed by blood and water. These data demonstrate that 810 nm wavelength light is within the optimal range for light penetration to tissues deep in the body (Byrnes *et al.,* 2005a).

Experiments in our laboratory also established that transcutaneous treatment parameters for a specific wavelength of light could be determined initially using *in vitro* models to identify effective laser parameters at the cellular level, and that these parameters could then be translated to pre-clinical research and clinical practice (Anders *et al.,* 2014). The translation of dose from *in vitro* to *in vivo* was accomplished by adjusting the *in vitro* parameters based on light penetration measurements. On average, 2.45% of infrared light (980 nm wavelength) applied to the skin reached the depth of the peroneal nerve in anesthetized white New Zealand rabbits. Based on our calculations, the following treatment parameters were used on the injured peroneal nerve: 980 nm wavelength; CW, output power: 1.5 W; treatment time: 43 seconds; scanned over an 8 cm^2 area, 65 J. This resulted in a significant improvement in the toe-spread reflex test compared to controls (Anders *et al.,* 2014).

Photoacceptors

Knowledge of the fundamental tenets of photobiology is essential to understanding the mechanistic basis of PBM and PBMT. The first law of photochemistry states that light must be absorbed for photochemistry to occur (Smith 1991). Therefore, for PBM to occur, there must be a molecule capable of absorbing light: a photoacceptor. Upon light absorption, an electronically excited state occurs, which alters the primary molecular processes that lead to biological effects at the cellular level by secondary biochemical reactions and cellular signaling (Passarella and Karu 2014). What wavelengths a photoacceptor will absorb can be determined by its absorption spectrum (Smith 1991).

The electron transport chain, embedded in the inner membrane of eukaryotic mitochondria, consists of four large membrane protein complexes. The function of the electron transport chain is to produce a transmembrane proton electrochemical gradient through redox reactions (Murray *et al.,* 2003). Two of the protein complexes contain photoacceptors: NADH dehydrogenase and cytochrome c oxidase (CCO). NADH dehydrogenase is located in complex 1, which is the first enzyme of the electron transport chain (Brandt 2006), and absorbs light in the violet to blue spectral region, with absorption maxima at 272, 372, and 448 nm wavelengths (Wakao *et al.,* 1987).

Mitochondrial CCO

CCO is located in complex IV of the electron transport chain, and its oxidized and reduced forms have absorption spectra in the red and near-infrared region (Figure 3.2) (UCL, 2016). It is a complex enzyme, consisting of a large number of polypeptide subunits (Figure 3.3). Subunits I, II, and III are mitochondrially encoded, and I and II are the catalytic core of the enzyme. Subunit I contains two heme groups (heme a, heme a3) and a redox-active copper site, Cu_B; subunit II contains another redox-active copper site, Cu_A, and the cytochrome c binding site (Cooper *et al.,*, 1991). Cytochrome c is the small protein that delivers electrons to CCO. CCO uses the metal ions to reduce

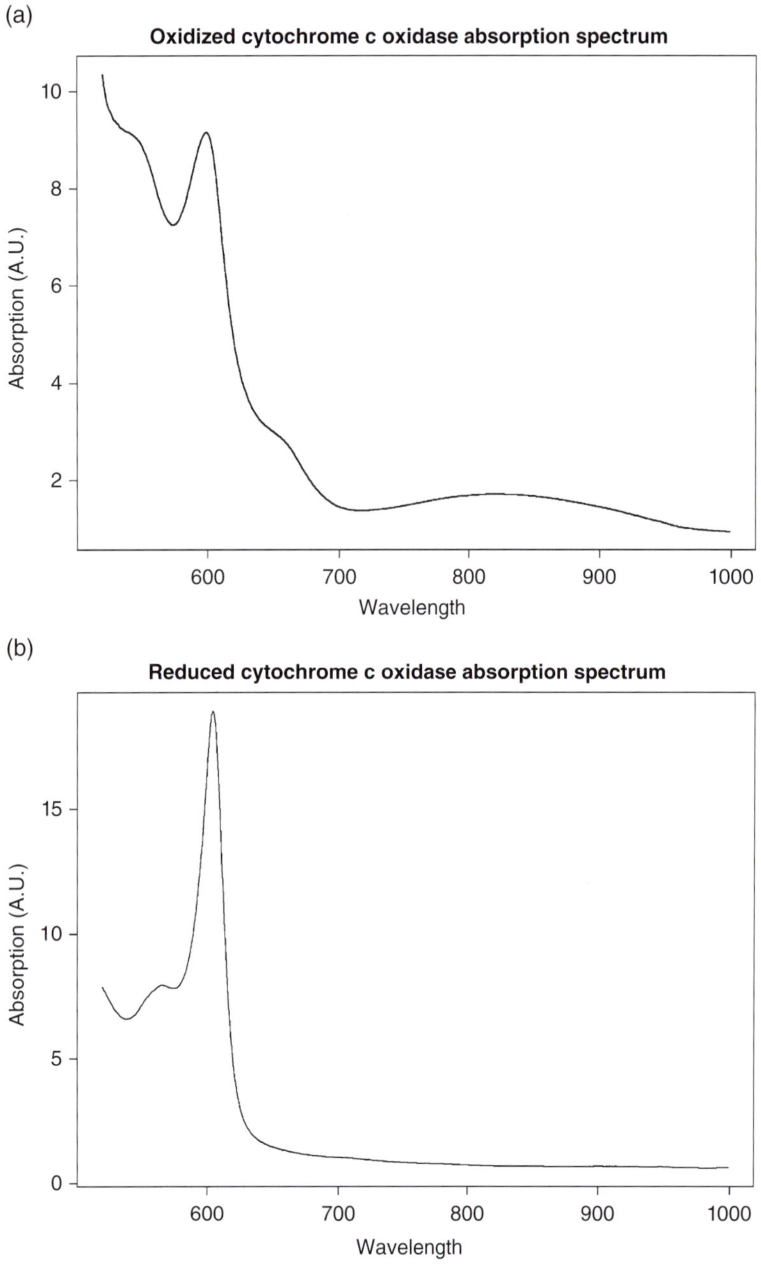

Figure 3.2 Oxidized (a) and reduced (b) CCO absorption spectra (converted to absorbance from extinction spectra data by Xingjia Wu).

molecular oxygen to water (Tsukihara *et al.*, 1995; Voet and Voet 2010).

Karu defined the action spectra for the DNA and RNA synthesis rate, adhesive properties, and proliferation rate of HeLa cells, and generated a generalized action spectrum in the range of 580–860 nm. This action spectrum had defined maxima at 620, 680, 760, and 820 nm (Karu 1998). Based on the premise that the action spectrum approximates the shape of the absorption spectrum of the photoacceptor (Hartmann 1983), Karu proposed that the bands of the generalized action spectrum may be related to CCO (Karu 1998). In fact, Karu had previously proposed that the photoacceptor for PBM was a component of the mitochondrial respiratory chain (Karu 1987). Based on comparative analysis of the generalized action spectrum and the spectroscopic data for CCO, Karu and Afanas'eva hypothesized that the 820 nm band correlated with the oxidized Cu_A, the 760 band with the reduced Cu_B, the 680 band with the oxidized Cu_B, and the 620 band with the reduced Cu_A (Figure 3.3) (Karu and Afanas'eva 1995). An experiment looking at the effect of 632.8 nm light on the purified CCO enzyme caused an increase in the oxidation of the enzyme and increased electron transfer, thus supporting Karu's conclusion (Pastore *et al.*, 2000).

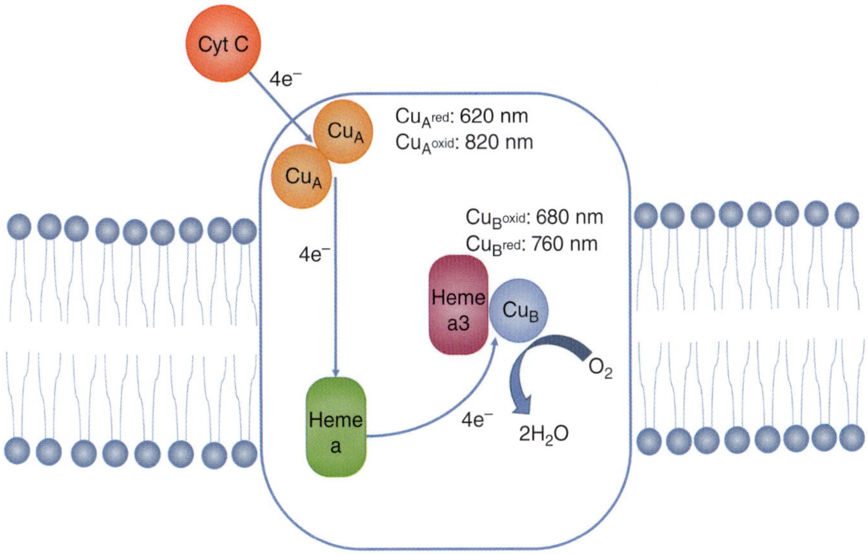

Figure 3.3 Subunit components of CCO and the wavelength maxima that correlate with the oxidized and reduced forms of the copper sites, as suggested by Karu. CCO uses the metal ions to reduce molecular oxygen to water. Subunit I contains heme a, heme a3, and a redox-active copper site, Cu_B; Subunit II contains the redox-active copper site (Cu_A) and the cytochrome c binding site. Cytochrome c is the small protein that delivers electrons to CCO.

Cellular Signaling Molecules

Excitation of CCO leads to an electronically excited state and acceleration of electron transfer reactions in mitochondria, which eventually leads to alteration of molecular and cellular changes through cellular signaling reactions. Increases in three signaling molecules are implicated in PBM activation of cellular signaling cascades. These molecules are adenosine triphosphate (ATP), reactive oxygen species (ROS), and nitric oxide (NO) (Hamblin and Demidova 2006; Karu 2010).

Adenosine Triphosphate

ATP is a nucleotide that performs many essential roles in the cell. It provides the energy for most of its energy-consuming activities and regulates many biochemical pathways. ATP levels control the level of cyclic adenosine monophosphate (cAMP)- and ATP-driven carriers for ions such as Na^+/K^+ ATPase and calcium ion pumps. ATP stimulates intracellular pathways such as mitogen-activated protein kinases (MAPKs) and can act in conjunction with growth factors such as fibroblastic growth factor 2 (FGF2), epidermal growth factor (EGF), and nerve growth factor (NGF) to elicit biological responses. Therefore, ATP levels can have profound effects on almost every important biochemical process (Karu 2010; Hamblin and Demidova 2006).

In 1984, Passarella demonstrated that irradiation of isolated rat liver mitochondria with 632.8 nm light increased ATP synthesis, mitochondrial membrane potential, and the electrochemical proton gradient (Passarella *et al.*, 1984). Increased ATP syntheses induced by various wavelengths of light have been reported not only in isolated mitochondria but also in various cell types (Passarella and Karu 2014; Karu 2007). Therefore, increasing cellular ATP and cellular metabolism can have beneficial effects on injured and diseased cells and tissues in which cellular metabolism is suppressed (Karu 2010).

It is now known that ATP is also an important intercellular signaling molecule (Burnstock 2009; Karu 2010; Khakh and Burnstock 2009; Novak 2003). The release of ATP from cells can affect the ATP-releasing cells or adjacent cells through purinergic receptors. A wide variety of purinergic receptors associated with many different cell types is now known (Novak 2003).

In 1978, Burnstock proposed that specific G-protein-linked receptors mediate the physiological effects of ATP, such as calcium mobilization and second messenger activation (Burnstock 1978; Abbracchio and Burnstock 1994). Abbracchio and Burnstock (1994) proposed that two families of purinoceptors be established: (i) a P2X family, which mediates fast receptor responses linked to an ion channel, and (ii) a P2Y family, which mediates slower responses through G-proteins. They further proposed that the P2-purinoceptors (ATP/ADP) that are G-protein-coupled should be incorporated into the P2Y family (Abbracchio and Burnstock 1994). G-protein-coupled receptors represent the largest superfamily of proteins in the body, with over 1000 different receptors identified. Interestingly, G-protein-coupled receptors mediate exogenous stimuli such as light, smell, and taste (Gether 2000). In 2008, our laboratory reported that P2Y receptors were involved in light-mediated neurite outgrowth of normal human neuronal progenitor cells (Figure 3.4). In this study, we used 810 nm-wavelength light and demonstrated that

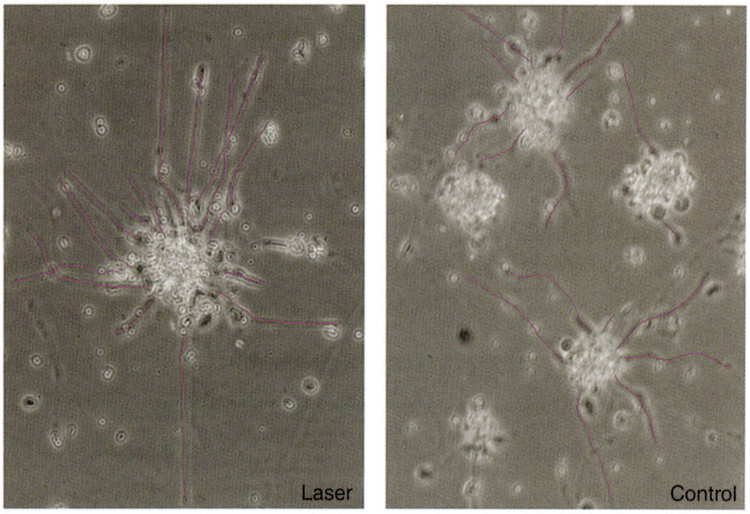

Figure 3.4 Photomicrographs of normal human progenitor cells (208×). Laser panel shows cells treated with a CW, 810 nm-wavelength diode laser with an output power of 150 mW at an irradiance of 50 mW/cm^2 an exposure time of 4 seconds, and a fluence of 0.2 J/cm^2. The control panel shows cells that were handled exactly like the laser-treated cells, except the laser was off. Neurite extensions are marked in pink using Neuron J in Image J (http://rsb.info.nih.gov/ij). Note that the irradiated cells have more neurites and longer total neurite length.

neurite outgrowth stimulated by PBM was caused by increased ATP acting as a signaling molecule through the P2Y receptors (Anders *et al.*, 2008). These findings suggest that G-protein-coupled membrane receptors may play a critical role in the response of cells to light.

Reactive Oxygen Species

Oxygen metabolism produces chemically reactive, oxygen-containing molecules known collectively as ROS (Chung *et al.*, 2012). High concentrations of ROS produced by chronic inflammatory processes, toxic chemical exposure, and environmental stresses can cause oxidative cell damage. However, in lower concentrations, these molecules (including peroxides, superoxide, hydroxyl radical, and singlet oxygen) have beneficial effects (Chung *et al.*, 2012; Farivar *et al.*, 2014; Tafur and Mills 2008). ROS have been shown to promote cell proliferation (Burdon 1995; Burdon *et al.*, 1995; Callaghan *et al.*, 1996; Murrell *et al.*, 1990), induce neuronal differentiation (Suzukawa *et al.*, 2000), protect cardiac cells (Das 2001; Vanden Hoek *et al.*, 1998), and serve as important signaling molecules for gene expression, cell growth, and transcription factor activation (Rhee 1999; Suzuki and Ford 1999).

ROS production *in vitro* by both visible and near-infrared light has been reported by various laboratories. Lubart and colleagues used a 780 nm diode laser to stimulate proliferation of cultured normal human keratinocytes with a single dose of 0.45–0.95 J/cm^2 and reported an increase in cell number and cell division. To determine the role of ROS in keratinocyte proliferation, they added a variety of ROS scavengers and antioxidants, which resulted in differing levels of reduction in proliferation (Grossman *et al.*, 1998; Lubart *et al.*, 2005). Experiments with skin fibroblasts have had similar results. In an elegant study carried out in conjunction with colleagues at the Food and Drug Administration (FDA), we used a specially designed nanoprobe to measure real-time transient ROS kinetics in fibroblasts exposed to 832.8 nm light. We found an increase in ROS production that was dependent on both laser intensity and total energy dose (Pal *et al.*, 2007). Using confocal laser-scanning microscopy, Alexandratou *et al.* (2002) illuminated single human fetal foreskin fibroblast cells with a 647 nm laser and reported ROS generation as monitored by specific fluorescent vital probes. Using both 810 and 980 nm light, the Hamblin laboratory reported dose-dependent ROS production in mouse embryonic fibroblasts; 0.03–0.3 J/cm^2 resulted in a positive effect, while 30 J/cm^2 reduced ROS production (Chen *et al.*, 2011)

Cells respond to ROS in a variety of ways, maintaining the tight balance between moderate oxidative stress and cytotoxic high concentrations of ROS. Various molecules with ROS-detection systems can initiate signal transduction pathways via transcription factors, resulting in production of scavenger antioxidants, protein modification, and gene expression (Chen *et al.*, 2011). Some of the transcription factors that are regulated by these changes in mitochondrial respiration are redox factor 1 (Ref-1), dependent activator protein 1 (AP-1, a heterodimer of c-Fos and c-Jun), nuclear factor kappa B (NF-KB), p53, activating transcription factor/cAMP response element-binding protein (ATF/CREB), hypoxia inducible factor 1 (HIF-1), and HIF-like factor (Chung *et al.*, 2012; Farivar *et al.*, 2014). Activation of these factors leads to synthesis of proteins that play roles in cell proliferation, tissue oxygenation, and cytokine modulation, as well as growth factors and other inflammatory mediators (Chung *et al.*, 2012; Hamblin and Demidova 2006).

Nitric Oxide

Robert F. Furchgott first described the relaxation of endothelial cells in blood vessels mediated by light in 1968 (Hamblin and Demidova 2006). His work led to the discovery of NO, a potent vasodilator that plays an important role in CCO activity. NO is a free-radical gas that regulates circulation and acts as an essential neurotransmitter (Hamblin and Demidova 2006). It is generated from the amino acid L-arginine by the enzyme nitric oxide synthase (NOS), which has three isoforms.

Two main pathways have been proposed to explain the ability of light to increase local production and release of NO (Chung *et al.,* 2012). The first is disassociation of NO from CCO by PBM. NO is well known to inhibit mitochondrial respiration through its competitive displacement of oxygen with the reduced binuclear center Cu_B/a3 of CCO (Farivar *et al.,* 2014). The "NO hypothesis" proposes that near-infrared light can cause NO to disassociate from CCO heme iron and copper centers, resulting in an increase in oxygen binding and leading to increased respiration (Hamblin and Demidova 2006).

Karu *et al.* (2005) were the first to provide evidence for the involvement of NO in PBM. They irradiated suspensions of HeLa cells with either 600–860 nm light or an 820 nm diode laser, then, after a 30-minute incubation, recorded the number of cells attached to the glass matrix. They added NO donors to the suspensions before or after irradiation and demonstrated that the addition of NO donors affected CCO binding by the NO molecules, and that the effect was dependent on both the wavelength and the fluence of the irradiation (Karu *et al.,* 2005).

Increased NO has also been reported in *in vivo* studies using a 780 nm laser to stimulate bone healing in rats (Guzzardella *et al.,* 2002) and an 804 nm laser to promote cardioprotection and angiogenesis following heart attacks in mice (Tuby *et al.,* 2006).

The second pathway that might explain the increase in NO bioavailability in response to PBM was proposed by Ball and colleagues, who demonstrated nitrite reductase enzymatic activity regulation by CCO in biological conditions where the oxygen concentration was low, such as in many disease states (Ball *et al.,* 2011; Poyton and Ball 2011; Poyton *et al.,* 2009). Conversely, other investigators reported reduced levels of NO in local tissues in response to PBM, and proposed that PBM in these cases reduced one of the isoforms of NOS (Leung *et al.,* 2002; Moriyama *et al.,* 2005). Research elucidating the different mechanisms of NO related to PBMT continues.

The NO produced by these proposed pathways can have effects both intracellularly, where it is involved in hypoxic signaling, and extracellularly (Ball *et al.,* 2011; Poyton *et al.,* 2009; Karu *et al.,* 2005). Beneficial effects of NO include pain relief, resolution of edema, improved lymphatic drainage, and improved wound healing via angiogenesis (Hamblin 2008).

PBMT Effects at the Molecular, Organelle, Cellular, and System Level

Molecular Level: Alteration of Gene Expression

There have been a number of reports on the effects of PBM on gene expression. It has been reported that red light increases expression of a number of growth factors by cells *in vitro*, including FGF-2, insulin-like growth factor (IGF), NGF, and vascular endothelial growth factor (VEGF) (Peplow and Baxter 2012). Gene expression profiles of normal human fibroblasts exposed to 632.8 nm-wavelength light were examined using a cDNA microarray (Zhang *et al.,* 2003), and 111 genes were altered by the light. This group included an up-regulation of genes related to energy metabolism and the respiratory chain, and cell proliferation. Other genes were down-regulated, including stress-induced phosphoprotein. Red light (660 nm) also caused an up-regulation of the genes coding for the subunits of enzymes involved in complexes I and IV of the mitochondrial electron transport chain and ATP synthase in *in vitro* fibroblasts (Masha *et al.,* 2013).

We examined the effects of PBM on gene expression in olfactory ensheathing cells (OECs) (Byrnes *et al.,* 2005b). OEC transplantation has been under investigation as a treatment for spinal cord injury. OECs were purified from adult rat olfactory bulbs and exposed to 810 nm light. Analysis of gene expression revealed statistically significant up-regulation of brain-derived neurotrophic factor (BDNF), glial-derived neurotrophic factor (GDNF), and collagen expression. These results demonstrate that PBM up-regulated neurotrophic growth factors and extracellular matrix (ECM) proteins known to support neurite outgrowth.

We also investigated gene expression in a rat model of spinal cord injury (dorsal hemisection at vertebral level T9 in adult female rats). The PBMT parameters used for the laser-treated group were: 810 nm CW diode laser, 150 mW output power, treatment time = 49 minutes, 57 seconds, spot size = 0.3 cm^2 fluence = 1589 J/cm^2. The treatment was done daily for 14 consecutive days. For microarray analysis, microarrays with over 1200 genes were run at 1, 6, and 48 hours post-injury and light treatment, or post-lesion and sham treatment. Expression of over 200 genes was significantly altered after PBMT and spinal cord injury. Many of the altered genes were involved in decreasing the inflammatory response, increasing receptor

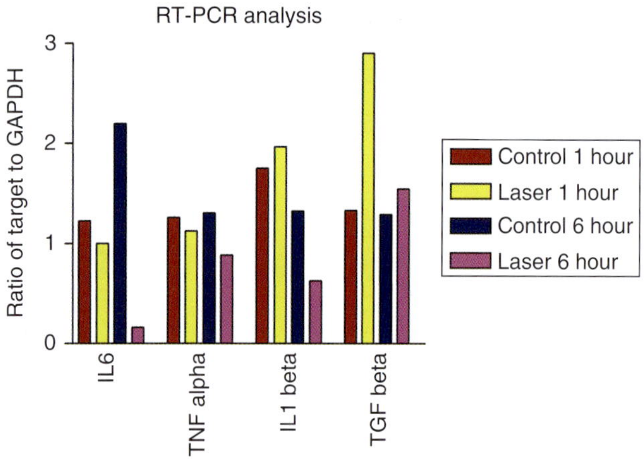

Figure 3.5 Bar graph showing the ratio of target to glyceraldehyde 3-phosphate dehydrogenase (GAPDH) based on RT-PCR analysis of control and irradiated injured spinal cord tissue at 1 and 6 hours postinjury. PBM caused a suppression of RNA expression of pro-inflammatory cytokine genes (TNFα, IL1β, and IL6) and an increase in RNA expression of the anti-inflammatory gene TGF-β.

expression for neurotrophic factors, decreasing receptor expression for glutamate and gamma-amino butyric acid (GABA) (which can induce cell death), and decreasing cell proliferation. Based on reverse transcription polymerase chain reaction (RT-PCR) analysis (Figure 3.5), PBMT caused suppression of interleukin 6 (IL6) expression at 6 hours (IL6's peak), suppression of tumor necrosis factor alpha (TNFα) expression at 6 hours (peak at 1 hour), suppression of IL1β at 6 hours (IL1β's peak), and an increase in expression of transforming growth factor beta (TGF-β) at 1 and 6 hours. TGF-β normally peaks at 7 days postinjury and is responsible for decreasing the inflammatory response. In summary, there was suppression of RNA expression of pro-inflammatory cytokine genes (TNFα, IL1β, and IL6) and an increase in RNA expression of the anti-inflammatory gene TGF-β. Our previous experiments established that PBMT increases axonal regrowth following injury and decreased inflammatory cell invasion/activation (Byrnes *et al.*, 2005a). These data demonstrate that PBMT also has a significant effect on altering gene expression in the injured spinal cord.

Organelle Level: Mitochondrial Function

The structure and function of mitochondria are affected by irradiation with visible and near-infrared light. Functional changes that occur in response to irradiation relate to oxidative phosphorylation, including modulation of the mitochondrial membrane potential and metabolism and calcium intake (Passarella and Karu 2014).

The effect of irradiation on membrane potential was first reported by the Passarella laboratory (Passarella *et al.*, 1984). *In vitro* rat liver mitochondria irradiated with a HeNe laser (15 mW/cm^2, J/cm^2) caused an increase in membrane potential and proton gradient difference compared to non-irradiated samples. However, Passarella and Yu further demonstrated that high membrane potential alone does not account for the effects of PBM (Passarella *et al.*, 1984; Passarella *et al.*, 1988; Yu *et al.*, 1997b). Further studies with 660 nm light demonstrated increased oxygen consumption, phosphate potential, energy charge, and electron chain enzymatic activity (Hermann and Shaw 1998).

Of the mitochondrial processes responsive to PBM, several involve Ca^{2+} activity, including modifying the shape of cytosolic Ca^{2+} pulses, oxidative phosphorylation rate, induction of the mitochondrial permeability transition, and possibly apoptotic cell death (Passarella and Karu 2014). Investigators have attempted to determine the role of Ca^{2+} in response to PBM. Lubart and colleagues (Breitbart *et al.*, 1996; Lubart *et al.*, 1997) tested to see whether PBM could influence Ca^{2+} transport across the mitochondrial membrane. They irradiated digitonin-treated spermatozoa or plasma membrane vesicles with a HeNe laser (fluence rate: 0.3–10.0 mW/cm^2 fluence: 0.04–0.8 J/cm^2) and measured Ca^{2+} uptake. For these experiments, cells were incubated in a medium with Ca^{2+} and immediately irradiated. The investigators determined that PBM at lower power caused an increased uptake of Ca^{2+} by mitochondria but not by membrane vesicles, while higher-power irradiation inhibited Ca^{2+} uptake (Breitbart *et al.*, 1996). Lubart also reported that irradiation with 780 nm light inhibited Ca^{2+} uptake by mitochondria, indicating the importance of dosing. Passarella reported increased mitochondrial membrane potential, along with increased cytosolic free Ca^{2+} and c-fos expression changes, when isolated hepatocytes were mixed with Ca^{2+} and irradiated with a HeNe laser (fluence rate: 12 mW/cm^2; fluence: 0.24 J/cm^2) (Vacca *et al.*, 1997).

Cellular Level

Cellular responses to PBMT have been determined using *in vitro* and *in vivo* models. They include increases in metabolism, proliferation, migration, synthesis, and secretion of proteins. This section will focus on cell proliferation in the treatment of tendinopathies and wound healing, to highlight these two important clinical PBMT applications. *In vitro* studies have demonstrated the proliferative effect of PBMT in a variety of human and animal cell types, including fibroblasts, keratinocytes, endothelial cells, lymphocytes, muscle cells, and stem cells (Hamblin and Demidova 2006; Peplow *et al.*, 2010a). Though the mechanisms for each cell type are not completely understood, in general, the increase of ROS by irradiated cells results in the expression of transcription factors such as NF-KB, which then activate a form of NOS and lead to proliferation (Alexandratou *et al.,* 2002; Lubart and Breitbart 2000).

PBMT has been used clinically to treat a variety of tendinopathies (Doyle *et al.,* 2016; Haslerud *et al.,* 2015; Nogueira Jr. and Junior Mde 2015), and one potential mechanism is the proliferation of tenocytes (Tsai *et al.,* 2014; Tsai *et al.,* 2012). Tenocyte migration and proliferation are largely responsible for the deposition of the extracellular matrix (ECM) required in the regenerative phase of tendon repair (Chen *et al.,* 2009). *In vitro* rat tenocytes were used to test the effects of PBMT on cellular proliferation in response to irradiation with 660 nm light (output power: 50 mW; energy densities: 1.0, 1.5, 2.0, or 2.5 J/cm^2) (Tsai *et al.,* 2014). These dosing parameters were similar to those used to increase Achilles tendon fibroblast proliferation in other experiments by the same investigators (Chen *et al.,* 2009). Proliferation was significantly elevated compared to controls in these studies. A recent systematic review of 50 animal studies and 5 human studies evaluated the effect of PBMT on tendon healing and reported positive impacts, though the lack of homogeneity of treatment parameters prevented meta-analysis of the reviewed data (He *et al.,* 2023). Differing levels of evidence demonstrated that PBMT contributed to tendon healing by suppressing inflammation, promoting collagen synthesis and re-organization, inhibiting pro-inflammatory cytokines and MMPs, stimulating growth factors secretion, and restoring biomechanical properties (He *et al.,* 2023).

PBMT has also been effectively used to accelerate wound healing; proliferation of fibroblasts and epithelial cells plays an important role in the multi-step wound-healing process. After the inflammatory phase of healing, fibroblast division and collection at wound edges occur, as fibroblasts are essential in the synthesis of connective-tissue proteins, such as collagen (Reddy 2004). Fibroblast proliferation has been demonstrated in response to PBMT for several decades, with the first experiments reporting a fivefold increase in mouse fibroblasts *in vitro* when irradiated by pulsed ruby laser, as compared to nonirradiated controls (Hardy *et al.,* 1967). More recently, Lucroy irradiated mouse fibroblasts and endothelial cells with a range of wavelengths: visible red light from 625 to 675 nm with a KTP-pumped tunable dye laser, and near-infrared light at 810 nm with a diode laser (power density: 5 mW/cm^2 energy density: 10 J/cm^2) (Moore *et al.,* 2005). They measured proliferation 72 hours post-irradiation using a colorimetric assay for viable cells. Compared to control cells, irradiated fibroblasts had increased proliferation in all visible red wavelengths studied, but near-infrared 810 nm light resulted in inhibition. Maximum proliferation was measured in those fibroblasts irradiated with red light. In endothelial cells, proliferation was recorded in all red and near-infrared wavelengths, with the maximum proliferation at 655 nm (Moore *et al.,* 2005). This study and others highlight the importance of well-designed PBM parameters and serve as precursors to preclinical and clinical studies (Peplow *et al.,* 2010b).

Results from our laboratory demonstrate that effective *in vitro* parameters can be translated into optimized parameters for preclinical wound-healing experiments (Wu *et al.,* 2015). An *in vitro* hyperglycemic, diabetic model of primary human dermal fibroblasts (HDFs) was irradiated with an organic light-emitting diode (OLED) (623 nm peak wavelength at either 7 or 10 mW/cm^2 with fluences of 0.2, 1.0, or 5.0 J/cm^2). The effects on ATP production, mitochondrial metabolism, and HDF proliferation were measured. Groups treated with 10 mW/cm^2 at all three fluences showed significant HDF proliferation compared to controls. The 5 J/cm^2 energy density was chosen for the *in vivo* experiments based on positive results in cell proliferation and mitochondrial metabolism. The Zucker diabetic fatty (ZDF) rats were used for the preclinical study. An 8 mm full-thickness biopsy punch wound was made on the left and right flanks. The right-side wounds were treated by direct contact with the OLED device or laser (635 nm) and the left-side wounds were untreated controls. Measures of wound closure were obtained at regular intervals, histological scoring was conducted using skin samples from day 13 postinjury, and immunohistochemistry was performed to measure macrophages (ED1) and FGF2. FGF2 was used to measure cell proliferation. The OLED- and laser-treated wounds had significantly higher percentages of wound closure than control wounds; histological scores were also significantly higher in the treated groups compared to controls. Additionally, OLED-treated wounds had significantly more macrophage (ED1) labelling and FGF2 expression than non-treated controls (Wu *et al.,* 2015).

System Level

The broad systemic effects of PBMT make it an ideal therapy to use to promote tissue healing, resolve inflammation, and treat pain (Chung *et al.,* 2012). This section will focus on the effect of PBM on inflammation and pain.

Decreased Inflammation

The immunological process of inflammation is controlled by a variety of mediators, including cytokines and chemokines, which regulate the process using complex signaling mechanisms (Viegas *et al.,* 2007). Immune cells can be triggered by certain wavelengths of light, resulting in the release of inflammatory mediators (Chung *et al.*, 2012). Inflammation plays an important role in wound healing, pain management, and peripheral and central nervous system (CNS) injuries, along with a number of other disease processes.

Muscle repair following acute injury involves regulation by inflammatory cytokines. PBMT has been used to speed recovery, presumably by modulation of the inflammatory process. The proinflammatory cytokine IL1β was decreased in PBM-treated groups (660 nm, 20 mW, 5 J/cm^2) of male Wistar rats with cryoinjury, but not in injured rats without PBM treatment 1 week after injury (Fernandes *et al.*, 2013).

The effect of PBMT on inflammatory joint diseases has been investigated. Following sub-plantar muscle-tissue carrageenan injection of rat paws, PBM with 660 or 684 nm wavelengths (30 mW, 7.5 J/cm^2) resulted in increased mRNA expression of IL1β, TNFα, and IL6 3 hours after treatment (Albertini *et al.*, 2008). Another study reported the IL1β, TNFα, and IL6 response to PBMT following papain solution (4%) injection into knee joints of male Wistar rats (osteoarthritis model). Two dose groups of 808 nm light were compared, a 50 mW and a 100 mW group. The 50 mW group had a power density of 1.78 W/cm^2, while the 100 mW group had a power density of 3.57 W/cm^2; both groups had a total energy of 4 J and an energy density of 142.4 J/cm^2. The 50 mW group had decreased cellular inflammation (as assessed by histological analysis) and, more significantly, decreased IL1β and IL6 expression compared to the 100 mW group (Alves *et al.*, 2013).

The effect of PBMT on inflammatory markers in neuropathic pain animal models has also been investigated. Masoumipoor *et al.* (2014) investigated the effect of PBM (660 nm light) on inflammatory markers in a neuropathic pain model (chronic constriction injury) in adult male Sprague–Dawley rats. Hsieh *et al.* (2012) reported a decrease in pro-inflammatory markers (TNF, IL1β, HIF-1α) at the injury site (sciatic nerve) in PBMT-treated animals compared to nontreated injured animals. Both studies provide evidence that PBMT effectively modulates the inflammatory response following nerve injury.

Immunohistochemistry and Western blot were used to characterize changes in activated macrophages promoting cytokine production following nerve injury. Treated animals also had reduced production of TNFα and IL1, reduced macrophage activation, and decreased accumulation of HIF-1α-positive cells compared to nontreated injured animals (Hsieh *et al.*, 2012). The reduction in these pro-inflammatory cytokines implicated in neuropathic pain initiation and maintenance may elucidate a mechanism for the effectiveness of PBM treatment in decreasing neuropathic pain and should be carefully characterized. Peripheral nerve injury caused region-specific macrophage and microglia activation along spinothalamic and dorsal-column medial lemniscus pathways. There was no difference between treated and nontreated groups in the expression of Iba-1, a general macrophage and microglial cell-surface protein. However, the pro-inflammatory microglial marker CD86 was expressed in the spinal cord of injured rats in contrast to the PBM-treated and sham groups. Additionally, the PBM-treated dorsal root-ganglion macrophages expressed the anti-inflammatory macrophage marker CD206 (Kobiela Ketz *et al.*, 2017).

Decreased Pain

PBMT has been used to reduce pain and improve function in a variety of musculoskeletal and neuropathic pain conditions. Evidence from animal studies and clinical trials provides insight into the multiple potential mechanisms involved in treating both acute and chronic pain. It is likely that multiple mechanisms are at play when treating complex issues such as pain.

Based on several studies, it has been proposed that local vasodilation and increased microcirculation from the release of NO contribute to musculoskeletal pain relief (Cidral-Filho *et al.*, 2014; Mitchell and Mack 2013; Samoilova *et al.*, 2008). Other groups have hypothesized that PBMT increases the nociceptive threshold by inhibiting Aδ and C nerve fibers, as evidenced by a group of studies demonstrating slowed conduction velocity in peripheral nerves. A systematic review of 44 studies indicated that PBM has a range of inhibitory neural effects across different peripheral nerve experimental models of pain (Chow *et al.*, 2011). Other data suggest that PBMT may increase endorphins, activate endogenous opioids, and recruit opioid-containing leukocytes to the site of injury (Cidral-Filho *et al.*, 2014). In one study utilizing the plantar incision model of postoperative pain in adult male Swiss mice, the animals were treated with a 950 nm light-emitting diode (LED) device (spot size: 1 cm^2; irradiance: 80 mW/cm^2; dose: 9 J/cm^2; time: 153 seconds) under different conditions. The investigators assessed the involvement of opioid receptors, recruitment of opioid-containing leukocytes to inflamed tissue, and activation of the L-arginine/NO pathway by injecting agonist or antagonist solutions intrathecally prior to LED treatment. Pain behavior was measured using mechanical hypersensitivity via von Frey filament. The results of behavioral testing indicated that pre-administration of L-arginine prevented the analgesic effect of the LED therapy. They also provided evidence that activation of peripheral, but not central, opioid receptors, along with recruitment of opioid-containing leukocytes to the injury site, is involved in the efficacy of LED therapy in decreasing mechanical hypersensitivity in this model (Cidral-Filho *et al.*, 2014).

The effect of PBM on neuropathic pain and functional recovery was investigated in rats with a chronic constriction injury (Hsieh *et al.*, 2012; Hsieh *et al.*, 2014). They treated four spots (spot size 0.2 cm^2) transcutaneously over the constriction site with a CW 660 nm laser beginning 7 days after injury. Each spot was treated at an energy density of 9 J/cm^2 for 60 seconds daily for 7 consecutive days. Mechanical allodynia was assessed with an electronic von Frey filament, and functional recovery was assessed using walking patterns. PBM-treated animals demonstrated significant improvements in neuropathic pain measures and functional recovery.

Daigo and colleagues recently studied the effect of PBMT on analgesia and associated microglial/astrocyte activation in rats with an inferior alveolar nerve injury model. They delivered PBMT at 8 J/cm^2 with a 940 nm diode laser daily for 7 days, and found pain behavior measures returned to baseline in the treatment group by 14 days postop, while they did not recover in the sham treatment group (Daigo *et al.*, 2023). Additionally, immunological analysis of microglia and astrocyte cell bodies demonstrated greater expression area, hypertrophy of cell bodies, and end-feet extensions in the PBMT group compared to the surgery alone group, indicating that PBMT may be related to preventing hyperalgesia and allodynia (Daigo *et al.*, 2023).

PBMT also altered microglial phenotypes across the M1/M2 spectrum *in vitro* in a dose-dependent manner (Von Leden *et al.*, 2013). Primary microglia and a microglial cell line were exposed *in vitro* to 808 nm light. Higher energy densities (4–30 J/cm^2) induced expression of the M1 (pro-inflammatory) phenotype, whereas lower densities (0.2–10.0 J/cm^2) induced M2 (anti-inflammatory) marker expression. Fernandes *et al.* (2015) demonstrated that both 660 and 780 nm light could reduce TNFα and inducible NOS (iNOS) expression and TNFα and cyclooxygenase 2 (COX-2) production in J774 cells activated to the M1 (pro-inflammatory) macrophage phenotype.

Two other studies compared different parameters for 660, 830, and 980 nm light on pain outcome measures in male Wistar rats. Bertolini *et al.* (2011) found that animals that received five daily treatments of 830 nm light at doses of 4 and 8 J/cm^2 following chronic constriction injury had significant improvements in the rat knee-joint incapacitation test. Another group compared control, 660 nm light, and 980 nm light for chronic constriction injury. The 660 nm irradiation group received 4 J/cm^2 (0.354 W/cm^2) and the 980 nm group received 4 J/cm^2 (0.248 W/cm^2). Both treatment groups were effective at reducing mechanical allodynia (Masoumipoor *et al.*, 2014).

Our laboratory has conducted a series of pilot studies using the spared nerve injury model to optimize laser parameters and treatment schedules for PBMT in neuropathic pain (unpublished). Parameters were selected based on results from light-penetration experiments and previous *in vivo* and *in vitro* experiments using 980 nm light and used in a study to characterize the activation of macrophages and microglia along ascending somatosensory pathways related to neuropathic pain. Adult male Sprague–Dawley rats underwent a spared nerve injury (SNI) model and were randomly assigned to three groups: sham injury, SNI with no treatment, and SNI with PBMT. Light was applied to affected hind paw (output power: 1 W; 20 seconds; 41 cm above the skin; power density: 43.25 mW/cm^2; dose: 20 J), dorsal root ganglia (output power: 4.5 W; 19 seconds; on-contact with skin; power density: 43.25 mW/cm^2; dose: 85.5 J), and spinal cord (output power: 1.5 W; 19 seconds; on-contact with skin; power density: 43.25 mW/cm^2; dose: 28.5 J) regions every other day from day 7–30 postoperatively. Mechanical hypersensitivity was measured by electron von Frey device, and immunohistochemistry was used to characterize macrophage and microglial activation. Injured groups demonstrated mechanical hypersensitivity 1–30 days postoperatively. PBM-treated animals began to recover after two treatments; at day 26, mechanical sensitivity reached baseline (Kobiela Ketz *et al.*, 2017). Though treatment parameters and behavioral measurements differ between these studies, the findings suggest that PBMT can be effective in decreasing neuropathic pain behavior and altering the inflammatory process associated with peripheral nerve injury (Hsieh *et al.*, 2012).

Conclusion

Since Mester's discovery in the 1960s that low-level light produces biostimulatory effects on cells, an incredible amount of work has been done to elucidate the mechanisms behind PBM. Though much is yet to be discovered, great strides have been made in understanding the effects of light on the primary photoacceptor, along with its effects at the molecular, organelle, cellular, and system levels. To further strengthen the science, future work must focus on a deeper understanding of molecular mechanisms and the biological contexts of treating conditions (Arany 2012). Of paramount importance is the establishment of device and dosing parameters to achieve desired clinical outcomes.

Acknowledgments

The opinions expressed herein are those of the authors. The information or content and conclusions do not necessarily represent the official position or policy of, nor should any official endorsement be inferred on the part of, USU, the Department of Defense, or the US government.

References

Abbracchio, M.P. and Burnstock, G. (1994). Purinoceptors: are there families of P2X and P2Y purinoceptors? *Pharmacol Ther.* 64:445–475.

Albertini, R. *et al.* (2008). Cytokine mRNA expression is decreased in the subplantar muscle of rat paw subjected to carrageenan-induced inflammation after low-level laser therapy. *Photomed Laser Surg.* 26:19–24.

Alexandratou, E. *et al.* (2002). Human fibroblast alterations induced by low power laser irradiation at the single cell level using confocal microscopy. *Photochem Photobiol Sci.* 1:547–552.

Alghamdi, K.M. *et al.* (2012). Low-level laser therapy: a useful technique for enhancing the proliferation of various cultured cells. *Lasers Med Sci.* 27:237–249.

Alves, A.C. *et al.* (2013). Effect of low-level laser therapy on the expression of inflammatory mediators and on neutrophils and macrophages in acute joint inflammation. *Arthritis Res Ther.* 15:R116.

Anders, J. *et al.* (2008). Light supports neurite outgrowth of human neural progenitor cells: the role of P2Y receptors. *IEEE J Sel Top Quantum Electron.* 14:118–125.

Anders, J.J. *et al.* (2014). In vitro and in vivo optimization of infrared laser treatment for injured peripheral nerves. *Lasers Surg Med.* 46:34–45.

Anders, J.J. *et al.* (2015). Low-level light/laser therapy versus photobiomodulation therapy. *Photomed Laser Surg.* 33:183–184.

Arany, P.R. (2012). Photobiomodulation: poised from the fringes. *Photomed Laser Surg.* 30:507–509.

Ball, K.A. *et al.* (2011). Low intensity light stimulates nitrite-dependent nitric oxide synthesis but not oxygen consumption by cytochrome c oxidase: implications for phototherapy. *J Photochem Photobiol, B.* 102:182–191.

Basford, J.R. (1993). Laser therapy: scientific basis and clinical role. *Orthopedics.* 16:541–547.

Basford, J.R. (1995). Low intensity laser therapy: still not an established clinical tool. *Lasers Surg Med.* 16:331–342.

Basford, J.R. *et al.* (1998). A randomized controlled evaluation of low-intensity laser therapy: plantar fasciitis. *Am J Phys Med Rehabil.* 79:249–254.

Bertolini, G.R. *et al.* (2011). Low-level laser therapy, at 830 nm, for pain reduction in experimental model of rats with sciatica. *Arq de Neuro-Psiquiatria.* 69:356–359.

Brandt, U. (2006). Energy converting NADH:quinone oxidoreductase (complex I). *Annu Rev Biochem.* 75:69–92.

Breitbart, H. *et al.* (1996). Changes in calcium transport in mammalian sperm mitochondria and plasma membrane irradiated at 633 nm (HeNe laser). *J Photochem Photobiol, B.* 34:117–121.

Burdon, R.H. (1995). Superoxide and hydrogen peroxide in relation to mammalian cell proliferation. *Free Radical Biol Med.* 18:775–794.

Burdon, R.H. *et al.* (1995). Hydrogen peroxide and the proliferation of BHK-21 cells. *Free Radical Res.* 23:471–486.

Burnstock, G. (1978). A basis for distinguishing two types of purinergic receptor. In: *Cell Membrane Receptors for Drugs and Hormones: A Multidisciplinary Approach.* (eds. R. Straub and L. Bolis). Raven Press, New York.

Burnstock, G. (2009). Purines and sensory nerves. *Handb Exp Pharmacol*:333–392.

Byrnes, K.R. *et al.* (2005a). Light promotes regeneration and functional recovery and alters the immune response after spinal cord injury. *Lasers Surg Med.* 36:171–185.

Byrnes, K.R. *et al.* (2005b). Low power laser irradiation alters gene expression of olfactory ensheathing cells in vitro. *Lasers Surg Med.* 37:161–171.

Calderhead, R.G. (1991). Watts a joule: on the importance of accurate and correct reporting of laser parameters in low reactive-level laser therapy and photobioactivation research. *Laser Therapy.* 3:177–182.

Callaghan, G.A. *et al.* (1996). Reactive oxygen species inducible by low-intensity laser irradiation alter DNA synthesis in the haemopoietic cell line U937. *Lasers Surg Med.* 19:201–206.

Chen, C.H. *et al.* (2009). Low-level laser irradiation promotes cell proliferation and mRNA expression of type I collagen and decorin in porcine Achilles tendon fibroblasts in vitro. *J Orthop Res.* 27:646–650.

Chen, A.C. *et al.* (2011). Low-level laser therapy activates NF-kB via generation of reactive oxygen species in mouse embryonic fibroblasts. *PLoS One.* 6:e22453.

Chow, R. *et al.* (2011). Inhibitory effects of laser irradiation on peripheral mammalian nerves and relevance to analgesic effects: a systematic review. *Photomed Laser Surg.* 29:365–381.

Chung, H. *et al.* (2012). The nuts and bolts of low-level laser (light) therapy. *Ann Biomed Eng.* 40:516–533.

Cidral-Filho, F.J. *et al.* (2014). Light-emitting diode therapy induces analgesia in a mouse model of postoperative pain through activation of peripheral opioid receptors and the L-arginine/nitric oxide pathway. *Lasers Med Sci.* 29:695–702.

Cooper, C.E. *et al.* (1991). Cytochrome c oxidase: structure, function, and membrane topology of the polypeptide subunits. *Biochem Cell Biol.* 69(9):586–607.

Craig, G. and Welch, A.J. (2001). *Optical and Thermal Response of Tissue to Laser Radiation. Lasers in Medicine.* CRC Press.

Daigo, E. *et al.* (2023). Photobiomodulation activates microglia/astrocytes and relieves neuropathic pain in inferior alveolar nerve injury. *Photobiomodulation Photomed Laser Surg.* 41:694–702.

Das, D.K. (2001). Redox regulation of cardiomyocyte survival and death. *Antioxid Redox Signaling.* 3:23–37.

Doyle, A.T. *et al.* (2016). The effects of low-level laser therapy on pain associated with tendinopathy: a critically appraised topic. *J Sport Rehabil.* 25:83–90.

Farivar, S. *et al.* (2014). Biological effects of low level laser therapy. *J Lasers Med Sci.* 5:58–62.

Fernandes, K.P. *et al.* (2013). Effect of photobiomodulation on expression of IL-1beta in skeletal muscle following acute injury. *Lasers Med Sci.* 28:1043–1046.

Fernandes, K.P. *et al.* (2015). Photobiomodulation with 660-nm and 780-nm laser on activated J774 macrophage-like cells: effect on M1 inflammatory markers. *J Photochem Photobiol, B.* 153:344–351.

Gether, U. (2000). Uncovering molecular mechanisms involved in activation of G protein-coupled receptors. *Endocr Rev.* 21:90–113.

Grossman, N. *et al.* (1998). 780 nm low power diode laser irradiation stimulates proliferation of keratinocyte cultures: involvement of reactive oxygen species. *Lasers Surg Med.* 22:212–218.

Guzzardella, G.A. *et al.* (2002). Laser stimulation on bone defect healing: an in vitro study. *Lasers Med Sci.* 17:216–220.

Hamblin, M.R. (2008). The role of nitric oxide in low level light therapy. In: *Proceedings of SPIE - the International Society for Optical Engineering.* (eds. M.R. Hamblin *et al.*). The International Society for Optical Engineering.

Hardy, L.B. *et al.* (1967). Effect of ruby laser radiation on mouse fibroblast culture. *Fed Proc.* 26:668.

Hartmann, K.M. (1983). Action spectroscopy. In: *Biophysics.* (eds. W. Hoppe *et al.*). Springer-Verlag, Berlin.

Haslerud, S. *et al.* (2015). The efficacy of low-level laser therapy for shoulder tendinopathy: a systematic review and meta-analysis of randomized controlled trials. *Physiother Res Inter.* 20:108–125.

He, K. *et al.* (2023). Histological, physiological and biomechanical effects of low-level laser therapy on tendon healing in animals and humans: a systematic review. *Ann Biomed Eng.* 51:2659–2707.

Hermann, G.J. and Shaw, J.M. (1998). Mitochondrial dynamics in yeast. *Annu Rev Cell Dev Biol.* 14:265–303.

Hsieh, Y.L. *et al.* (2012). Low-level laser therapy alleviates neuropathic pain and promotes function recovery in rats with chronic constriction injury: possible involvements in hypoxia-inducible factor 1alpha (HIF-1alpha). *J Comp Neurol.* 520:2903–2916.

Hsieh, Y.L. *et al.* (2014). Fluence-dependent effects of low-level laser therapy in myofascial trigger spots on modulation of biochemicals associated with pain in a rabbit model. *Lasers Med Sci.* 30(1):209–216.

Jenkins, P.A. and Carroll, J.D. (2011). How to report low-level laser therapy (LLLT)/photomedicine dose and beam parameters in clinical and laboratory studies. *Photomed Laser Surg.* 29:785–787.

Karu, T. (1987). Photobiological fundamentals of low-power laser therapy. *IEEE J Quantum Electron.* 23:1703–1717.

Karu, T. (1998). Primary and secondary mechanisms of the action of monochromatic visible and near infrared radiation on cells. In: *The Science of Low Power Laser Therapy.* (ed. T. Karu). Gordon and Breach Science Publishers, London.

Karu, T. (2007). *Ten Lectures on Basic Science of Laser Phototherapy.* Sweden, Prima Books AB, Grangesberg.

Karu, T. (2010). Mitochondrial mechanisms of photobiomodulation in context of new data about multiple roles of ATP. *Photomed Laser Surg.* 28:159–160.

Karu, T.I. and Afanas'eva, N.I. (1995). Cytochrome c oxidase as the primary photoacceptor upon laser exposure of cultured cells to visible and near IR-range light. *Dokl Akad Nauk.* 342:693–695.

Karu, T.I. *et al.* (2005). Cellular effects of low power laser therapy can be mediated by nitric oxide. *Lasers Surg Med.* 36:307–314.

Khakh, B.S. and Burnstock, G. (2009). The double life of ATP. *Sci Am.* 301(84–90):92.

Kobiela Ketz, A. *et al.* (2017). Characterization of macrophage/microglial activation and effect of Photobiomodulation in the spared nerve injury model of neuropathic pain. *Pain Med.* 18:932–946.

Leung, M.C. *et al.* (2002). Treatment of experimentally induced transient cerebral ischemia with low energy laser inhibits nitric oxide synthase activity and up-regulates the expression of transforming growth factor-beta 1. *Lasers Surg Med.* 31:283–288.

Lubart, R. and Breitbart, H. (2000). Biostimulative effects of low-energy lasers and their implications for medicine. *Drug Dev Res.* 50:471–475.

Lubart, R. *et al.* (1997). Changes in calcium transport in mammalian sperm mitochondria and plasma membranes caused by 780 nm irradiation. *Lasers Surg Med.* 21:493–499.

Lubart, R. *et al.* (2005). Low-energy laser irradiation promotes cellular redox activity. *Photomed Laser Surg.* 23:3–9.

Maiman, T.H. (1960). Stimulated optical radiation in ruby. *Nature.* 187:493–494.

Masha, R.T. *et al.* (2013). Low-intensity laser irradiation at 660 nm stimulates transcription of genes involved in the electron transport chain. *Photomed Laser Surg.* 31:47–53.

Masoumipoor, M. *et al.* (2014). Effects of 660- and 980-nm low-level laser therapy on neuropathic pain relief following chronic constriction injury in rat sciatic nerve. *Lasers Med Sci.* 29:1593–1598.

Mcguff, P.E. *et al.* (1964). Surgical applications of laser. *Ann Surg.* 160:765–777.

Mester, E. *et al.* (1968a). The stimulating effect of low power laser rays on biological systems. *J Name: Laser Rev.* 1:3 (Mar. 1968).; Other Information: Orig. Receipt Date: 31-DEC-69; Bib. Info. Source: UK (United Kingdom (sent to DOE from)), Medium: X.

Mester, E. *et al.* (1968b). The stimulating effect of low power laser rays on biological systems. *Laser Rev.* 1.

Mester, E. *et al.* (1968c). On the effect of laser beams on bacterial phagocytosis of leukocytes. *Acta Biol Med Ger.* 21:317–321.

Mester, E. *et al.* (1971). Effect of laser rays on wound healing. *Am J Surg.* 122:532–535.

Mester, E. *et al.* (1985). The biomedical effects of laser application. *Lasers Surg Med.* 5:31–39.

Mick, J. 2014. Study Silences Controversy, Illuminates the Biochemistry of Laser Healing. *DailyTech* [Online]. Available from: http://www.dailytech.com/Study+Silences+Controversy+Illuminates+the+Biochemistry+of+Laser+Healing/article34991.htm 2016].

Mitchell, U.H. and Mack, G.L. (2013). Low-level laser treatment with near-infrared light increases venous nitric oxide levels acutely: a single-blind, randomized clinical trial of efficacy. *Am J Phys Med Rehabil.* 92:151–156.

Moore, P. *et al.* (2005). Effect of wavelength on low-intensity laser irradiation-stimulated cell proliferation in vitro. *Lasers Surg Med.* 36:8–12.

Moriyama, Y. *et al.* (2005). In vivo study of the inflammatory modulating effects of low-level laser therapy on iNOS expression using bioluminescence imaging. *Photochem Photobiol.* 81:1351–1355.

Murray, R.K. *et al.* (2003). *Harper's Illustrated Biochemistry.* McGraw-Hill Medical.

Murrell, G.A. *et al.* (1990). Modulation of fibroblast proliferation by oxygen free radicals. *Biochem J.* 265:659–665.

Nogueira, A.C. Jr. and Junior Mde, J. (2015). The effects of laser treatment in tendinopathy: a systematic review. *Acta Ortop Bras.* 23:47–49.

Novak, I. (2003). ATP as a signaling molecule: the exocrine focus. *Physiology.* 18:12–17.

Ohshiro, T. (1989). Editorial. *Laser Therapy.* 1:5.

Pal, G. *et al.* (2007). Effect of low intensity laser interaction with human skin fibroblast cells using fiber-optic nano-probes. *J Photochem Photobiol, B.* 86:252–261.

Passarella, S. and Karu, T. (2014). Absorption of monochromatic and narrow band radiation in the visible and near IR by both mitochondrial and non-mitochondrial photoacceptors results in photobiomodulation. *J Photochem Photobiol, B.* 140:344–358.

Passarella, S. *et al.* (1984). Increase of proton electrochemical potential and ATP synthesis in rat liver mitochondria irradiated in vitro by helium-neon laser. *FEBS Lett.* 175:95–99.

Passarella, S. *et al.* (1988). Increase in the ADP/ATP exchange in rat liver mitochondria irradiated in vitro by helium-neon laser. *Biochem Biophys Res Commun.* 156:978–986.

Pastore, D. *et al.* (2000). Specific helium-neon laser sensitivity of the purified cytochrome c oxidase. *Int J Radiat Biol.* 76:863–870.

Peplow, P.V. and Baxter, G.D. (2012). Gene expression and release of growth factors during delayed wound healing: a review of studies in diabetic animals and possible combined laser phototherapy and growth factor treatment to enhance healing. *Photomed Laser Surg.* 30:617–636.

Peplow, P.V. *et al.* (2010a). Laser photobiomodulation of proliferation of cells in culture: a review of human and animal studies. *Photomed Laser Surg.* 28(Suppl 1):S3–S40.

Peplow, P.V. *et al.* (2010b). Laser photobiomodulation of wound healing: a review of experimental studies in mouse and rat animal models. *Photomed Laser Surg.* 28:291–325.

Poyton, R.O. and Ball, K.A. (2011). Therapeutic photobiomodulation: nitric oxide and a novel function of mitochondrial cytochrome c oxidase. *Dis Med.* 11:154–159.

Poyton, R.O. *et al.* (2009). Mitochondria and hypoxic signaling: a new view. *Ann N Y Acad Sci.* 1177:48–56.

Reddy, G.K. (2004). Photobiological basis and clinical role of low-intensity lasers in biology and medicine. *J Clin Laser Med and Surg.* 22:141–150.

Rhee, S.G. (1999). Redox signaling: hydrogen peroxide as intracellular messenger. *Exp Mol Med.* 31:53–59.

Samoilova, K.A. *et al.* (2008). Role of nitric oxide in the visible light-induced rapid increase of human skin microcirculation at the local and systemic levels: II. Healthy volunteers. *Photomed Laser Surg.* 26:443–449.

Smith, K.C. (1991). The photobiological basis of low level laser radiation therapy. *Laser Therapy.* 3:19–24.

Suzukawa, K. *et al.* (2000). Nerve growth factor-induced neuronal differentiation requires generation of Rac1-regulated reactive oxygen species. *J Biol Chem.* 275:13175–13178.

Suzuki, Y.J. and Ford, G.D. (1999). Redox regulation of signal transduction in cardiac and smooth muscle. *J Mole and Cell Cardiol.* 31:345–353.

Tafur, J. and Mills, P.J. (2008). Low-intensity light therapy: exploring the role of redox mechanisms. *Photomed Laser Surg.* 26:323–328.

Tsai, W.C. *et al.* (2012). Low-level laser irradiation stimulates tenocyte migration with up-regulation of dynamin II expression. *PLoS One.* 7:e38235.

Tsai, W.C. *et al.* (2014). Low-level laser irradiation stimulates tenocyte proliferation in association with increased NO synthesis and upregulation of PCNA and cyclins. *Lasers Med Sci.* 29:1377–1384.

Tsukihara, T. *et al.* (1995). Structures of metal sites of oxidized bovine heart cytochrome c oxidase at 2.8 a. *Science.* 269:1069–1074.

Tuby, H. *et al.* (2006). Modulations of VEGF and iNOS in the rat heart by low level laser therapy are associated with cardioprotection and enhanced angiogenesis. *Lasers Surg Med.* 38:682–688.

Tuner, J. and Hode, L. (1998). It's all in the parameters: a critical analysis of some well-known negative studies on low-level laser therapy. *J Clin Laser Med and Surg.* 16:245–248.

UCL. (2016). Tissue spectra. Available from: http://www.ucl.ac.uk/medphys/research/borl/intro/spectra (accessed November 30, 2016).

Vacca, R.A. *et al.* (1997). The irradiation of hepatocytes with He-Ne laser causes an increase of cytosolic free calcium concentration and an increase of cell membrane potential, correlated with it, both increases taking place in an oscillatory manner. *Biochem Mol Biol Int.* 43:1005–1014.

Vanden Hoek, T.L. *et al.* (1998). Reactive oxygen species released from mitochondria during brief hypoxia induce preconditioning in cardiomyocytes. *J Biol Chem.* 273:18092–18098.

Viegas, V.N. *et al.* (2007). Effect of low-level laser therapy on inflammatory reactions during wound healing: comparison with meloxicam. *Photomed Laser Surg.* 25:467–473.

Voet, D. and Voet, J.G. (2010). *Biochemistry*. John Wiley & Sons, New York.

Von Leden, R.E. *et al.* (2013). 808 nm wavelength light induces a dose-dependent alteration in microglial polarization and resultant microglial induced neurite growth. *Lasers Surg Med.* 45:253–263.

Wakao, H. *et al.* (1987). Purification and properties of NADH dehydrogenase from a thermoacidophilic archaebacterium, Sulfolobus acidocaldarius. *J Biochem.* 102:255–262.

Weersink, R. *et al.* (2007). Light dosimetry for low-level laser therapy: accounting for differences in tissue and depth. In: *Proceedings of SPIE - the International Society for Optical Engineering*. (eds. M.R. Hamblin *et al.*). The International Society for Optical Engineering, SPIE.

Wu, X. *et al.* (2015). Organic light emitting diode improves diabetic cutaneous wound healing in rats. *Wound Repair Regener.* 23:104–114.

Yu, W. *et al.* (1997a). Improvement of host response to sepsis by photobiomodulation. *Lasers Surg Med.* 21:262–268.

Yu, W. *et al.* (1997b). Photomodulation of oxidative metabolism and electron chain enzymes in rat liver mitochondria. *Photochem Photobiol.* 66:866–871.

Zhang, Y. *et al.* (2003). cDNA microarray analysis of gene expression profiles in human fibroblast cells irradiated with red light. *J Invest Dermatol.* 120:849–857.

Part III

Practical Applications of Laser Therapy

4

General Principles of Laser Therapy

Lisa A. Miller

Companion Animal Health, New Castle, DE, USA

1st Edition Contributor:

Jeffrey J. Smith

Middletown Animal Hospital, Middletown, CA, USA

Introduction

Photobiomodulation (PBM) (laser therapy) has three broad physiologic effects on tissues: it decreases inflammation, it decreases pain, and it accelerates healing. When training staff, using the mnemonic reminder of pointing two fingers down (decreased inflammation and pain) and the thumb upward (increased healing) is an easy way to keep the entire team conveying the same information. Further, these effects are not the result of heating or warming the tissue (photothermal). Instead, they are the result of a photobiochemical change akin to the events that occur with photosynthesis or vitamin D synthesis: biological changes in chemistry at the cellular level, caused by light.

"Photobiomodulation" is the best term to describe the effects of near-infrared laser light in tissue (Anders *et al.*, 2015), since some parts of the healing process are accelerated (organization and proliferation), while other parts are diminished (inflammation). The initial effect of near-infrared laser light is stimulation of production of adenosine triphosphate (ATP), reactive oxygen species (ROS), and nitric oxide (NO) (Karu, 2010; Farivar *et al.*, 2014; Sommer *et al.*, 2015). In turn, these bioactive substances cause the cascade of effects for each of the three mechanisms of action involving inflammation, pain, and healing (Chung *et al.*, 2012). These cascades are well documented, and are summarized in Chapter 3.

Therapeutic Dosing

Much of the successful evolution of laser therapy is the direct result of understanding the dose-dependent nature of tissue response to infrared light. In other words, the intended target tissue must receive the appropriate dose of light energy to manifest the effects of laser therapy. This phenomenon is analogous to dosing tissue with antibiotics (mg/kg) or radiation (J/kg = Gy), but for laser therapy the dosing in the literature is usually described in terms of the range of fluence, or energy density (J/cm^2), administered to the surface of a specific treatment area measured in square centimeters. If suboptimal doses are administered, then the effects will also be suboptimal, or may not even be apparent.

Multiple current publications recommend different dosing for superficial tissues (those that are visible to the eye) versus deep tissues (below the skin or mucosa). Some older publications recommend dosing differently based on acute-versus-chronic conditions, and this seems to be based on historic recommendations for other physical modalities (such as therapeutic ultrasound), since dosing in this manner does not take into account the different amounts of light reaching superficial vs. deep tissues. The doses are different because there is a loss of light energy in the interposing tissue on the way to the deeper target tissues due to reflection, scatter, and absorption (Lister *et al.*, 2012). Superficial dose ranges are usually between 1 and 5 J/cm^2

Laser Therapy in Veterinary Medicine: Photobiomodulation, Second Edition. Edited by Christopher J. Winkler and Lisa A. Miller.

(Peplow *et al.*, 2010), while dosing for most deep tissues is in the 8–20 J/cm^2 range, scaling up with the size of the patient and subsequent depth of the target tissue (Bjordal *et al.*, 2003; Roberts *et al.*, 2013; Looney *et al.*, 2018). Further dosing recommendations are described in relevant chapters to follow.

To facilitate delivering proper doses of laser therapy in a real-world setting, other factors that impact clinical efficacy, such as estimating the proper treatment size area, wavelength, power (W), and patient characteristics must also be understood (Sommer *et al.*, 2015). Light penetration, absorption, and scattering may be affected by method of beam delivery (on vs off contact), tissue type, tissue depth, species (there are likely differences in absorption between mammalian skin and reptile scales as an example), haircoat color and length, skin color, and body condition (Weersink, 2007; Enwemeka, 2009; Anders *et al.*, 2014). As such, dosing should be adjusted accordingly taking all of these factors into account. Effective dosing intervals (again, just like with antibiotic or radiation therapy) are critical to achieving positive clinical outcomes. Factors such as patient preparation, application techniques, frequency of administration, and proper patient management are also essential for optimal results.

Appropriate Treatment Area Estimation

As fluence or energy density is described in terms of the amount of energy (J) administered to the surface of a specific treatment area (measured in square centimeters), and a large part of the effectiveness of PBM is achieved through not only autocrine but paracrine tissue effects (de Freitas and Hamblin, 2016), an important concept in proper dosing is the inclusion of all the tissue associated with a lesion or area, and not just the visible pathology. For example, when treating pyotraumatic dermatitis or a wound, one should include a wide margin around the visible lesion, which in most cases nearly doubles the size of the area being treated. Similarly, if one is treating the hip, it is important to treat all the associated anatomical structures and soft tissues around the entire hip joint. This means treating the joint from 360º and at least half the distance to the stifle and all the way to the midline.

Manual Dose Calculation

It is helpful to conceptualize laser therapy dosing by calculating or confirming dosing manually. A 7.5 × 12.7 cm index card or a CD is almost exactly 100 cm^2 and because 100 is an easy multiplier, one can determine approximate dosages by visualizing the area to be treated relative to one of these objects. For example, if one wanted to treat the hip of a dog (360º around the joint), and the area approximated that of five index cards, one would multiply the desired fluence (10 J/cm^2) by the area (500 cm^2) to calculate the total amount of energy to be delivered (5000 J). On the other hand, if a pyotraumatic dermatitis lesion was half the size of an index card, one would multiply the target fluence (4 J/cm^2) by the area (50 cm^2) to calculate the total amount of energy to be delivered (200 J).

The inverse of this concept is also helpful. When given a dose to administer, an understanding of where to administer that dose can be helpful. For example, for deep tissue being dosed at 10 J/cm^2 every 1000 J should be spread over an area of 100 cm^2 Therefore, a dose of 4500 J would be administered over an area of 4.5 index cards. For superficial tissue being dosed at 4 J/cm^2 every 400 J should be administered over an area of 100 cm^2. Therefore, a superficial dose of 200 J would be administered over an area of half an index card.

Software Automatic Dose Calculation

Fortunately, many lasers are now programmed with very specific and detailed dosing information in their software. However, it is important to note that these are not standardized across laser devices or manufacturers, so the therapist should be comfortable inquiring with the laser manufacturer to gain a more thorough understanding of the basis for dosing in their device's protocols. For most automatic protocols, laser operators enter patient-specific data and anatomical information, and the software calculates the dose according to the science and experience incorporated in its algorithms. Software-calculated doses are usually in the accepted 1–5 J/cm^2 range for superficial conditions. Software-calculated doses for deep-tissue conditions typically fall in the 8–20 J/cm^2 range, scaling up with the size of the patient and depth of the target tissue. The laser operator is encouraged to double check that software calculations are approximately the same as what they would have calculated manually for the patient, condition, and area(s) being treated.

Adjusting Calculated Doses

Software in newer-generation therapy lasers provides a starting point for most conditions, and the dosing delivered will be successful in the majority of cases. Still, it is important to have a working knowledge of how dosing is calculated, in much the same way that it is important to understand the readings on patient monitoring devices. Some patients and conditions require adjustment of the dose for the best effect on an individual case-to-case basis.

Lesions that have both a superficial and a deep component – like degloving injuries, postsurgical fractures, and advanced otitis – should be treated with a higher dose. Superficial target tissues within this treatment area will be treated simultaneously.

Refractory conditions often respond to higher dosing. For example, if a canine patient has a particularly chronic pain that is not responding to 10 J/cm^2, then doubling the dose to 20 J/cm^2 will often achieve a better outcome. As an example, a dose of 37.5 J/cm^2 has been validated in the application of laser therapy for chronic lower back pain in humans (Vallone *et al.*, 2014).

Practicing clinicians anecdotally reported that certain difficult conditions or lesions may require higher doses (upwards of 20–30 J/cm^2) in order to see consistent clinical responses. These can include lick granulomas, degenerative myelopathy, treatment of equine spinal structures, and feline eosinophilic complex lesions.

Power and Irradiance

The power of therapeutic lasers determines the rate of energy delivery and is measured in watts (W), where 1 W = 1 J/sec. This means that a 1 W laser can deliver 60 J/min while operating in continuous wave delivery (CW), while a 10 W laser can deliver 600 J/min. Power does not determine depth of penetration (that is a function of wavelength) but does determine the concentration of photons reaching the depth to which a particular wavelength can penetrate, in a particular tissue, in a fixed amount of time. As already mentioned, laser medical procedures usually describe recommended dosing in terms of the fluence or energy density (J/cm^2) administered to the surface of a specific treatment area measured in square centimeters. The most practical reason for recommending doses in this manner is that it is possible to achieve the same energy density in a nearly infinite number of ways by adjusting either the treatment time or the irradiance (also known as power density, measured in W/cm^2).

For example, photobiomodulation therapy (PBMT) applied to the hip joint of a medium-sized dog with a hip area of approximately 250 cm^2 (the joint itself, as well as surrounding biomechanically associated soft tissues, both medially and laterally) and a target fluence (energy density) of 10 J/cm^2 would be calculated in the following manner:

$$10\ \text{J/cm}^2 \times 250\ \text{cm}^2 = 2500\ \text{J total dose over the entire hip area}$$

The question of what combination of treatment time and irradiance is ideal for these treatments is slightly more complicated. Irradiance is determined by the power (W) setting of the laser device as well as the laser beam spot size/area of the handpiece or treatment head (in cm^2). The practitioner may conclude, for example, that this dose can be delivered in either of the following combinations:

$$100\ \text{mW(or 0.1 W)} \times 25000\ \text{sec(416 minutes, 40 seconds)} = 2500\ \text{J total}$$

$$12\ \text{W} \times 208\ \text{sec(3 minutes, 28 seconds)} = 2500\ \text{J total}$$

Clearly, the second combination is a more efficient use of time, and allows the opportunity to treat multiple affected areas during one treatment session. However, it is more important when treating various conditions to remember there is also a minimum irradiance required that will create a clinically meaningful effect. That is, there is a certain threshold of power density at the target tissue required to ensure a therapeutic result. Below this threshold, no matter how long the treatment time, no clinical effect will be seen. Similarly, international safety standards are based on the laser parameters of wavelength, time, and irradiance, because above a certain threshold for power density, thermal or other damage may be created. Therefore, the ideal goal for treatment is to utilize a dose that is in a window above the minimum irradiance that will produce a clinically meaningful effect and below a maximum irradiance that would produce damage (Sommer *et al.*, 2001). In order to calculate irradiance, the laser operator must know not only the power (W) setting but also the spot area (in cm^2) of the laser handpiece. Laser devices may have handpieces with either a fixed or an adjustable spot area, and it is important that the operator know which type their device has in order to be familiar with the irradiance(s) of which it is capable.

Due to the percentage of light lost in transmission from the skin surface to deeper tissues, the irradiance required to produce a therapeutic effect is higher for so-called "deep-tissue" conditions, including musculoskeletal disorders, than it is for "superficial" conditions, including wounds, burns, and other dermatological conditions. This is why good clinical outcomes may be appreciated with lower irradiance when treating superficial conditions, but the results are inconsistent when treating deep-tissue conditions, even with longer treatment times.

Many studies have examined the relationship between irradiance, light penetration, and effectiveness in treating various conditions (Oron *et al.*, 2006, Anders *et al.*, 2014, Morries *et al.*, 2015). The optimal irradiance also varies for different wavelengths, and it is important that this be taken into account when interpreting PBM research, but the critical parameter is the dose delivered to target tissue. A recent *in vivo* review study (Zein *et al.*, 2018) identified that the two factors of most importance in PBM for determining clinical success are *both* fluence (J/cm^2) and irradiance (W/cm^2) and not merely the total quantity of photons absorbed by target tissues as previously surmised. Factors including the overall depth of the target tissue being treated, the presence or absence of melanin in the skin, the presence or absence of blood vessels (and the blood contained within) in the tissues, the thickness of any bone present, and tissue hydration all play a role in the penetration of photons to the target tissue and ultimately in the clinical success of the PBM treatment. Further, these factors help explain the disparity of results in early *in vitro* vs. *in vivo* PBM studies when dosages that were effective for positive results in a cell culture model did not show the same results when applied to tissues in a living animal. Further discussion on searching through laser literature and interpreting results may be found in Chapter 11.

Calculations for clinical dosimetry, especially for deeper tissue conditions, should take as many of these factors into account as possible. Software for "preset" protocols in many commercially available PBMT units may take only some (or none) of these into account, and the clinician should feel comfortable inquiring with the laser manufacturer to gain a more thorough understanding of the basis for dosing in protocols and changes based on patient characteristics in their individual PBMT devices.

Wavelength

Chapter 2 has discussed wavelength in depth. As a brief review, wavelengths between 600 nm (visible light) and 1100 nm (infrared light) are within the "therapeutic window," so called because these wavelengths are able to both penetrate tissues better than other wavelengths and stimulate PBM via their absorption by the main chromophore for PBM found in the mitochondria of cells, cytochrome c oxidase (CCO) (Kim, 2014; Passarella and Karu, 2014). No particular wavelength in this range has any significantly unique biological effects, though there are differences in absorption depending on the amount of other nonbiologically active pigments present in the treated tissue. These nonactive chromophores include hemoglobin (both oxyhemoglobin and deoxyhemoglobin.), myoglobin, and most importantly, melanin. These incidental absorbers can in effect "block" light from penetrating deeper into tissue; they should thus be considered when determining which wavelengths should be used for treating certain patients and how dosing should be adjusted to compensate for light's losses as it travels through tissue layers. Though numerous studies have been published using multiple wavelengths, there is no consensus that one wavelength of light has an optimal effect in all patient types or all conditions.

Delivery Method

The delivery method of the laser beam is an often-overlooked component of the therapeutic dose, but is critical especially for delivering this dose to deeper tissues. The loss of light due to reflection is significant at PBMT wavelengths, but when a handpiece is placed in firm contact with the skin, this loss is minimized and significantly more photons can be delivered to the deeper structures (Enwemeka, 2009, Zein *et al.*, 2018). One study looking at transmission of light into the spinal canal of large-breed dog cadavers showed an almost 70% increase in light penetration when an in-contact delivery method was utilized (Piao *et al.*, 2018). Treating in contact and applying pressure to the skin also creates blanching and disperses blood from the dermis and underlying tissues (Chien and Wilhelmi, 2012). Since blood absorption is a barrier to photon penetration via hemoglobin acting as the main absorber of light in the dermis (Lister *et al.*, 2012), blanching improves light penetration to deeper tissues. This enhanced delivery also reduces the distance to the target tissue by compression, and parting or pushing the hair coat out of the way. In addition, using a handpiece in contact with the tissue delivers an added, independent, massaging benefit that may also aid in treating myofascial trigger points. Laser devices can vary significantly in their handpieces and treatment head options. The laser operator is encouraged to educate themselves about these options and know when different delivery methods may be necessary or preferred based on the condition and patient being treated.

Pulsing

The frequency or pulsing of therapeutic infrared light was at one time thought to have an effect on the different mechanisms of PBM, and there is some evidence that pulsed light has effects that are different from those of CW delivered light. However, further work is needed to define these effects for various disease conditions and frequencies. A comprehensive review of literature publications indicates that there is little consensus about the effect of pulsing in different clinical conditions (Hashmi *et al.*, 2010). To many laser therapists, this review supports the concept that light should be delivered continuously (continuous wave, CW). This intuitively makes sense, since the cellular effect is the direct result of photons stimulating CCO, and not the result of some spacing or "blinking" of the photons as they arrive at the mitochondria. In addition, any pulsing (whether at 50 or 5000 Hz) results in the laser light being on some of the time and off some of the time. This results in a lower overall average power output than the highest power the device is capable of emitting at any given moment (the so-called peak power). If the beam is pulsed, then the reported power (used for determining dose) should be the average power, calculated as follows:

$$\text{peak power (W)} \times \text{pulse width (s)} \times \text{pulse frequency (Hz)} = \text{average power (W)}.$$

Therapeutic laser devices that pulse usually utilize a variable pulse frequency with a fixed duty cycle, the amount of time the laser is actually emitting (Barrett and Pack, 2006). For example, a 10 Hz pulse with a 50% duty cycle has a pulse width of a 50-ms on and a 50-ms off period

(1/10 × 0.5 = 0.05 s [50 ms]). If the pulse frequency is increased, the average power remains the same, so a 10 W peak-power laser will deliver an average power of 5 W.

"Super-pulsed" lasers (usually 904- or 905-nm devices) typically use a different format, a fixed pulse width and variable pulse frequency. In this format, if the pulse is 200 ns and the frequency is 1000 Hz, then there are 1000 pulses, each 200 ns long. If the peak power were 10 W, then the average power would be 10 W × 200 ns × 1000 Hz = 2 mW (0.002 W) average power. In this case, increasing the pulse frequency increases the average power. For example, If the pulse frequency were increased to 10 000 Hz, the average power would increase to 20 mW (0.02 W), and so on. It should be mentioned that claims of better light penetration from super-pulsed lasers have been discredited in the laser literature (Hashmi *et al.*, 2010, Hamblin *et al.*, 2018) even though this is a popular marketing claim of many super-pulsed devices.

Pulsing means that more time is required to deliver the same dose. Thus, treating a large dog's lumbar region with 6000 J of energy would take 10 minutes with a 10 W laser in CW, but would take 20 minutes with the same 10 W laser pulsing at a 50% duty cycle. Therefore, it is always important that the laser operator confirm the dosing in automatic protocols, as shorter, faster protocols do not usually deliver the same amount of total energy that a laser operator may desire for a certain area or patient.

Application Frequency

Though therapy laser software provides the proper dosing for most conditions, it does not provide any information about the frequency of treatment or interval between treatments. Determining and prescribing the number and frequency of laser therapy sessions is the responsibility of the prescriber. Most conditions fall into one of three categories: postprocedure, acute, or chronic. Less frequently are acute on chronic or relapsed conditions that warrant additional consideration. In addition, multimodal management, as opposed to laser therapy alone, will influence dosing intervals (AAHA, 2015).

Postprocedure Conditions

Postprocedure treatments are applied once or twice with the goal of mitigating or managing postoperative or post-traumatic pain and swelling. Since these treatments are not sustained over a long period of time, no increase in healing times is necessarily expected, however some veterinary studies have shown an improved cosmetic appearance in PBM treated surgical incisions (Wardlaw *et al.*, 2019). Nonetheless, laser therapy should be part of a multimodal pain management plan according to the American Animal Hospital Association (AAHA) and American Association of Feline Practitioners (AAFP) Pain Management Guidelines for Dogs and Cats (AAHA, 2015). Laser therapy will dramatically reduce edema, pain, self-mutilation, and acute inflammation. These treatments are typically very short (1–2 minutes) and are applied during the anesthetic recovery period. If animals are hospitalized overnight, they benefit from a second application the following day. The cost of these treatments is often incorporated into the procedure or pain-management fees for the patient.

Acute Conditions

Acute conditions are typically treated daily or every other day, and then at decreasing intervals until resolution of the condition. In addition to the postprocedure benefits, wounds will heal and resolve noticeably faster (Avci *et al.*, 2013) and the pain-modulating effect will be more sustained. In most cases, the more acute the injury or inflammation, the more important it is to try to treat it daily. In some cases, treating daily for 3 days and then every other day until the condition resolves is efficacious. When pets are hospitalized, daily treatments are both beneficial and practical. If owners have their pets treated on an outpatient basis, then sometimes a compromise between ideal medical care (daily treatments) and reasonable client compliance (every 2–3 days) must be worked out. In most cases, treating more than once a day does not provide substantially improved outcomes. The fees for treating these conditions are usually based on the treatment time.

Chronic Conditions

Chronic conditions are more complicated to treat than postprocedure or acute conditions. These are primarily conditions for which there is no complete resolution (i.e., an ongoing painful and/or degenerative condition), but in which the practitioner's goal in treating with PBM is to reduce the severity of symptoms of the condition and/or manage chronic pain. In general, one should expect chronic conditions to respond "chronically" (after a series of treatments), unlike acute conditions, which usually respond "acutely" (after one or two treatments). Chronic conditions are managed in three phases:

1) **Induction phase:** Treatments administered two to three times a week until significant improvements are noted.
2) **Transition phase:** One or two treatments a week for 2–3 weeks.
3) **Maintenance phase:** One treatment every 2–4 weeks, keeping symptoms at a "minimum" for that patient.

Patients will often show significant improvement after three treatments and remarkable improvement after six treatments, but induction should continue until significant improvement in clinical symptoms is noted. Some particularly advanced conditions will require up to 9–12 treatment sessions to show significant improvement.

Like fees for acute conditions, fees for treatment of chronic conditions are usually based on the treatment time.

Relapsed Conditions

Patients that have done well with laser therapy can exacerbate their controlled condition with a burst of overactivity. These pets can sometimes be rescued with a series of three to six sessions of daily or every-other-day treatments. Another scenario is the pet that responded well to laser therapy, but has stopped returning for its maintenance therapy. Often, after several months without laser therapy, the pet's symptoms will begin to recur. In these cases, the patient needs to restart the entire chronic condition protocol (induction phase first) to control their symptoms. This is an important point to make clients aware of beforehand, to encourage compliance with the maintenance phase of their pet's laser therapy.

Multimodal Management vs. Laser Therapy Alone

Laser therapy is a very effective modality, but it is even more effective when used as a component of a multimodal management strategy. There are many excellent pharmaceutical and non-pharmaceutical options when treating pain and delayed healing. New standards of care call for incorporating multiple modalities for maximum effectiveness and minimum side effects.

When laser therapy is used as a sole modality, it is likely to require more frequent use while delivering less than optimal results, especially with advanced conditions and pathology. When multiple modalities are used to manage pain, inflammation, and healing at different points along the healing and pain pathways, superior outcomes are the logical and scientifically proven result (AAHA, 2015).

Preparation for Laser Therapy

Preparing the Laser Therapy Room

Ideally, the laser therapy room should be a quiet, separate, relaxing space designed for the comfort of the patient, as well as the owner and therapist (Figure 4.1). In the limited confines of some hospitals, this is not possible, and other rooms may be tasked to serve a dual function. Many post-procedure treatments can be performed in the treatment or surgery room. In mobile practices, laser therapy can be performed in a huge variety of settings, though these sometimes present extra challenges.

The room should be equipped with comfortable dog beds or possibly a single large (120 × 200 cm) platform table to make the therapy sessions both comfortable and ergonomic. Small, low, rolling stools can also be very helpful for the laser operator and/or pet owner. In most cases, the pets will assume a prone position for laser therapy, though positioning is ultimately a question of patient comfort and compliance.

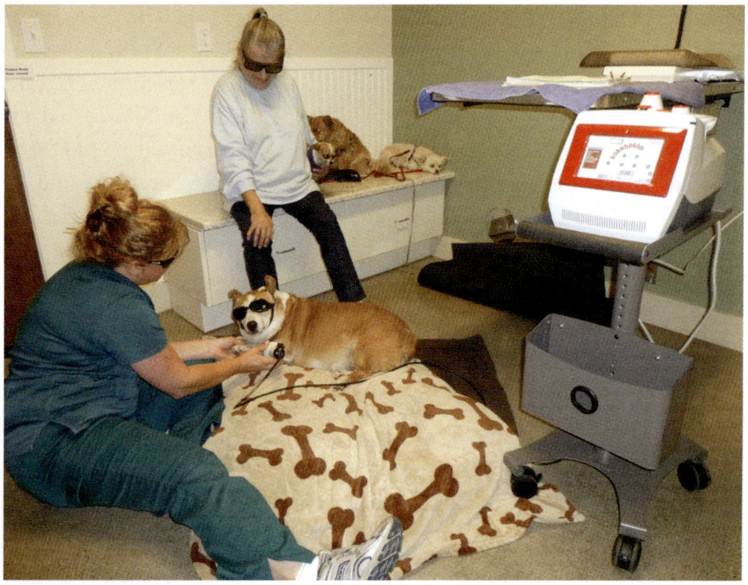

Figure 4.1 Laser therapy-appropriate room with appropriate bedding. Client, patient, and laser therapist are all comfortable, and the patient can easily be moved to access treatment areas.

Preparing for Laser Safety

Safe operation of the laser equipment is a function of both good training and compliance with that training. Regulators require two main safety measures: appropriate eye protection for humans and patients, and "Laser in Use" signage (ANSI, 2011a, 2011b). See Chapter 5 for a complete discussion of laser therapy safety.

Other than eye safety, the central objective in applying laser therapy safely is to introduce the energy into the tissues without excessive or uncomfortable warming. This is accomplished primarily by proper choice of delivery handpiece, proper movement of the handpiece, and proper choice of power (often determined by the laser's software). When appropriate, monitoring the patient's skin temperature with a trailing finger is good practice. If a temperature other than a pleasant, gentle warming is detected, the speed of movement of the handpiece should be increased.

Preparing the Laser Equipment

The laser itself should be prepared and programmed in advance, if possible. In addition, the cleanliness, integrity, and functionality of the laser should be checked.

Preparing the Patient for Laser Therapy

Laser therapy should not cause discomfort. Most pets come to accept and appear to enjoy their laser therapy sessions. Naturally soothing or calming methods such as dog-appeasing pheromone dispensers, feline pheromone diffusers, quiet music, special treats, and low lighting may be utilized to make the laser treatment room more relaxing if possible. The impulse to get started treating a patient needs to be balanced with the benefits of being well-prepared to administer laser therapy. Following the same routine or checklist every time will ensure proper technique, positive outcomes, and a pleasant experience for the patient and client. Laser therapy is unique among the services that veterinarians offer to clients in that clients usually remain with the pet during the treatment. Furthermore, the pet has a less fearful experience because it is not experiencing anything painful like an injection, venipuncture, or a nail trim. As a result, clients and pets can have an entirely new experience at the veterinarian's office, which leads to clients becoming very bonded to the practice.

Laser Therapy Treatment Procedure

Laser therapists should develop a routine that ensures all appropriate steps are included in sessions (Box 4.1). Begin by preparing the client and the patient. Explain why laser therapy is being prescribed, and outline the expected results.

Box 4.1 Ten-step Laser Therapy Treatment Procedure

1) Briefly explain to the owner what laser therapy does and communicate the expectations for results.
2) Take a few 4- to 5-second videos of the patient moving if they are exhibiting lameness, or a before-photo if a visual lesion is being treated.
3) Position the patient comfortably in the laser therapy treatment environment.
4) Program the laser and enter the patient's details into the laser software.
5) Provide protective eyewear to all people in the room or area.
6) Place laser-safe goggles or eye protection (soft black Elizabethan collars) on the patient or ensure the patient's eyes are orientated away from the treatment area.
7) Approach the patient briefly with the handpiece without turning the laser on. This allows the patient to adapt to the sensation of the handpiece prior to the addition of laser therapy itself.
8) Activate the laser and apply the laser therapy to all of the prescribed treatment areas.
9) Pause as needed.
10) Record the laser therapy treatment details and relevant progress notes.

Take several 4- to 5-second videos of the pet moving or trotting, if they are lame. When incorporated into the patient's record, these videos can be an important reference for evaluating progress during future sessions.

If the therapy laser software has an individual record-keeping system, enter the patient's pertinent information. If the software has condition-specific protocols, select the prescribed protocol and prepare for the administration of therapy. If the therapy laser does not have software, or has only limited software, calculate the total energy to be administered and select an appropriate power setting.

As discussed in Chapter 5, the number-one safety concern with the use of any therapy laser is the protection of the eyes of the patient, the laser therapist, and anyone in the immediate treatment vicinity. For this reason, everyone should be equipped with and wear laser-safe eyewear, marked with the appropriate optical density for the wavelengths of light emitted by the laser unit being used. When treating around the head and neck, the patient should also be wearing laser-safe "doggles," or alternatively should have their eyes covered with a dark cloth or shielded through the use of an opaque, soft Elizabethan collar. Photos of the patient wearing their doggles for the owner to share with friends and their online community through social media are also a nice secondary marketing tool (see Chapter 37).

Approach the patient briefly without turning the laser on to allow them to adapt to the sensation of the handpiece prior to the addition of laser therapy itself. Activate the laser and administer the laser therapy. Pause as needed during the treatment to reposition and allow the patient to reposition. Proceed sequentially through the prescribed areas to be treated. After the treatment is completed, record treatment parameters, observations, and progress notes in the patient's record.

Record Keeping

Good record keeping is important for the same reasons as for other medical procedures. The most important information to record is the dose administered, in J/cm^2 and the total amount of energy (total joules) administered to any specific area. Other information, such as application method, power (wattage), surface area in cm^2, handpiece aperture size, treatment response, pain score, and owner comments can also be included.

Records can be in electronic or written form. Some lasers will record (and export) treatment records, facilitating the continuation of a patient's treatment across different veterinary practices. These lasers have the added benefit of allowing quick, repeatable access to previous treatments, which provides added efficiency and reproducibility.

Photos, Videos, Radiographs, and Digital Thermal Images

Records can also include visual formats like photographs, videos, radiographs, and digital thermal images. These types of imaging are helpful to both the veterinarian and the owner, as they provide excellent before-and-after documentation of the progress being made with the laser therapy. Photographs are particularly valuable for wounds, incisions, and dermatitis. Videos are very helpful for lameness and neurologic conditions. Radiographs are appropriate for fractures and bony lesions. Digital thermal imaging is a simple and effective method of producing an image that reveals changes in temperature and circulation in injured and healing tissue (Figure 4.2).

Anesthesia

Patients will sometimes be under anesthesia when laser therapy is administered, and this requires extra attention to be paid to the warmth of the tissue being treated. Since an unconscious patient cannot respond to excessive warmth, continually checking the tissue temperature with a trailing finger or using a lower power setting is appropriate. Thorough instruction of support staff in these cases is essential.

Hair Coat Challenges

In practice, PBMT may be applied with minimal patient preparation. The hair coat may be clipped or shaved for optimal light penetration, but it is not absolutely necessary, depending on the power capabilities of the device. PBMT units may have built-in software that can calculate a dose of energy that will help compensate for additional light losses in thick or long hair coats. Alternatively, adjustment can be made manually when calculating a dose for administration (see Chapter 11). The hair coat should be free of excessive debris, and any lotions, sprays, or ointments that may have been applied to the treatment area should be rinsed off completely with water prior to treatment. Water will not significantly reduce laser therapy penetration, so treatments can be administered to pets emerging from underwater treadmill therapy, following bathing, or coming in from the rain as well, however the laser therapist should attempt to towel-dry the patient as much as possible prior to beginning treatment. If the coat is matted, crusted, or dirty, then clipping, debriding, or cleaning may be needed.

Bandages, Splints, Casts, and Pet Clothing

Laser therapy should not be administered through any sort of clothing, bandage, splint, or cast. The amount of light scattered by these materials is highly variable, and in some cases so complete that the dose of light reaching the target tissue is unknown and therefore unreliable. Remove any intervening clothing and collars or harnesses the pet is wearing. If a bandage is being used, administer laser therapy during bandage changes. If a splint or cast is being used, create a window of clear plastic over the area to be treated, and cover the window with material that can be easily removed for successive laser therapy treatments (Figure 4.3).

Laser Therapy Application Techniques

In general, two different application techniques can be utilized, depending on the power of the laser being used (Pryor and Millis, 2015). For lower-powered devices, typically those less than 500 mW (0.5 W), a point-to-point treatment is usually used. Multiple individual points within the

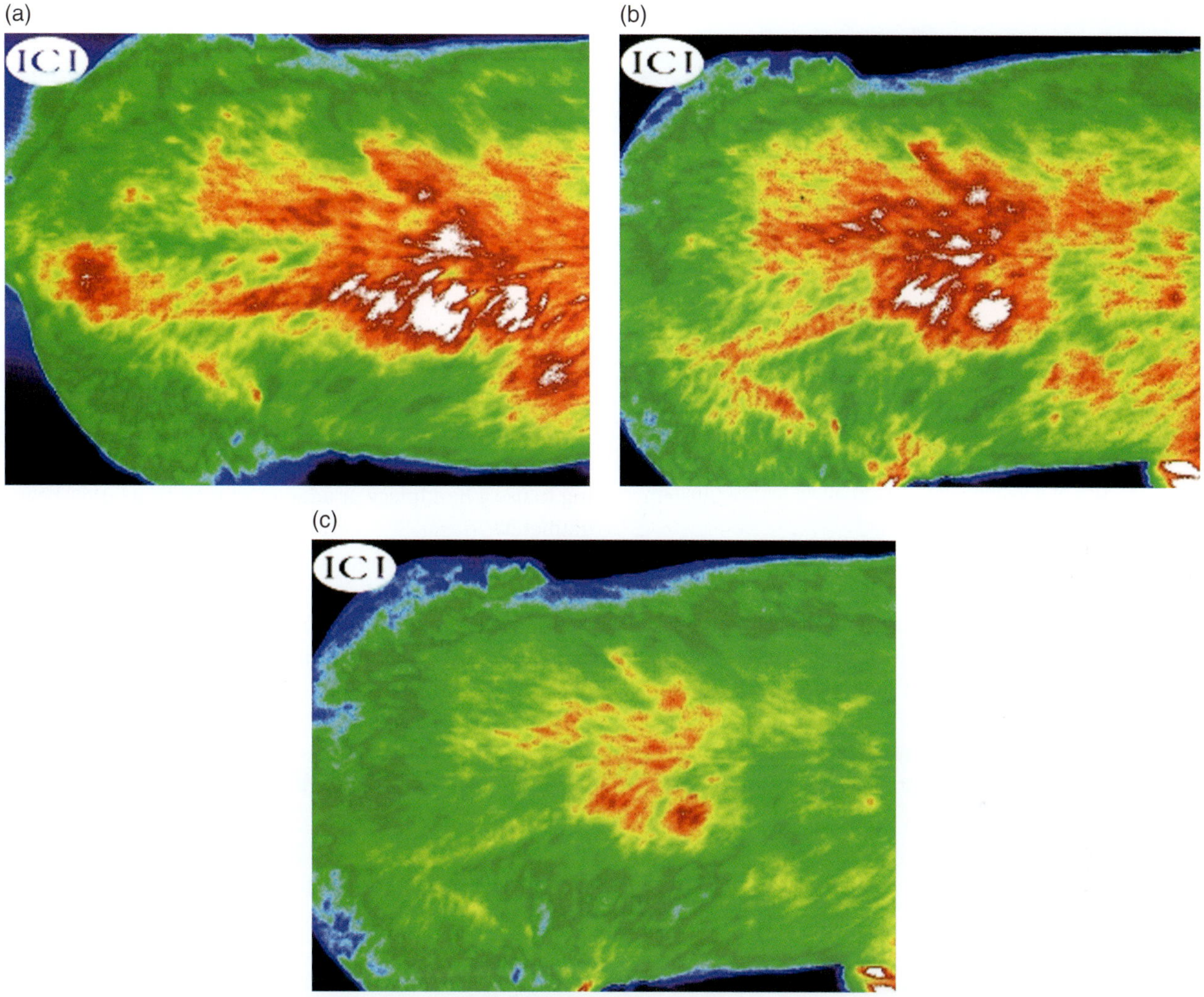

Figure 4.2 (a) Initial digital thermal image of a 9-year-old MN Scottish terrier presenting with bilateral pain along the spine. The white and red areas in the image are areas of increased thermal gradient. Using a combination of 810 and 980 nm, 8 J/cm^2 of laser therapy was administered with a contact scanning technique. No medication was administered. (b) Digital thermal image taken 24 hours after the initial laser therapy. Clinically, the patient was not in as much pain and was moving a great deal more easily. This image indicates a drop in thermal gradient of 34%. This is a very close approximation of the progress of the therapy and is a guide as to where to direct the next therapy session. Laser therapy was repeated with a slightly higher dose to all areas still exhibiting higher thermal gradients. (c) Digital thermal image taken 72 hours after the initial therapy and 48 hours after the second treatment, depicting a 92.5% decrease within the initial increased thermal gradients. Clinically, the patient was not in pain on palpation and was ready to play.

treatment area must be treated in order to deliver the appropriate target dose to tissues beneath the surface. Depending on the size of the area, or when dealing with multiple treatment areas in the same patient, this may become challenging from a time perspective and also varies from device to device as to the recommended duration to stay "on" each point. Point-to-point treatment also requires the laser operator to have the ability to precisely identify and locate the exact area(s) of deeper soft tissue structures that they wish to treat with this technique; they will not be treating over a regional area and saturating the tissues evenly with photons. Additionally, as previously discussed, irradiance (W/cm^2) plays an important role in therapeutic outcome, especially when dealing with deep-tissue conditions. For this reason, higher-powered devices may be able to achieve better results, in addition to being more time-efficient. For these devices (those lasers emitting more than 500 mW), a scanning technique should always be used. Even though these lasers generally have a larger spot size (depending on the optics of the treatment handpiece or head being used), thereby mitigating some of the increased power density, caution should always be used to ensure continuous movement during laser emission and good monitoring of both hair coat temperature and patient

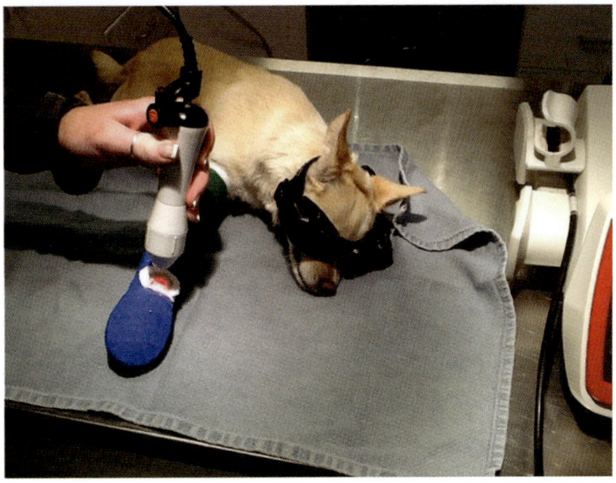

Figure 4.3 Use of a window in a cast to allow for laser therapy treatment.

behavior during treatment. A scanning speed that maintains irradiance and fluence within the recommended safety ranges for the treatment handpiece, and therefore the beam being used, is recommended. For devices above 500 mW, a scanning speed of 3–7 cm/s is usually appropriate; however, the laser operator should confirm with the manufacturer.

Handpiece Selection and Contact vs. Noncontact Application

Many higher-powered therapy lasers come with a choice of handpiece sizes, or a choice of small or large treatment heads, in both contact and noncontact designs. Others have handpieces that allow for manual adjustment of the diameter of the emitted laser beam. These choices improve application ergonomics and allow the option of spreading higher-power laser beams over a larger area of application.

As a general rule, handpieces or adapters that produce a beam diameter <2 cm should be used with a power of 3 W or less. These are most useful when treating small patients or small areas at those lower power settings.

Larger handpieces or adapters that produce a beam diameter >2 cm can be used with lower or higher power settings since they spread the energy over a much larger area (thus managing the irradiance of the beam) than the smaller handpieces. When a higher power setting is selected, some therapy laser software will provide a warning to use a handpiece or adapter that emits a larger beam diameter.

As previously mentioned, a contact handpiece should be used for any deep tissue condition (pathology that is not visible to the eye, or is below the skin or mucosa). Examples are musculoskeletal conditions, abdominal conditions, thoracic conditions, middle- or inner-ear conditions, and conditions within the closed mouth. Handpieces designed to be in contact with the tissue surface can also be designated as deep-tissue applicators if the lens introduces the light directly into the tissue (Figure 4.4).

Handpieces designed not to be in contact with the tissue surface are designated for superficial conditions (those conditions where the pathology is visible to the eye, or is not below the skin or mucosa) (Figure 4.5). These applicators are used to treat tissue 2–5 cm away and are also preferred for areas that are infected or have exudate, areas that are

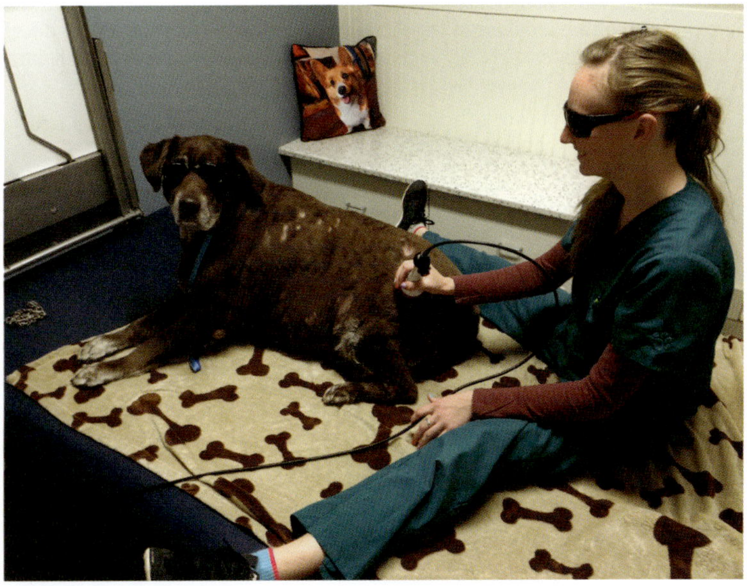

Figure 4.4 Proper positioning for treatment with a handpiece designed for deep-tissue treatment. The handpiece is in contact with, and held perpendicular to, the tissue surface.

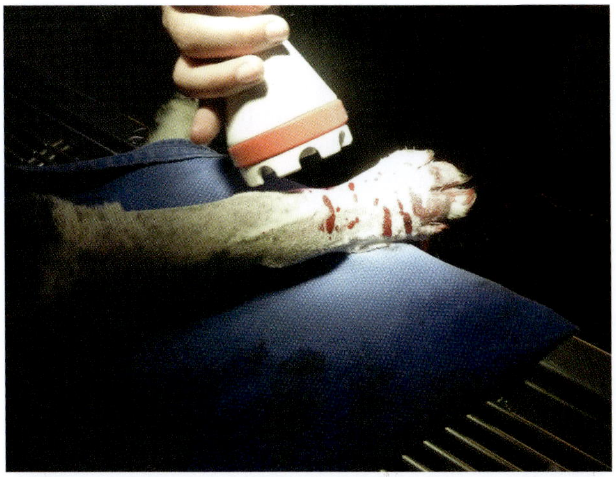

Figure 4.5 Treatment with a handpiece designed for noncontact treatment of superficial tissue conditions.

hypersensitive to physical touch, or areas that the laser operator wishes to remain sterile. Examples are dermatitis, wounds, incisions, the outer ear, the open mouth, and intraoperative applications.

Combination Contact and Noncontact Application

Otitis, oral applications, and some extensive wounds like degloving injuries may benefit from a combination of both contact and noncontact treatment, since they have components of both pathologies. For example, when treating otitis externa, the authors recommend using a noncontact application for the pinnae and outer ear, then changing to contact application for the middle and inner ear and the surrounding tissues. This allows the entire associated anatomy to be treated and provides superior results to a focused or limited application.

Treating Through Passive Range of Motion for Articular Areas

When treating articular areas, it is recommended to move the targeted tissue through a passive range of motion (try for at least two different positions) if possible, to aid in light penetration to various soft tissue structures and intra-articular surfaces. At the start of a course of therapy, the patient may be hypersensitive to pain, and movement of the area being treated may not be possible during the first few laser sessions. In these cases, it is best to first treat in a passive position, and then to attempt gentle movement for passive range of motion during subsequent treatments. This is described in further detail in Chapter 11.

Training and Expertise

All laser operators should be fully trained in the safe and effective delivery of therapeutic treatments. Each practice should develop a training protocol and finalize a training checklist, ensuring the operators are comfortable with the concepts outlined, prior to treating patients (Box 4.2).

Box 4.2 Therapy Laser Training Checklist

Equipment Care

- Assembly and disassembly of the laser for travel
- Proper care and insertion of the fiber into the laser
- Proper cleaning of the end of fiberoptic cable
- Proper cleaning of handpiece and attachments
- Application of the emission and fiber caps
- Maximum bending radius for the fiber and handpiece
- Shutdown of the laser device

General Laser Therapy Guidelines

- Versatility and goals of laser therapy in practice
- Software safety features and messages
- Proper recording of laser therapy treatments in the patient record

Safety First

- Safety features of the laser device
- Emergency shutdown switch or icon
- Standby, ready, and emission modes
- Safety interlock
- Power on/off visual indicator
- Laser emission indicator
- Eye protection
- Device-specific safety glasses for humans
- Patient eye protection: goggles, dark cloth, dark soft Elizabethan collars, therapist's hand
- "Laser in Use" safety sign
- Pigment levels in hair, skin, and tattoos
- Safe location for use of the laser device
- Contraindications, special considerations, and precautions

General Therapy Protocols

- Correct dosage for a given area and condition
- Calculation of dosage for therapy
- Positioning of the patient for the administration of the therapy
- Handpiece selection
- Noncontact handpiece for superficial tissue conditions
- Contact handpiece for deep-tissue conditions
- Maximum power for small versus large handpieces or beam diameters

(Continued)

Box 4.2 (Continued)

- Treatment settings concerning skin and coat color
- Number and frequency of therapy sessions required for therapeutic outcomes:
  - **Postprocedure:** One to two treatments
  - **Acute conditions:** Three to six treatments, daily or every other day
  - **Chronic conditions:** Open-ended number of treatments through three phases:
    - **Induction phase:** Every other day, or three times a week until significant improvement noted
    - **Transition phase:** Gradual reduction in frequency of treatments
    - **Maintenance phase:** Treatments as needed to maintain effect

General Treatment Principles

- Holding handpiece perpendicular to tissue
- Treatment from 360° or multiple directions
- Movement of handpiece at 2–7 cm/sec
- "Grid-like" application pattern evenly over treatment area(s)
- Treatment of joints through range of motion
- Avoiding splint, casting, and bandage material

Laser Therapy Treatment Plans

Treatment plans should incorporate all information provided in this chapter. It is helpful to "under promise" and "overdeliver" when communicating expectations for laser therapy. Photos, videos, objective outcome measures such as pain questionnaires, etc. will often help the owner see the progress being made with therapy and enforce the validity of the treatment plan.

Prescribing Treatment Packages for Compliance

For acute and chronic conditions, laser therapy may be prescribed as a multiple-treatment "package." Like antibiotics, a full course of therapy is commonly needed to achieve the optimal outcome, so providing treatments one at a time can be counterproductive and does not encourage compliance. Prescribing a package of three, six, or nine treatments is a convenient way to maximize clinical success, and because most owners will see satisfying progress after a few sessions, acceptance and continued compliance (in the case of further maintenance treatments needed) is generally very high.

Conclusion

Mastering the techniques of laser therapy is like mastering the techniques of dental prophylaxis. Like dentistry, laser therapy is largely a technician-administered modality that offers veterinarians the opportunity to provide a service that produces excellent results, endears strong client bonding, and adds an entirely new revenue stream. Attention to the principles and methods described in this chapter will optimize outcomes, improve consistency, and ensure both safety and efficiency.

References

AAHA (2015). 2015 AAHA/AAFP Pain Management Guidelines for Dogs and Cats. Available from: https://www.aaha.org/professional/resources/pain_management.aspx (accessed November 30, 2016).

Anders, J.J. *et al.* (2014). In vitro and in vivo optimization of infrared laser treatment for injured peripheral nerves. *Lasers Surg Med.* 46(1):34–45.

Anders, J. *et al.* (2015). Low-level light/laser therapy versus photobiomodulation therapy. *Photomed Laser Surg.* 33(4):183–184.

ANSI. (2011a) *American National Standard for Safe Use of Lasers in Health Care Facilities ANSI Z136.3 – 2011.* American National Standards Institute, Washington, DC.

ANSI. (2011b). *American National Standard for Environmental and Facility Safety Signs ANSI Z535.2 – 2011.* American National Standards Institute, Washington, DC.

Avci, P. *et al.* (2013). Low-level laser (light) therapy (LLLT) in skin: stimulating, healing, restoring. *Semin Cutan Med Surg.* 32(1):41–52.

Barrett, S.F. and Pack, D.J. (2006). Timing subsystem. In: *Microcontrollers Fundamentals for Engineers and Scientists*, pp. 51–64. Morgan and Claypool, San Rafael, CA.

Bjordal, J. *et al.* (2003). A systematic review of low level laser therapy with location specific doses for pain from chronic joint disorders. *Aust J Physiother.* 49(2):107–116.

Chien, S. and Wilhelmi, B.J. (2012). A simplified technique for producing an ischemic wound model. *J Vis Exp.* 2(63):e3341.

Chung, H. *et al.* (2012). The nuts and bolts of low-level laser (light) therapy. *Ann Biomed Eng.* 40(2):516–533.

Enwemeka, C.S. (2009). Intricacies of dose in laser phototherapy for tissue repair and pain relief. *Photomed Laser Surg.* 3:387–393.

Farivar, S. *et al.* (2014). Biological effects of low level laser therapy. *J Lasers Med Sci.* 5(2):58–62.

de Freitas, L.F. and Hamblin, M.R. (2016). Proposed mechanisms of photobiomodulation or low-level light therapy. *IEEE J Sel Top Quantum Electron.* 22(3): 7000417.

Hamblin, M. *et al.* (2018). Introduction. In: *Low-Level Light Therapy: Photobiomodulation*, p. 11. SPIE, Bellingham, WA.

Hashmi, J. *et al.* (2010). Effect of pulsing in low-level light therapy. *Lasers Surg Med.* 42(6):450–466.

Karu, T. (2010). Mitochondrial mechanisms of photobiomodulation in context of new data about multiple roles of ATP. *Photomed Laser Surg.* 28(2):159–160.

Kim, H.P. (2014). Lightening up light therapy: activation of retrograde signaling pathway by photobiomodulation. *Biomol Ther (Seoul).* 22(6):491–496.

Lister, T. *et al.* (2012). Optical properties of human skin. *J Biomed Opt.* 17(9):90901.

Looney, A.L. *et al.* (2018). A randomized blind placebo-controlled trial investigating the effects of photobiomodulation therapy (PBMT) on canine elbow osteoarthritis. *Can Vet J.* 59(9):959–966 http://www.ncbi.nlm.nih.gov/pubmed/30197438.

Morries, L.D. *et al.* (2015). Treatments for traumatic brain injury with emphasis on transcranial near-infrared laser phototherapy. *Neuropsychiatr Dis Treat.* 11:2159–2175.

Oron, A. *et al.* (2006). Low-level PBMT applied transcranially to rats after induction of stroke significantly reduces long-term neurological deficits. *Stroke.* 37(10):2620–2624.

Passarella, S. and Karu, T. (2014). Absorption of monochromatic and narrow band radiation in the visible and near IR by both mitochondrial and non-mitochondrial photoacceptors results in photobiomodulation. *J Photochem Photobiol B.* 140:344–358.

Peplow, P.V. *et al.* (2010). Laser photobiomodulation of wound healing: a review of experimental studies in mouse and rat animal models. *Photomed Laser Surg.* 28(3):291–325.

Piao, D. *et al.* (2018). Flexible nine-channel photodetector probe facilitated intraspinal multisite transcutaneous photobiomodulation therapy dosimetry in cadaver dogs. *J Biomed Opt.* 23(1):010503.

Pryor, B. and Millis, D. (2015). Therapeutic Laser in veterinary medicine. *Vet Clin North An Small Anim Pract.* 45(1):45–56.

Roberts, D.B. *et al.* (2013). The effectiveness of therapeutic class IV (10 W) laser treatment for epicondylitis. *Lasers Surg Med.* 45(5):311–317.

Sommer, A.P. *et al.* (2001). Biostimulatory windows in low-intensity laser activation: lasers, scanners, and NASA's light-emitting diode array system. *J Clin Laser Med Surg.* 19(1):29–33.

Sommer, A.P. *et al.* (2015). Tuning the mitochondrial rotary motor with light. *Ann Transl Med.* 3(22):346.

Vallone, F. *et al.* (2014). Effect of diode laser in the treatment of patients with nonspecific chronic low back pain: a randomized controlled trial. *Photomed Laser Surg.* 32(9):490–494.

Wardlaw *et al.* (2019). Laser therapy for incision healing in 9 dogs. *Front Vet Sci.* 5(349):1–8.

Weersink, R. (2007). Light dosimetry for low level laser therapy: accounting for difference in tissue and depth. *Proc SPIE.* 6428:642803.

Zein, R. *et al.* (2018). Review of light parameters and photobiomodulation efficacy: dive into complexity. *J Biomed Opt.* 23(12):1–17.

5

Therapy Laser Safety

Christopher J. Winkler

Suffolk Veterinary Group Animal Wellness and Laser Surgery Center, Selden, NY, USA

1st Edition Contributors:

Chapter 4 Kenneth E. Bartels

Professor Emeritus, Department of Veterinary Clinical Sciences, Oklahoma State University, Stillwater, OK, USA

Chapter 7 John C. Godbold, Jr.[1] and Ronald J. Riegel[2]

[1] Stonehaven Veterinary Consulting, Jackson, TN, USA
[2] American Institute of Medical Laser Applications, Marysville, OH, USA

Introduction

Theodore Maiman, working at the Hughes Research Laboratory in California, is credited for the announcement and publication of work shining a high-power pulsed flash lamp on a ruby rod with silver-coated surfaces to produce laser light. His announcement included a prediction that lasers would see applications in medicine and surgery (Hecht, 2005). Other physicists and engineers, including Charles Townes, Charles Schalow, Peter Sorokin, Mirek Stevenson, Ali Javen, William Bennett, Donald Harriott, Kumar C. Patel, and Robert Hall, from research and development companies including IBM, Bell Labs, and General Electric, were also involved in the concept of "a solution looking for a problem." In other words, there was tremendous interest in potentially using this new technology to advance communications, industrial applications, systems, and medical devices. In the development of these technologies, concepts of energy absorption, transmission, reflection, and material ablation to minimize potential harm to operators or patients were considered potentially serious limiting problems (Bartels, 2002; Fry, 2002).

Since Endre Mester and his colleagues first reported what we now know as photobiomodulation (PBM) in 1968 (Mester *et al.*, 1968), those using lasers for therapeutic purposes have sought to use them safely. Researchers, industry, and laser therapists have published contraindications for laser therapy in an effort to "do no harm." Texts and journal articles have published lengthy lists of contraindications (Navratil & Kymplova, 2002; Houghton *et al.*, 2010; Tuner & Hode, 2010), some of which have been reproduced in veterinary therapy laser user manuals. Safety hazards associated with improper use of medical lasers need to be understood and observed, since they are related to many state, national, and international mandated guidelines (Barat, 2014a). The safe use of medical lasers is essential for the use of high-power surgical lasers (Sliney, 1995). It is also an essential aspect of using medical lasers designated for PBM therapy.

Significant inconsistency remains among the recommendations in publications, texts, and user manuals. Some conditions originally considered contraindications for PBM now require special consideration before treatment, while some simply require precaution when treating. Other conditions are no longer contraindications. Historical contraindications for PBM should continue to be appropriately reevaluated in light of publications continuing to appear as laser therapy is used and analyzed in numerous bench-top studies, animal-model studies, and clinical trials.

Proper training is a requirement for treating veterinary patients with a therapy laser. Many veterinarians, including new graduates, have had little or no training regarding the clinical and safe use of medical lasers. The curricula of most veterinary schools until the last several years often did not cover this topic, and current content

Laser Therapy in Veterinary Medicine: Photobiomodulation, Second Edition. Edited by Christopher J. Winkler and Lisa A. Miller.

in core didactic course work is still minimal. To that end, many veterinarians begin using this technology following limited exposure during corporate-sponsored weekend short-courses, or at state, regional, national, or international continuing-education meetings that include a minimum of "hands-on" experience and a brief discussion of medical laser safety. Only with proper training and knowledge can contraindications, special considerations, and precautions be evaluated and appropriately applied in each patient's treatment alongside the safe utilization of the laser therapy unit itself.

Function of the American National Standards Institute and the Laser Institute of America

Laser safety is a part of the multi-mission task of the American National Standards Institute (ANSI). Founded in 1918, ANSI remains a private, nonprofit membership organization supported by both private industry and public-sector organizations. It helps to facilitate specific American National Standards by working with constituent groups composed of organizational bodies and individuals from manufacturers, government agencies, medical institutions, and the academic community. It maintains basic requirements for openness, balance, consensus, and due process in order to develop voluntary national consensus standards that relate to products, processes, services, systems, and safety. It ensures that standards undergo public review. Consensus must be reached by representatives from affected businesses and companies. Comments from the consensus body and public review must be reported in good faith, and an appeals process is a requirement. An estimated 10,000 American National Standards exist today. ANSI promotes standardization efforts in the United States, but also advocates for these policies and technical positions to the international community as international standards are adopted (ANSI, 2014).

The Laser Institute of America (LIA) was founded in 1968 as the professional society for laser applications and safety. Its mission is to foster lasers as a useful technologic advancement, encourage useful laser applications, and promote laser safety worldwide. It represents the core of the profession and includes a group of academic scientists, engineers, physicist, manufacturers, and medical specialists who are passionate about growing the technology, as well as turning it into a viable industry that is both safe and efficacious for many uses. Further, to enhance this mission, it serves as the secretariat and publisher of the ANSI Z136 series of laser safety standards (www.lia.org). Its standards are the foundation of laser safety programs throughout the United States and in most of the world.

The American Veterinary Medical Association (AVMA) saw the need for the veterinary profession to become a part of the ANSI group in 1999, to ensure the profession met the standards for safe use of medical lasers and to collaborate in the standardization of safety guidelines by the ANSI Z136 Laser Safety Committee. This membership has been crucial in ensuring veterinary medicine has been included in discussions over the writing of new guidelines as the technology has grown, including the use of high power surgical lasers and, more recently, the use of therapy lasers in PBM therapy.

The ANSI documents are definitive in outlining the safe use of lasers in veterinary medicine (ANSI, 2011a, 2014). The Z136 guidelines represent general agreement among manufacturers, sales personnel, and users regarding the best current practices. ANSI Z136.3 addresses the "Safe Use of Lasers in Health Care Facilities," whereas ANSI Z136.1, "American National Standard for Safe Use of Lasers," covers the much broader topic of laser safety in general, including in industrial and research environments. These standards are guidelines (not regulations) for the safe use of laser systems. Currently, use of medical lasers in veterinary medicine is included in both standard sections and as an appendix within the Z136.3 guideline. It must also be assumed that the Occupational Safety and Health Administration (OSHA) and state regulatory agencies will use these same guidelines as safety issues arise in veterinary medicine. It is up to the veterinary profession to be proactive and to provide the safest possible use of medical lasers, both for the sake of patient care and for the health of the veterinarian and technical assistants. Both of these laser safety documents are continuously under review, and it is likely that new versions of Z136.3 will continue to be released in the future.

Additional federal regulations regarding lasers as medical devices fall under the authority of the Food and Drug Administration (FDA) Center for Devices and Radiological Health (CDRH) via enforcement of the Federal Laser - Product Performance Standard and the Medical Devices Amendment to the Food, Drug, and Cosmetic Act (FDA, 2015a). All laser products sold in the United States since August 1976 must be certified by the manufacturer as meeting safety standards, and each laser must bear a label indicating compliance with the standards and giving its laser hazard classification (Class 1–4). Operating manuals must be included with the device and must contain adequate instructions for assembly, calibration (especially for Class 3 and 4 lasers), operation, and maintenance, including necessary precautions to avoid potentially hazardous exposure to direct laser and collateral radiation.

Laser Hazard Classification

The ANSI standard laser hazard classifications are used to indicate the level of hazard associated with a laser system and the degree of safety control required. Lasers are classified based on the ability of the beam to cause histologic damage to the eye and skin. The relevant parameters include laser output energy or power, radiation wavelengths, exposure duration, and the cross-sectional area of the laser beam at the tissue target area. Laser hazard classification is also based on the accessibility of the laser radiation or accessible emission limit within a particular laser hazard class.

A Class 1 laser system (Class 1/1M) is considered not able to produce tissue damage during operation, so is exempt from control measures. Class 1M laser systems are considered incapable of producing a hazardous beam exposure during normal operation unless the beam is viewed with an optical eye-loupe or telescope. The safety goal is to prevent potentially hazardous optically aided viewing. Examples of Class 1 lasers are grocery store price-scanning devices and laser printers (LIA, 2000).

A Class 2 laser system (Class 2/2M) emits a visible portion of the light spectrum (400–700 nm). Ocular protection is usually provided by the aversion response, which includes the blink reflex (<0.25 seconds), eye or head movement, and pupillary constriction. A Class 2M laser system also emits a similar visible light spectrum and is considered hazardous if viewed with optical aids. In considering this laser classification, the concept of maximum permissible exposure (MPE) is introduced. MPE is defined as the level of laser radiation to which an unprotected person may be exposed without adverse biological changes in the eye or skin. In the case of a Class 2M system, MPE equals the 0.25 second eye-aversion response time (LIA, 2000).

Class 3 laser systems (3R/3B) are not considered a fire hazard or a significant hazard to the skin. Class 3B laser systems (medium-power lasers) can be dangerous under direct and indirect or specular (mirror-like) viewing conditions, but are usually not a hazard through diffuse reflection or a fire hazard.

Class 4 laser systems (high-power visible and invisible wavelengths) are potentially an acute hazard to the eye and skin via both direct intrabeam exposure and diffuse or scattered reflection. Class 4 lasers also potentially present a hazard for ignition (fire) and byproduct production via ablated (vaporized) laser-generated airborne contaminants (LGACs), which include gaseous toxic compounds, dead and live cellular components, and viruses (LIA, 2000; ANSI, 2011a).

For the ANSI Z136.1 and Z136.3 guidelines, the ANSI 136 Committee made an extreme effort to have classification guidelines be identical or as close as possible to the FDA Code of Federal Regulations Title 21, Part 1040 – Performance Standards for Light-Emitting Products (FDA, 2015c) and Part 878 – Medical Devices: General and Plastic Surgery Devices (FDA, 2015a), FDA guidance regarding low-level laser systems for aesthetic use (FDA, 2011), FDA laser hazard classes (FDA, 2015b), the International Electrotechnical Commission guidelines (FDA, 2007), and OSHA regulations regarding laser hazards (OSHA, 2015).

Though some US states and the international community may rewrite them to include a different approach, including laser registration processes, the ANSI guidelines usually are closely utilized to "harmonize" documents so as not to create confusion among laser users and institutional entities, such as national laboratories and universities. In the past few years, the major change that has been considered is a reclassification of laser classes to align with ocular hazards related to actual hazards detectable from beams enclosed in a protective housing, as well as to include classes of lasers that may be hazardous under direct or specular reflection but pose minimal hazard for fire or do not generate LGACs.

Administrative Controls

Each veterinary facility utilizing any medical laser should appoint a laser safety officer (LSO) with primary responsibility for all aspects of the institution's laser safety program (Barat, 2006b; Oleson, 2016). In a general practice or private specialty practice, the LSO's duties may be fulfilled by either a veterinarian or a technician. The LSO is responsible for laser system classification (Classes 1–4), hazard evaluation, control measures, standard operating procedure development, protective equipment use, appropriate signage and labels, and facility modification to follow manufacturer's guidelines for safe laser installation. Of utmost importance for the LSO, is the establishment and maintenance of laser safety training programs for all individuals in the practice. The programs should ensure that all Class 3B and 4 laser users and observers are properly instructed and know how to maintain personnel and patient safety. Though clinical experience with one class of medical laser can be beneficial, it is important that those using the lasers be thoroughly familiar with each specific device, especially regarding its wavelength and absorption characteristics. Familiarity with state requirements for LSO establishment and responsibilities, as well as established guidelines, local, state, and federal regulations, advisory standards, and professional recommended practices on the use of medical lasers within veterinary facilities, is extremely important.

In this author's experience, veterinary technicians are as interested as veterinarians in learning basic laser science, how it affects their patients, and aspects of laser safety; delegation of the LSO position to an interested and trained Licensed Veterinary Technician (LVT) should therefore be strongly considered (Winkler, 2019).

Laser Use Environment

Use of high-power medical lasers (Class 4) of various wavelengths and in different operational modes (CW vs. pulsed) for tissue vaporization presents a very different spectrum of beam hazards compared to therapy lasers. Therapy lasers vary from low-power (Class 1–3B, sometimes colloquially called "cold lasers"), to high-power (Class 4), and include wavelengths ranging from the ultraviolet to the infrared, as previously outlined.

The nominal hazard zone (NHZ) is defined by ANSI as the space within which the level of direct-beam, reflected, or scattered laser radiation during treatment (especially Class 3B or 4) exceeds the applicable MPE and presents potential detrimental laser effects to the laser operator, surgical assistants, and casual observer. Even with use of Classes 1M, 2, 2M, and 3R lasers, if there is potential for any direct beam exposure, proper signage should be considered. In practice, the NHZ is considered the room in which the procedure is performed. Often, therapy lasers are used in a treatment or exam room, which can be acceptable if proper warning signage is used and any potential observation windows are blocked with an opaque laser-safe material or appropriate filter glass (which is often quite expensive). Another option is to use portable laser-safe barriers or curtains, which can be purchased from laser manufacturers.

Appropriate laser radiation warning signage for use on doors or access areas for laser therapy treatment zones needs to be in accordance with ANSI Z535.2 – "Environmental and Facility Safety Signs" (ANSI, 2011b). Understanding the need for warning signs is essential (Henderson, 1997; Barat, 2006a). Laser manufacturers should, and usually do, provide the appropriate signage with the device. The warning sign needs to conform to the specifications designated for the class of laser, as given by the ANSI Z136.1 or ANSI Z136.3 guidelines, which also comply with the OSHA Technical Manual for Laser Hazards (OSHA, 2015). Some laser surgery or therapy areas may have illuminated signage that is used when laser radiation is being emitted. More common is temporary signage, which is posted on the entry door of the laser treatment area, and removed when a laser therapy is not being conducted. The sign should clearly indicate the danger of laser radiation, all eye safety requirements, the wavelength(s) of laser light, and the highest power emission available to the specific device (Figure 5.1).

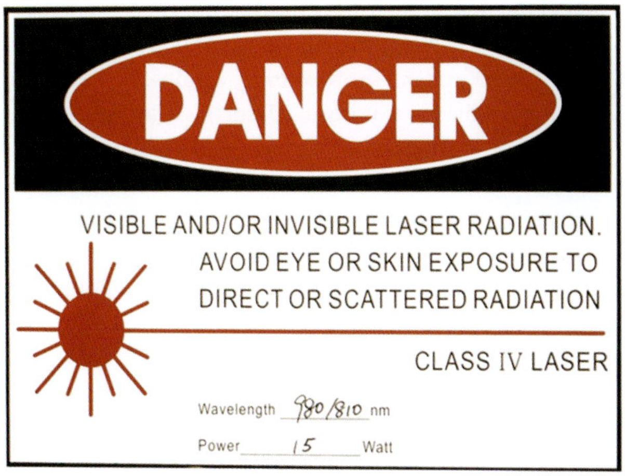

Figure 5.1 Laser safety temporary warning/danger sign with laser classification and precautions for use with all Class 3B and 4 lasers. The sign is removed from the laser control environment after the procedure is completed.

In some rare cases, especially with high-power Class 4 surgical or industrial lasers, safety interlocks may be used to interrupt laser emission if the entry door is opened during a procedure. Their use is somewhat problematic, however, since interrupting a procedure could be detrimental to the patient's health and safety.

Operating room protocol should never be casual, particularly when a laser is in use. Laser warning signs should be in full view on the doors, and all windows and doors need appropriate laser-safe covers. Prior to laser activation, the attending clinician should observe all attendant personnel for proper eye safety wear; it is particularly important when multiple laser wavelengths are in use in the NHZ to be certain that the safety eyewear worn is of the proper optical density (OD) for the wavelength currently in use. The clinician should then announce, "laser on," so that no one is uncertain about beam activation. When not in use, standby modes are appropriate to avoid inadvertent laser radiation exposure.

Laser Beam-Related Hazards and Hazard Prevention

Primary hazard assessment of medical lasers includes concerns over eye safety and skin exposures (Winburn, 1990). MPE values have been calculated based on laser wavelength for both skin and eye exposures

(Henderson & Schulmeister, 2004b). MPEs depend on laser wavelength, exposure time, and mode of delivery: continuous-wave (CW) or pulsed repetition. Values are expressed as either radiant exposure (J/cm^2), also known as "fluence," or as irradiance (W/cm^2), also known as "power density." Values for each laser are published in the ANSI documents. Any value higher than the MPE can cause tissue damage. In general, the longer the laser wavelength, the higher the MPE, and the longer the exposure time, the lower the MPE (ANSI, 2011a, 2014).

Nonbeam Hazards

Electrical Hazards

Since most lasers utilize high-voltage power supplies, the possibility of electric shock does exist. Medical laser manufacturers are required to build in many safety features to reduce the chances of shock, electrocution, or inadvertent laser beam exposure, and to comply with FDA manufacturer guidelines. These features include protective housings, key control, laser door interlocks, shutters or attenuators, radiation emission indicators, error-sensing programs, fail-safe circuitry and shutter design, power output monitoring, and appropriate classification labeling. Other features include guarded foot or hand switches to prevent inadvertent laser exposure, low-power visible lasers (diode or helium neon devices) that emit aiming beams to ensure accurate tissue targeting, and emergency-off switches (Fry, 2002).

The probability of electrical shock is minimal if operation is in compliance with instructional manuals and common precautions are exercised with any electrical device. However, removal of the exterior housing for servicing may dramatically increase the risk of serious injury. Only authorized professional service personnel should ever attempt to remove the housing and perform maintenance on the laser.

Fire Hazards and Controls

As with concern over LGACs, the likelihood of fire hazard due to the thermal effects of therapy laser devices is minimal. Use of Class 4 therapy laser devices at recommended power and pulse settings for PBM purposes should not involve the creation of a plume of smoke associated with surgical laser tissue ablation. In rare instances, ignition of the hair in the target area is possible. This phenomenon only occurs when proper application techniques are not utilized.

However, if there is a malfunction of a laser therapy handpiece, an undetected broken laser fiber or cable, or accidental laser beam exposure due to improper use, especially with a Class 4 device used at maximum power, the potential for ignition of protective drapes or other accessories becomes possible, though still extremely unlikely. The availability of a fire extinguisher should always be considered, in case a fire does occur.

Beam Hazards and Contraindications

The list of absolute contraindications for exposure to therapeutic laser light is remarkably short, with only one item (Box 5.1).

Eye Exposure

The one absolute clinical contraindication for veterinary laser therapy is direct or reflected exposure through the pupil on to the retina. The hazards inherent in laser interaction with ocular structures are the historical basis for laser classifications by regulatory bodies, and present the greatest threat to the laser therapist, support staff, patient, and those who accompany the patient.

Hazardous effects to the eye associated with therapy lasers and high-power surgical lasers consist of corneal and lenticular opacities and retinal damage, both of which depend on laser wavelength, expressed in nanometers (Sliney & Freasier, 1973). Other factors that also affect the amount and type of tissue damage include tissue volume and circulation, beam energy, and length of exposure (LIA, 2000).

Box 5.1 Laser Therapy Contraindications, Special Considerations, and Precautions

Absolute contraindication

- Eye exposure

Special considerations

- Malignancy
- Locally injected medication
- Pregnancy

Precautions

- Active epiphyses
- Hemorrhage
- Testicles
- Thyroid gland

False contraindications

- Hyperpigmentation and tattoos
- Implants
- Microbial infection
- Photosensitizing medications

Visible-wavelength (400–780 nm) and near-infrared (IR-A; 780–1400 nm) energy will pass through the cornea and lens and directly induce thermal damage to the retina, causing loss of color vision, night blindness, and potentially complete loss of vision. As a result, visible and near-infrared wavelengths are known as the "retinal hazard region" of the light spectrum. Within this retinal hazard zone (440–1400 nm), the retina is 100 000 times more vulnerable to injury than the skin (LIA, 2000). Veterinary medical lasers such as the Nd:YAG lasers (1064 nm) and some diode lasers (808 and 980 nm) may induce retinal damage, resulting in decreased vision or potential blindness. This damage is increased with longer-duration exposures and pupillary dilation. In human medicine, near-infrared diode laser wavelengths are deliberately applied to the retina to destroy tumors such as melanoma; such applications may become more mainstream for veterinary medicine in the future (B. Marr, MD, personal communication May 16, 2023).

Near-ultraviolet wavelengths (UV-A; 315–400 nm) pass through the cornea and are absorbed by the lens, resulting in photochemical denaturation of lens proteins, which potentially causes cataract formation. Far-ultraviolet wavelength energy (UV-B, UV-C; 100–315 nm) will be absorbed by the corneal epithelium, resulting in photokeratitis due to denaturation of corneal proteins. Conjunctivitis is also a possible result. Far-infrared wavelengths (IR-B, IR-C; 1400–10 600 nm) will result in corneal damage due to selective tissue water absorption inducing protein denaturation on the corneal surface, which results in corneal burns. Wavelengths from 1400 to 3000 nm may penetrate deeper and lead to cataracts, due to heating of lens proteins. Minimal temperature rise is necessary for these changes to occur (LIA, 2000).

Class 2 and 3R lasers powered by AAA and AA batteries marketed as laser pointers are restricted within the United States to 0.1–0.5 mW of laser radiation. Used improperly, laser pointers are potentially hazardous; even with an aversion response, temporary flash blindness or "welder's glare" can result. Instances of permanent damage to the retina can potentially occur from direct beam viewing of Class 3R laser pointers. Some illegally imported laser pointers have visible wavelengths ranging from 532 nm green light to 690 nm red light generate in excess of 0.5 mW. These are classified as Class 3B, and require additional considerations regarding eye safety.

It is mandatory that the eyes of all personnel present during laser therapy be protected by wavelength-specific safety eyewear or other shielding devices. Safety eyewear for humans will be supplied by any responsible veterinary therapy laser manufacturer. The patient's eyes can be protected by wavelength-specific goggles made for animals, dark soft Elizabethan collars, or covering with a dark cloth or a hand. The patient should not be allowed to investigate the target area while the treatment is being administered. Restraint, food treats, or attention should be used to distract the patient from the treatment site as required.

For safe use of medical lasers, eyewear must match the conditions of potential exposure during treatment (Barat, 2014b). Most manufacturers of both high-power and therapy devices provide appropriate eyewear for diffuse, accidental beam exposure. Specifically for therapy lasers, an essential understanding of power (laser class) and wavelength is required to avoid potential accidents to the operator, assistant, and patient. Class 3B and 4 devices are of major safety concern. Instructions provided by the manufacturer and ANSI guidelines must be followed. As explained previously, Classes 1 through 3R lasers need to be used with care to avoid direct exposure to the eye, but Classes 3B and Class 4 devices can and will damage the eye if used carelessly and safety guidelines are ignored.

In deciding what type of eye protection is needed, two important factors must be determined: laser wavelength and the maximum viewing duration for the specific procedures. MPE limits are used to determine guidelines for protecting personnel from three types of viewing conditions: (i) unintentional accidental exposure to a visible beam where the MPE may exceed 0.25 seconds – the blink-aversion reflex; (ii) unintentional, accidental viewing of a near-infrared laser beam for up to 10 seconds; and (iii) intentional viewing of diffuse reflection for up to 600 seconds. In order to choose the most appropriate set of safety glasses for a specific device designed for a specific procedure, OD should be employed. OD is a mathematical–physics logarithmic calculation that factors attenuation of the laser beam input radiance divided by the transmittance radiance. Tabular values are provided in ANSI guidelines and other references. The bottom line is that the OD of the filtration medium (glass or polycarbonate plastic) should match the exposure condition for diffuse or intrabeam viewing conditions.

Design of laser-safe eyewear is a factor that must be considered in order to afford the best compliance for proper use. If eyewear is heavy, uncomfortable, or restricts visualization of the target tissue due to the color of the optical filter, its use may be ignored. Even with newer designs of glasses and goggles designated for specific devices, administrative controls or requirements implemented by the practice or institution for appropriate use must be seriously applied. The choice between glass and plastic (polycarbonate) lenses should be considered: glass-lensed eyewear is heavier and more expensive, but usually more robust and resistant to scratches and breakage. For laser therapy, and even high-power laser surgery, eyewear is designed

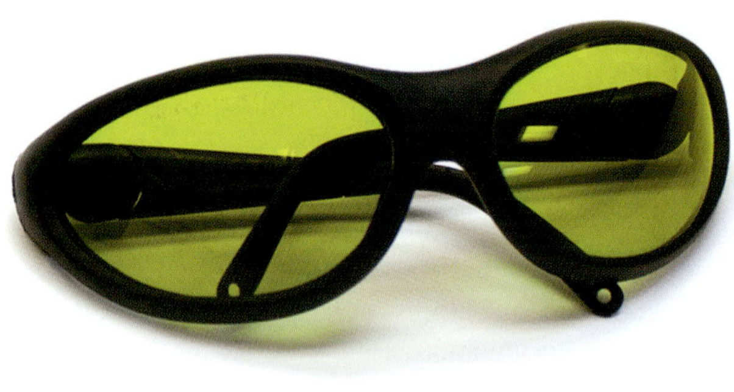

Figure 5.2 Laser-protective glasses.

with appropriate OD requirements to protect the wearer against specular reflection but not direct beam impact. Side shields are also recommended, to protect against unnoticed reflection, which could potentially cause ocular damage (Figure 5.2).

With the tunability of some surgical lasers and the manufacture of laser therapy devices delivering multiple wavelengths at the same time, additional caution must be considered when selecting safe eyewear for clinical use. A pair of single-wavelength protective eyewear is obviously not appropriate for multiple-wavelength delivery. Most manufacturers providing proper eyewear for their own product take care to supply dual-wavelength protection, but it is still the operator's responsibility to ensure the appropriate laser-safe eyewear has been provided. All laser eyewear must be distinctly marked on the bows, frames, or lenses regarding the protective OD designation and the wavelengths covered (LIA, 2000) (Figure 5.3).

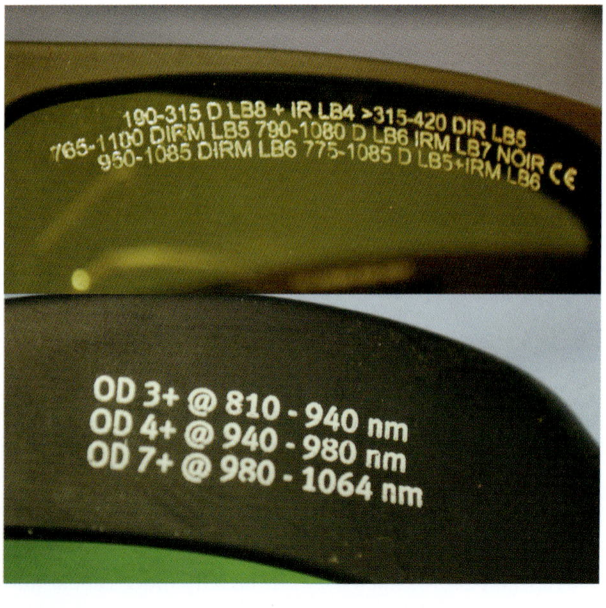

Figure 5.3 Specification of wavelength and OD on the lens (top) and frame (bottom).

Laser-safe eyewear must be properly fitted (Henderson & Schulmeister, 2004a). It should be maintained to protect against breakage and scratches. If utilized appropriately, laser-safe eyewear can provide many years of use. Eyewear always needs to be carefully examined prior to laser therapy and surgery. If it is damaged in any way (broken frames, scratched or cracked lenses), it must be replaced.

One can adapt the environment in which the therapy laser is used to reduce the possibility of direct or reflected accidental laser beam exposure of eyes. Reflective surfaces, such as stainless steel veterinary treatment tables, should be covered with patient-comfortable, nonreflective material. Mirrors, jewelry, and other potential sources of reflected laser energy must also be evaluated for potential harm.

Patient eye protection is also essential. Potential options for shielding include saline-moistened sponges, pieces of black felt, wavelength-specific laser eye-shields, corneal shields, and laser-safe eyewear fitted for animals (Fry, 2002; Riegel, 2008).

Ocular hazards stem from the therapy laser beam penetrating the cornea and pupil, and being focused by the lens on the retina. Scattered photons reaching the retina after transmission through other tissues do not pose an optical hazard. Thus, careful laser therapy application to the periorbital tissues is possible, as long as direct or reflected beam penetration through the pupil is avoided.

Skin Hazards

Far-ultraviolet radiation (UV-B, UV-C) falls in the actinic or photochemical ultraviolet zone. Exposures may result in erythema or blistering of skin due to epidermal absorption. A common source of UV-B is sunlight, which has been implicated in skin carcinogenesis. Devices emitting the shorter wavelengths of ultraviolet light (180–200 nm) are used for their potential germicidal effects in some laser therapy devices. Skin effects may occur in all regions of the infrared spectrum (IR-A, IR-B, IR-C), being influenced by hyperpigmentation and photosensitization from certain drugs. With extreme exposure, they can include blistering or charring of the tissue.

Skin hazards need to be considered with higher-powered visible or infrared lasers (Class 4), which includes all surgical lasers and some laser therapy devices. Lower-power lasers (Classes 1–3B), though potentially hazardous to the eye, are not usually considered as hazardous to the skin. Some Class 4 therapy laser devices have potential to cause photothermal skin injury if not used according to manufacturer's recommendations. Even then, factors such as the laser power emitted, the beam diameter of the delivery device, pulsed versus continuous beam delivery, the patient's skin pigmentation, hair length and color, and the depth of beam penetration can potentially cause blistering and perhaps photothermal skin necrosis. There are many recommendations regarding treatment regimens for multiple conditions, including pain relief and wound healing, that must be considered on an individual patient basis in order to ensure appropriate exposure and medical benefit.

Laser therapy protocols are recommended from many sources, including research papers and case reports, as well as technical representatives of companies. Computerized programs installed in some devices, as well as manuals provided with the devices, make the use of therapeutic lasers seem easy for most amenable conditions. Treatments provided to animals that are not anesthetized or lightly sedated may cause them to react to uncomfortable photothermal sensitivity, providing the operator with the necessary reaction to adjust the treatment dosage and/or technique appropriately. The potential advantages of using higher-power therapeutic laser devices include providing treatment protocols using higher radiant energy over a shorter time interval and, potentially, allowing deeper penetration of that energy. However, the operator must be aware that a "set recipe" treatment protocol for a specific condition may not be appropriate for every patient treated for that specific condition. Close clinical observation of the patient and the use of the laser as an extension of the veterinarian's other treatment modalities is most prudent.

Special Considerations

Historically, a lack of knowledge and a healthy dose of prudence resulted in a long list of conditions being considered contraindications to laser therapy. Increased knowledge of the mechanisms of PBM brings an increased understanding that most of those conditions are not absolute contraindications. Rather, some are conditions that merit special consideration before being treated (see Box 5.1).

Patients with special consideration conditions will most often not be appropriate candidates for therapy. These are patients with conditions for which the risk of laser therapy, or the perceived risk, outweighs the benefit. Properly trained and knowledgeable veterinary laser therapists will evaluate each patient, communicate the special considerations to the patient's owner, obtain owner consent, and then deliver laser therapy treatment only when appropriate.

Malignancy

A significant number of contradictory data exist concerning the effect of laser therapy on malignant tissue. Most of the data continues to come from *in vitro* studies using malignant human cell lines.

Strong arguments have been made for a new understanding of the role of PBM in the treatment of cancer (Karu, 2010; Lanzafame, 2011; Santana-Blank *et al.*, 2012b). A 2012 systematic literature review presented existing data on the potential application of PBM in the treatment of solid tumors (Santana-Blank *et al.*, 2012a). This review proposed that PBM might help restore homeostasis and homeokinesis in cancer patients. It suggested that by reestablishing physiological rhythms and inducing physiologically reparative effects for disease reversal in cancer and other complex diseases, PBM might, with minimal or no adverse effects, provide significant improvements in quality of life, even in patients with advanced neoplasms. Using various wavelengths and parameters, laser application has been demonstrated to induce increased proliferation in human leukemic cells (Dastanpour *et al.*, 2015) and increased proliferation and invasion in human oral squamous cell carcinoma (SCC) cells (Gomes *et al.*, 2014). Seemingly contradictory is the demonstration of laser application having no significant effect on human breast adenocarcinoma cells (Cialdai *et al.*, 2015) and having a selective cytotoxic effect on human oral cancer cells (Liang *et al.*, 2015). A recent study analyzed the effect of PBM on the modulation of the osteoclastogenic potential of a cell line derived from human lingual SCC (Dias Schalch *et al.*, 2016). Using parameters for mucositis treatment, the study demonstrated a reduced osteoclastogenic effect on the tumor cells and suggested that PBM might represent a potential useful side effect while treating mucositis.

A more recent publication argued that PBM can raise the standard of care and improve the quality of life of patients with cancer and other complex diseases (Santana-Blank *et al.*, 2016). Subsequent follow-up studies to this continued to indicate the safety, efficacy, and benefits of PBM in cancer patients, while still concluding that more randomized controlled trials are needed to inform clinical guidelines and routine practice (Bensadoun *et al.*, 2020; Wang *et al.*, 2022).

Another study noted arrested tumor growth, improved clinical condition, decreased lung metastases, and enhanced survival in triple-negative breast cancer-bearing mice when PBM was applied (Silva, 2021). Special considerations for the application of PBM in the presence of malignancy in animals will likely continue to be reevaluated as further evidence emerges. Until more data specific to veterinary species are available, laser therapy should not be applied directly over a malignancy or the surgical site from which a malignancy has just been removed.

Special consideration should be given to a surgical site from which a malignancy has been removed and surgical margins have been submitted for histopathological review. A positive margin report is a contraindication for laser therapy and an indication for further surgical resection. Less obvious is whether laser therapy is appropriate after a negative or clear margin report. In generating negative margin reports, pathologists look at a very small percentage of the entire margin, and there is often not a standard definition of how wide a negative margin should be. Thus, even with a negative margin report, a possibility remains that some malignant cells have not been removed. That possibility should be discussed with the owner before instituting laser therapy.

Consideration must also be given to the safety of treating sites in close-proximity or distant to a malignancy. A pilot study indicated an improved quality of life when PBM was used in the management of radiation dermatitis in human breast cancer patients (Censabella *et al.*, 2016). Though PBM does result in some systemic effects, current data indicate it is safe to apply laser therapy to veterinary patients in areas distant to known malignancies. The safety of treating at a distant site is illustrated by use of laser therapy to treat chemotherapy-induced oral mucositis in human cancer patients (Ottaviani *et al.*, 2013).

Another special consideration regarding laser therapy and malignancy exists for terminal veterinary patients. PBM can be effective in reducing the pain and inflammation in tissue around a malignancy, so it should be considered a part of hospice management for terminal cancer patients. Owners should be involved in the decision to add laser therapy for pain management in terminal malignancies, after being informed about the potential effect on the malignancy. Anecdotal reports from practitioners support the concept that laser therapy can increase the duration and quality of the lives of veterinary hospice patients with terminal malignancy.

A more detailed discussion of PBM applications in the veterinary oncology patient continues in Chapter 19 of this text.

Locally Injected Medication

Laser therapy should not be applied over local vaccine or medication injection sites until sufficient time has passed for the injected substance to be absorbed and translocated from the site. Laser-induced vasodilation may alter pharmacologically ideal absorption and trans location rates, and no information exists about how various wavelengths of light might interact with vaccine components or medications.

If an injection is going to be made, and the area is going to be treated with laser therapy, first treat with laser therapy and then administer the injection.

A good understanding of the pharmacodynamics of any vaccine or medication will help the veterinarian properly schedule therapy laser treatments. If, for example, a medication administered by intramuscular injection induces a myositis, and if that medication is renally cleared in 24 hours, then laser therapy of the myositis is appropriate after 24 hours.

Pregnancy

Applying laser therapy directly over a gravid uterus is almost always listed as a contraindication. The historical basis for pregnancy being a contraindication is lack of knowledge of the potential effect on the fetus, in addition to studies demonstrating changes in chicken embryo tissue after application of visible red laser wavelengths through a window opened in the eggshell (Avila *et al.*, 1999).

A rational analysis would indicate that fetal tissue within a gravid uterus will not be harmed by visible or near-infrared light photons. These wavelengths lack any mutagenic or teratogenic effect. Further, the fetus is well-protected from exposure to photons, being surrounded by a significant thickness of tissues rich in the chromophores that most readily absorb the wavelengths being used. A recent study concluded the safe and effective use of laser therapy on humans during pregnancy for the treatment of several different disorders (Allameh *et al.*, 2021).

Yet, despite evidence to the contrary, unless a special consideration exists that warrants direct treatment over a gravid uterus, the prudent veterinary laser therapist will avoid such treatment. As with some other modalities used during pregnancy, no proof exists of potential harm to the fetus. But no proof exists that there is not a potential harm. Absence of proof does not legally constitute proof of absence. Thus, if laser therapy is applied over the gravid uterus, and an unrelated pregnancy complication or fetal deformity occurs, the burden of proof will be on the veterinarian to demonstrate that laser therapy did not cause the complication (Tuner & Hode, 2010).

A valid consideration is whether pregnant veterinary laser therapists (or other pregnant females present during treatment) are at risk. Clothing reflects, scatters, and absorbs visible and infrared photons, significantly reducing the number reaching underlying skin. Thus, clothing gives an additional layer that blocks photons from reaching the fetus. There is no evidence that the well-protected fetus of a pregnant and clothed female is at risk during a veterinary therapy laser application.

Precautions

Veterinary patients often present with conditions mentioned as contraindications for laser therapy for which strong evidence now indicates the risk, or the perceived risk, is significantly outweighed by the benefits of therapy. These conditions require precautions in prescribing and administering laser therapy (see Box 5.1).

Active Epiphyses

Epiphyses and open fontanels have been listed as contraindications because these are areas of rapid growth, with rapidly dividing cells. The reasoning has been that if metabolic rate is increased by laser therapy, and osteogenesis is stimulated, then perhaps premature closure or asynchronous bone growth might occur.

Dozens of studies demonstrate that laser light has a stimulatory effect on osteogenesis (Son *et al.*, 2012; Jawad *et al.*, 2013). Yet, confusing data exist about the effect of laser therapy on active epiphyses. Studies have demonstrated different effects, depending on wavelength and different treatment parameters in animals.

Daily application for 21 days of 10 J/cm^2 of 830 nm laser light to the distal epiphysis of rat femurs negatively influenced growth plates and reduced longitudinal length (Oliveira *et al.*, 2012). Application every other day for 20 days of 5 and 15 J/cm^2 of 830 nm laser light induced changes in epiphyseal cartilage, and increased the number of chondrocytes present, but the changes were insufficient to induce changes in bone length (Cressoni *et al.*, 2010). Daily application for 10 days of 4, 8, and 16 J/cm^2 of 670 nm laser light induced no changes in the epiphyseal cartilage or final bone length of rat tibias (de Andrade, 2012).

Common to these studies is multiple applications of laser light over a period of several weeks. What these studies do not suggest is that application of laser therapy over a few days, for acute conditions in the area of active epiphyses, will induce the same negative consequences.

Prudent application of laser therapy, several times over 3–4 days, to an acute epiphysitis would be below the parameters used in the studies mentioned, and is indicated. Prolonged and repeated treatment over multiple weeks is not indicated.

Another consideration is the possible effect that laser therapy will have on an epiphysis if applied in close proximity. Though systemic effects are noted with laser therapy, animal studies indicate that while there is a local biostimulative effect on bone in the area being treated, this effect is not observed distant to the treated area (Batista *et al.*, 2015).

Hemorrhage

It has been clearly demonstrated, using a variety of wavelengths, energy densities, and delivery modes, that laser therapy induces a transient vasodilation (Maegawa *et al.*, 2000; Chung *et al.*, 2012; Larkin *et al.*, 2012). Since any induced vasodilation is unwanted during active hemorrhage, laser therapy should not be applied to tissue that is bleeding.

This precaution does not apply to tissue in which active hemorrhage is no longer present. No data suggest laser therapy will reactivate hemorrhage. Anecdotal reports from veterinary practices using laser therapy during and after invasive procedures, and for treatment of wounds, confirm that hemorrhage is not reactivated once hemostasis has been achieved.

Testicles

Though application of laser therapy to the testes has been listed as a possible contraindication in some sources, treatment in the area of the testes and of scrotal skin should be considered safe. The wavelengths of light used for veterinary laser therapy are not mutagenic.

In vitro studies have demonstrated increased motility in human sperm after irradiation with 830 and 905 nm laser light (Firestone *et al.*, 2012; Salman *et al.*, 2014). In an *in vivo* study using an animal model, a cumulative dose of approximately 28 J/cm^2 of 830 nm laser light over 15 days resulted in increased spermatogenesis, while a cumulative dose of approximately 47 J/cm^2 over the same time had a destructive effect on the seminiferous epithelium (Taha & Valojerdi, 2004). Another animal model study in mice using low energy densities of PBM demonstrated increases in Sertoli and Leydig cell counts, increased sperm counts, and elevated sperm motility compared to a control group (Dadras *et al.*, 2018).

These studies suggest that normally recommended doses of laser therapy light applied to the skin of the scrotum or the tissues around the testicles will, at worst, increase spermatogenesis and sperm motility. They also suggest that excessively high doses should not be applied directly into the testicle.

Thyroid Gland

Early animal studies on the effect of laser irradiation of the thyroid gland demonstrated increased mitotic activity of follicular cells and changes in the thyroid parenchyma (Parrado *et al.*, 1990, 1999). Using 904 nm laser light, these studies delivered cumulative doses of up to 140 J/cm^2 over 10 sessions. Understandably, reports like these suggest that laser therapy application over the thyroid glands should be contraindicated.

Subsequent studies indicated that lower total doses, delivered with fewer applications, result in no histological changes in the thyroid parenchyma. Three daily applications of 780 nm laser light at 4 J/cm^2 produced no morphological alteration in the thyroid glands of mice (Azevedo *et al.*, 2005). This study also demonstrated that irradiation of the thyroid has a stimulatory effect on thyroid hormone levels.

More recent studies suggest that laser therapy can be used for chronic autoimmune thyroiditis in humans, reducing dependence on medication (Höfling, 2010; Höfling *et al.*, 2013). A follow-up study indicated that thyroid function was better in those patients treated with PBM, and advocated for PBM treatment during subclinical and early stages of hypothyroidism, while advising safety practices toward the thyroid whenever surrounding tissues are treated with PBM (Höfling *et al.*, 2018).

An objective analysis indicates that repetitive, high-dose treatment directly over the glands should be avoided. It also indicates that occasional inadvertent exposure of the thyroid glands when treating nearby tissue is not contraindicated.

As more is learned about dosing, frequency of treatment, and effect on the thyroid gland in animal-model studies, it is possible that laser therapy may be indicated for veterinary species that experience reduced thyroid function.

False Contraindications

Conditions once thought to be contraindications for laser therapy that have been clearly disproved are false contraindications (see Box 5.1). Veterinary laser therapists should be able to explain to their patients' owners why these conditions are no longer contraindicated.

Hyperpigmentation and Tattoos

Increased presence of pigments in the form of melanin or tattoo pigment, such as an identification tattoo in a spayed or neutered patient, is not a contraindication for laser therapy. Increased pigments will result in more superficial photon absorption, so when pigments are increased, treatment parameters need to be adjusted accordingly (Anderson & Parrish, 1981).

To ensure proper dosing for deep-tissue conditions, those patients with darker skin and hair coats should be treated with longer wavelengths in the therapeutic spectrum when possible, and the total dose for which their conditions are treated should be increased. When using higher power density in such patients, monitoring the patient's skin temperature with a trailing finger is good practice. If a temperature other than a pleasant, gentle warming is detected, the speed of movement of the handpiece should be increased. Faster movement of the laser beam across the surface of the tissue can help avoid accumulation of unpleasant warmth, even with a laser delivering a higher power-density beam.

Implants

Therapy laser wavelengths do not have a detrimental effect on metal or synthetic implants, suture material, or tissue adhesives used in veterinary medicine. Use in the presence of implants is not contraindicated.

PBM has been demonstrated to improve the health of soft tissue around implants in a number of animal models and in human dental patients (Tang & Arany, 2013; Aoki *et al.*, 2015). Since implant success is dependent on the health of the surrounding soft tissue, laser therapy may actually improve the chances of implant success.

The presence of a reflective metal implant does change the recommended parameters of treatment when the implant is only covered by a thin layer of tissue. Since the implant will reflect photons back into the overlying tissue, any dose delivered to the overlying tissue should be reduced. In most cases, this is accomplished simply by delivering only a small amount of the entire laser treatment directly over the implant.

Microbial Infection

In vitro, some wavelengths of light have been shown to stimulate the growth of cultures of some bacterial species and to inhibit others (Nussbaum *et al.*, 2003). Reliance on this information would indicate that microbial infection is a contraindication for laser therapy. On the contrary, however, other studies indicate that laser therapy, when applied *in vivo*, has a variety of immune-stimulating responses that help overcome microbial infection.

An animal-model investigation into the PBM effects of 1072 nm light on the immune response involved in antibacterial and wound-healing processes (Lee *et al.*, 2011) demonstrated enhancement of cutaneous immune response and higher vascular endothelial growth factor (VEGF) levels associated with more favorable clinical outcomes.

A study involving human patients showed the positive fungicidal effects of 830 nm laser light on oral stomatitis in a clinical setting (Maver-Biscanin *et al.*, 2004). Following laser irradiation at both 685 and 830 nm, statistically significant effects were observed *in vitro* on the turbidimetric growth kinetics of *Candida albicans* cultures and *in vivo* on the survival rate of infected mice (Seyedmousavi *et al.*, 2014).

In an animal-model study to see whether 780 nm laser light would stimulate host immunity in fighting fungal infection, neutrophils from mice that received laser therapy were more active metabolically and had higher fungicidal activity (Burger *et al.*, 2015).

A study to investigate the effects of laser therapy on a rat model of mastitis demonstrated that the number of polymorphonuclear cells in the mammary alveolus and the myeloperoxidase activity (an indicator of mastitis in dairy cattle) were decreased after therapy. The authors suggested that laser therapy might be beneficial in decreasing the somatic cell count and improving milk nutritional quality in cows with an intramammary infection (Wang *et al.*, 2014).

In vivo, PBM produces a complex, immune-enhancing effect that improves response to microbial infection. Laser therapy is indicated for use in microbial infections in veterinary patients.

Photosensitizing Medications

Numerous medications, both topical and systemic, are reported as being photosensitizers. A photosensitivity occurs when a chemical in a medication is photoactivated by light and a cutaneous manifestation arises. It has been suggested that photosensitization might be possible with the wavelengths and treatment parameters used in laser therapy, and thus treatment of both human and veterinary patients on these medications has historically been contraindicated.

In 2014, a review of publications for any report of adverse effects from laser therapy in patients on photosensitizing medication was conducted (Kerstein *et al.*, 2014). Only four publications linked the search term "laser therapy" with multiple terms for photosensitive reactions. No adverse effects were reported.

In the absence of any published evidence that laser therapy-induced photosensitization occurs in veterinary patients, this should be considered a false contraindication.

Conclusion

Used improperly, therapeutic lasers have the potential to be hazardous to the eyes and skin. Many historical contraindications for laser therapy are inconsistent, inaccurate, and outdated. Knowledge from five decades of research and clinical application has rewritten the recommendations against using laser therapy on many conditions and anatomical sites once thought to be contraindicated. Some historical contraindications now require special consideration before treatment can be indicated, others simply require precaution when treating, and still others have been demonstrated to be false. Whatever the application, safety is a critical component in any laser therapy program, and each laser user has the obligation to establish and comply with a laser safety program, as outlined by ANSI and implemented by their facility's LSO. It is essential, even with therapeutic laser devices, that potential beam hazards be recognized and precautions be taken to ensure the use of laser-safe eyewear within the establishment of a controlled laser operational environment, with appropriate signage and security precautions. Direct eye exposure continues to remain an absolute contraindication for all veterinary providers, patients, and owners. Practitioners are encouraged to periodically update their use of laser PBM with current knowledge about contraindications, special considerations, and precautions.

References

Allameh, F. *et al.* (2021). A systematic review of elective laser therapy during pregnancy. *J Lasers Med Sci.* 12:e50. doi:10.34172/jlms.2021.50.

Anderson, R.R. and Parrish, J.A. (1981). The optics of human skin. *J Invest Dermatol.* 77(1):13–19.

ANSI (2011a). *American National Standard for Safe Use of Lasers in Health Care Facilities ANSI Z136.3 - 2011.* American National Standards Institute, Washington, DC.

ANSI (2011b). *American National Standard for Environmental and Facility Safety Signs ANSI Z535.2 - 2011.* American National Standards Institute, Washington, DC.

ANSI (2014). *American National Standard for Safe Use of Lasers ANSI Z136.1 - 2014.* American National Standards Institute, Washington, DC.

Aoki, A. *et al.* (2015). Periodontal and peri-implant wound healing following laser therapy. *Periodontol.* 68(1):217–269.

Avila, R. *et al.* (1999). Structural changes induced by He-Ne laser on the chick embryo ovary. *Rev Fac Cien Med Univ Nac Cordoba.* 50(1):7–10.

Azevedo, L.H. *et al.* (2005). Evaluation of low intensity laser effects on the thyroid gland of male mice. *Photomed Laser Surg.* 23(6):567–570.

Barat, K. (2006a). Warning signs and labels. In: *Laser Safety Management*, p. 58. Taylor & Francis, Boca Raton, FL.

Barat, K. (2006b). Laser safety officer or advisor. In: *Laser Safety Management*, p. 9. Taylor & Francis, Boca Raton, FL.

Barat, K. (2014a). Laser safety – where are we? In: *Laser Safety: Tools and Training*, 2 edn, pp. 1–2. CRC Press, Boca Raton, FL.

Barat, K. (2014b). Laser eyewear. In: *Laser Safety: Tools and Training*, 2 edn, pp. 243–262. CRC Press, Boca Raton, FL.

Bartels, K. (2002). Lasers in veterinary medicine – where have we been, and where are we going? *Vet Clin North Am Small Anim Pract.* 32(3):495–515.

Batista, J.D. *et al.* (2015). Low-level laser therapy on bone repair: is there any effect outside the irradiated field? *Lasers Med Sci.* 30(5):1569–1574.

Bensadoun, R.-J. *et al.* (2020). Safety and efficacy of photobiomodulation therapy in oncology: a systematic review. *Cancer Med.* 9(22):8279–8300.

Burger, E. *et al.* (2015). Low-level laser therapy to the mouse femur enhances the fungicidal response of neutrophils against *Paracoccidioides brasiliensis. PLoS Negl Trop Dis.* 9(2):e0003541.

Censabella, S. *et al.* (2016). Photobiomodulation for the management of radiation dermatitis: the DERMIS trial, a pilot study of MLS® laser therapy in breast cancer patients. *Support Care Cancer.* 24(9):3925–3933.

Chung, H. *et al.* (2012). The nuts and bolts of low-level laser (light) therapy. *Ann Biomed Eng.* 40(2):516–533.

Cialdai, F. *et al.* (2015). In vitro study on the safety of near infrared laser therapy in its potential application as postmastectomy lymphedema treatment. *J Photochem Photobiol B.* 151:285–296.

Cressoni, M.D. *et al.* (2010). Effect of GaAlAs laser irradiation on the epiphyseal cartilage of rats. *Photomed Laser Surg.* 28(4):527–532.

Dadras, S. *et al.* (2018). Photobiomodulation improved stereological parameters and sperm analysis factors in streptozotocin-induced type 1 diabetes mellitus. *J Photochem Photobiol B.* 186:81–87.

Dastanpour, S. *et al.* (2015). The effect of low-level laser therapy on human leukemic cells. *J Lasers Med Sci.* 6(2):74–79.

de Andrade, A.R. (2012). The effects of low-level laser therapy, 670 nm, on epiphyseal growth in rats. *ScientificWorldJournal.* 2012:231723.

Dias Schalch, T. *et al.* (2016). Photomodulation of the osteoclastogenic potential of oral squamous carcinoma cells. *J Biophotonics.* doi:10.1002/jbio.201500292.

FDA. (2007). Laser Products – Conformance with IEC 60825-1 and IEC 60601-2-22 (Laser Notice No. 50). Available from: http://www.fda.gov/MedicalDevices/DeviceRegulationandGuidance/GuidanceDocuments/ucm094361.htm (accessed November 30, 2016).

FDA. (2011). Guidance for industry and FDA staff – Class II special controls guidance document: low level laser system for aesthetic use. Available from: http://www.fda.gov/RegulatoryInformation/Guidances/ucm251260.htm (accessed November 30, 2016).

FDA. (2015a). Federal Laser Product Performance Standard and the Medical Devices Amendment to the Food, Drug, and Cosmetic Act. FDA 21 CFR Part 878. Available from: https://www.accessdata.fda.gov/scripts/cdrh/cfdocs/cfcfr/CFRSearch.cfm?fr=878.4810 (accessed November 30, 2016).

FDA. (2015b). Laser hazard classes. Available from: http://www.accessdata.fda.gov/scripts/cdrh/cfdocs/cfcfr/CFRSearch.cfm?FR=1040.10 (accessed November 30, 2016).

FDA. (2015c). Performance standards for light emitting products. FDA 21 CFR Part 1040. Available from: https://www.accessdata.fda.gov/scripts/cdrh/cfdocs/cfCFR/CFRSearch.cfm?CFRPart=1040 (accessed November 30, 2016).

Firestone, R. *et al.* (2012). The effects of low-level laser light exposure on sperm motion characteristics and DNA damage. *J Androl.* 33(3):469–473.

Fry, T. (2002). Laser safety. *Vet Clin North Am Small Anim Pract.* 32(3):535–547.

Gomes, H. *et al.* (2014). Low-level laser therapy promotes proliferation and invasion of oral squamous cell carcinoma cells. *Lasers Med Sci.* 29(4):1385–1395.

Hecht, J. (2005). *Beam: The Race to Make the Laser*, Chapters 15 and 16, pp. 169–194. Oxford University Press, New York, NY.

Henderson, A.R. (1997). Signs and warning labels. In: *A Guide to Laser Safety*, pp. 26–27. Springer Science and Business Media, Bioptica, Cambridge.

Henderson, A.R. and Schulmeister, K. (2004a). Eye protection. In: *Laser Safety*, pp. 403–419. Taylor & Francis, New York.

Henderson, A.R. and Schulmeister, K. (2004b). The concepts of exposure limits (MPE). In: *Laser Safety*, pp. 74–101. Taylor & Francis, New York.

Höfling, D.B. (2010). Low-level laser therapy in chronic autoimmune thyroiditis: a pilot study. *Lasers Surg Med.* 42(6):589–596.

Höfling, D.B. *et al.* (2013). Low-level laser in the treatment of patients with hypothyroidism induced by chronic autoimmune thyroiditis: a randomized, placebo-controlled clinical trial. *Lasers Med Sci.* 28(3):743–753.

Höfling, D.B. *et al.* (2018). Safety and efficacy of low-level laser therapy in autoimmune thyroiditis: long-term follow-up study. *Int J Endocrinol.* 2018, Article ID 8387530, 9 pages https://doi.org/10.1155/2018/8387530.

Houghton, P. *et al.* (2010). Electrophysical agents – contraindications and precautions: an evidence-based approach to clinical decision making in physical therapy. *Physiother Can.* 62(5):1–80.

Jawad, M.M. *et al.* (2013). Effect of 940 nm low-level laser therapy on osteogenesis in vitro. *J Biomed Opt.* 18(12):12800.

Karu, T. (2010). Mitochondrial mechanisms of photobiomodulation in context of new data about multiple roles of ATP. *Photomed Laser Surg.* 28(2):159–160.

Kerstein, R.L. *et al.* (2014). Laser therapy and photosensitive medication: a review of the evidence. *Lasers Med Sci.* 29(4):1449–1452.

Lanzafame, R.J. (2011). Photobiomodulation and cancer and other musings. *Photomed Laser Surg.* 29(1):3–4.

Larkin, K. *et al.* (2012). Limb blood flow after class 4 laser therapy. *J Athl Train.* 47(2):178–183.

Lee, S.Y. *et al.* (2011). Enhancement of cutaneous immune response to bacterial infection after low-level light therapy with 1072 nm infrared light: a preliminary study. *J Photochem Photobiol B.* 105(3):175–182.

LIA (2000). *LIA Guide for the Selection for Laser Eye Protection*, 5 edn. Laser Institute of America, Orlando, FL.

Liang, W.Z. *et al.* (2015). Selective cytotoxic effects of low-power laser irradiation on human oral cancer cells. *Lasers Surg Med.* 47(9):756–764.

Maegawa, Y. *et al.* (2000). Effects of near-infrared low-level laser irradiation on microcirculation. *Lasers Surg Med.* 27(5):427–437.

Maver-Biscanin, M. *et al.* (2004). Fungicidal effect of diode laser irradiation in patients with denture stomatitis. *Lasers Surg Med.* 35(4):259–262.

Mester, E. *et al.* (1968). The effect of laser beams on the growth of hair in mice. *Radiobiol Radiother.* 9(5):621–626.

Navratil, L. and Kymplova, J. (2002). Contraindications in noninvasive laser therapy: truth and fiction. *J Clin Laser Med Surg.* 20(6):341–343.

Nussbaum, E.L. *et al.* (2003). Effects of low-level laser therapy (LLLT) of 810 nm upon in vitro growth of bacteria: relevance of irradiance and radiant exposure. *J Clin Laser Med Surg.* 21(5):283–290.

OSHA. (2015). Occupational Safety and Health Administration Section III: Chapter 6, Laser Hazards. Available from: https://www.osha.gov/dts/osta/otm/otm_iii/otm_iii_6.html (accessed November 30, 2016).

Oleson, S. (2016). Laser safety officer information. Available from: https://www.lia.org/subscriptions/safety_bulletin/laser_safety_info/#The Laser Safety Officer (accessed November 30, 2016).

Oliveira, S.P. *et al.* (2012). Low-level laser on femoral growth plate in rats. *Acta Cir Bras.* 27(2):117–122.

Ottaviani, G. *et al.* (2013). Effect of class IV laser therapy on chemotherapy-induced oral mucositis: a clinical and experimental study. *Am J Pathol.* 183(6):1747–1757.

Parrado, C. *et al.* (1990). Quantitative study of the morphological changes in the thyroid gland following IR laser radiation. *Lasers Med Sci.* 5(1):77–80.

Parrado, C. *et al.* (1999). A quantitative investigation of microvascular changes in the thyroid gland after infrared (IR) laser radiation. *Histol Histopathol.* 14(4):1067–1071.

Riegel, R. (2008). *Laser Therapy in the Companion Animal Practice*, pp. 39–43. LiteCure, Newark, NJ.

Salman, Y.R. *et al.* (2014). Effect of 830-nm diode laser irradiation on human sperm motility. *Lasers Med Sci.* 29(1):97–104.

Santana-Blank, L. *et al.* (2012a). Solid tumors and photobiomodulation: a novel approach to induce physiologically reparative homeostasis/ – review. *J Solid Tumors.* 2(6):623–635.

Santana-Blank, L. *et al.* (2012b). Concurrence of emerging developments in photobiomodulation and cancer. *Photomed Laser Surg.* 30(11):615–616.

Santana-Blank, L. *et al.* (2016). "Quantum leap" in photobiomodulation therapy ushers in a new generation of light-based treatments for cancer and other complex diseases: perspective and mini-review. *Photomed Laser Surg.* 34(3):93–101.

Seyedmousavi, S. *et al.* (2014). Effects of low-level laser irradiation on the pathogenicity of *Candida albicans*: in vitro and in vivo study. *Photomed Laser Surg.* 32(6):322–329.

Silva, C. (2021). Photobiomodulation therapy combined with radiotherapy in the treatment of triple-negative breast cancer-bearing mice. *J Photochem Photobiol B Biol.* 220:112215.

Sliney, D.H. (1995). Laser safety. *Lasers Surg Med.* 16(3):215–225.

Sliney, D.H. and Freasier, B.C. (1973). Evaluation of optical radiation hazards. *Appl Opt.* 12(1):1–24.

Son, J. *et al.* (2012). Bone healing effects of diode laser (808 nm) on a rat tibial fracture model. *In Vivo.* 26(4):703–709.

Taha, M.F. and Valojerdi, M.R. (2004). Quantitative and qualitative changes of the seminiferous epithelium induced by Ga. Al. As. (830 nm) laser radiation. *Lasers Surg Med.* 34(4):352–359.

Tang, E. and Arany, P. (2013). Photobiomodulation and implants: implications for dentistry. *J Periodontal Implant Sci.* 43(6):262–268.

Tuner, J. and Hode, L. (2010). Contraindications. In: *The New Laser Therapy Handbook*, pp. 473–481. Prima Books, Coeymans Hollow, NY.

Wang, Y. *et al.* (2014). Low-level laser therapy attenuates LPS-induced rats mastitis by inhibiting polymorphonuclear neutrophil adhesion. *J Vet Med Sci.* 76(11):1443–1450.

Wang, Y. *et al.* (2022). The effectiveness and safety of low-level laser therapy on breast cancer-related lymphedema: an overview and update of systematic reviews. *Lasers Med Sci.* 37:1389–1413.

Winburn, D.C. (1990). Laser damage mechanisms. In: *Practical Laser Safety*, 2 edn, p. 16. Marcel Dekker, New York.

Winkler, C.J. (2019). Laser safety in the operating theater. In: *Laser Surgery in Veterinary Medicine*, Chapter 6. (ed. C.J. Winkler), p. 53. Wiley-Blackwell.

Part IV

Clinical Applications of Laser Therapy in Companion Animals

6

Laser Therapy and Pain Management

Michael C. Petty

Dogtor Consulting, Plymouth, Michigan, USA

Introduction

The ability to experience pain is universally shared by not only dogs and cats but all vertebrates and invertebrates. Physiological and behavioral observations show that animals experience the sensory aspect of pain but also the unpleasantness, averseness, and negative emotions attached to that experience, just as humans do. As veterinary health professionals, we have a moral and ethical duty to mitigate suffering from pain to the best of our ability. The use of photobiomodulation therapy (PBMT) can and should be an important part of that responsibility.

Mechanism of Action

PBMT works by administering to tissue a low level of red or near-infrared light. Therapeutically, it works by promoting healing, reducing inflammation and edema, and treating the pain of osteoarthritis (Bjordal, *et al.*, 2003), traumatic and postsurgical damage (Posten *et al.*, 2005), and neurological disorders (Gigo-Benato *et al.*, 2005). There are contradicting trials showing the efficacy (or lack thereof) of PBMT, because these trials are impacted by many factors including wavelength, laser power output, and the number and duration of treatments (Rayegani *et al.*, 2017). However, PBMT has been shown to be effective in treating musculoskeletal disorders as long as proper treatment protocols are adhered to (Clijsen *et al.*, 2017). This underlines the ability of using PBMT as an alternative to medications to control pain (Lutfallah *et al.*, 2023).

Reducing inflammation and edema is an important mechanism in the relief of pain. Inflammation is a physiological response in tissue to injury, whether it is intentional (surgery) or unintentional (trauma) or due to a pathological condition such as infection or osteoarthritis. The responding action is that immune cells (such as macrophages, mast cells, and neutrophils) release mediators and cytokine molecules, which in turn attach to receptors on the nociceptor, causing pain sensitization. Specific anti-inflammatory effects of PBMT have been demonstrated in several different experimental models (e.g., suppression of IL 6 following tendon injury in rats and decreased mRNA expression of kinin receptors and inflammatory cytokines, reduced COX-2 expression in a similar model (Chow, 2018)). In conditions where inflammation is central to the pathophysiology, PBMT can effectively reduce pain, which in some studies is equivalent to anti-inflammatory drugs (Albertini *et al.*, 2004). Edema is a normal response to acute and chronic inflammation. Fluid moves into the interstitial space in response to the above inflammatory mediators. Although there may be an immediate or adaptive response to injury, preventing the full use of an injured area, it becomes maladaptive as it persists, contributing to pain and even causing tissue scarring as fibrin in the interstitial fluid becomes organized. PBMT reduces edema in experimentally induced arthritis (Pallotta *et al.*, 2011) and in carrageenan-induced inflammation in rat paws (Ferreira *et al.*, 2005), and improves macromolecular clearance via lymph nodes (Shimotoyodome *et al.*, 2001).

Tissue repair benefits from PBMT both in acute tissue damage and when there is delayed healing. Much of the research in this area relates to chronic wound healing (Mester *et al.*, 1972). Other conditions where repair is critical to return to normal function, such as tendinopathies, can benefit from PBMT as well; laser therapy stimulates the migration and activation of cells to the injured area (Hemvani *et al.*, 1998), decreases inflammatory cytokine production by neutrophils (Alves *et al.*, 2013), increases the phagocytosis of neutrophils (Chen *et al.*, 2008), improves microvasculature and endothelial cell proliferation (Damante *et al.*, 2009), and increases the production of growth factors and procollagen by fibroblasts (Rico *et al.*, 1996).

Laser Therapy in Veterinary Medicine: Photobiomodulation, Second Edition. Edited by Christopher J. Winkler and Lisa A. Miller.

Decreases in nociceptive signaling can be attributed to inhibitory actions by the laser. Most of the benefits of PBMT occur secondary to laser-induced stimulation, such as that seen in increased time of wound healing. However, there are several mechanisms by which inhibition can decrease nociception. Peripheral nerves that have been damaged undergo negative cytoskeletal changes wherein varicosities are formed along the nerve. Varicosities are identified as multiple swellings or beading occurring at regular intervals along an affected axon. PBMT causes disruption of the cytoskeleton, and blockade of fast axonal flow (Chow *et al.*, 2007). Near-infrared (NIR) light treatment on the skin over the affected nerve can cause cytoskeletal and varicosity changes resulting in a conduction block in the nociceptive nerves to decrease the transmission of pain signals (Holanda *et al.*, 2017; Liebert *et al.*, 2016). The cytoskeletal disruptions reported in these studies only further support a mechanism of light-induced analgesia in which nociceptive transmission is hampered (Cheng *et al.*, 2021). Suppression of bradykinin by PBMT (Chow *et al.*, 2011) is another inhibitory effect that reduces pain. Bradykinin is a pro-inflammatory peptide and is a key element in pain and the associated inflammation. Substance P, another neuropeptide associated with nociception, was inhibited by laser irradiation (Ohno, 1997).

Another inhibitory effect is light-gated channels. One of the best-defined signaling events occurring after light-activation of opsins is the opening of light-gated ion channels such as members of the transient receptor potential (TRP) family of calcium channels (Poletini *et al.*, 2015). TRP channels are now known to be pleiotropic cellular sensors mediating the response to a wide range of external stimuli (heat, cold, pressure, taste, smell), and involved in many different cellular processes (Caterina & Pang 2016). Activation of TRP causes nonselective permeabilization (mainly of the plasma membrane) to calcium, sodium, and magnesium (Montell, 2011). TRP channels such as TRPV1 are responsible for the release of inflammatory mediators. PBMT has been shown to inactivate TRP channels (de Freitas & Hamblin, 2016).

Photobiomodulation as Part of a Multimodal Approach

PBMT should be considered for any animal in pain. It is common to approach pain therapy with a pharmaceutical intervention, then take a wait-and-see approach prior to implementing anything else. PBMT is a great therapeutic to consider adding on to *any* noncancerous pain treatment. For those patients that have cancer, please refer to Chapter 19. Any kind of infection, ear, anal sac, skin, etc. can be added to standard treatments of antibiotics to bring relief to the suffering animal. A dog or cat that has been newly diagnosed with osteoarthritis can receive PBMT when an anti-NGF or NSAID is given, while waiting for those drugs to reach maximum efficacy. Instead of using only analgesics for postoperative or trauma pain, start PBMT right away for an immediate reduction in pain.

Osteoarthritis

Osteoarthritis (OA) is a major cause of debilitation in dogs and cats of any age. In the case of dogs, most cases of osteoarthritis are secondary to confirmational abnormalities, injury, and obesity. Confirmational abnormalities include such risk factors as hip or elbow dysplasia, luxating patellas, and chondrodystrophy to name a few (Anderson *et al.*, 2020). As such, OA that is secondary to confirmational abnormalities is not only unavoidable, but it can also be considered a young dog disease as the mechanisms for its development are in place at birth. OA that is secondary to obesity can certainly be avoided with owner education. OA that is secondary to injury can also be lessened by proper animal husbandry, but is impossible to avoid altogether, especially in the cases of sporting and working dogs. Less is known about the etiology of OA in cats, but in one cross-sectional study it was found that cats of any age have a prevalence of 92% showing radiographic evidence of OA, which increased with the age of the cat (Lascelles *et al.*, 2010). It is felt that OA in cats is often secondary to an underlying cause such as trauma or obesity (Bonecka *et al.*, 2023).

Diagnosis of OA in Dogs

The definitive diagnosis of OA in dogs depends on radiographic evidence. This is most commonly seen as osteophytes, enthesophytes, effusion, soft tissue swelling, subchondral sclerosis, and intra-articular mineralization. It is not always possible to diagnose OA through physical examination. However, findings such as decreased range-of-motion or joint crepitus and swelling can increase the likelihood that OA will be found on radiographs. Additionally, there could be other issues causing pain such as a fracture, osteosarcoma, and bone cysts, that could be ruled out by an x-ray study.

It is important to quantify the pain of OA by providing the caregiver with a validated chronic pain metric, so as to measure the degree of pain both before treatment and as an ongoing evaluation of the treatment's efficacy. The author prefers the Canine Brief Pain Inventory (www.vet.upenn.edu/research/clinical-trials-vcic/our-services/pennchart/cbpi-tool) as it is easy to use and understand. This provides invaluable information to the clinician (is the treatment helpful?) and to the client; often, progress can be slow enough that there might be a question as to whether or not the treatment is helpful at all. Treatment outcome is especially important in the case of dogs, as owners often have an expectation of what the treatment end-point might look like – sometimes these expectations are unreasonable, depending on the severity of the OA. It is best to have a discussion prior to any therapy to ask the caregiver what outcome measure they hope to attain. The clinician may want to see a reasonable outcome such as being able to use stairs, stand up more easily, or jump onto a couch. The owner may be hoping for more such as competitive sports. Having a discussion of expectations while looking at the severity of the OA can prevent future disappointment in the outcome of the treatment.

Diagnosis of OA in Cats

As in dogs, definitive diagnosis of OA depends on radiographic evidence; in cats the radiographic appearance can be markedly different than it is in dogs. Although they can have osteophytes, enthesophytes, effusion, soft tissue swelling, subchondral sclerosis, and intra-articular mineralization, it is also common to see areas of calcification in the vicinity of the joint and not on the joint itself. As in dogs, a radiographic study would help rule out the presence of other causes of pain, such as a fracture.

It is important to quantify the pain of OA in cats just as in dogs above. As of this publication date, the author finds that the Feline Musculoskeletal Pain Index Questionnaire available at North Carolina State University is a very good option for cat owners (cvm.ncsu.edu/research/labs/clinical-sciences/comparative-pain-research).

Pain metrics should not be administered less than a few weeks apart and the caregiver should not be allowed to see the answers to the previous questionnaire, so as not to influence the answers given.

Caregiver videos of cats can be very helpful in diagnosing lameness and assisting in determining which body part is affected. The three best videos to have the caregiver take are (i) walking across a floor both toward and away from the camera, (ii) jumping up and down from a height, such as a chair or windowsill, and (iii) climbing and descending stairs. Depending on the source and severity of lameness, the cat will most likely exhibit an abnormality on at least one, if not all, of the videos. It is often necessary to use software to slow the videos down so as to better observe for any gait abnormality.

General Considerations on the Treatment of Osteoarthritis

As with any type of pain, it is common to have to use some kind of polytherapy in order to adequately control the pain, and photobiomodulation is not any exception. It is not within the scope of this part of the book to discuss other therapies, but it should be noted that photobiomodulation is safe to use with any pain medications. The clinician should look for contributing factors that might worsen the impact of the osteoarthritis (such as obesity, poor diet, and a home environment where the dog may have to use stairs or walk across slippery floors), and consider diet or alterations to improve the outcome of the laser therapy.

Finally, consider the resources the owner has – not only financial, but time (Can the caregiver bring the dog in for regular therapies?), physical (Is the caregiver able to load and unload a large dog into the car to bring it in?), and emotional (Does the caregiver have an overwhelming situation at home, such as taking care of an elderly or disabled family member?). Outlining the treatment, not only with reference cost but also with consideration of these other issues, can precipitate a discussion wherein the clinician and caregiver can modify a treatment plan that works for the caregiver, the patient, and the clinician.

For complete dosing information, please see Chapter 11 on Musculoskeletal Disorders and Osteoarthritis. In general, the target dose is 8–20 J/cm^2.

Treatment of Osteoarthritis

In general, PBMT of any joint must have an adequate application of energy in order to be effective. As a general rule of thumb, the delivery of 10–20 $joules/cm^2$ is adequate, but many devices will provide different dosing, depending on the joint in question. For example, elbow OA responds to higher doses of photobiomodulation therapy than many other joints (Looney *et al.*, 2018). Those lasers that have built-in software for determining treatments are obviously easier and quicker to administer the proper therapy, but the reader needs to research the laser company to be certain that they are updating their software as new treatment protocols are discovered.

It is also important to understand the anatomy of the joint when applying PBMT. For example, both a dorsal (Figure 6.1) and a ventral (Figure 6.2) approach to the coxofemoral joint is necessary to get full coverage. The evidence

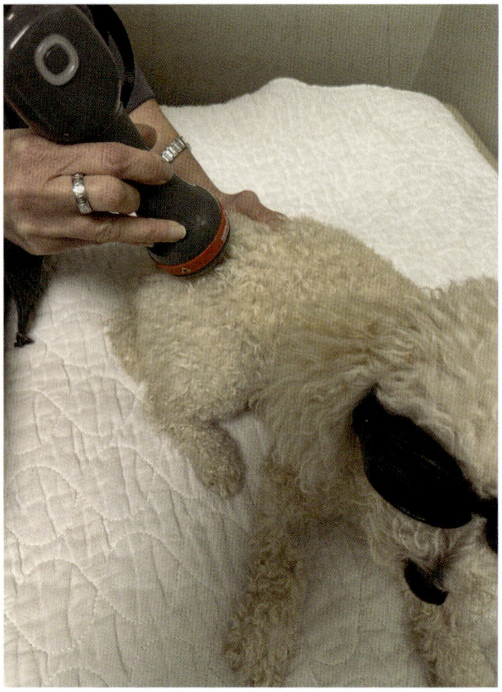

Figure 6.1 Hip OA dorsal approach. It is important to cover not only the region directly over the hip but also the structures (tendons, ligaments, musculature, etc.) immediately around the hip, or any affected joint.

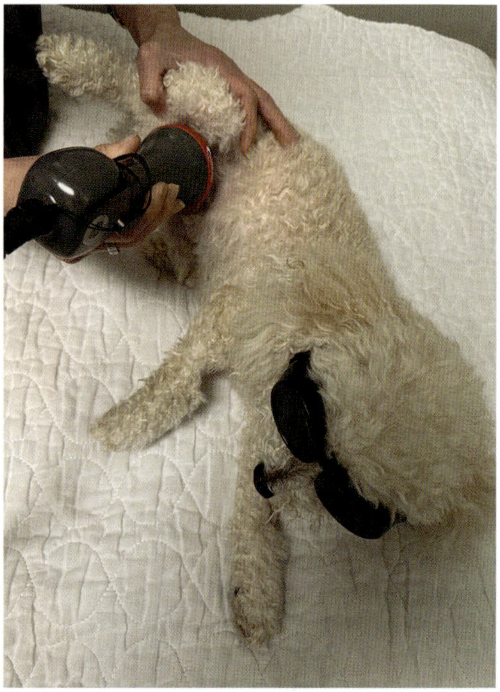

Figure 6.2 Hip OA ventral approach. In order to get complete coverage of the hip (and other joints) it is important to access all sides of the joint with the laser beam.

is strong: one study (Alves *et al.*, 2022) comparing a PBMT-treated group to a control group receiving meloxicam for three weeks showed that there was an improvement in pain scores and range-of-motion in the PBMT group that was both faster and superior to the NSAID group. The laser therapy group also had a reduction in pain that lasted longer than the NSAID group after the discontinuation of therapy.

Neuropathic Pain

Neuropathic pain in people is often reported as diffuse burning, or pricking pain, sometimes as feelings of electric shock, or even a wet feeling. Neuropathic pain, a self-reporting issue in people, must have other issues ruled out in order to be considered the definitive diagnosis (Widerstrom-Noga *et al.*, 2017). In most cases of dogs and cats, the diagnosis of neuropathic pain is at best an educated guess. There are exceptions, such as a dog with intervertebral disc disease (IVDD) that is also exhibiting lameness in a leg. This is often radicular or neuropathic pain secondary to the spinal cord damage. We can also assume that dogs with any nervous system injury will probably develop neuropathic pain during recovery. It is often thought that dogs with longstanding osteoarthritis may develop neuropathic pain as well. There is a reason for this: Nerve growth factor concentrates in areas of osteoarthritis, and a sequelae of this is that it encourages neurogenic sprouting of a-delta (pain) fibers and recruitment of a-beta (touch) fibers as pain fibers. The end result is neurogenic inflammation, which can be a factor in the development of neuropathic pain.

PBMT has been used to successfully treat neuropathic pain. However, the basis for the beneficial outcomes may vary, depending on the level of irradiance and fluence used. Studies indicate that treatment with an irradiance of 270 mW/cm^2 or higher at the level of the nerve can rapidly block pain transmission. In rat models with nerve injury surgery, decreased sensitivity to cold and pin prick was found within 1 hour of PBMT and lasted for 5 days. This same study suggested that a combination therapy could be used to treat neuropathic pain: initial high irradiance/fluence rates for fast pain relief followed by low irradiance/fluence rates for prolonged pain relief by altering chronic inflammation (Holanda *et al.*, 2017).

Intervertebral Disc Disease

Classically, the treatment of IVDD has been through surgical intervention by various methods. With the advent of physical modalities (including PBMT, acupuncture, and rehabilitation), noninvasive options for treating IVDD have gained acceptance. The evidence for using PBMT as either a sole therapy or as part of a polytherapy regimen has shown that this is an alternative to surgery. One human study comparing PBMT to lidocaine injections showed that laser irradiation caused an immediate decrease in low back pain similar to pain reduction following a lidocaine injection (Holanda *et al.*, 2016). Another review looking at 16 randomized controlled trials found that in acute neck pain there was a 95% improvement when compared to placebo (Chow and Johnson, 2009).

Myofascial Pain

Myofascial pain syndrome (MPS) is likely one of the most common comorbidities in animals with musculoskeletal pain, but it is a poorly understood and largely unknown problem in veterinary medicine. MPS is a chronic pain condition originating from a localized area within a muscle, muscle group, or fascia. The pathophysiology of MPS is not fully understood; an energy crisis of a muscle band is one of the most accepted theories, based on overuse by repetitive or prolonged activity causing overload and consequent muscle hypoxia. It is beyond the scope of this writing to discuss the etiology of trigger points, but there are several excellent sources for the reader to pursue (Gerwijn *et al.*, 2004; Petty, 2018).

When a cat or dog has OA, a traumatic injury, or is recovering from musculoskeletal surgery, the propensity to avoid use of the affected limb can lead to an abnormal prolonged use of the muscles of that limb by carrying it or not bearing full weight on it. Other limbs in the body are affected as weight is shifted from the painful limbs to the less- or nonpainful limbs. An example is when a dog has a cruciate injury. As the dog avoids putting weight on that leg, it will use various muscles such as the iliopsoas muscle to draw the leg up and lessen pain in the knee. Another example is a dog with hip OA. Where a dog may normally carry about 60% of its weight on the front legs, this percentage increases in the OA dog, putting additional stress on the front legs, especially the triceps and infraspinatus muscles. This weight shift can also affect other muscles, such as the epaxial muscles of the back.

Myofascial pain should be considered in animals with any pain issue, but especially those animals with appendicular pain. MPS is most often diagnosed by palpation of one of the affected taut bands (Wall, 2014). Failure to recognize and treat MPS in a patient in pain could mean the difference between a successful outcome and a disappointing outcome. There are several methods of treating MPS, including dry-needling (Gattie *et al.*, 2017), extracorporeal shockwave (Ji *et al.*, 2012), local heating (Petrofsky *et al.*, 2020), ischemic compression (Hains *et al.*, 2010), and PBMT (Ahmed *et al.*, 2020).

PBMT has been shown to be an effective method for treatment of MPS (Ahmed *et al.*, 2020; Kiraly *et* al., 2018; Lee *et al.*, 2013; Sobral *et al.*, 2021) in human medicine. However, there is a lack of well-done studies in veterinary medicine. As the mechanistic basis is the same across all animals, it is the author's conclusion that PBMT is a reliable method for treating MPS in dogs and cats. The suggested dose is 8–20 J/cm^2.

Postsurgical Pain

Most studies of photobiomodulation therapy have looked at reduction of chronic pain such as from OA, and subacute pain such as IVDD. However, PBMT can also be used in the immediate postoperative period for treatment of incisional pain. Although it can help reduce pain postoperatively, it should be part of a multimodal analgesic regimen, not used as a sole source of analgesia. One study looked at the use of PBMT to treat the sternal incision following coronary artery bypass surgery in people and found that PBMT was very effective in reducing the pain score after both the first and second treatment. No people in the study required a third dose (Karlekar *et al.*, 2015). Considering the noninvasive and effective nature of PBMT on surgical wounds, it should be considered for postoperative treatment in all surgical patients, with the exception of those patients that received Nocita (bupivacaine liposome injectable suspension) because of the unknown effect of laser on the bupivacaine-containing liposomes. Consider delivering a dose of 4–6 J/cm^2.

Other Pain Conditions

Although not researched for this book, it is common to consider the use of PBMT for other conditions that cause pain. Otitis externa (Figure 6.3), anal sacculitis (Figure 6.4), stomatitis, and acute moist dermatitis should be treated with doses of 4–6 J/cm^2. Urinary cystitis and Pandora syndrome should be treated as deep tissue at 8–20 J/cm^2.

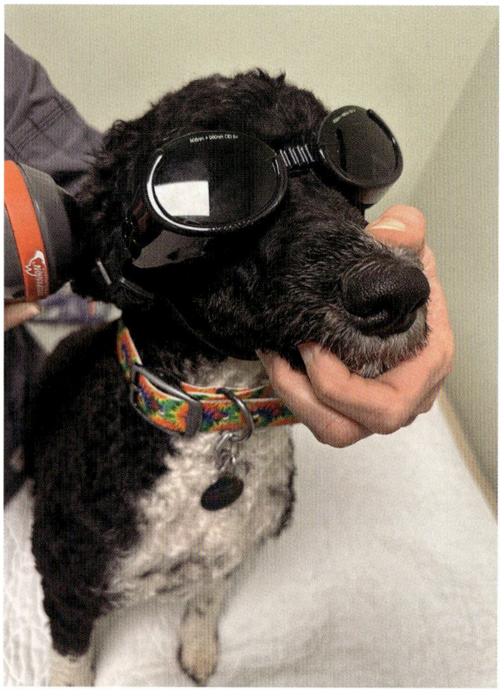

Figure 6.3 PBMT and otitis. Many dogs will not tolerate ear cleaning and instillation of medication. Not only does PBMT help with the pain and inflammation of otitis, but it also allows the owner to more readily treat the infection at home as it is then easier to handle the ear and put in prescribed medications.

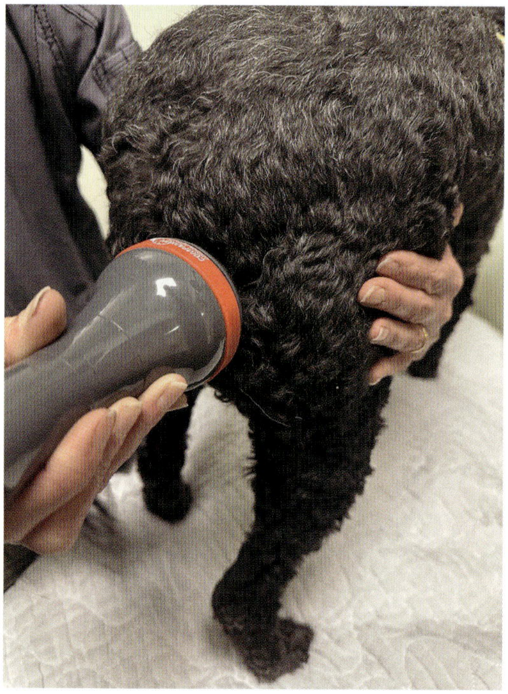

Figure 6.4 PBMT and anal sacculitis. The pain and inflammation of anal sacculitis is readily treated by PBMT – in this case, using an offset head to avoid direct contact with the area.

References

Ahmed, H. *et al.* (2020). High intensity laser therapy on pain in patients with myofascial trigger points. *Egypt J Phys Ther.* 3:1–8.

Albertini, R. *et al.* (2004). Effects of diferent protocol doses of low power gallium-aluminum-arsenate laser radiation on carrageenan induced rat Paw oedema. *J Photochem and Photobiol B Biol.* 27:101–107.

Alves, S.C. *et al.* (2013). Effect of low-level laser therapy on the expression of inflammatory mediators and on neutrophils and macrophages in acute joint inflammation. *Arthritis Res Ther.* 15:R116.

Alves, J. *et al.* (2022). A randomized double-blinded controlled trial on the effects of photobiomodulation therapy in dogs with osteoarthritis. *AJVR.* 83(8):1–8.

Anderson, K.L. *et al.* (2020). Risk factors for canine osteoarthritis and its predisposing arhtropathies: a systematic review. *Front Vet Sci.* 7:200.

Bjordal, J.M. *et al.* (2003). A systematic review of low level laser therapy with location-specific doses for pain from chronic joint disorders. *Austral J Physiother.* 49 (2):107–116.

Bonecka, J. *et al.* (2023). Knee joint osteoarthritis in overweight cats: the clinical and radiographic findings. *Animals.* 13(15):2427.

Caterina, M.J. and Pang, Z. (2016). TRP channels in skin biology and pathophysiology. *Pharmaceuticals.* 9:77.

Chen, C.H. *et al.* (2008). Low-energy laser irradiation increases endothelial cell proliferations, migration and eNOS gene expression possibly via P13k signal pathway. *Lasers Surg Med.* 40:46–54.

Cheng, K. *et al.* (2021). Mechanisms and pathways of pain photobiomodulation: a narrative review. *J Pain.* 22(7):771.

Chow, R. *et al.* (2011). Inhibitory effects of laser irradiation on peripheral mammalian nerves and relevance to analgesic effects: a systematic review. *Photomed Laser Surg.* 10(10):1–17.

Chow, R. (2018). LLLT Treatment of Pain: Clinical applications. *Low-level light Ther: Photobiomodul.* 17:258.

Chow, R. *et al.* (2007). 830-nm laser irradiation induces varicosity formation, reduces mitochondrial membrane potential and blocks fast axonal flow in small and medium diameter rat dorsal rood ganglion neurons; implications for the analgesic effects of 830-nm laser. *J Peripher Nerv Syst.* 12:28–39.

Chow, R. and Johnson, M. (2009). Efficacy of low-level laser therapy int he management of neck pain; a systematic review and meta-analysis of randomised placebo or active-treatment controlled trials. *Lancet.* 374:1897–1908.

Clijsen, R. *et al.* (2017). Effects oaf low-level laser therapy on pain in patients with musculoskeletal disorders: a systematic review and meta-analysis. *Eur J Phys Rehabil Med.* 53(4):603–610.

Damante, C.A. *et al.* (2009). Effect of laser phototherapy on the release of fibroblast growth factors by human gingival fibroblasts. *Lasers Med Sci.* 24:885–891.

de Freitas, L.F. and Hamblin, M.R. (2016). Proposed Mechanisms of Photobiomodulation or Low-Level Light Therapy. *IEEE J Sel Top Quantum Electron.* 22(3).

Ferreira *et al.* (2005). Analgesic effect of He-Ne Low-level laser therapy on acute inflammation pain. *Photomed Laser Surg.* 23:117–181.

Gattie, E. *et al.* (2017). The effectiveness of trigger point dry needling for musculoskeletal conditions by physical therapists: a systematic review and meta-analysis. *J Orthopaedic & Sports Phys Ther.* 47:133–149.

Gerwijn, R.D. *et al.* (2004). An expansion of Simons' integrated hypothesis of trigger point formation. *Curr Pain Headache Rep.* 8:468–475.

Gigo-Benato, D. *et al.* (2005). Phototherapy for enhancing peripheral nerve repair: a review of the literature. *Muscle & Nerve: Official Journal of the American association of electrodiagnostic Medicine.* 31(6):694–701.

Hains, G. *et al.* (2010). Chronic shoulder pain of myofascial origin: a randomized clinical trial using ischemic compression therapy. *J Manipul Physiol Ther.* 33:362–369.

Hemvani, N. *et al.* (1998). Effect of helium-neon laser on cultured human macrophages. *Laser Ther.* 10:159–164.

Holanda, V. *et al.* (2016). *Photobiomodulation of the Dorsal Root Ganglion for the Treatment of Low Back Pain: A Pilot Study.* Wiley Online Library. doi:10.1002/lsm.2252.

Holanda, V.M. *et al.* (2017). The mechanistic basis for photobiomodulation therapy of neuropathic pain by near infrared laser light. *Lasers Surg Med.* 49:516–524.

Ji, H. *et al.* (2012). Extracorporeal shock wave therapy in myofascial pain sydrome of upper trapezius. *Annals of Rehabil Med.* 36:675–680.

Karlekar, A. *et al.* (2015). Assessment and feasibility and efficacy of Class IV laser therapy for postoperative pain relief in off-pump coronary artery bypass surgery patients: a pilot study. *Ann Card/Anaesth.* 18(3):317.322.

Kiraly, M. *et al.* (2018). Comparative study of shockwave therapy and low-level laser therapy effects in patients with myofascial pain syndrome of the trapezius. *Rheumatol Internat.* 38:2045–2052.

Lascelles, B.D. *et al.* (2010). Cross-sectional study of the prevalence of radiographic degenerative joint disease in domesticated cats. *Vet Surg.* 39(5):535–544.

Lee, E. *et al.* (2013). A pilot study to determine the efficacy of therapeutic class IV laser treatment on local muscle spasm associated with myofascial pain syndrome in patients with neck pain. In: *Proceedings 2013 AAPM Annual Meeting.* AAPM, Fort Lauderdale, FL (April 11–14, 2013).

Liebert, A. *et al.* (2016). Neuroprotective effects against POCD by photobiomodulation: evidence from assembly/disassembly of the cytoskeleton. *J Exp Neurosci.* 10:1–19.

Looney, A. *et al.* (2018). A randomized blind placebo-controlled trial investigating the effecgts of photobiomodulation therapy on canine elbow osteoarthritis. *Can Vet J.* 59:959–966.

Lutfallah, S. *et al.* (2023). Low-level laser therapy for acute pain: a comprehensive review. *Curr Pain and Different Rep.* 27:607–613.

Montell, C. (2011). The history of TRP channels, a commentary and reflection. *Pflugers Arch.* 461:499–506.

Mester, E. *et al.* (1972). Stimulation of wound healing by laser rays. *Acta Chirugica Academiae Scientiarum Hugari.* 13:315–324.

Ohno, T. (1997). Pain suppressive effect of low power laser irradiation: a quantitative analysis of substance P in the rat spinal dorsal root ganglion. *J Nippon Med Sch.* 64:395–400.

Pallotta, R.C. *et al.* (2011). Infrared low-level laser therapy on rat experimental knee inflammation. *Lasers Med. Sci. Laser Surg.* 27:71–78.

Petrofsky, J. *et al.* (2020). Local heating of trigger points reduces neck and plantar fascia pain. *J Back Musculoskelet Rehabil.* 33:21–28.

Petty, M. (2018). Unbundling myofascial pain syndrome in your veterinary patients. DVM 360. July 9. https://www.dvm360.com/view/unbundling-myofascial-pain-syndrome-your-veterinary-patients.

Poletini, M.O. *et al.* (2015). TRP Channels: a missing bond in the entrainment mechanism of peripheral clocks throughout evolution. *Temperature.* 2:522–534.

Posten, W. *et al.* (2005). Low-level laser therapy for wound healing: mechanism and efficacy. *Dermatol Surg.* 31 (3):334–340.

Rayegani, S.M. *et al.* (2017). Safety and effectiveness of lowe-level laser therapy in patients with knee osteoarthritis: a systematic review and meta-analysis. *J Lasers Med Sci.* 8(Supp 1):S12.

Rico, A.F. *et al.* (1996). Beta endorphin response in the blood and cerebrospinal fluid after single and multiple irradiation with HeNe and GaAs low-power laser. *J Clin Laser Med Surg*. 12:1–6.

Shimotoyodome, S. *et al*. (2001). Improvement of macromolecular clearance via lymph flow in hamster gingiva by low-power carbon dioxide laser-irradiation. *Lasers Surg Med*. 29:442–447.

Sobral, A.P. *et al*. (2021). Photobiomodulation and myofascial temporomandibular disorder: systemic review and meta-analysis flowed by cost-effectiveness analysis. *J Clin Exp Dent*. 13:e724–e732.

Wall, R. (2014). Introduction to myofascial trigger points in dogs. *Topics in Comp Ani Med*. 191(29):43–48.

Widerstrom-Noga, E. *et al*. (2017). AAPT Diagnostic criteria for central neuropathic pain. *J Pain*. 18:1417–1426.

7

Intra- and Postoperative Laser Therapy

Christopher J. Winkler

Suffolk Veterinary Group Animal Wellness and Laser Surgery Center, Selden, NY, USA

1st Edition Contributors:

Steven Buijs[1] and John C. Godbold, Jr.[2]

[1] *Dierenhospitaal Visdonk, Roosendaal, Netherlands*
[2] *Stonehaven Veterinary Consulting, Jackson, TN, USA*

Introduction

This chapter describes the incorporation of photobiomodulation with surgical procedures, performed at Dierenhospitaal Visdonk, in Roosendaal, the Netherlands, and elsewhere. During the postoperative phase, it is expected to encounter predictable, minor surgical complications such as edema, pain, inflammation, time required for return of function, and occasional wound problems. The addition of laser therapy does not significantly increase the overall time required for surgeries (as most laser therapy sessions are only minutes in duration) and significantly decreases complications. The use of laser therapy and photobiomodulation (PBM) in conjunction with surgery has been previously reported for both human and veterinary patients (Draper *et al.*, 2012; Karlekar *et al.*, 2015; Nesioonpour *et al.*, 2014). The therapeutic use of PBM, which is aimed at alleviating pain and inflammation, modulating immune responses, and promoting wound healing and tissue regeneration, continues to be reviewed (Arany 2016; Pryor and Millis 2015).

Treating surgery patients with laser therapy offers the opportunity to observe those patients while they are hospitalized, witness their improvement, and appreciate how laser PBM is helping to assist them with their recovery. Laser therapy leads to increased comfort in patients and to more satisfied owners, who often readily accept the technology.

Overview

Surgical interventions are selected to give expected outcomes for patients. For example, treatment of a ruptured cruciate ligament involves selecting a procedure that will stabilize the stifle joint and provide a return of function of the stifle, involving tissue handling, which results in unwanted responses from the body. The more invasive the procedure, the more tissue is disrupted and the greater the response that follows. These responses cause most of the unwanted side effects of surgery. Inflammation will occur, swelling will develop, changes in vasculature are unavoidable, and suture materials will cause enzymatic processes that will absorb the materials. All these processes result in pain, inflammation, and discomfort, and affect the speed of healing. Goals for successful perioperative and postoperative integration of photobiomodulation are to minimize undesirable responses of the body, increase those desirable, increase patient comfort, and decrease healing time.

The first patients treated perioperatively with photobiomodulation at Dierenhospitaal Visdonk were dogs with cruciate ligament ruptures. Our surgical procedure for these patients before that point was usually tibial tuberosity advancement (TTA), by KYON (n.d. c). Due to swelling and inflammation at the surgical site, the development of edema in the distal part of the hind limb was often seen, occurring in all patients within 2 days following surgery

Laser Therapy in Veterinary Medicine: Photobiomodulation, Second Edition. Edited by Christopher J. Winkler and Lisa A. Miller.

and causing discomfort and delaying use of the leg. The swelling can sometimes be massive and require additional treatment, including diuretic medication, massage, and pressure bandaging. Use of a therapeutic laser commenced immediately after these surgeries 3 years prior to the publication of this text's first edition, and it was observed that in the majority of these patients there was hardly any edema formation, and that most patients returned to weight-bearing use of the affected hind limb within 2 days.

Treating these patients with photobiomodulation therapy every other day for the first 10 days significantly improved the speed of their return to function. Monitoring and comparing their pain scores verified that laser-treated patients are more comfortable than expected. It was also observed that these patients show less interest in the wound, with fewer cases of wound complications occurring due to licking. We recognized that an important part of patients assuming more rapid weight bearing and return to function was better management of pain and postoperative complications with the application of laser therapy. Our observations of reduced pain in postoperative patients following laser therapy mirror what has been reported in bench-top studies and in animal-model and human studies (Bjordal *et al.*, 2006; Enwemeka *et al.*, 2004; Fulop *et al.*, 2010; Hawkins and Abrahamse 2006; Sprouse-Blum *et al.*, 2010).

We have now started using laser therapy intraoperatively during ruptured cranial cruciate stabilization, as well as postoperatively. Photobiomodulation can be applied effectively without touching the tissue during surgery, maintaining asepsis. Laser therapy is now applied to closed arthrotomy wounds, before closure of the subcutis and skin. This technique is more efficient, since the laser light is delivered directly to the surgical site, without any absorption of photons by chromophores within the skin.

Because of the success experienced with this group of patients, the perioperative use of laser therapy was expanded to all of our surgical procedures (Table 7.1).

Table 7.1 Examples of procedures in which intraoperative or postoperative treatment is indicated.

Procedure	Intraoperative laser therapy	Postoperative laser therapy
Amputation (leg, tail, claws, etc.)		×
Arythenoid lateralization	×	×
Arthroscopy		×
Arthrotomy	×	×
Aural hematoma (othematoma)		×
Brachycephalic obstructive syndrome	×	×
Caudectomy		×
Coeliotomy (laparotomy)		×
Corrective osteotomy (TTA, TPLO, TPO, etc.)	×	×
Cystotomy	×	×
Dorsal hemilaminectomy	×	×
Enterectomy	×	×
Enterotomy	×	×
Enucleation of the eye		×
Episioplasty		×
Femoral head excision	×	×
Gastric dilation and volvulus	×	×
Gastrotomy	×	×
Laparoscopy		×
Orchiectomy		×
Osteosynthesis (fracture stabilization)	×	×
Ovario(hyster)ectomy		×
Promotion of secondary healing	×	×
Thoracoscopy		×
Thoracotomy	×	×
Total ear canal ablation	×	×
Total hip prosthesis	×	×
Urethrostomy (perineal or scrotal)	×	×
Ventral slot	×	×

Intraoperative Laser Therapy

There are multiple advantages of the intraoperative use of a therapeutic laser, the most obvious being that laser light can be delivered much earlier in the healing process. A 2015 study of human dental patients reported the effectiveness of immediate versus delayed photobiomodulation therapy (PBMT) in reducing the severity of postoperative inflammation (Abdel-Alim *et al.*, 2015). When applying laser therapy almost immediately after tissue trauma, PBMT will result in a decrease in the release of cytokines and a reduction in inflammatory cell activity. Healing will be stimulated very quickly. The therapy laser beam can be pinpointed to localized areas we want to treat, such as an arthrotomy wound, or an enterotomy or cystotomy wound. Since this technique allows treatment directly on the deeper tissues, photon absorption by more superficial tissues are avoided.

During surgery, the surgical staff must take care not to interfere with the aseptic environment and technique.

Laser therapy can easily be delivered intraoperatively without touching the tissue. When treating intraoperatively, the tissues being targeted are in clear sight and do not require a deep-tissue dose and technique; contact with the tissue is not necessary. To maintain asepsis, the laser therapist must be a well-trained member of the surgery team. There must be good coordination between the therapist and the surgeon so there is no unwanted touching of tissue with the laser handpiece.

Before surgery, the handpiece and cable should be thoroughly cleaned to avoid particles or dust falling into the surgical field. The laser therapist should wear sterile surgical gloves for the same purpose. The therapist must make sure that both handpiece and cable remain clear of the surgical field and do not touch any part of the patient (Figure 7.1).

The surgeon should present the organ or surgical wound to the therapist, manipulating it to expose the target tissues to the laser light so a maximal exposure can be achieved. Whenever the surgeon is going to move the patient or tissue, this should be communicated so that the therapist can avoid accidental touching. When treating intraoperatively and the target tissue can be visualized, the laser settings should deliver a dose of 3–4 J/cm^2. The tissue being targeted is often sensitive and traumatized, so it is recommended not to exceed a power of 4 W. Since the tissue areas being treated are relatively small, and the dose being delivered is relatively low, using a lower power setting does not increase the treatment time significantly.

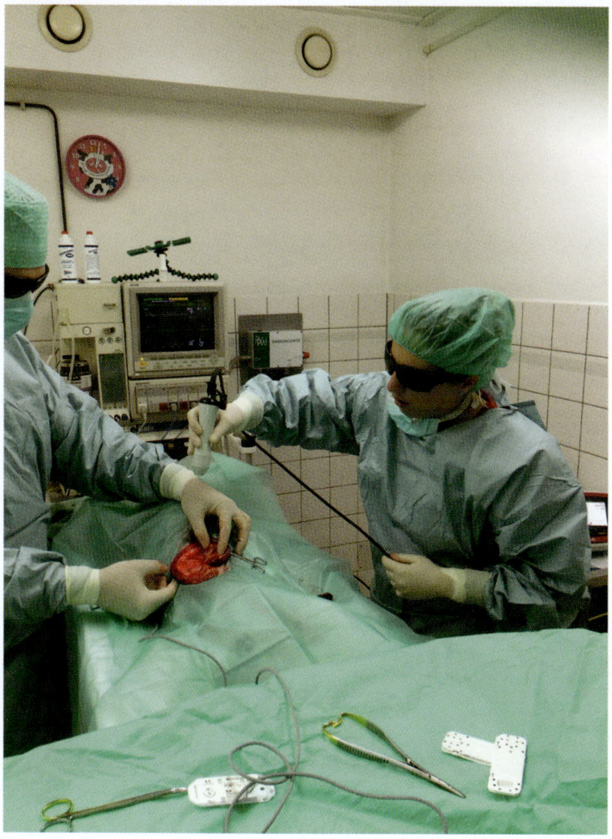

Figure 7.1 Intraoperative application of a therapy laser, maintaining aseptic technique.

Postoperative Laser Therapy

It is ideal to treat the wound and the surrounding tissues with the therapy laser immediately following closure of the surgical wound without interfering with sterility. A member of the surgical team should treat the wound(s) and tissues as soon as surgery has finished. The tissue can be touched with the laser handpiece, using a contact delivery. Since we are treating the skin, subcutis, and deeper tissues in this application, the laser settings should deliver 8–10 J/cm^2. A well-trained laser therapist will apply a gentle pressure with the handpiece and will treat from all directions to facilitate photon permeation of the tissue. When treating a wound where the skin and more superficial tissues have been affected, such as a coeliotomy wound, the treatment area should include the immediate wound area, including the skin, subcutis, and underlying musculature, as well as a margin of normal tissue around the wound. Following procedures resulting in a greater degree of tissue damage and disruption, a larger area should be treated. For example, following a stifle surgery, the tissue being treated should include the surgical wound, the entire stifle, the musculature associated with the stifle, and the vasculature caudal to the stifle.

It is recommended that patients be scheduled to return to the hospital daily or every other day to repeat laser therapy following invasive procedures. The main goals are to reduce pain, reduce edema by improving blood flow and reducing swelling, reduce inflammation, promote healing, and promote quicker return of function. When patients have reached a point of expected healing and return to function, laser therapy can be discontinued. The effects of PBMT on wound healing are outlined in Chapter 10 and are well-established in current publications (Avci *et al.*, 2013; Hawkins and Abrahamse, 2006; Medrado *et al.*, 2003; Silveira *et al.*, 2007). Other studies and literature reviews verify the effective pain-reduction mechanisms of PBMT (Chow *et al.*, 2007, 2011; Fulop *et al.*, 2010).

Clinical Examples of Intra- and Postoperative Laser Therapy Application

The following procedures are examples of how laser therapy can be used intra- and postoperatively to effectively impact overall patient care.

Rhytidectomy

Excessive facial folds are common in breeds such as the Chow Chow and Basenji, and they contribute to significant and even debilitating periocular dermatitis, entropion, and corneal lesions. Conditions such as stenotic nares can coincide and contribute to patient distress. Several clinical examples of treatment combining rhytidectomy with photobiomodulation have been reported (Knollinger *et al.*, 2023; Winkler, 2018). Removal of facial fold tissue should be sufficient to improve facial and eyelid contours so as to minimize tissue removal required for entropion correction. This author endorses a fluence of 8–30 J/cm^2 over rhytidectomy sites due to the (usually considerable) skin thickness and increased pigmentation in the treatment area. Postsurgical laser therapy doses for entropion are typically much less (4–7 J/cm^2); the administering therapist should take great care protecting the eyes from direct exposure during entropion site treatment.

Ruptured Cruciate Ligament

The majority of canine patients with a ruptured cranial cruciate ligament seen at Dierenhospitaal Visdonk are treated with a correctional osteotomy to neutralize the forces associated with the ligament dysfunction. The goals with this type of surgery are to regain comfortable function as soon as possible and to have a very low complication rate. Laser therapy is a very useful adjunct to surgery in accomplishing these goals. Neither surgery nor laser therapy can replace the other, but when used together properly, they can enhance the outcome.

The first step in surgery is an arthrotomy or arthroscopy to confirm the diagnosis, examine for possible meniscal injury, remove the remnants of the ruptured cruciate ligament, and, if a meniscal tear is present, remove the loose border or body of the meniscus. In addition to confirming the diagnosis, the purpose of this part of the surgery is to reduce the inflammatory response of the body. If remnants of the cruciate ligament are left in the joint, the body will attempt to absorb them. The accompanying joint inflammation will be an onset for the development of osteoarthritis and an increased effusion of synovial fluid, which will distend the joint capsule and cause more discomfort and pain. After inspection of the joint, removal of cruciate ligament remnants, and possible meniscectomy, the joint capsule is closed in two layers, incorporating the patellofemoral ligament if it was severed with an open approach.

Due to the tissue damage when opening the joint, the handling of instruments in the joint, and suture placements in the joint capsule, significant tissue disruption is induced, which will induce an inflammatory response in return. The inflammatory response can be tempered with laser therapy. In 2014, a study demonstrated that laser therapy, using an 808 nm laser and doses of 10 and 50 J/cm^2 prevented features related to the articular degenerative process, such as increased release of inflammatory mediators, in the knees of rats after anterior cruciate ligament transection (Bublitz *et al.*, 2014).

After closure of the joint capsule, the laser therapist will take up the prepared laser handpiece and focus the laser beam using a noncontact delivery on the joint only, with emphasis on the surgical wound (Figure 7.2).

A correct laser therapy dose is delivered by estimating the surface area to be treated and setting the laser to deliver 3–4 J/cm^2. It is recommended to not exceed a laser power setting of 4 W to minimize any potential heating of the tissues. The time required for laser therapy treatment of this area is no more than 1–2 minutes. The benefits of administering laser therapy at this point are that PBMT can be started as soon as possible in order to reduce inflammation, and that the target tissues can be exactly located without any intervening skin.

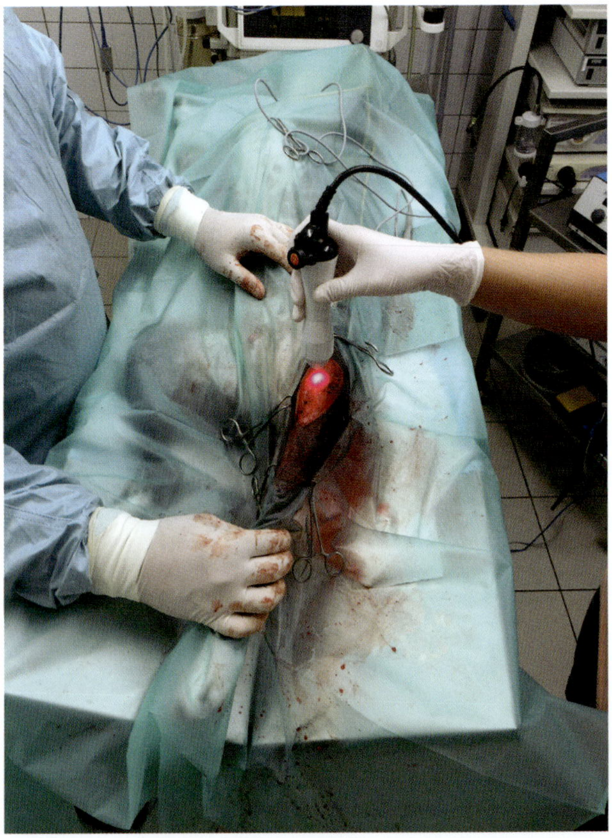

Figure 7.2 Intraoperative photobiomodulation therapy during a stifle surgery, following closure of an arthrotomy wound, maintaining aseptic technique.

The laser therapist may then change gloves and rejoin the surgery aseptically if needed to continue with the procedure. The medial side of the proximal tibia is approached to perform a tibial plateau leveling osteotomy (TPLO) (KYON, n.d. b), TTA, or other correctional technique. At Dierenhospitaal Visdonk, we have performed mostly TTA (KYON, n.d. c), but more recently we have added TTA-2 (KYON, n.d. c) to our possibilities for treating this condition.

In performing these surgeries, tissue damage can be extensive. All techniques involve performing an osteotomy, cutting through soft tissues on the medial side of the tibia before cutting the bone itself. The osteotomy is either circular with a TPLO, or curved with a TTA. Securing the implants requires bone screws (except in TTA-2). Drilling screw holes and placing screws inflicts further tissue damage. Closing and restoring the medial soft tissue is important in order to fully cover the implants and provide added support in reducing cranial thrust of the tibia. Due to the extensive damage to these tissues during surgery, swelling of the entire stifle area is expected. The swelling puts pressure on the saphenous vein, reducing venous return, and promotes accumulation of fluid and edema in the distal area of the limb.

To help reduce postoperative swelling and edema after medial closure of the subcutis and skin, laser therapy is administered again. Since this is a postoperative application, maintaining asepsis is no longer required. Gentle delivery in contact with the tissue is recommended, with a fluence of 3–4 J/cm^2 to the superficial soft tissues. To address all the affected superficial soft tissue, the laser therapist should treat the entire stifle area from all directions. Treatment should extend distal and medial to the stifle to include all soft tissues over the osteotomy site.

To facilitate continued applications of laser therapy, it is recommended not to apply a bandage after surgery. When required, the surgical site can be protected with wound-protection sleeves or an Elizabethan collar. Patients are scheduled for their next postoperative laser therapy treatment 24 hours after surgery.

Patients treated with laser therapy intra- and postoperatively at Dierenhospitaal Visdonk in this manner are observed to be weight bearing, either at release the day of surgery or within 24 hours. A moderate amount of edema at the distal tibia and hock region is occasionally observed. When this occurs, laser therapy is administered using contact delivery and gentle massage, starting in the stifle area to enhance venous return. Gentle handpiece massage is accompanied by the therapist massaging the hock and distal tibia with the other hand. Halfway through the treatment, the therapist will move to the distal part of the leg and treat over the edematous area. During the treatment, the edema will visibly reduce, and rapid pain reduction results in an immediate improvement in weight bearing (Figure 7.3).

It is recommended the postoperative patient return for laser therapy every other day for the first 10 days. At each return visit, the stifle, proximal tibia, and the associated soft tissues are treated with contact delivery, gentle massage, movement of the stifle through passive range of motion, and laser settings delivering 8–10 J/cm^2. Beginning at the second visit, edema is not normally seen in the distal parts of the limb. Laser therapy treatments may be discontinued 10 days postoperatively if the pet is responding

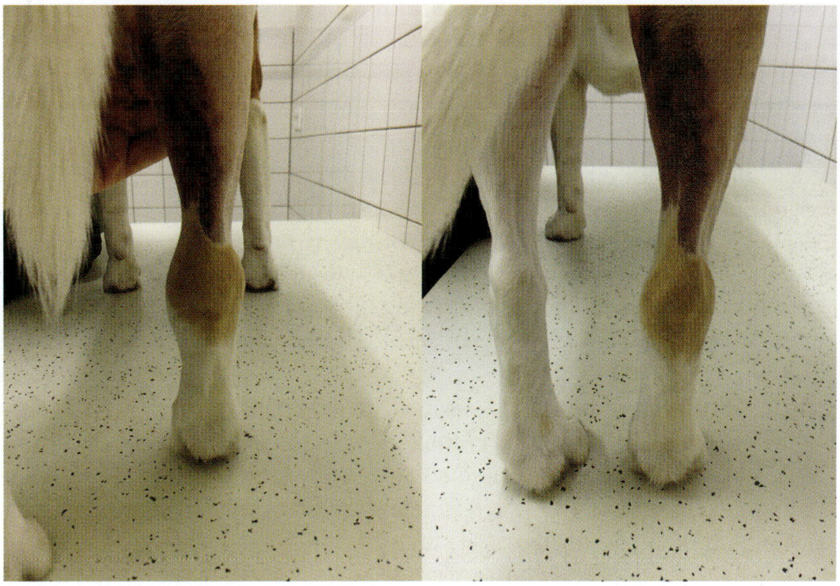

Figure 7.3 Left: Marked swelling of the hock 2 days after TTA, with patient placement of the leg more cranially to avoid weight bearing. Right: Reduced edema and normal weight bearing immediately after laser therapy treatment.

satisfactorily, or continued twice-weekly until better function is noted.

Using this combination of surgery and intense laser therapy treatment, canine cranial cruciate ligament rupture patients can have a 99% chance of having a successful outcome, without any minor or major complications, and a much quicker return to full function.

Medial-Compartment Disease in the Elbow Joint

At Dierenhospitaal Visdonk, medial-compartment disease in the elbow joint is treated with arthroscopy. This developmental condition most often affects the medial coronoid process of young to middle-aged patients and is a result of an overload of pressure on the medial aspect of the elbow joint. In many cases, it will be the result of a limb malalignment that develops during bone growth. Symptoms such as joint distention, osteoarthritis, and reduced range of motion of the elbow joint may recur if treatment is focused only on the intra-articular fragment without addressing the underlying cause, Two different approaches are required to properly manage these patients: arthroscopy alone or limb-realignment osteotomy to correct the predisposing cause of the condition.

Arthroscopy is very useful in verifying the diagnosis and can be helpful in providing treatment at the same time. It allows visual inspection of the joint, an evaluation of the degree of inflammation, and visualization of collateral damage caused by the fragment in kissing lesions on the medial humeral condyle. In an affected joint, the medial coronoid process may have a fissure, a nondisplaced fragment, a displaced fragment, or worn cartilage in complete medial-compartment disease.

Whenever applicable, loose fragments should be removed during arthroscopy to minimize iatrogenic damage to the joint and surrounding soft tissue. If successful, the only wounds will be 3–4 mm arthroscopy puncture wounds, which can be closed with a simple suture. Immediately after the arthroscopy, a laser therapy treatment is administrated to the elbow joint using a contact delivery and fluence of 8–10 J/cm^2. The laser therapist will treat the joint from all directions and through a full passive range of motion. This first postoperative treatment helps reduce the pain and inflammation caused by the arthroscopy, and begins to address any chronic arthritic caused by the condition.

In order to reduce joint inflammation, reduce pain, improve function, and promote healing of the cartilage defects, it is recommended to continue laser therapy every other day (Assis *et al.*, 2016). The treatment protocol is the same as that used immediately after surgery, delivering a deep-tissue target dose of 8–10 J/cm^2.

For most patients, a limb-correction alignment surgery is recommended following arthroscopy. Conservative management can be implemented to slow degenerative joint disease and improve function should owners decline this option.

After an induction phase of five or six every-other-day laser therapy treatments following the arthroscopy, a transition phase of treatments is then commenced, tapering the frequency by treating twice a week for 2 weeks and then once a week for 2 weeks. Long-term maintenance-phase treatments are prescribed every 2–4 weeks and continued lifelong. In these conservatively managed patients, progressive degenerative joint disease is expected; however, with continued laser therapy, the progression occurs at a slower pace (Wang *et al.*, 2014).

When patients require limb alignment correction and the owners accept the recommendation, a proximal abducting ulnotomy (PAUL) (KYON, n.d. a) surgery is scheduled 1–2 weeks after the arthroscopy. Laser therapy is continued between the arthroscopy and the alignment correction. and continued as part of overall patient management as with other osteosynthesis.

Osteosynthesis

Every patient that is subject to a fracture is confronted with hematoma, edema, pain, and dysfunction. The majority of patients will be treated with some form of osteosynthesis, in order to repair the damage to the bones (and the soft tissue, if necessary). In addition to its important effects on soft tissue, PBMT plays an important role in activating osteogenic factors, stimulating osteoblastic cells, and accelerating bone healing (Barbosa *et al.*, 2014; Chang *et al.*, 2014; Ebrahimi *et al.*, 2012; Jawad *et al.*, 2013; Mota *et al.*, 2013; Son *et al.*, 2012; Tim *et al.*, 2014). There is thus a definite indication to treat these patients with a therapeutic laser, before and after surgery.

The way laser therapy is used in managing fractures is the same whether in treatment of traumatic fractures or in elective surgeries such as corrective osteotomies. Examples of elective, corrective osteotomies are distal femoral osteotomy, proximal tibial osteotomy, PAUL, and proximal sliding ulnotomy.

Patients with traumatic fractures are presented with an instability, accompanied by a hematoma, profuse swelling, and even skin wounds. If fracture fixation is delayed by the presence of other injuries and the need to stabilize the patient, the surgeon is often confronted with massive soft-tissue swelling. To help prevent and control swelling before surgery, the application of a splint or bandaging is recommended. Laser therapy is administered before bandage or splint application and during each change of the bandage or splint. Laser therapy cannot be administered through bandage or splint material as even very thin layers of bandage material will produce massive scattering of the coherent laser beam and significant reduction of the percentage of photons reaching the target tissue. Repeat laser therapy as often as twice a day if possible until surgery for osteosynthesis is performed. A combination of bandaging, support, and laser therapy will result in a markedly decreased amount of swelling and edema, and improved visualization for the surgeon during surgery.

After osteosynthesis, regardless of the indication or location, laser therapy is commenced immediately after closure of the wounds with a contact delivery and fluence of 8–10 J/cm^2. This deep-tissue target dose is appropriate for treating both the osteosynthesis sites and the more superficially damaged soft tissue. During this treatment, the laser is applied to the fracture site, circumferentially around the fractured bone, moving from proximal to distal. This laser therapy treatment will help reduce swelling and pain, and at the same time promote soft-tissue healing and ostoegenesis.

Laser therapy will then be repeated every day for the first 3–5 days, then every other day until 10–14 days after surgery. Depending on the functional result, the degree of swelling, and the progression of wound healing, laser therapy can be discontinued at that time or be continued with weekly treatments for as long as needed. If a patient has any risk of a delayed healing, as for example with a fracture of the proximal ulna, laser therapy is continued twice weekly until the fracture is stable.

Femoral Head Excision

Femoral head excision is primarily indicated in cats with trauma to the acetabulum, femoral head, or femoral neck. In dogs, excision is most often required in toy breeds with similar trauma or with hereditary diseases of the femoral head, such as avascular femoral head necrosis. After femoral head excision, patients are dependent on the development of a neoarthrosis to regain a fully functional hind limb with a normal range of motion. Managing postoperative pain in these patients is critical, since they should begin using their leg as soon as possible after surgery to facilitate a return to function. If the surgical area is painful, the patient will be reluctant to use the leg, leading to a lengthening of functional healing time.

Laser therapy should commence in the surgical theater immediately after the femoral head excision is completed and the surgical wound has been closed using a contact delivery with laser settings that deliver a deep-tissue target dose of 8–10 J/cm^2. Direct the laser beam toward the acetabulum, circling around the major trochanter, and into the surgical site from the medial aspect of the proximal femur. Move the femur through passive range of motion, through flexion and extension, as the treatment is delivered.

Continue daily laser therapy until weight bearing is comfortable for the patient. Use the same laser settings and delivery as used immediately after the surgery. At Dierenhospitaal Visdonk, we see much better and quicker results when we incorporate laser therapy in the rehabilitation of femoral head excision patients compared to similar patients in which laser therapy is not used. A return to full function is expected in 2–3 weeks after surgery when incorporating laser therapy. Laser therapy is continued twice a week for 6 weeks after surgery to facilitate healing and increased formation of connective tissue between the acetabulum and proximal femur.

Coeliotomy (Laparotomy)

Laser therapy is indicated for every abdominal surgery that does not involve a malignancy. At Dierenhospitaal Visdonk, it was noted after applying laser therapy to the abdominal wall and surgical wounds following coeliotomy that the reduction in pain and swelling resulted in patients showing less interest in, and engaging in less licking of and biting at, their wounds. The application of laser therapy after an abdominal surgery is quick, easy, and efficacious (Figure 7.4). Use either a contact or a noncontact delivery with a fluence of 3–4 J/cm^2.

Regardless of the reason for the laparotomy single laser therapy application is prescribed for a normal approach into the abdomen through healthy tissue. If conditions within the abdomen warrant continued treatment (such as when enteritis, cystitis, or peritonitis are present), laser therapy is applied immediately after surgery and then continued daily or twice-daily until the intra-abdominal condition has resolved, using a contact delivery and a fluence of 8–10 J/cm^2.

Enterotomy and Enterectomy

The most common indication for enterotomy or enterectomy (intestinal resection and anastomosis) is a foreign object too large to pass through the lumen of the small intestine with normal peristaltic movements. If the foreign object can't move, the damage to the intestinal wall may be minor, or it may result in significant pressure necrosis, vascular impairment, and perforation. Similar vascular compromise, necrosis, and perforation are also seen with intussusception.

If vascular supply has not been compromised, a foreign object can be removed with an enterotomy. If there is doubt about the vascular integrity, or if tissue changes show the

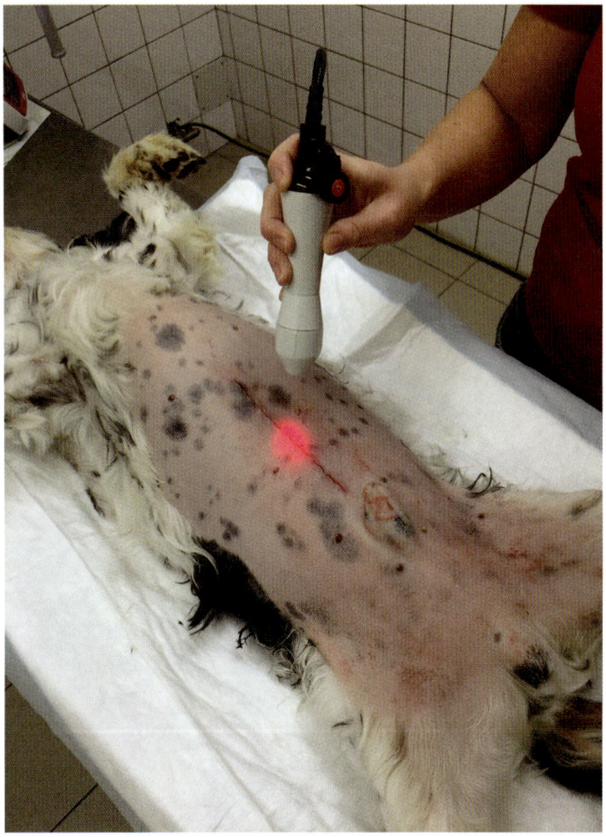

Figure 7.4 Laser therapy treatment of a coeliotomy incision immediately after closure.

vascular supply is compromised, an enterectomy is indicated. Regardless of the procedure, laser therapy is indicated immediately after closure of the small intestines with suturing or stapling. The sterile- gloved laser therapist will take the cleaned, prepared laser handpiece, their hands becoming nonsterile at this point. The size of the intestinal tract area to be treated will be estimated and the laser will be set to deliver a dose of 3–4 J/cm^2. It is helpful for the surgeon to "present" and move the intestines during treatment to maximize photon penetration from as many different directions as possible while maintaining and insuring sterility (Figure 7.5). Communication between the surgeon and the laser therapist is important in order that unpredictable movements and inadvertent contamination of the tissue do not occur. In this application, it is not unusual to be able to actually visualize the effect of PBMT on the tissues. Visible improvement in tissue color and motility can frequently be seen within a few minutes as tissue perfusion improves. Laser therapy has been demonstrated to cause potent dilation in rat mesenteric arterioles *in vivo*, which leads to a marked increase in the arteriolar blood flow (Maegawa *et al.*, 2000). If ischemia and reperfusion injury are present, laser therapy will reduce their impact on distant organs (Kirkby *et al.*, 2012).

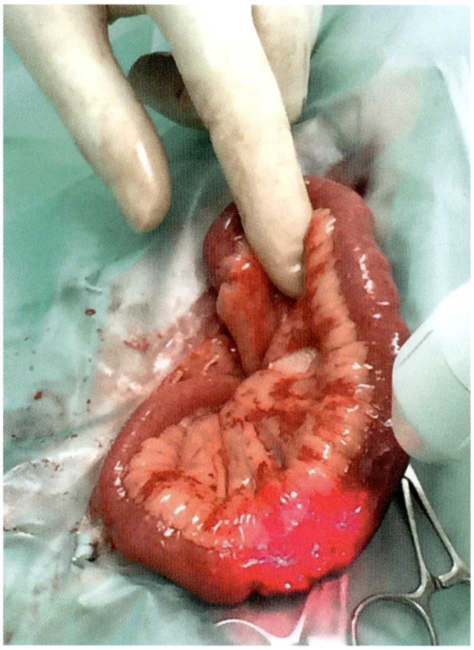

Figure 7.5 Intraoperative treatment of an enterotomy wound. The surgeon is presenting the jejunum, and the laser therapist is aiming the handpiece, making sure to maintain aseptic technique.

After direct laser therapy of the intestinal wound, closure of the coeliotomy is performed in the routine manner. As previously described for coeliotomies, the abdominal incision and abdominal wall are also treated with laser therapy, with a fluence of 3–4 J/cm^2. If the surgery encounters focal or generalized peritonitis, laser therapy treatment through the body wall is repeated after 24 hours, using a contact delivery and with the laser set to deliver 8–10 J/cm^2. Daily treatments should be continued until the problem is resolved.

At Dierenhospitaal Visdonk, with the addition of laser therapy in this described manner, improved patient comfort has been observed following gastrointestinal surgery, with reduced healing time and reduced frequency of leakage and dehiscence of enterotomy and enterectomy wounds.

Cystotomy

Cystotomy is most often performed to remove bladder stones, polyps, or masses from the urinary bladder – false-positive results of urine antigen tests for tumors such as transitional cell carcinoma make confirmation via biopsy of bladder tissue even more valuable diagnostically while avoiding percutaneous tumor seeding (Winkler, 2017).

The technique of administering laser therapy intraoperatively, directly to the target tissue, can be very beneficial in cystotomy patients, reducing or eliminating postoperative hematuria and patient discomfort while urinating.

Cystotomy surgical wounds should be treated immediately after their closure, prior to returning the bladder to the abdomen. As with other intraoperative applications, a cleaned, prepared handpiece is used by a laser therapist wearing sterile gloves. The surface area of the bladder to be treated is estimated and the laser is set to deliver 3–4 J/cm^2. As seen in intestinal tissue during the treatment of enterotomy and enterectomy surgery sites, the bladder wall and serosa show immediate response to therapy laser treatment, with improved perfusion. Closure of the abdominal wall is performed routinely, and the incisional area is treated immediately after surgery as previously described.

Since virtually all cystotomy patients have some degree of cystitis, laser therapy is administered to the bladder through the abdominal wall daily for 3–5 days following surgery. A contact delivery is used to deliver a fluence of 8–10 J/cm^2. Since the bladder is in a predictable position in the caudal abdomen, treatment can be delivered from the ventral and both lateral directions. Cystotomy patients appear to be more comfortable when laser therapy is added to their management, and many display a return to normal frequency of urination within 24 hours.

Urethrostomy

Though the combination of medical and dietary management can reduce the incidence of urinary calculi, male cats continue to be susceptible to blockage of the distal urethra, and male dogs can have calculi lodge in the distal urethra caudal to the bone of the penis (baculum).

In both cats and dogs, the success rate of displacing the urethral blockage or calculi with retrograde flushing will be higher if laser therapy is administered before passing a catheter. Using a contact delivery and a laser setting that delivers 6–8 J/m^2, the suspected location of the obstruction and the surrounding tissue are treated to decrease edema and swelling, and to help relax muscle spasms in the urethra. In most cases, subsequent passage of a urinary catheter and retrograde flushing of urethral contents will then be easier.

If it is impossible to dislodge the obstruction, surgery is required. If frequent recurrence of a blockage occurs, surgery to reroute the urethra is indicated. The mucosal lining of the urethra is sensitive tissue and develops inflammation rapidly. Performing a urethrotomy to remove calculi or a urethrostomy to reroute the urine passage requires delicate handling of tissue. In addition to preexisting and intraoperative tissue damage, the urethral mucosa will be damaged during the suturing process. The responses to tissue damage and the presence of sutures will be pain, swelling, and inflammation, all of which can cause urinary straining and patient self-trauma.

Important to this procedure is the delicate handling of the urethral mucosa to minimize trauma. In both perennial urethrostomy in the cat and scrotal urethrostomy in the dog, the diameter of the stoma is of great importance. Prevention of licking of the urethral surgical wounds is critical to a successful result. Laser therapy is indicated to reduce swelling, inflammation, and pain immediately after creating the stoma and placing sutures. For this treatment, a noncontact delivery is recommended, with laser settings that deliver 3–4 J/cm^2. Laser therapy is repeated daily for 5–10 days. Laser therapy markedly decreases swelling at the stoma, and patients are observed to be more comfortable and less tempted to lick the site.

Thoracotomy

Because of the invasiveness of thoracotomies, and the level of patient discomfort postoperatively, laser therapy can play an important role in a patient's return to function following surgery. Whether the approach is intercostal or sternal, there is a lot of postoperative pain. Respirations produce more motion of the cut tissues and increased pain compared to other surgeries. Use of the therapy laser intra- and postoperatively is an important adjunct to other pain-management modalities.

At Dierenhospitaal Visdonk, the most common reasons for performing thoracotomies are lung lobe removal, pericardiectomy, vascular ring anomaly, persistent ductus arteriosus (duct of Botalli), thymoma removal, and biopsy. All these thoracotomy patients will benefit from laser therapy. After closure of the ribs or sternum, and after reestablishing negative pressure in the thorax, laser therapy is administered prior to skin closure. Using noncontact delivery, and maintaining aseptic technique as in other intraoperative applications, the laser therapy treatment is delivered to the closed entrance to the thorax. The size of the area is estimated before delivering a dose of 3–4 J/cm^2. Following this treatment, the overlying muscle, subcutis, and skin are closed routinely. When all the soft tissues have been closed, the incision is treated using a contact delivery with laser settings delivering a dose of 3–4 J/cm^2. Laser therapy is repeated every day for 3–5 days. The result of incorporating laser therapy for these patients is much less postoperative discomfort and less frequent seroma formation.

Stimulation of Secondary Healing

When trauma or surgical intervention results in a large area of skin loss, laser therapy is certainly indicated (Peplow *et al.*, 2010; Skopin and Molitor, 2009; Takashi, 1988).

Addressing the wound surgically is the first step, to remove all devitalized tissue, clean the remaining tissue as well as possible, and begin to prevent movement of loose skin by suturing it to underlying tissues. Regardless of whether open healing by second intention or support and healing of skin grafts is the goal, laser therapy will contribute to faster healing (Calisto *et al.*, 2015; Hodjati *et al.*, 2014; Hopkins *et al.*, 2004; Kovacs, 2015; Kuffler, 2016).

An excellent example is a Belgian shepherd that presented with a large area of necrosis, which was caused by a wound inflicted by a cat. There was a small, extremely painful area of necrosis visible through the fur 5 days after the incident. Under full anesthesia, the area was clipped and a much larger area of involvement became visible (Figure 7.6a). This kind of wound is not a candidate for closure or grafting,

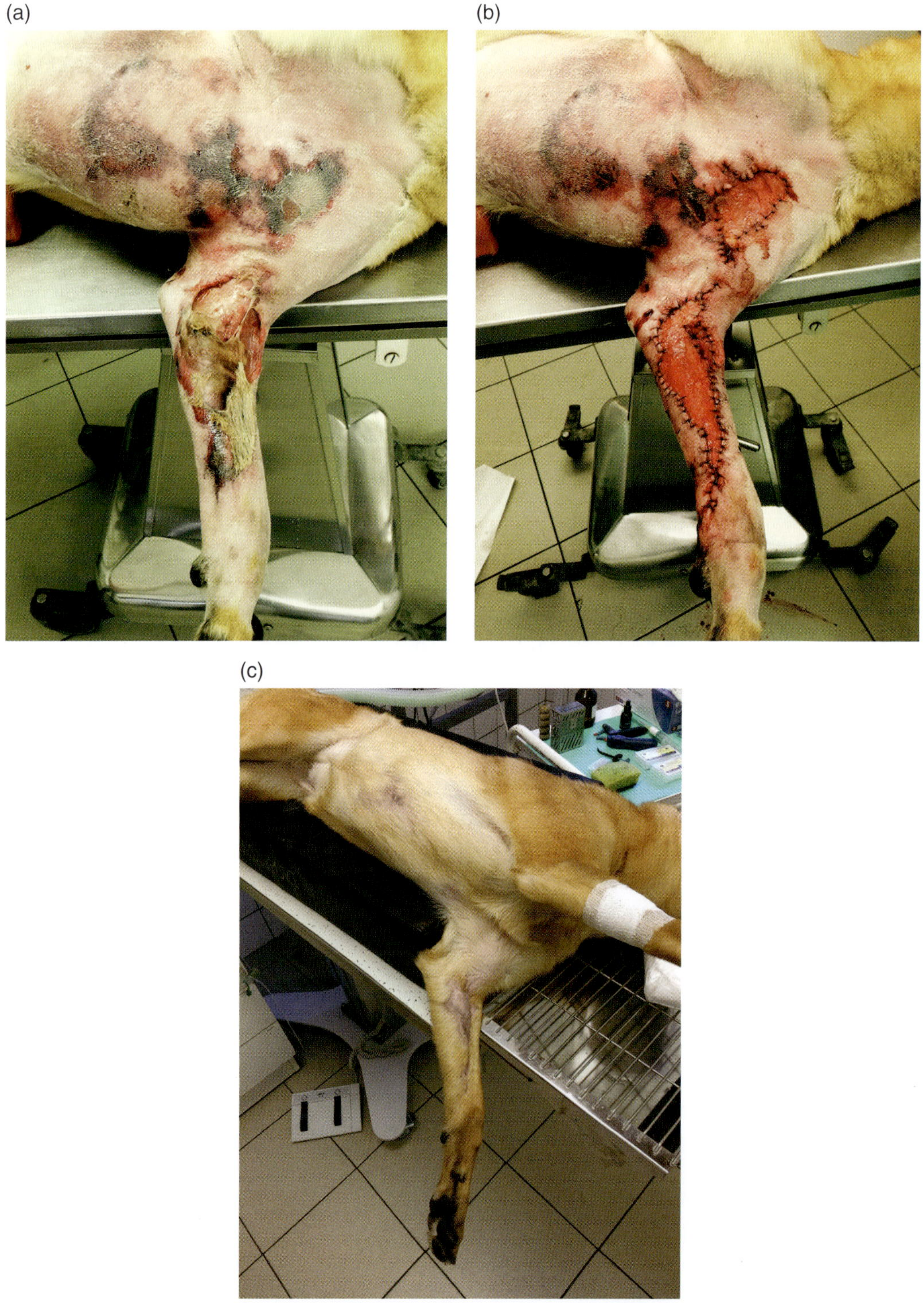

Figure 7.6 (a) Necrotic wound at initial presentation. (b) Necrotic wound after cleaning and suturing at the starting point of secondary healing. (c) Necrotic wound 45 days after starting laser therapy treatment. Note the complete healing, hair regrowth, and relatively small scars.

and needs to be treated, at least initially, in a conservatively manner to encourage granulation formation.

Necrotic tissue was debrided and the wound cleaned with sterile physiologic fluids. Simple interrupted sutures were placed to fix the skin edge to the underlying tissue. Suturing is necessary to limit the exposed area and prevent movement of skin in relation to the underlying tissue, as movement will delay healing (Figure 7.6b).

Applying bandages or dressings was impossible with this particular patient. It removed any dressing within hours after placement, and preventing it from licking the wound was very difficult. After 5 days, it was decided to leave the wounds open and uncovered, without any bandage or dressing, and began laser therapy treatment with a laser setting delivering 3–4 J/cm^2 to the affected area via a noncontact delivery. Immediately after the first treatment, the patient showed decreased interest in the wounds. The wound was treated with laser therapy twice a day for the first week, then every day for the next week. After the initial 2 weeks of laser therapy, the wounds were fully granulated and an epithelial margin was noted around all wound edges.

Since the patient was not showing interest in the wound, we decided to continue conservative treatment and wait for secondary healing. At this point, surgery was considered again to use skin grafts to cover the wounds, but the owner saw the rapid closure of the wounds and elected to continue with secondary healing.

The frequency of laser therapy treatments was tapered down to every other day until complete healing was noted 45 days after starting the laser therapy treatments (Figure 7.6c).

Measurements of the rate of wound healing indicated a closure rate of approximately 1.4 mm/day, which is significantly faster than expected without laser therapy. In this case, in addition to an accelerated rate of healing, laser therapy provided the important benefit of creating noninterest in the wound for the dog. Scar formation was observed to be very limited; the scars that did form were flexible and did not limit motion of the foreleg.

Conclusion

The procedures described in this chapter are examples of how laser therapy and PBM can be used as a valuable adjunct to other modalities in generating better surgical outcomes. By adopting the laser therapy application techniques described here, administering appropriate laser therapy doses, and prescribing an appropriate schedule of treatments intra- and postoperatively, laser therapy can be made a successful part of virtually all veterinary surgeries.

References

Abdel-Alim, H.M. *et al.* (2015). A comparative study of the effectiveness of immediate versus delayed photobiomodulation therapy in reducing the severity of postoperative inflammatory complications. *Photomed Laser Surg.* 33(9):447–451.

Arany, P.R. (2016). Craniofacial wound healing with photobiomodulation therapy: new insights and current challenges. *J Dent Res.* 95(9):977–984.

Assis, L. *et al.* (2016). Aerobic exercise training and low-level laser therapy modulate inflammatory response and degenerative process in an experimental model of knee osteoarthriti in rats. *Osteoarthritis Cartilage.* 24(1): 169–177.

Avci, P. *et al.* (2013). Low-level laser (light) therapy (LLLT) in skin: stimulating, healing, restoring. *Semin Cutan Med Surg.* 32(1):41–52.

Barbosa, D. *et al.* (2014). Laser therapy in bone repair in rats: analysis of bone optical density. *Acta Ortop Bras.* 22(2):71–74.

Bjordal, J.M. *et al.* (2006). Low-level laser therapy in acute pain: a systematic review of mechanisms of action and clinical effects in randomized placebo-controlled trials. *Photomed Laser Surg.* 24(2):158–168.

Bublitz, C. *et al.* (2014). Low-level laser therapy prevents degenerative morphological changes in an experimental model of anterior cruciate ligament transection in rats. *Lasers Med Sci.* 29(5):1669–1678.

Calisto, F.C. *et al.* (2015). Use of low-power laser to assist the healing of traumatic wounds. *Acta Cir Bras.* 30(3):204–208.

Chang, W. *et al.* (2014). Therapeutic outcomes of low-level laser therapy for closed bone fracture in the human wrist and hand. *Photomed Laser Surg.* 32(4):212–218.

Chow, R.T. *et al.* (2007). 830 nm laser irradiation induces varicosity formation, reduces mitochondrial membrane potential and blocks fast axonal flow in small and medium diameter rat dorsal root ganglion neurons: implications for the analgesic effects of 830 nm laser. *J Peripher Nerv Syst.* 12(1):28–39.

Chow, R. *et al.* (2011). Inhibitory effects of laser irradiation on peripheral mammalian nerves and relevance to analgesic effects: a systematic review. *Photomed Laser Surg.* 29(6):365–381.

Draper, W. *et al.* (2012). Laser therapy reduces time to ambulation in dogs after hemilaminectomy. *J Small Anim Pract.* 53(8):465–469.

Ebrahimi, T. *et al.* (2012). The influence of low-intensity laser therapy on bone healing. *J Dent (Tehran).* 9(4):238–248.

Enwemeka, C.S. *et al.* (2004). The efficacy of low-power lasers in tissue repair and pain control: a meta-analysis study. *Photomed Laser Surg.* 22(4):323–329.

Fulop, A. *et al.* (2010). A meta-analysis of the efficacy of laser phototherapy on pain relief. *Clin J Pain.* 26(8):729–736.

Hawkins, D. and Abrahamse, H. (2006). The role of laser fluence in cell viability, proliferation, and membrane integrity of wounded human skin fibroblasts. *Lasers Surg Med.* 38(1):74–83.

Hodjati, H. *et al.* (2014). Low-level laser therapy: an experimental design for wound management: a case-controlled study in rabbit model. *J Cutan Aesthet Surg.* 7(1):14–17.

Hopkins, T.J. *et al.* (2004). Low-level laser therapy facilitates superficial wound healing in humans: a triple-blind, sham-controlled study. *J Ath Train.* 39(3):223–229.

Jawad, M.M. *et al.* (2013). Effect of 940 nm low-level laser therapy on osteogenesis in vitro. *J Biomed Opt.* 18(12):128001.

Karlekar, A. *et al.* (2015). Assessment of feasibility and efficacy of class IV laser therapy for postoperative pain relief in off-pump coronary artery bypass surgery patients: a pilot study. *Ann Card Anaesth.* 18(3):317–322.

Kirkby, K. *et al.* (2012). The effects of low-level laser therapy in a rat model of intestinal ischemia-reperfusion injury. *Lasers Surg Med.* 44(7):580–587.

Knollinger, A. *et al.* (2023). Treatment of canine periocular dermatitis with rhytidectomy (surgical face lift) and fluorescence photobiomodulation: a case report. *Vet Derm.* 34(5):478–482.

Kovacs, K. (2015). Low level laser therapy of serious wounds of dogs. Poster presentation. ASLMS Annual Meeting, April 24–26. Orlando, FL.

Kuffler, D.P. (2016). Photobiomodulation in promoting wound healing: a review. *Regen Med.* 11(1):107–122.

KYON. (n.d.) (a). Proximal Abducting ULnar Osteotomy (PAUL). Available from: http://www.kyon.ch/current-products/proximal-abducting-ulnar-osteotomy-paul (accessed November 30, 2016). (b) Tibial Plateau Leveling Osteotomy (TPLO). Available from: http://www.kyon.ch/current-products/tibial-plateau-leveling-osteotomy-tplo (accessed November 30, 2016). (c) TTA surgery. Available from: http://www.kyon.ch/current-products/tibial-tuberosity-advancement-tta (accessed November 30, 2016).

Maegawa, Y. *et al.* (2000). Effects of near-infrared low-level laser irradiation on microcirculation. *Lasers Surg Med.* 27(5):427–437.

Medrado, A.R. *et al.* (2003). Influence of low level laser therapy on wound healing and its biological action upon myofibroblasts. *Lasers Surg Med.* 32(3):239–244.

Mota, F.C. *et al.* (2013). Low-power laser therapy for repairing acute and chronic-phase bone lesions. *Res Vet Sci.* 94(1):105–110.

Nesioonpour, S. *et al.* (2014). The effect of low-level laser on postoperative pain after tibial fracture surgery: a double-blind controlled randomized clinical trial. *Anesth Pain Med.* 4(3):e17350.

Peplow, P.V. *et al.* (2010). Laser photobiomodulation of wound healing: a review of experimental studies in mouse and rat animal models. *Photomed Laser Surg.* 28(3):291–325.

Pryor, B. and Millis, D.L. (2015). Therapeutic laser in veterinary medicine. *Vet Clin North Am Small Anim Pract.* 45(1):45–56.

Silveira, P.C. *et al.* (2007). Evaluation of mitochondrial respiratory chain activity in wound healing by low-level laser therapy. *J Photochem Photobiol B.* 86(3):279–282.

Skopin, M.D. and Molitor, S.C. (2009). Effects of near-infrared laser exposure in a cellular model of wound healing. *Photodermatol Photoimmunol Photomed.* 25(2): 75–80.

Son, J. *et al.* (2012). Bone healing effects of diode laser (808 nm) on a rat tibial fracture model. *In Vivo.* 26(4):703–709.

Sprouse-Blum, A.S. *et al.* (2010). Understanding endorphins and their importance in pain management. *Hawaii Med J.* 69(3):70–71.

Takashi, K. (1988). Low level diode laser treatment for hematomas under grafted skin and its photobiological mechanisms. *Keio J Med.* 37(4):415–428.

Tim, C.R. *et al.* (2014). Low-level laser therapy enhances the expression of osteogenic factors during bone repair in rats. *Lasers Med Sci.* 29(1):147–156.

Wang, P. *et al.* (2014). Effects of low-level laser therapy on joint pain, synovitis, anabolic, and catabolic factors in a progressive osteoarthritis rabbit model. *Lasers Med Sci.* 29(6):1875–1885.

Winkler, C. (2017). CO_2 laser excision of a bladder mass. *Veterinary Practice News.* 29(5):40–41.

Winkler, C. (2018). CO_2 laser entropion and stenotic nares correction in a shar pei. *Veterinary Practice News.* 30(6):50–51.

8

Wounds

David S. Bradley

Summus Medical Laser, Franklin, TN, USA

Introduction

Photobiomodulation (PBM) for improved wound healing and other dermatologic conditions is still one of the most studied and widely used veterinary applications of the technology. It was first described in 1968 as the founding concept behind PBM, when Dr. Endre Mester was experimenting with the effects of laser light on recalcitrant cancer cells he implanted in rats. Though the proposed experiment was a failure, he observed that the implantation sites healed faster, and the hair grew back faster, on those rats that received laser exposure (Mester *et al.*, 1968).

Proper wound applications integrate all available laser parameters for optimal results. These include the proper wavelength or wavelengths. A nonstatic delivery mode. And proper dosage based not only on the size of the wound but the chronicity and severity. This chapter will provide a brief review of wound healing and discuss the adjustment of these PBM factors in order to obtain the best, most efficient, and safest clinical results.

Wound Healing

Wound healing is a multistage process. For optimal results, a well-orchestrated series of events needs to unfold, including clotting, inflammation, granulation tissue formation, collagen synthesis, epithelialization, and tissue remodeling. An inappropriate inflammatory response, poor angiogenesis, or defects in collagen production and differentiation can lead to delayed healing and an increased risk of infection (Meireles *et al.*, 2008).

Important processes that occur in wound healing are:

- Formation of a platelet- and fibrin-containing plug at the wound site.
- Invasion of the wound by neutrophils, monocytes, and macrophages.
- Proliferation and migration of keratinocytes from the wound edge to begin re-epithelization of the wound.
- Proliferation of fibroblasts at the dermal edge.
- Formation of granulation tissue, comprising fibroblasts, macrophages, lymphocytes, plasma cells, and an extracellular matrix (ECM) containing collagen fibers and macromolecular components such as glycoproteins, as well as the formation of new blood vessels.
- Maturation of granulation tissue and collagen fibers and vascularization of wound tissue.

The processes involved in inflammation, re-epithelization, granulation tissue, ECM formation, angiogenesis, and tissue remodeling are controlled by growth factors and cytokines produced by the cellular elements present in the wounds and in blood. Cytokines regulate inflammatory cells during the early stages of wound healing and influence the gene expression and release of growth factors important in the proliferation and differentiation of cells and the synthesis of ECM. The presence of receptors or binding proteins for specific growth factors on cells is also important in determining cellular responses (Pavletic, 2010; Stadelman *et al.*, 1998).

There are a variety of cells integral to proper wound healing. For example, mast cells release histamine, which reacts with collagen and interleukin 4 (IL4) to stimulate fibroblasts to proliferate and migrate. New investigations show that skin mast cells modulate the inflammatory response in healing wounds, play a role in angiogenesis, and may participate in tissue remodeling in the late phase of wound healing. Recent evidence has shown that skin mast cells are important for the formation of granulation tissue and for the synthesis of collagen fibers at the edge of a wound (Vasheghani *et al.*, 2008).

Laser Therapy in Veterinary Medicine: Photobiomodulation, Second Edition. Edited by Christopher J. Winkler and Lisa A. Miller.

Effects of Photobiomodulation on Wound Healing

It is important to emphasize that PBM enhances normal cell function. It enables the cell to do its job better. This does not mean it makes normal cells super cells. It does not just ramp everything up or turn everything down. It allows the cell to do its proper job, which sometimes means doing nothing! *In vitro* studies demonstrate that part of a cell's normal function is to recognize normal cell-to-cell contact inhibition once cell cultures approach confluence (Martz and Steinberg, 1972). This is analogous, *in vivo*, to a healthy organism, which will regenerate healing tissue, but stop further growth when healing is complete. It is important to note that laser treatment accelerates normal healing and tissue regeneration without producing overgrowth or neoplastic transformation.

PBM aims to restore and enhance the normal biological function of injured or stressed cells. "Normalization" is the key word when it comes to laser therapy (Tuner and Hode, 2002). The cellular effects of photobiomodulation therapy (PBMT) can be classified as either primary effects, which are light-induced, or secondary effects, which occur in response to the primary effects (Hawkins and Abrahamse, 2007).

In primary effects, a direct photochemical reaction occurs when photons emitted by the laser reach the mitochondria and membranes of cells (e.g., fibroblasts, keratinocytes, and endothelial cells) and the photonic energy is absorbed by their endogenous chromophores (mitochondrial cytochromes, porphyrins, and flavoproteins) and converted into a chemical kinetic energy. This causes an improved efficiency of the respiratory chain within the mitochondria, due to changes in membrane permeability, improved signaling between mitochondria, nucleus, and cytosol, and increased oxidative metabolism, which enables more adenosine triphosphate (ATP) to be produced (Karu, 1989). In addition, reactive oxygen species (ROS) such as nitric oxide (NO) and superoxide dismutase (SOD) are produced, and there is a shift in the redox state.

Secondary effects lead to amplification of the previously mentioned primary photoreactions. Calcium is released from the mitochondria into the cytoplasm with changes in intracellular calcium levels (Tuner and Hode, 2002), which stimulates cell metabolism and regulation of the signaling pathways responsible for events required for wound repair, such as cell migration, DNA and RNA synthesis, cell mitosis, protein secretion, and cell proliferation. A cascade of metabolic effects results in various physiological changes at the cellular level, such as activation of fibroblasts, macrophages, and lymphocytes, growth factor release, neurotransmitter release, vasodilation, collagen synthesis, and improvement of cell membrane permeability and the function of the Na^+/K^+ pump. PBM has a positive effect on prostaglandin production, mediating neutrophil activation, lymphocyte accumulation, and other inflammatory effects. Increased metabolic activity increases oxygen and nutrient availability, leading to enhanced protein and enzyme production. These factors ultimately lead to normalization of cell function. They stimulate and accelerate cell reproduction and growth, leading to faster repair of damaged tissues and moderation of the inflammatory response. Concurrently, a sequence of cellular events provides analgesia (Hamblin and Demidova, 2006; Karu, 1989, 1999; Karu and Kolyakov, 2005; Martin, 2003; Peavy, 2002; Wray *et al.*, 1988).

In laboratory animals, biostimulation of the wound-healing process through PBM, results in the stimulation of fibroblast proliferation, significant increases in re-epithelialization, increased collagen synthesis and granulation tissue formation, acceleration of wound closure, improved tensile strength of scars, and faster healing of burns (Calisto *et al.*, 2015; Gal *et al.*, 2006; Hodjati *et al.*, 2014). In rodent skin-wound models, PBM leads to earlier regression of the inflammatory phase, faster re-epithelization, and acceleration of the maturation phase. The production of growth factors increases, including vascular endothelial growth factor (VEGF), keratinocyte growth factor (KGF), transforming growth factor (TGF), and platelet-derived growth factor (PDGF) (Stadler *et al.*, 2001). The photochemical effects of red and near-infrared exposure on human fibroblast growth rates in an *in vitro* model of wound healing demonstrate that PBM, at appropriate exposure levels, accelerates cell growth (Skopin and Molitor, 2009).

PBM stimulates a better alignment and organization of collagen fibers. Collagen organization is important to the strength and elasticity of healing wounds (Doillon *et al.*, 1988). Similarly, there is a linear relationship between the tensile strength of a tendon and both the content and the arrangement of collagen fibers. In a study analyzing cutaneous wounds in the dorsum of Wistar rats, irradiated subjects showed increased collagen production and organization when compared to non-irradiated controls (Mendez *et al.*, 2004). PBM stimulates a more normal distribution of type I and III collagen during healing in wounds, as well as in tendons (Paraguassu *et al.*, 2014; Wood *et al.*, 2010).

As a general mechanism, enhancing blood flow and oxygenation to a diseased area will help tissue healing (Larkin *et al.*, 2012). The effect of laser light on blood flow is extended after the exposure to the light has finished. It is supported by an increased angiogenesis promoted by basic fibroblastic growth factor (FGF) and VEGF. These benefits in wound healing apply to clean surgical wounds, second-intention healing, graft and flap survival, and contaminated and infected wounds (Kubota, 2002).

The increased oxygenation also helps with infections since many pathogenic microorganisms grow poorly in an oxygen-rich environment. Laser therapy also helps treat infection by enhancing macrophage function and modulating immune response and ROS production (Burger *et al.*, 2015).

There is also a potential direct effect on microorganisms. *In vitro* studies have not fully elucidated the underlying mechanisms of the antimicrobial effect and have provided variable results. Most experiments seem to show a decreased microbial growth after exposure to laser light, including common pathogenic and opportunistic species such as *Staphylococcus aureus*, *Escherichia coli*, *Pseudomonas aeruginosa*, and *Candida albicans* (Redondo, 2015). It is important to realize that some bacteria show no effect, or even experience increased growth, from exposure to laser light. However, decreased microbial growth after PBM *in vivo* is almost universally accepted, and *in vivo* experiments (as well as case reports) have provided consistent and encouraging results to support laser use in infected tissues (Nussbaum *et al.*, 2003). In addition, these results seem to be consistent despite the different technical parameters encountered when comparing *in vivo* studies.

Due to the problem of increasing antibiotic resistance worldwide, PBMT has been explored as a nonpharmacological antimicrobial tool. Laser therapy, using a dose of 5 J/cm^2 on both the intact skin and wounds of rats infected with methicillin-resistant *S. aureus* (MRSA), has been shown to reduce bacterial proliferation (Silva *et al.*, 2013). In another animal study using rats, laser therapy showed promise as an adjunct or alternative to pharmacological agents in the treatment of osteomyelitis experimentally induced by MRSA (Kaya *et al.*, 2011).

Optimal Parameters for Photobiomodulation

The variety of mechanisms behind the photochemical and physiologic effects of PBMT on specific chromophores is becoming better understood every day (Assis *et al.*, 2012; Emanet *et al.*, 2010; Joensen *et al.*, 2012; Longo *et al.*, 1987; Moriyama *et al.*, 2009). Certainly, there is still more to learn, but the question, "Does laser therapy work?" is no longer relevant. The more pertinent questions today, and where most research is now being focused, are how to optimize laser therapy and expand the applications of this remarkable modality. Let us review the parameters found in today's therapy lasers and their software and discuss how they can be modified to enhance the clinical response. Again, these parameters include wavelength, delivery mode, and dosage.

Wavelength

Wavelength is what determines the best function of any particular laser. Laser therapy works by a wavelength-specific form of PBM. Cellular chromophores within blood and tissue mitochondria absorb laser energy and a series of direct biochemical processes are stimulated or enhanced, along with a broad cascade of secondary and tertiary effects.

The most important target chromophores are: superficial chromophores such as melanin, which absorb wavelengths in the visible red range (630–660 nm); water, which has a nice peak of absorption in the 970–980 nm range; hemoglobin, which has a broad absorption peak at 890–990 nm; and cytochrome c oxidase (CCO), which has a peak absorption at 790–830 nm (Anderson and Parrish, 1981).

Though shorter wavelengths (630–660 nm) do not have the ability to penetrate deeper layers as readily as longer wavelengths, they are absorbed superficially and are very beneficial in wound healing (Al-Watban *et al.*, 2007). The wavelengths near the 970–980 nm range have a moderately increased absorption by water. This produces a mild warming effect in local tissues when higher-powered therapy lasers are used, creating a thermal gradient. Blood tends to flow along thermal gradients from warm to cool or from higher to lower pressure, increasing circulation in these areas. Wavelengths near 800 nm (750–830 nm) are at the peak of absorption for the CCO enzyme. As a rate-limiting step in the conversion of oxygen to ATP within the electron transport chain, CCO that has absorbed photonic energy can accelerate steps to improve ATP and NO production.

Many therapy laser manufacturers now construct single devices that simultaneously deliver multiple wavelengths; their goal is to produce a synergistic effect and a wider range of treatment options, leading to improved clinical outcomes.

Delivery Mode

How laser light is delivered to the tissue has clinical significance. The delivery modes used in laser applications can be modified and tailored to optimize laser therapy across a broad range of applications and patient parameters. Laser light can be delivered in continuous wave (CW), pulsed (modulated or gated), or superpulsed modes.

Different tissue culture types respond differently to different frequencies, or pulse rates (Karu *et al.*, 1997), and adjusting the pulse rate of a laser's modulated delivery technique can have differing physiologic effects on cell-tissue structures (Cheida *et al.*, 2002). In cell cultures, lower pulse rates and CW impart a better effect on pain-modulation processes, while higher frequencies have more anti-inflammatory and biostimulatory effects (Tuner and Hode,

2004). These *in vitro* effects in tissue cultures may not be as simple as the rate of pulsing; they might also include the time for which the laser is on versus off (Karu *et al.*, 1999).

The literature continues to show that adding pulse delivery modes to treatment protocols may have an effect on overall long-term results. For example, pulsing may improve outcomes by mitigating the filtration effects of cutaneous melanin (Brondon, 2009). Another example is a 2009 study in a transgenic murine model, which demonstrated that different wavelengths and CW versus pulsed delivery mode resulted in different effects in an induced inflammatory process (Moriyama *et al.*, 2009). The importance of evaluating the effects of pulsing was addressed in a 2014 guest editorial in *Photomedicine and Laser Surgery*, in which it was noted, "The PW (pulsed) LLLT (low-level laser therapy) device has more laser (illumination) parameters, such as peak and average power outputs, pulse frequency, and pulse duration, than CW LLLT, all of which add to the medical applicability of this technique. It is assumed that by investigating different values of these parameters, researchers can select better protocols and achieve more satisfactory outcomes with PW LLLT devices than with CW LLLT devices" (Bayat, 2014).

A 2010 review analyzed relevant laser literature from 1970 to 2010 regarding the effects of pulsing versus CW in laser therapy. This review suggested that though CW light has been the gold standard and has been used for all types of laser therapy application, pulsed light may be superior, particularly for wound healing and post-stroke management. As noted in the review, there is unfortunately no consensus on the very best pulsing parameters for specific diseases or pathologies, due to inconsistent reporting of parameters in studies. It is suggested that future researchers record all laser parameters in order to help determine optimal protocols for a wider variety of conditions (Hashmi *et al.*, 2010).

A recent unpublished study conducted by the International Centre for Genetic Engineering and Biotechnology (ICGEB) in Trieste, Italy, showed a more consistent and prolonged stimulation of cellular ATP production using pulsed versus CW delivery modes (Ottaviani *et al.*, 2015). This study was done subsequent to several other studies from the University of Trieste illustrating the profound beneficial effects of laser therapy in resolving oral mucositis secondary to chemotherapy and radiation therapy in human patients with head and neck cancer (Chermetz *et al.*, 2014; Gobbo *et al.*, 2014; Ottaviani *et al.*, 2013).

Superpulse is another laser delivery mode that is available for some surgical, therapeutic, and industrial lasers. Superpulsing in therapeutic lasers can mitigate the thermal and absorption effects of pigmented tissue. In theory, it may therefore improve penetration and, with proper parameters, increase the number of photons that reach the target tissue. Data on depth of penetration using superpulsing with different wavelengths vary considerably, and more recent work challenges the notion (Anders and Wu, 2015; Joensen *et al.*, 2012).

The peak power capability of a pulsing or superpulsing laser device do not equate to an increased average power. It is very important to keep in mind the average power and the total joules per minute being delivered for effective results.

Another concept related to delivery mode is administering therapy in a contact or noncontact method. Though in wound healing almost all treatments will be performed while not touching the tissue (noncontact mode), this is still an important concept to discuss (Enwemeka, 2009). No laser fiber directly touches the patient during laser therapy; all lasers transmit their energy through a type of delivery handpiece. This is especially important in veterinary patients, because with many of the conditions that we treat (other than wounds), laser energy is often administered through a hair coat. In human treatments, clothing is removed from the treatment area. Hair can be just as much an impediment to laser energy as clothing, but to shave all our patients for every treatment would greatly decrease client compliance. By using a delivery handpiece (and proper dosage), hair can be displaced adequately to allow enough photons to reach our target tissue.

No study shows any delivery system or handpiece design is superior to any other. The most pertinent features of a delivery handpiece, therefore, are related to ease of use, cleaning and sanitization, durability, and adjustability. Since most wounds will probably have lost hair due to trauma or are otherwise shaved as part of the treatment process, the delivery handpiece should be held perpendicular to, and just a centimeter or two above, the target tissue and the area to be treated.

Dosage

The last parameter to discuss is dosage and how it relates to the average power delivered by laser devices. Dosage is one of the primary factors that will determine the success of laser therapy. It also seems to be one of the more confusing issues among clinicians beginning to use laser therapy.

Let us start with some basic laser terminology:

- Power is the rate of delivery of energy and is measured in watts (W), where 1 W = 1 J/sec.
- Energy is the total number of joules (J) delivered and is simply calculated by multiplying power (W) by time (sec).
- Irradiance (W/cm^2) is the amount of power (W) delivered to a specific area (cm^2).
- Fluence (J/cm^2) is the total amount of energy (J) delivered to a given area (cm^2).

Credible studies of PBMT in the literature should list the exact parameters used, including dosage. It is possible to accurately calculate the dosage delivered to the specific area (fluence), whether holding the handpiece stationary or using a scanning technique. Confusion in varying dosage recommendations can arise, not from the physics of laser energy delivery, but rather from not taking into consideration the principles related to the optics of animal tissue. Photons of light are constantly scattered, reflected, and absorbed within tissue, causing attenuation or "decay" of the laser beam as it travels through the tissue. While this must be considered when calculating the number of photons needed to elicit the desired direct photochemical effect on a structure not on the surface, such math behind this is quite complicated, taking into account Beer's law and the Kubelka–Munk theory, which incorporates scatter coefficients, the absorption coefficients found in Boltzmann's equation, and other diffusion constants (Anderson and Parrish, 1981).

Power dictates the rate of delivery and is an important component when determining efficiency, efficacy, and safety. Being able to adjust the power should be one of the critical features looked for when selecting a therapy laser. If power is too high, with too many photons delivered too rapidly, especially to a very small area (high irradiance), then superficial tissue heating may occur. If power is too low, with too few photons delivered too slowly (low irradiance), there will be too much superficial absorption and scatter to allow the photons to saturate large volumes of deep tissue. If delivered at an appropriate irradiance, all the positive effects will be experienced safely. This can be tailored to properly stimulate small or superficial conditions, or for direct tissue stimulation of a large volume of tissue. The total energy delivered to a tissue or body part (fluence) will be a direct measure of the irradiance (power delivered per unit area) times the length of exposure.

Dosages listed and recommended in the literature range from 1 to 10 J/cm^2 (or higher), depending on the size and depth of the lesion, severity, and chronicity (Al-Watban *et al.*, 2007; Hawkins and Abrahamse, 2007; Peplow *et al.*, 2010; Tuner and Hode, 2002).

A simple wound of 3 × 3 cm has an area of roughly 10 cm^2. To deliver 1 J/cm^2 requires delivery of 10 J. With a 1 W laser, that takes 10 seconds. With a 500 mW laser, it takes 20 seconds. With a 5 mW laser, it takes 2000 seconds, or over 30 minutes.

The classification of lasers is dictated by ANSI Standards and relates to the maximum *average* laser output (ANSI 2014). Maximum average laser output is calculated by the total average power (J/sec), not a single burst or peak power. A laser that has a broad range of power adjustability will give the best results on the widest range of conditions, from small patients and superficial wounds to larger patients and deep musculoskeletal or neurologic conditions. Most high-powered lasers can still be turned down to 500 mW or less when needed for small patients, delicate tissue, or very superficial lesions.

Understanding the science and physics of laser–tissue interactions is just as important as understanding the physiology and biochemistry. As we increase our understanding, we can more accurately quantify minimum desired dosages, and lasers can then be preset to deliver these dosages safely and accurately in order to simplify treatments. Realize, though, that there is no perfect dosage.

Many patient variables affect dose: coat length and color, skin color, hydration, vascularity, chronicity, severity, and even individual patient response. Minimum dosages can be calculated and preset for ease of use (see Boxes 8.1 and 8.2), but keep in mind two principles: (i) the only thing we can say for sure is that if you give too little a dosage, you will produce little to no response; and (ii) there is a very wide margin of safety.

Box 8.1 Laser Therapy Dosage Recommendations

Acute Superficial Wounds or "Hot" Inflammatory Conditions
1–4 J/cm^2
Chronic Superficial Conditions or Chronic Wounds
4–30 J/cm^2
Acute Superficial Pain or Injury
2–4 J/cm^2
Acute Deep Pain or Injury
4–8 J/cm^2
Chronic Deep Pain or Injury
6–20 J/cm^2

Adapted from Hawkins and Abrahamse (2007) and Peplow *et al.* (2010).

Box 8.2 Pulse Frequency Recommendations based on *in vitro* Cell Studies

The following recommendations are based on cell studies.
Pain/Neuralgia
2–20 Hz or CW
Edema/Swelling
1,000 Hz
General Stimulation
500 Hz
Inflammation
5,000 Hz
Infection
10,000 Hz

Adapted from Tuner and Hode (2002).

Fluorescence Biomodulation

There is another novel PBM device that is specific for wound treatments. It is labeled commercially as Phovia and is a type of fluorescent light therapy approved for domestic canine and feline treatments at the time of this publication. The product uses a blue light to stimulate a topically applied gel, causing the gel to emit fluorescent light directly over the wound site in a combination of mainly blue (405–495 nm), green (495–570 nm), and yellow (570–600 nm) wavelengths. The product is another form of direct PBM making use of other wavelengths outside the IR spectrum, and differs from photodynamic therapy (PDT), which uses a sensitizing chromophore activated by light to have a direct effect on its target through heat or ROS.

Blue light has been shown to have direct antibacterial effects on some species when delivered at the appropriate dose. Green, yellow, and orange wavelengths do have biostimulatory properties that target additional chromophores in the cell and have been shown to have positive effects on cellular metabolism and function. Light from the gel is not coherent or collimated as is laser therapy, and the depth of tissue penetration is not expected to be great but may yet be greater with the gel than using the light alone. The treatment may remain useful for superficial wound healing and the treatment and prevention of superficial infections if the dosage threshold of blue light is reached to have its intended clinical effect on target chromophores.

This treatment is not recommended in patients with any photosensitivity or if the patient is receiving drugs known to induce photosensitivity. The blue light is quite intense, and eye protection is therefore highly warranted, with additional measures taken by administering personnel to protect the patient's eyes in the absence of supplied protective pet eyewear. Caution is also indicated over cutaneous cancers.

Clinically, the site/wound should be clipped. The gel is applied, and the light therapy is then administered directly over the site for 2 minutes, offering a coverage of approximately 50 cm^2. Treatments are recommended twice weekly for optimum results.

Studies done by the company indicate that Phovia as a sole therapy can speed healing by 36% in canine superficial pyoderma as compared to dogs receiving oral antibiotics alone, or as much as 50% in deep pyoderma when used in conjunction with antibiotics. In another study carried out by the manufacturer on canine surgical wounds, fluorescence PBM was found to increase the expression of factors that play a role in epithelial growth and collagen deposition. These included factor VIII, epidermal growth factor, and collagen III while increasing the pro-inflammatory marker-TNF alpha. Histologically, the skin was found to have increased collagen deposition and neoangiogenesis with inflammation having been reduced. The use of Phovia in conjunction with laser PBM may stimulate additional chromophores outside the IR spectrum, lending additional benefits to wound healing and antibacterial effects to challenging sequelae such as highly resistant cases of pyoderma.

Basic Principles of Laser Wound Therapy

Delivery Methods

Though the principles behind laser therapy can be very intricate and seem complicated, they are becoming more and more well-understood. Software protocols already set up in most therapeutic lasers simplify the parameters described above. Because of the wide margin of safety, laser therapy can be instituted quickly and easily. It can and should be delegated to the veterinary staff for the most efficient and economic benefits. Initial training is essential, and continuing education is necessary to fully realize the benefits of laser therapy.

There are two basic delivery methods for laser therapy: direct contact of the delivery handpiece with the tissue, and delivery with the handpiece not in contact with the tissue. Direct contact is rarely used for wound therapy but is the technique of choice when treating most nonwound conditions. It can be done on light-coated, short-haired, or shaved patients (Enwemeka, 2009). It is especially important to separate hairs on long-coated animals wherever possible. You can use your other hand to do this, while monitoring for superficial warmth.

The thermal effect of laser therapy varies with coat color and skin pigmentation. Darker colors absorb more. If you notice patient sensitivity due to heavy pigmentation and unexpected tissue warming, as evidenced by a withdrawal response or aversion reactions, try using the following techniques:

- Increase your hand speed.
- Increase the distance between the laser handpiece and the patient.
- Decrease the power density (use a larger-diameter spot size).
- Decrease the power (the time must be increased as well to maintain proper dosage).

Whether in contact with the tissue or not, treat either in a grid pattern or a scanning technique. Treat the area of interest, as well as a border of surrounding healthy tissue. Treatment can be administered in conjunction with stretching or range-of-motion movement if indicated.

A grid-pattern delivery technique involves holding the handpiece in a fixed spot for 1–3 seconds then moving it in a uniform pattern every 1–3 seconds to cover the entire area. It is important to try not to immediately overlap with this technique.

A scanning delivery technique in contact or noncontact mode employs a slow, steady movement of the laser handpiece in a pattern that uniformly covers the desired treatment area. This could be large and even parallel strokes, small expanding circles, large concentric circles, or any pattern that thoroughly covers the area. The area can be treated in a methodical process with repeat passages until the total calculated dosage is delivered. Move at a rate that is not too slow or too fast and is comfortable for the patient. About 3 cm/sec is adequate.

Noncontact delivery is how most wounds will be treated. This is usually done using a scanning technique with the handpiece perpendicular to the surface. Scan 1–2 cm from the surface with slow passage over the affected area. This delivery is used for open wounds, incisions, or any area with discharge or exudates. It is also used on very painful or sensitive areas. Use the other hand to separate hair if needed.

Always apply the laser to a 2–5 cm border of healthy tissue surrounding the area of greatest concern. Include any other structures that may be injured or are adding stress to the injured area. If treating for edema/congestion, swelling, ischemia, or large and severe wounds, start treating proximally and work distally. Laser the major draining lymph nodes in the axilla or groin and the associated lymphatic and blood supply.

Some wounds will only need one to three treatments to help stimulate rapid, improved healing. Most will need at least six. It is always warranted to begin laser therapy as soon as possible after the initial injury. Acute injuries and wounds should be treated daily for 2–5 days, then every other day for three to five treatments. Twice weekly or even weekly intervals may be adequate if patient or client compliance dictates. In very severe trauma or compromised tissues, treating twice daily for the first 1–2 days may be beneficial. If further treatment is needed, continue twice weekly (or at least weekly) until the condition plateaus or is resolved.

Chronic conditions and wounds can initially be treated on an every-other-day basis for the first three to five treatments. Then continue twice weekly (or at least weekly) until the condition plateaus, has resolved, or is healed. Some conditions with underlying factors (allergies, autoimmune disorders, immunocompromised patients, or repetitive stress or trauma) will need ongoing maintenance treatments at least monthly. Shorter intervals may be warranted and are perfectly safe if owner compliance allows.

PBM effects are cumulative. Observable response, or the duration of response, should increase with each treatment until the condition plateaus or is healed. PBMT has a wide margin of safety. It is prudent to start with a more conservative dosage with acute lesions. Injured tissue is very responsive to laser therapy. Most patients will show at least a mild positive response within the first few treatments. If a positive response is not noted within three or four treatments with a standard protocol, re-evaluate the condition, diagnosis, or treatment protocol. If the diagnosis is correct and other underlying contributing factors are being addressed, make sure you are delivering at least the minimum recommended dose. You can then begin to increase the delivered dosage by 25–50% per treatment until a positive response is being noted. Do this by first adjusting the time, and then the power if the time is becoming too prolonged (Lanzafame *et al.*, 2007).

Wound Classification and Treatment

The types of wound to be discussed will start with simple, acute clean wounds and progress to more extensive, infected, and chronic wounds. This discussion will encompass post-operative wounds, minor abrasions, pressure sores and ulcers, burns, degloving injuries, grafts, and flaps. The same principles apply whether the wound was caused by surgical intervention, external trauma, self-trauma, thermal injury, ischemic injury, tissue toxins, or envenomation. Any underlying or predisposing pathology or repetitive trauma needs to be addressed appropriately. PBM will almost always be an adjunct treatment, with other standard protocols being implemented simultaneously. These will include proper cleaning, debridement, lavage, topical treatments, dressing, systemic therapies, Elizabethan collars or other preventive mechanisms, wraps, and bandages. It is important to note that laser energy will not penetrate wraps or bandage material of any kind. If laser therapy is warranted more frequently than a bandage will be changed, consideration must be made when applying the bandage. A window that can be easily unwrapped and rewrapped without disrupting the integrity of the bandage or support should be included over the area to be treated. When treating large wounds or extremely compromised or infected tissue, it is recommended to always start by treating the vasculature and lymphatic vessels proximal or central to the area and then progress distally.

Surgical Incisions and Clean Wounds

Simple, clean wounds and postoperative incisions in healthy patients will benefit from a single laser therapy treatment administered during recovery. If the patient is staying overnight, a second treatment may be administered the following day. Larger incisions, incisions with undue tension or stress on them, incisions near or involving compromised tissue, and incisions in older or debilitated patients should all receive a minimum of three treatments. Keep in mind the general principles of wound treatment and be sure to include a margin of healthy tissue surrounding the incision as part of the treatment area. Though cases of acute pyotraumatic dermatitis (hot spots) are usually infected, they can be included in this category and treated in a similar fashion.

Measure the incision or wound area and the surrounding margin of healthy tissue. This margin may be as small as 1 cm for wounds on very small animals or 3 cm or more for large or severe wounds. Follow the basic treatment principles and dosages as outlined earlier in this chapter. Deliver an initial dosage of 2–4 J/cm^2. Treat daily for 2–3 days if possible, then every other day.

Figure 8.1 shows sibling patients. These two dogs were from the same breeder, owned by the same person, and both had an ovariohysterectomy on the same day, performed by the same surgeon. The patient on the left did not receive laser therapy postoperatively. The patient on the right received one laser therapy treatment immediately postoperatively. The patients were otherwise not managed differently. There is an observable reduction in the tissue swelling and reaction to the sutures in the laser-treated incision. There also appears to be less papular and macular reaction in the surrounding skin. Using laser therapy will not guarantee that your patients never experience postoperative incisional complications or reactions, but it will decrease the incidence and severity of these reactions.

Chronic, Granulomatous, and Infected Wounds

Chronic, granulomatous, and infected wounds will often require a prolonged and aggressive treatment regimen (Figure 8.2). It is recommended to start with daily treatments, along with standard adjunct therapies. High dosages of laser therapy will often be needed to resolve these lesions. If wound healing is not progressing, do not hesitate to increase the dosage significantly based on the guidelines in Box 8.1. With consistent treatment, a high number of these wounds can be resolved. It is important to persevere and continue all measures until complete resolution.

Measure the incision or wound area and the surrounding margin of healthy tissue. This margin may be as small as 1 cm for wounds on very small animals or 3 cm or more on large or severe wounds. Follow the basic treatment principles and dosages as outlined earlier in this chapter. Deliver a starting dosage of 4–10 J/cm^2. Treat daily for 2–5 days, if possible, then every other day. If no improvement is noted within the first two to four treatments, increase the dosage (joules) by an additional 25–50% per treatment until a positive response is noted. Do this by first adjusting the treatment time, then by increasing the power if the treatment time is becoming too long. In very large wounds such as degloving injuries or lick granulomas, you can decrease treatment intervals to twice weekly or even weekly once the wound is showing strong positive clinical response, usually after 10–20 days.

Traumatic Wounds and Burns

Traumatic wounds encompass a wide range of potential complicating factors. Many traumatic wounds will appear worse several days after the incident. This is

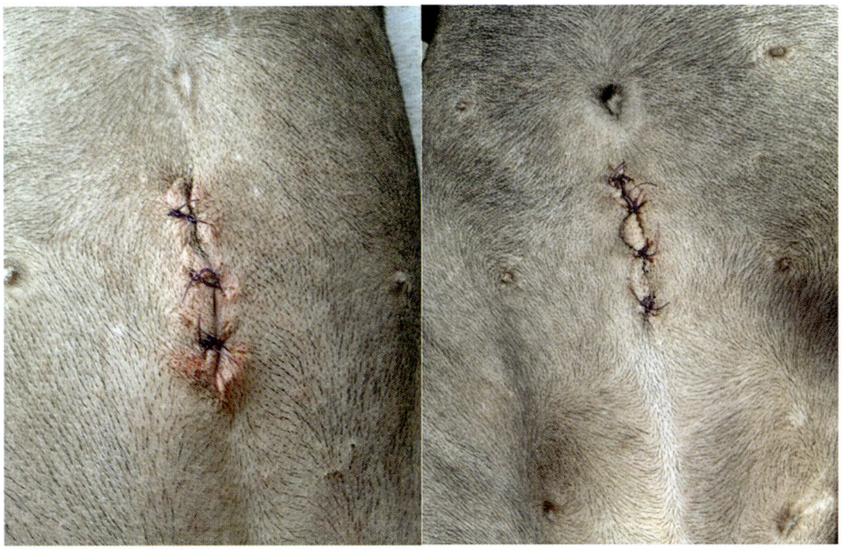

Figure 8.1 Postoperative ovariohysterectomy incisions. The patient on the left did not receive laser therapy postoperatively. The patient on the right did receive laser therapy immediately postoperatively. Images courtesy of Dr. Susan Kelleher.

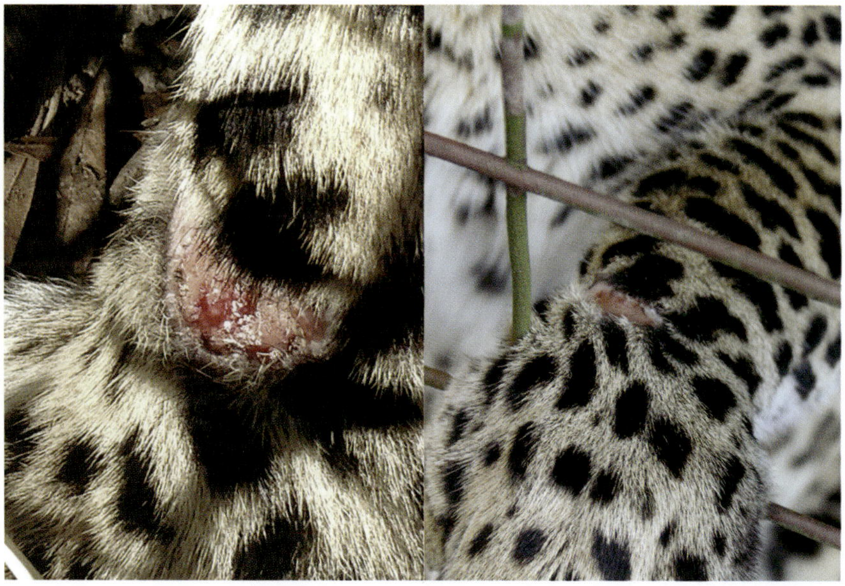

Figure 8.2 Chronic granulomatous lesion on the front paw of a leopard at a rescue sanctuary. Multiple therapies had been attempted prior to PBMT, along with environmental enrichment with no success at reducing continued self-trauma. Laser therapy was instituted (left) and improvement was noted (right).

due to the unseen damage from crushing and pressure injuries or from thermal insults. It can also result from disruption to the integrity of the blood supply. Ongoing damage due to a tissue toxin such as snake or insect envenomation will also result in delayed onset of the full extent of tissue damage. To improve results, these possibilities should be anticipated during initial evaluation. Proper laser therapy protocols should be utilized to treat the wider margin of potential injury, as well as the vasculature supplying or draining the injured area (Kovacs, 2015).

Measure the wound area and the surrounding margin of healthy tissue. As with other types of wounds, this margin may be as small as 1 cm for wounds on very small animals or 3 cm or more on large or severe wounds. Follow the basic treatment principles and dosages as outlined earlier in this chapter. For burns, it is recommended to initially begin with low power, and a fluence of approximately 2 J/cm^2. For all other traumatic wounds, plan on delivering an initial dosage of 4–6 J/cm^2. Treat daily for 2–3 days if possible, then every other day. If no improvement is noted within the first two to four treatments, begin increasing the dosage (joules) by 25–50% per treatment until a positive response is being noted. Do this by first adjusting the treatment time, then, if the treatment time is becoming too long, adjust the power upward. In very large or severe wounds, decrease the treatment intervals to twice weekly once the wound is showing strong positive clinical response, usually after 10–20 days.

Figure 8.3 shows a patient with severe bite wounds following being attacked by another dog. The top picture shows the wounds following initial treatment and repair at an emergency facility 4 days earlier, with severe swelling, bruising, and copious drainage of serosanguinous fluid. Laser therapy treatment was instituted daily for 3 days. Antibiotics were continued, but no other therapy was used. The swelling, bruising, and discharge improved measurably over the next 2 days.

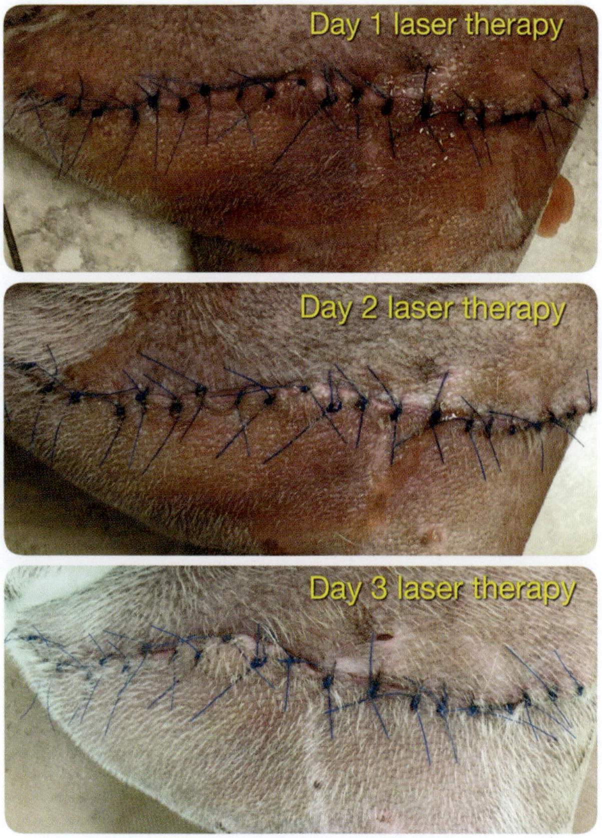

Figure 8.3 Soft-tissue wound prior to laser therapy (top), and 1 day (middle) and 2 days (bottom) after starting laser therapy. Images courtesy of Dr. Boaz Man.

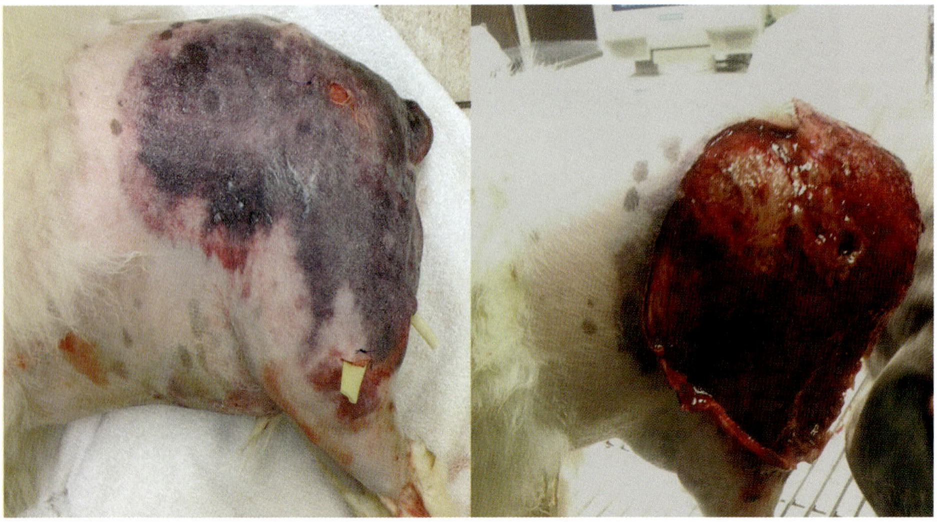

Figure 8.4 Initial tissue changes from fight wounds (left) and substantial sloughing of tissue 7 days later (right). Images courtesy of Dr. Daniel M. Core.

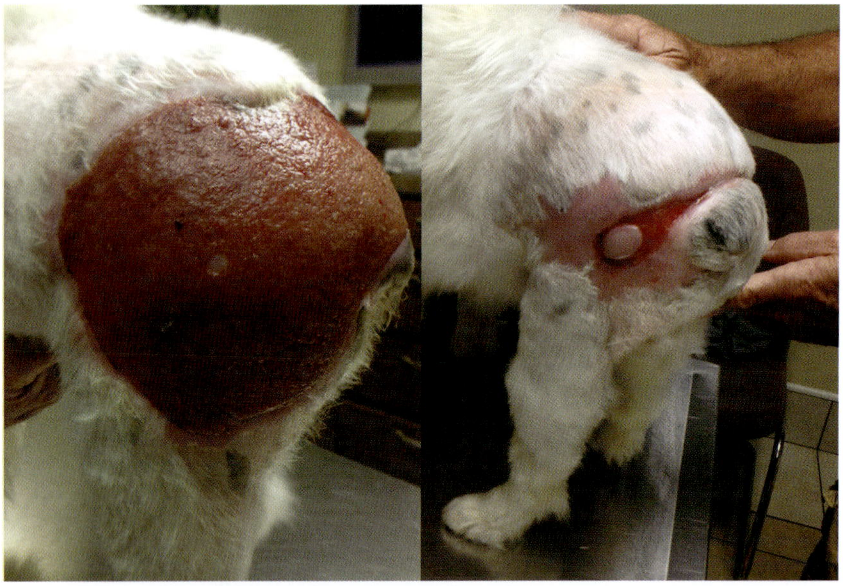

Figure 8.5 Progression of healing of the wound in Figure 8.4 at days 28 (left) and 56 (right) following standard open-wound management and laser therapy. Images courtesy of Dr. Daniel M. Core.

Figure 8.4 shows a patient with substantial sloughing of tissue over the left hip region 7 days after sustaining fight wounds. Laser therapy was initiated along with standard management appropriate for open wound healing by second intention. Figure 8.5 shows the healing wound at 28 and 56 days.

Degloving Injuries

Degloving injuries often require weeks of therapy to heal. PBMT will improve the granulation bed, the rate and quality of epithelialization, and help prevent infection. Regular laser therapy treatments, with proper bandaging and other management protocols, will greatly improve the success of full coverage, with minimal scarring. If tissue grafts or flaps are employed, laser therapy will enhance the survival and proliferation of the grafted tissue and heal the donor sites. Treat the entire area, as well as a generous margin of healthy tissue surrounding the denuded area. Stimulation of the contributing vasculature will be beneficial to tissue proliferation and graft survival. This can be accomplished by applying laser energy to the proximal or central blood supply. Begin at the axilla or groin, or at least one joint above the area of injury.

Follow the basic treatment principles and dosages as outlined earlier in this chapter. Deliver a starting dosage of 4–6 J/cm^2. Treat daily for 2–3 days if possible, then every other day. If no improvement is noted within the first two to four treatments, start increasing the dose by 25–50% per treatment until a positive response is noted. Do this by first adjusting the treatment time, then, if the treatment time is becoming too long, adjust the power upwards. In very large or severe wounds, treatment intervals may be decreased to twice weekly once the wound is showing strong positive clinical response, usually after 10–20 days.

Figure 8.6 shows a degloving injury to the distal medial aspect of the left front limb of a canine patient. There was also rupture and avulsion of the extensor carpi radialis tendon. Laser therapy was instituted after proper cleaning. Topical dressing with bandaging and a splint were applied. The progression of a healthy wound bed and rapid epithelial migration in the early stages are evident in the images. This wound healed completely within 6 weeks. The carpal joint also regained full strength and integrity.

Figures 8.7 and 8.8 are from a 20-year-old Morgan mare. Ten years prior, the mare degloved the entire anterior aspect of the right hind cannon region. This injury took 1 year and skin grafts for complete healing. The mare degloved the same area in the pictured case study. This new wound was managed in a similar fashion with the inclusion of laser therapy.

Vasculitis and Ischemia

Some wounds and tissue damage result from vasculitis or vascular damage and lead to tissue ischemia. Etiologies include infections, autoimmune disease, trauma, vascular occlusion, clotting disorders, and cardiovascular disease. Alternatively, the etiology may be idiopathic. The underlying pathology and contributing factors must be addressed with proper treatment. PBM is indicated, since it improves blood flow and circulation via the mechanisms discussed earlier: thermal gradients, vasodilation, and angiogenesis (Kubota, 2002). Laser therapy will also help regulate the inflammatory response and have a positive immunomodulating effect. Treat the affected area and the entire vascular branch involved, starting centrally and working peripherally.

Measure the wound area and the surrounding margin of healthy tissue. Follow the basic treatment principles and dosages as outlined earlier in this chapter. Deliver a starting dosage of 4–6 J/cm^2. Treat daily for 2–3 days if possible, then every other day. If no improvement is noted within the first two to four treatments, start increasing the dose (joules) by 25–50% per treatment until a positive response is noted. In very large or severe wounds, treatment intervals may be decreased to twice weekly once the wound is showing strong positive clinical response, usually after 10–20 days.

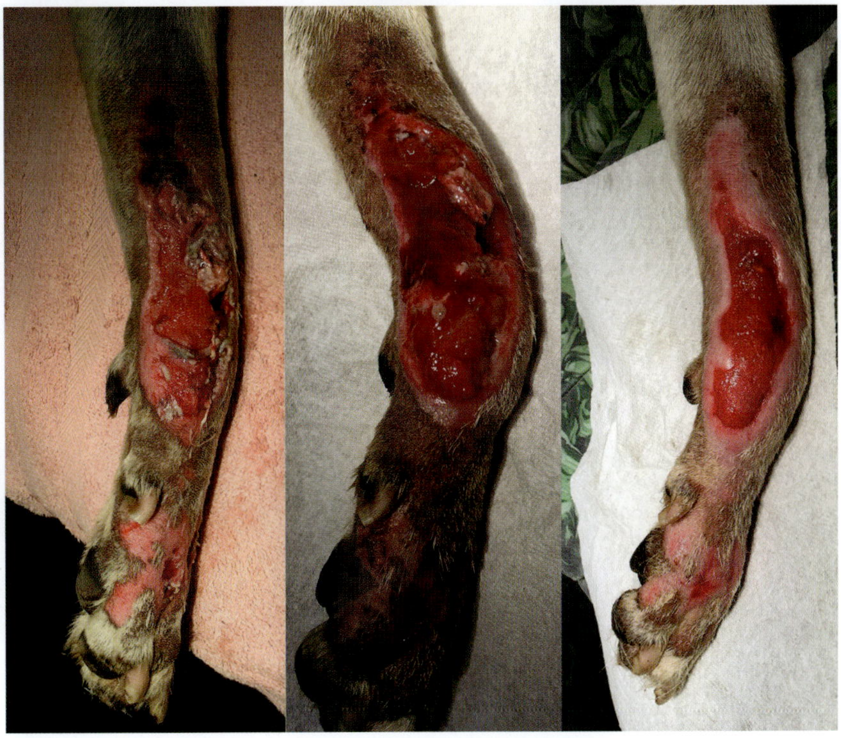

Figure 8.6 Degloving injury to the medial aspect of the distal foreleg at presentation (left), at 7 days (middle), and at 14 days (right). Images courtesy of Dr. Azeddine Menighed and Sandy Skouras, RVT.

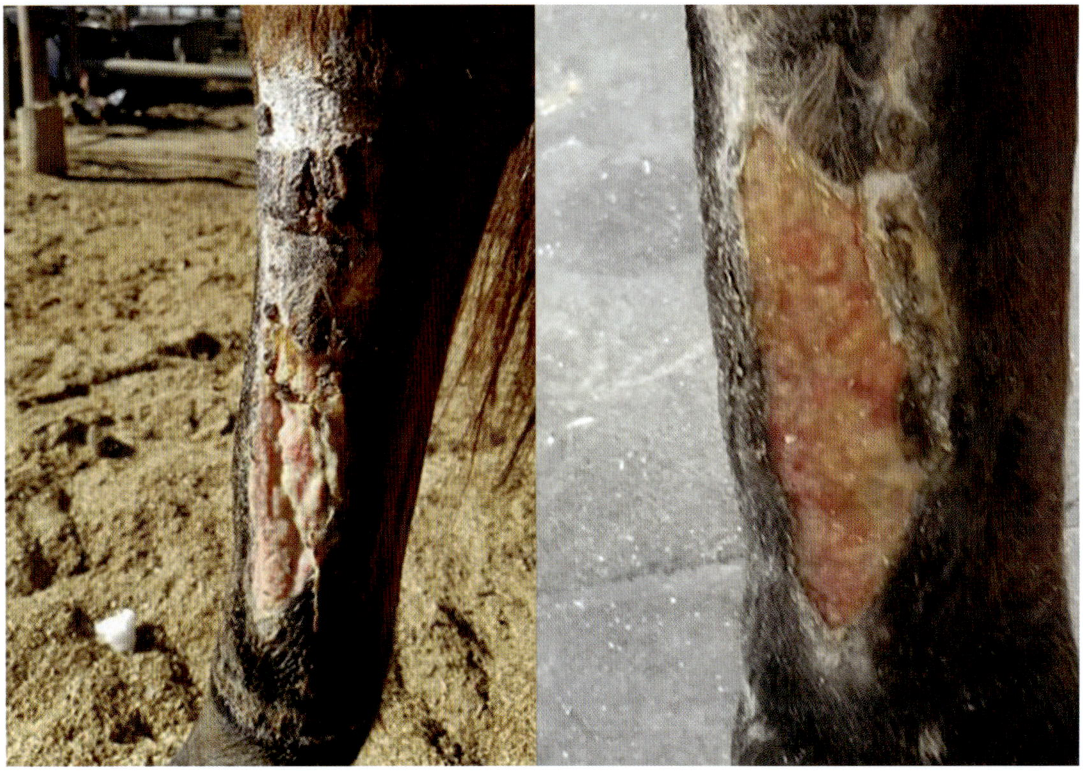

Figure 8.7 A traumatic wound that stripped the skin from the cannon bone (left). Traditional wound management was initiated along with laser therapy. The figure on right is just 2 days later. Images courtesy of Dr. Jody Hallstrom.

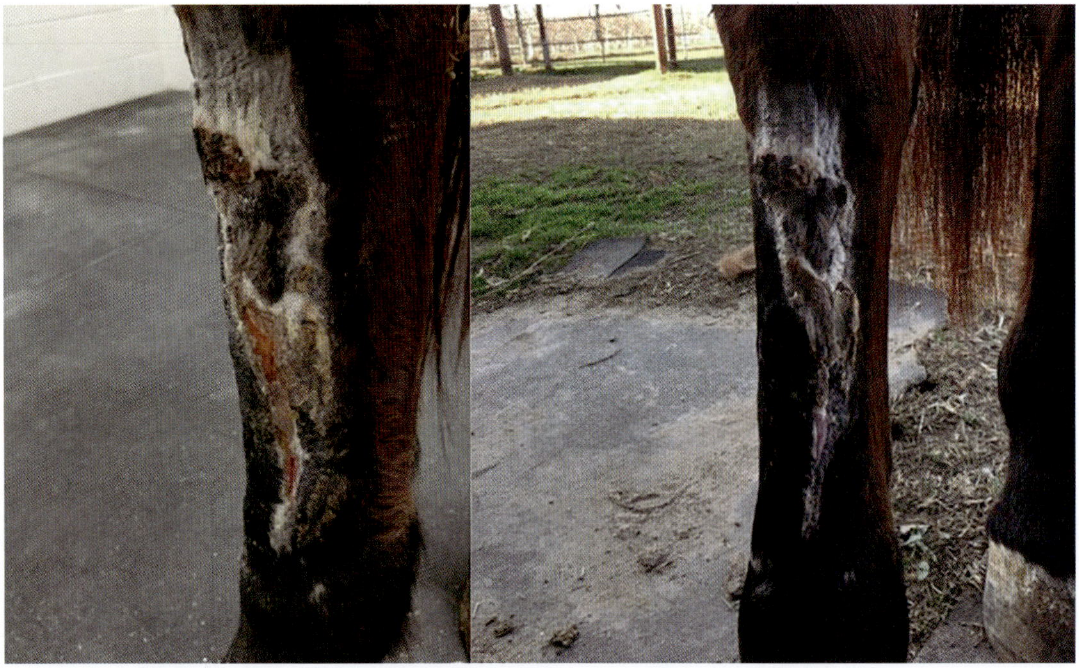

Figure 8.8 The same traumatic wound 6 weeks and 8 laser treatments later (left). The picture on the right shows the wound healed after only 8 weeks. Images courtesy of Dr. Jody Hallstrom.

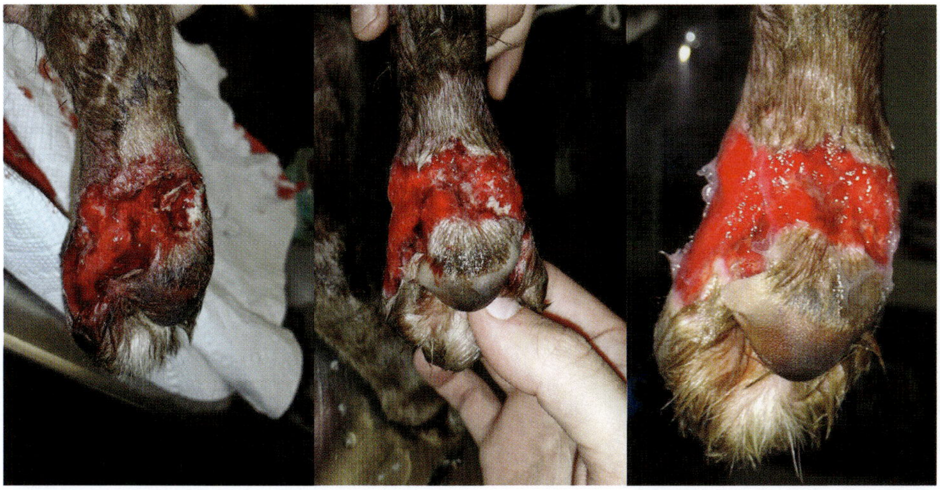

Figure 8.9 Traumatic wound that has been closed and dehisced (left). Traditional open-wound management and laser therapy were instituted. Rapid improvement was noted 1 (center) and 4 (right) days later, with the formation of a healthy granulation bed and significant epithelial migration. Images courtesy of Dr. Seth Narwold.

Figure 8.9 shows the early stages of healing in a fence trauma wound. The wound was initially debrided and sutured upon presentation. Due to vascular compromise, the wound devitalized and dehisced 5 days later. After cleaning and further debriding, laser therapy was instituted. The figure shows a rapid improvement, with the formation of a healthy granulation bed and improved epithelial margins. The wound progressed satisfactorily and was completely healed within 3 weeks.

Autoimmune, Allergic Conditions, Photosensitivity

Many autoimmune diseases have a dermatologic component as their primary clinical complaint or as part of the disease complex. Allergic reactions often manifest as a dermatologic problem. Systemic therapy is always warranted to help regulate the immune system, and laser therapy can be used to mitigate local dermatologic effects. Other topical and immunomodulating treatments should be used in conjunction with laser therapy (Gobbo *et al.*, 2012).

Photosensitivity is an immune system reaction triggered by the sun or other forms of UV radiation. Photosensitivity can develop as a result of certain drugs or medications, a medical condition or genetic disorder, or even topically applied products. Some plants contain compounds that, once absorbed into the blood stream, can react to UV exposure, and stimulate a photosensitivity reaction.

There are two distinct types of photosensitivity reactions: phototoxic and photoallergic. The phototoxic reaction is most common. As described above, an oral or topical medication is activated by exposure to UV light and causes damage to the skin. A photoallergic reaction is related to a topical product that the body recognizes as foreign. The immune system responds by producing antibodies which then attack the substance, causing a reaction.

Photosensitivity is universally associated with UV light. Although photosensitivity is listed as a precaution in many laser therapy texts, no problems have been encountered when delivering PBM using red and infrared wavelengths, making laser therapy an excellent adjunct in managing dermatologic photosensitivity reactions.

Follow the basic treatment principles and dosages as outlined earlier in this chapter. Treatment is initiated by delivering a starting dosage of 4–6 J/cm^2. Many outbreaks will improve or resolve completely. Recurrences are common if the underlying allergy or immune system dysfunction has not been corrected. Therefore, two options for ongoing treatment are recommended. For severe or frequent reactions, a routine prophylactic treatment can be performed every 2–4 weeks, depending on patient response. This will decrease the frequency and/or severity of future flareups. The owner can also be counseled to be vigilant in monitoring for any signs of recurrence; at the first sign of a flare-up, medications, and laser therapy are resumed to suppress the reaction and minimize the length and severity of outbreak.

Figure 8.10 shows the immediate anti-inflammatory effects that a laser can provide to an acute pyotraumatic dermatitis lesion.

Figures 8.11 and 8.12 are from a 6-year-old paint gelding that was presented initially with severe facial swelling and petechiation after ingesting stinging nettles. The patient

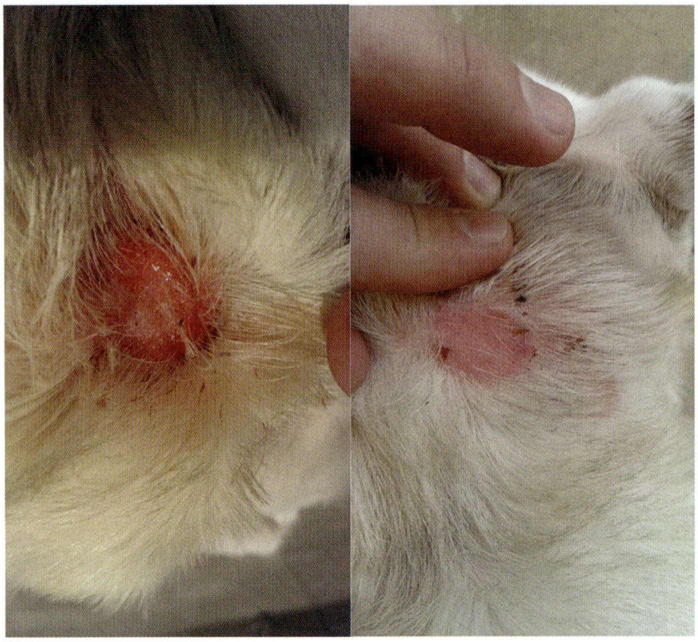

Figure 8.10 Acute pyotraumatic dermatitis lesion on presentation (left) and after therapy laser treatment (right). Images courtesy of Claus Walther.

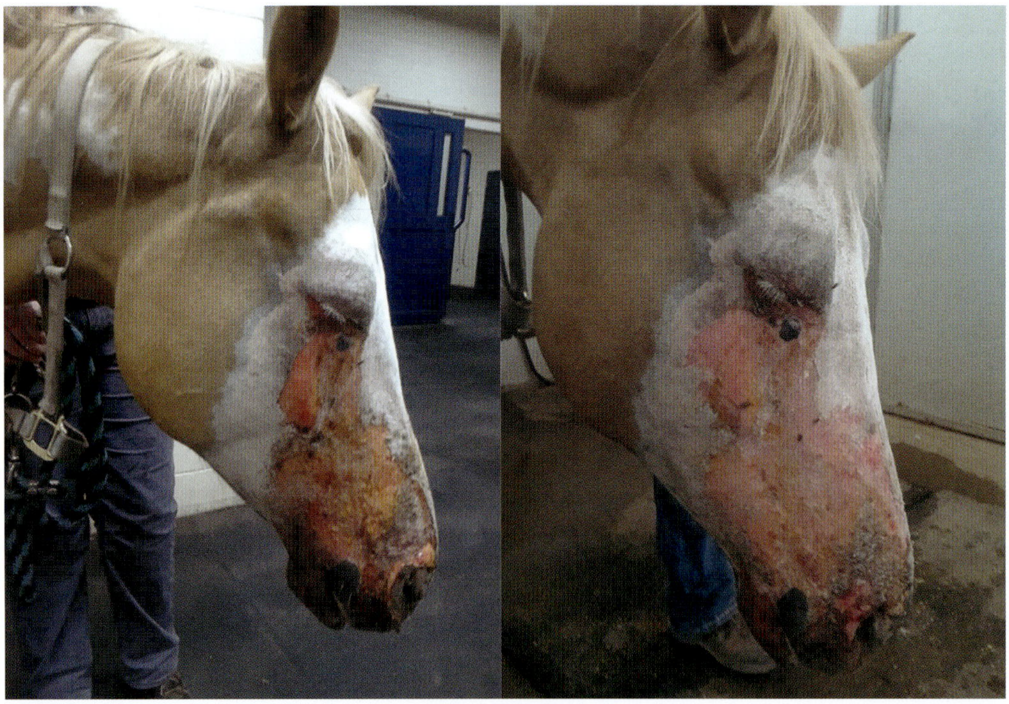

Figure 8.11 Photosensitivity reaction postexposure to stinging nettles, before laser therapy treatment (left), and one day post-initial laser treatment (right). Images courtesy of Dr. Jody Hallstrom.

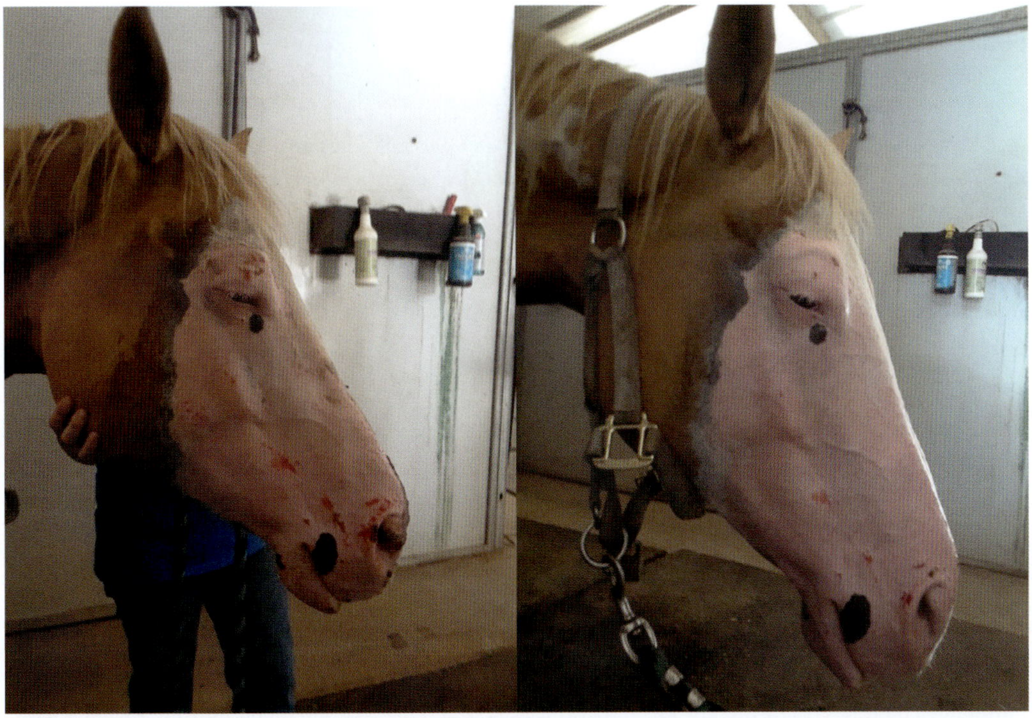

Figure 8.12 The same horse with photosensitivity reaction 6 days (left) and 8 days later (right). Images courtesy of Dr. Jody Hallstrom.

was violently uncomfortable, striking, and rolling on the ground. The patient was treated, responded well, and was returned to pasture. One week later, the patient presented again with a severe photosensitivity reaction confined strictly to the white-haired areas of the body. Liver enzymes were within normal limits. The patient was confined to a shady stall with daily cleaning and debriding of affected areas, and laser therapy was initiated.

Conclusion

Laser therapy can be a tremendous adjunct to your armamentarium for wound therapy (Hopkins *et al.*, 2004). When used appropriately, it can help both acute and chronic wounds heal more efficiently, with fewer complications. Keep in mind all the parameters and principles needed for optimal results, and your success rate will continue to grow.

References

Al-Watban, F.A.H. *et al.* (2007). Low-level laser therapy enhances wound healing in diabetic rats: a comparison of different lasers. *Photmed Laser Surg.* 25(2):72–77.

Anders, J.J. and Wu, X. (2015). Comparison of light penetration of 810 nm and 904 nm wavelength light in anesthetized rats. *Lasers Med Sci.* 30(8):2041.

Anderson, R.R. and Parrish, J.A. (1981). The optics of human skin. *J Invest Dermatol.* 77(1):13–19.

ANSI (2014). *American National Standard for Safe Use of Lasers. ANSI Z136.1 - 2014.* American National Standards Institute, Washington, DC.

Assis, L. *et al.* (2012). Low-level laser therapy (808 nm) reduces inflammatory response and oxidative stress in rat tibialis anterior muscle after cryolesion. *Lasers Surg Med.* 44(9):726–735.

Bayat, M. (2014). The necessity for increased attention to pulsed low-level laser therapy. *Photomed Laser Surg.* 32(8):1–2.

Brondon, P. (2009). Pulsing influences photoradiation outcomes in cell culture. *Lasers Surg Med.* 41(3):222–226.

Burger, E. *et al.* (2015). Low-level laser therapy to the mouse femur enhances the fungicidal response of neutrophils against *Paracoccidioides brasiliensis*. *PLoS NeglTrop Dis.* 9(2):e0003541.

Calisto, F.C. *et al.* (2015). Use of low-power laser to assist the healing of traumatic wounds. *Acta Cir Bras.* 30(3):204–208.

Cheida, A.A. *et al.* (2002). Resonance response of cell tissue structures to impulse frequency of infrared laser radiation of low intensity. *Vopr Kurortol Fizioter Lech Fiz Kult.* 6:33–35.

Chermetz, M. *et al.* (2014). Class IV laser therapy as treatment for chemotherapy-induced oral mucositis in onco-haematological paediatric patients: a prospective study. *Int J Paediatr Dent.* 6:441–449.

Doillon, C.J. *et al.* (1988). Relationship between mechanical properties and collagen structure of closed and open wounds. *J Biomech Eng.* 110(4):352–356.

Emanet, S.K. *et al.* (2010). Investigation of the effect of GaAs laser therapy on lateral epicondylitis. *Photomed Laser Surg.* 28(3):397–403.

Enwemeka, C.S. (2009). Intricacies of dose in laser phototherapy for tissue repair and pain relief. *Photomed Laser Surg.* 3:387–393.

Gal, P. *et al.* (2006). Histological assessment of the effect of laser irradiation on skin wound healing in rats. *Photomed Laser Surg.* 24(4):480–488.

Gobbo, M. *et al.* (2012). Acneifrom rash due to epidermal growth factor receptor inhibitors: high-level laser therapy as an innovative approach. *Lasers Med Sci.* 27(5): 1085–1090.

Gobbo, M. *et al.* (2014). Evaluation of nutritional status in head and neck radio-treated patients affected by oral mucositis: efficacy of class IV laser therapy. *Support Care Cancer.* 7:1851–1856.

Hamblin, M.R. and Demidova, T.N. (2006). Mechanisms of low level light therapy. *Proc of SPIE.* 6140(612001):1–12.

Hashmi, J. *et al.* (2010). Effect of pulsing in low-level light therapy. *Lasers Surg Med.* 42(6):450–466.

Hawkins, D. and Abrahamse, H. (2007). Phototherapy – a treatment modality for wound healing and pain relief. *African J Biomed Res.* 10:99–109.

Hodjati, H. *et al.* (2014). Low-level laser therapy: an experimental design for wound management: a case-controlled study in rabbit model. *J Cutan Aesthet Surg.* 7(1):14–17.

Hopkins, T.J. *et al.* (2004). Low-level laser therapy facilitates superficial wound healing in humans: a triple-blind, sham-controlled study. *J Ath Train.* 39(3):223–229.

Joensen, J. *et al.* (2012). Skin penetration and time-profiles for continuous 810nm and superpulsed 904nm lasers in a rat model. *Photomed Laser Surg.* 30(12):688–694.

Karu, T. (1989). *Photobiology of Low Power Laser Therapy.* Harwood Academic Publishers, London.

Karu, T. (1999). Primary and secondary mechanisms of action of visible to near-IR radiation on cells. *J Photochem Photobiol B.* 49(1):1–17.

Karu, T. and Kolyakov, S.F. (2005). Exact action spectra for cellular responses relevant to phototherapy. *Photomed Laser Surg.* 23(4):355–361.

Karu, T. *et al.* (1997). Nonmonotomic behavior of the dose dependence of the radiation effect on cells in vitro exposed to pulsed laser radiation at 820 nm. *Lasers Surg Med.* 21(5):485–492.

Karu, T. *et al.* (1999). Studies into the action specifics of a pulsed GaAlAS laser (820 nm) on a cell culture. *Lasers Life Sci.* 9:211–219.

Kaya, G.Ş. *et al.* (2011). The use of 808-nm light therapy to treat experimental chronic osteomyelitis induced in rats by methicillin-resistant *Staphylococcus aureus. Photomed Laser Surg.* 29(6):405–412.

Kovacs, K. (2015). Low level laser therapy of serious wounds of dogs. Poster presented at the ASLMS Annual Meeting, Orlando, FL (April 24–26, 2015).

Kubota, J. (2002). Effects of diode laser therapy on blood flow in axial pattern flaps in the rat model. *Lasers Med Sci.* 17(3):146–153.

Lanzafame, R.J. *et al.* (2007). Reciprocity of exposure time and irradiance on energy density during photoradiation on wound healing in a murine pressure ulcer model. *Lasers in Surg Med.* 39(6):534–542.

Larkin, K.A. *et al.* (2012). Limb blood flow after class 4 laser therapy. *J Ath Train.* 47(2):178–183.

Longo, L. *et al.* (1987). Effects of diode-laser silver arsenide-aluminum (Ga-Al-As) 904 nm on healing of experimental wounds. *Lasers Surg Med.* 7(5):444–447.

Martin, R. (2003). Laser accelerated inflammation/pain reduction and healing. *Pract Pain Manag.* 3(6):20–25.

Martz, E. and Steinberg, M.S. (1972). The role of cell-cell contact in "contact" inhibition of cell division: a review and new evidence. *J Cell Physio.* 79(2):189–210.

Meireles, G.C. *et al.* (2008). Effectiveness of laser photobiomodulation at 660 or 780 nanometers on the repair of third-degree burns in diabetic rats. *Photomed Laser Surg.* 26(1):47–54.

Mendez, T.M. *et al.* (2004). Dose and wavelength of laser light have influence on the repair of cutaneous wounds. *J Clin Laser Med Surg.* 22(1):19–25.

Mester, E. *et al.* (1968). The effect of laser beams on the growth of hair in mice. *Radiobiol Radiother (Berl).* 9(5):621–626.

Moriyama, Y. *et al.* (2009). In vivo effects of low level laser therapy on inducible nitric oxide synthase. *Lasers Surg Med.* 41(3):227–231.

Nussbaum, E.L. *et al.* (2003). Effects of low-level laser therapy (LLLT) of 810 nm upon in vitro growth of bacteria: relevance of irradiance and radiant exposure. *J Clin Laser Med Surg.* 21(5):283–290.

Ottaviani, G. *et al.* (2013). Effect of class IV laser therapy on chemotherapy-induced oral mucositis: a clinical and experimental study. *Am J Pathol.* 183(6):1747–1757.

Ottaviani, G. *et al.* (2015). *Study on Human Skin Fibroblasts and Data Related to ATP Content after Laser Exposure*

Compared to a Control Group. International Centre for Genetic Engineering and Biotechnology and the University of Trieste, Unpublished.

Paraguassu, G. *et al.* (2014). Effect of laser phototherapy (660nm) on type I and III collagen expression during wound healing in hypothyroid rats: an immunohistochemical study in a rodent model. *Photomed Laser Surg*. 32(5): 281–288.

Pavletic, M.M. (2010). *Basic principles of wound healing*. In: *Atlas of Small Animal Wound Management and Reconstructive Surgery*, 3 edn, pp. 18–28. Wiley-Blackwell, Hoboken, NJ.

Peavy, G.M. (2002). Lasers and laser-tissue interaction. *Vet Clin Small Anim*. 32(3):517–534.

Peplow, P.V. *et al.* (2010). Laser photobiomodulation of wound healing: a review of experimental studies in mouse and rat animal models. *Photomed Laser Surg*. 28(3):291–325.

Redondo, M.S. (2015). Laser therapy approach to wound healing in dogs. Available from: www.vettimes.co.uk/article/laser-therapy-approach-to-wound-healing-in-dogs/ (accessed November 30, 2016).

Silva, D.C. *et al.* (2013). Low level laser therapy (AlGaInP) applied at 5J/cm2 reduces the proliferation of *Staphylococcus aureus* MRSA in infected wounds and intact skin of rats. *An Bras Dermatol*. 88(1):50–55.

Skopin, M.D. and Molitor, S.C. (2009). Effects of near-infrared laser exposure in a cellular model of wound healing. *Photodermatol Photoimmunol Photomed*. 25(2):75–80.

Stadelman, W.K. *et al.* (1998). Physiology and healing dynamics of chronic cutaneous wounds. *Am J Surg*. 176(2A Suppl):26S–38S.

Stadler, I. *et al.* (2001). 830-nm irradiation increases the wound tensile strength in a diabetic murine model. *Lasers Surg Med*. 28(3):220–226.

Tuner, J. and Hode, L. (2002). Some basic laser physics. In: *Laser Therapy – Clinical Practice and Scientific Background*, pp. 12, 21–22. Prima Books AB, Grängesberg.

Tuner, J. and Hode, L. (2004). *The Laser Therapy Handbook*, pp. 78–80. Prima Books AB, New York.

Vasheghani, M.M. *et al.* (2008). Effect of low-level light therapy on mast cells in second-degree burns in rats. *Photomed Laser Surg*. 26(1):1–5.

Wood, V.T. *et al.* (2010). Collagen changes and realignment induced by low-level laser therapy and low-intensity ultrasound in the calcaneal tendon. *Lasers Med Surg*. 42(6):559–565.

Wray, S. *et al.* (1988). Characterization of the near infrared absorption spectra of cytochrome aa3 and haemoglobin for the non-invasive monitoring of cerebral oxygenation. *Biochim Biophys Acta*. 933(1):184–192.

9

Dermatological and Non-musculoskeletal Soft-Tissue Conditions

Christopher J. Winkler

Suffolk Veterinary Group Animal Wellness and Laser Surgery Center, Selden, NY, USA

1st Edition Contributors:

Daniel M. Core[1] *and John C. Godbold, Jr.*[2]

[1] *Airline Animal Health and Surgery Center, Bossier City, LA, USA*
[2] *Stonehaven Veterinary Consulting, Jackson, TN, USA*

Introduction

Early use of therapy lasers in veterinary medicine focused on the treatment of musculoskeletal disorders. The clinical success of veterinary practitioners treating musculoskeletal disorders with laser therapy (photobiomodulation therapy, PBMT) mirrors the evidence-based data being published about similar responses in animal-model studies and clinical trials with human patients (Bjordal *et al.*, 2008; Chow *et al.*, 2009; Jang and Lee, 2012; Assis *et al.*, 2016; de Carvalho *et al.*, 2016). As veterinarians have grown confident in the successful application of PBMT to the musculoskeletal system, they have begun to treat conditions involving other organ systems. Wounds and other skin and soft-tissue conditions are commonly used experimental models for ongoing research into the effects of photobiomodulation (PBM) (Hodjati *et al.*, 2014; Calisto *et al.*, 2015; Kovacs, 2015; Kuffler, 2016). Laser therapy has now become a standard of care for many practices in the treatment of many conditions involving the skin and other non-musculoskeletal soft tissues. Not surprisingly, the current experience of practitioners treating these disorders mirrors evidence being published (Peplow *et al.*, 2010; Avci *et al.*, 2013).

Skin makes up 12–24% of the total body weight and is the largest organ of the body. Dermatological complaints are the number one reason patients are presented for small-animal consultations (Hill *et al.*, 2006). Skin disorders, including ear problems, skin allergies, and pyoderma, are the top reasons for insurance claims in dogs, and number five in cats (PRNewswire, 2015). Patients with disorders of the skin and other non-musculoskeletal soft tissues thus make up a significant number of those that are candidates for laser therapy. In practices that are fully utilizing the capabilities of a therapeutic laser, these types of cases should represent a significant percentage of the overall number of cases treated with PBMT.

This chapter will focus on the most common conditions involving dermatological and non-musculoskeletal soft-tissue conditions for which laser therapy is indicated, with the exclusion of traumatic wounds, discussed in Chapter 8.

Laser therapy is indicated for virtually any condition that requires healing, reduction of pain, modulation of inflammation, acceleration of healing, and restoration of function (Chung *et al.*, 2012). It is compatible with traditional protocols for the treatment of skin and soft-tissue disorders, is noninvasive, and has minimal side effects if used properly. The complex mechanisms by which PBMT exerts these effects are discussed in detail in Chapter 3. This chapter will focus on the practical clinical application of PBMT in common, everyday conditions affecting dermatological and non-musculoskeletal soft tissues.

Acral Lick Dermatitis

Acral lick dermatitis, also known as lick granuloma, acral pruritic nodule, or canine neurodermatitis, is a common skin disorder in dogs. The lesions are the result of obsessive self-licking. The licking is a stereotypic behavior, a pattern of repetitive licking, repeated without variation, without any apparent purpose (Knol and Wisselink, 1996).

Laser Therapy in Veterinary Medicine: Photobiomodulation, Second Edition. Edited by Christopher J. Winkler and Lisa A. Miller.

Acral lick dermatitis usually begins as an area of inflamed alopecia. As the licking continues, the lesion increases in size and becomes thickened, and secondary bacterial infections are common. Acral lick dermatitis lesions can become deeply ulcerated and can range in size from small lesions a few centimeters in diameter to large masses. Lesions most commonly occur in the distal, dorsal surface of the fore and hind legs, but can occasionally occur on the flank and near the tail base (Ackerman, 2008a).

The etiology of acral lick dermatitis is not completely understood but is thought to be multifactorial. Potential causes include atopy, food allergy, bacterial folliculitis, behavior disorders, boredom, foreign-body penetration, local trauma, underlying musculoskeletal disorder, and peripheral neuropathy (Ackerman, 2008a; Rosychuk, 2011). Those individuals with behavioral- or psychogenic-induced acral lick dermatitis may have other accompanying behavioral disorders, such as separation anxiety or storm anxiety. Canine acral lick dermatitis has served as an animal model of obsessive–compulsive disorder (OCD) (Rapoport *et al.,* 1992). Secondary bacterial infections are common, with a 50% incidence of multi-drug-resistant organisms (Shumaker *et al.,* 2008).

Acral lick dermatitis is best managed with a multimodal therapeutic protocol. Treatment should be preceded by detailed diagnostics, including radiography, to try to determine the etiology. Extended use of an appropriate antibiotic based on culture and sensitivity is required, since lesions usually develop a deep pyoderma component with microabscesses and fistulas. Allergy testing and treatment with hyposensitization, avoidance, and anti-inflammatory drugs such as corticosteroids are often warranted. Bandages, Elizabethan collars, and leggings can be beneficial in limiting patient access to the lesions. Behavioral modification with medications, therapy, and change of environment can be helpful in those individuals suspected of having a behavioral etiology.

Laser therapy for acral lick dermatitis is most appropriately added to other forms of therapy. Practitioner experience indicates these dense, complex lesions require higher doses of laser therapy than are used for most conditions, and that treatment is required over an extended period of time. Laser settings that deliver 30–40 J/cm^2 are recommended. Treatment with the delivery handpiece in contact with the lesion will increase photon penetration into the tissue (Enwemeka, 2009).

Lesions should be treated through an induction phase, every other day or twice a week, with treatments coinciding with bandage changes. Note that laser therapy cannot be administered through a bandage: photons are absorbed and scattered by bandaging materials, resulting in an unpredictable dose reaching the target tissue.

Once a clinical response has been noted, treatment frequency can be reduced, through a transition phase. A complete resolution of acral lick dermatitis is not always possible. Lesions that persist should continue to be treated indefinitely, with maintenance-phase treatments every 3–4 weeks.

Moist Dermatitis, Hot Spots, and Pyotraumatic Dermatitis

Lesions of acute moist dermatitis, also known as pyotraumatic dermatitis or hot spots, result from self-trauma and are characterized by focal, moist, erythematous wounds with partial alopecia. There are multiple causes, including hypersensitivity due to flea allergy or atopy, trauma in the form of abrasions, foreign bodies, and in some cases behavior disorders. Heat and moisture act to exacerbate this condition. Progressive self-trauma often leads to rapidly enlarging lesions (Ackerman, 2008b).

Acute moist dermatitis can occur on any part of the body. In one study in 2004, males were overrepresented and 25 of 27 cases cultured grew *Staphylococcus intermedius* (Holm *et al.,* 2004). Traditional treatment includes clipping hair from the lesions and a border of normal skin around the lesion, local cleansing with a topical antimicrobial solution or shampoo, systemic corticosteroids, appropriate systemic antibiotics, and topical anti-inflammatory and antibiotic medications. The efficacy of a topical preparation containing a bacteriostatic antibiotic and a corticosteroid was compared to systemic therapy (comprising a combination of parenteral corticosteroid and an oral antibiotic) in the treatment of 104 dogs with acute moist dermatitis. Significant improvement was evident after 7 days in both treatment groups, and there was no significant difference in the overall response between the two groups (Cobb *et al.,* 2005).

Laser therapy can be a valuable adjunct to traditional topical or systemic therapeutics for acute moist dermatitis. In the authors' experience, when PBMT is used as an adjunct to topical or systemic therapy, or a combination of both, the lesions appear to resolve more quickly than with traditional therapy alone. Laser therapy rapidly reduces how painful these lesions are, and thus reduces patient obsession with the lesions and self-trauma. Edema, swelling, and inflammation are reduced. Complex photobiomodulatory mechanisms may also result in enhanced macrophage and neutrophil response against any microorganisms present (Burger *et al.,* 2015).

Acute moist dermatitis is normally treated, as its name implies, as an acute condition. Laser treatment normally follows clipping and cleaning during the initial patient presentation (Figure 9.1). Laser settings that deliver 3–4 J/cm^2 are

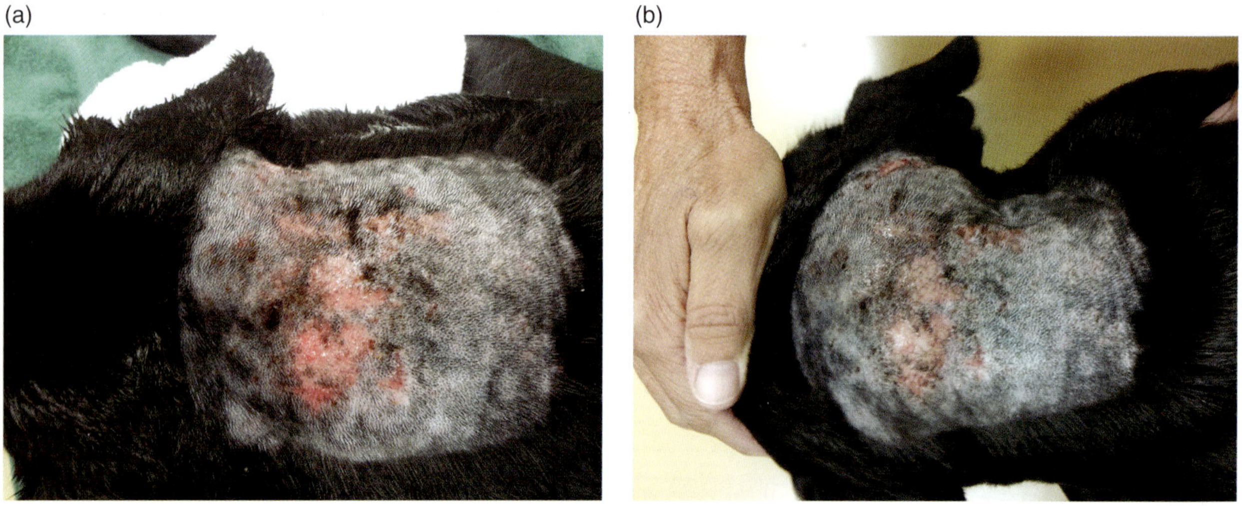

Figure 9.1 (a) Acute moist dermatitis after clipping and rinsing with sterile saline solution. (b) Reduced inflammation and dryness 3 hours after clipping, rinsing with sterile saline solution, and treating with laser therapy at 4 J/cm^2. Traditional pharmacological agents were withheld for 3 hours for observation of the effects of laser therapy.

recommended. The treatment should be delivered in a non-contact manner, with the delivery handpiece not touching the inflamed and contaminated tissue. Since the lesion is superficial, contact delivery, preferred for best photon penetration when treating deep-tissue conditions, is not necessary.

In most cases, clipping, cleaning, laser therapy, and an appropriate medical protocol result in rapid resolution. If the patient continues to self-traumatize, repeat laser therapy treatments are recommended every 24 hours until resolution. If areas of deeper pyoderma or cellulitis are noted, two to four additional every-other-day treatments are indicated.

Though laser therapy is recommended as an addition to traditional therapeutics for acute moist dermatitis, many practitioners find that its addition eliminates or reduces the need for systemic and topical corticosteroids. Practitioners are encouraged to monitor the effects of adding laser therapy to their traditional protocol and to adjust the protocol accordingly.

Anal Sacculitis and Anal Sac Abscess

The anal sacs, sometimes erroneously referred to as "anal glands," are a pair of sacs lined with sebaceous glands located between the internal and external anal sphincter muscles at the 4 and 8 o'clock positions. They are connected to the exterior via the anal sac ducts, which empty at the 3 and 9 o'clock positions near the anal mucocutaneous junction.

The exact function of the anal sacs is not completely understood. Normal anal sac secretions are liquid, clear to translucent, and often pale yellow in color. Abnormal secretions are thicker in consistency, dark brown in color when impaction has occurred, and pus-colored when infection is present (Halnan, 1976a). The secretions are thought to be involved in territory marking, serving as a form of communication.

Anal sacs are normally emptied by compression of the anal sphincter muscles during a bowel movement, depositing a small amount of anal sac secretion on the feces. Clinical problems usually occur when there is incomplete emptying of the sacs during bowel movement. This results in anal sac impaction and discomfort. A survey of over 3000 dogs presented to two practices, one in England and one in Australia, indicated that 12.5% were affected with some degree of anal sac disease (Halnan, 1976b).

Possible causes of anal sac impaction are hypersecretion of sebaceous glands, constipation, chronic diarrhea, laxity of anal sphincters, narrowing of the anal sac ducts, imperforate ducts, and food allergy (van Duijkeren, 1995). Untreated anal sac impaction can lead to pain, constipation, and self-trauma in the form of licking and rubbing or dragging the perineum. Diagnosis of anal sacculitis is based on history and physical examination. Physical examination should include a rectal examination, with expression of the anal sacs and examination of their contents, as well as careful palpation for masses (Culp, 2012). Findings from analysis of anal sac secretions show no statistically significant cytological differences between secretions from normal dogs and those with anal sac disease. Thus, cytology appears to be an ineffective tool for diagnosing anal sac disease (James *et al.*, 2011).

Acute anal sacculitis, usually a result of short-term impaction, often responds to simple expression of the affected sac. In addition to the discomfort and inflammation present in the anal sac area, patients presenting with acute anal sacculitis may have superficial perianal abrasions from scooting and self-trauma, and may have localized areas of skin irritation around the tail base from licking and chewing. Manual expression of the sacs during rectal palpation may induce increased discomfort and inflammation.

Laser therapy can significantly reduce the pain and inflammation of acute anal sacculitis, and is an excellent alternative to corticosteroids in preventing continued symptoms. Laser settings that deliver 6–8 J/cm^2 are recommended, using either contact or noncontact delivery. This dose is appropriate for secondary, superficial lesions, as well as for somewhat deeper anal sacs and the tissue that surrounds them. Most acute anal sac impactions resolve quickly after expression and treatment, and require no further treatment. Anecdotal information from practitioners indicates that performing laser therapy prior to anal sac expression may reduce patient discomfort and resistance, facilitating easier expression.

Chronic anal sacculitis presents a far more difficult therapeutic challenge. Cases often present intermittently with impaction, marked inflammation, bacterial infection of the sacs, and large amounts of noxious, purulent secretions. Systemic antibiotics, anti-inflammatories, and pain medications are indicated, along with repeated manual expression, flushing, and packing of the sacs. Laser therapy should be added to recommended medical protocols for chronic anal sacculitis. As with acute anal sacculitis, laser settings that deliver 6–8 J/cm^2 are recommended, using either contact or noncontact delivery.

Chronic cases should be treated through an induction phase, every other day or twice a week, with treatments coinciding with expression of the sacs. Once a clinical response has been noted, treatment frequency can be reduced through a transition phase, gradually extending the time between treatments. A complete resolution of anal sacculitis is not always possible. Patients with symptoms that persist or reoccur frequently should continue to be treated indefinitely, with maintenance- phase treatments every 3–4 weeks. Administration of maintenance-phase PBMT long-term treatments can, in some cases, control symptoms and flare-ups sufficiently to avoid surgical excision of the sacs.

If anal sac impaction is not resolved, abscess formation can result, accompanied by cellulitis and fistulous tracts. Anal sac abscesses should be managed with traditional incision and drainage, debridement and flushing, and systemic and topical medications (Figure 9.2). Additionally, as with any abscess or deep-tissue infection, treatment with laser therapy is recommended. Because deeper and more extensive tissues are usually affected when anal sacs abscess, laser settings that deliver 8–10 J/cm^2 are recommended. Treatment should be administered daily for 2–3 days, then on alternate days for three or four more sessions, or until the cellulitis and fistulous tracts have healed.

(a) (b)

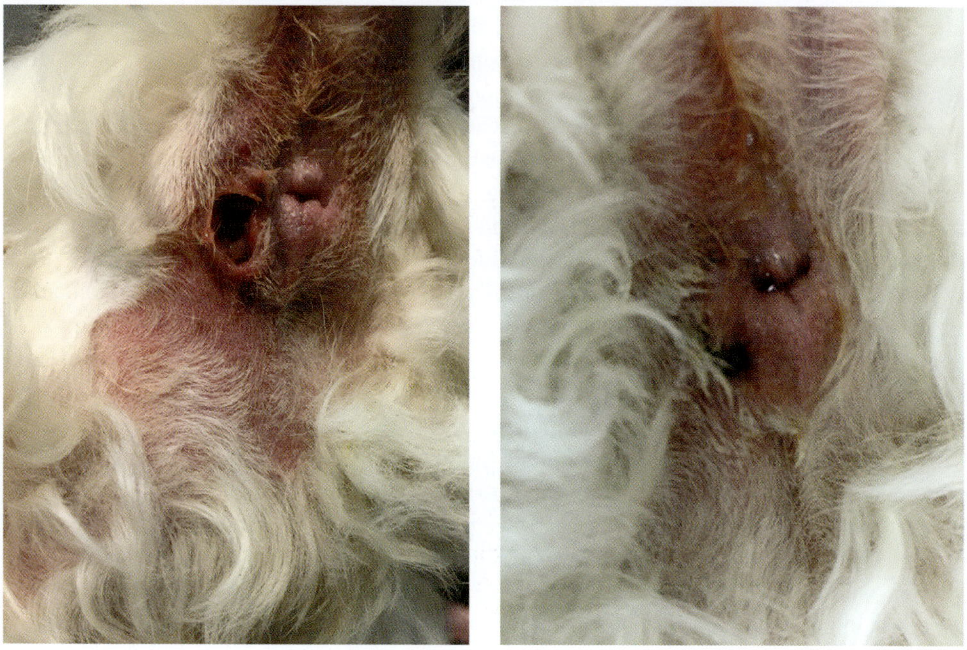

Figure 9.2 (a) Anal sac abscess on initial presentation. In addition to traditional therapeutics, anal sac abscesses should be treated with laser therapy daily for 2–3 days, with laser settings that deliver 8–10 J/cm^2. (b) Anal sac abscess 7 days after initial laser therapy treatment.

Aural Hematoma

Aural hematoma is a collection of blood between the cartilage of the pinna and the skin. The exact cause of this condition is unknown; however, it is often observed in conjunction with acute or chronic otitis. Excessive head shaking and scratching accompanying otitis can result in an aural hematoma, as can direct trauma to the pinna.

Predisposing otitis must be addressed when treating aural hematomas. Untreated, aural hematomas undergo a slow healing process in which the hematoma clot is absorbed and fibroses and the pinna heals with a classical cauliflower appearance (MacPhail, 2016).

The list of therapeutic options for treating aural hematomas reflects the ingenuity of veterinary practitioners. Historically, these hematomas have been treated by incision and drainage, with an incision from proximal to distal along the full length of the hematoma, followed by multiple suture placements through the full thickness of the ear and over-the-head bandaging for 2–3 weeks (Brown, 2010). This technique is successful, but the slow healing and extended bandaging time are uncomfortable for both the patient and the owner, and make addressing predisposing otitis difficult. Partial-thickness suture placement has been suggested as an alternative closure (Győrffy and Szijártó, 2014).

Other therapeutic approaches have resulted in varying degrees of success. The application of fibrin sealant between the cartilage layers has been successful in humans, but proved unsuccessful in a reported canine case (Blättler, 2007). Use of the CO_2 laser to produce a drain hole, followed by multiple punctate incisions over the hematoma surface to stimulate adhesions, has been reported (Dye *et al.*, 2002). Incision and laterally placed vacuum drains resulted in excellent cosmetic results in four of five patients (Pavletic, 2015). Treatment with parenteral drainage and intralesion injection of corticosteroids is sometimes attempted with variable success.

The reported effect of laser therapy on other types of hematomas suggests that it can be a valuable tool in managing aural hematomas. Laser therapy improves circulation, enhances hematoma absorption, and accelerates degradation of fibrin in post-surgical hematomas (Takashi, 1988). Anecdotal reports from practitioners indicate that laser therapy appears to be efficacious when added to a number of different aural hematoma management protocols. Laser therapy can be combined with traditional drainage and surgical tacking with or without bandaging. If a bandage is employed, it must be removed prior to laser treatment.

One author (Core) combines laser therapy with surgical placement of a drain at the most dependent portion of the hematoma. A small, round incision, 3–5 mm in diameter, is created with a CO_2 laser at the most dependent portion of the hematoma. The contents are drained and the hematoma is flushed with sterile saline. A small tube, such as a 16–18-gauge polypropylene catheter or teat tube, is inserted in the drain hole and secured with stay sutures. The pinna is treated with laser therapy at a dose of 3–6 J/cm^2 immediately after surgery, and then every third day until healing is complete. Patients seldom require a bandage. The drain tube is usually removed 10 days post-surgically. Healing with minimal fibrosis and a pleasant cosmetic appearance is expected.

Another author (Godbold) recommends a similar technique in lieu of drain tube placement. In this technique, drainage is accomplished by aspiration with a 16–18-gauge needle, a 5–7 mm biopsy punch, or a 5–7 mm CO_2 laser incision at the most dependent portion of the hematoma, followed by laser therapy (3–6 J/cm^2) and a light pressure bandage. The bandage is changed every 2–3 days, with repeated aspiration as required, and laser therapy while the bandage is off. With this technique, healing is expected in 10–14 days.

Bacterial Folliculitis

Bacterial folliculitis is the most frequently encountered form of pyoderma in dogs (Lloyd, 2012). It is more common in dogs than any other mammalian species. The etiology in the majority of cases is *Staphylococcus pseudoepidermititis*. Infection is a result of disruption of the skin barrier. Located within the hair follicle, this bacterial infection causes inflammation in and around the follicle, and appears as multifocal areas of alopecia, follicular papules or pustules, epidermal collarettes, and serous crusts. Pruritus is frequently present. There are a multitude of underlying conditions that lower the skin's defense to bacterial infection. Cushing's disease, diabetes mellitus, hypothyroidism, anatomical disorders such as skin folds, immune deficiencies, allergies, and parasites such as *Demodex canis* and *Sarcoptes scabiei* can adversely predispose individuals to bacterial folliculitis.

Historically, the first-line response to bacterial folliculitis has been systemic administration of a potentiated amoxicillin, a first-generation cephalosporin, or a potentiated sulfonamide. Currently, methicillin-resistant *Staphylococcus pseudintermedius* and *Staphylococcus aureus* (MRSA) are becoming more prevalent in canine bacterial folliculitis (Sousa, 2013). Regrettably, the emergence of these multiresistant bacteria means that multimodal management of bacterial folliculitis is indicated (Bloom, 2014). Recent updated guidelines have been published for the diagnosis and antimicrobial therapy of canine bacterial folliculitis (Hillier *et al.*, 2014).

As practitioners adopt more comprehensive, multimodal protocols to treat bacterial folliculitis, PBMT should be included. Laser treatment will reduce inflammation and pruritus, reducing self- trauma. Additionally, multiple studies, using multiple laser wavelengths, suggest laser therapy application is indicated for bacterial infections (Nussbaum *et al.*, 2002, 2003; Silva *et al.*, 2013). In a 2009 study, a near-infrared (870 and 930 nm) laser was demonstrated to produce photoinactivation of *S. aureus*, *Escherichia coli*, *Candida albicans*, and *Trichophyton rubrum* at physiologic temperatures (Bornstein *et al.*, 2009). Equally promising, though not yet available clinically, is the use of lasers with photosensitizers to photodeactivate bacteria (St. Denis *et al.*, 2011; Alves *et al.*, 2014).

Research has also shown that laser therapy enhances healing. A 2016 review indicated that wound healing is stimulated by many different wavelengths and powers, but that optimal parameters are still being identified (Kuffler, 2016). In patients with an endocrinopathy (diabetes mellitus), laser therapy has been shown to increase the rate of healing (Al-Watban *et al.*, 2007; Minatel *et al.*, 2009). As practitioners turn to multimodal management of bacterial folliculitis, any possible laser therapy effect is welcome.

Multimodal therapy for bacterial folliculitis includes culture and sensitivity, treatment with an appropriate systemic antibiotic, topical therapeutics, identification and management of any underlying disorders, and laser therapy. Laser settings that deliver 3–4 J/cm^2 are recommended, using a noncontact delivery to reduce the possibility of contamination of the handpiece and subsequent nosocomial infections. Since large areas of skin may be involved, treatment times can become prolonged. The laser power may be increased to reduce treatment time as long as the speed of movement of the handpiece and laser beam increases. Likewise, to reduce treatment time, pulsed delivery can be turned off by setting the laser in a continuous delivery mode. Initial treatment daily or every other day for three to five treatments should be followed by twice-weekly treatments until the folliculitis is resolved.

Canine Noninflammatory Alopecia

Canine noninflammatory alopecia is a heterogeneous group of skin disorders with different underlying pathogeneses. In a significant deviation from normal canine hair follicle physiology, the basis of noninflammatory alopecia is a defect in the formation of the hair follicle or a failure of the follicle to continually cycle (Welle *et al.*, 2016). The alopecia results as hair is gradually lost, follicles remain inactive, and no new hair grows. The common and distinguishing histological characteristic is a marked increase in kenogen follicles, indicating that the induction of the new anagen phase is impaired (Müntener *et al.*, 2012). Seasonal flank alopecia, alopecia X, color-mutant alopecia, and other causes of follicular dysplasia are examples of canine noninflammatory alopecia. The therapeutic approach is challenging, and new treatment options are desirable.

As is noted elsewhere in this book, the first report of what we now know as PBM was in 1968, when Endre Mester and his colleagues reported their observations of the effect of laser beams on the growth of hair in mice (Mester *et al.*, 1968). More-rapid-than-expected hair growth is often reported by veterinarians after treating patients in which hair has been clipped and the area treated with laser therapy.

Current publications support these anecdotal observations by veterinarians, as well as the observations published by Mester and his colleagues nearly 50 years ago, that laser light stimulates hair growth. Laser therapy treatment accelerated hair regrowth in a rat model of chemotherapy-induced alopecia (Wikramanayake *et al.*, 2013). A 2016 evidence-based review analyzed studies reporting the effects of laser therapy on hair regrowth, finding positive responses (Zarei *et al.*, 2016). A 2015 pilot study reported promising results of laser therapy on hair regrowth in canine noninflammatory alopecia (Olivieri *et al.*, 2015). Patients were treated twice a week for a maximum of 2 months with a combination of 470, 685, and 830 nm laser light at a dose of 3 J/cm^2. At the end of the study, hair regrowth was significantly improved in six of seven animals and showed some improvement in the remaining one. Treatment using photobiomodulation in a case of hair cycle arrest in a Pembroke Welsh Corgi has also been reported (Bello *et al.*, 2022).

Enough evidence exists to warrant clinical treatment of canine noninflammatory alopecia by practitioners. A suggested protocol is twice-weekly treatment at a dose of 3 J/cm^2, with treatments continued until hair growth is noted. Since deep-photon penetration is not required, treatment using a noncontact delivery, with the laser beam spread out over a larger area, is appropriate.

Deep-Tissue Infections, Abscesses, and Cellulitis

Skin and soft-tissue infections are common, with complicated, deep-tissue infections being the most extreme and presenting the greatest challenge. Deep-tissue infections, abscesses, and cellulitis frequently begin with some degree of dermatological involvement or penetration, followed by extension of the infection into the deeper tissues. A variety of bacterial and fungal agents may be involved.

As an abscess develops, the abscess wall that is formed by adjacent healthy cells (in an attempt to keep pus from infecting neighboring structures) creates an encapsulation. If not contained to a focal area and encapsulated, infection spreads between tissue planes, producing cellulitis. Draining fistulous tracts may or may not develop. Pain, erythema, swelling, and edema increase as the infection spreads.

Successful management involves prompt recognition, timely surgical drainage, appropriate antimicrobial therapy, and pain management. In addition to this traditional management protocol, laser therapy is indicated to help reduce the pain, swelling, and edema, to stimulate host response to the microbial infection, and to accelerate the healing process. The mechanisms by which laser therapy exert PBM effects are similar in deep-tissue infections to those in more superficial infections. These mechanisms have been mentioned previously in this chapter.

Deep-tissue infections generally require a higher laser therapy dose and a longer course of therapy, due to the depth of the involved tissue and the degree of inflammatory changes present. While more superficial infections require laser settings that deliver 3–5 J/cm^2, infections involving the subcutaneous tissue require a higher dose of 6–8 J/cm^2, and infections extending even deeper into tissue require 8–10 J/cm^2 (Box 9.1). Treatment should be administered daily for 2–3 days, and then on alternate days until the infection is resolved. If bandages are being used, treatment should coincide with bandage removal. If the infection is open and draining, use a noncontact delivery to reduce the possibility of contamination of the handpiece and subsequent nosocomial infections. Use a contact delivery if drainage is not present, contamination of the handpiece is not a concern, and patient sensitivity allows touching of the affected area.

Though not a result of microbial infection, juvenile cellulitis is a candidate for the immune-modulating effects of PBM (Figure 9.3). This uncommon granulomatous and pustular disorder of the face, pinnae, and submandibular lymph nodes is most often seen in puppies (White *et al.*, 1989). Aspirates of lesions usually reveal pyogranulomatous inflammation with no microorganisms (Reimann *et al.*, 1989). Cultures are negative. Since the condition responds to high, short-term doses of corticosteroids, an immune etiology is suspected (Hutchings, 2003). Treat affected areas of the skin with laser therapy doses of 6–8 J/cm^2, as the lesions frequently coalesce and become deep. Treat the affected regional lymph nodes with deep-tissue doses of 8–10 J/cm^2 (Box 9.1). Early treatment is important to reduce long-term scarring. Daily treatments should be administered until the lesions and lymphadenopathy resolve.

Box 9.1 Dermatological and Non-musculoskeletal Soft-tissue-condition Treatment Doses

Acral Lick Dermatitis
30–40 J/cm^2

Acute Moist Dermatitis
3–4 J/cm^2

Anal Sacculitis
6–8 J/cm^2

Anal Sac Abscess
8–10 J/cm^2

Aural Hematoma
3–6 J/cm^2

Bacterial Folliculitis
3–4 J/cm^2

Canine Noninflammatory Alopecia
3 J/cm^2

Deep-Tissue Infections, Abscesses, and Cellulitis
Superficial: 3–5 J/cm^2
Subcutaneous: 6–8 J/cm^2
Deep tissue: 8–10 J/cm^2

Elbow Hygroma
30–40 J/cm^2

Otitis Externa
Superficial component: 3–4 J/cm^2
Deep component: 8–10 J/cm^2
Deep component with severe hyperplasia: 10–20 J/cm^2

Perianal Fistulas
12–14 J/cm^2

Pododermatitis
6–8 J/cm^2

Elbow Hygroma

A hygroma is a fluid-filled cavity surrounded by a connective-tissue capsule over a bony prominence or pressure point. The elbow is the most common location, but hygromas can occur over any bony prominence. In younger individuals, elbow hygromas are thought to be a response to trauma. In older patients, hygromas tend to occur with impaired ambulation and excessive time spent in recumbency on hard surfaces. A soft, fluctuant, fluid-filled swelling develops, which, with continued trauma, can develop ulceration, infection, abscess formation, fistulous tracts, and proliferative granulomatous tissue.

The pathogenesis of elbow hygroma formation and a number of management protocols have been well reported.

(a) (b)

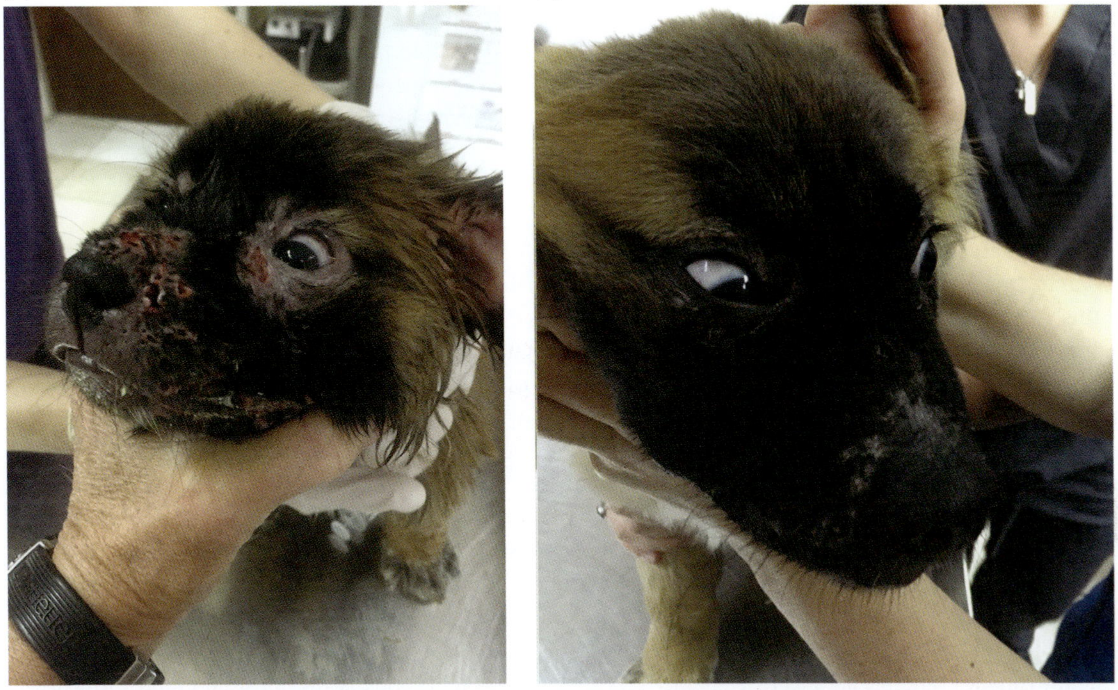

Figure 9.3 (a) Juvenile cellulitis, a candidate for the immune-modulating effects of PBM (affected areas of the skin are treated with laser therapy doses of 6–8 J/cm^2, and the affected regional lymph nodes with doses of 8–10 J/cm^2). (b) Resolution of juvenile cellulitis after 12 days of prednisone (2.2 mg/kg/day) and the immune-modulating effect of PBM. Early resolution of lesions helps reduce scarring.

Aspiration, injection with anti-inflammatory medications, surgical drainage, excision, and a variety of protective bandaging options have been recommended (Newton *et al.*, 1974; Johnston, 1975; Canapp *et al.*, 2012). Treatment is often frustrating, and surgical options are usually avoided as they result in frequent complications. Recently, closed suction drain management was reported to be a simple, economical, and successful method of collapsing an elbow hygroma (Pavletic and Braum, 2015).

Laser therapy can aid in the management of elbow hygroma. Lasers reduce inflammation and edema and stimulate healing processes. As in laser therapy treatment of hematomas, increased circulation, and fibrin degradation should contribute to improvement (Takashi, 1988).

Laser therapy for elbow hygromas is most appropriately added to other forms of therapy. The use of padded bandages and laser therapy is indicated well before surgical intervention is considered. Practitioner experience indicates these dense, complex lesions require higher doses of laser therapy than are used for most conditions, and that treatment is required over an extended period of time. Laser settings that deliver 30–40 J/cm^2 are recommended. Treatment with the delivery handpiece in contact with the hygroma will increase photon penetration into the tissue.

Hygroma should be treated through an induction phase, every other day or twice a week, with treatments coinciding with removal and change of the padded bandage. Once a clinical response has been noted, treatment frequency can be reduced, through a transition phase, gradually extending the time between treatments. A complete resolution of an elbow hygroma is not always possible. Lesions that persist should continue to be treated indefinitely, with maintenance-phase treatments administered every 3–4 weeks, along with continued protection of the elbow.

Otitis Externa

Otitis is one of the most common reasons for small-animal veterinary consultations. Though acute otitis is often treated successfully with quick results, chronic otitis can be very difficult to manage successfully. Laser therapy can be an important adjunct in the management of both acute and chronic otitis.

Otitis has multiple factors that can contribute to, promote, and predispose individuals to ear infection. In dogs, the ear anatomy, with a long external ear canal and an "L" shape, makes them prone to otitis. The primary and secondary causes of otitis have been well identified in ear-disease texts (Gotthelf, 2004), as well as general dermatology texts.

In virtually all cases of acute otitis, the inflammatory changes produce edema and swelling of the epithelium of the ear canal. The canal narrows, moisture and debris are retained, and infections by bacteria, yeast, and fungi quickly follow. Chronic otitis causes hyperplastic changes within and around the ear canal that result in a permanently narrowed meatus. Traditional diagnostics include identification of primary and secondary causes, physical examination, otoscopy, and cytology.

Often, the ear canal is occluded with wax, hair, and inflammatory debris. The narrowed meatus and debris can make otoscopy and sample collection for cytology painful and difficult. Using laser therapy to reduce pain and swelling in the canal can facilitate otoscopic procedures that visualize, flush, and clean the ear in anesthetized patients. This allows better visualization of the tympanic membrane, to rule out middle- or inner-ear infection or a space-occupying mass. Laser therapy, along with improved otoscopic instrumentation and advanced imaging with radiographs and computed tomography (CT) scans, can contribute to a more accurate diagnosis.

Following a complete diagnostic workup, a multimodal management is recommended for otitis. A number of topical and systemic medications have been recommended that address the pain, swelling, and microbial infections normally present. Laser therapy can be a valuable adjunct to available medical protocols. The rapid reduction of pain from laser therapy increases patient tolerance of topical treatment, and the reduction of epithelial swelling allows more effective penetration of topical medication to the target tissue.

When treating otitis with a therapy laser, two components – or anatomical areas – must be addressed. The first is the affected portion of the pinna and the visible, more distal portion of the ear canal. These tissues should be treated with a laser setting that delivers 3–4 J/cm^2 and are most commonly treated with a noncontact delivery. The second component is the more proximal portion of the ear canal, including most of the vertical and the entire horizontal canal. This deeper tissue component requires a higher target dose of 8–10 J/cm^2 and is treated with a contact delivery (see Box 9.1).

With acute presentations of otitis externa, laser therapy can be incorporated into the initial visit, facilitating diagnostics and enhancing the overall management protocol. Laser therapy treatments are short enough (8–10 minutes) that treatment can be included during an outpatient consultation. Response to initial treatment is often sufficient that further treatment is not required. If pain and swelling persist, continue laser therapy treatments daily until resolved.

With chronic otitis, thickening of the ear canal epithelium and hyperplastic changes in the cartilage dictate a more prolonged management and a much poorer prognosis. Laser therapy is indicated in these cases, but the long-term goal becomes one of pain reduction and improved quality of life, rather than complete resolution. In these cases, because of the dense and chronic tissue changes, treatment of the deep-tissue component requires a laser setting that delivers 10–20 J/cm^2.

Chronic otitis should be treated through an induction phase, every other day or twice a week, until a reduction in pain and an improvement of quality of life are noted. Once a clinical response is noted, treatment frequency can be reduced, through a transition phase, gradually extending the time between treatments. Long-term maintenance-phase treatments are recommended every 3–4 weeks.

Pemphigus

Pemphigus is an autoimmune disease that results in the formation of bullous lesions of the skin or mucous membranes, or both (Figure 9.4). Patients form autoantibodies against desmogleins that are transmembrane glycoproteins. The breakdown of desmogleins disrupts the adhesion between keratinocytes and results in the formation of detached keratinocytes called "acanthylotic cells." This disruption of the normal connections between the squamous cells of the epidermis causes fragile, superficial, intraepidermal bullae.

Pemphigus foliaceous is the most common form of the disease in dogs and cats. It causes crusts and large pustules, primarily on the face, ears, and feet. The lesions are usually bilaterally symmetrical. Pemphigus vulgaris is much less common in dogs, and has only rarely been reported in cats. It differs from pemphigus foliaceous in that the lesions involve mucous membranes and mucocutaneous junctions. Pemphigus vulgaris is usually more difficult to treat (Olivry and Linder, 2009; Blair *et al.,* 2015).

Treatment of pemphigus requires immune suppression, which normally begins with high doses of glucorticosteroids (Bizikova and Olivry, 2015). Multimodal pharmacological therapy is recommended for long-term maintenance, to help reduce the reliance on glucorticosteroids. The analgesic and immune-modulating effects of PBM suggest that laser therapy should be part of the multimodal management of pemphigus patients. Prompt analgesia and accelerated healing of oral and cutaneous lesions have been reported in humans with pemphigus vulgaris when laser therapy has been added to treatment with systemic glucorticosteroids (Minicucci *et al.,* 2012; Pavli *et al.,* 2014).

The successful response in human patients suggests that laser therapy should be added to other management modalities for pemphigus in dogs and cats. Laser settings that deliver 3–4 J/cm^2 are recommended, using a noncontact delivery to reduce the possibility of contamination of the handpiece and subsequent nosocomial infections. Lesions should be treated through an induction phase, every other day or twice a week. Once a clinical response has been noted, treatment frequency can be reduced through a transition phase, gradually extending the time between treatments. Patients with symptoms that persist or reoccur

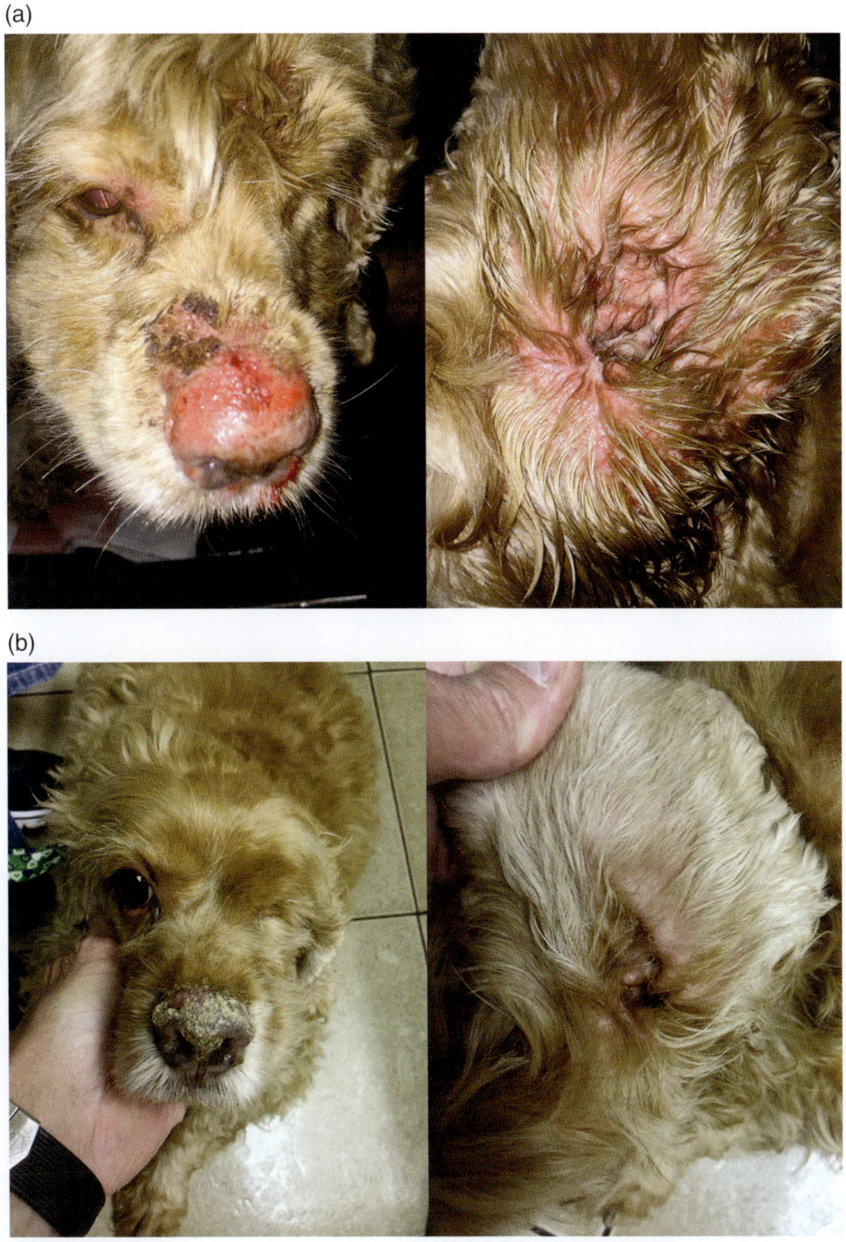

Figure 9.4 (a) Pemphigus foliaceous lesions on the face and pinna prior to laser therapy as an adjunct to immunomodulating pharmacological agents and antibiotics for a resistant bacterial infection. (b) Improvement in pemphigus foliaceous lesions 10 weeks after beginning prednisone, azathioprine, chloramphenicol, and laser therapy.

frequently should continue to be treated indefinitely, with maintenance-phase treatments every 3–4 weeks.

Perianal Fistulas

Perianal fistulas are a chronic, debilitating, inflammatory condition that results in fistulous tracts in the perianal and perirectal tissues and the surrounding perineum (Figure 9.5). They are rare in cats, more common in dogs, and most commonly seen in German shepherds, as well as in Irish setters and Labrador retrievers. The etiology was once thought to be related to the tail conformation of German shepherds, but it is now believed to be immune-mediated (Craven, 2010). Comparisons have been made to Crohn's disease in humans.

Patients present with a history of excessive grooming of the perianal area, tenesmus, hematochezia, and dyschezia. As the condition worsens, malodorous, mucopurulent discharge is often present around the anus, and elevation of the tail is extremely painful. Inappetence, lethargy, and weight loss may occur in severe cases.

Though surgical excision was once thought to present the best option for resolution, medical management, using different combinations of immunomodulating drugs such as cyclosporine, prednisone, azathioprine, and topical tacrolimus, is now recommended (Patricelli *et al.*, 2002; House, 2006; Stanley and Hauptman, 2009; Craven, 2010; Pieper and McKay, 2011).

(a) (b)

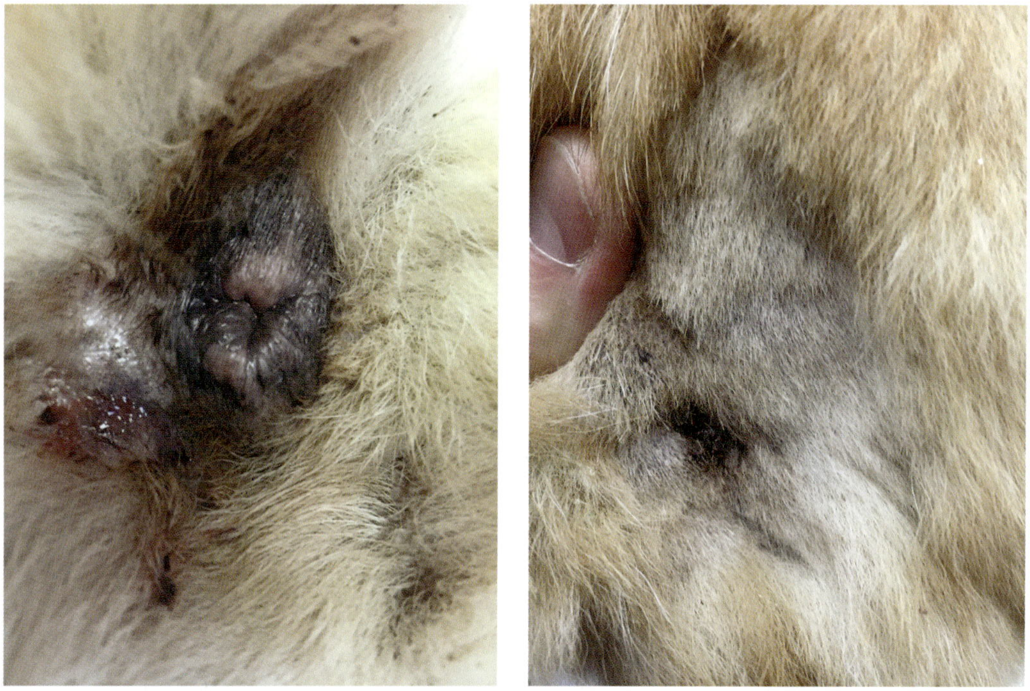

Figure 9.5 (a) Perianal fistula with dorsally draining tract prior to therapy. (b) Reduction in inflammation and swelling 7 days after laser therapy, with the laser set to deliver 12–14 J/cm^2.

Laser therapy is recommended as an adjunct to medical protocols. The reduction of pain and inflammation that laser therapy gives can have a significant effect on patient quality of life. Higher doses of laser therapy are required to successfully target the depth of the fistulas and the extensive secondary inflammatory changes. Laser settings that deliver 12–14 J/cm^2 are recommended, using a noncontact delivery.

Patients should be treated through an induction phase, every other day or twice a week. Initially, patients may be resistant to elevation of the tail for treatment, but as discomfort is reduced through successive treatments, tail elevation normally becomes better tolerated. Once a clinical response has been noted, treatment frequency can be reduced through a transition phase, gradually extending the time between treatments. Prognosis is guarded; complete resolution of perianal fistulas is often not possible, and reoccurrence is common. Patients with symptoms that persist or reoccur frequently should continue to be treated indefinitely, with maintenance-phase treatments every 3–4 weeks.

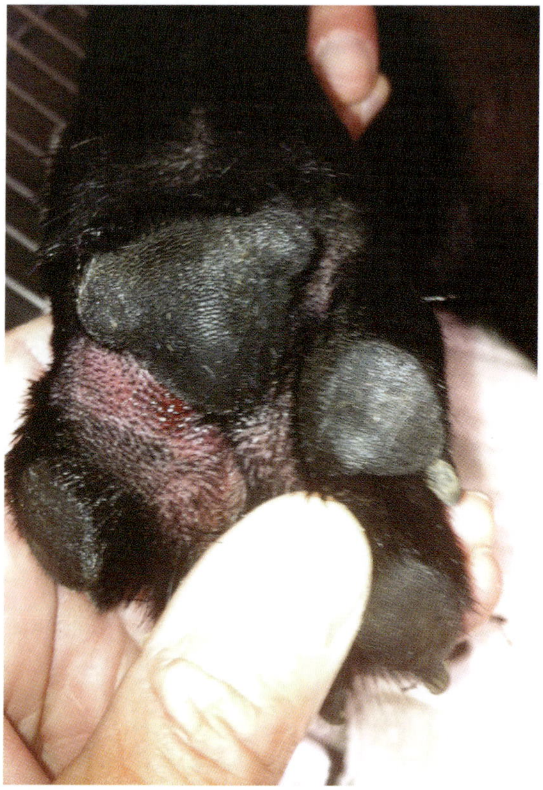

Figure 9.6 Pododermatitis. This may affect multiple tissues, including interdigital spaces, foot pads, nail folds (paronychia), claws, and other tissues of the foot.

Pododermatitis

Pododermatitis, by definition, and as the term is commonly used by veterinary practitioners, refers to any inflammation of the skin of the foot (Figure 9.6). Affected tissues may include interdigital spaces, foot pads, nail folds (paronychia), claws, or other tissues of the foot. There are many potential causes, and therefore many presentations of inflammatory foot disease.

Some veterinary texts use the term "pododermatitis" to refer to pedal folliculitis and furunculosis (Miller *et al.*, 2012), while others use it to refer to the group of as many as a dozen of the most common skin diseases that cause lesions on the canine paw (Duclos, 2013). The etiology of the various presentations of pododermatitis includes trauma, irritants, allergies (food allergy, atopy, contact dermatitis), infections (bacterial, fungal, and viral), parasites (demodectic mange), and osteomyelitis, as well as immune-mediated (pemphigus), nutritional (zinc deficiency), neoplasia, behavioral, metabolic (hepatic cutaneous syndrome), and inherited and congenital factors (Rosychuk, 2002). Some cases have been classified as idiopathic and are now identified as immunomodulatory-responsive lymphotic-plasmocytic pododermatitis (Breathnach *et al.,* 2008).

Pododermatitis, regardless of etiology, is often chronic and painful. Management includes identifying and treating the primary etiology and contributing causes. Therapy includes an appropriate antimicrobial agent, elimination or hyposensitization allergy therapy, immune-modulating medications, pain control, topical therapy, and bandages.

Regardless of the etiology or the management plan, when added as an adjunct, laser therapy can facilitate a reduction in pain, edema, swelling, and inflammation in affected feet.

Though both superficial and deeper tissues may be affected in pododermatitis, because of the anatomy of the foot, the depths of all of the target tissues are relatively shallow. Laser settings that deliver 6–8 J/cm^2 are recommended. The complex anatomy and limited surface area of the foot usually require a noncontact delivery. Treatment of the foot should be administered from all directions (360°).

Acute, superficial inflammations of the tissues of the feet may be treated a single time with laser therapy, during the initial outpatient consultation. If inflammation does not respond to medical and laser therapy, treatments can be repeated daily or every other day.

Chronic and deeper involvement of the tissues of the feet should be treated through an induction phase, every other day or twice a week. Once a clinical response has been noted, treatment frequency can be reduced, through a transition phase, gradually extending the time between treatments. Patients with symptoms that persist or reoccur frequently should continue to be treated indefinitely, with maintenance-phase treatments every 3–4 weeks.

Conclusion

As the various conditions summarized in this chapter indicate, laser therapy can be an important tool in the management of dermatological and non-musculoskeletal soft-tissue conditions. In almost all cases, the effects of PBM will be added to an overall, multimodal management plan for these conditions.

The conditions discussed in this chapter are examples of dermatological and non-musculoskeletal conditions for which laser therapy is indicated. Many other conditions affecting the same tissues will also be candidates for laser therapy treatment. Practitioners are encouraged to extrapolate the principles detailed in this chapter and apply them to the diversity of other conditions seen every day in practice.

References

Ackerman, L. (2008a). Acral lick dermatitis. In: *Atlas of Small Animal Dermatology*, pp. 322–326. Inter-Médica, Buenos Aires.

Ackerman, L. (2008b). Pyotraumatic dermatitis (hot spots). In: *Atlas of Small Animal Dermatology*, pp. 8–14. Inter- Médica, Buenos Aires.

Alves, E. *et al.* (2014). An insight on bacterial targets of photodynamic inactivation. *Future Med Chem.* 6(2):141–164.

Al-Watban, F.A. *et al.* (2007). Low-level laser therapy enhances wound healing in diabetic rats: a comparison of different lasers. *Photomed Laser Surg.* 25(2):72–77.

Assis, L. *et al.* (2016). Aerobic exercise training and low-level laser therapy modulate inflammatory response and degenerative process in an experimental model of knee osteoarthritis in rats. *Osteoarthr Cartil.* 24(1):169–177.

Avci, P. *et al.* (2013). Low-level laser (light) therapy (LLLT) in skin: stimulating, healing, restoring. *Semin Cutan Med Surg.* 32(1):41–52.

Bello, K. *et al.* (2022). The use of photobiomodulation therapy in the treatment of hair cycle arrest in a Pembroke Welsh corgi. *Vet Rec Case Rep.* 10(2):e299.

Bizikova, P. and Olivry, T. (2015). Oral glucocorticoid pulse therapy for induction of treatment of canine pemphigus foliaceus – a comparative study. *Vet Dermatol.* 26(5):354–358.

Bjordal, J.M. *et al.* (2008). A systematic review with procedural assessments and meta-analysis of low level laser therapy in lateral elbow tendonopathy (tennis elbow). *BMC Musculoskelet Disord.* 9:75.

Blair, R.V. *et al.* (2015). Pathology in practice. *Pemphigus vulgaris. J Am Vet Med Assoc.* 246(4):419–421.

Blättler, U. (2007). Fibrin sealant as a treatment for canine aural haematoma: a case history. *Vet J.* 173(3):697–700.

Bloom, P. (2014). Canine superficial bacterial folliculitis: current understanding of its etiology, diagnosis and treatment. *Vet J.* 199(2):217–222.

Bornstein, E. *et al.* (2009). Near-infared photoinactivation of bacteria and fungi at physiologic temperatures. *Photochem Photobiol.* 85(6):1364–1374.

Breathnach, R.M. *et al.* (2008). Canine pododermatitis and idiopathic disease. *Vet J.* 176(2):146–157.

Brown, C. (2010). Surgical management of canine aural hematoma. *Lab Anim (NY).* 39(4):104–105.

Burger, E. *et al.* (2015). Low-level laser therapy to the mouse femur enhances the fungicidal response of neutrophils against *Paracoccidioides brasiliensis. PLoS NeglTrop Dis.* 9(2):e0003541.

Calisto, F.C. *et al.* (2015). Use of low-power laser to assist the healing of traumatic wounds. *Acta Cir Bras.* 30(3):204–208.

Canapp, S. *et al.* (2012). Orthopedic coaptation devices and small-animal prosthetics: elbow hygroma. In: *Veterinary Surgery: Small Animal*, pp. 638–639. Saunders, St. Louis, MO.

de Carvalho, P.K. *et al.* (2016). Analysis of experimental tendinitis in rats treated with laser and platelet-rich plasma therapies by Raman spectroscopy and histometry. *Lasers Med Sci.* 31(1):19–26.

Chow, R. *et al.* (2009). Efficacy of low-level laser therapy in the management of neck pain: a systematic review and meta-analysis of randomized placebo or active-treatment controlled trials. *Lancet.* 374(9705):1897–1908.

Chung, H. *et al.* (2012). The nuts and bolts of low-level laser (light) therapy. *Ann Biomed Eng.* 40(2):516–533.

Cobb, M.A. *et al.* (2005). Topical fusidic acid/ betamethasone-containing gel compared to systemic therapy in the treatment of canine acute moist dermatitis. *Vet J.* 169(2):276–280.

Craven, M. (2010). Rectoanal disease: perianal fistula. In: *Textbook of Veterinary Internal Medicine*, 7 edn, pp. 1602–1604. Saunders, St. Louis, MO.

Culp, W.T.N. (2012). Anal sac disease. In: *Small Animal Soft Tissue Surgery*, pp. 399–405. John Wiley & Sons, Chichester.

Duclos, D. (2013). Canine pododermatitis. *Vet Clin North Am Small Anim Pract.* 43(1):57–87.

van Duijkeren, E. (1995). Disease conditions of canine anal sacs. *J Small Anim Pract.* 36(1):12–16.

Dye, T.L. *et al.* (2002). Evaluation of a technique using the carbon dioxide laser for the treatment of aural hematomas. *J Am Anim Hosp Assoc.* 38(4):385–390.

Enwemeka, C.S. (2009). Intricacies of dose in laser phototherapy for tissue repair and pain relief. *Photomed Laser Surg.* 3:387–393.

Gotthelf, L. (2004). *Small Animal Ear Diseases: An Illustrated Guide*, 2 edn. Saunders, Philadelphia, PA.

Győrffy, A. and Szijártó, A. (2014). A new operative technique for aural haematoma in dogs: a retrospective clinical study. *Acta Vet Hung.* 62(3):340–347.

Halnan, C.R.E. (1976a). The diagnosis of anal sacculitis in the dog. *J Small Anim Pract.* 17(8):527–535.

Halnan, C.R.E. (1976b). The frequency of occurrence of anal sacculitis in the dog. *J Small Anim Pract.* 17(8): 537–541.

Hill, P.B. *et al.* (2006). Survey of the prevalence, diagnosis and treatment of dermatological conditions in small animals in general practice. *Vet Rec.* 158(16):533–539.

Hillier, A. *et al.* (2014). Guidelines for the diagnosis and antimicrobial therapy of canine superficial bacterial folliculitis (antimicrobial guidelines working Group of the International Society for companion animal infectious diseases). *Vet Dermatol.* 25(3):163–175.

Hodjati, H. *et al.* (2014). Low-level laser therapy: an experimental design for wound management: a case-controlled study in rabbit model. *J Cutan Aesthet Surg.* 7(1):14–17.

Holm, B.R. *et al.* (2004). A prospective study of the clinical findings, treatment and histopathology of 44 cases of pyotraumatic dermatitis. *Vet Dermatol.* 15(6):369–376.

House, A.K. (2006). Evaluation of the effect of two dose rates of cyclosporine on the severity of perianal fistulae lesions and associated clinical signs in dogs. *Vet Surg.* 35(6):543–549.

Hutchings, S.M. (2003). Juvenile cellulitis in a puppy. *Can Vet J.* 44(5):418–419.

James, D.J. *et al.* (2011). Comparison of anal sac cytological findings and behaviour in clinically normal dogs and those affected with anal sac disease. *Vet Dermatol.* 22(1):80–87.

Jang, H. and Lee, H. (2012). Meta-analysis of pain relief effects by laser irradiation on joint areas. *Photomed Laser Surg.* 30(8):405–417.

Johnston, D.E. (1975). Hygroma of the elbow in dogs. *J Am Vet Med Assoc.* 167(3):213–219.

Knol, B.W. and Wisselink, M.A. (1996). Lick granuloma in dogs; an obsession for dogs, owners and veterinarians. *Tijdschr Diergeneeskd.* 121(1):21–23.

Kovacs, K. (2015). Low Level Laser Therapy of Serious Wounds of Dogs. Poster presentation. ASLMS Annual Meeting. April 24–26. Orlando, FL.

Kuffler, D.P. (2016). Photobiomodulation in promoting wound healing: a review. *Regen Med.* 11(1):107–122.

Lloyd, D.H. (2012). Antimicrobial therapy of bacterial folliculitis in dogs. *Proc Am College Vet Int Med Forum.* May 30–June 1. New Orleans, LA.

MacPhail, C. (2016). Current treatment options for auricular hematomas. *Vet Clin North Am Small Anim Pract.* 46(4):635–641.

Mester, E. *et al.* (1968). The effect of laser beams on the growth of hair in mice. *Radiobiol Radiother (Berl).* 9(5):621–626.

Miller, W. *et al.* (2012). Bacterial skin diseases: pedal folliculitis and furunculosis. In: *Muller and Kirk's Small Animal Dermatology*, 7 edn, p. 201. Saunders, St. Louis, MO.

Minatel, D.G. *et al.* (2009). Phototherapy promotes healing of chronic diabetic leg ulcers that failed to respond to other therapies. *Lasers Surg Med.* 41(6):433–441.

Minicucci, E.M. *et al.* (2012). Low-level laser therapy on the treatment of oral and cutaneous pemphigus vulgaris: case report. *Lasers Med Sci.* 27(5):1103–1106.

Müntener, T. *et al.* (2012). Canine noninflammatory alopecia: a comprehensive evaluation of common and distinguishing histological characteristics. *Vet Dermatol.* 23(3):206–e44.

Newton, C.D. *et al.* (1974). Surgical closure of elbow hygroma in the dog. *J Am Vet Med Assoc.* 164(2):147–149.

Nussbaum, E.L. *et al.* (2002). Effects of 630-, 660-, 810-, and 905-nm laser irradiation delivering radiant exposure of 1–50 J/cm^2 on three species of bacteria in vitro. *J Clin Laser Med Surg.* 20(6):325–333.

Nussbaum, E.L. *et al.* (2003). Effects of low-level laser therapy (LLLT) of 810 nm upon in vitro growth of bacteria: relevance of irradiance and radiant exposure. *J Clin Laser Med Surg.* 21(5):283–290.

Olivieri, L. *et al.* (2015). Efficacy of low-level laser therapy on hair regrowth in dogs with noninflammatory alopecia: a pilot study. *Vet Dermatol.* 26(1):35–39.

Olivry, T. and Linder, K.E. (2009). Dermatoses affecting desmosomes in animals: a mechanistic review of acantholytic blistering skin diseases. *Vet Dermatol.* 20(5–6):313–326.

Patricelli, A.J. *et al.* (2002). Cyclosporine and ketoconazole for the treatment of perianal fistulas in dogs. *J Am Vet Med Assoc.* 220(7):1009–1016.

Pavletic, M.M. and Braum, D.E. (2015). Successful closed suction management of canine elbow hygroma. *J Small Anim Pract.* 56(7):476–479.

Pavletic, M.M. (2015). Use of laterally placed vacuum drains for management of aural hematomas in five dogs. *J Am Vet Med Assoc.* 246(1):112–117.

Pavli, V. *et al.* (2014). *Pemphigus vulgaris* and laser therapy: crucial role of dentists. *Med Pregl.* 67(1–2):38–42.

Peplow, P.V. *et al.* (2010). Laser photobiomodulation of wound healing: a review of experimental studies in mouse and rat animal models. *Photomed Laser Surg.* 28(3):291–325.

Pieper, J. and McKay, L. (2011). Perianal fistulas. *Compend Contin Educ Vet.* 33(9):E4.

PRNewswire. (2015). Top 10 most common medical conditions for dogs and cats. Available from: http://www.prnewswire.com/news-releases/top-10-most-common-medical-conditions-for-dogs-and-cats-300065935.html (accessed November 30, 2016).

Rapoport, J.L. *et al.* (1992). Drug treatment of canine acral lick. An animal model of obsessive-compulsive disorder. *Arch Gen Psychiatry.* 49(7):517–521.

Reimann, K.A. *et al.* (1989). Clinicopathologic characterization of canine juvenile cellulitis. *Vet Pathol.* 26(6):499–504.

Rosychuk, R. (2002). Pododermatitis in dogs and cats. In: *Proc Am College Vet Int Med Forum*, pp. 494–496. ACVIM, Dallas, TX (May 29–June 1).

Rosychuk, R. (2011). Canine lick granuloma. In: *World Small Animal Veterinary Association World Congress Proceedings.* WSAVA, Jeju (October 14–17).

Shumaker, A.K. *et al.* (2008). Microbiological and histological features of acral lick dermatitis. *Vet Dermotol.* 19(5):288–298.

Silva, D.C. *et al.* (2013). Low level laser therapy (AlGaInP) applied at 5J/cm^2 reduces the proliferation of *Staphylococcus aureus* MRSA in infected wounds and intact skin of rats. *An Bras Dermotol.* 88(1):50–55.

Sousa, C.A. (2013). Staphylococcal pyoderma in the world of methicillin resistance. *Proc Atlantic Coast Veterinary Conference*, Atlantic City, NJ (October 14–17).

St. Denis, T.G. *et al.* (2011). All you need is light: antimicrobial inactivation as an evolving and emerging discovery strategy against infectious disease. *Virulence.* 2 (6):509–520.

Stanley, B.J. and Hauptman, J.G. (2009). Long-term prospective evaluation of topically applied 0.1% tacrolimus ointment for treatment of perianal sinuses in dogs. *J Am Vet Med Assoc.* 235(4):397–404.

Takashi, K. (1988). Low level diode laser treatment for hematomas under grafted skin and its photobiological mechanisms. *Keio J Med.* 37:415–428.

Welle, M.M. *et al.* (2016). A comparative review of canine hair follicle anatomy and physiology. *Toxicol Pathol.* 44(4):564–574.

White, S.D. *et al.* (1989). Juvenile cellulitis in dogs: 15 cases (1979–1988). *J Am Vet Med Assoc.* 195 (11):1609–1611.

Wikramanayake, T.C. *et al.* (2013). Low-level laser treatment accelerated hair regrowth in a rat model of chemotherapy-induced alopecia (CIA). *Lasers Med Sci.* 28 (3):701–706.

Zarei, M. *et al.* (2016). Low level laser therapy and hair regrowth: an evidence-based review. *Lasers Med Sci.* 31(2):363–367.

10

Snakebites

Christopher J. Winkler

Suffolk Veterinary Group Animal Wellness and Laser Surgery Center, Selden, NY, USA

1st Edition Contributor:

Barbara R. Gores

Veterinary Specialty Center of Tucson, Tucson, AZ, USA

Introduction

Pit vipers (Crotalinae) form the largest group of venomous snakes in the United States and are involved in an estimated 150,000 bites of dogs and cats annually (Armentano and Schaer, 2011; Peterson, 2006a,b). Rattlesnakes, copperheads, and cottonmouth water moccasins are all pit vipers. At our large multi-specialty 24-hour veterinary emergency and critical care hospital in Tucson, Arizona, we treat an average of 395 rattlesnake envenomation cases each year.

The toxicity of rattlesnake venom varies widely, and envenomation is diagnosed primarily as a focal site with a rapid onset of severe swelling, hemorrhage, pain, and local tissue necrosis. Crotalid venom consists of 90% water and has a minimum of 10 enzymes and 3–12 nonenzymatic proteins and peptides. Envenomation results in potentially severe soft-tissue damage and necrosis, vasculotoxicity, cytotoxicity, and coagulopathy (Armentano and Schaer, 2011; Peterson, 2006a). Specifically, hyaluronidase and collagenase work to break down connective tissues, while proteases contribute to coagulopathy and cellular necrosis. Phospholipases are likely the cause of cell-membrane damage and the resultant echinocytosis observed with rattlesnake envenomation. The venom also contains anticoagulants, which contribute to platelet dysfunction and margination of platelets along the vessel wall. Clinically, these patients often have significant prolongation of coagulation times (prothrombin and activated partial thromboplastin times), so hemorrhage is common (Wells, 2012; Witsil *et al.*, 2015).

The clinical manifestations of rattlesnake envenomation depend on the type of snake, anatomical location of the bite, amount of venom injected, age of the snake, and size of the patient. The common presenting signs in dogs and cats include pain, swelling, petechiation, or ecchymosis (or both), weakness, hypotension, and local tissue necrosis. In the Mojave rattlesnake, neuromuscular signs such as ataxia, seizures, and respiratory muscle paralysis predominate. The majority of bites occur on the nose and facial region in dogs (Figure 10.1), and secondarily on the extremities in dogs and cats. Cats are more resistant to the effects of rattlesnake venom on a weight basis, but they typically present with more severe clinical signs, due to their smaller body size resulting in a larger relative dose of venom (Wells, 2012; Witsil *et al.*, 2015).

The less-frequent coral snake (Elapoidea) envenomation has been described by human patients as a painful paresthesia. Accompanying local inflammation is common (Greene et al., 2021). Characterized as primarily neurotoxic and similar to curare, elapid venom may cause little pain or local tissue reaction in the canine patient, though hemolysis, anemia, hemoglobinuria, and progressive fasciculations and paralysis have been reported. Longer coral snakes are associated with increased envenomation. A delay in onset of clinical signs of as much as 10–18 hours could lead to a false sense of security for the pet owner; once clinical signs become apparent, they can become difficult to reverse (Peterson, 2006b).

Snakebite patients should be rapidly transported to a veterinary critical care facility as soon as possible for hospitalization and treatment, and closely monitored for both the

Laser Therapy in Veterinary Medicine: Photobiomodulation, Second Edition. Edited by Christopher J. Winkler and Lisa A. Miller.

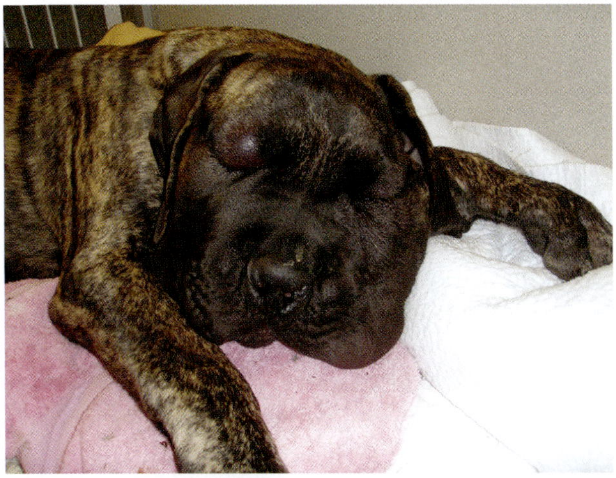

Figure 10.1 Severe swelling, edema, and ecchymosis in a mastiff puppy that suffered multiple snakebite envenomations to the muzzle and periocular regions.

development of any neuromuscular signs and to determine the degree of envenomation. The only proven, specific therapy against snake envenomation is the administration of antivenin. The mainstays of treatment include antivenin, intravenous crystalloid fluid therapy, and analgesic medications. In our experience, most dogs and cats require one to three vials of antivenin over 24–36 hours for crotalid envenomation.

Treatment for elapid envenomation also includes compression bandage, antiemetics, and respiratory support (including assisted ventilation up to 72 hours) as needed (Peterson, 2006b). Antimicrobial therapy and blood products are used if clinically indicated (Armentano and Schaer, 2011). Lab work should initially be run and then monitored closely throughout hospitalization to determine the response to systemic therapies. However, antivenin and other systemic therapies are ineffective in neutralizing the severe, rapid, local tissue damage following snakebite envenomation.

In 2006, our hospital began implementing photobiomodulation (PBM) as an adjuvant therapy for crotalid envenomation in conjunction with the standard accepted systemic treatment (including antivenin) just described. We felt there were numerous clinical case studies utilizing laser therapy technology that supported the beneficial effects of PBM on tissues and cells post-wounding (see Chapter 3). These effects include the local mechanisms of anti-inflammation (via an anti-edema effect, as it causes vasodilation, activation of the lymphatic drainage system, and subsequent reduction in swelling and bruising), analgesia (via decreasing nerve sensitivity and production of endorphins and enkephalins), accelerated tissue repair and cell growth (via increasing cellular metabolism), and improved vascular activity (via neovascularization and angiogenesis.) It seemed that these effects would prove beneficial in actively treating the local tissue damage in snakebite envenomation cases in our veterinary center.

At the time we launched laser photobiomodulation therapy (PBMT) for snakebite envenomation cases, there was only one clinical study in the scientific literature (Dourado *et al.*, 2003). We made an educated guess at the laser treatment protocol and have adapted it over time as we observed the clinical response to therapy. In the past decade since we started using laser therapy as an adjuvant treatment in our snakebite patients, the scientific literature has greatly expanded in the area of PBMT in general, and specifically in regard to Crotalinae envenomation wounds. There are now many other published studies that support our clinical findings over the past decade in utilizing PBMT for snake envenomation.

Literature Review

A review of the literature for studies on the effects of PBMT on the changes induced in tissue by snake venom reveals a number of recent publications. These publications indicate that laser therapy irradiation has a significant effect on the inflammatory response and myonecrosis of mice gastrocnemius muscles injected with Bothrops (a genus of pit viper endemic to Central and South America) snake venom. While the principal treatment for Bothrops envenomation remains antivenom therapy, antivenin is ineffective in neutralizing envenomation's local tissue effects (Silva *et al.*, 2018).

Laser irradiation does not alter the venom toxicity, but laser therapy does significantly reduce myonecrosis of the envenomed muscle and the neuromuscular transmission-blocking effect of the pit viper venom (Barbosa *et al.*, 2009; Doin-Silva *et al.*, 2009). Studies have demonstrated that PBM induces an inhibition of the ability of the venom myotoxins to rapidly disrupt the integrity of the cellular plasma membrane, thereby decreasing the amount of edema, leukocyte influx, and myonecrosis following venom inoculation (Barbosa *et al.*, 2008; Dourado *et al.*, 2003; Nadur-Andrade *et al.*, 2012, 2014). Laser therapy combined with antivenin therapy was more efficient than either therapy alone, indicating that PBMT is a potentially therapeutic approach to minimizing the severity of snakebite envenomation and to treating the local tissue effects caused by envenomation (Barbosa *et al.*, 2008, 2009; Nadur-Andrade *et al.*, 2012, 2014).

In a 2016 *in vitro* study, the effect of laser irradiation was examined on cytotoxicity induced by crotoxin in C2C12 mouse myoblast cell line cells. The mouse myoblast cells were exposed to crotoxin, and then irradiated with PBMT at either red (685 nm) or infrared (830 nm) light at energy densities of 2.0, 4.6, and 7.0 J/cm^2. As demonstrated in other studies, irradiation had no effect on the venom itself. In non-irradiated cells, the venom caused a decrease in cell viability and a massive release of creatine kinase and lactate dehydrogenase, indicating myonecrosis. At the energy densities tested, both infrared and red laser light were able to cause a protective effect against the crotoxin, considerably decreasing venom-induced cytotoxicity (Silva *et al.*, 2016). A subsequent study at closely similar red (660 nm) and infrared (780 nm) wavelengths showed PBMT delayed myotoxicity, reduced edema formation, and promoted anti-hypernociception (Lauria *et al.*, 2021).

PBMT has also been shown to increase angiogenesis by the promotion of vascular endothelial growth factor receptor 1 (VEGFR-1) expression at 3 days postinjection of venom into mouse gastrocnemius muscle. This is the first time that VEGFR-1 expression, and its modulation by PBM, has been demonstrated in endothelial and nonendothelial cells of snake-envenomed skeletal muscle (Dourado *et al.*, 2011).

Laser PBMT of crotoxin-damaged mouse cranial tibialis muscles at a dose of 3 J resulted in an increased cross-sectional area of regenerating myofibers and a reduction in the previously injured muscle area compared to controls and mice receiving lower doses of 1.5 J. This suggests that laser PBMT improves skeletal muscle regeneration by accelerating the recovery of myofiber mass (Silva *et al.*, 2012). An increase of myogenin mRNA expression following PBMT of Bothrops-envenomated mouse muscle suggests that laser therapy also stimulates satellite cells, enhancing the repair of damaged muscle tissue via improved myogenic differentiation (Vieira *et al.,* 2021).

Treatment

Our PBMT protocol for snakebite envenomation is currently to initiate laser therapy (810 and 980 nm, 7.2–8.0 J/cm^2) every 24 hours beginning 6–8 hours post-hospital admission. We have been reluctant to initiate laser therapy immediately in snake-envenomation patients out of concern for local vasodilation created by the laser resulting in a worsening of the myotoxic effect on the tissues. The delay in commencing laser therapy allows us to better stabilize the patient with systemic crystalloids and opioids, which improves patient comfort and tolerance to any movement or positioning needed to administer the laser treatments, as well as to monitor for early onset of possible neuromuscular signs indicative of a more severe Mojave rattlesnake envenomation that could markedly worsen the overall patient prognosis. However, we are currently in the process of reevaluating the time to commence and the frequency of laser treatments based on the current literature already cited.

We vary the PBMT dose slightly based on size and location of the wound and patient size. For example, smaller patients, smaller wounds, or areas with less tissue density such as the carpus or muzzle, will receive doses at the lower end of the range. Plastic templates allow us to accurately measure surface area for calculations without having to overmanipulate the already damaged and painful tissues.

Periocular bites can be challenging to treat in terms of adequately shielding the patient's eyes. Likewise, lingual-based bites, commonly seen in dogs, are difficult to perform PBMT on, due to the limitations of intraoral access in awake or mildly sedated patients. Many of these patients can experience significant swelling and edema of the tongue, to the point of obstructing their airway, necessitating the performance of tracheostomies until the swelling resolves.

Most snakebite-envenomation patients remain hospitalized for 2–3 days, and subsequently receive two to four laser treatments (see Figure 10.2). About 30% of patients return for continued laser treatments every 24–48 hours for two to four more sessions over the next week postenvenomation if they have wounds that are more extensive.

Anecdotally, over the past 10 years since initiating PBMT for rattlesnake envenomation, our results have shown a significant decrease in the clinical morbidity associated with the local tissue-necrosis effects of snakebite wounds. We now very rarely must perform major surgical reconstruction (consisting of extensive skin wound management, skin flaps, and grafts) of snakebite wounds, and almost never perform amputations of appendages as we did routinely in the past, pre-laser therapy. The most severe cases of tissue necrosis tend to occur in those patients that delay seeking veterinary care, or are treated at other veterinary facilities with antivenin but without PBMT.

Conclusion

Laser PBMT alone has made a significant impact not only on the overall prognosis and outcome of snakebite patients, but also on reducing the duration and financial costs of treatment. Laser PBMT of snakebites is comfortable and well-tolerated by the patient, and is easy for technical staff to administer. It is an extremely cost-effective therapy when considering the high success rates in preventing the more extensive, complicated, and expensive surgeries required to treat the high degree of wound necrosis so characteristic of snakebite envenomation. PBMT truly is an exciting and rewarding therapy that can be offered with confidence to these patients in order to ensure the best outcomes, with the most rapid return to health.

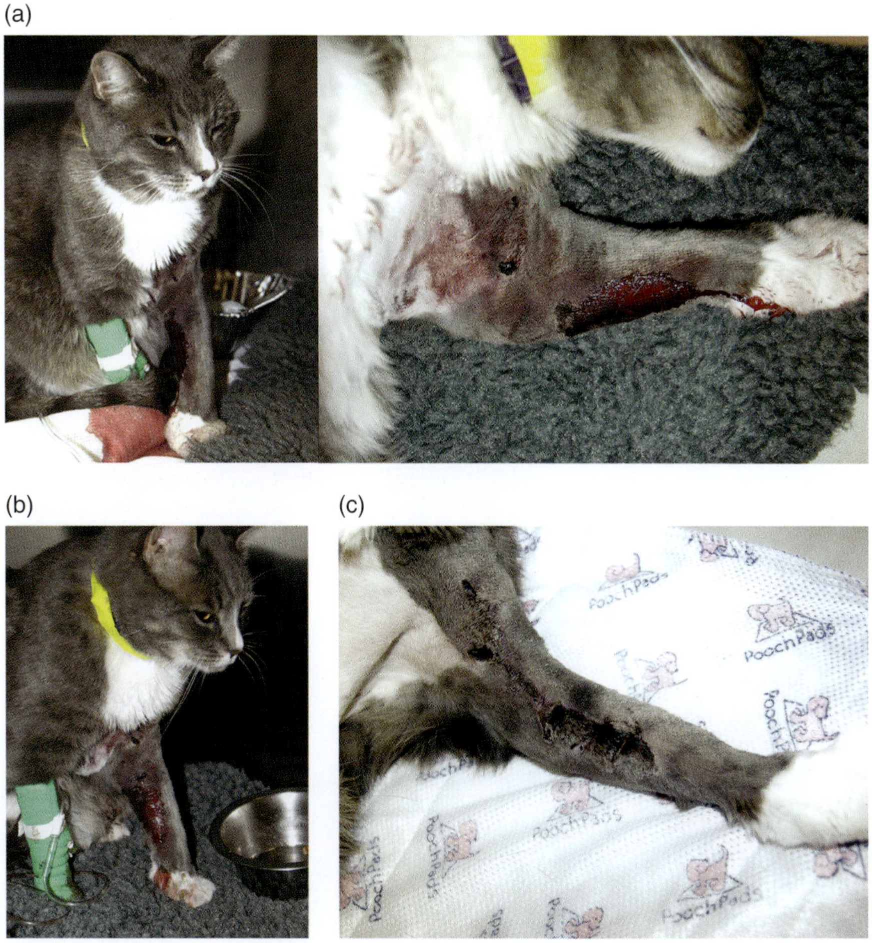

Figure 10.2 (a) Cat snakebite envenomation of the left antebrachium before PBMT. Note severe limb and paw edema and local ecchymosis. (b) Cat snakebite envenomation 12 hours after first PBMT. Note reduction of paw swelling, limb and paw edema, and ecchymosis. (c) Cat snakebite 5 days post-envenomation, after receiving three PBMTs. Limb edema and bruising have resolved. The envenomation wound is healing without complications or the need for surgical intervention.

References

Armentano, R. and Schaer, M. (2011). Overview and controversies in the medical management of pit viper envenomation in the dog. *J Vet Emerg Crit Care*. 21(5):461–470.

Barbosa, A.M. *et al.* (2008). Effect of low-level laser therapy in the inflammatory response induced by Bothrops jararacussu snake venom. *Toxicon*. 51(7):1236–1244.

Barbosa, A.M. *et al.* (2009). Effect of low-level laser therapy in the myonecrosis induced by Bothrops jararacussu snake venom. *Photomed Laser Surg*. 27(4):591–597.

Doin-Silva, R. *et al.* (2009). The ability of low level laser therapy to prevent muscle tissue damage induced by snake venom. *Photochem Photobiol Sci*. 85(1):63–69.

Dourado, D. *et al.* (2003). Effects of the Ga-As laser irradiation on myonecrosis caused by Bothrops Moojeni snake venom. *Lasers Surg Med*. 33(5):352–357.

Dourado, D. *et al.* (2011). Low-level laser therapy promotes vascular endothelial growth factor receptor-1 expression in endothelial and nonendothelial cells of mice gastrocnemius exposed to snake venom. *Photochem Photobiol Sci*. 87(2):418–426.

Greene, S. *et al.* (2021). Epidemiology, Clinical Features, and Management of Texas Coral Snake (Micrurus tener) Envenomations Reported to the North American Snake Bite Registry. *J Med Toxicol*. 17(1):51–56.

Lauria, P.S. *et al.* (2021). Effects of photobiomodulation therapy on the local experimental envenoming by Bothrops leucurus snake. *J Photochem Photobiol B*. 214:112087.

Nadur-Andrade, N. *et al.* (2012). Effects of photobiostimulation on edema and hemorrhage induced by Bothrops moojeni venom. *Lasers Med Sci*. 27(1):65–70.

Nadur-Andrade, N. *et al.* (2014). Photobiostimulation reduces edema formation induced in mice by Lys-49 phospholipases A2 isolated from Bothrops moojeni venom. *Photochem Photobiol Sci*. 13(11):1561–1567.

Peterson, M. (2006a). Snake bite: Pit Vipers. *Clin Tech Small Anim Pract*. 21(4):174–182.

Peterson, M. (2006b). Snake bite: Coral Snakes. *Clin Tech Small Anim Pract*. 21(4):183–186.

Silva, L.H. *et al.* (2012). GaAs 904-nm laser irradiation improves myofiber mass recovery during regeneration of skeletal muscle previously damaged by crotoxin. *Lasers Med Sci.* 27(5):993–1000.

Silva, L.M. *et al.* (2016). Photobiomodulation protects and promotes differentiation of C2C12 myoblast cells exposed to snake venom. *PLoS One.* 11(4):e0152890.

Silva, L.M. *et al.* (2018). Photobiomodulation therapy on bothrops snake venom-induced local pathological effects: A systematic review. *Toxicon.* 152:23–29.

Vieira, W.F. *et al.* (2021). Exploring the ability of low-level laser irradiation to reduce myonecrosis and increase Myogenin transcription after Bothrops jararacussu envenomation. *Photochem Photobiol Sci.* 20(4):571–583.

Wells, R. (2012). Rattlesnake envenomation. In: *Proceedings of 84th Annual Western Veterinary Conference. February*, pp. 19–23. Las Vegas, NV.

Witsil, A. *et al.* (2015). 272 cases of rattlesnake envenomation in dogs: demographics and treatment including safety of F(ab′)2 antivenom use in 236 patients. *Toxicon.* 105: 19–26.

11

Musculoskeletal Disorders and Osteoarthritis

Lisa A. Miller[1] *and João C. Alves*[2]

[1] *Companion Animal Health, New Castle, DE, USA*
[2] *Clinica Veterinária de Cães, Guarda Nacional Republicana, Lisbon, Portugal*

Introduction

Osteoarthritis is a progressive, complex syndrome involving the interaction of a multitude of factors, both biochemical and biomechanical in nature, which results in the degenerative disease of the synovial joints. The disease accounts for at least 80% of the lameness diagnosis and affects around 20% of adult dogs in the United States and 200,000 dogs in the United Kingdom. Over 90% of elderly dogs show clinical signs of osteoarthritis (Johnston, 1997; Venable *et al.*, 2008; Anderson *et al.*, 2018). In cats, a similar scenario is observed. Up to 40% of animals present with clinical signs of osteoarthritis, and the disease has a prevalence of over 90% in animals over 12 years (Lascelles, 2010; Lascelles *et al.*, 2012). The prevalence is expected to increase due to increased life expectancy and obesity rates (Anderson *et al.*, 2020).

Regardless of the origin of the disease process, once started, the interactions of these biomechanical and biochemical factors ultimately affect all components of the joints, leading to cartilage degradation, osteophyte and enthesiophyte formation, subchondral bone sclerosis, synovial membrane inflammation, and synovial fluid alterations, as well as further changes to periarticular tissues. These changes include a thickening and increased fibrosis of the joint capsule, which results in the stiffness, pain, and decreased range of motion often observed in osteoarthritic patients. The low-grade inflammation in osteoarthritis drives disease progression, and controlling inflammation and predisposing factors are paramount in the management of osteoarthritis (Alves *et al.*, 2022a,b,c). Inflammation of the synovial membrane and a secondary influx of leukocytes into the joint space further facilitate the release of prostaglandins, cytokines, free radicals, and other destructive enzymes, including metalloproteinases, all of which can change cartilage metabolism, create further inflammation, or damage cartilage matrix, perpetuating the vicious cycle (McLaughlin, 2000).

Different guidelines for managing osteoarthritis and pain have recently become available (Mosley *et al.*, 2022; Cachon *et al.*, 2023; Monteiro *et al.*, 2023). Current treatment strategies in veterinary medicine are aimed primarily toward controlling pain, improving joint function, and minimizing functional incapacity in patients through pet owner education and home environmental management. Multimodal management of patients with osteoarthritis includes a therapeutic approach involving the use of a proper weight-management program (when indicated), nutraceutical supplementation, pharmacological therapy, rehabilitation therapy (including physical modalities and therapeutic exercise), and, when necessary, surgical intervention or regenerative medicine (including the use of platelet-rich plasma [PRP] or stem-cell therapy).

Increasingly, pet owners and practitioners are seeking nonpharmacological adjuncts or alternatives to standard-of-care medical therapies for the treatment of chronic painful conditions, including osteoarthritis and other musculoskeletal conditions. Photobiomodulation therapy (PBMT), delivered with a therapeutic laser, may be utilized along with any or all these therapies, and though it may often be used as a standalone therapy, its results are better appreciated as part of a multimodal approach to pain management and rehabilitation. Utilizing PBMT for its analgesic and anti-inflammatory effects is especially important, as it may reduce or eliminate the need for medications, and the concomitant side effects that can come with their use. While useful at all stages of the disease, PBMT can be particularly effective in the earlier stages, helping to control the disease-driving low-grade inflammation, and while the disease is more "localized," where compensation mechanisms and central sensitization are still not present (Alves *et al.*, 2022a,b,c).

Laser Therapy in Veterinary Medicine: Photobiomodulation, Second Edition. Edited by Christopher J. Winkler and Lisa A. Miller.

Physiological Effects of PBMT

The photochemical processes initiated on a cellular level by PBMT have been described in detail in previous chapters; however, some of the analgesic and anti-inflammatory physiological effects that make this modality particularly useful in treating osteoarthritis and other musculoskeletal conditions should be reviewed. Literature supporting the use of PBMT for specific musculoskeletal conditions is detailed in the individual condition sections that follow; here, the general physiologic principles will be discussed. Unlike other physical modalities used in rehabilitation, PBMT has biomodulating effects. Several different mechanisms of action result in a reduction of inflammation and pain (Pryor and Millis, 2015), making it versatile for both short- and long-term effects.

Following PBMT application, the synthesis and secretion of inflammatory prostaglandins are inhibited (Mizutani *et al.*, 2004), and cytokines and growth factors with antioxidative, anti-inflammatory, and antiapoptotic actions are stimulated (Zhang *et al.*, 2003). PBMT has been shown to significantly reduce cyclooxygenase 2 (COX-2) production (Prianti *et al.*, 2014), as well as to reduce bradykinin levels (Jimbo *et al.*, 1998). Bradykinin is important in chronic pain states as it elicits pain by stimulating nociceptive afferents in the skin and viscera, as well as sensitizing them through the production of prostanoids or the release of other mediators (Dray and Perkins, 1993). It also reduces the production of interleukin 1 (IL1) (Lopes-Martins *et al.*, 2005) and prostaglandin E2 (PGE2) (Mizutani *et al.*, 2004).

Photobiomodulation (PBM) blocks depolarization of C-afferent fiber peripheral nerves (Wakabayashi, 1993), improves nerve cell action potential (Cambier *et al.*, 2000), promotes regeneration and recovery of injured peripheral nerves (Anders *et al.*, 2004), and promotes axonal sprouting (Rochkind *et al.*, 2009). The localized and systemic increase of beta endorphins after therapy laser irradiation has been clinically reported in multiple studies (Labajos, 1988; Montesinos, 1988), with subsequent pain reductions, and there is also PBMT-mediated analgesia via enhancement of peripheral endogenous opioids (Hagiwara *et al.*, 2007).

Increased microcirculation, and secondarily increased tissue oxygenation, are also achieved with PBMT via dilation of microvessels of all orders, effects on arteriolar vasomotions, an opening of "reserved" capillaries, and a metabolism rise in parenchymatous cells (Skobelkin *et al.*, 1990). Vasodilation is accomplished by an increase in nitric oxide (NO) in the treated area (Shiva and Gladwin, 2009), as well as an increase in serotonin release (Walker, 1983), which also plays an important role in analgesia. Acceleration of neoangiogenesis occurs via release of cytokines and growth factors into the circulation, and numerous studies have examined the relationship between PBMT and vascular endothelial growth factor (VEGF) (Silva *et al.*, 2010; Góralczyk *et al.*, 2015).

The control of inflammations is central to disease management. It has been shown that the inflammatory state created by fat tissue or by shifts in the gut microbiome has a role in the development and progression of osteoarthritis. Controlling this inflammation positively affects a patient's clinical signs (Barić Rafaj *et al.*, 2017; Schott *et al.*, 2018). There is increasing evidence that conditions characterized by an intense local or systemic inflammatory response, which can lead to maladaptive pain states if not appropriately managed, may be associated with abnormal ion transport (Schomberg *et al.*, 2012; Waxman and Zamponi, 2014). Calcium, sodium, and potassium concentrations, as well as the proton gradient over the mitochondrial membrane, are positively influenced by PBM (Karu *et al.*, 1997; Ignatov *et al.*, 2005; Chow *et al.*, 2011). After PBMT, there is an integrated and rapid modulation of ion channels. This is achieved through both direct action on photo-acceptors (such as cytochrome c oxidase, CCO) and indirect modulation via enzymes (Liebert *et al.*, 2014).

Searching for Evidence and Understanding the Literature

Literature regarding the use of PBMT in treating musculoskeletal conditions (including osteoarthritis) is prevalent, though at first glance not in the journals that might regularly come across the desk of a veterinarian in general practice. Additionally, many studies have been conducted in induced disease models or with a combination of different interventions (e.g., PBMT and exercise programs). Further complicating any search for evidence are the numerous terms that have been used to describe PBM in the body of research publications. Older terms may be used, such as "cold laser," "low-level laser therapy" (LLLT), or simply "laser therapy" in order to differentiate the modality from so-called "hot" lasers used to thermally cut, ablate, or coagulate tissue.

We currently have studies available in different species, from lab animals with experimentally induced arthritis (Carlos *et al.*, 2014; Peimani and Sardary, 2014; Assis *et al.*, 2016), to human studies in naturally occurring disease models (Alfredo *et al.*, 2012; Ammar, 2014; Baltzer *et al.*, 2016; Fukuda *et al.*, 2015; Ip and Fu, 2015a) and in clinical settings (Gendron and Hamblin, 2019; Pinto *et al.*, 2022). Veterinary studies in companion animals are also available (Looney *et al.*, 2018; Alves *et al.*, 2022a,b,c).

Despite the increasing body of evidence surrounding PBMT, searching through the scientific literature for studies related to PBMT and effectiveness in veterinary conditions, including musculoskeletal disorders and osteoarthritis, presents challenges. The true effectiveness of the modality for pain relief and other benefits in these conditions continues to be debated in the literature, though the authors believe this is more due to poor study design(s), inadequate parameters used, and misreporting parameters than it is a failure of the modality itself. It is important to take into account the possible reasons for the varying outcomes reported in some papers, which are not limited to the osteoarthritis studies alone, but also apply to much of the published research in the field of PBMT. Outcome measures used for similar conditions have varied. The laser parameters used, including wavelength, pulse frequency (Hz), energy density (fluence [J/cm^2]), and power density (irradiance [mW/cm^2]) have not always been reported clearly, and in many cases they are misreported entirely. In addition, the method of application (on-contact versus off-contact administration), anatomic areas treated (treatment of "pain points" alone versus involved periarticular soft tissues), tissue type selection (amount of melanin in treated tissue), and frequency of treatments have also varied widely and have not always been clearly reported. This variability of methods has led to mixed, sometimes contradictory, results. Though there have been meta-analyses examining the multitude of studies concluding efficacy for treating pain in osteoarthritis (Jang and Lee, 2012) and other musculoskeletal conditions (Chow *et al.*, 2009), further studies should be encouraged using consistent reported parameters to optimize outcomes and elucidate the factors necessary for effectiveness, particularly since the growing body of evidence indicates efficacy in the management of musculoskeletal conditions, allied with an almost total lack of side effects (Gendron and Hamblin, 2019).

Of the parameters just mentioned, the differences in therapeutic outcomes with varying fluence (J/cm^2) and irradiance (W/cm^2) reported in the literature seem to be the most significant, as long as wavelengths within the therapeutic window are being used. Some studies have demonstrated clear fluence-dependent biochemical effects with PBMT (Hsieh *et al.*, 2014). Others, including a meta-analysis of studies on tendinopathy (Tumilty *et al.*, 2010), also support the existence of a fluence-dependent dosing window in those trials that have had positive results. Additionally, a seminal review on PBMT for neck pain published in the *Lancet* (Chow *et al.*, 2009) concluded that when studies that utilized low doses or demonstrated flaws in treatment procedure were excluded, statistical heterogeneity in results disappeared.

Most importantly, when examining the literature and the dosing reported within it, one should also take into consideration whether the study described is *in vitro* or *in vivo*. As demonstrated in a 2014 study on peripheral nerve injury, doses optimized for each wavelength *in vitro* must then be translated for optimal *in vivo* parameters due to the percentage of light lost in transmission to deeper tissues from the skin surface (Anders *et al.*, 2014). A recent review study looking at efficacious *in vitro* and *in vivo* PBM research concluded that the parameters of most importance in PBM treatment success are *both* irradiance and fluence (Zein *et al.*, 2018). Other important conclusions of this study were that ineffective *in vivo* studies are more likely to be due to underdosing and that inconsistency of (and incorrect) reporting laser parameters is a major source of contradictory research findings and has done much to hinder the acceptance of PBM effects in the scientific community. As always, in order to optimize treatment, further studies should be encouraged using consistent reported parameters to truly examine the factors necessary for real world clinical efficacy.

Importance of Proper Examination and Diagnostics

As for all therapeutic protocols, it should be emphasized that a proper diagnosis must be established prior to beginning treatment. This is even more important in patients with musculoskeletal pain as a large part of the success or failure of treatment will rely on the local application of the correct dose of PBMT to the correct area(s) of tissue. All veterinary patients should undergo a thorough orthopedic and neurologic examination, as well as an investigation of their clinical history, prior to being prescribed PBMT, or, indeed, any other pharmacologic or therapeutic interventions for their osteoarthritis. The presence of comorbidities should be considered when tailoring a treatment plan for the patient, including not only the presence of other systemic or local diseases but also any localized pain (not just in the joint being treated) due to compensatory changes in biomechanics. Pain examinations should be repeated regularly on all patients, to evaluate for improvement after therapy has started and to ensure there are no "new" issues that should be treated. In the case of lack of an improvement or a worsening, pain examinations can also help to determine whether further diagnostics are indicated. It is also important to remember that the degree of radiographic or pathologic change discovered may not necessarily be consistent with the amount of lameness displayed by the patient or the severity of their discomfort.

Prescribed treatment areas should primarily be based on the orthopedic and pain-assessment examinations. As part of the initial pain evaluation, and for purposes of follow-up and objective outcome measures for any treatment plan, the use of validated owner questionnaires for assessing pain in veterinary patients is strongly encouraged. Different client-reported outcome measures have been developed for companion animals with osteoarthritis. In dogs, these include the Canine Brief Pain Inventory (Brown *et al.*, 2008), the Liverpool Osteoarthritis in Dogs (B. Walton *et al.*, 2018; M. B. Walton *et al.*, 2013), the Canine Orthopedic Index (COI) (Brown, 2014), and the Helsinki Chronic Pain Index (HCPI) (Hielm-Björkman *et al.*, 2009). For cats, there are four client-reported outcome measures available, including the Feline Musculoskeletal Pain Index (FMPI), Client Specific Outcome Measure (CSOM), Montreal Instrument for Cat Arthritis Testing (MI-CAT), and the Feline Physical Function Formula (FPFF) (Lascelles *et al.*, 2007; Benito *et al.*, 2013; Gruen *et al.*, 2015; Stadig *et al.*, 2019). Objective measures, as stance analysis platforms are also becoming more readily available, and have been reported as sensitive for detecting lameness in dogs, with a pressure-sensitive walkway as a reference (Clough *et al.*, 2018), and in the assessment of response to treatment (Alves *et al.*, 2022a,b,c). Patients may not undergo as many trials at the required velocity in some conditions like OA to obtain valid trials on a force plate. Still, they may be able to stand long enough to collect data using a stance analyzer (Cole and Millis, 2017).

Not only do these evaluation tools provide the practitioner with information on the patient's behavior, demeanor, and locomotion as observed by the pet owner, but they also serve to allow the pet owners themselves to evaluate improvement or decline in their pet's quality of life with regards to their chronic pain status. Other pain-scoring systems and scales exist and may also be utilized by the practitioner for evaluation of veterinary patients. The use of one or more of these systems is in keeping with the guidelines set forth in the American Animal Hospital Association (AAHA)/American Association of Feline Practitioners (AAFP) Pain Management Guidelines for Dogs & Cats (AAHA/AAFP, 2007).

Patient Preparation and Treatment Techniques

In practice, PBMT may be applied for musculoskeletal disorders with minimal patient preparation. Patients generally experience a calming, warm sensation and relaxation during therapy, negating the need for sedation. The hair coat may be clipped or shaved for optimal light penetration, but it is not absolutely necessary, depending on the power capabilities of the device. PBMT units may have built-in software that can calculate a dose of energy that will compensate for additional light losses in thick or long hair coats; alternatively, adjustment can be made manually when calculating a dose for administration (see section on "Dosimetry for Musculoskeletal Conditions"). The hair coat should be free of excessive debris, and any lotions, sprays, or ointments that may have been applied to the treatment area should be rinsed completely off with water prior to PBMT.

A comfortable surface for the pet to lie on should be provided, such as a dog bed or pad placed on the floor or exam table. This is particularly important for patients that are geriatric or in pain. A treatment platform may be constructed slightly elevated off the floor, to allow for comfortable seating during therapy sessions for both the laser therapist and pet owner (Figure 11.1). Laser treatment should be performed in whatever position the pet is most comfortable that also allows access to the anatomic areas being treated. Laser operators should be educated that "posture breaks" may be necessary and that repositioning from side to side should be minimized to maintain maximum patient comfort. For example, with a patient lying in lateral recumbency, the laser therapist can treat both the cranial, lateral, and caudal aspects of any joints on the "upside" limbs and the medial aspects of any joints on the "downside" limbs, without having to turn over the patient repeatedly (Figure 11.2).

As discussed in Chapter 5, the number-one safety concern with the use of any therapy laser is the protection of the eyes of the patient, the laser therapist, and anyone in the immediate treatment vicinity. For this reason, everyone should wear laser-safe eyewear, marked with the appropriate optical density for the wavelengths of light emitted by the laser unit being used. When treating around the head and neck, the patient should also be wearing laser-safe "doggles" (Figure 11.3), or should have their eyes covered with a dark cloth (Figure 11.4) or by the hand of someone assisting in the treatment.

The patient should never be allowed to stare at the treatment area. A dark-colored Elizabethan collar may serve as a shielding device when treating caudal to the head if the patient cannot be distracted with food treats or attention, or otherwise restrained to avoid directly investigating the laser treatment area.

In general, there are two different application techniques that can be utilized, depending on the power of the laser being used (Pryor and Millis, 2015). For lower-powered devices, typically those less than 500 mW (0.5 W), a point-to-point treatment is usually used.

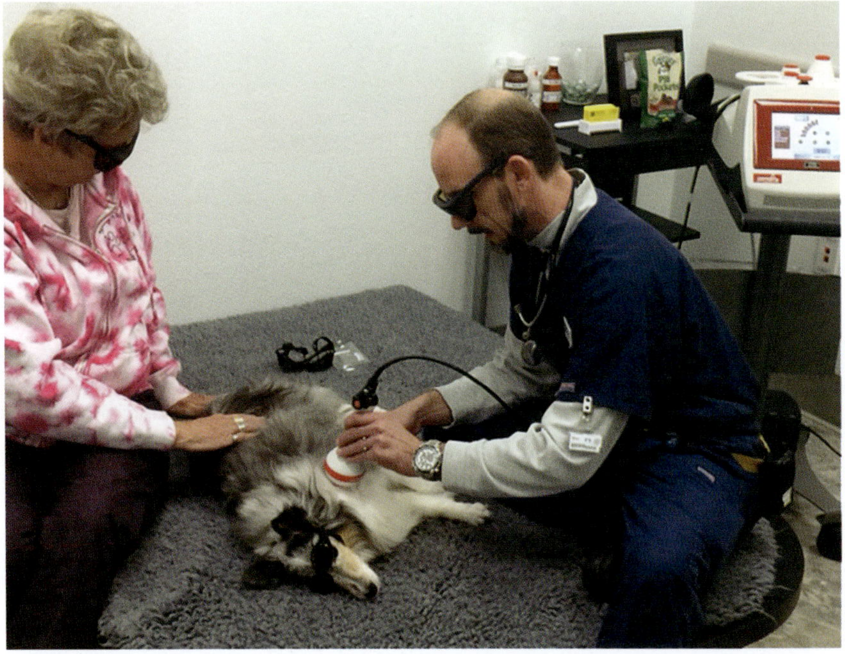

Figure 11.1 Laser therapist and patient seated comfortably on a raised laser-treatment platform.

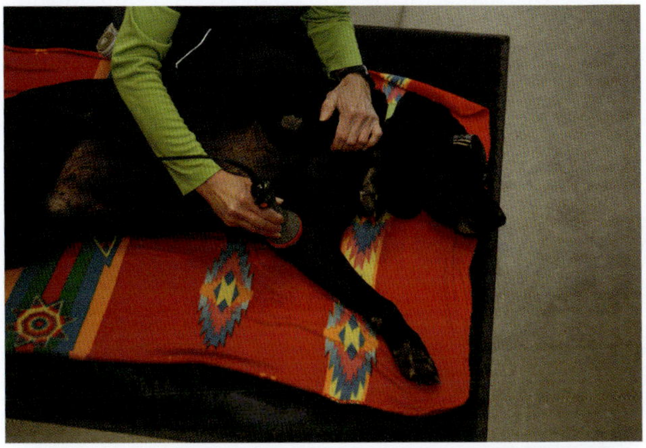

Figure 11.2 Laser therapist treating the medial aspect of the elbow on the "downside" limb.

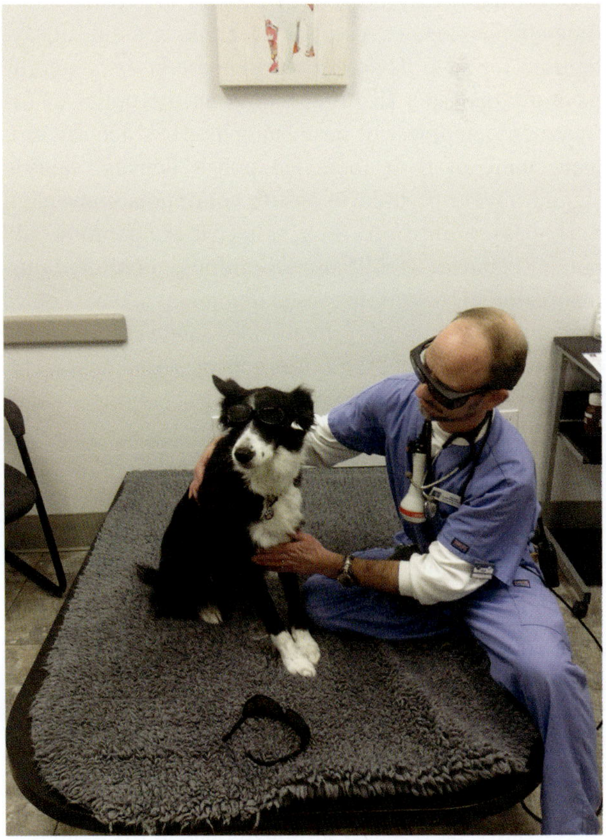

Figure 11.3 Patient and laser therapist wearing laser-safe eyewear.

Multiple individual points within the treatment area must be treated in order to deliver the appropriate target dose to tissues beneath the surface. Depending on the size of the area, or when dealing with multiple treatment areas in the same patient, this may become challenging from a time perspective. Point-to-point treatment also requires the laser operator to have the ability to precisely identify and locate the exact area(s) of deeper soft tissue structures that they wish to treat with this technique. While this may not be a challenge for those that have further training or

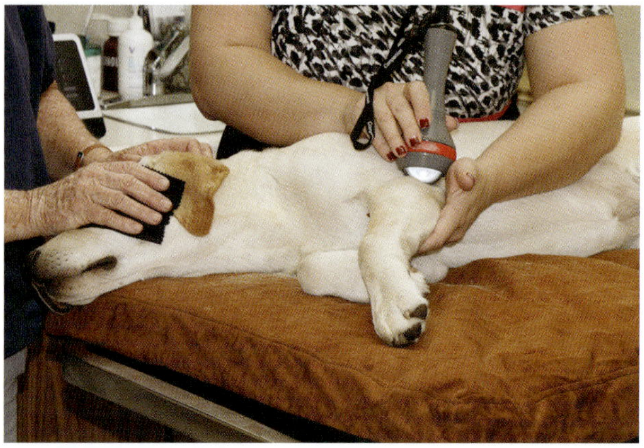

Figure 11.4 Assistant covering the patient's eyes with a dark cloth in lieu of laser-safe goggles.

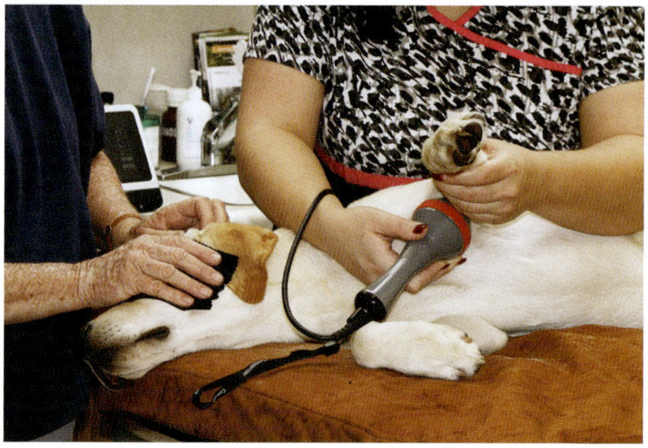

Figure 11.5 Laser therapist keeping the treatment head perpendicular to the surface of the medial aspect of the elbow.

expertise in rehabilitation therapy or orthopedic disease, it can certainly pose a potential roadblock to success for the laser operator that may be less knowledgeable in these areas. As previously discussed, irradiance (W/cm^2) plays an important role in therapeutic outcome, especially when dealing with deep-tissue conditions such as osteoarthritis. For this reason, higher-powered devices (emitting 500 mW or more) may be able to achieve better and more time-efficient results. A scanning technique should always be used for such devices. Though these lasers generally have a larger spot size (depending on the optics of the treatment handpiece or head being used), which can mitigate some of their increased power density, caution should always be used to ensure continuous movement during laser emission. Both hair coat temperature and patient behavior should also be carefully monitored during treatment. A scanning speed that maintains irradiance and fluence within the recommended safety ranges for the treatment handpiece and beam being used is recommended. For devices above 500 mW, a scanning speed of 3–7 cm/sec is usually appropriate; the laser operator should confirm this with the manufacturer. Some modern equipment offers a handpiece with sensors that detect and inform the operator when the scanning speed is higher or lower than intended.

A "trailing finger" through the patient's fur may be used when treating with the hand on the treatment handpiece, or the laser therapist may follow the path of the handpiece with their other hand to monitor for excessive thermal build-up, and adjust treatment speed or lower treatment power as needed. If, signs of potential discomfort are noted at any time during treatment (patient vocalizing, withdrawing the limb, or suddenly turning to look at the treatment area), the laser therapist should check that the technique and settings being utilized are appropriate.

The laser treatment handpiece should be held perpendicular to the surface being treated (Figure 11.5) and moved in a consistent, systematic motion, such as a grid pattern evenly covering the entire area to be treated. As outlined before, osteoarthritis is a disease of the whole joint organ; surrounding tissues are also involved and are a source of pain. It is recommended to treat all the soft-tissue structures associated with the joint biomechanically, encompassing 360º around the limb and utilizing landmarks approximately half the distance to the next joint on the limb, both proximal and distal, to demarcate a comprehensive area of treatment. For example, in Figures 11.6 and 11.7, the laser therapist is shown treating both the cranial and caudal aspects of the stifle joint. A common mistake in treating the coxofemoral joint is for the laser therapist to not include the ventral, medial aspect of the hip joint in the treatment area (Figure 11.8), an omission that risks less than optimal therapeutic outcomes. A smaller, more

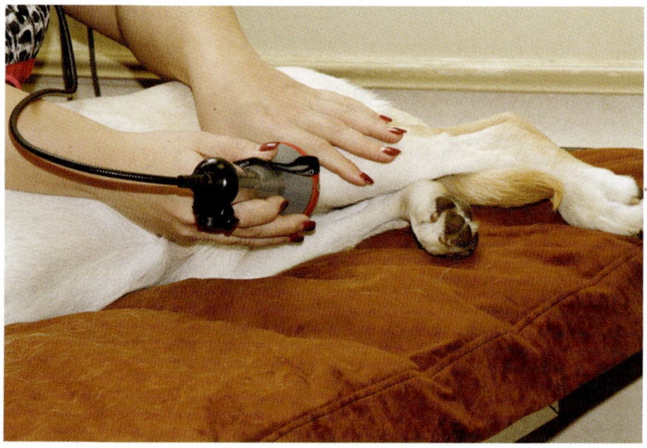

Figure 11.6 Laser therapist treating the cranial aspect of the patient's stifle joint.

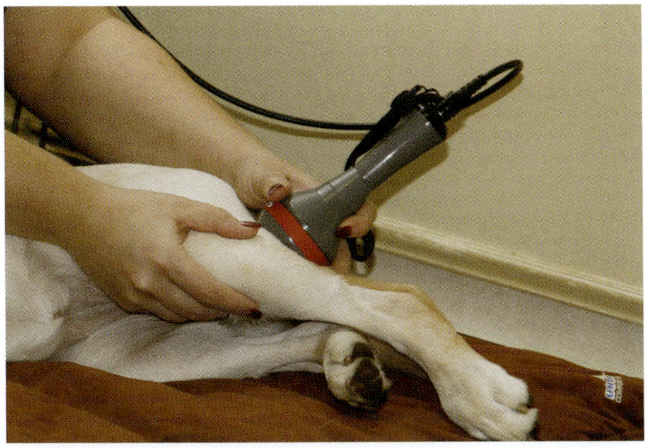

Figure 11.7 Laser therapist treating the caudal aspect of the patient's stifle joint.

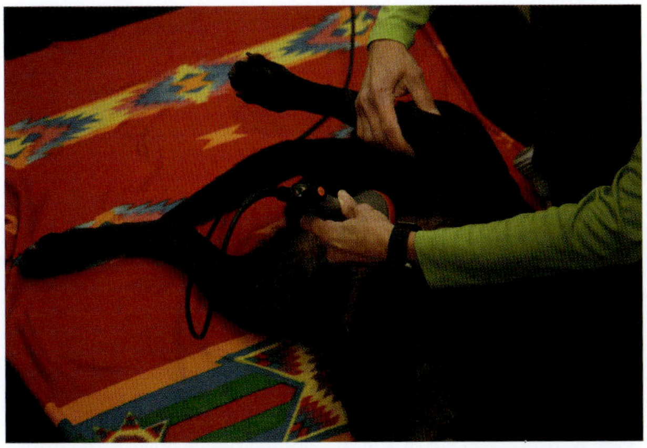

Figure 11.8 Laser therapist treating the ventral, medial aspect of the patient's coxofemoral joint.

specific anatomic area of focus may of course be treated if desired, based on the anatomic knowledge of the laser therapist and utilization of appropriate dosing (see section on Dosimetry for Musculoskeletal Conditions).

Treatment is optimally applied in direct contact with the skin, using a contact handpiece or a treatment head that has been specifically designed for deep-tissue conditions. Treating on-contact and applying pressure to the skin creates blanching and disperses blood from the dermis and underlying tissues (Chien and Wilhelmi, 2012). Since blood absorption is a barrier to photon penetration via hemoglobin acting as the main absorber of light in the dermis (Lister *et al.*, 2012), blanching improves light penetration to deeper tissues. Due to differences in the refractive index between air and skin, a large amount of light may be lost due to reflection off the skin when treating in an off-contact manner. Treating on-contact minimizes these losses (Zein *et al.*, 2018).

Providing passive tissue massage is another benefit of treating on-contact, though it is important to note that some patients in pain may be hypersensitive to such physical contact. This is particularly true over bony prominences and in areas of thinned skin, especially over the elbow and stifle. In these patients, as well as in any patient with a wound in the treatment area, treating in an off-contact manner may be necessary.

Particularly when administering PBMT over a joint, the limb should be placed through a gentle passive range of motion during treatment to maximize light penetration to the articular surfaces and associated soft-tissue structures. At the start of a course of therapy the osteoarthritic pet may often be very stiff and painful, and passive range of motion may not be possible during the first few visits or in the early stages of a given treatment session. In these cases, it is best to first address the patient's pain and discomfort by treating the limb in a passive position, before attempting gentle manipulation of the limb for passive range of motion during the later stages of the treatment session or a subsequent visit.

Use of PBMT with Metal Implants and Sutures

A commonly asked question regarding PBMT in musculoskeletal conditions is, "Can it be applied in patients that have metal surgical hardware, including plates, pins, and screws?" Diffuse near-infrared light will be primarily reflected by smooth metal implant surfaces, including staples. While this means the practitioner need not be concerned about such implants heating up, there are several special considerations to be aware of:

1) Be careful when treating over implants in small patients or anywhere there is a superficial implant, such as a tibial plateau leveling osteotomy (TPLO) or other type of plate that is only covered by thinner layers of tissue. These areas will effectively receive an increased dose as the light reflects back off the implant into the surrounding tissue overlying and adjacent to it. The laser therapist should quickly pass over these areas when treating in a "grid-pattern" movement in order to disperse the dose evenly throughout the area. Adjustments may also be made to lower the treatment power (W) slightly for patient comfort.
2) Because the light does not penetrate through the metal hardware, it is equally important to treat 360º around the limb, to ensure that the light is penetrating to all the associated soft tissues the therapist wishes to target.

This is particularly important for osteotomy sites, such as in TPLO patients, and in fracture-repair situations.

3) When treating over staples, treatment should include several inches of margin around the incision as well as the incision line itself. The laser therapist should quickly cross the incision line instead of "hovering" or treating back and forth directly over the line itself.
4) When treating an incision closed with sutures, the incision and the area immediately adjacent to the incision itself should be treated with the same technique described above. However, unless the optical properties of the suture itself are known, the practitioner should be aware that some darker suture materials may absorb light and heat up. Therefore, the laser operator is reminded again to continue a scanning pattern crossing the incision line and never to "hover" directly over the sutures themselves.

Dosimetry for Musculoskeletal Conditions

Laser medical procedures for musculoskeletal conditions, including osteoarthritis, usually describe recommended dosing in terms of the fluence or energy density (J/cm^2) administered to the surface of a specific anatomical area. The most practical reason for recommending doses in this manner is that it is possible to achieve the same energy density in a number of ways by adjusting either treatment time or power density (irradiance, W/cm^2). An in-depth discussion of ideal dose calculation and the relationship between irradiance, light penetration, and effectiveness in treating various conditions (especially deep-tissue musculoskeletal conditions) is included in Chapter 4.

As a brief summary, due to the percentage of light lost in transmission from the skin surface to deeper tissues, the irradiance required to produce a therapeutic effect is higher for "deep-tissue" conditions than it is for "superficial" conditions, such as wounds, burns, and other dermatological conditions. This is why good clinical outcomes may be appreciated with lower irradiance when treating superficial conditions, while results may be inconsistent when treating deep-tissue conditions, even with longer treatment times. The optimal irradiance also varies for different wavelengths, but the critical parameter is the dose delivered to the target tissue. As previously mentioned, a recent *in vivo* review study (Zein *et al.*, 2018) identified that the two factors of most importance in PBM for determining clinical success are both fluence (J/cm^2) and irradiance (W/cm^2) and not merely the total quantity of photons absorbed by target tissues as previously surmised. Factors including the overall depth of the target tissue being treated, the presence or absence of melanin in the skin, the presence or absence of blood vessels (and the blood contained within) in the tissues, the thickness of any bone present, and tissue hydration all play a role in the penetration of photons to the target tissue. Calculations for clinical dosimetry for deep-tissue or musculoskeletal conditions should take as many of these factors into account as possible. Software for "preset" protocols in many commercially available PBMT units may take some (or none) of this into account, and the clinician should feel comfortable inquiring with the laser manufacturer to gain a more thorough understanding of the basis for dosing in protocols and changes based on patient characteristics in their individual PBMT devices.

When calculating clinical dosimetry for musculoskeletal conditions, a general range of energy densities of 8–20 J/cm^2 is recommended, scaling up with the size of the patient and subsequent depth of the target tissue in the treatment area(s) (Bjordal *et al.*, 2006; Roberts *et al.*, 2013; Gaynor, 2015; Looney *et al.*, 2018; Alves *et al.*, 2022a,b,c). Though the specifics are device- and design-dependent, the power used to achieve the desired fluence should be lower for smaller patients, areas with increased sensitivity, or areas with either very little soft tissue present (e.g., over bony prominences), or relatively shallow target tissue (e.g., the Achilles tendon versus the coxofemoral joint). Table 11.1 provides a range of recommended power settings for musculoskeletal conditions in veterinary patients of various sizes. These doses should be effective and safe for most commercially available laser units, but the practitioner should *always* confirm with the laser manufacturer regarding safety specifications.

Table 11.1 The recommended range of power (W) settings for treating musculoskeletal conditions in canine and feline patients. These are ranges and adjustments should be made accordingly with clinical judgment, patient body type, observation of patient comfort level, consideration of anatomic area being treated, spot area of the laser handpiece being used and/or concurrent issues.

Patients weight (kg)	Power settings (W)
<4.5	2.5–6.0
4.5–9.0	3–7
9.1–18.0	5–10
18.1–27.0	6–12
27.1–36.0	7–15
36.1–45.0	8–16
>45.0	10–18

Patient comfort should be continuously monitored during treatment (see section on "Patient Preparation and Treatment Techniques"), and adjusted as necessary. It should be noted that for conditions that are nonresponsive to this standard dosing, or for those that reach a plateau in improvement, increasing the target energy density as discussed in Chapter 4 may be appropriate, by either increasing treatment time or increasing irradiance itself. However, prior to increasing the dose of PBMT being applied, the practitioner should ensure that a proper diagnosis is in place, and that common reasons for perceived treatment failure are not present (see section on "Common Reasons for Perceived Treatment Failure or Inconsistent Results").

Following these guidelines, various anatomic areas may be measured in square centimeters (cm^2) or estimated with experience. Given a target energy density (J/cm^2), the total energy required to treat the area can then be calculated. Provided the power chosen is within the therapeutic range of irradiance discussed earlier, delivery of the dose will determine the treatment time. The practitioner is encouraged to check with the laser manufacturer to confirm that chosen parameters are within this range, as this is dependent on each device's design. For example, compare the calculations for treating the carpus of a 4 kg feline patient and a 40 kg canine patient in Box 11.1.

"Preset" protocols in various laser units vary from manufacturer to manufacturer. The practitioner should have a thorough understanding of the size of the areas to be treated once they are selected in the laser software. While preset guidelines are helpful for beginner laser users, they should not replace a thorough understanding of dosimetry. They should always be checked against the practitioner's calculations or estimates to ensure that an effective treatment dose is being delivered.

Box 11.1 Dosage

The dose to be delivered (total joules) is easy to calculate manually, by multiplying the size of the area to be treated (cm^2) by the target energy density (J/cm^2).

4 kg Feline Carpus

50 cm^2 total area × 6 J/cm^2 = 300 J total
Treated at 2.5 W in continuous wave (CW)
Treatment time = 120 seconds (2 minutes)

34 kg Canine Carpus

125 cm^2 total area × 15 J/cm^2 = 1875 J total
Treated at 8 W in continuous wave (CW)
Treatment time = 234 seconds (3 minutes, 54 seconds)

Treatment Session Frequency

For any acute or chronic painful condition such as osteoarthritis, an "induction phase" of initial, more frequent treatment sessions is recommended (i.e., every-other-day treatments until a significant effect is seen). For patients in acute pain that may be experiencing an overuse injury or flare-up of their arthritis pain, treating daily is optimal for faster results (Riegel, 2008). Each patient must be evaluated and treated as an individual; some take longer to respond than others. Though significant improvement may be appreciated sooner for some patients with osteoarthritis, it is usually noted between four and six treatment sessions. However, for those with severe osteoarthritis or multiple joint involvements, improvement may not be noted for 7–10 sessions. It is helpful for the practitioner to set expectations with pet owners, to avoid their becoming discouraged when they do not see immediate results. Once a significant improvement is noted in clinical signs, a "transition phase" of treatment sessions is begun. During transition, treatments are decreased to twice weekly, then once weekly, and so on as the patient improves, until either the condition resolves (e.g., resolution of a soft-tissue injury) or a "maintenance phase" of treatment is established (for chronic conditions such as osteoarthritis). The maintenance phase's commencement and interval between treatments should be based on the patient's response to therapy.

Pet owners should also be counseled that while PBMT may help alleviate their pet's pain and decrease other clinical symptoms, it will not change anatomical biomechanical defects (such as osteochondritis dissecans lesions or dysplastic changes) or "cure" the osteoarthritic disease process permanently. PBMT is part of a long-term treatment plan for pain management. Owners should be aware that their pet will require ongoing maintenance therapy based on their clinical signs. Maintenance treatments should be scheduled before the pet experiences any deterioration in the improvements seen with their induction-phase treatments. Owners can be encouraged to schedule follow-up visits for maintenance treatments at the first sign of returning discomfort or difficulties with their pet's daily activities (e.g., decreased activity, hesitation to go up or down stairs, or difficulty laying down or getting up from the floor). The available client-reported outcome measures can be used to this end, for example, by scheduling regular follow-up completions of the questionnaires. Alternatively, a regular maintenance treatment session may be scheduled, at a time interval established by the practitioner and the owner. It is not uncommon, if maintenance visits are missed or delayed, to require a "mini re-induction" phase of several more frequent sessions in order to reestablish patient comfort, and then to wean the treatment sessions back out to a maintenance-phase interval.

It should be noted that one of the potential benefits of PBMT is the ability to decrease the dosage or frequency of administration of chronic pain medications, especially nonsteroidal anti-inflammatory drugs (NSAIDs). The weaning of chronic medications is not recommended until a patient is on a regular schedule of maintenance treatments with PBMT that seems to best control their symptoms. In this way, the practitioner may appreciate changes in the patient's response and comfort level while changing only one factor at a time.

Variations in the treatment frequencies recommended here may be noted in the individual musculoskeletal condition sections that follow.

Osteoarthritis and Rheumatoid Arthritis

One of the most common uses of PBMT in veterinary medicine today is for the treatment of chronic pain associated with osteoarthritis. Many different animal and human trials have been performed that show the modulatory effect of PBMT on inflammatory markers (IL1β, PGE2, tumor necrosis factor alpha [TNFα]) and other aspects of the inflammatory process (reducing edema and influx of neutrophils) (Bjordal *et al.,* 2006). Others have shown the ability of PBMT to significantly reduce the total number of leukocytes and neutrophils in a treated arthritic joint cavity, as well as the concentration of IL1β and IL6 in joint fluid (Pallotta *et al.,* 2012). These results are important, since leukocyte influx to the joint is a hallmark of arthritis and IL1β and IL6 have been implicated in cartilage degradation and the stimulation of metalloproteinases, respectively. Treatment with laser therapy has also been shown to reduce the activity of metalloproteinases 2 and 9 in an experimental model involving rats with induced knee arthritis (Carlos *et al.,* 2014). Several studies have been published looking at the use of PBMT in treating humans with Bouchard's and Heberden's osteoarthritis (Baltzer *et al.,* 2016) and knee osteoarthritis (Fukuda *et al.,* 2015). As a whole, laser-treated patients experienced a significant reduction in pain and swelling, as well as a decrease in stiffness and increase in joint mobility and function. PBMT has been evaluated alone and in combination with other therapeutic approaches to osteoarthritis. The effect of PBMT was superior to placebos and some exercise programs, and the combination of PBMT with other therapeutic approaches improved overall results (Ahmad *et al.,* 2022; Alqualo-Costa *et al.,* 2021; de Paula Gomes *et al.,* 2018; Nazari *et al.,* 2019; Pinto *et al.,* 2022; Stausholm *et al.,* 2019; Vassão *et al.,* 2021). PBMT has also been used successfully to treat the pain and stiffness associated with rheumatoid arthritis (Brosseau *et al.,* 2000). More recently, clinical studies on canine osteoarthritis have become available in veterinary patients, focusing on hip and elbow osteoarthritis, the latter of which can be particularly challenging to manage. Over a period of 6 weeks, 980 nm PBMT at 10 to 20 J/cm^2 improved lameness and pain scores in dogs with elbow osteoarthritis while reducing the need or dose for NSAIDs (Looney *et al.,* 2018). A randomized controlled clinical study evaluated the effect of 980 nm PBMT on military working dogs with moderate to severe hip osteoarthritis with a power of 6.5–8 W, an irradiance of 4.5–5.2 W/cm^2, and a fluence of 14.3–19.5 J/cm^2 over the hip area. PBMT reduced pain levels and improved client-report outcome measure scores and joint ranges of motion compared to NSAID administration (meloxicam) alone (Alves *et al.,* 2022a,b,c).

Temporomandibular Joint Disorders

The temporomandibular joint (TMJ) is a unique anatomic area that can cause a range of clinical symptoms in veterinary patients when affected, including difficulty opening the mouth, dysphagia, pain, and performance problems in canine and equine athletes. These symptoms can have a major impact on the patient's overall quality of life, affecting adequate feeding, drinking, and involvement in some types of play. It is important when treating the TMJ that all structures typically associated with pain and dysfunction in this area are treated and included when calculating dose. These structures include the TMJ itself, periarticular tissues, and masticatory muscles (Figure 11.9). Human

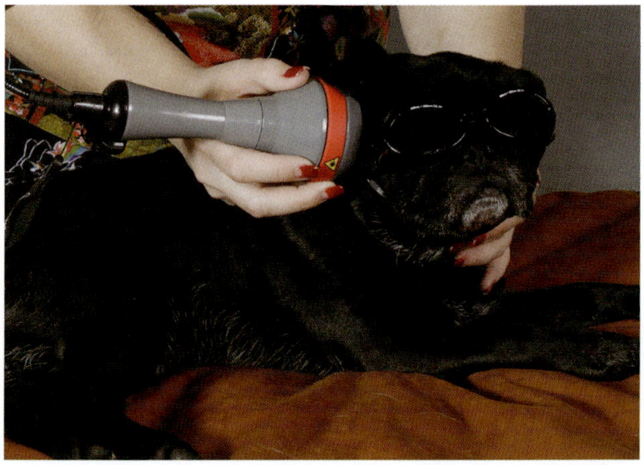

Figure 11.9 Laser therapist treating the TMJ.

reports show that PBMT has been used to treat disorders of the TMJ, alone or in combination with other modalities, with the aim of relieving pain and improving function (Brochado *et al.,* 2018; Chellappa and Thirupathy, 2020; Nadershah *et al.,* 2020; Melis *et al.*, 2012). Different systematic reviews show that PBMT effectively relieves pain and improves functional outcomes in patients with TMD (S. A. Ahmad *et al.,* 2021; Chellappa and Thirupathy, 2020; Xu *et al.,* 2018). In many cases, pain-relieving effects lasted beyond the treatment period and into 1- to 2-year follow-up (Ayyildiz *et al.,* 2015). Little animal information is available, and reports are restricted to animal models. In induced inflammation on TMJ of rats, induced PBMT inhibited leukocyte chemotaxis, and reduced the concentration of pro-inflammatory mediators, specifically TNF-α, IL-1β and CINC-1, while increasing the levels of the anti-inflammatory cytokine IL-10 (de Mazuqueli Pereira *et al.,* 2021). Similarly, PBMT inhibited the local inflammatory response in the masseter muscle by a central inhibition of fractalkine observed in the trigeminal ganglion (Ferrara-Jr *et al.,* 2019).

As with all treatments performed on or around the face, head, and neck, special care should be taken and appropriate protection for the patient's eyes should be provided (see section on "Patient Preparation and Treatment Techniques").

Myopathies and Myositis

PBMT for muscle injury rehabilitation and for use in myositis caused by snakebite envenomation is covered in Chapters 23 and 10, respectively. When examining the literature with regard to myositis in general, PBMT has been used to treat experimentally induced myositis in rats, resulting in a significant reduction in the presence of inflammatory cells and in the amount of edema present in tissue after treatment (de Carvalho *et al.,* 2015; Oliveira *et al.,* 2020). Additional studies on experimental myopathy show significant changes in inflammatory biomarkers and oxidative stress (decreased levels of fibrinogen, L-citrulline, and superoxide dismutase [SOD]) and significant muscle recovery (Servetto *et al.,* 2010), as well as a notable reduction in the area occupied by inflammatory infiltrates (Dávila *et al.,* 2011). In humans, reports show that PBMT reduced symptoms in a patient with focal myositis nonresponsive to NSAIDs and local corticosteroid injection (Ghanbarnasab *et al.,* 2019). Though most inflammatory myopathies in dogs and cats are either idiopathic (e.g., masticatory myositis, idiopathic polymyositis) or secondarily associated with other diseases (e.g., Rickettsial or parasitic infections), both types are the result of inflammatory cells infiltrating striated muscles (Podell, 2002). The muscle cell degeneration and necrosis seen in idiopathic inflammatory myopathies are thought to be caused by lymphocyte-mediated cytotoxic mechanisms. In particular, many of the cytokines involved in the process (including IL1β and TNFα) were mentioned in the literature review sections as those downregulated by the application of PBMT.

Current therapies for idiopathic inflammatory myopathies in veterinary medicine are aimed at reducing pain and inflammation with systemic immunosuppression and analgesics, followed by either maintenance anti-inflammatory or immune-modulatory medications when necessary. In the author's subjective experience, PBMT may be very effective, especially in managing pain in patients affected by masticatory myositis, and it has been used in several veterinary patients without any harmful sequelae noted. Dosing has been similar to that used for treating TMJ or other deep-tissue musculoskeletal disorders. Again, precautions should be taken to protect the patient's eyes during treatment around the face. Similarly, the author recommends treating all the affected muscles of mastication (temporalis, digastricus, and masseter), any painful facial muscles, as well as the muscles in the cranial cervical area for any associated spasm or soreness. Daily treatment is recommended initially for optimal pain management, tapering as for other chronic conditions as the patient improves. PBMT should always be used as an adjunct alongside standard-of-care treatment until further research is done to examine its effectiveness in treating these disorders in veterinary patients in a clinical setting.

Tendinopathies

Other chapters cover the treatment of acute tendon and ligament injuries with PBMT and regenerative medicine; the same mechanisms of action apply to the effectiveness of the modality for chronic tendinopathies that occur following damage to a tendon. Histopathology of common overuse tendon conditions includes discontinuous and disorganized collagen fibers, abnormal neovascularization, and necrosis. Pain, edema, crepitus, and impaired function may be diagnosed clinically in patients with these conditions (Jozsa and Kannus, 1997; Khan *et al.,* 1999). The etiology is not completely understood.

Treating chronic tendinopathies can be frustrating, as they are difficult to heal due to the nature of their blood supply, making it difficult to manage proinflammatory mediators and delivery of needed healing support. Even though most improve with rest, a certain percentage of patients will experience recurrence of symptoms as soon as activities are resumed. Not unexpectedly, reports exist demonstrating a reduction in the proinflammatory mediators IL6, TNFα, TGFβ cytokines, COX-2, and matrix metalloproteinase 1 and 13 enzyme following PBM application in a tendonitis model (Pires *et al.*, 2011; Fernandes de Jesus *et al.*, 2019). While there is still a need for standardization of treatment parameters and proper reporting, most *in vitro* studies show that PBMT increases cell proliferation and migration, allied to a higher protein and gene expression of tendon biomarkers (da Silva *et al.*, 2022). Fibroblast metabolism and proliferation are also enhanced, with an increase in mesenchymal cell proliferation and the synthesis of collagen type II, collagen fibril size, and biomechanical strength (Ng *et al.*, 2004; Akamatsu *et al.*, 2021; Alzyoud *et al.*, 2022).

In a randomized, placebo-controlled, double-blinded clinical trial, 16 human subjects with chronic tendinopathy of the extensor carpi radialis brevis tendon (lateral epicondylitis) received eight treatments with either a sham or a real therapy laser over a period of 18 days. The laser-treated group demonstrated improvement in handgrip strength, function, and reduction in pain continuously over a 12-month period, despite return to normal activity (Roberts *et al.*, 2013). In contrast, pain, strength, and functional impairment in the sham group remained unchanged until 12 months, when there was partial improvement in these outcomes, consistent with resolution of clinical signs of tendinopathy following 12 months of reduced use (Jozsa and Kannus, 1997). Systemic reviews and meta-analysis concluded that PBMT leads to improved function and greater decreases in pain levels when compared to other therapeutic modalities such as exercise (Martimbianco *et al.*, 2020; Tripodi *et al.*, 2021). PBMT can also improve the results obtained with other therapeutic modalities (Martins *et al.*, 2022).

Treatment of tendinopathies in veterinary patients is optimally performed in conjunction with an excellent rehabilitation therapy program. Dosing and frequency of treatment are typical for deep-tissue musculoskeletal conditions, with consideration given to the location and depth of the tendon being treated and of its associated soft tissues when selecting power parameters. It should be noted that patients experiencing an acute exacerbation of tendinitis or tendinopathy may be very hypersensitive to pressure, temperature, or both, and that adjustments in treatment power and a choice between on- or off-contact treatment be made according to the practitioner's clinical judgment.

Cranial Cruciate Ligament Injuries

Though literature specific to ligament injuries is described in other chapters, some studies specifically examine injury of the cranial cruciate ligament (CCL) and the progression of subsequent osteoarthritis in the knee. In one rodent model, laser treatment started immediately after cruciate ligament transection was shown to prevent certain features related to articular degeneration of the knee following transection (Bublitz *et al.*, 2014). A similar rabbit model showed that at least 6 weeks of intermittent laser treatment could relieve knee pain and control synovium inflammation and cartilage damage (Wang *et al.*, 2014).

Unsurprisingly, one of the most common uses for PBMT in daily veterinary practice is in the conservative pain management of partial CCL tears. But does application of PBMT to these injuries contribute to healing or prevent further injury? Though supporting literature is more common regarding calcaneal tendon models, the principles of potential efficacy are the same. Studies have demonstrated the exertion of an anti-inflammatory effect over injured tendons, with reduction of the release of pro-inflammatory cytokines such as TNFα (Da Ré Guerra *et al.*, 2016), improvement in the remodeling of extracellular matrix (ECM) during the healing process in tendons through activation of matrix metalloproteinase 2 (MMP2), and stimulation of collagen synthesis (Guerra *et al.*, 2013). Improvement of collagen fiber organization (Oliveira *et al.*, 2009) and increased neovascularization in injured tendons exposed to PBMT (Salate *et al.*, 2005) have also been demonstrated. Additionally, PBMT attenuates joint capsule contracture by inhibiting inflammation and fibrosis (Kaneguchi *et al.*, 2022).

There are also some veterinary studies specifically examining injury of the CCL and outcomes when PBMT was used postoperatively. In dogs, Renwick et al. utilized PBM for three treatments postoperatively following TPLO surgery and found a greater improvement in the gait section of the adjusted Canine Orthopedic Index questionnaire (Renwick *et al.*, 2018). Rogatko and colleagues investigating the use of PBM as a single preoperative treatment for the same surgery and found a significant difference in peak vertical force (PVF) in the PBM treated group as well as a greater proportion of patients that were healed at 8 weeks postop (Rogatko *et al.*, 2017). Neither of these studies showed significant differences in bone healing; however, this author would refer back to previous comments regarding increased dosing needed for deep tissue conditions. In the former canine study, doses listed within its appendix section on laser settings are less than 50% that suggested for deep tissue conditions (including bone healing), suggesting perhaps that dosimetry, while adequate for some benefits to be appreciated from pain relief, were not sufficient for other outcomes to be significant. Similarly, Chavez *et al.* (2023) performed a post-TPLO study in which dogs received either a single PBM treatment or sham treatment preoperatively and four treatments postoperatively at various time periods and evaluating various outcome measures including measuring C-reactive protein (CRP), percentage weight bearing (%WB), lameness using a short form of a composite measure pain scale (CMPS-SF) evaluated by the clinician and owners, and surgical site infection (SSI). No statistically significant differences were found between treatment groups when evaluating CRP, % WB, and CMPS-SF by the clinician and weekly evaluation of the CMPS-SF by owners. Although no statistically significant differences were found in patients developing SSIs between treatment groups, SSI was only observed in patients in the control group (5/30, 16.6%). Most were minor/superficial infections (4/30 13.3%), and a single dog (1/30, 3.3%) had a major/deep SSI. Chavez et al. concluded that with "promising but not statistically significant differences between groups, SSIs may be reduced after PBMT application." The chapter authors here again emphasize that the dose used in this study (5 J/cm^2) was also half of what would have been typically recommended for deep tissue dosing of the stifle joint, though adequate for superficial wound healing recommendations.

For conservative management of partial CCL tears, typical dosing for deep-tissue musculoskeletal conditions should be used. It is recommended that both stifles be treated due to compensatory weight shifting and that treatment of the lower back be considered as well, paying particular attention to the iliopsoas muscle for any pain or spasm (Figure 11.10). Treatment for the stifle should include a large area (see section on "Patient Preparation and Treatment Techniques"), incorporating all important soft-tissue structures, including the patellar ligament and insertion of the hamstring muscles. As with all chronic conditions, treatment should be administered at least three times weekly until significant improvement is noted with continuous reassessment, and should optimally be utilized along with an appropriate physical rehabilitation program.

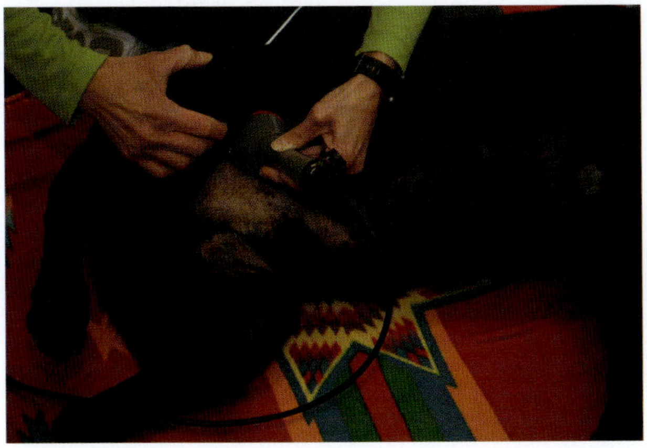

Figure 11.10 Treating the iliopsoas.

Additional uses of PBMT with regards to the CCL deal with its application postoperatively for many of the surgeries used to address complete CCL tears, as well as for those pets that have not had surgery due to the owner's decision, other medical conditions, or other factors preventing surgery. It should be emphasized that PBMT is most beneficial for managing pain and decreasing inflammation associated with these conditions. Though it may also contribute to tendon healing in partial CCL tear situations, its application will not correct the structural instability in cases of complete CCL tears. It is always best utilized in combination with an appropriate physical rehabilitation program.

Treatment with PBMT should begin immediately after surgery to address pain and inflammation and to assist in wound healing. The incisional area and superficial soft tissues disrupted during surgery may be treated with a more superficial target energy density of 4–6 J/cm^2 and with a lower power setting than would be used in a deep-tissue musculoskeletal dose. The deeper soft tissues of the anatomic region, which are often painful, swollen, or bruised after surgery, should be treated with a dose typical for musculoskeletal disorders (target energy density 8–20 J/cm^2, depending on the size of the patient). The entire treatment area mentioned for partial CCL tear management (including the contralateral stifle and lower back) should be treated in post-operative cases as well. Treatment should ideally be performed daily for the first 3 days if possible, and then twice to three times weekly as with other chronic conditions, tapering as the patient improves. Please note that if the patient is placed in a soft bandage after surgery, the application of PBMT should be performed during bandage changes, as PBMT cannot be performed through bandage, splint, or casting material.

Fractures and Bone Healing

PBMT may also be used to address fractures, whether freshly surgically fixated or delayed/nonunion. In addition to the pain-relieving aspects that PBMT brings to these cases, there is quite a lot of evidence in both animal and human studies for its use in situations where bone healing is desired, despite a need for refinement of treatment parameters. In rat models of bone healing, histological analysis showed that groups treated with PBMT exhibited faster bone healing, bone tissue matrix production, and mineralization in the alveolar region than in control groups (da Fonseca *et al.*, 2022; Kuzu *et al.*, 2022; Ribeiro *et al.*, 2022). In a review of 25 relevant articles regarding the use of PBMT in bone healing (13 *in vitro* and 12 animal studies), 11 of the *in vitro* studies showed positive results with regard to acceleration of cell proliferation and differentiation. All animal studies showed improved bone healing in laser-treated sites (Ebrahimi *et al.*, 2012). In human studies, particularly dentistry procedures, PBMT improved bone healing and increased bone density, neoformation, regeneration, and mineralization while promoting anti-inflammatory and analgesic effects (Kulkarni *et al.*, 2019; Lopes de Lopes *et al.*, 2022; Noba *et al.*, 2018).

There is ample evidence that PBMT acts in the first two stages of bone healing, the inflammatory and reparative stages (Asteinza Castro *et al.*, 2023). Another study showed that while PBM's effects were more prominent when treatment started during the acute phase of the injury, it still aided the bone consolidation process and favored the physiopathologic mechanisms involved in bone tissue repair when used in the chronic phase as well (Mota *et al.*, 2013).

Osteopenic patients, or those with compromised bone healing, have also been examined in research. A study investigating bone healing of the femur in both osteopenic and normal rats with titanium implants showed an improved osseointegration process in both groups, particular in the initial phase of bone formation (de Vasconcellos *et al.*, 2014). Another study, looking at bone healing in diabetic rats with a tibial defect, showed that all laser-treated groups had a better histological pattern and a higher amount of newly formed bone than control groups in both histological and morphometric evaluation (Magri *et al.*, 2015). A human systematic review showed that PBMT can improve bone density in maxillofacial bony defects (dos Santinoni *et al.*, 2017).

Further controlled studies should be performed in veterinary patients to characterize the optimal dosing and effects for bone healing, but at this time it is recommended that treatment be performed immediately after stabilization and then every other day, for a total of six to eight treatments (Godbold and Arza, 2011). Fracture healing should be reassessed at this time, and treatments continued if healing is not progressing.

Please note that if the patient is placed in a soft bandage or other covering after surgery, the application of PBMT should be performed during bandage changes, as PBMT cannot be performed through bandage, splint, or casting material. Alternatively, a "window" can be created in the bandage material, through which PBMT can be performed over part of the fracture site; the window can then be re-bandaged to keep the overall bandage intact (though this is less than ideal, since the entire area may not be treated). A target energy density of 8–20 J/cm^2 is recommended (scaling up with the size of the patient and depth of target tissue(s)), and the entire area to be measured or estimated for treatment should include not only the fractured area itself, but also several square centimeters of adjacent normal bone, both proximal and distal. Any areas that have open wounds should receive a more superficial dose for wound healing, treated in an off-contact manner to avoid contamination. When possible, the deep tissue dose listed above should be utilized in an on-contact manner, circumferentially to treat the deeper fracture sites for better light penetration to these tissues. Please note the information regarding the use of PBMT with metal implants given earlier.

Osteomyelitis

Based on *in vivo* and *in vitro* studies, which initially reported that laser energy in differing wavelengths had potential bactericidal effects on certain infections such as *Staphylococcus aureus*, another study looked at its effects on chronic osteomyelitis induced experimentally in the rat tibia. Methicillin-resistant *S. aureus* (MRSA) was used to induce osteomyelitis in the rats' tibias. After 3 weeks, rats with evidence of osteomyelitis were treated with debridement alone, treated with debridement plus laser irradiation, or not treated at all. Irradiation commenced immediately after debridement surgery with an 808 nm, 100 mW continuous-wave (CW) diode laser with an irradiance of 127.3 mW/cm^2 and was applied daily for 5 consecutive days at three different energy densities ranging from 7.64 to 22.93 J/cm^2. Following sacrifice, tibias were removed and analyzed histopathologically, radiographically, and microbiologically. Histopathology showed that infection levels had decreased by 37%, 67%, 81%, and 93% in the groups treated by debridement and by debridement plus 7.64, 15.29, and 22.93 J/cm^2 of light therapy, respectively, compared to the negative control group (Kaya *et al.*, 2011). Further studies should be done in veterinary patients if practitioners wish to attempt the use of PBMT as an adjunct to other standard-of-care osteomyelitis treatments. Deep-tissue musculoskeletal dosing similar to that used for bone healing should be sufficient to achieve energy densities in this range for infections in the same anatomic areas.

Neck and Back Pain

One of the most common causes of neuropathic pain in veterinary medicine is intervertebral disk disease (IVDD). Acute IVDD is discussed in depth in Chapter 16. Here we will discuss chronic neck and back pain in veterinary patients, as these can have a variety of causes, including IVDD and other orthopedic conditions.

In the human literature, one study followed 26 human patients diagnosed with chronic neck pain caused by cervical disk herniation who were treated twice weekly for 4 weeks with laser irradiation over the painful area. A visual analog scale was used to determine the effects of laser therapy on chronic pain. After the end of the treatment regimen, a significant improvement was observed (Takahashi *et al.,* 2012). These findings and others from similar studies involving the use of PBMT in treating cervical pain are consistent with conclusions from a meta-analysis of 16 randomized controlled trials (RCTs), including 820 patients treated with PBMT for neck pain (Chow *et al.,* 2009). This review showed that laser treatment reduced pain immediately after treatment in acute neck pain and up to 22 weeks after completion of treatment in chronic neck pain. Lower back pain (LBP) also commonly affects human patients. PBMT of the dorsal root ganglion of the second lumbar spinal nerve resulted in a pain reduction of at least 50% immediately post-procedure (Holanda *et al.,* 2016). In a double-blind prospective RCT, PBMT reduced pain and improved function and quality of life (Lin *et al.,* 2020). PBMT associated with other treatment modalities contributed to improved outcomes compared to their isolated use (Nambi *et al.,* 2019). A systematic review concluded that it effectively relieves pain in patients with chronic LBP (Hwang *et al.,* 2015).

In patients with discogenic back pain, PBMT effectively treats neck and back pain caused by disk hernia (Takahashi *et al.,* 2012; Yilmaz *et al.,* 2020). Compared to other therapies, PBMT had a longer effect on some parameters (Boyraz *et al.,* 2015). Even patients who failed to respond to a conventional physical therapy program to avoid recourse to surgical intervention have been shown to benefit from treatment with PBMT. One paper reported on the long-term mean 5-year prospective follow-up of a group of 50 unselected patients visiting a referral pain center for discogenic back pain. Each patient had a single-level lesion documented by magnetic resonance imaging (MRI) followed by discography to confirm the affected disk was the source of pain. All the patients who entered the study had failed response to a combination of NSAIDs, and all had at least 3 months of conventional physical therapy prior to being treated with three laser therapy treatment sessions per week for 12 consecutive weeks. At the end of treatment at 12 weeks, 49 of 50 patients had significant improvement in their Oswestry Disability Index score, which was maintained at long-term follow-up assessments 1 and 5 years later (Ip and Fu, 2015b).

One recent publication has examined whether treatment of LBP could improve the clinical signs of acquired, non-neurologic urinary incontinence (UI) in dogs (Lane & Hill de Lopes *et al.,* 2022). Urethral sphincter mechanism incompetency (USMI) is the most common non-neurogenic acquired cause of UI in dogs (Chew *et al.,* 2011; Byron *et al.,* 2017) and Lane and Hill reported on therapeutic outcomes in 39 patients treated over a 6-year period for LBP using combined acupuncture and manual therapy (with 33/39 patients also having received concurrent PBM therapy). Treated patients showed a statistically significant reduction in both the frequency ($p < 0.01$) and volume ($p < 0.01$) of UI episodes. Treatment responses ranged from no improvement to complete resolution of the USMI clinical signs. Lane and Hill logically concluded that the reduction of USMI clinical signs following LBP treatment suggested a relationship between the two conditions, and that combined acupuncture, manual therapy, with or without PBM was shown to be an effective treatment for USMI. PBM parameters reported to be utilized in the treatment of these patients were varied and were not described in detail in the publication.

Current deep-tissue musculoskeletal dosing is appropriate for treating the cervical, thoracic, lumbar, and sacral spine. Treatment surface areas used for calculating dose should take into consideration the cause of the back pain. For example, if discogenic in origin, a few spinal segments both cranial and caudal to the suspected area of intervertebral disk extrusion or protrusion are included, as well as any descending nerve tracts that may be affected and any paraspinal muscles that have trigger points or spasm(s). If any spasms in the paraspinal muscles are noted further caudally or if neurological deficits are present in the limbs, it is recommended to treat the remainder of the spine as well. For thoracolumbar pain, treatment should be applied directly over the spine (Figure 11.11), as well as a few inches to either side, aiming toward the spine through the paraspinal musculature. In the neck area, a lateral and ventral approach is recommended, and the laser therapist is reminded that, in order to effectively treat the caudal cervical area (Figure 11.12), manipulation of the front leg may be necessary, which may be painful for the patient due to radicular pain. This should be done with care, and a good knowledge of anatomy is critical to treating the correct areas in these patients. Patients with back and neck pain should be treated in the position that is most comfortable for them, which may involve standing, sitting, or lying down in various positions.

For chronic neck or back pain in patients that are experiencing an acute flare-up or episode, standard recommendations for neurological workup and further treatment(s)

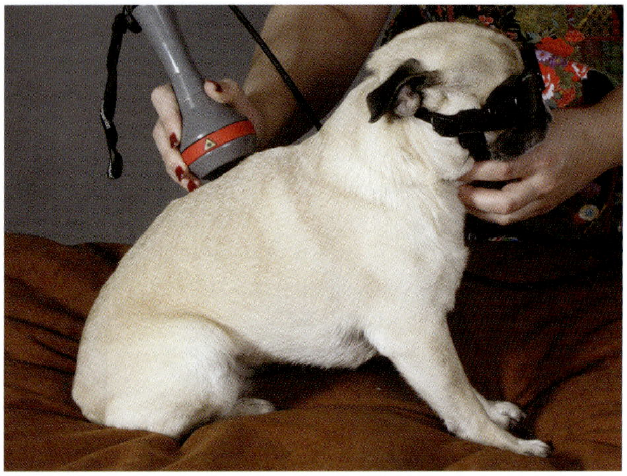

Figure 11.11 Laser therapist treating the spine.

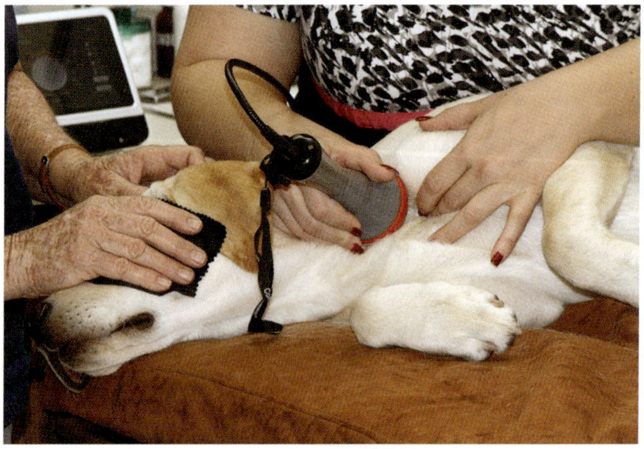

Figure 11.12 Laser therapist treating the caudal cervical area.

(including potentially surgery) still apply. However, PBMT may be applied in the acute situation to help resolve any muscle spasms and relieve pain while decisions regarding further workup and treatment are made. Further recommendations for postsurgical IVDD cases are discussed in chapter 16. For all other acute-on-chronic situations, including conservative treatment of neck or back pain, PBMT should begin immediately and continue daily, if possible, until significant improvement is seen. At that time, weaning to a transition phase of less-frequent treatments (twice per week, then once per week) is recommended, followed by a continued maintenance-therapy treatment once every 2–4 weeks, depending on severity of clinical signs and frequency of "flare ups," as in patients with osteoarthritis. As always, results with PBMT are optimized when used in conjunction with an excellent physical rehabilitation program and other supportive care for neurologic patients.

Common Reasons for Perceived Treatment Failure or Inconsistent Results

In general, PBMT should produce consistent, reliable improvement if used in the appropriate manner (see sections describing "Patient Preparation and Treatment Techniques" and "Dosimetry for Musculoskeletal Conditions"). As with any treatment modality, however, certain factors may influence its effectiveness. The most common reasons for a lack of efficacy or inconsistent results include:

1) **Treating the incorrect area.** Ensure that a recent, complete orthopedic, neurologic, and pain examination has been performed to confirm the source of the problem. Often, a patient may be referred for PBMT for osteoarthritis of a specific joint, which may or may not be the primary source of discomfort. Additionally, as previously mentioned, the degree of pathologic change noted on radiographs alone may not necessarily be consistent with the amount of lameness displayed by a patient or the severity of their discomfort. To ensure that a therapeutic dose is delivered properly, ensure that the laser therapist performing the treatment knows the correct anatomical landmarks to delineate the proper treatment area, and that these are the same as those used by the veterinarian prescribing the treatment.
2) **Not treating all problem areas.** Ensure that all sources of pain or anatomic dysfunction identified on examination are being addressed. Compensatory biomechanical changes commonly occur with chronic, painful conditions, and if they are not therapeutically addressed with PBMT and additional rehabilitation therapy, the patient may continue to experience discomfort and exhibit lameness or difficulties. For example, most animals with stifle or hip osteoarthritis usually have some degree of back pain and pain in the contralateral joint from weight shifting if both sides are not being addressed.
3) **A change in patient activity or medications.** Though more commonly seen after an initial improvement and subsequent worsening, make sure to inquire with the pet owner about any changes in medication or activity level at home. Oftentimes after improvement with PBMT, pet owners will wean or discontinue other medications, even if this has not yet been recommended. They might also take their pet for a run or play session at the local dog park, which can result in increased soreness or, worse, an overuse injury. Animals can also increase their spontaneous activity level, so some awareness and care should be taken to manage this possibility.
4) **Exacerbation of the condition.** Also more commonly seen after initial improvement and subsequent

worsening. Some conditions, such as osteoarthritis, typically have periods of naturally increased or decreased complaints and clinical signs (e.g., motivated by weather changes), and may require additional pain management and further diagnostics. It is not uncommon in some areas for loose or damaged pieces of articular cartilage or small pieces of osteophytes to break off with normal activity and further irritate the joint. Some anatomical areas, particularly the elbow joint, are notoriously difficult to treat, and may require higher doses of PBMT alongside other medications or therapeutics in order to bring about improvement. Further examination and diagnostics should always be performed any time a patient presents with acute-on-chronic pain.

5) **Presence of an undiagnosed problem.** Ensure that there is not another pathologic process affecting the anatomic area of concern. Repeat radiographs and examinations are recommended to rule out malignancy if joint or bone pain is present and does not improve with PBMT.

6) **Inappropriate "induction phase" or the need for a "mini re-induction phase."** While a treatment interval of three treatments during week 1, two treatments during week 2, and one treatment during week 3 may be effective for some patients, others will not respond unless a more intensive and frequent induction phase is used. Patients may also fail to respond if transition- or maintenance-phase treatments have been missed due to poor owner compliance. Ensure that an appropriate induction phase has been administered before weaning the frequency of treatments to a transition or maintenance phase (see section on "Treatment Session Frequency").

References

AAHA/AAFP (2007). AAHA/AAFP pain management guidelines for dogs & cats. *J Am Anim Hosp Assoc.* 43(5):235–248.

Ahmad, S.A. *et al.* (2021). Low-level laser therapy in temporomandibular joint disorders: a systematic review. *J Med and Life.* 14(2):148–164. doi:10.25122/jml-2020-0169.

Ahmad, M.A. *et al.* (2022). Effects of low-level and high-intensity laser therapy as adjunctive to rehabilitation exercise on pain, stiffness and function in knee osteoarthritis: a systematic review and meta-analysis. *Physiotherapy.* 114:85–95. doi:10.1016/j.physio.2021.03.011.

Akamatsu, F.E. *et al.* (2021). Photobiomodulation therapy increases collagen II after tendon experimental injury. *Histol Histopathol.* 36(6):663–674. doi:10.14670/HH-18-330.

Alfredo, P.P. *et al.* (2012). Efficacy of low level PBMT associated with exercises in knee osteoarthritis: a randomized double-blind study. *Clin Rehab.* 26(6):523–533.

Alqualo-Costa, R. *et al.* (2021). Interferential current and photobiomodulation in knee osteoarthritis: a randomized, placebo-controlled, double-blind clinical trial. *Clin Rehab.* 35(10):1413–1427. doi:10.1177/02692155211012004.

Alves, J.C. *et al.* (2022a). A randomized double-blinded controlled trial on the effects of photobiomodulation therapy in dogs with osteoarthritis. *Am J Vet Res.* 83(8). doi:10.2460/ajvr.22.03.0036.

Alves, J.C. *et al.* (2022b). Characterization of weight-bearing compensation in dogs with bilateral hip osteoarthritis. *Topics in Comp Anim Med.* 49:100655. doi:10.1016/j.tcam.2022.100655.

Alves, J.C. *et al.* (2022c). The influence of IL-1 and C-reactive protein levels in synovial fluid of companion dogs with bilateral hip osteoarthritis on various clinical disease parameters. *Am J Vet Res.* 1–10. doi:10.2460/ajvr.22.05.0079.

Alzyoud, J.A.M. *et al.* (2022). Photobiomodulation for tendinopathy: a review of preclinical studies. *Photobiomodulation Photomed Laser Surg.* 40(6):370–377. doi:10.1089/photob.2021.0192.

Ammar, T.A. (2014). Monochromatic infrared photo energy versus low level PBMT in patients with knee osteoarthritis. *J Lasers Med Sci.* 5(4):176–182.

Anders, J.J. *et al.* (2004). Phototherapy promotes regeneration and functional recovery of injured peripheral nerve. *Neurol Res.* 26(2):233–239.

Anders, J.J. *et al.* (2014). In vitro and in vivo optimization of infrared laser treatment for injured peripheral nerves. *Lasers Surg Med.* 46(1):34–45.

Anderson, K.L. *et al.* (2018). Prevalence, duration and risk factors for appendicular osteoarthritis in a UK dog population under primary veterinary care. *Sci Rep.* 8(1):5641. doi:10.1038/s41598-018-23940-z.

Anderson, K.L. *et al.* (2020). Risk factors for canine osteoarthritis and its predisposing Arthropathies: a systematic review. *Front Vet Sci.* 7. doi:10.3389/fvets.2020.00220.

Assis, L. *et al.* (2016). Aerobic exercise training and low-level PBMT modulate inflammatory response and degenerative process in an experimental model of knee osteoarthritis in rats. *Osteoarthritis Cartil.* 24(1):169–177.

Asteinza Castro, I.M. *et al.* (2023). Photobiomodulation therapy combined with static magnetic field in tibial fracture healing of a dog: a case report. *Vet Med Sci.* 9(2):591–599. doi:10.1002/vms3.1071.

Ayyildiz, S. *et al.* (2015). Evaluation of low-level PBMT in TMD patients. *Case Reports in Dent.* 2015:424213.

Baltzer, A.W.A. *et al.* (2016). Positive effects of low level PBMT (LLLT) on Bouchard's and Heberden's osteoarthritis. *Lasers Surg Med.* 48(5):498–504.

Barić Rafaj, R. *et al.* (2017). Plasma markers of inflammation and hemostatic and endothelial activity in naturally overweight and obese dogs. *BMC Vet Res.* 13(1):13. doi:10.1186/s12917-016-0929-8.

Benito, J. *et al.* (2013). Feline musculoskeletal pain index: responsiveness and testing of criterion validity. *J Vet Intern Med.* 27(3):474–482. doi:10.1111/jvim.12077.

Bjordal, J.M. *et al.* (2006). Photoradiation in acute pain: a systematic review of possible mechanisms of action and clinical effects in randomized placebo-controlled trials. *Photomed Laser Surg.* 24(2):158–168.

Boyraz, I. *et al.* (2015). Comparison of high-intensity laser therapy and ultrasound treatment in the patients with lumbar discopathy. *Biomed Res Int.* 2015:1–6. doi:10.1155/2015/304328.

Brochado, F.T. *et al.* (2018). Comparative effectiveness of photobiomodulation and manual therapy alone or combined in TMD patients: a randomized clinical trial. *Brazilian Oral Res.* 32(0). doi:10.1590/1807-3107bor-2018.vol32.0050.

Brosseau, L. *et al.* (2000). Low level PBMT for osteoarthritis and rheumatoid arthritis: a metaanalysis. *J Rheumatol.* 27(8):1961–1969.

Brown, D.C. (2014). The canine orthopedic index. Step 2: psychometric testing. *Vet Surg.* 43(3):241–246. doi:10.1111/j.1532-950X.2014.12141.x.

Brown, D.C. *et al.* (2008). Ability of the canine brief pain inventory to detect response to treatment in dogs with osteoarthritis. *J Am Vet Med Assoc.* 233(8):1278–1283 http://www.ncbi.nlm.nih.gov/pubmed/19180716.

Bublitz, C. *et al.* (2014). Low-level PBMT prevents degenerative morphological changes in an experimental model of anterior cruciate ligament transection in rats. *Lasers Med Sci.* 29(5):1669–1678.

Byron, J.K. *et al.* (2017). Urethral sphincter mechanism incompetence in 163 neutered female dogs: diagnosis, treatment, and relationship of weight and age at neuter to development of disease. *J. Vet. Intern. Med.* 31:442–448. doi:10.1111/jvim.14678.

Cachon, T. *et al.* (2023). COAST development group's international consensus guidelines for the treatment of canine osteoarthritis. *Front Vet Sci.* 10. doi:10.3389/fvets.2023.1137888.

Cambier, D. *et al.* (2000). The influence of low intensity infrared laser irradiation on conduction characteristics of peripheral nerve: a randomised, controlled, double blind study on the sural nerve. *Lasers Med Sci.* 15(3):195–200.

Carlos, F.P. *et al.* (2014). Protective effect of low-level PBMT (LLLT) on acute zymosan-induced arthritis. *Lasers Med Sci.* 29(2):757–763.

de Carvalho, A.F.M. *et al.* (2015). The low-level laser on acute myositis in rats. *Acta Cirurgica Brasileira.* 30(12):806–811. doi:10.1590/S0102-865020150120000003.

Chavez, O.A. *et al.* (2023). Photobiomodulation therapy in dogs undergoing TPLO after cranial cruciate ligament rupture shows promise but no statistically significant difference in a randomized trial. *Am J Vet Res.* 85(2). doi:10.2460/ajvr.23.06.0138 PMID: 38039628.ajvr.23.06.0138

Chellappa, D. and Thirupathy, M. (2020). Comparative efficacy of low-level laser and TENS in the symptomatic relief of temporomandibular joint disorders: a randomized clinical trial. *Indian J Dent Res.* 31(1):42. doi:10.4103/ijdr.IJDR_735_18.

Chew, D.J. *et al.* (2011). Disorders of micturition and urinary incontinence. In: *Canine and Feline Nephrology and Urology.* (eds. R.E. Raskin *et al.*), 2 edn, 409–433. W.B. Saunders, Saint Louis, MI. doi:10.1016/B978-0-7216-8178-8.10013-2.

Chien, S. and Wilhelmi, B.J. (2012). A simplified technique for producing an ischemic wound model. *J Visualized Exp.* 2(63):e3341.

Chow, R.T. *et al.* (2009). Efficacy of low level PBMT in the management of neck pain: a systematic review and meta-analysis of randomized placebo or active-treatment controlled trials. *Lancet.* 374(9705):1897–1908.

Chow, R.T. *et al.* (2011). Inhibitory effects of laser irradiation on peripheral mammalian nerves and relevance to analgesic effects: a systematic review. *Photomed Laser Surg.* 29(6):365–381.

Clough, W. *et al.* (2018). Sensitivity and specificity of a weight distribution platform for the detection of objective lameness and orthopaedic disease. *Vet Comp Orthop Traumatol.* 31(06):391–395. doi:10.1055/s-0038-1667063.

Cole, G. and Millis, D. (2017). The effect of limb amputation on standing weight distribution in the remaining three limbs in dogs. *Vet Comp Orthop Traumatol.* 30(01):59–61. doi:10.3415/VCOT-16-05-0075.

Da Ré Guerra, F. *et al.* (2016). Low-level PBMT modulates pro-inflammatory cytokines after partial tenotomy. *Lasers Med Sci.* 31(4):759–766.

Dávila, S. *et al.* (2011). Low level PBMT on experimental myopathy. *PBMT.* 20(4):287–292.

Dray, A. and Perkins, M. (1993). Bradykinin and inflammatory pain. *Trends Neurosci.* 16(3):99–104.

Ebrahimi, T. *et al.* (2012). The influence of low-intensity PBMT on bone healing. *J Dent (Tehran).* 9(4):238–248.

Fernandes de Jesus, J. *et al.* (2019). Photobiomodulation of matrix metalloproteinases in rat calcaneal tendons.

Photobiomodulation Photomed Laser Surg. 37(7):421–427. doi:10.1089/photob.2019.4633.

Ferrara-Jr, J.I. *et al.* (2019). Photobiomodulation-induced analgesia in experimental temporomandibular disorder involves central inhibition of fractalkine. *Lasers Med Sci.* 34(9):1841–1847. doi:10.1007/s10103-019-02785-6.

da Fonseca, G.A.M.D. *et al.* (2022). Laser-photobiomodulation on titanium implant bone healing in rat model: comparison between 660- and 808-nm wavelength. *Lasers Med Sci.* 37(4):2179–2184. doi:10.1007/s10103-021-03481-0.

Fukuda, V.O. *et al.* (2015). Short term efficacy of low level PBMT in patients with knee osteoarthritis: a randomized, placebo-controlled, double-blind clinical trial. *Revista Brasileira de Ortopedia*. 46(5):526–533.

Gaynor, J. (2015). Energy modalities, therapeutic laser and pulsed electromagnetic field therapy. In: *Handbook of Veterinary Pain Management*, 3 edn, pp. 357–362. Mosby, St. Louis, MO.

Gendron, D.J. and Hamblin, M.R. (2019). Applications of photobiomodulation therapy to musculoskeletal disorders and osteoarthritis with particular relevance to Canada. *Photobiomodulation Photomed Laser Surg.* 37(7):408–420. doi:10.1089/photob.2018.4597.

Ghanbarnasab, M. *et al.* (2019). The effect of high-intensity laser therapy on trapezius focal myositis: a rare case report. *J Lasers in Med Sci.* 10(4):346–349. doi:10.15171/jlms.2019.56.

Godbold, J. and Arza, R. (2011). *Reference Guide to Common Conditions for CTC.* CTS. LiteCure, Newark, DE.

Góralczyk, K. *et al.* (2015). Effect of LLLT on endothelial cells culture. *Lasers Med Sci.* 30(1):273–278.

Gruen, M.E. *et al.* (2015). Criterion validation testing of clinical metrology instruments for measuring degenerative joint disease associated mobility impairment in cats. *PLoS One.* 10(7):e0131839. doi:10.1371/journal.pone.0131839.

Guerra, F.R. *et al.* (2013). LLLT improves tendon healing through increase of MMP activity and collagen synthesis. *Lasers Med Sci.* 28(5):1281–1288.

Hagiwara, S. *et al.* (2007). GaAlAs (830 nm) low-level laser enhances peripheral endogenous opioid analgesia in rats. *Lasers Surg Med.* 39(10):797–802.

Hielm-Björkman, A.K. *et al.* (2009). Psychometric testing of the Helsinki chronic pain index by completion of a questionnaire in Finnish by owners of dogs with chronic signs of pain caused by osteoarthritis. *Am J Vet Res.* 70 (6):727–734. doi:10.2460/ajvr.70.6.727.

Holanda, V.M. *et al.* (2016). Photobiomodulation of the dorsal root ganglion for the treatment of low back pain: a pilot study. *Lasers Surg Med.* 48(7):653–659. doi:10.1002/lsm.22522.

Hsieh, Y.L. *et al.* (2014). Fluence-dependent effects of low-level PBMT in myofascial trigger spots on modulation of biochemicals associated with pain in a rabbit model. *Lasers Med Sci.* 30(1):209–216.

Hwang, M.H. *et al.* (2015). Low level light therapy modulates inflammatory mediators secreted by human annulus fibrosus cells during intervertebral disc degeneration in vitro. *Photochem Photobiol.* 91(2):403–410.

Ignatov, Y. *et al.* (2005). Effects of helium–neon laser irradiation and local anesthetics on potassium channels in pond snail neurons. *Neurosci Behav Physiol.* 35:871–875.

Ip, D. and Fu, N.Y. (2015a). Can combined use of low-level lasers and hyaluronic acid injections prolong the longevity of degenerative knee joints? *Clin Interv Aging.* 10:1255–1258.

Ip, D. and Fu, N.Y. (2015b). Can intractable discogenic back pain be managed by low-level PBMT without recourse to operative intervention? *J Pain Res.* 8:253–256.

Jang, H. and Lee, H. (2012). Meta-analysis of pain relief effects by laser irradiation on joint areas. *Photomed Laser Surg.* 30(8):405–417.

Jimbo, K. *et al.* (1998). Suppressive effects of low-power laser irradiation on bradykinin evoked action potentials in cultured murine dorsal root ganglion cells. *Neurosci Lett.* 240(2):93–96.

Johnston, S.A. (1997). Osteoarthritis. Joint anatomy, physiology, and pathobiology. *The Vet Clin of North Am Small Anim Pract.* 27(4):699–723. doi:10.1016/S0195-5616(97)50076-3.

Jozsa, L.G. and Kannus, P. (1997). *Human Tendons: Anatomy, Physiology, and Pathology.* Human Kinetics, Champaign, IL.

Kaneguchi, A. *et al.* (2022). Low-level laser therapy attenuates Arthrogenic contracture induced by anterior cruciate ligament reconstruction surgery in rats. *Physiol Res*:389–399. doi:10.33549/physiolres.934796.

Karu, T. *et al.* (1997). He–Ne laser radiation influences single-channel ionic currents through cell membranes: a patch-clamp study. *Proc SPIE.* 3198:57–66.

Kaya, G.Ş. *et al.* (2011). The use of 808-nm light therapy to treat experimental chronic osteomyelitis induced in rats by methicillin-resistant *Staphylococcus aureus. Photomed Laser Surg.* 29(6):405–412.

Khan, K.M. *et al.* (1999). Histopathology of common tendinopathies. Update and implications for clinical management. *Sports Med.* 27(6):393–408.

Kulkarni, S. *et al.* (2019). Efficacy of photobiomodulation on accelerating bone healing after tooth extraction: a systematic review. *Lasers Med Sci.* 34(4):685–692. doi:10.1007/s10103-018-2641-3.

Kuzu, T.E. *et al.* (2022). Effect of photobiomodulation therapy on peri-implant bone healing in extra-short implants in a rabbit model: a pilot study. *Photobiomodulation Photomed Laser Surg.* 40(6):402–409. doi:10.1089/photob.2021.0098.

Labajos, M. (1988). Beta-endorphin levels modification after GaAs and HeNe laser irradiation on the rabbit. Comparative Study. *Invest Clin*. 1–2:6–8.

Lascelles, B.D.X. (2010). Feline degenerative joint disease. *Vet Surg*. 39(1):2–13. doi:10.1111/j.1532-950X.2009.00597.x.

Lascelles, B.D.X. *et al.* (2007). Evaluation of client-specific outcome measures and activity monitoring to measure pain relief in cats with osteoarthritis. *J Vet Intern Med*. 21(3):410–416. doi:10.1892/0891-6640(2007)21[410:eocoma]2.0.co;2.

Lascelles, B.D.X. *et al.* (2012). Relationship of orthopedic examination, goniometric measurements, and radiographic signs of degenerative joint disease in cats. *BMC Vet Res*. 8:10. doi:10.1186/1746-6148-8-10.

Liebert, A.D. *et al.* (2014). Protein conformational modulation by photons: a mechanism for laser treatment effects. *Med Hypotheses*. 82(3):275–281.

Lin, Y.-P. *et al.* (2020). Light-emitting diode photobiomodulation therapy for non-specific low back pain in working nurses. *Medicine*. 99(32):e21611. doi:10.1097/MD.0000000000021611.

Lister, T. *et al.* (2012). Optical properties of human skin. *J Biomed Opt*. 17(9):90901.

Looney, A.L. *et al.* (2018). A randomized blind placebo-controlled trial investigating the effects of photobiomodulation therapy (PBMT) on canine elbow osteoarthritis. *The Canad Vet J*. 59(9):959–966 http://www.ncbi.nlm.nih.gov/pubmed/30197438.

de Lopes, C.C.A. *et al.* (2022). Effectiveness of photobiomodulation therapy on human bone healing in dentistry: a systematic review. *Photobiomodulation Photomed Laser Surg*. 40(7):440–453. doi:10.1089/photob.2021.0092.

Lopes-Martins, R.A. *et al.* (2005). Spontaneous effects of low-level PBMT (650 nm) in acute inflammatory mouse pleurisy induced by carrageenan. *Photomed Laser Surg*. 23(4):377–381.

Magri, A.M. *et al.* (2015). Photobiomodulation and bone healing in diabetic rats: evaluation of bone response using a tibial defect experimental model. *Lasers Med Sci*. 30 (7):1949–1957.

Martimbianco, A.L.C. *et al.* (2020). Photobiomodulation with low-level laser therapy for treating Achilles tendinopathy: a systematic review and meta-analysis. *Clin Rehab*. 34(6):713–722. doi:10.1177/0269215520912820.

Martins, J.P.S. *et al.* (2022). Analysis of pain relief and functional recovery in patients with rotator cuff tendinopathy through therapeutic ultrasound and photobiomodulation therapy: a comparative study. *Lasers Med Sci*. 37(8):3155–3167. doi:10.1007/s10103-022-03584-2.

de Mazuqueli Pereira, E., S.B. *et al.* (2021). Photobiomodulation inhibits inflammation in the temporomandibular joint of rats. *J Photochem Photobiol, B*. 222:112281. doi:10.1016/j.jphotobiol.2021.112281.

McLaughlin, R. (2000). Management of chronic osteoarthritic pain. *Vet Clin North Am Small Anim Pract*. 30(4):933–949.

Melis, M. *et al.* (2012). Low level laser therapy for the treatment of temporomandibular disorders: a systematic review of the literature. *Cranio*. 30(4):304–312.

Mizutani, K. *et al.* (2004). A clinical study on serum prostaglandin E2 with low-level PBMT. *Photomed Laser Surg*. 22(6):537–539.

Monteiro, B.P. *et al.* (2023). 2022 WSAVA guidelines for the recognition, assessment and treatment of pain. *J Small Anim Pract*. 64(4):177–254. doi:10.1111/jsap.13566.

Montesinos, M. (1988). Experimental effects of low power laser in encephalin and endorphin synthesis. *J Eur Med Laser Assoc*. 1(3):2–7.

Mosley, C. *et al.* (2022). Proposed Canadian consensus guidelines on osteoarthritis treatment based on OA-COAST stages 1–4. *Front Vet Sci*. 9. doi:10.3389/fvets.2022.830098.

Mota, F.C.D. *et al.* (2013). Low-power PBMT for repairing acute and chronic-phase bone lesions. *Res Vet Sci*. 94(1):105–110.

Nadershah, M. *et al.* (2020). Photobiomodulation therapy for myofascial pain in temporomandibular joint dysfunction: a double-blinded randomized clinical trial. *J Maxillofac and Oral Surg*. 19(1):93–97. doi:10.1007/s12663-019-01222-z.

Nambi, G. *et al.* (2019). Spinal manipulation plus laser therapy versus laser therapy alone in the treatment of chronic non-specific low back pain: a randomized controlled study. *Europ J Phys and Rehab Med*. 54(6). doi:10.23736/S1973-9087.18.05005-0.

Nazari, A. *et al.* (2019). Efficacy of high-intensity laser therapy in comparison with conventional physiotherapy and exercise therapy on pain and function of patients with knee osteoarthritis: a randomized controlled trial with 12-week follow up. *Lasers Med Sci*. 34(3):505–516. doi:10.1007/s10103-018-2624-4.

Ng, G.Y.F. *et al.* (2004). Comparison of single and multiple applications of GaAlAs laser on rat medial collateral ligament repair. *Lasers Surg Med*. 34(3):285–289.

Noba, C. *et al.* (2018). Laser for bone healing after oral surgery: systematic review. *Lasers Med Sci*. 33(3):667–674. doi:10.1007/s10103-017-2400-x.

Oliveira, F.S. *et al.* (2009). Effect of low level PBMT (830 nm) with different therapy regimes on the process of tissue repair in partial lesion calcaneous tendon. *Lasers Surg Med*. 41(4):271–276.

Oliveira, C.G. *et al.* (2020). Photobiomodulation reduces nociception and edema in a CFA-induced muscle pain model: effects of LLLT and LEDT. *Photochem Photobiol Sci*. 19(10):1392–1401. doi:10.1039/d0pp00037j.

Pallotta, R.C. *et al.* (2012). Infrared (810-nm) low-level PBMT on rat experimental knee inflammation. *Lasers Med Sci.* 27(1):71–78.

de Paula Gomes, C.A.F. *et al.* (2018). Incorporation of photobiomodulation therapy into a therapeutic exercise program for knee osteoarthritis: a placebo-controlled, randomized, clinical trial. *Lasers Surg Med.* 50(8):819–828. doi:10.1002/lsm.22939.

Peimani, A. and Sardary, F. (2014). Effect of low-level laser on healing of temporomandibular joint osteoarthritis in rats. *J Dent (Tehran).* 11(3):319–327.

de Pinto, N.C., M.V.P. *et al.* (2022). Customized photobiomodulation modulates pain and alters thermography pattern in patients with knee osteoarthritis: a randomized double-blind pilot study. *Photobiomodulation Photomed Laser Surg.* 40(10):698–707. doi:10.1089/photob.2022.0067.

Pires, D. *et al.* (2011). Low-level PBMT (LLLT; 780 nm) acts differently on mRNA expression of anti- and pro-inflammatory mediators in an experimental model of collagenase-induced tendinitis in rat. *Lasers Med Sci.* 26(1):85–94.

Podell, M. (2002). Inflammatory myopathies. *Vet Clin North Am Small Anim Pract.* 32(1):147–167.

Prianti, A.C.G. *et al.* (2014). Low-level PBMT (LLLT) reduces the COX-2 mRNA expression in both subplantar and total brain tissues in the model of peripheral inflammation induced by administration of carrageenan. *Lasers Med Sci.* 29(4):1397–1403.

Pryor, B. and Millis, D.L. (2015). Therapeutic laser in veterinary medicine. *Vet Clin North Am Small Anim Pract.* 45(1):45–56.

Renwick, S.M. *et al.* (2018). Influence of class IV laser therapy on the outcomes of tibial plateau leveling osteotomy in dogs. *Vet Surg.* 47(4):507–515. doi:10.1111/vsu.12794.

Ribeiro, L.N.S. *et al.* (2022). Low-level laser therapy (LLLT) improves alveolar bone healing in rats. *Lasers Med Sci.* 37(2):961–969. doi:10.1007/s10103-021-03340-y.

Riegel, R. (2008). General therapy guidelines. In: *Laser Therapy in the Companion Animal Practice*, 3 edn, p. 7. LiteCure, Newark, DE.

Roberts, D.B. *et al.* (2013). The effectiveness of therapeutic class IV (10 W) laser treatment for epicondylitis. *Lasers Surg Med.* 45(5):311–317.

Rochkind, S. *et al.* (2009). Increase of neuronal sprouting and migration using 780 nm laser phototherapy as procedure for cell therapy. *Lasers Surg Med.* 41(4):277–281.

Salate, A.C. *et al.* (2005). Effect of in-Ga-Al-P diode laser irradiation on angiogenesis in partial ruptures of Achilles tendon in rats. *Photomed Laser Surg.* 23(5):470–475.

dos Santinoni, C.S. *et al.* (2017). Influence of low-level laser therapy on the healing of human bone maxillofacial defects: a systematic review. *J Photochem Photobiol, B.* 169:83–89. doi:10.1016/j.jphotobiol.2017.03.004.

Schomberg, D. *et al.* (2012). Neuropathic pain: role of inflammation, immune response, and ion channel activity in central injury mechanisms. *Ann Neurosci.* 19(3): 125–132.

Schott, E.M. *et al.* (2018). Targeting the gut microbiome to treat the osteoarthritis of obesity. *JCI Insight.* 3(8). doi:10.1172/jci.insight.95997.

Servetto, N. *et al.* (2010). Evaluation of inflammatory biomarkers associated with oxidative stress and histological assessment of low-level PBMT in experimental myopathy. *Lasers Surg Med.* 42(6):577–583.

Shiva, S. and Gladwin, M.T. (2009). Shining a light on tissue NO stores: near infrared release of NO from nitrite and nitrosylated hemes. *J Mol Cell Cardiol.* 46(1):1–3.

Silva, T.C. *et al.* (2010). *In vivo* effects on the expression of vascular endothelial growth factor-A165 messenger ribonucleic acid of an infrared diode laser associated or not with a visible red diode laser. *Photomed Laser Surg.* 28 (1):63–68.

da Silva, M.R. *et al.* (2022). Light stimulation on tenocytes: a systematic review of in vitro studies. *Porto Biomed J.* 7(4): e176. doi:10.1097/j.pbj.0000000000000176.

Skobelkin, O. *et al.* (1990). Blood microcirculation under laser physiotherapy and reflexotherapy in patients with lesions in vessels of low extremities. *Laser Ther.* 2(2):69–77.

Stadig, S. *et al.* (2019). Evaluation and comparison of pain questionnaires for clinical screening of osteoarthritis in cats. *Vet Record.* 185(24):757. doi:10.1136/vr.105115.

Stausholm, M.B. *et al.* (2019). Efficacy of low-level laser therapy on pain and disability in knee osteoarthritis: systematic review and meta-analysis of randomised placebo-controlled trials. *BMJ Open.* 9(10):e031142. doi:10.1136/bmjopen-2019-031142.

Takahashi, H. *et al.* (2012). Low level PBMT for patients with cervical disk hernia. *PBMT.* 21(3):193–197.

Tripodi, N. *et al.* (2021). The effect of low-level red and near-infrared photobiomodulation on pain and function in tendinopathy: a systematic review and meta-analysis of randomized control trials. *BMC Sports Sci Med Rehabil.* 13(1):91. doi:10.1186/s13102-021-00306-z.

Tumilty, S. *et al.* (2010). Low level laser treatment of tendinopathy: a systematic review with meta-analysis. *Photomed Laser Surg.* 28(1):3–16.

de Vasconcellos, L.M.R. *et al.* (2014). Healing of normal and osteopenic bone with titanium implant and low-level PBMT (GaAlAs): a histomorphometric study in rats. *Lasers Med Sci.* 29(2):575–580.

Vassão, P.G. *et al.* (2021). Association of photobiomodulation therapy (PBMT) and exercises programs in pain and functional capacity of patients with knee osteoarthritis

(KOA): a systematic review of randomized trials. *Lasers Med Sci.* 36(7):1341–1353. doi:10.1007/s10103-020-03223-8.

Venable, R.O. *et al.* (2008). Examination of synovial fluid hyaluronan quantity and quality in stifle joints of dogs with osteoarthritis. *Am J Vet Res.* 69(12):1569–1573. doi:10.2460/ajvr.69.12.1569.

Wakabayashi, H. (1993). Effect of irradiation by semiconductor laser on responses evoked in trigeminal caudal neurons by tooth pulp stimulation. *Lasers Surg Med.* 13(6):605–610.

Walker, J.B. (1983). Relief from chronic pain by low-power laser irradiation. *Neurosci Lett.* 43:339–344.

Walton, M.B. *et al.* (2013). Evaluation of construct and criterion validity for the 'Liverpool osteoarthritis in dogs' (LOAD) clinical metrology instrument and comparison to two other instruments. *PLoS One.* 8(3):e58125. doi:10.1371/journal.pone.0058125.

Walton, B. *et al.* (2018). 'How do I know my animal got better?' – measuring outcomes in small animal orthopaedics. *In Practice.* 40(2):42–50. doi:10.1136/inp.k647.

Wang, P. *et al.* (2014). Effects of low-level PBMT on joint pain, synovitis, anabolic, and catabolic factors in a progressive osteoarthritis rabbit model. *Lasers Med Sci.* 29(6):1875–1885.

Waxman, S.G. and Zamponi, G.W. (2014). Regulating excitability of peripheral afferents: emerging ion channel targets. *Nat Neurosci.* 17(2):153–163.

Xu, G.-Z. *et al.* (2018). Low-level laser therapy for temporomandibular disorders: a systematic review with Meta-analysis. *Pain Res Manage.* 2018:1–13. doi:10.1155/2018/4230583.

Yilmaz, M. *et al.* (2020). Comparison of high-intensity laser therapy and combination of ultrasound treatment and transcutaneous nerve stimulation on cervical pain associated with cervical disc herniation: a randomized trial. *Complement Therap in Med.* 49:102295. doi:10.1016/j.ctim.2019.102295.

Zein, R. *et al.* (2018). Review of light parameters and photobiomodulation efficacy: dive into complexity. *J Biomed Opt.* 23(12):1–17. doi:10.1117/1.JBO.23.12.120901.

Zhang, Y. *et al.* (2003). cDNA microarray analysis of gene expression profiles in human fibroblast cells irradiated with red light. *J Invest Dermatol.* 120(5):849–857.

Rogatko, C.P. *et al.* (2017). Preoperative low level laser therapy in dogs undergoing tibial plateau levelling osteotomy: a blinded, prospective, randomized clinical trial. *Vet Comp Orthop Traumatol.* 30(01):46–53. doi:10.3415/VCOT-15-12-0198.

12

Upper and Lower Respiratory Conditions

Michael C. Petty

Dogtor Consulting, Plymouth, Michigan, USA

1st Edition Contributor:

Chapter 14 Ray A. Arza

RSA Veterinary Technologies, Taylorsville, KY, USA

Introduction

More than a decade of studies have shown the beneficial effects of photobiomodulation therapy (PBMT) on upper and lower respiratory function. Most recently, it has shown the potential for treating COVID through its effects of reducing pulmonary inflammation and increasing the number of T-cells (Sohelifar *et al.*, 2021). These studies indicate that PBMT is an effective modality in reducing pain, modulating the inflammatory response, improving the immune response, and increasing microcirculation in both upper and lower respiratory conditions with virtually no side effects, thus alleviating symptoms and hastening recovery. Anecdotal results reported in the veterinary profession have been consistent with these findings. The addition of this modality when treating upper and lower airway disease has proven to minimize inflammatory symptoms, expedite recovery, potentiate the effects of conventional therapies, and decrease the need for pharmaceuticals with potential side effects, such as corticosteroids and non-steroidal anti-inflammatories. Practitioners are encouraged to add PBMT to their therapeutic regimens when treating conditions in the upper and lower respiratory tracts.

Upper Respiratory Conditions

The major passages and structures of the upper respiratory tract include the nose or nostrils, nasal cavity, mouth, pharynx, and larynx. Conditions affecting the mouth in relation to its function as part of the alimentary tract are discussed in Chapter 13.

General Guidelines

There are several things to consider when treating a patient in the area of the head. Of utmost importance is patient eye safety. Eye protection is recommended anytime a patient is treated, but is most important when treating in close proximity to the eyes (Figure 12.1). Exposure of direct or indirect laser light through the pupil and lens to the retina is the primary concern, so proper eye protection is vital. This may be provided by goggles (with lenses appropriate for the specific wavelengths being used) or simply by covering both eyes with dark (preferably black), dense cloth.

The second consideration is treating with a proper dose of light energy, delivering an effective dose to the target tissue. The dose must be delivered in a way and at a rate that is comfortable to the patient and does not induce excessive heat. Some treatment areas will be relatively small (e.g., the nose or sinuses in feline patients). When treating small areas, the laser power settings should be adjusted low enough so as not to create any thermal build-up in the tissues. It is beyond the scope of this chapter to make specific recommendations for every laser device, so it is crucial to not only discuss settings with the laser manufacturer but to be vigilant for apparent discomfort by the patient.

It is important to note that some upper respiratory conditions may be treated as superficial conditions, through the open mouth, with direct exposure of the laser beam to the target tissue. Other conditions must be treated transcutaneously as deep-tissue conditions, increasing the total dose to account for the loss of irradiance as photons travel through various tissue densities to the target tissue.

Laser Therapy in Veterinary Medicine: Photobiomodulation, Second Edition. Edited by Christopher J. Winkler and Lisa A. Miller.

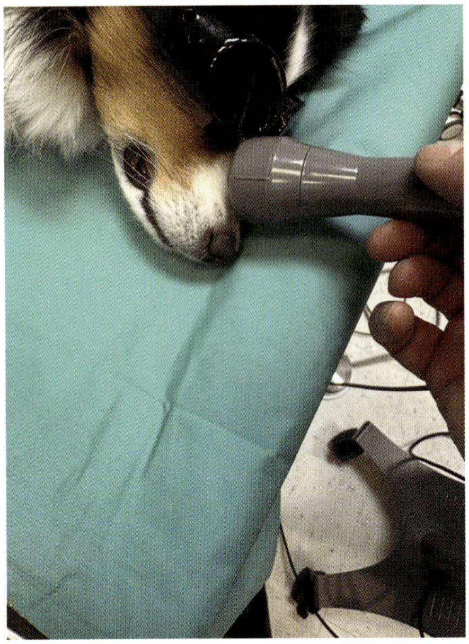

Figure 12.1 Treating the nasal cavity from a dorsal direction. Exposure of direct or indirect laser light through the pupil and lens to the retina is the primary concern, so proper eye protection is vital.

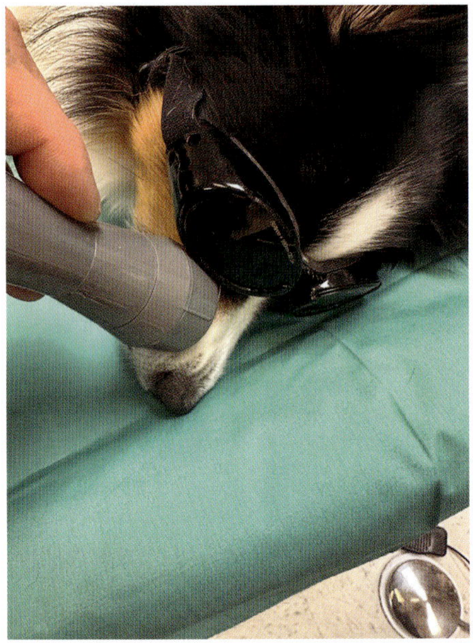

Figure 12.2 Treating the nasal cavity from a lateral direction. Treatment is optimally applied in direct contact with the skin, using a contact handpiece or a treatment head that has been specifically designed for deep tissue conditions. This will decrease reflection of light from the tissue surface, reduce potential exposure to the patient's eyes, and increase penetration of the light deep into the tissues.

Some upper respiratory structures are contained within bone, requiring treatment through that bone. Multiple studies have verified that transcranial therapy with near-infrared laser light is possible. Transcranial near-infrared laser transmission of 800 nm laser light was demonstrated by Lapchak *et al.,* (2015) in four mammalian species. As expected, they found an inverse relationship between the thickness of bone and the percentage of photonic transmission through it. In another study using intact human cadaver heads, measurement of transcranial transmission confirmed the penetration of measurable 808 nm wavelength light through the scalp, skull, and meninges to a brain depth of 40–50 mm (Tedford *et al.,* 2015).

Since conditions being treated transcutaneously require much deeper penetration of light energy, treatment is optimally applied in direct contact with the skin, using a contact handpiece or treatment head specifically designed for deep-tissue conditions (Figure 12.2). This will decrease reflection of light from the tissue surface, reduce potential exposure to the patient's eyes, and increase penetration of the light deep into the tissues (Enwemeka 2009). Treating in contact and applying gentle pressure creates blanching and disperses blood from the skin and underlying tissues. Since hemoglobin is the main absorber of light in the dermis (Lister *et al.,* 2012; Ilko *et al.,* 2003), blanching will improve light penetration to deeper tissues.

Treat with the handpiece perpendicular to the tissue. Deliver photonic energy with movement of the handpiece so there is a uniform irradiation of the target tissues. The laser therapist should monitor the temperature of the patient's skin and hair coat with a finger placed adjacent to the handpiece on the skin, or by placing the other hand in direct proximity to the treatment area. If anything other than a gentle warming is noted, the therapist should pause and adjust the laser and treatment parameters.

Rhinitis and Sinusitis

Rhinitis is defined as any inflammation of the nasal mucous membranes. It is often associated with sinusitis, which is an inflammation of the lining of the sinuses. Both conditions are commonly presented to veterinary clinics. Of particular concern are patients with chronic rhinitis and sinusitis, since they are often challenging to treat.

In dogs, chronic nasal disease is often caused by neoplasia, followed by lympho-plasmacytic rhinitis, fungal infections, and foreign bodies. Other, less common etiologies include nasal polyps, granulomatous rhinitis, oro-nasal fistula, and naso-pharyngeal stenosis (Cohn 2014; Lobetti 2009; Windsor and Johnson 2006).

In cats, as in dogs, the most common cause is neoplasia. The second most common cause, accounting for approximately 35% of feline cases, is the chronic rhino-sinusitis that follows feline herpesvirus 1 infection (Reed 2014).

Due to the prevalence of malignancies, especially with chronic rhinitis, appropriate diagnostics with radiography, rhinoscopy, cultures, and histopathology is always recommended before PBMT is added to the therapeutic regimen. However, there has been successful treatment of intranasal malignancies in both the dog and cat when used as part of photodynamic therapy (Lucroy *et al.,* 2003).

Once a diagnosis that does not include any malignancies is established, there is sound basis for including laser therapy in the clinical management of rhinitis and sinusitis. A recent pilot study showed that patients had significant improvement in symptoms from chronic rhino-sinusitis when treated with laser therapy three times per week for 10 total treatments (Naghdi *et al.,* 2013). Another pilot study demonstrated that phototherapy is an effective modality for treating perennial allergic rhinitis in humans and is an option in the steroid-free management of immune-mediated mucosal diseases (Lee *et al.,* 2013). In an animal-model study, positive effects were noted after laser therapy treatment of an ovalbumin-induced model of allergic rhinitis in mice (Choi 2013).

The role of microorganisms in rhinitis and sinusitis may be significant. Viral infections in cats are often followed by secondary bacterial infections (Reed 2014). Sinonasal fungal infections with aspergillosis are increasingly diagnosed in both dogs (Sharman and Mansfield 2012) and cats (Barrs and Talbot 2014).

Studies indicate that incorporating laser therapy into therapeutics when microorganisms are present is warranted. Neutrophils from mice that received laser therapy have been shown to be more active metabolically, and to have higher fungicidal activity *in vivo* and *in vitro* (Burger *et al.,* 2015).

Laser-assisted nasal decolonization of *Staphylococcus aureus*, including methicillin-resistant *S. aureus* (MRSA), was demonstrated in human patients (Krespi and Kizhner 2012). The study concluded that laser therapy could eradicate MRSA and potentially resensitize the bacteria to the antimicrobial effect of erythromycin.

All these studies are consistent with clinical reports from veterinarians using laser light as an adjunct to conventional therapy for rhinitis and sinusitis in companion pets.

When developing a protocol for incorporating PBMT into the management of rhinitis and sinusitis, severity and chronicity should be considered, as should response after initiation of treatment. In acute conditions, a typical induction phase of daily or every-other-day treatment is indicated, with a gradual transition to less-frequent treatment until the condition resolves. When treating chronic rhinitis or sinusitis, the author recommends three phases of treatment, as for other chronic conditions: an induction phase, a transition phase, and a maintenance phase. The induction phase will usually start with every-other-day treatment, followed, as symptoms improve, by a gradual decrease in frequency through a transition phase of treatments twice weekly, once weekly, every other week, and so on. With severe symptoms, starting with three to four daily treatments is recommended. If the condition persists, a maintenance phase may be necessary, with treatments at a frequency that maintains the clinical response achieved during the induction and transition phases. A word of caution: Do not decrease treatment frequency too quickly; rather, tailor it to the patient's improvement.

The recommended target dose for treating rhinitis and sinusitis is 8–10 J/cm^2. The higher end of this range is recommended for larger patients with thicker bones, as the thickness of the bone affects the penetration of light. When treating small dogs or cats, especially when skin and coat color is dark, the author recommends adjusting the laser power setting to no more than 3 W to prevent excessive heat buildup. Though the area of skin overlying the nose and sinuses is small, the laser handpiece should move during treatment. When treating larger dogs, power settings may be increased to 10–12 W as long as there is constant movement of the handpiece over the entire area for the duration of treatment.

The author recommends always treating the entire area covering both nasal passages and frontal and maxillary sinuses. It is helpful to have a template to use when estimating the size of the area to be treated, in square centimeters. A 7.5×12.7 cm index card is almost exactly 100 cm^2, and because 100 is an easy multiplier, one can determine approximate dosages by visualizing the area to be treated in terms of the number of index cards. Once the area is known, the total dose in joules can be easily calculated.

Tonsillitis

Tonsillitis is common in dogs, mostly in brachycephalic or small breeds (Kaplan 1981, Fasanella *et al.,* 2010). Though rare in cats, it has been reported (Prescott 1968). It seldom occurs as a primary disease; instead, it is usually secondary to other nasal, oral, or pharyngeal disorders. In brachycephalic dogs, it is thought to be associated with chronic inflammation due to elongation of the soft palate.

Clinical signs of tonsillitis are associated with pain and inflammation, and with the physical presence of the enlarged tonsils in the pharynx. Treatment is typically aimed at resolving the underlying disease. Analgesics and antibiotics are often indicated.

Laser therapy appears to be a good adjunct therapy for treating tonsillitis. Among 445 human children and teenagers (aged 2–15 years) with pollinosis (68), adenoiditis and rhino-sinusitis (198), tonsillitis (64), or otitis (115), treatment was carried out simultaneously with infrared and red laser irradiation (Gogeliia *et al.,* 2006). Positive results were achieved in 85% of patients. Another controlled study evaluated the effects of laser irradiation on reduction of pain following tonsillectomy in human adults. In the treated group, the tonsil beds were irradiated at the end of surgery with a 980 nm laser at a dose of 4 J/cm^2. The reductions in both pain and analgesic consumption were significantly more pronounced in patients who received postoperative laser therapy treatment than in those who did not (Aghamohammadi *et al.,* 2013).

Like other oropharyngeal conditions, tonsillitis may be treated as a superficial condition, with the mouth open so the light directly treats the tonsil (as in Aghamohammadi *et al.,* 2013). This is easiest if the patient is sedated or under anesthesia. Most awake patients will not tolerate prolonged opening of the mouth and displacement of the tongue, so the tonsils can be treated as deep tissues if the patient is not sedated or under anesthesia.

When treating with open mouth and direct access to the tonsils, a treatment protocol that delivers 4–6 J/cm^2 is recommended.

If treating with the mouth closed, a laser setting that delivers 6–10 J/cm^2 is recommended. The treatment should be aimed at the pharynx from the caudal border of the mandible, with the handpiece on-contact with the skin. The power setting should not exceed 3–4 W, as this is a relatively small area and movement of the handpiece will be limited. Initial treatments may be administered daily to decrease the severity of pain and inflammation, then every other day until resolution.

Brachycephalic Syndrome

Animals with brachycephalic obstructive airway syndrome (BOAS) suffer from obstruction of the airways at a number of levels within the respiratory tract. The anomalies include stenotic nares, abnormally conformed turbinates, soft-palate elongation and hyperplasia, and less often hypoplastic trachea. As the condition worsens, the laryngeal saccules may evert and a secondary structural collapse of the larynx and left bronchus may occur (Dupré and Heidenreich 2016). Secondary tonsillitis is common.

The pathological changes accompanying the syndrome result from a decrease in the lumen of the airways, which increases respiratory effort, especially on inspiration. Poiseuille's law states that as lumen radius decreases in size, the resistance to flow through the lumen increases fourfold (Sutera and Skalak 1993). This means that even relatively small changes in the radius of the airways cause large changes in airway resistance. Thus, the significant resistance in airflow caused by the stenotic nares and elongated soft palate lead to the devastating secondary changes (Dupré *et al.,* 2012).

Most surgeons believe that early surgical intervention helps prevent development of the secondary complications (Meola 2013). The author of the current chapter believes that this syndrome is best approached by early rhinoplasty and palatoplasty using a carbon dioxide (CO_2) surgical laser, and has performed surgical (CO_2) soft-palate and stenotic nares correction in over 350 dogs. The technique has been described in multiple publications (Clark and Sinibaldi 1994; Davidson *et al.,* 2001; Dunié-Mérigot *et al.,* 2010). However, PBMT may play an adjunctive role in brachycephalic syndrome as a means of bringing about postoperative reduction of inflammation and pain, as well as of managing the inflammatory changes that occur if early surgical intervention is not accomplished.

When laser therapy is used to treat immediately after surgical correction of brachycephalic syndrome, attention should be given to all potential areas of inflammation, including the nares, pharyngeal and laryngeal areas, and the trachea. Perioperative treatment should be administered while the patient is under anesthesia so the pharyngeal area can be treated directly through the open mouth. Depending on the degree of postoperative pain and swelling, closed-mouth treatments may be administered daily or twice daily for 3–4 days.

For the nares, a laser setting that delivers 3–4 J/cm^2 using a power not greater than 2 W and a noncontact technique is recommended. The nasal cavity can be treated with the protocols described in the section on "Rhinitis and Sinusitis." Prior to recovery from anesthesia, the visible areas of the pharynx and larynx can be treated through the open mouth with 3–4 J/cm^2 at 2–3 W, followed by closed-mouth treatment delivering 6–10 J/cm^2 at 4–8 W using on-contact technique over all the pharyngeal and laryngeal areas and the proximal trachea.

When using therapy laser as an adjunct to conventional medical therapy for the treatment of brachycephalic symptoms in lieu of surgery, the author recommends the standard three phases of laser therapy for chronic conditions. The induction phase should start with daily or every-other-day treatments until symptoms subside, with a gradual decrease in treatment frequency through a transition phase, followed by maintenance-phase treatments every 2–4 weeks at a frequency sufficient to maintain effect.

Laryngitis

Laryngitis, an inflammation of the larynx, may result from upper respiratory tract infection, foreign bodies, or irritant inhalants such as dust, smoke, or other gases. Excessive barking or trauma from endotracheal tubes may also be a culprit. Any breed is susceptible, but as described in the section on

"Brachycephalic Syndrome," brachycephalic breeds are predisposed to general upper respiratory inflammation, including of the larynx. Patients with laryngeal paralysis will suffer laryngeal inflammation as well.

Treatment should address the underlying etiology, but symptomatic treatment to decrease laryngeal edema and swelling of the mucous membranes is often indicated. In addition to pharmacological agents, PBMT may be a helpful adjunctive therapy, and it is indicated for any form of laryngitis, except where malignancy is the underlying etiology. Studies in laboratory animals have demonstrated that laser therapy can successfully modulate the inflammatory response in experimental laryngitis and that it may therefore be a useful tool for the treatment of laryngitis (Marinho *et al.,* 2013a,b).

A treatment protocol that delivers 6–10 J/cm^2 (lower doses for smaller patients and higher doses for larger patients) is recommended for the treatment of the larynx. Treatment with the handpiece on-contact with the skin is indicated, and a maximum power setting of 4–8 W is recommended. Depending on the degree of inflammation, laryngeal swelling, and severity of symptoms, treatments should start daily or twice daily and then decrease to every other day until resolution.

Laryngeal Collapse and Laryngeal Paralysis

Laryngeal collapse occurs when the laryngeal cartilage loses rigidity, causing the larynx to fold and fall in. This structural abnormality results in an obstruction of the normal movement of air through the larynx. Laryngeal collapse can occur following trauma to the neck, but is more commonly seen in BOAS patients secondary to their longstanding upper respiratory conditions.

Laryngeal paralysis differs in that it is a functional abnormality of the nerves that control the muscles and cartilage of the larynx. The paralysis results in voice changes and difficulty with eating and breathing (MacPhail 2014).

Both conditions can result in severe respiratory distress. Surgical intervention with unilateral arytenoid lateralization is most commonly used to treat laryngeal paralysis. The same technique can be used to treat laryngeal collapse, though some severely affected patients may require a permanent tracheostomy (Monnet 2016; Monnet and Tobias 2012).

As described earlier, PBMT reduces pain, inflammation, and edema in the larynx regardless of the cause. Laser therapy treatment of the larynx is indicated in pre- and postoperative patients undergoing surgery for collapse or paralysis, or in patients with milder symptoms that are not deemed immediate surgical candidates (Figure 12.3).

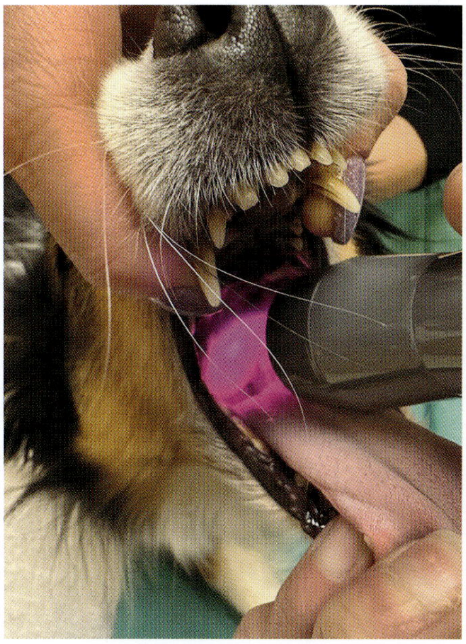

Figure 12.3 A small, noncontact handpiece should be used at power setting of 2–3 W. Treatment may be somewhat easier if the handpiece collimates the laser beam and allows treatment at a greater distance from the target area.

Lower Respiratory and Thoracic Conditions

General Guidelines

Laser therapy treatment of lower respiratory conditions should be administered with the laser handpiece on-contact with the skin, to maximize penetration of photons deep into the target areas. When treating diffuse conditions of the lower respiratory tract, the dose should be calculated based on the entire surface area of the thorax. If the trachea is involved in the condition being treated, then the neck should be considered part of the treatment area. Treatment of either the thorax or the neck should be applied from 270º (from a ventral direction, as well as both lateral sides) (Figure 12.4). Penetration into the thorax can be facilitated by following the intercostal spaces as much as possible with the handpiece. In larger patients, all treatment of the thoracic walls can be directed through the intercostal spaces.

When considering laser therapy for a lower respiratory or thoracic condition of unknown etiology, a complete physical exam and proper diagnostic workup of the patient are strongly recommended, to rule out possible underlying malignancies.

When treating the neck, caution should be exercised to avoid prolonged, repeated treatments over the thyroid glands. Some early studies showed high dose laser irradiation of the thyroid gland could cause changes in the thyroid

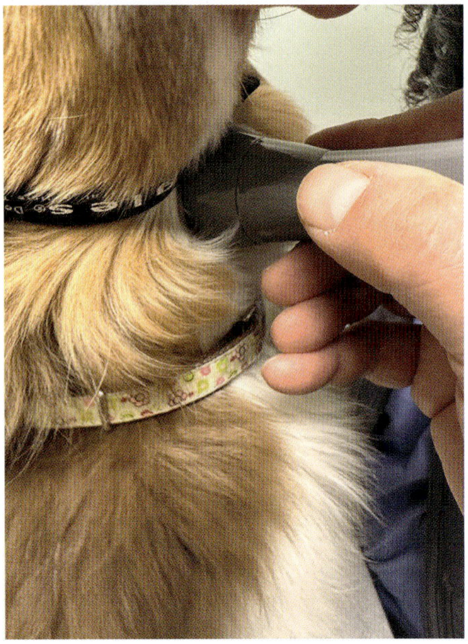

Figure 12.4 Laser therapy treatment of the larynx is indicated for laryngitis, for reduction of edema in laryngeal collapse or paralysis, and for pre- and postoperative patients undergoing surgery for laryngeal collapse or paralysis. Treatment should be administered with the laser handpiece in contact with the skin, to maximize penetration of photons deep into the target areas.

parenchyma (Parrado *et al.*, 1990). Other studies indicated that lower total doses, delivered with fewer applications, result in no histological changes in the thyroid parenchyma (Azevedo *et al.*, 2005). These studies indicate that repetitive, high-dose treatment directly over the glands should be avoided. They also indicate that occasional inadvertent exposure of the thyroid glands when treating nearby tissue is not contraindicated.

Chronic Obstructive Pulmonary Disease

Chronic obstructive pulmonary disease (COPD), also known as chronic bronchitis, is a condition that affects the lower airways of dogs and cats. It tends to be irreversible and progressive (Rozanski 2014). Though the etiology is not totally understood, the chronic inflammation may be caused by many factors, including inhaled irritants, allergens, and recurrent infections. As with the other respiratory conditions described in this chapter, a complete diagnostic workup is always indicated prior to starting treatment with laser therapy.

PBMT should be considered a helpful adjunctive therapy to conventional treatment protocols for COPD. A study involving 89 human patients with chronic obstructive bronchitis showed that adding laser therapy to other therapeutic modalities accelerated elimination of clinical symptoms, increased respiratory efficiency, promoted drainage function of the bronchi, and facilitated normalization of the patient's immune status (Kashanskaia and Fedorov 2009).

Since COPD affects all the lower airways, treatment with PBMT should be administered over the entire thorax using a treatment protocol delivering 6–10 J/cm^2. Power settings will vary depending on the size of the patient, and may be as low as 4 W for smaller patients and as high as 15 W for the giant canine breeds. The calculated dose should be delivered via on-contact handpiece within the intercostal spaces, using a dorsal-to-ventral application technique (Figures 12.5–12.7). Since COPD is a chronic disease, the treatment should start with an induction phase of daily or every-other-day treatments, depending on the severity of symptoms, followed by a transition phase with a very gradual decrease in frequency of treatments, as dictated by the improvement of symptoms. Long-term maintenance-phase treatments will be required at a frequency dictated by the patient's response. The goal of adding PBMT to conventional therapy should be to help decrease symptoms to a tolerable degree, as well as to decrease the dose and frequency of pharmacological agents that may have adverse effects on the patient.

Feline Asthma

Feline asthma is a challenging lower airway disease that can be difficult to distinguish because of the similarity of its symptoms to those of other lower airway diseases. Confirming a diagnosis of feline asthma is important because

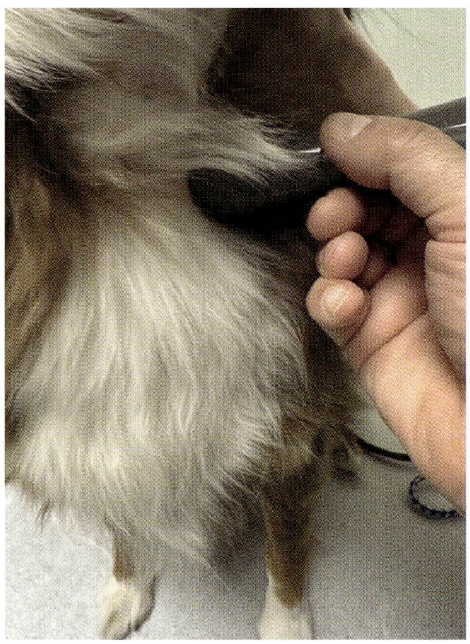

Figure 12.5 In any respiratory condition, if the trachea is involved, the neck should be considered part of the treatment area. Treatment of the cervical portion of the trachea cannot be achieved with the laser perpendicular to the trachea as intervening structures would not allow adequate penetration of the beam. Instead it should be administered from 270° (from a ventral direction, as well as both lateral sides) and into the cranial thoracic trachea through the thoracic inlet.

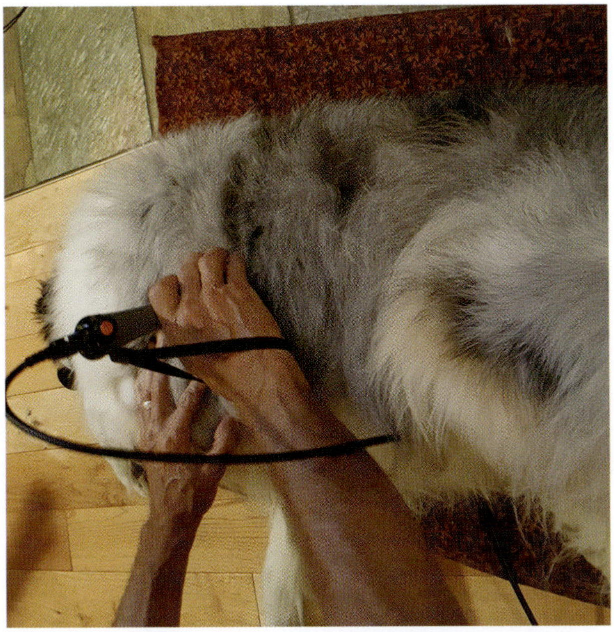

Figure 12.6 The laser handpiece should be maintained in contact with the skin when treating the lower respiratory tract with transthoracic laser application. The entire area of the thoracic walls should be treated from 270°. In this image, treatment is beginning dorsally and the treatment handpiece is moved in an arc, along the lines of the ribs, in a ventral direction.

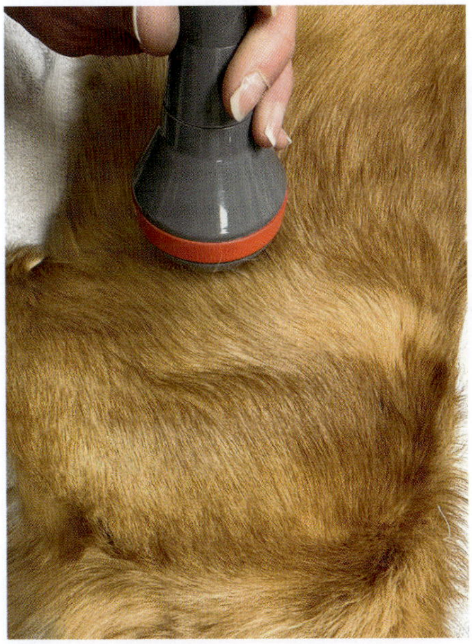

Figure 12.7 Once the handpiece has reached the ventral edge of the thoracic cavity, it should be moved back dorsally. Both sides of the thorax should be covered with a series of dorsal-to-ventral and ventral-to-dorsal movements along the lines of the ribs. The handpiece should be maintained perpendicular to the skin.

treatment and prognosis differ from those of other lower airway diseases (Reinero 2011).

Standard pharmacological therapies for feline asthma include glucocorticoids and bronchodilators. These medications are not ideal treatments, since some cats are nonresponsive and the therapies do not stop chronic airway remodeling, which leads to declining pulmonary function (Trizil and Reinero 2014).

The application of the anti-inflammatory and immunomodulatory effects of PBMT in treating asthma is sound because of the inflammatory nature of the disease and the less-than-ideal pharmacological options. Recent studies of the effects of laser therapy on allergic asthma have shown encouraging results. One compared the effects of laser therapy on asthma in rats to that of the glucocorticoid budesonide and found they were similar (Wang 2014). The findings suggest that the mechanism of laser therapy treatment of asthma is similar to that of budesonide, involving the adjustment of Th1/Th2 imbalance, which is postulated in many studies to play a major role in the pathogenesis of asthma. Another study, using mice, showed that laser therapy inhibits bronchoconstriction, Th2 inflammation, and airway remodeling in experimentally induced allergic asthma (Silva *et al.,* 2014). The results of these laboratory studies are similar to those observed in human asthma patients treated with laser therapy in clinical settings (Ailioaie and Ailioaie 1997; Ostronosova 2006).

The animal-model and human studies have definite cross-species application. The results are consistent with reported observations of efficacy from the veterinary community. The treatment recommendations for asthma parallel those discussed for COPD.

Chronic Idiopathic Pulmonary Fibrosis in West Highland White Terriers (Westie Lung)

Chronic idiopathic pulmonary fibrosis (IPF) is a disease seen most often in West Highland white terriers, but has been reported in other terriers including Jack Russel, Staffordshire, and Cairn (Corcoran, Cobb *et al.,* 1999a; Corcoran, Dukes-McEwan *et al.,* 1999b; Tilley and Smith 2000). These dogs commonly present with signs of lethargy and exercise intolerance, with or without a productive cough. Physical exam usually reveals generalized, marked crackles and wheezes on auscultation of the thorax, along with marked respiratory effort and "bellows" breathing. Other diseases, such as neoplasia, infection and other causes of bronchitis, should be considered in the differential diagnosis.

The mean age of onset of IPF is 9 years, and life expectancy is approximately 18 months after the onset of clinical signs, or approximately 11 months following diagnosis. Symptomatic treatment of IPF involves corticosteroids, bronchodilators, and oxygen therapy (Corcoran et al., 1999a,b).

Similar to COPD, treatment with PBMT for IPF should be administered over the entire thorax using a treatment protocol that delivers 6–10 J/cm^2. On larger dogs, treatment should be delivered with the handpiece on-contact within the intercostal spaces, using a dorsal-to-ventral application technique (Figures 12.5–12.9). On smaller dogs, the operator may treat over the ribs as well. Treatment area(s) should include the lung fields bilaterally as well as at the thoracic inlet. Mirroring other chronic disease treatments, the frequency of laser sessions should begin with an induction phase of daily or every-other-day treatments depending on the severity of symptoms, followed by a transition phase with a very gradual decrease in frequency of treatments, as dictated by the improvement of symptoms. Long-term maintenance-phase treatments will be required at a frequency dictated by the patient's response.

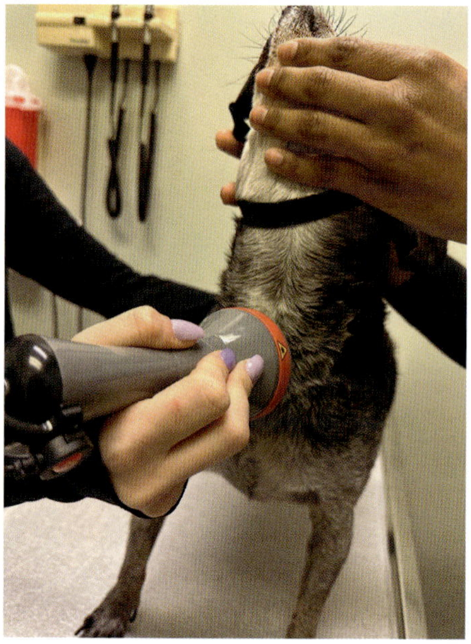

Figure 12.9 In addition, the upper trachea should be targeted by treating the entire ventral neck area, and by aiming into the thoracic inlet.

Tracheal Collapse

This condition, seen most often in small breeds of dogs, occurs when the C-shaped cartilage rings weaken and begin to collapse, and the trachealis muscle on the dorsal surface stretches. The collapse can extend all the way into the bronchi, resulting in severe airway compromise (Maggiore 2014). Just as in brachycephalic syndrome, the restriction of airflow results in inflammation of the respiratory tissues. As the condition worsens, excitement or exercise will usually induce a characteristic hacking or honking cough. Treatment may include weight control, behavioral alterations (to decrease anxiety), medical treatments, and, in more severe cases, surgical intervention (Herrtage 2009).

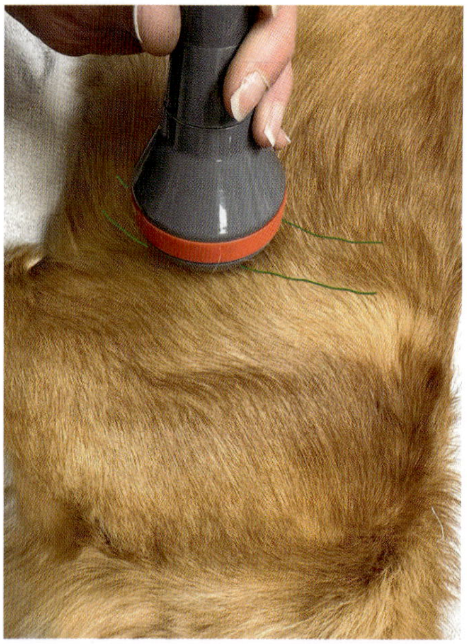

Figure 12.8 In patients of sufficient size, transthoracic treatment should be delivered through the intercostal spaces as the handpiece is moved along the lines of the ribs. The green lines represent the caudal and cranial margins of the ribs with the head of the laser in the intercostal space.

Though the use of laser therapy will not do anything for the anatomical abnormalities of a collapsed trachea, practitioners should consider PBMT as an adjunct to other therapies. The intent would be to help decrease the inflammatory component. The reduction of lower respiratory inflammation that results from the application of laser therapy has been demonstrated in multiple studies (Aimbire *et al.*, 2005, 2007, 2008; Miranda da Silva *et al.*, 2015; Oliveira *et al.*, 2014). Inflammation is reduced via multiple complex mechanisms, without any impairment of pulmonary function (Cury 2015).

Because bronchi may be involved, the inflammation resulting from the anatomical abnormality will extend into deeper pulmonary tissue. It is therefore important to treat the entire lower respiratory tract with laser therapy. A contact technique should be used to deliver 6–10 J/cm^2 over both thoracic walls.

The power setting will depend on the size of the patient and the area to be treated. When treating smaller dogs, the author recommends not exceeding 4–6 W.

Pneumonia

Bacterial pneumonia is much more commonly seen in dogs than in cats. New evidence suggests a complex relationship between respiratory viruses and the development of bacterial pneumonia in dogs (Dear 2014). Respiratory viruses are frequently found in dogs with bacterial pneumonia and may be important in its pathogenesis (Viitanen 2015).

The COVID-19 pandemic yielded new information on the beneficial effects of PBMT for people with pneumonia. Following LLLT a patient showed improvement over a few days in respiratory indices, radiological findings, inflammatory markers, and patient outcomes (Sigman *et al.,* 2020). Although this is not an animal study, consideration should be given to use PBMT in dogs and cats with pneumonia.

One study concluded that transcutaneous laser therapy of elderly human patients with pneumonia shows an undeniable positive impact, with earlier regression of clinical symptoms and sound recovery of functional parameters (Lutaĭ 2001). It suggested that in the absence of side effects, PBMT should be considered for rehabilitation of elderly patients with pneumonia.

In another study, laser therapy was demonstrated to be an effective method of pneumonia treatment that can be included in relevant combined schemes (Amirov 2002). Human pneumonia patients were randomly divided into two groups: those treated with drugs and laser therapy and those treated with drugs alone. Response in the group treated with both drugs and laser therapy was more positive.

When PBMT is being considered as adjunctive therapy in the treatment of pneumonia, a complete diagnostic workup is recommended to rule out malignancy. Note that a benefit of this modality is its compatibility with any other form of treatment for pneumonia, with essentially no known side effects.

A treatment protocol that delivers 6–10 J/cm^2 is recommended, and the author suggests treating the entire thoracic cavity. If a protocol for treating the thorax is not available in the therapy laser software, an approximate dosage can be determined by visualizing the area to be treated relative to the size of an index card, as described in the section on "Rhinitis and Sinusitis." On-contact treatment technique is recommended, with the handpiece following the intercostal spaces. A power setting of 6–15 W is recommended.

Tracheobronchitis

Tracheobronchitis is an acute or chronic inflammatory condition of the trachea and bronchial airways. The etiology is diverse, and may include viral or bacterial infection, parasites, smoke aspiration, and noxious chemical fumes. As with other airway conditions, appropriate diagnostic workup is always very important in determining the best course of therapy, though identification of a specific etiology or pathogen may not be possible in each case (Priestnall 2014).

Tracheobronchitis is yet another condition in which laser therapy may play an adjunctive role in ameliorating the inflammatory component. The author recommends considering this modality as part of the therapeutic approach when treating tracheobronchitis in any companion pet. As with other lower respiratory conditions, laser settings that deliver 6–10 J/cm^2 should be used to treat all of the trachea and the entire thorax. The treatment design will be similar to that described in the section on COPD. When treating acute tracheobronchitis, daily or every-other-day treatments are indicated until the desired effects are obtained. Treatment of chronic tracheobronchitis will necessitate treating through the three phases of induction, transition, and maintenance.

Smoke Inhalation

The complex pathophysiology of smoke inhalation injury has been described in both dogs and cats (Drobatz *et al.,* 1999a,b; Farrow 1975). The formation of reactive oxygen and nitrogen species (ROS and RNS) and procoagulant and antifibrinolytic factors results in alveolar imbalance. Cast formation, bronchospasm, increased bronchial circulation, and transvascular fluid lead to massive airway obstruction (Rehberg *et al.,* 2009). Neurological signs such as stupor or nonambulatory tetraparesis have been reported in dogs after smoke (and presumably carbon monoxide, CO) inhalation injury (Mariani 2003). Delayed neurological sequela may be seen after the initial response to treatment.

Changes seen in the upper and lower airways following inhalation of smoke and other noxious gases may benefit from adding laser therapy to conventional treatment. A study in mice established that laser therapy reduces acute lung inflammation without provoking any deleterious effects in pulmonary function (Cury 2015). This study concluded that transthoracic laser application reduces inflammation in acute lung injury, even when the therapy is applied after the inflammatory process is established. The reduction in inflammation occurs through inhibition of cytokine and chemokine secretion and leads to a marked decrease in immune-cell infiltration in inflamed lungs.

Troxel (2012) reported the initial successful management of a dog with smoke inhalation. Treatment included oxygen administered via intranasal tube, intravenous (IV) lactated Ringer's solution, short-acting glucocorticoids, furosemide, theophylline, ophthalmic ointment, and infrared treatment.

Though the patient recovered from the initial respiratory distress, it subsequently developed neurological signs that led to euthanasia. Necropsy and histopathology demonstrated delayed post-hypoxic leukoencephalopathy.

Anecdotal reports from small-animal practitioners indicate that in the first 24–48 hours after presentation, smoke-inhalation patients appear to breathe more comfortably following laser therapy treatments. Twice-a-day treatments are recommended, and should be dosed and applied as per the recommendations in the section on COPD.

Ischemia Reperfusion Injury-Induced Pulmonary Inflammation

Like smoke inhalation, ischemia reperfusion injuries result in complex pathophysiology (Kalogeris *et al.,* 2012). The pathophysiology may have a delayed effect on distant organs, including the lungs. Pulmonary inflammation following ischemia reperfusion injuries can be an issue in companion animals following gastrointestinal or limb ischemia. Studies in lab animals have demonstrated that PBMT can ameliorate remote-organ lung injury induced by hind-limb (Ashrafzadeh Takhtfooladi *et al.,* 2015) and gut (de Lima *et al.,* 2013a,b) ischemia and reperfusion. These studies suggest that proactive treatment of the pulmonary fields is indicated following any ischemia reperfusion injury. Again, these patients should be treated twice a day with treatments dosed and applied as per the recommendations in the section on COPD.

Conclusion

PBMT is playing an ever-increasing role in thousands of veterinary practices and in the management of a variety of conditions in millions of patients. The anti-inflammatory effects of PBMT have been well-established and are now being incorporated into the therapeutic approach to many inflammatory conditions in the upper and lower respiratory tracts. Based on the general and condition-specific treatment concepts presented in this chapter, veterinarians are encouraged to consider the addition of PBMT to the treatment of these conditions whenever possible.

References

Aghamohammadi, D. *et al.* (2013). Effect of low level laser application at the end of surgery to reduce pain after tonsillectomy in adults. *J Lasers Med Sci.* 4(2):79–85.

Ailioaie, C. and Ailioaie, L. (1997). The treatment of bronchial asthma with LLLT in attack-free period in children. *Ter Arkh.* 69(12):49–50.

Aimbire, F. *et al.* (2005). Effect of LLLT Ga-Al-as (685 nm) on LPS-induced inflammation of the airway and lung in the rat. *Lasers Med Sci.* 20(1):11–20.

Aimbire, F. *et al.* (2007). Effect of low-level laser therapy on hemorrhagic lesions induced by immune complex in rat lungs. *Photomed Laser Surg.* 25(2):112–117.

Aimbire, F. *et al.* (2008). Low level laser therapy (LLLT) decreases pulmonary microvascular leakage, neutrophil influx and IL-1beta levels in airway and lung from rat subjected to LPS-induced inflammation. *Inflammation.* 31(3):189–197.

Amirov, N.B. (2002). Parameters of membrane permeability, microcirculation, external respiration, and trace element levels in the drug-laser treatment of pneumonia. *Ter Arkh.* 74(3):40–43.

Ashrafzadeh Takhtfooladi, M. *et al.* (2015). Effect of low-level laser therapy on lung injury induced by hindlimb ischemia/reperfusion in rats. *Lasers Med Sci.* 30(6):1757–1762.

Azevedo, L.H. *et al.* (2005). Evaluation of low intensity laser effects on the thyroid gland of male mice. *Photomed Laser Surg.* 23(6):567–570.

Barrs, V.R. and Talbot, J.J. (2014). Feline aspergillosis. *Vet Clin North Am Small Anim Pract.* 44(1):51–43.

Burger, E. *et al.* (2015). Low-level laser therapy to the mouse femur enhances the fungicidal response of neutrophils against *Paracoccidioides brasiliensis. PLoS Negl Trop Dis.* 9(2):e0003541.

Choi, B. (2013). Effects of low level laser therapy on ovalbumin-induced mouse model of allergic rhinitis. *Complement Alternat Med.* 2013:753829.

Clark, G.N. and Sinibaldi, K.R. (1994). Use of a carbon dioxide laser for treatment of elongated soft palate in dogs. *J Am Vet Med Assoc.* 204(11):1779–1781.

Cohn, L.A. (2014). Canine nasal disease. *Vet Clin North Am Small Anim Pract.* 44(1):75–89.

Corcoran, B.M. *et al.* (1999a). *Chronic pulmonary disease in West Highland white terriers Vet Rec*:1.

Corcoran, B.M. *et al.* (1999b). Idiopathic pulmonary fibrosis in a Stafforshire bull terrier with hypothyroidism. *J. Small Anim Pract.* 40:185–188.

Cury, V. (2015). Low level laser therapy reduces acute lung inflammation without impairing lung function. *J Biophotonics.* doi:10.1002/jbio.201500113.

Davidson, E.B. *et al.* (2001). Evaluation of carbon dioxide laser and conventional incisional techniques for resection of soft palates in brachycephalic dogs. *J Am Vet Med Assoc.* 219(6):776–781.

Dear, J.D. (2014). Bacterial pneumonia in dogs and cats. *Vet Clin North Am Small Anim Pract.* 44(1):143–159.

Drobatz, K.J. *et al.* (1999a). Smoke exposure in dogs: 27 cases (1988–1997). *J Am Vet Med Assoc.* 215(9):1306–1311.

Drobatz, K.J. *et al.* (1999b). Smoke exposure in cats: 22 cases (1986–1997). *J Am Vet Med Assoc.* 215(9):1312–1316.

Dunié-Mérigot, A. *et al.* (2010). Comparative use of CO_2 laser, diode laser and monopolar electrocautery for resection of the soft palate in dogs with brachycephalic airway obstructive syndrome. *Vet Rec.* 167(18):700–704.

Dupré, G. and Heidenreich, D. (2016). Brachycephalic syndrome. *Vet Clin North Am Small Anim Pract.* 46(4):691–707.

Dupré, G. *et al.* (2012). Brachycephalic airway syndrome. In: *Small Animal Soft Tissue Surgery*, pp. 167–183. Wiley-Blackwell, Ames, IA.

Enwemeka, C.S. (2009). Intricacies of dose in laser phototherapy for tissue repair and pain relief. *Photomed Laser Surg.* 27(3):387–393.

Farrow, C.S. (1975). Smoke inhalation in the dog: current concepts of pathophysiology and management. *Vet Med Small Anim Clin.* 70(4):404–414.

Fasanella, F.J. *et al.* (2010). Brachycephalic airway obstructive syndrome in dogs: 90 cases (1991-2008). *J Am Vet Med Assoc.* 237(9):1048–1051. doi:10.2460/javma.237.9.1048 PMID: 21034343.

Gogeliia, A. *et al.* (2006). Experience on treatment of children with otorhinolaryngological diseases by low intensity laser irradiation. *Georgian Med News.* 130:84–86.

Herrtage, M.J. (2009). Medical management of tracheal collapse. In: *Kirk's Current Veterinary Therapy XIV*, pp. 630–635. Saunders Elsevier, St. Louis, MO.

Ilko, K. *et al.*, (2003). *In vivo* spectral transmission measurements through single and multiple tissue layers and blood ***Conference on Lasers and Electro-Optics***

Kalogeris, T. *et al.* (2012). Cell biology of ischemia/reperfusion injury. *Int Rev Cell Mol Biol.* 298:229–317.

Kaplan, B. (1981). Evaluation and management of tonsillitis & pharyngitis in dogs. *Vet Med Small Anim Clin.* 76(11):1599–1603.

Kashanskaia, E.P. and Fedorov, A.A. (2009). Low-intensity laser radiation in the combined treatment of patients with chronic obstructive bronchitis. *Vopr Kurortol Fizioter Lech Fiz Kult.* 2:19–22.

Krespi, Y.P. and Kizhner, V. (2012). Laser-assisted nasal decolonization of *Staphylococcus aureus*, including methicillin-resistant *Staphylococcus aureus*. *Am J Otolaryngol.* 33(5):572–575.

Lapchak, P.A. *et al.* (2015). Transcranial near-infrared laser transmission (NILT) profiles (800 nm): systematic comparison in four common research species. *PLoS One.* 10(6):e0127580.

Lee, H.M. *et al.* (2013). A comparative pilot study of symptom improvement before and after phototherapy in Korean patients with perennial allergic rhinitis. *Photochem Photobiol.* 89(3):751–757.

de Lima, F.M. *et al.* (2013a). Suppressive effect of low-level laser therapy on tracheal hyperresponsiveness and lung inflammation in rat subjected to intestinal ischemia and reperfusion. *Lasers Med Sci.* 28(2):551–564.

de Lima, F.M. *et al.* (2013b). Low-level laser therapy restores the oxidative stress balance in acute lung injury induced by gut ischemia and reperfusion. *Photochem Photobiol.* 89(1):179–188.

Lister, T. *et al.* (2012). Optical properties of human skin. *J Biomed Opt.* 17(9):90901.

Lobetti, R.G. (2009). A retrospective study of chronic nasal disease in 75 dogs. *J S Afr Vet Assoc.* 80(4):224–228.

Lucroy, M. *et al.* (2003). Photodynamic therapy for the treatment of intranasal tumors in 3 dogs and 1 cat. *J Vet Intern Med.* 17:727–729.

Lutaĭ, A.V. (2001). Laser therapy of elderly patients with pneumonia. *Vopr Kurortol Fizioter Lech Fiz Kult.* 3:15–18.

MacPhail, C. (2014). Laryngeal disease in dogs and cats. *Vet Clin North Am Small Anim Pract.* 44(1):19–31.

Maggiore, A.D. (2014). Tracheal and airway collapse in dogs. *Vet Clin North Am Small Anim Pract.* 44(1):117–127.

Mariani, C.L. (2003). Full recovery following delayed neurologic signs after smoke inhalation in a dog. *J Vet Emerg Crit Care.* 13(4):235–239.

Marinho, R.R. *et al.* (2013a). Potentiated anti-inflammatory effect of combined 780 nm and 660 nm low level laser therapy on the experimental laryngitis. *J Photochem Photobiol B.* 121:86–93.

Marinho, R.R. *et al.* (2013b). Potential anti-inflammatory effect of low-level laser therapy on the experimental reflux laryngitis: a preliminary study. *Lasers Med Sci.* 29(1):239–243.

Meola, S.D. (2013). Brachycephalic airway syndrome. *Top Companion Anim Med.* 28(3):91–96.

Miranda da Silva, C. *et al.* (2015). Low level laser therapy reduces the development of lung inflammation induced by formaldehyde exposure. *PLoS One.* 10(11):e0142816.

Monnet, E. (2016). Surgical treatment of laryngeal paralysis. *Vet Clin North Am Small Anim Pract.* 46(4):709–719.

Monnet, E. and Tobias, K.M. (2012). Larynx. In: *Veterinary Surgery Small Animal*, p. 1724. Elsevier, St, Louis, MO.

Naghdi, S. *et al.* (2013). A pilot study into the effect of low-level laser therapy in patients with chronic rhinosinusitis. *Physiother Theory Pract.* 29(8):596–603.

Oliveira, M.C. Jr. *et al.* (2014). Low level laser therapy reduces acute lung inflammation in a model of pulmonary and extrapulmonary LPS-induced ARDS. *J Photochem Photobiol B.* 134:57–63.

Ostronosova, N.S. (2006). Outpatient use of laser therapy in bronchial asthma. *Ter Arkh.* 78(3):41–44.

Parrado, C. *et al.* (1990). Quantitative study of the morphological changes in the thyroid gland following IR laser radiation. *Lasers Med Sci.* 5:77–80.

Prescott, C.W. (1968). A case of tonsilitis in the cat. *Aust Vet J.* 44(7):331–332.

Priestnall, S.L. (2014). New and emerging pathogens in canine infectious respiratory disease. *Vet Pathol.* 51(2):492–504.

Reed, N. (2014). Chronic rhinitis in the cat. *Vet Clin North Am Small Anim Pract.* 44(1):33–50.

Rehberg, S. *et al.* (2009). Pathophysiology, management and treatment of smoke inhalation injury. *Expert Rev Respir Med.* 3(3):283–297.

Reinero, C.R. (2011). Advances in the understanding of pathogenesis, and diagnostics and therapeutics for feline allergic asthma. *Vet J.* 190(1):28–33.

Rozanski, E. (2014). Canine chronic bronchitis. *Vet Clin North Am Small Anim Pract.* 44(1):107–116.

Sharman, M.J. and Mansfield, C.S. (2012). Sinonasal aspergillosis in dogs: a review. *J Small Anim Pract.* 53(8):434–444.

Sigman, S. *et al.* (2020). Adjunct low level laser therapy (LLLT) in a morbidly obese patient with severe COVID-19 pneumonia: a case report. *Can J Respir Ther.* 56:52–56.

Silva, V.R. *et al.* (2014). Low-level laser therapy inhibits bronchoconstriction, Th2 inflammation and airway remodeling in allergic asthma. *Respir Physiol Neurobiol.* 194:37–48.

Sohelifar, S. *et al.* (2021). Photobiomodulation therapy as a high potential treatment modality for COVID-19. *Lasers in Medical Science.* 36:935–938.

Sutera, S.P. and Skalak, R. (1993). The history of Poiseuille's law. *Annu Rev Fluid Mech.* 25:1–20.

Tedford, C.E. *et al.* (2015). Quantitative analysis of transcranial and intraparenchymal light penetration in human cadaver brain tissue. *Lasers Surg Med.* 47(4):312–322.

Tilley, L.P. and Smith, F.W.K. (2000). Pulmonary fibrosis. In: *The 5 Minute Veterinary Consultant.* (eds. L.P. Tilley and F.W.K. Smith). Williams and Wilkins, Philadelphia Lippincott 2000:1126.

Trizil, J.E. and Reinero, C.R. (2014). Update on feline asthma. *Vet Clin North Am Small Anim Pract.* 44(1):91–105.

Troxel, M. (2012). Smoke inhalation in a dog: clinician's brief (capsule). Available from: http://www.cliniciansbrief.com//column/category/column/capsules/smoke-inhalation-dog (accessed November 30, 2016).

Viitanen, S.J. (2015). Co-infections with respiratory viruses in dogs with bacterial pneumonia. *J Vet Intern Med.* 29(2):544–551.

Wang, X.Y. (2014). Effect of low-level laser therapy on allergic asthma in rats. *Lasers Med Sci.* 29(3):1043–1050.

Windsor, R.C. and Johnson, L.R. (2006). Canine chronic inflammatory rhinitis. *Clin Tech Small Anim Pract.* 21(2):76–81.

13

Oral Conditions

Ashton B. Thompson

Companion Animal Health, New Castle, DE, USA

1st Edition Contributor:

Ray A. Arza

RSA Veterinary Technologies, Taylorsville, KY, USA

Introduction

The number of veterinary practices using therapeutic lasers has increased significantly and photobiomodulation therapy (PBMT) has become an important treatment modality in veterinary medicine. There is now overwhelming evidence that PBMT helps control pain, modulates inflammation, and stimulates healing and tissue regeneration (Avci *et al.*, 2013; Bjordal *et al.*, 2006; Chung *et al.*, 2012). The mechanisms by which PBMT has such far-reaching effects are detailed in Chapter 3.

Veterinarians first used therapy lasers to treat musculoskeletal conditions based on the success reported in the treatment of similar conditions in human patients (Bjordal *et al.*, 2008; Chow *et al.*, 2009; Jang and Lee 2012). Successful treatment of wounds soon became commonly reported (Al-Watban *et al.*, 2007; Peplow *et al.*, 2010), as did the use of laser therapy for the treatment of painful conditions (Chow *et al.*, 2011; Fulop *et al.*, 2010). Veterinarians have subsequently expanded the use of this modality to treat a wide variety of medical applications, including those involving the oral cavity.

Much has been learned about the roles that proper application and dosing play in the expected results from laser therapy (Enwemeka 2009; Zein 2018). Increased knowledge of proper dosing and application allows practitioners to design successful treatment protocols for the oral cavity. As with other conditions that veterinarians treat with PBMT, the successful treatment of oral conditions in veterinary patients mirrors what is being reported in the treatment of human oral conditions (Arany 2016; Boras 2013; Kalhori *et al.*, 2019; Kathuria *et al.*, 2015; Khan and Arany 2015; Ross 2016). This chapter will focus on some of the common conditions that affect the oral cavity in canine and feline patients, and will demonstrate how PBMT is utilized in the management of these conditions.

Oral Inflammatory Conditions

Use of laser therapy to reduce oral inflammation in both humans and animals has been widely reported (Ahmed *et al.*, 2015; Bjordal *et al.*, 2011; Chermetz *et al.*, 2014; Freire *et al.*, 2014; Ottaviani *et al.*, 2013). A pair of comprehensive review articles examined the use of PBMT in the management of the side effects of radiation and chemoradiation therapy in human head and neck cancer patients (Zecha *et al.*, 2016a, 2016b). The articles state that among the few supportive care measures available for the treatment of the side effects of radiation therapy or chemoradiotherapy in human patients, PBMT has shown the most promise. These publications emphasize the important role that laser therapy can play in the management of oral inflammatory conditions.

A 2016 review notes that PBM “effectively modulates biological function is supported by a plethora of clinical and laboratory studies” (Zecha *et al.*, 2016a). It “elicits several potentially beneficial effects, including reduction of inflammation and pain, promotion of tissue repair, reduction of fibrosis, and protection and regeneration of nerves” (Zecha *et al.*, 2016b).

Publications reporting the successful application of PBMT in oral inflammatory conditions in humans give cross-species evidence that treatment of similar conditions

Laser Therapy in Veterinary Medicine: Photobiomodulation, Second Edition. Edited by Christopher J. Winkler and Lisa A. Miller.

is indicated in veterinary patients. Regardless of the cause of inflammation (and with careful consideration for malignancy), therapy lasers can be used in the oral cavity with promising results and very little evidence of side effects.

Inflammation of oral tissues may be primary or secondary, and may affect many soft tissues in the mouth, including the oral mucosa (stomatitis), the gingiva (gingivitis), the periodontium (periodontitis), the alveolar mucosa (alveolar mucositis), the mucosa of the tongue (glossitis), and the mucosa of the pharynx (pharyngitis) (Gorrel *et al.*, 2013a). Periodontal disease is the most common oral condition presenting to veterinarians (Gorrel *et al.*, 2013b). Other causes of oral inflammation include infectious agents, trauma, autoimmune disease, chemical agents, metabolic disease, and burns. Traumatic stomatitis is sometimes seen when an animal has oral exposure to toxic plants or other toxic substances.

Periodontal Disease

Periodontal disease is typically an inflammatory response to the presence of bacterial plaque on adjacent tooth surfaces. It responds well when treated with PBMT and should be the most common oral condition treated with it. Periodontal disease is widespread in canine patients and is often associated with serious systemic diseases. It is more common in small breeds than large breeds and increases with advancing age (Marshall *et al.*, 2014). Periodontal disease includes gingivitis (inflammation of the gums) and periodontitis (loss of soft tissue and bone around the teeth). It can cause significant pain and secondary healthy issues, often undetected by clients, leading to a decreased quality of life for companion animals (Bellows *et al.*, 2019).

The diagnostic criteria and grading of gingivitis and periodontal disease have been well established in publications (Harvey *et al.*, 2008) and are specified by the American Veterinary Dental College (AVDC, n.d.). Even the earliest diagnosis and the lowest grading (grade I gingivitis) merit attention, which should include laser therapy. Adding PBMT to the overall management plan for periodontal disease, including after dental prophylaxis, will help reduce the patient's inflammation (Alves *et al.*, 2023; Watson and Brundage, 2019) and oral pain. A 2023 study in canines showed significantly lower gingivitis scores when evaluated from +1 to +15 days after one half of the mouth received a single PBMT treatment following dental prophylaxis (Alves *et al.*, 2023).

Periodontal disease may be treated as a superficial condition (when treatment can be administered with the mouth open) or through the lips as a deep tissue condition (if the patient will not allow the mouth to be opened). Treatments are usually initiated in conjunction with dental procedures, under sedation or anesthesia. When treating with the mouth open, a laser setting that delivers 3–4 J/cm^2 is

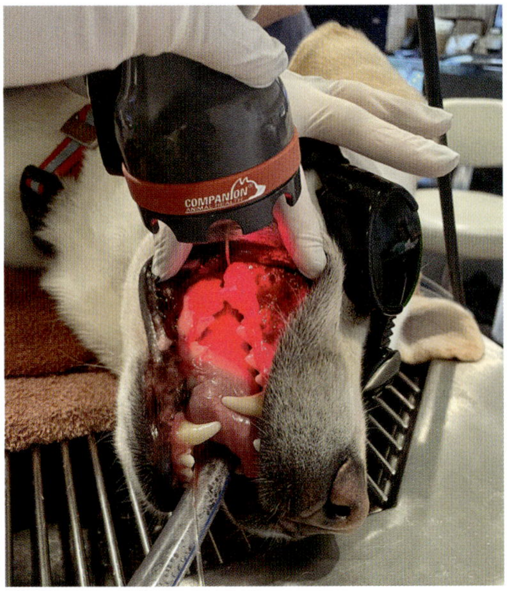

Figure 13.1 Treating periodontal disease with the mouth open.

recommended (Figure 13.1). Since the laser light does not have to penetrate through other tissues to get to the target site, this is the preferred method of delivery.

The author recommends positioning the handpiece 3–5 cm from the target area. If available, a handpiece that collimates the laser beam and allows treatment at an even greater distance from the tissue may be used, though hand speed should be increased with this technique (Figure 13.2). The laser power settings should be adjusted according to patient size but not exceed 5 W or an irradiance of 2 W/cm^2.

Treating the entire mouth, including upper and lower arcades and both the left and right halves is recommended for most periodontal disease. If the gums appear excessively dry during treatment, the area can be misted with water.

When treating with the mouth closed, laser settings that deliver 6–8 J/cm^2 are recommended (Figure 13.3), as a higher dose is required in order to deliver a clinically relevant quantity of photons to the target tissue. The laser power settings should be adjusted according to patient size but not exceed 8 W or an irradiance of 2 W/cm^2. The author recommends treating with the handpiece in contact with the skin using a light pressure and continually moving. The treatment area should include the entire dental arcades and from the ventral aspect through the intermandibular space (Figure 13.4). If the patient cannot be touched due to pain, treating with the handpiece held 3–5 cm from the skin can be substituted during initial visits until patient comfort improves. For any laser treatment of oral conditions, since treatment is being applied around the face, eye protection using laser-safe doggles or a dark cloth must be utilized.

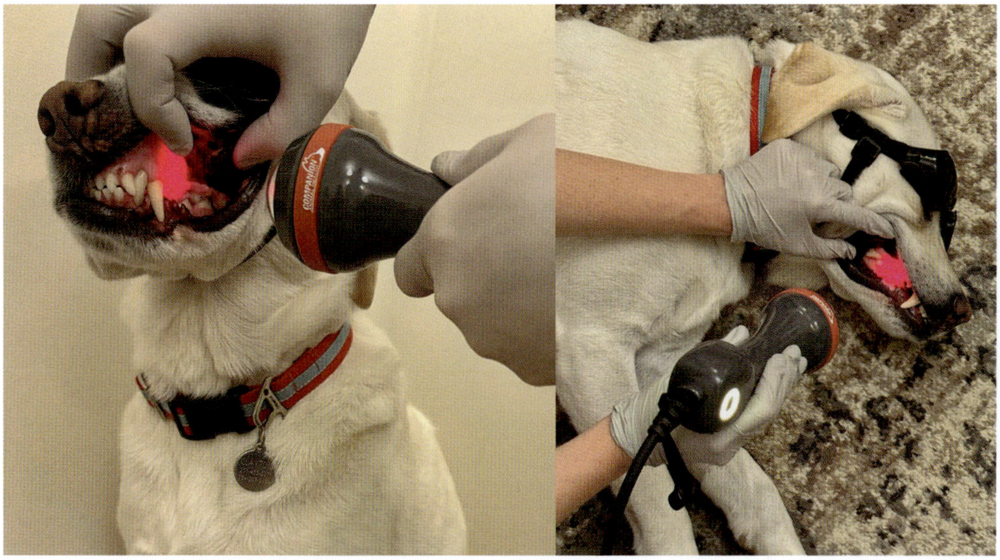

Figure 13.2 Use of a collimated beam to treat periodontal disease with the mouth open.

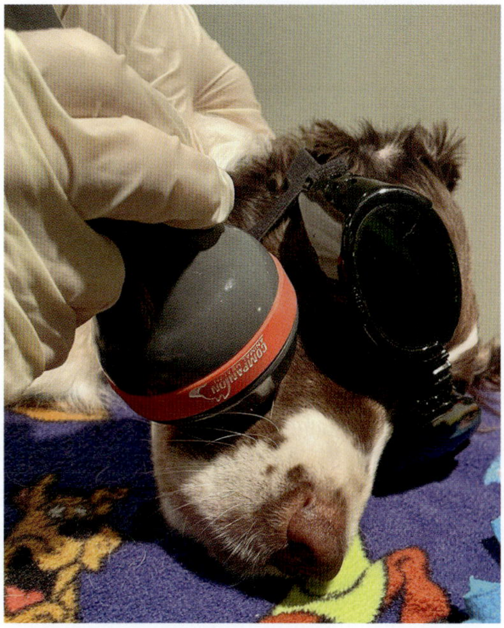

Figure 13.3 Treating periodontal disease with the mouth closed.

Severity, chronicity, and the patient's degree of discomfort should dictate how often the patient is treated. If the patient is there for routine dental prophylaxis, a single treatment will be beneficial in the reduction of gingivitis scores (Alves *et al.,* 2023). If the patient has low-grade periodontal disease that responds to multimodal care, therapy laser treatments may only be necessary as part of that care for a limited time.

More often, periodontal disease becomes a chronic condition and requires long-term, open-ended treatment. When periodontal disease is chronic, three phases of treatment should be implemented: an induction phase, a transition phase, and a long-term maintenance phase. The induction phase usually starts with every-other-day treatments and continues until a desirable clinical response is noted. When improvement is noted, the frequency of treatment can be reduced gradually through a transition phase, with the goal of finding a maintenance schedule that will keep the patient at the desired level of comfort. Most conditions can be maintained with one treatment every 2–4 weeks, but treatment frequency must be based on patient response.

Feline Stomatitis

Though uncommon and seen in only 3.9% of feline patients (Kornya *et al.,* 2014), feline stomatitis causes patients to experience severe discomfort, making it both very serious and difficult to manage. Affected cats present with inflammation of oral mucosal tissues that often worsens with time and becomes refractory to treatment. Typical findings are severely ulcerated and inflamed tissues, most commonly affecting the caudal aspect of the oral cavity, involving the fauces and pharyngeal areas. Severe bilateral ulceroproliferative inflammation of these areas is considered pathognomonic for feline stomatitis (Crawford 2013). The etiology of feline stomatitis is not completely understood, but a high percentage of affected cats are chronic carriers of feline calicivirus. There is also evidence that an overreaction of the immune system to antigens in dental plaque may play a role in these pathological changes (Robson and Crystal 2011).

(a) (b)

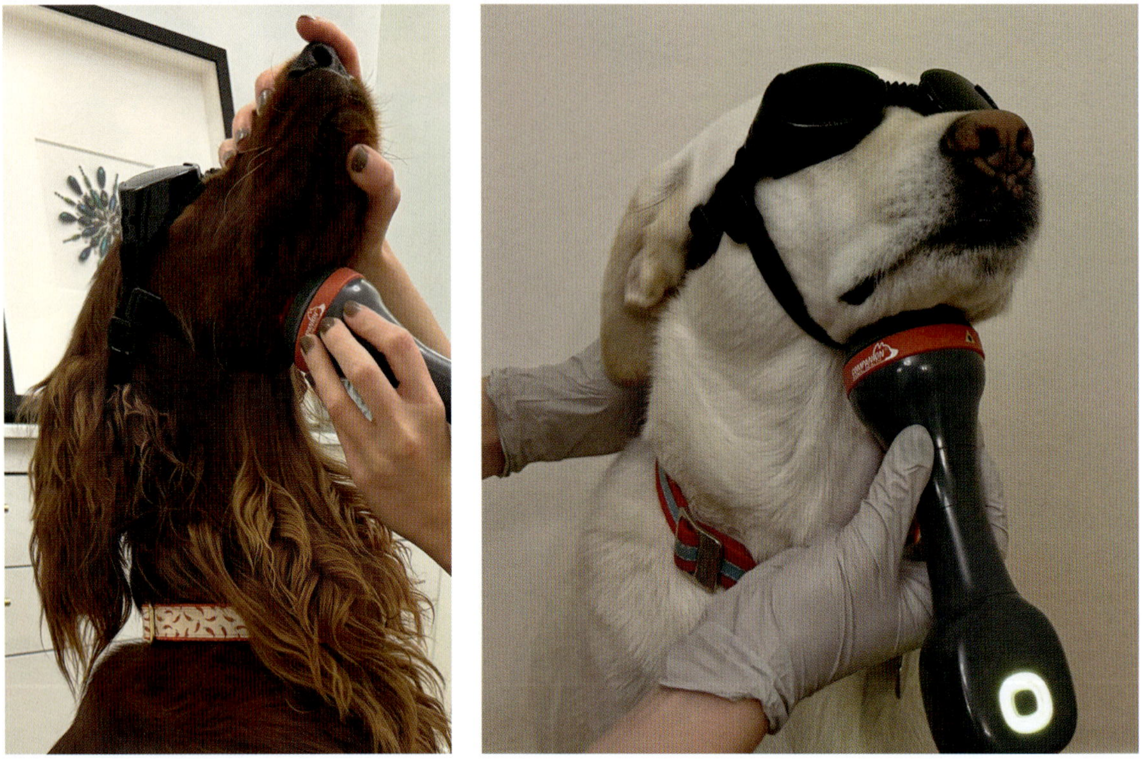

Figure 13.4 (a) Treatment through the intermandibular space with the mouth closed. (b) The handpiece should be placed in contact with the skin with light pressure for more effective penetration of photons.

The most common symptom is severe pain when opening the mouth. As the condition worsens, halitosis and dysphagia may be seen, and weight loss may be evident with time. Examination of the oral cavity is often difficult without sedation, due to patient discomfort and severe pain.

Diagnosis of feline stomatitis is usually made by observation of bilateral inflammation of the caudal oral cavity. However, attempts to isolate calici and herpes viruses, as well as to evaluate other potential problems such as renal failure, are recommended. Biopsy generally reveals a predominance of lymphocytes and plasma cells.

Management of this condition requires a multimodal approach. Published data indicate that early partial or full mouth extraction is the best choice to provide long-lasting improvement (Jennings *et al.,* 2015). Medical therapy focuses on controlling inflammation, infection, and pain. This includes the use of corticosteroids, other immunosuppressants (e.g., cyclosporine or chlorambucil), antibiotics (e.g., amoxicillin-clavulanic acid, clindamycin, or azithromycin), and pain medications (e.g., buprenorphine or fentanyl). Ablating the abnormal tissue with a CO_2 surgical laser has been reported as an adjunctive treatment for caudal stomatitis (Lewis *et al.,* 2007).

Evidence that PBMT reduces oral pain and inflammation, and the experience of veterinary practitioners, support using laser therapy as an adjunct to medical and dental protocols for feline oropharyngeal inflammation. The possibility should be explored that the antiviral effects of laser therapy reported in humans may contribute to better patient outcomes in cats if viral etiologies are a factor (Navarro *et al.,* 2007).

Though practitioners report that lesions often do not improve in appearance following laser therapy, patients frequently display significantly improved clinical signs related to appetite, grooming, and attitude. Treatment of this chronic and insidious condition must be tailored to the severity of the case and the patient's response to treatment.

Feline stomatitis may be treated as a superficial condition (when treatment can be administered with the mouth open) or as a deep condition (if the patient will not allow the mouth to be opened). Some practitioners recommend a combination of both open- and closed-mouth protocols each time a patient is treated – a practice this author believes should be considered for the presentation of any severe oral disease.

When treating with the mouth open, dosages in the range of 3–4 J/cm^2 are recommended, since the laser light does not have to penetrate through other tissues to get to the target site. The author recommends using a handpiece held 3–5 cm from the target area. If available, a handpiece that collimates the laser beam and allows treatment at a greater distance from the tissue can be used. The laser power setting should be no more than 3 W and the handpiece should move over the entire affected area until the total dose of 3–4 J/cm^2 is delivered.

When treating with the mouth closed, dosages in the range of 6–8 J/cm^2 are recommended. The area to be treated should run from the temporomandibular joint on one side, across the front of mouth to the temperomandibular joint on the other side, as well as from the ventral aspect through the intermandibular space. The power setting should be 4–5 W and the handpiece held in contact with the skin if possible, continually moving over the entire area to be treated until the total dose of 6–8 J/cm^2 has been delivered.

As when treating periodontal disease, the severity, chronicity, and degree of patient discomfort should dictate how often the patient is treated. Because feline stomatitis is a chronic condition, the management plan should include induction and transition phases followed by long-term maintenance treatments. The induction phase usually starts with every-other-day treatments. It should continue until a desirable clinical response has been noted. With severely painful presentations, the author recommends treating 3–4 days in a row before moving to every-other-day treatments. When improvement is noted, the frequency of treatment can be reduced gradually through a transition phase of less frequent treatments, with the goal of finding a maintenance schedule that will keep the patient at the desired level of comfort.

It is important to note that proper, continued management of a chronic condition like feline stomatitis is critical to success. A common mistake in the management of these cases is a premature reduction in the frequency of treatment, which leads to a perceived failure of PBMT.

Canine Stomatitis

Canine patients can present with severe, chronic, ulcerative, oral inflammatory lesions known as chronic ulcerative paradental stomatitis (CUPS, also known as canine chronic ulcerative stomatitis, idiopathic stomatitis, ulcerative stomatitis, or lymphocytic-plasmacytic stomatitis). As the name implies, paradental disease should be differentiated from periodontal disease (Lyon 2005). Periodontal disease affects the tissues that attach the tooth in the socket (gingiva, alveolar bone, periodontal ligament, and cementum of the root). These structures often remain normal in the presence of paradental disease, which affects the other soft tissues in the oral cavity, including the buccal and palatal mucosa, lips, and tongue.

Many breeds may present with CUPS, but the Maltese and Cavalier King Charles spaniel appear to be over-represented. Clinical signs usually include halitosis, inappetence or anorexia, drooling, lip-fold dermatitis, and oral pain. While diagnosis is often made by clinical observation of lesions, it is important to note that other conditions can present with similar signs and history. Other conditions which should be ruled out include immune-mediated diseases such as pemphigus and bullous pemphigoid, erythema multiforme and epitheliotropic T-cell lymphoma (Nemec *et al.,* 2012), and Wegener's granulomatosis (Krug *et al.,* 2006). Proper diagnosis is important, since treatment of these other conditions is very different from treatment of CUPS.

The etiology of CUPS is not completely understood, but it is evident these animals have an abnormal immune-system response and appear to be intolerant of the presence of bacterial plaque. Even small amounts of plaque lead to an abnormal ulcerative inflammatory response in mucous membranes in contact with the teeth (Lobprise 2012; Niemiec 2010).

Management of this chronic condition can be very frustrating to both the veterinarian and the patient's owner. The focus of management should be scrupulous plaque control. Teeth with concurrent periodontal disease should be extracted and home dental health care should be instituted. Medical treatment is occasionally required, with the use of appropriate antibiotics and prudential use of corticosteroids. Pain control should be considered, since these patients are often very uncomfortable.

Given the established ability of PBMT to prevent and ameliorate pain and inflammation associated with oral mucositis, laser therapy should be used in the treatment of this condition. The goal is to utilize laser therapy as part of a multimodal approach to reduce pain and inflammation, while minimizing potential adverse effects. Laser therapy should not be the sole treatment for this condition.

Laser therapy is used in the management of CUPS similar to how it is used in the management of feline stomatitis, and should include induction, transition, and maintenance phases of treatment. As with feline stomatitis, the frequency of treatments should be dictated by the severity of the condition and the response to treatment.

Canine patients may be treated with the mouth open, which is the author's preference, or with the mouth closed. When treating the buccal or labial mucosal tissues, lifting of the lips without opening the jaws will often be tolerated (Figure 13.5). This technique allows direct delivery of the

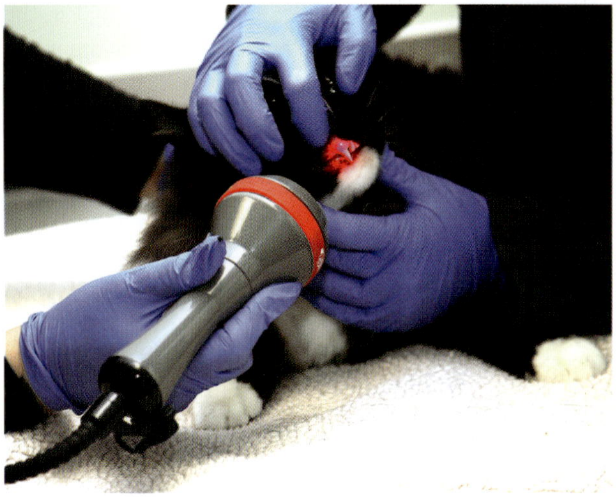

Figure 13.5 Lifting the patient's lips without opening the jaws. This technique allows direct delivery of therapeutic light to the target tissue.

therapeutic light to the target tissue. When treating with the mouth open, directly on the target tissue, administer a dose of 3–4 J/cm^2 with a power setting of 3–5 W. This should be accomplished with the treatment handpiece held 3–5 cm from the target tissue. The handpiece should move over the entire affected area until the total dose of 3–4 J/cm^2 has been delivered.

If a patient does not tolerate treatment with the mouth open, treatment can be delivered over the entire affected area through the facial tissues, at a dose of 6–8 J/cm^2 and a power setting of 4–8 W. The dose should be adjusted according to the size of the patient and the thickness of the facial tissues. If possible, treat with the handpiece in contact with the facial tissues to increase photon penetration.

Oral Wounds

PBMT has been shown to enhance wound repair and tissue regeneration by influencing the three phases of injury resolution: inflammatory, proliferative, and maturation (remodeling) (Hawkins and Abrahamse 2006). Additionally, there is initial evidence that PBMT reduces the bacterial load of contaminated wounds (Rico-Holgado *et al.*, 2021). The benefits of laser therapy application specifically regarding oral wound healing has also been demonstrated (Arany 2016; Khan and Arany 2015; Ebrahimi *et al.*, 2021; Wagner *et al.*, 2016). The well-established beneficial effects of PBMT on wound healing should make laser therapy a standard part of wound management in the oral cavity.

Traumatic Wounds

Though a problem in both canine and feline patients, their affinity for chewing sticks, bones, and other inanimate objects makes dogs more susceptible to oral injuries. Common presentations include punctures, abrasions, lacerations, burns, stings, and other traumatic wounds. Both soft and hard tissues are sometimes involved, and each need to be addressed appropriately. The rich blood supply to the oral cavity lends to an environment not only susceptible to profuse bleeding, but also tending to heal rapidly. In some cases, minor injuries heal quickly without medical intervention.

As with other oral conditions, treatment of oral wounds using laser therapy may be accomplished with the mouth open or closed. The author recommends treating these wounds with direct exposure to the target tissue whenever possible. When treating with direct exposure to tissue (open mouth), administer a dose of 3–4 J/cm^2 with a power setting of 1–4 W. A lower power setting is recommended for small wounds and a higher setting for larger ones. If the patient does not allow direct treatment of the wound, then treating with the mouth closed will require higher doses of 6–8 J/cm^2 depending on the thickness of the tissue and the location of the wound. Power settings of 4–8 W can be used.

Traumatic wounds that involve fractures of the mandible or maxilla may also benefit from PBMT. Beneficial effects regarding fracture healing, including that in dentistry, are well established (Kazem *et al.*, 2010; Medalha *et al.*, 2016; Lopes *et al.*, 2022; Son *et al.*, 2012). PBMT has also been shown to improve neurosensory recovery following mandibular fracture (Salari *et al.*, 2022). The author recommends treating traumatic oral conditions immediately upon presentation to decrease inflammation and pain, then again after fracture repair, to enhance healing.

There are essentially no contraindications for the use of lasers with surgical implants. The success of fixation implants will always increase if the health of surrounding soft tissues is improved by application of PBMT (Tang and Arany 2013). Since photons are reflected by metal, the metal is not heated; however, if there is only a small amount of soft tissue superficial to the implant, one should avoid or cross the area of the implant quickly to prevent heating of superficial tissues. Reducing the power (W) is also indicated if thermal discomfort is noted.

Dosages of 6–10 J/cm^2 should be used to treat oral fractures, with 2–8 W of power, depending on the size of the patient and the area to be treated. Current protocols recommend applying laser therapy at the time of fracture fixation and then two to three times a week for 3–4 weeks. After several weeks, the fracture should be assessed radiographically, and treatment should be continued for several more weeks if active healing is not noted.

Surgical Wounds

In many practices, laser therapy has become a standard of care as part of the multimodal approach to decreasing pain and inflammation in postoperative management. Studies in human medicine have shown that treating postsurgical wounds with PBMT has analgesic and anti-inflammatory effects (Karlekar 2015). Surgical wounds in the mouth, with either soft- or hard-tissue involvement, or both, will receive the same PBMT benefits (Hadad *et al.,* 2022; Le *et al.,* 2022). With routine soft-tissue surgery or minor extractions, the author recommends one treatment immediately postoperatively. Immediate treatment has been demonstrated to reduce postoperative inflammatory complications when compared to delayed treatment (Abdel-Alim *et al.,* 2015). With more extensive soft-tissue surgery, or with more involved extractions, multiple daily (or at least every-other-day) treatments should be considered. Repeat treatments have been shown to significantly increase bone density following premolar extraction (Abdel Hamid *et al.,* 2021). With acute inflammation and pain, daily treatments are recommended until patient comfort improves. In some cases, treatments should be continued two to three times a week until the wound has healed.

Laser settings for surgical wounds will be the same as described for inflammatory conditions. Intraoral treatment, with the mouth open at the time of surgery, is indicated. Subsequent treatments can be extraoral, with the mouth closed (Sierra *et al.,* 2016). While an individual surgical or extraction site may be treated (Figure 13.6), if the patient has other concurrent oral disease, treatment of the entire mouth is the author's preference.

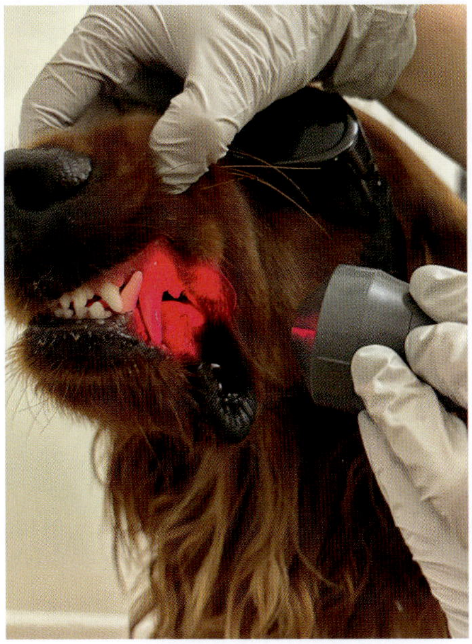

Figure 13.6 Treatment of an individual surgical site. Use of a handpiece with a small spot size may be considered. Power should be reduced to accommodate the smaller treatment area.

Other Oral Conditions

Eosinophilic Granuloma Complex

According to William H. Miller, VMD, Professor of Dermatology at Cornell University College of Veterinary Medicine, eosinophilic granuloma complex includes three distinctly different clinical presentations that are grouped together "because all three show the activity of eosinophils and have an apparent allergic condition as the triggering event" (Cornell University College of Veterinary Medicine, 2016). The three different forms are eosinophilic granuloma, eosinophilic ulcer (indolent ulcer), and eosinophilic plaque (Buckley and Nuttall 2012). This chapter will only discuss the first two, since eosinophilic plaque does not occur in the oral cavity.

Treatment is dependent on the severity and the underlying cause (the source of the apparent allergic reaction), but may include corticosteroids, antibiotics (for secondary infection), antihistamines, and other immunosuppressive drugs (e.g., cyclosporine or chlorambucil).

Eosinophilic granuloma is the most commonly presented form, with a wide variation in clinical appearances that can present anywhere on the body. It is commonly seen in the oral cavity and on the hind legs. Lesions may vary, but typically are nodular or linear raised thickened areas, red or yellow in color, sometimes with loss of hair and ulcerations. In the oral cavity, the lesions are usually found on the tongue or palate.

Eosinophilic ulcers typically occur toward the edge of the upper lips, often close to the midline (philtrum) on one or both sides. Generally, they are well-defined ulcerated lesions with raised borders, which may become disfiguring and bleed over time. Severe lesions may cause pain and inappetence (Rees 2011).

PBMT has been used as an adjunct to conventional medical therapy based on anecdotal reports from practitioners. The recommended dose of laser therapy for this complex of conditions has changed dramatically over the past 10 years. When a low dose (e.g., 3–4 J/cm^2 as is traditionally utilized for superficial conditions) is used to treat eosinophilic granulomas and ulcers, there is no appreciable clinical improvement. However, when a dosage of 30–40 J/cm^2 is applied, significantly better clinical results are observed. Since lesions in the mouth are usually relatively small, the power setting should not exceed 2 W. Lesions should be treated two to three times a week until resolved.

Lip-Fold Dermatitis in Dogs

Lip-fold dermatitis or lip-fold pyoderma is most commonly seen in breeds with large, saggy, floppy lips, such as St. Bernards, bloodhounds, springer spaniels, shar peis, Neapolitan mastiffs, and bulldogs. Accumulation of saliva and food debris in the lip fold creates an environment that leads to irritation, inflammation, and, if left untreated, infection with bacteria or yeast. Treatment will depend on severity and underlying cause, but often includes medicated shampoos, topical ointments, or oral antibiotics. In severe unresponsive cases, surgical reconstruction of the lip folds may be indicated.

As with moist dermatitis found elsewhere on the body, laser therapy may play an adjunctive role in decreasing inflammation and discomfort and promoting healing. Laser settings that deliver a dosage of 3–4 J/cm^2 should be used, with a power setting of 1–4 W, depending on the size of the area to be treated. Lesions should be treated two to three times a week until resolved. In frequently reoccurring cases, long-term maintenance treatments every 7–10 days may help avoid acute exacerbations.

Conclusion

PBMT is an important component of the multimodal approach to decreasing both pain and inflammation while stimulating healing in oral tissues. Many oral conditions result in similar changes in the mouth, with some variations due to the severity, chronicity, and size and thickness of the involved tissue. Regardless, all oral conditions are treated with similar laser therapy protocols. With special consideration for malignancies, practitioners are encouraged to utilize PBMT on any condition in the mouth that presents with inflammation, pain, or tissue damage.

References

Abdel Hamid, M.A. *et al.* (2021). Efficacy of flat-top hand-piece using 980 nm diode laser photobiomodulation on socket healing after extraction: Split-mouth experimental model in dogs. *Photochem Photobiol.* 97(3):627–633.

Abdel-Alim, H.M. *et al.* (2015). A comparative study of the effectiveness of immediate versus delayed photobiomodulation therapy in reducing the severity of postoperative inflammatory complications. *Photomed Laser Surg.* 33(9):447–451.

Ahmed, K. *et al.* (2015). Evaluation of low level laser therapy in the management of chemotherapy induced oral mucositis in pediatric and young cancer patients: a randomized clinical trial. *Eur Sci Journ.* 11(27):209–222.

Alves, J.C. *et al.* (2023). The effect of photobiomodulation therapy on inflammation following dental prophylaxis. *J Vet Dent.* doi:10.1177/08987564221150.

Al-Watban, F.A. *et al.* (2007). Low-level laser therapy enhances wound healing in diabetic rats: a comparison of different lasers. *Photomed Laser Surg.* 25(2):72–77.

Arany, P.R. (2016). Craniofacial wound healing with photobiomodulation therapy: new insights and current challenges. *J Dent Res.* 95(9):977–984.

Avci, P. *et al.* (2013). Low-level laser (light) therapy (LLLT) in skin: stimulating, healing, restoring. *Semin Cutan Med Surg.* 32(1):41–52.

AVDC. (n.d.). AVDC nomenclature. https://avdc.org/avdc-nomenclature/(accessed 02 October 2023).

Bellows, J. *et al.* (2019). 2019 AAHA dental care guidelines for dogs and cats. *J Am Anim Hosp Assoc.* 55(2):49–69.

Bjordal, J.M. *et al.* (2006). Low-level laser therapy in acute pain: a systematic review of mechanisms of action and clinical effects in randomized placebo-controlled trials. *Photomed Laser Surg.* 24(2):158–168.

Bjordal, J.M. *et al.* (2008). A systematic review with procedural assessments and meta-analysis of low level laser therapy in lateral elbow tendonopathy (tennis elbow). *BMC Musculoskeletal Disord.* 9:75.

Bjordal, J.M. *et al.* (2011). A systematic review with meta-analysis of the effect of low-level laser therapy (LLLT) in cancer therapy-induced oral mucositis. *Support Care Cancer.* 19:1069–1077.

Boras, V.V. (2013). Applications of low level laser therapy. In: *A Textbook of Advanced Oral and Maxillofacial Surgery.* InTech, Rijeka.

Buckley, L. and Nuttall, T. (2012). Feline eosinophilic granuloma complex(ities): some clinical clarification. *J Feline Med Surg.* 14(7):471–481.

Chermetz, M. *et al.* (2014). Class IV laser therapy as treatment for chemotherapy-induced oral mucositis in onco-haematological paediatric patients: a prospective study. *Int J Paediatr Dent.* 6:441–449.

Chow, R. *et al.* (2009). Efficacy of low-level laser therapy in the management of neck pain: a systematic review and meta-analysis of randomized placebo or active-treatment controlled trials. *Lancet.* 374(9705):1897–1908.

Chow, R. *et al.* (2011). Inhibitory effects of laser irradiation on peripheral mammalian nerves and relevance to analgesic effects: a systematic review. *Photomed Laser Surg.* 29:365–381.

Chung, H. *et al.* (2012). The nuts and bolts of low-level laser (light) therapy. *Ann Biomed Eng.* 40(2):516–533.

Cornell University College of Veterinary Medicine. (n.d.). Eosinophilic granuloma complex. Available from: http://www.vet.cornell.edu/fhc/Health_Information/eosinophilic.cfm (accessed November 30, 2016).

Crawford, J. (2013). Gingivostomatitis. In: *Small Animal Dental Procedures for Veterinary Technicians and Nurses*, pp. 145–140. Wiley-Blackwell, Hoboken, NJ.

Ebrahimi, P. *et al.* (2021). Effect of photobiomodulation in secondary intention gingival wound healing – a systemic review and meta-analysis. *BMC Oral Health.* 21(1) 258.

Enwemeka, C.S. (2009). Intricacies of dose in laser phototherapy for tissue repair and pain relief. *Photomed Laser Surg.* 3:387–393.

Freire, M. *et al.* (2014). LED and laser photobiomodulation in the prevention and treatment of oral mucositis: experimental study in hamsters. *Clin Oral Investig.* 18(3):1005–1013.

Fulop, A. *et al.* (2010). A meta-analysis of the efficacy of laser phototherapy on pain relief. *Clin J Pain.* 26(8):729–736.

Gorrel, C. *et al.* (2013a). Common oral conditions. In: *Veterinary Dentistry for the General Practitioner*, 2 edn, pp. 81–95. Elsevier, Philadelphia, PA.

Gorrel, C. *et al.* (2013b). Periodontal disease. In: *Veterinary Dentistry for the General Practitioner*, 2 edn, pp. 97–119. Elsevier, Philadelphia, PA.

Hadad, H. *et al.* (2022). Photobiomodulation therapy improves postoperative pain and edema in third molar surgeries: a randomized, comparative, double-blind, and prospective clinical trial. *J Oral Maxillofac Surg.* 80(1):37.

Harvey, C.E. *et al.* (2008). Scoring the full extent of periodontal disease in the dog: development of a total mouth periodontal score (TMPS) system. *J Vet Dent.* 25(3):176–180.

Hawkins, D. and Abrahamse, H. (2006). The role of laser fluence in cell viability, proliferation, and membrane integrity of wounded human skin fibroblasts following helium-neon laser irradiation. *Lasers Surg Med.* 38(1):74–83.

Jang, H. and Lee, H. (2012). Meta-analysis of pain relief effects by laser irradiation on joint areas. *Photomed Laser Surg.* 30(8):405–417.

Jennings, M.W. *et al.* (2015). Effect of tooth extraction on stomatitis in cats: 95 cases (2000–2013). *J Am Vet Med Assoc.* 246(6):654–660.

Kalhori, K.A.M. *et al.* (2019). Photobiomodulation in oral medicine. *Photobiomodul Photomed Laser Surg.* 37(12):837–861.

Karlekar, A. (2015). Assessment of feasibility and efficacy of class IV laser therapy for postoperative pain relief in off-pump coronary artery bypass surgery patients: a pilot study. *Ann Card Anaesth.* 18(3):317–322.

Kathuria, V. *et al.* (2015). Low level laser therapy: a panacea for oral maladies. *Laser Ther.* 24(3):215–223.

Kazem, S.S. *et al.* (2010). Effect of low-level laser therapy on the fracture healing process. *Lasers Med Sci.* 25(1):73–77.

Khan, I. and Arany, P.R. (2015). Biophysical approaches for oral wound healing: emphasis on photobiomodulation. *Adv Wound Care (New Rochelle).* 4(12):724–737.

Kornya, M.R. *et al.* (2014). Association between oral health status and retrovirus test results in cats. *J Am Vet Med Assoc.* 245(8):916–922.

Krug, W. *et al.* (2006). Diagnosis and management of Wegener's granulomatosis in a dog. *J Vet Dent.* 23(4):231–236.

Le, H.T. *et al.* (2022). Effect of photobiomodulation therapy on reducing acute pain and inflammation following surgical removal of impacted mandibular third molars: a randomized, split-mouth clinical trial. *Photobiomodul Photomed Laser Surg.* 40(4):245–225.

Lewis, J.R. *et al.* (2007). Use of CO_2 laser as an adjunctive treatment for caudal stomatitis in a cat. *J Vet Dent.* 24(4):240–249.

Lobprise, H.B. (2012). Oral ulceration and chronic ulcerative paradental stomatitis. In: *Blackwell's Five-Minute Veterinary Consult Clinical Companion – Small Animal Dentistry*, 2 edn, pp. 243–247. Wiley-Blackwell, Ames, IA.

Lopes, C.C.A. *et al.* (2022). Effectiveness of photobiomodulation therapy on human bone healing in dentistry: a systemic review. *Photobiomodul Photomed Laser Surg.* 40(7):440–453.

Lyon, K.F. (2005). Gingivostomatitis. *Vet Clin North Am Small Anim Pract.* 35(4):891–911.

Marshall, M.D. *et al.* (2014). A longitudinal assessment of periodontal disease in 52 miniature schnauzers. *BMC Vet Res.* 10:166.

Medalha, C.C. *et al.* (2016). Low level laser therapy accelerates bone healing in spinal cord injured rats. *J Photochem Photobiol B.* 59:179–185.

Navarro, R. *et al.* (2007). Low-level-laser therapy as an alternative treatment for primary herpes simplex infection: a case report. *J Clin Pediatr Dent.* 31(4):225–228.

Nemec, A. *et al.* (2012). Erythema multiforme and epitheliotropic T-cell lymphoma in the oral cavity of dogs: 1989 to 2009. *J Small Anim Pract.* 53(8):445–452.

Niemiec, B.A. (2010). Chronic ulcerative paradental stomatitis. In: *Small Animal Dental, Oral and Maxillofacial Disease: A Color Handbook*, pp. 189–191. Manson Publishing, London.

Ottaviani, G. *et al.* (2013). Effect of class IV laser therapy on chemotherapy-induced oral mucositis: a clinical and experimental study. *Am J Pathol.* 183(6):1747–1757.

Peplow, P.V. *et al.* (2010). Laser photobiomodulation of wound healing: a review of experimental studies in mouse and rat animal models. *Photomed Laser Surg.* 28(3):291–325.

Rees, C.A. (2011). Eosinophilic granuloma complex. In: *The Feline Patient*, pp. 154–156. Wiley-Blackwell, Hoboken, NJ.

Rico-Holgado, S. *et al.* (2021). Effect of low-level laser therapy on bacterial counts of contaminated traumatic wounds in dogs. *J Lasers Med Sci.* doi:10.34172/jlms.2021.78.

Robson, M. and Crystal, M.A. (2011). Gingivitis-stomatitis-pharyngitis. In: *The Feline Patient*, pp. 199–201. Wiley-Blackwell, Hoboken, NJ.

Ross, G. (2016). Evidence based use of photobiomodulation in periodontics – a literature search. In: *Abstract #129 presented to the American Society for Laser Medicine and Surgery Conference.* ASLMS, Boston, MA, (April 3, 2016).

Salari, B. *et al.* (2022). Effect of delayed photobiomodulation therapy on neurosensory recovery in patients with mandibular nerve neurotmesis following traumatic mandibular fracture: a randomized triple-blinded clinical trial. *J Photochem Photobiol B.* doi:10.1016/j.jphotobiol.2022.112460.

Sierra, S.O. *et al.* (2016). Choosing between intraoral or extraoral, red or infrared laser irradiation after impacted third molar extraction. *Lasers Surg Med.* 48(5):511–518.

Son, J. *et al.* (2012). Bone healing effects of diode laser (808 nm) on a rat tibial fracture model. *In Vivo.* 26(4):703–709.

Tang, E. and Arany, P. (2013). Photobiomodulation and implants: implications for dentistry. *J Periodontal Implant Sci.* 43(6):262–268.

Wagner, V.P. *et al.* (2016). Photobiomodulation regulates cytokine release and new blood vessel formation during oral wound healing in rats. *Lasers Med Sci.* 31(4):665–671.

Watson, A.H. and Brundage, C.M. (2019). Photobiomodulation as an inflammatory therapeutic following dental prophylaxis in canines. *Photomed Laser Surg.* 37(5):276–281.

Zecha, J. *et al.* (2016a). Low-level laser therapy/photobiomodulation in the management of side effects of chemoradiation therapy in head and neck cancer. Part 1: mechanisms of action, dosimetric, and safety considerations. *Support Care Cancer.* 24(6):2781–2792.

Zecha, J. *et al.* (2016b). Low-level laser therapy/photobiomodulation in the management of side effects of chemoradiation therapy in head and neck cancer. Part 2: proposed applications and treatment protocols. *Support Care Cancer.* 24(6):2793–2805.

Zein, R. (2018). Review of light parameters and photobiomodulation efficacy: dive into complexity. *J Biomed Opt.* 23(12):1–17.

14

Abdominal Conditions

Richard L. Godine

Ruckersville Animal Hospital and Veterinary Laser Therapy Center, Ruckersville, VA, USA

Introduction

The effects of photobiomodulation (PBM) to decrease inflammation, increase microcirculation, promote tissue regeneration, modulate the immune system, and control pain makes it a useful modality for the treatment of a number of gastrointestinal and urinary tract diseases of small animals. This is particularly true when treating cats and smaller dogs. The stomach, pancreas, intestines, and urinary tract of larger dogs and humans are more difficult to reach with transcutaneous light therapy. As inflammation is a common symptom of most gastrointestinal and urinary diseases of small animals, photobiomodulation therapy (PBMT) can be a useful modality in the treatment armamentarium. The aim of most protocols is to apply a biostimulatory dose (1–4 J/cm^2) at the level of the affected organ. Also applying a biostimulatory dose to the regional lymph nodes will aid in decreasing inflammation and stimulating tissue regeneration.

Gastrointestinal Disorders

A dearth of published literature exists about the treatment of the alimentary system with PBM. Much comes out of Russia, where both transcutaneous and intravenous light therapy have been in clinical use since the 1980s. One emerging area of interest is the manipulation of the microbiome with PBMT in order to effect various clinical outcomes. By virtue of treating smaller patients, veterinarians can lead the medical community in discovering the applications and efficacy of using PBMT to treat diseases of the gastrointestinal system.

Oropharynx

Conditions of the oral cavity are covered in more detail in Chapter 13.

Stomatitis and gingivostomatitis are common painful inflammatory conditions seen primarily in cats but also in dogs. Feline gingivostomatitis is an incompletely understood multifactorial disease and is thought to involve a hyperreactive immune response against certain pathogenic periodontal bacteria (Crawford and Losey 2013; Robson and Crystal 2011). Best clinical results are achieved when affected teeth are extracted; it is not uncommon for whole-mouth extractions to be necessary (Jennings *et al.*, 2015). The use of a CO_2 ablative laser can also be extremely helpful in eliminating residual bacteria and involved tissue following full-mouth extractions (Lewis *et al.*, 2007).

The management of other types of stomatitis can be improved by incorporating PBMT in the overall care (Santoso *et al.*, 2023). Laser therapy has been shown to downregulate the expression of inflammatory cytokines related to oral mucositis (tumor necrosis factor alpha, TNFα; interleukins 6 and 8, IL6 and IL8) (Basso *et al.*, 2015). It has been well established that PBM can be used prophylactically to prevent or substantially decrease the formation of oral mucositis in human cancer patients being treated with either chemotherapy and/or oral radiation (Ahmed *et al.*, 2015; Zadik *et al.*, 2019). For patients in which PBM has not been used prophylactically, therapeutic treatment can still be successful (Muñoz-Corcuera *et al.*, 2013).

Stomatitis in cats and dogs that is not related to the hypersensitivity reaction to periodontal bacteria can be greatly helped by PBM. Biostimulatory doses can be applied transcutaneously through the oral labia at a dose of 8–10 J/cm^2 or into an open mouth at 1–4 J/cm^2. The submandibular and prescapular lymph nodes should be treated with biostimulatory doses, as well. Treatment frequency should be every 24–48 hours until the stomatitis has resolved. Both red and near-infrared wavelengths can be used, and both work well. A large clinical study by Russian ear, nose,

Laser Therapy in Veterinary Medicine: Photobiomodulation, Second Edition. Edited by Christopher J. Winkler and Lisa A. Miller.

and throat physicians demonstrated 85% efficacy in the treatment of pharyngeal inflammatory conditions with PBM (Gogeliia *et al.*, 2006).

Salivary mucocele is another disease that can be helped by PBM. Light therapy has been shown to decrease pain and swelling of the salivary glands, making it useful for treating patients prior to corrective surgery (Simões *et al.*, 2009; Ahad A *et al.*, 2017). The affected salivary gland and associated lymph nodes should be treated with biostimulatory doses of either red or infrared light.

Application of light to a tooth extraction site has been shown to improve new bone trabeculae formation and communication yielding an increase in bone surface (Rosera *et al.*, 2020). This can be particularly useful when extractions requiring extensive bone removal make fractures more possible.

Stomach

Light therapy can be useful in the treatment of gastric reflux, gastric ulcers, and gastritis. Most of the published literature is from Russia and involves the use of intravenous delivery of 405 nm laser light. Intravenous laser therapy uses low doses (<5 mW) of blue, green, yellow, red and infrared light delivered through a fiberoptic catheter placed inside an intravenous catheter (Figure 14.1). Depending on the wavelength chosen, white blood cells, red blood cells, or platelets can be modulated.

Intravenous blue light (405 nm) has been successfully used in gastroesophageal reflux disease (GERD) to normalize gastric pH, increase microcirculation, and decrease inflammation of damaged esophageal tissue (Burduli and Tadtaeva 2012a, 2012b, 2014). Benefits can also be achieved through transcutaneous application of light directed toward the gastroesophageal junction.

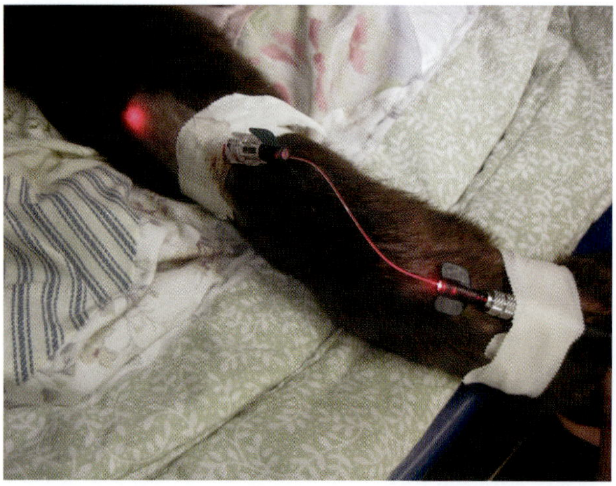

Figure 14.1 Intravenous laser therapy. The fiberoptic cable is attached to a fiberoptic intravenous catheter in a cephalic vein.

Researchers have shown that chronic atrophic gastritis in rats can be successfully treated with PBM. They demonstrate a marked decrease in inflammatory cells of the gastric mucosa, as well as a return to normal gastric mucosal thickness and cellular function following laser therapy (Shao *et al.* 2005; Yang *et al.* 2005). This represents an opportunity for veterinarians to treat cases of chronic gastritis with light therapy when neoplasia has been ruled out as the underlying cause. Several publications have shown that the healing time of gastric ulcers can be significantly shortened through the use of endoscopic laser application, intravenous laser therapy, or transcutaneous PBM (Alebastrov and Butov 2005; Burduli and Gutnova 2008). The beneficial systemic stimulation of the immune system by transcutaneous light application or intravenous laser therapy plays as much of a role in the healing of the gastric ulcer as does direct stimulation via endoscopic application of light (Alebastrov *et al.*, 2004).

Pancreatitis

Pancreatitis is a common, potentially serious disease encountered frequently in small-animal veterinary hospitals. Mild cases of edematous pancreatitis often resolve spontaneously or with medical treatment and dietary modification. Severe necrotizing pancreatitis is a life-threatening condition that can affect multiple organs. Treatment involves hospitalization, fluid and electrolyte therapy, analgesics, antiemetics, antibiotics, nutritional support, and, sometimes, surgical intervention (Steiner 2010). It is not uncommon for these patients to be hospitalized for up to a week.

Pancreatitis is painful and involves severe inflammation and decreased microcirculation of the pancreas. PBM is known to promote analgesia, increase microcirculation, decrease inflammation, reduce oxidative stress, and regenerate tissue, including Beta cells (Burduli and Gutnova, 2009; Huang L *et al.*, 2015). It is an extremely important adjunct to the conventional treatment of pancreatitis. Not only will PBM increase the chances of a successful outcome in pancreatitis treatment but it also often reduces the hospital stay down to 2–3 days.

The treatment involves transcutaneous application of light directed over the pancreas and surrounding organs in the right and mid-cranial abdomen every 12–24 hours (Figure 14.2). Initially, bioinhibitory doses (24–30 J/cm^2) of NIR light are used to control pain and decrease inflammation. The dose can be decreased to the biostimulatory range (4–16 J/cm^2) once the patient is no longer in pain. Treating the sublumbar and inguinal lymph nodes with

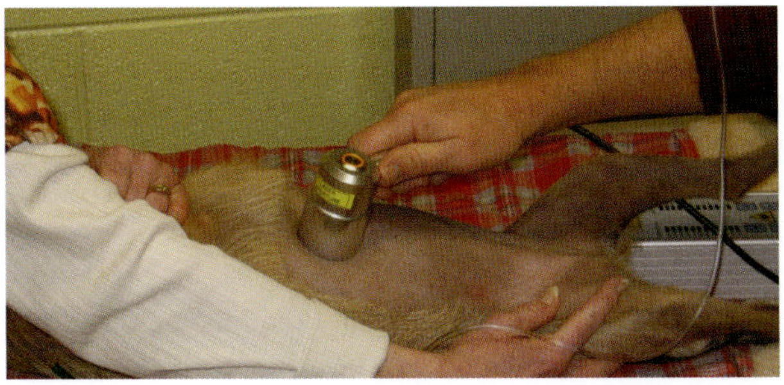

Figure 14.2 An 810 nm 500 mW × 4 multiprobe applied over the pancreas of a dog with pancreatitis.

biostimulatory doses (4–16 J/cm^2) helps speed recovery. The concurrent use of intravenous laser will also improve chances of success and hasten recovery (Geĭnits *et al.*, 2011). In cases of chronic pancreatitis, PBM has been shown to increase exocrine function (Gutnova 2011).

Intestines

Inflammatory bowel disease (IBD) is a frustrating problem for the veterinarian and owner. This is because the etiology for idiopathic IBD is not completely understood and the clinical course often waxes and wanes with treatment. For those cases that do not respond to dietary modification or antibiotic therapy, immunosuppressive drugs become the hallmark for successful treatment. These drugs can have undesirable side effects and can cause other diseases with long-term use.

Zigmond *et al.* (2014) showed that PBMT can induce mucosal healing in colitis of mice while de Paula-Silva *et al.* (2020) demonstrated that transcutaneous PBMT of colitis in mice modulated the immune response and promoted structural protection. Rodriques *et al.* (2023) compared transcutaneous abdominal PBMT to transcutaneous venous PBMT in ulcerative colitis of rats. It has been shown that irradiating over superficial blood vessels has a similar effect to intravenous laser therapy (Dos Santos Malavazzi *et al.*, 2023). Both methods were effective in decreasing mast cell degranulation, decreasing inflammatory cytokines, increasing pro-inflammatory cytokines, and increasing mucus production. However, only the transcutaneous abdominal PBMT was able to mitigate the histological changes associated with inflammatory cell migration to the mucosa and submucosa. It is well documented that PBM will decrease inflammation and edema of targeted tissues. It makes sense, therefore, to use light therapy to help control inflamed bowel. This is easy to do in cats and small dogs, since the abdominal cavity is small and shallow, making the intestines accessible to light. Alves *et al.* (2022) compared PBMT with psyllium husk PO in the treatment of large bowel diarrhea in canines. PBMT showed improvement over oral fiber supplementation in all statistical categories and clinical signs as well as increases in body weight and body condition scores.

The author has had several cases of short-term success in treating feline IBD with PBMT. It does resolve diarrhea and improve appetite, but must be repeated once or twice a week, in order to maintain clinical efficacy. This becomes a logistical problem for the owner, who will often want a pharmaceutical solution that will better fit their schedule and budget.

In cases where immunosuppressive drugs are not tolerated or are contraindicated, PBMT becomes the management solution of choice. For cats, a dose of 8–32 J/cm^2 will provide biostimulatory doses to the bowel. Dogs may require two to three times that dose, depending on their size and pigmentation. The abdomen can usually be accessed with the patient in a standing position. Special attention to the mesenteric lymph nodes, as well as the sublumbar and inguinal lymph nodes, will improve efficacy, as will intravenous or transcutaneous venous laser treatment.

An interesting new hypothesis for the beneficial effects of PBM in the treatment of metabolic and inflammatory diseases, including those of the intestines, has to do with light's interaction with the microbiome. It is well known that the gut microbiome is inextricably linked with the health and disease status of an individual. We know there exists a microbiome/gut/brain axis, a microbiome/gut/heart axis and possibly relationships between the gut and the lungs, muscle and skin. Liebert *et al.* (2019) and Bicknell *et al.,* (2019) demonstrated that PBM increases beneficial microbes in mice such as Allobaculum spp. over a sham device. In the conventional treatment of a woman for breast cancer, PBM was shown to be able to increase a number of beneficial gut microbes (*Akkermansia*, *Faecalibacterium*, and *Roseburia spp*) while decreasing the number of pathogenic microbes (Bicknell *et al.* 2022). This implies that PBMT of the gut can been very helpful with cases of intestinal dysbiosis and perhaps many other chronic diseases.

Liver

Clinically, the author has observed that PBMT has a very positive effect on patients with both acute and chronic liver disease. Light therapy has been shown to bring down and normalize biochemical markers such as alanine transaminase (ALT), aspartate aminotransferase (AST), alkaline phosphatase (ALP), gamma glutamyl transferase (GGT), direct bilirubin, and total bilirubin (Babaev *et al.* 2012; Takhtfooladi *et al.,* 2014). It also has been shown to reduce the pro-inflammatory cytokines ILβ1, IL6, and TNFα while increasing the anti-inflammatory cytokine IL4 (Burduli and Krifarid, 2011), leading to a reduction in hepatic inflammatory infiltrates (Oliveira-Junior *et al.*, 2013). A reduction in hepatic oxidative stress caused by nitric oxide (NO) free-radical metabolites was demonstrated by Burduli and Gutnova (2009) in 120 human patients with viral hepatitis, while Lim *et al.* (2009) demonstrated that PBM induces hepatic antioxidant defense in acute and chronic diabetic rats. PBM has also been shown to recruit mesenchymal stem cells, induce angiogenesis, improve microcirculation, and stimulate hepatocyte regeneration in injured livers (Burduli *et al.*, 2015; Oron *et al.*, 2010). In a large blinded clinical trial of humans comparing the post-laparoscopic cholecystectomy treatment of the liver with red light for 2 minutes vs no treatment, postoperative liver injury was markedly attenuated by PBMT (Redkin *et al.*, 2017).

In small-animal veterinary medicine, PBM can be used alongside traditional medical treatment options to enhance the resolution of acute hepatic insults, as well as to improve the clinical outcomes for chronic liver conditions. In the cat and very small dog, red light can be used. In most patients, however, near-infrared (NIR) light will provide optimal transcutaneous penetration to the liver. One should strive for biostimulatory doses (1–4 J/cm^2) at the target tissue level 1–4 cm below the skin surface. Depending on the size of the patient, this may be 4–30 J/cm^2 to the skin surface. Applying a similar dose to the inguinal and sublumbar lymph nodes prior to treating the liver is beneficial, as is the application of intravenous laser (if available). Acute cases can be treated every 24–48 hours until resolved, while chronic cases can be titrated down to being treated every other week indefinitely.

Anorectal

PBM is useful in the treatment of anal sac disease, rectal prolapse, and perianal fistulas. Anal gland abscessation and rupture causes severe subcutaneous inflammation and infection (Culp 2012). Administration of laser therapy can cause rapid resolution of pain and inflammation when used alongside traditional medical management. PBM results in stimulation of tissue healing, leading to a faster resolution of this painful condition. Biostimulatory doses of red or infrared light (1–6 J/cm^2) are applied transcutaneously over the inflamed anal gland, as well as to the inguinal and popliteal lymph nodes.

Perianal fistulas are notoriously difficult to treat and manage. They are believed to be an immune-mediated disorder and respond best to a combination of systemic immunosuppressive drugs, topical immunosuppressive drugs, and antibiotics (Craven, 2012; House 2006; Patricelli *et al.*, 2002; Pieper and McKay 2011; Stanley and Hauptman 2009). High doses of immunosuppressive medications are often needed initially and can cause unwanted side effects. The fistulous lesions will often return when immunosuppressive therapy is withdrawn. PBM seems to have mixed results when treating this condition. It does help control the pain and inflammation associated with the disease. In some cases, it can cause a dramatic resolution of the problem. More often, it is another useful tool in the multimodal approach to treatment. It does seem to enable the patient to improve on lower doses of immunosuppressive drugs, thereby reducing or eliminating potentially undesirable side effects. Imtiaz *et al.* (2024) successfully treated a case of solitary rectal ulcer syndrome in a human using bioinhibitory doses of red light (635 nm) at 85 J/cm^2 while Dos Santos *et al.* (2021) had mixed success treating anofistulous tracts in mice with 4 J/cm^2 of red light. One can try using bioinhibitory doses of either red or infrared light (8–30 J/cm^2) directly over the lesion, followed by biostimulatory doses (1–4 J/cm^2) to the popliteal and inguinal lymph nodes.

Medical management of a rectal prolapse involves cleansing of the exposed mucosal lining, immediate reduction of the swelling in the rectal mucosa, and reduction of the prolapse followed by a perianal purse string suture that will allow the passage of feces but hold the prolapse in normal anatomical position. After the prolapse has been rinsed clean, PBM can be applied to the swollen mucosa with 4–8 J/cm^2 of red or infrared light. The sublumbar and inguinal lymph nodes may also be treated. This will assist in reducing edema from the prolapse and make it easier to reduce.

Urinary Disorders

The urinary system is quite accessible to light therapy. The kidneys, ureters, urinary bladder, and urethra usually lie 1–3 cm beneath the skin surface. Most acute and chronic conditions of the urinary system can be helped by PBM.

Kidneys

Both acute and chronic kidney disease (CKD) will benefit from PBM. It is especially helpful in the treatment of CKD, but can also be of significant aid in the treatment of acute renal perfusion injuries (Oron *et al.* 2014). The roles of the vascular and tubular components of renal function are tightly intertwined, and the cause of onset of CKD often cannot be identified. Tubulointerstial nephritis is the most common histopathological diagnosis in cats; however, glomerular damage usually exists as well. The overall process is marked by inflammation and fibrosis of the nephrons.

We know that the kidney's initial autoregulatory response to decreasing glomerular filtration rate (GFR) is to dilate afferent arterioles and constrict efferent arterioles, as well as to contract mesangial cells. The resulting nephron hypertrophy leads to GFR homeostasis. However, over time, the increased hydrostatic pressure within the glomerular corpuscle leads to glomerular capillary damage and plasma protein leakage. These causes further subsequent glomerular and tubulointerstial damage and scarring. Central regulatory mechanisms kick in as autoregulatory mechanisms fail to maintain normal GFR. The renin–angiotensin system (RAS) is activated in the juxtaglomerular complex, with subsequent increases in antidiuretic hormone and aldosterone, as well as activation of the sympathetic nervous system.

CKD is one of the most common diseases veterinarians encounter in aging animals. Traditional management involves nutritional modifications to lower azotemia and phosphorus, improving hydration, decreasing acid secretion in the stomach, and stimulating appetite and the formation of new red blood cells. The author has noted that adding PBM to the traditional treatment protocols for CKD will decrease azotemia by 10–20% and stimulate both appetite, energy levels, and well-being. The PBM protocol for treating CKD involves applying a biostimulatory dose to the kidney, regional lymph nodes, and bone marrow of a long bone or sternum (Figure 14.3). It has been suggested that treatment of the gut may also benefit CKD patients through manipulation of the gut-renal axis (Bian *et al.*, 2022; Rukavina Mikusic *et al.*, 2020).

Based on the work of Uri Oron's lab, 1–4 J/cm^2 can also be applied to the bone marrow of the humerus or femur to stimulate the release of mesenchymal stem cells into circulation. These cells have been shown to migrate to the kidney lesions, increasing mesenchymal stem cell count 2.4-fold. Oron *et al.* (2014) found that this alone will decrease azotemia and pathological features in postischemic reperfusion injuries in the rat.

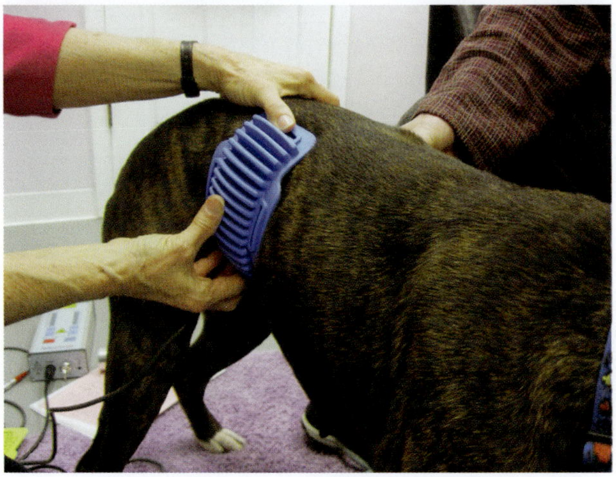

Figure 14.3 A canine patient with CKD being treated over the right kidney with a 1000 mW 840 nm superluminescent diode array.

Other potential beneficial mechanisms of PBM on CKD include the following:

- Increasing microcirculation within the kidney, modulating oxidative stress
- Decreasing proinflammatory cytokines – IL1β, TNFα (Yamota et al., 2013)
- Decreasing fibrotic factors – fibroblast-specific protein 1, FSP1; alpha smooth-muscle actin, αSMA (Oliveira et al., 2012)
- Decreasing renal hypertension (Ucero et al., 2013; Schiavon MDSC et al., 2023)
- Decreasing the progression of glomerular injuries (Lutoshkin et al., 1993; Ucero et al., 2013; Yamota et al., 2013)

The modulation of nephron inflammation and fibrosis by PBM allows autoregulatory mechanisms to control GFR longer, delaying the onset of central control mechanisms, and leading to improved clinical conditions and a longer and more vibrant life. It is therefore recommended that PBMT begin as early as possible (International Renal Interest Society [IRIS] stage 1 or 2) with these patients.

The frequency of treatments starts with biweekly applications for 2 weeks, then weekly applications for 2 weeks, then finally a continuous regimen of once every 2–3 weeks. The kidneys and sublumbar lymph nodes are treated along with the mid-femur or mid-humerus, or sternum for mesenchymal stem cell stimulation. Patients that experience an acute prerenal dehydration or uremic crisis can have the frequency of PBM increased to daily while they are hospitalized for intravenous fluid therapy. Concurrent intravenous laser irradiation of the blood (if available) has also been shown to be beneficial in a uremic crisis (Razzaghi *et al.*, 2021) It is also recommended to administer PBM during each outpatient subcutaneous fluid (SCF) treatment visit until the crisis has passed.

Urinary Bladder

Feline idiopathic cystitis (FIC) is a common and frustrating problem seen daily in most small-animal hospitals. This multifactorial disease involves genetic predisposition, nutritional factors, home stressors, and a chronic pain cycle (Forrester and Roudebush 2007; Forrester and Towell 2015). PBM can be quite useful in helping to downregulate the pain and inflammation associated with FIC. The target tissues are the bladder itself and the dorsal root ganglia of the hypogastric nerve (L2–4) and the pelvic and pudendal nerves (S1–3). Inflammation in the urinary bladder can be reduced with biostimulatory doses of NIR light; for example, 4–16 J/cm^2 of 810 nm laser light applied over the skin of the caudal abdomen will yield approximately 1–4 J/cm^2 to the bladder wall. Wind-up of neuropathic pain is thought to play a role in the persistent and recurring nature of FIC. PBM of the sympathetic, parasympathetic, and somatic dorsal root ganglia of the urinary bladder will help downregulate the acute and chronic pain associated with FIC. A bioinhibitory dose of 16–32 J/cm^2 of infrared light over the skin of the DRGs for L2–3, L3–4, and over the sacrum would be appropriate.

Transitional cell carcinoma (TCC) of the canine urinary bladder is a commonly encountered cancer in small-animal practice. In the author's experience, PBM offers an excellent palliative treatment for nonsurgical candidates. PBM initially shrinks the tumor by 10–20% and then helps manage the hematuria, pollakiuria, and stranguria associated with the disease. Breakthroughs of hematuria commonly respond quickly to antibiotics. PBM can be used in combination with piroxicam, but the author prefers to solely use PBM to avoid the potential gastrointestinal and renal side effects of piroxicam. Optimal results begin with treatment twice a week for 2 weeks, then once a week for 2 weeks, then every other week indefinitely. Survival times range from 8 to 30 months, with most patients living 12–18 months of good-quality life. The protocol involves applying 16–64 J/cm^2 of NIR light (depending on the size of the dog) to the bladder tumor, from as many angles as possible, and then 4–8 J/cm^2 to skin over the superficial inguinal lymph node. Interestingly, the author has found that PBM does not seem to be very effective for leiomyosarcoma of the urinary bladder. For most tumors, PBM has many benefits in modulating paraneoplastic symptoms.

Urethra

Urethral blockage of the male cat by grit and uroliths is a common sequela to untreated FIC (Marshall 2011). Distal blockages of grit can often be unobstructed by application of laser therapy and gently milking out the obstruction, thus avoiding the passing of a urethral catheter. After the patient is sedated, the penis can be extruded from the prepuce and 4 J/cm^2 of red or near-infrared light can be applied over and around it. This causes a decrease in the periurethral inflammation, making it possible in some cases to un-obstruct the cat. After 2–5 minutes, an attempt can be made to milk out the grit. If a good urine stream does not result after 1 minute of manipulation, a urethral catheter should be passed.

Prostate

The anti-inflammatory effects of PBM are very effective in treating benign prostatic hyperplasia of the canine. Infrared doses of 10–12 J/cm^2 aimed at the right and left lobe of the prostate will result in biostimulatory doses to the prostate, reducing inflammation and size. One can also apply 1–4 J/cm^2 of near infrared light to the superficial inguinal lymph nodes to assist with prostate reduction. This can be quite helpful in managing dysuria until the full benefits of castration are realized. Treat daily for 2–3 days, then twice weekly for 2 months following castration. It is also possible to use a laser catheter to irradiate from the center of the prostate (Figure 14.4). This protocol is beneficial for ancillary treatment of prostatitis. Care should be taken to rule out prostatic neoplasia, though PBM can be a useful palliative treatment for this condition when the owner elects not to pursue surgery, radiation, or chemotherapy.

Infections

PBM for bacterial infections of the urinary bladder and kidneys can be a useful ancillary treatment to antimicrobial therapy (Neimark *et al.*, 2007). It aids in stimulating the immune response and reducing associated inflammation and pain. The principal is to apply biostimulatory doses of NIR light (2–4 J/cm^2) at the target tissue to the affected organs and associated lymph nodes. Dose is important, and one should take care not to overdose and create bioinhibition, which can potentially make the infection worse. Treat every other day until resolution. Low-dose intravenous laser (5 mW) has been shown to be a potent stimulator of

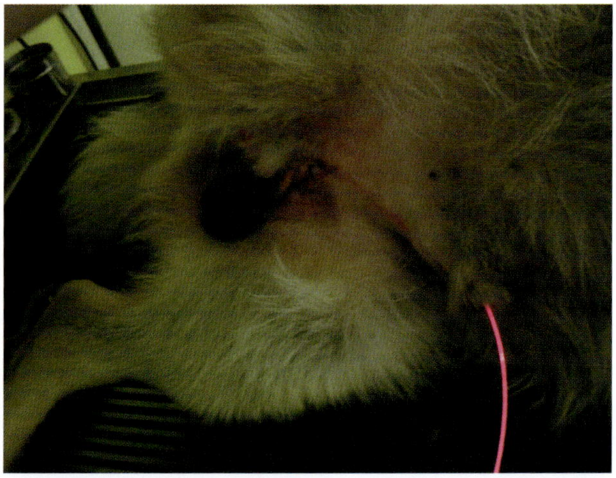

Figure 14.4 Canine prostatitis being treated post-castration with a 660 nm 100 mW laser fiberoptic catheter passed proximal through a urethral catheter to the level of the center of the prostate.

the immune system and can be used for pyelonephritis (Driianskaia 1997; Weber *et al.*, 2015).

Case Studies

Canine CKD

Signalment

"Savannah," 17-year-old FS Jack Russell terrier, 5.1 kg.

Client Complaint

The owner had recently moved to town. Savannah's previous veterinarian had diagnosed CKD 8 months previously and had been treating her for neck and shoulder pain.

History

Savannah was on 25 mg of tramadol q8h, laser therapy for neck pain, and SCF for CKD q3d. Lab parameters from the previous veterinarian 1 week prior showed a moderate azotemia.

Physical Examination

Bilateral shoulder tenderness, as well as cervical pain in the C3–4 area, a grade III/VI heart murmur, and grade III/IV periodontal disease.

Diagnosis

CKD, shoulder and neck pain, nonclinical heart murmur, periodontal disease.

Treatment Plan

Tramadol 25 mg was reduced from q8h to PRN, and famotidine 2.5 mg SID and a renal support diet were prescribed. PBM was initiated with twice weekly treatments for 2 weeks, followed by once a week for 2 weeks, and then every 2 weeks. The kidneys were treated with 660, 810, and 840 nm. The shoulder and dorsal root ganglia (C1–T1) were treated with 810 nm (Table 14.1).

Outcome

The shoulder and neck tenderness resolved after 2 months of treatments (eight treatments total) and PBM was discontinued for those conditions. PBM for the kidneys continued every other week until Savannah was euthanized 18 months after treatment began. After 5 months, Savannah developed dementia and a brain protocol was added to each PBM session, which effectively reversed the signs of dementia. Her elevated renal parameters fell gradually after 5 months and remained lower until her death. Savannah developed hypertension with mild syncopal episodes toward the end of her life and the owner requested humane euthanasia.

Canine Pancreatitis

Signalment

"Mickie," 15.5-year-old MN longhaired Dachshund, 10.7 kg.

Client Complaint

Ate two knee socks; vomiting and bloody diarrhea.

History

CKD and dementia being managed with PBM and a renal support diet; elbow luxation and surgical repair in the previous year; intervertebral disk disease 2 years ago.

Physical Examination

T = 38.2 °C (100.8 °F), overweight, dull coat, non-pliable doughy abdomen.

Table 14.1 PBMT protocol for treating a 17-year-old Jack Russell terrier with CKD and shoulder and neck pain.

Target tissue	Wavelength (nm)	Power (mW)	Emission and time	Power density (mW/cm^2)	Energy density (J/cm^2)	Total fluence (J)
Kidney	660	500	Continuous-wave (CW) 6 minutes	15	5.4	419
	840	1000	50 Hz 50% duty cycle 6 minutes			418
	810	250	CW 20 seconds	2.5	50	20/kidney
Shoulder	810	250 (4× multiprobe)	CW 30 seconds	2.5 × 12 points	60 × 12 points	180/shoulder
Dorsal root ganglion: C1–T1	810	500 (4× multiprobe)	CW 30 seconds	2.5 × 24 points	60 × 24 points	180/side × 2 sides

Differential Diagnosis

Dietary indiscretion gastroenteritis, metabolic disease, neoplasia, foreign body, pancreatitis.

Diagnostic Imaging

Abdominal radiographs showed increased radio opaqueness in the right cranial abdomen and gas in the colon. Abdominal ultrasound showed peripancreatic hyperechogenicity, multifocal hypoechoic pancreatic lesions, a distended gall bladder, and patches of hyperechogenicity in the liver.

Laboratory Data

A complete blood count (CBC) showed mild neutrophilia and mild lymphopenia. Amylase and lipase were very high and were accompanied by an azotemia and mild hyperkalemia.

Diagnosis

The primary problem appeared to be pancreatitis secondary to dietary indiscretion, with a secondary azotemia from prerenal exacerbation of the patient's chronic renal disease.

Treatment Plan

An intravenous catheter was placed and intravenous fluids were administered to correct the dehydration. Ampicillin (200 mg q12h) and famotidine (10 mg q24h) were administered intravenously. PBM was administered once a day: 810 nm, 500 mW × 4 multiprobe, continuous wave (CW), 60 seconds per point × five points over the pancreas; per point: 30 J, 2.5 W/cm^2, 35 mm spot size, 150 J/cm^2; total fluence: 600 J (30 J × 4 multiprobe × 5 points) (Table 14.2).

Outcome

Mickie improved daily, had no vomiting or diarrhea in the hospital, ate the morning of day 3 and tolerated the intake, and was discharged on metronidazole, sucralfate, and a low-fat gastrointestinal diet. PBM was repeated on days 2 and 4 following discharge, with no further symptoms of gastroenteritis. Maintenance PBM for CKD and dementia was resumed.

Canine Transitional Cell Carcinoma of the Urinary Bladder and CKD

Signalment

"Rudy," 13-year-old MN bichon frise, 14.5 kg.

History

Rudy presented at 11.5 years old with hematuria and was subsequently diagnosed with a bladder tumor. Histopathology after initial excision indicated the tumor was a transitional cell carcinoma with clean margins, and no further treatment was prescribed. The bladder was normal on ultrasound 2 months later, but 7 months after that the tumor reappeared. Thirteen pedunculated, friable masses were removed from the bladder. Piroxicam and misoprostol were prescribed. Symptoms returned 8 months later, and an ultrasound demonstrated diffuse infiltration of the tumor into the bladder wall. A week later, Rudy developed acute renal failure.

Treatment Plan

Medication was discontinued and Rudy was admitted for emergency intravenous fluid diuresis and PBM. Nine PBM treatments were administered over the kidneys and bladder every 4–6 days for 6.5 weeks. Doses averaged 5.85 J/cm^2 with 660 nm, 11.7 J/cm^2 with 840 nm, and 81 J/cm^2 with 830 nm. Rudy improved significantly after the first PBM treatment, and after nine treatments the bladder wall was less thick and Rudy was eating well. After 6 months, PBM was restarted at once every 5 weeks at average doses of 7 J/cm^2 with 660 nm, 18.7 J/cm^2 with 840 nm, and 64.8 J/cm^2 with 830 nm. Thirteen treatments were administered over the next 9 months, after which time Rudy rapidly deteriorated and was euthanized.

Outcome

The clinical results of using laser therapy on Rudy suggest it may be as effective as piroxicam in palliative treatment of transitional cell carcinoma of the canine urinary bladder, without any harmful side effects (Figure 14.5). In this case, piroxicam following debulking surgery resulted in 8 months (240 days) of good-quality life for Rudy, but ultimately caused acute renal failure while the mass continued to

Table 14.2 PBMT protocol for treating a 15.5-year-old longhaired Dachshund with acute pancreatitis.

Target tissue	Wavelength (nm)	Power (mW)	Emission and time	Power density (mW/cm^2)	Energy density (J/cm^2)	Total fluence (J)
Pancreas	810	500 (4× multiprobe)	CW 60 seconds	2.5 × 5 points	150 × 5 points	600

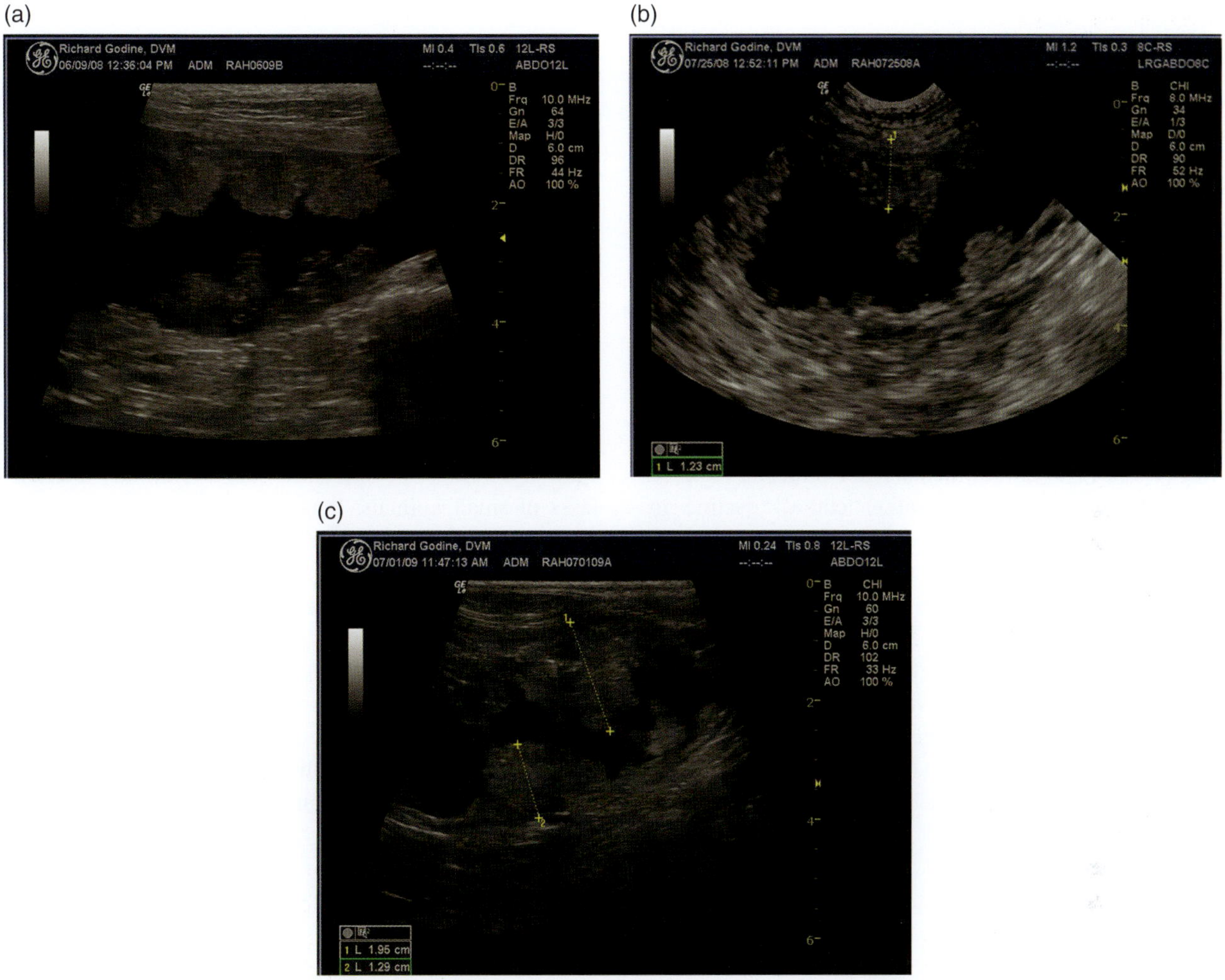

Figure 14.5 Ultrasound images showing the progression of transitional cell carcinoma of a canine urinary bladder being treated with PBMT. (a) 8 months after starting piroxicam and misoprostol therapy (ultrasound shows significant regrowth of the transitional carcinoma). (b) 8 weeks after discontinuing medication and starting PBMT. (c) 54 weeks after starting PBMT.

grow. Subsequent PBM alone resulted in 15 months (465 days) of good-quality life after piroxicam was discontinued and seemed to be beneficial in the treatment of both acute and chronic renal failure.

It is hypothesized that PBM has a beneficial biostimulatory effect on the immune system, which results in delay of tumor growth, decreased inflammation of the tumor and surrounding tissue, decreased pain, modulation of paraneoplastic syndromes, and possibly delay of metastasis. This is due in part to a systemic immunomodulating effect, as well as the direct effect of the laser on the bladder tumor.

Case Report

Signalment

"Teensy," 10 years old, Feline DSH F/S,

History

Teensy was diagnosed with CKD in July of 2016 at the age of 10. Four years prior, her right kidney had been removed due to a nephrolith being stuck in her uretero-pelvic junction.

Treatment and Outcome

A PBM protocol (Table 14.3) was begun twice weekly for 2 weeks, then once weekly for 2 weeks, then every other week for 1 month, then every 3 weeks.

Six months later (January 2017), her creatinine jumped to 4.0, and Teensy was hospitalized for IVF and daily PBM therapy. PBMT was increased to once per week with SQF for a month, and then every other week indefinitely. Teensy stabilized on this protocol, with her creatinine being between 2.9 and 3.5 until December of 2020, when she

Table 14.3 PBM protocol for Feline CKD case.

Location	Wavelength nm	Power Density mW/cm2	Time Seconds	Fluence J/cm^2
Kidney	660/850	45	60	3
Kidney	810	100	40	4
Inguinal LN	660/850	45	6	3
Femur BM	810	500	20	4
L2–3 DRG	810	500	20	4

became inappetent, and needed to be hospitalized again with IVF and IV laser treatments. Afterward, she received weekly PBMT and SQFs. Another clinical decline in November of 2021 was treated once more with IVFs and IV laser therapy, again with a very good clinical response. Teensy developed hypercalcemia in August of 2018, and was put on Alendronate 10 mg every 3 days.

After 2020, Teensy took Cerenia, Mirtazapine, and Ondansetron as needed. She lived another 2 years with a good-quality life, maintaining her weight and energy while being in mid-stage 3 IRIS CKD (see Figure 14.6). Teensy's demise was quick in December of 2022. Altogether, she lived 6 years with a good-quality of life, in spite of having only one kidney and being in stage 3 renal failure.

This case is a good example of how PBMT can significantly benefit feline CKD patients. It highlights how adjustments to protocols are part of the long-term plan and how more intensive PBMT (whether IV laser therapy or more frequent transcutaneous therapy) while hospitalized can jumpstart worsening azotemia, inappetence, and malaise.

Conclusion

The ability of PBM to decrease inflammation and stimulate tissue regeneration makes it a useful component in the treatment of a number of gastrointestinal and urinary tract diseases of small animals. It is particularly effective in the treatment of pancreatitis and liver diseases. One must be able to manipulate the parameters of the laser or light-emitting diode (LED) unit such that the desired power density at the level of the target tissue will be achieved. Treatment of the associated lymph nodes with biostimulatory doses will also enhance efficacy. By virtue of the accessibility of light to the internal organs of small animals, veterinarians can lead the medical community in the clinical applications of PBM for gastrointestinal and urinary tract disorders.

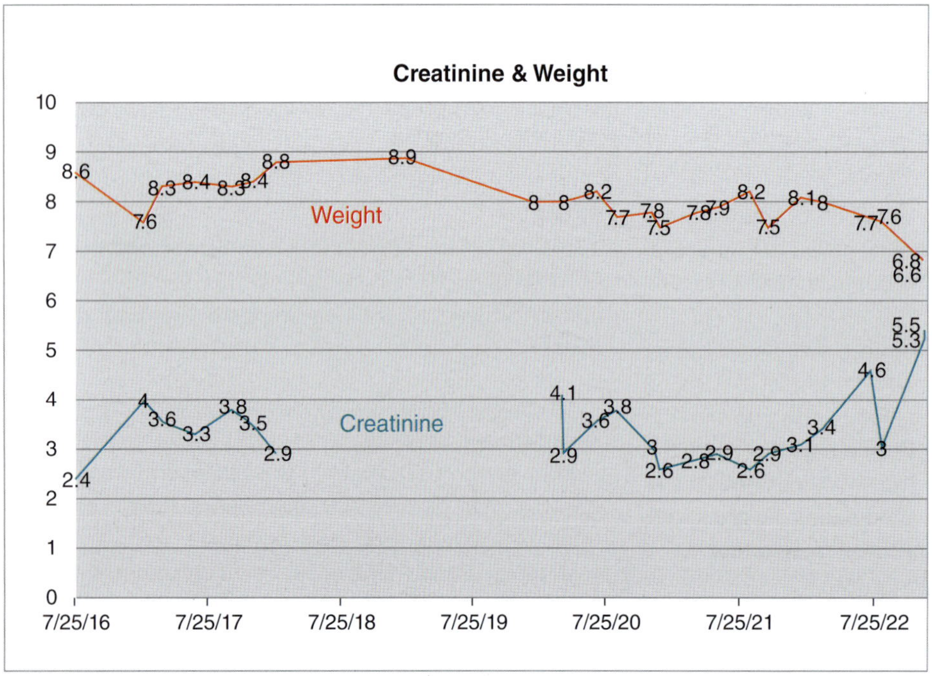

Figure 14.6 Measures of creatinine and weight over time for feline with CKD treated with PBMT.

References

Ahad, A. *et al.* (2017). Diode laser assisted excision and low level laser therapy in the management of mucus extravasation cysts: a case series. *J Lasers Med Sci.* 8(3):155–159.

Ahmed, K. *et al.* (2015). Evaluation of low level laser therapy in the management of chemotherapy induced oral mucositis in pediatric and young cancer patients: a randomized clinical trial. *Eur Sci Journ.* 11(27):209–222.

Alebastrov, A.P. and Butov, M.A. (2005). Potentialities of alternative non-drug therapy of gastric ulcer. *Klin Med (Mosk).* 83(11):69–71.

Alebastrov, A.P. *et al.* (2004). Clinical and immunological aspects of low-intensity laser irradiation in patients with gastroduodenal ulcers. *Esksp Klin Gastroentero.* 4:33–35.

Alves, J.C. *et al.* (2022). The effect of photobiomodulation therapy on the management of chronic idiopathic large-bowel diarrhea in dogs. *Lasers Med Sci.* 37(3):2045–2051.

Babaev, A.V. *et al.* (2012). Effect of intravenous low intensity laser irradiation of the blood on clinical and laboratory parameters of hepatocellular insufficiency. *Bull Exp Biol Med.* 153(5):754–757.

Basso, F.G. *et al.* (2015). Biomodulation of inflammatory cytokines related to oral mucositis by low-level laser therapy. *Photochem Photobio.* 91(4):952–956.

Bian, J. *et al.* (2022). Therapeutic potential of Photobiomodulation for chronic kidney disease. *Int J Mol Sci.* 23(14):8043.

Bicknell, B. *et al.* (2019). Photobiomodulation of the microbiome: implications for metabolic and inflammatory diseases. *Lasers Med Sci.* 34(2):317–317.

Bicknell, B. *et al.* (2022). Modifying the microbiome as a potential mechanism of photobiomodulation: a case report. *Photobiomodul Photomed Laser Surg.* 40(2):88–97.

Burduli, N.M. and Gutnova, S.K. (2008). Efficacy of different laser treatments in combined therapy of patients with gastroduodenal ulcer. *Ter Arkh.* 80(2):30–33.

Burduli, N.M. and Gutnova, S.K. (2009). Types of microcirculation and laser therapy and chronic pancreatitis. *Klin Med (Mosk).* 87(8):56–61.

Burduli, N.M. and Krifaridi, A.S. (2011). The influence of low-intensity laser radiation on the vascular endothelium function in the cytokine system in patients with chronic viral hepatitis. *Vopr Kurortol Fizioter Lech Fiz Kult.* 92(4):25–29.

Burduli, N.M. and Tadtaeva, D.Y. (2012a). The influence of intravenous laser therapy on PGE2 and F2-α dynamics and the state of microcirculation in the patients presenting with gastroesophageal reflux disease. *Vopr Kurortol Fizioter Lech Fiz Kult.* 6:17–20.

Burduli, N.M. and Tadtaeva, D.Y. (2012b). Impact of laser therapy on PGE2 level, 24-hour pH-metry changes, and quality of life in patients with gastroesophageal reflux disease. *Ter Arkh.* 84(12):58–61.

Burduli, N.M. and Tadtaeva, D.Y. (2014). The effect of low level laser therapy on gastric mucosa microcirculation in patients with gastroesophageal reflux diseases. *Eksp Klin Gastroenterol.* 9:35–38.

Burduli, N.M. *et al.* (2015). The influence of the low frequency laser radiation on microcirculatory disorders in the patients presenting with chronic viral hepatitis. *Vopr Kurotol Fizioter Lech Fiz Kult.* 92(4):25–29.

Craven, M. (2012). Rectoanal disease: perianal fistula. In: *Textbook of Veterinary Internal Medicine*, 7 edn, pp. 1602–1604. Saunders, St. Louis, MO.

Crawford, J. and Losey, B.J. (2013). Feline dentistry. In: *Small Animal Dental Procedures for Veterinary Technicians and Nurses*, pp. 143–160. Wiley-Blackwell, Hoboken, NJ.

Culp, W.T.N. (2012). Anal sac disease. In: *Small Animal Soft Tissue Surgery*, pp. 399–405. John Wiley & Sons, Chichester.

de Paula-Silva, M. *et al.* (2020). Red light-emitting diode treatment improves tissue recovery in DSS-induced colitis in mice. *J Photochem Photobiol B.* 212:112018. doi:10.1016/j.jphotobiol.2020.112018.

Dos Santos Malavazzi, T.C. *et al.* (2023). Effects of the invasive and non-invasive systematic photobiomodulation using low-level laser in experimental models: a systematic review. *Lasers Med Sci.* 38(1):137.

Dos Santos, C.H.M. *et al.* (2021). Efficacy of low-level laser therapy on fistula-in -Ano treatment. *Arq Bras Cir Dig.* 34(1):e1572.

Driianskaia, V. (1997). The clinico-immunological effects of immunotherapy in patients with acute pyelonephritis. *Lik-Sprava.* 4:89–92.

Forrester, S.D. and Roudebush, P. (2007). Evidence-based management of feline lower urinary tract disease. *Vet Clin North Am Small Anim Pract.* 37(3):533–558.

Forrester, S.D. and Towell, T.L. (2015). Feline idiopathic cystitis. *Vet Clin North Am Small Anim Pract.* 45(4):783–806.

Geĭnits, A.V. *et al.* (2011). The use of laser beam irradiation on acute destructive pancreatitis. *Khirurgiia (Mosk).* 7:56–61.

Gogeliia, A.L. *et al.* (2006). Experience on treatment of children with otorhinolaryngological diseases by low intensity laser irradiation. *Georgian Med News.* 130:84–86.

Gutnova, S.K. (2011). The evaluation of exocrine function of pancreas in patients with chronic pancreatitis. *Klin Lab Diagn.* 12:44–45.

House, A.K. (2006). Evaluation of the effect of two dose rates of cyclosporine on the severity of perianal fistulae lesions and associated clinical signs in dogs. *Vet Surg.* 35 (6):543–549.

Huang, L. *et al.* (2015). Photoactivation of Akt1/GSK3β isoform-specific signaling axis promotes pancreatic β-cell regeneration. *L Cell Biochem.* 116(8):1741–1754s.

Imtiaz, S. *et al.* (2024). Effective treatment of solitary rectal ulcer syndrome by using photobiomodulation therapy: A case report. *Photobiomod, Photomed Laser Surg.* 42(2):182–185. doi:10.1089/photob.2023.0117.

Jennings, M.W. *et al.* (2015). Effect of tooth extraction on stomatitis in cats: 95 cases (2000–2013). *J Am Vet Med Assoc.* 246(6):654–660.

Lewis, J.R. *et al.* (2007). Use of CO_2 laser as an adjunctive treatment for caudal stomatitis in a cat. *J Vet Dent.* 24(4):240–249.

Liebert, A. *et al.* (2019). "Photobiomics": can light, including Photobiomodulation, Alter the microbiome? Photobiomodul. *Photomed Laser Surg.* 37(11):681–693.

Lim, J. *et al.* (2009). Effects of low-level light therapy on hepatic antioxidant defense in acute and chronic diabetic rats. *J Biochem Mol Toxicol.* 23(1):1–8.

Lutoshkin, M. *et al.* (1993). Application of helium-neon laser for the correction of renal function in patients with chronic glomerulonephritis. *Uro Nefrol (Mosk).* 2:17–20.

Marshall, R. (2011). Urethral obstruction. In: *The Feline Patient*, 4 edn, pp. 530–534. Wiley-Blackwell, Hoboken, NJ.

Mikusic, N.L.R. *et al.* (2020). Gut microbiota and chronic kidney disease: evidence and mechanisms that mediate a new communication in the gastrointestinal-renal axis. *Pflugers Arch.* 472(3):303–320. doi:10.1007/s00424-020-02352-x.

Muñoz-Corcuera, M. *et al.* (2013). Use of laser for the prevention and treatment of oral mucositis induced by radiotherapy and chemotherapy for head and neck cancer. *Med Clin (Barc).* 143(4):170–175.

Neimark, A.I. *et al.* (2007). Efficacy of low-intensity laser irradiation and antibacterial therapy in the treatment of chronic prostatitis in the presence of sexually transmitted infections. *Urologlia.* 6(3):50–56.

Oliveira, F.A. *et al.* (2012). Low-level laser therapy decreases renal interstitial fibrosis. *Photomed Laser Surg.* 30(12):705–713.

Oliveira-Junior, M.C. *et al.* (2013). Low-level laser therapy ameliorates CC14-induced liver cirrhosis in rats. *Photochem Photobiol.* 89(1):173–178.

Oron, U. *et al.* (2010). Enhanced liver regeneration following acute hepatectomy by low-level laser therapy. *Photomed Laser Surg.* 28(5):675–678.

Oron, U. *et al.* (2014). Autologous bone marrow stem cells stimulation reverses post-ischemic reperfusion kidney injury in rats. *Am J Nephrol.* 40(5):425–433.

Patricelli, A.J. *et al.* (2002). Cyclosporine and ketoconazole for the treatment of perianal fistulas in dogs. *J A-M Vet Med Assoc.* 220(7):1009–1016.

Pieper, J. and McKay, L. (2011). Perianal fistulas. *Compend Contin Educ Vet.* 33(9):E4.

Razzaghi, M.R. *et al.* (2021). Intravenous laser therapy in patients with acute kidney injury: a randomized clinical trial. *J Lasers Med Sci.* 12:e49.

Redkin, A.V. *et al.* (2017). Reduce adverse effects of laparoscopic cholecystectomy with pulse width modulated LED light (625 nm, 76 Hz, 23% duty cycle). *Photomed Laser Surg.* 35(6):293–299.

Robson, M. and Crystal, M.A. (2011). Gingivitis-stomatitis-pharyngitis. In: *The Feline Patient*, pp. 199–201. Wiley-Blackwell, Hoboken, NJ.

Rodriques, V.M.M. *et al.* (2023). Comparison between local abdominal and transcutaneous tail vein photobiomodulation in experimental rat model of ulcerative colitis. *Lasers Med Sci.* 38(1):247.

Rosera, K.A.V. *et al.* (2020). Photobiomodulation as an adjunctive therapy for alveolar socket preservation: a preliminary study in humans. *Lasers Med Sci.* 35 (8):1711–1720.

Santoso, A.W. *et al.* (2023). Effectiveness of photobiomodulation in reducing pain of oral mucosal diseases: a case series. *Int Med Case Rep J.* 16(7):407–417.

Schiavon, M.D.S.C. *et al.* (2023). Chronic red laser treatment induces hypotensive effect in two-kidney-one clip model of renovascular hypertension in rat. *Lasers Med Sci.* 38(1):252.

Shao, X.H. *et al.* (2005). Effects of He-Ne laser irradiation on chronic atrophic gastritis in rats. *World J Gastroenterol.* 11(25):3958–3961.

Simões, A. *et al.* (2009). Laser as a therapy for dry mouth symptoms in a patient with Sjögren's syndrome: a case report. *Spec Care Dentist.* 29(3):134–137.

Stanley, B.J. and Hauptman, J.G. (2009). Long-term prospective evaluation of topically applied 0.1% tacrolimus ointment for treatment of perianal sinuses in dogs. *J Am Vet Med Assoc.* 235(4):397–404.

Steiner, J.M. (2010). Canine pancreatic disease. In: *Textbook of Veterinary Internal Medicine: Diseases of the Dog and the Cat*, pp. 1695–1703. Elsevier, St. Louis, MO.

Takhfooladi, M.A. *et al.* (2014). The effects of low-level laser therapy on hepatic ischemia-reperfusion injury in a rat model. *Lasers Med Sci.* 29(6):1887–1893.

Ucero, A.C. *et al.* (2013). Laser therapy in metabolic syndrome-related kidney injury. *Photochem Photobiol.* 89(4):953–960.

Weber, M. *et al.* (2015). Medical low-level laser therapy foundations and clinical applications. *Int Soc Med Laser App.* 2:283–297.

Yamota, M. *et al.* (2013). Low-level laser therapy improves crescentic glomerulonephritis in rats. *Laser Med Sci.* 28(4):1189–1196.

Yang, Y. *et al.* (2005). Effects of He-Ne laser on gastric mucosa in rat with chronic atrophic gastritis. *World J Gastroenterol.* 22(5):926–929.

Zadik, Y. *et al.* (2019). Systematic review of photobiomodulation for the management of oral mucositis in cancer patients and clinical guidelines. *Support Care Cancer.* 27(10):3969–3983.

Zigmond, E. *et al.* (2014). Low-level light therapy induces mucosal healing in a murine model of dextran-sodium sulfate induced colitis. *Photomed Laser Surg.* 32(8):450–457.

15

Laser Therapy for Urinary Conditions

Lisa A. Miller

Companion Animal Health, New Castle, DE, USA

Use of Photobiomodulation in Lower Urinary Tract Disease

For almost 50 years, laser devices have been used in humans to diagnose and treat various diseases of the genitourinary tract. Used in the management of menometrorrhagia and other conditions or to ablate and/or excise various lesions, this has included procedures in both normal and cancerous tissues (Lanzafame, 2019). Though many of these procedures have utilized fractional ablative CO_2 lasers or Er:Yag lasers to treat symptoms associated with genitourinary syndrome of menopause (GSM), such as vaginal dryness, atrophy, pain and incontinence, true photobiomodulation therapy (PBMT) has been suggested in the human medical realm as an alternative for managing GSM, interstitial cystitis/bladder pain syndrome (IC/BPS), and stress urinary incontinence (SUI) in women. The pathophysiology, symptoms, and management of these conditions easily lend themselves to the rationale for using PBMT as a possible treatment, and devices designed for these applications in humans have demonstrated beneficial clinical and histologic changes in recent studies (de la Torre & Miller, 2017; Gaspar & Leibaschoff, 2018; Kohli *et al.*, 2021).

In 2017, a randomized study using photobiomodulation (PBM) in female patients with provoked vestibulodynia demonstrated overall improvement compared to a sham group (Leg Sagie *et al.*, 2017). More recently, a novel system for the temporary relief of pelvic muscle pain and spasm in women clinically significantly improved pelvic pain and decreased pain with urination in 65% of participants in a clinical study, and follow-up data has indicated that the therapeutic effect may last several months (Kohli *et al.*, 2021; Zipper *et al.*, 2021). An observational cohort study of female patients with IC/BPS from 17 US practices who received photobiomodulation examined their pain as measured using a numeric rating scale (NRS) of 0–10. Minimal clinical important difference (MCID) was the primary outcome and was defined as reduction of the overall pelvic pain severity by at least 2 NRS points from baseline to after 8 treatments. Of the nearly 150 patients with IC/BPS who chose to start PBM therapy, almost 90% completed four treatments and 60% completed all treatments. In addition, 73.5% reported improvement of at least 1 NRS point and improvement of ≥2 points was reported by 64% of at treatment series completion. In this group, patients with moderate or severe pain decreased from 83% to 39% and overall both pain with urination and pelvic pain decreased with a MCID of −2.6 and −2.7, respectively. The researchers concluded that in realistic clinical settings, two of three women experiencing IC/BPS who were treated with PBM therapy experienced significant decrease in dysuria and pelvic pain (Butrick & Lamvu, 2022).

Feline Interstitial Cystitis

Based on the noninvasiveness of the modality and its ease of use for feline patients in particular, PBMT may also be a possible therapeutic intervention for certain lower urinary tract disorders in cats. Feline idiopathic (or interstitial) cystitis (FIC) has also been called feline urologic syndrome and idiopathic feline lower urinary tract disease (FLUTD). Having a multifactorial etiology that has not been completely elucidated, FIC appears to arise from interactions between the urinary bladder, adrenal glands, nervous system, and environmental factors. In response to stressful episodes or environmental changes, affected cats may have decreased adrenocortical function along with an excitatory sympathetic nervous system response and an associated increase in bladder wall permeability (Forrester & Towell, 2015). This abnormal degree of urothelial permeability, also found in human IC patients, allows increased potassium ions and

Laser Therapy in Veterinary Medicine: Photobiomodulation, Second Edition. Edited by Christopher J. Winkler and Lisa A. Miller.

protons from urine to penetrate through to the submucosa, which cause irritation and stimulation of sensory neurons (Lavelle *et al.*, 2000; Westropp *et al.*, 2006; Parsons, 2007). The positive effects noted in the aforementioned human studies are consistent with the mechanism of action of PBM, and the potential impact on multiple pelvic and bladder pain generators (Cotler *et al.*, 2015).

Pain research has demonstrated that PBM results in analgesia through numerous mechanisms. However, a large part of the mechanism of action is exerted through its reduction in C fiber and A-delta activity, modification of growth factors, and pro-inflammatory cytokines and chemokines. A major contributor to the development of the allodynia that causes the symptom of urinary frequency and bladder pain, C-fiber activation is prevalent in human patients with IC/BPS (Gao *et al.*, 2018). Cats with FIC have C-fiber sensory neurons in the bladder that are also more sensitive compared to normal cats, contributing to altered activation of neural pathways. Research has also indicated that in afferent neurons, abnormal transient receptor potential (TRP) vanilloid receptor 1 responses may contribute to this enhanced bladder sensitivity in FIC (Sculptoreanu *et al.*, 2005). The ability to potentially mediate the activation of TRP (Freitas and Hamblin, 2016) and/or reduce the sensitivity of C-fiber sensory neurons in the bladder of these patients could be a potential target for PBMT to exert antinociceptive effects.

Cats with FIC may present in a variety of ways, including those that experience frequent recurrent episodes, chronic persistent signs, or even urethral obstruction (Houston *et al.*, 2003). PBMT may be of potential benefit in all these situations as a part of the multimodal management, decreasing the severity of clinical signs by providing analgesia, and decreasing urethral spasm during episodes of acute pain. When urethral obstruction does occur, many veterinarians (including the author) have also found PBMT helpful for decreasing swelling, spasm, and pain prior to and/or during the placement of a urinary catheter to alleviate any obstruction, and in providing pain management for unblocked cats whether discharged home or remaining in hospital with indwelling urinary catheters (Lavallee and Olson, 2017).

Urinary Incontinence

While research in humans has determined that there is a relationship between lower back pain (LBP) and urinary incontinence (UI) (Zhang *et al.*, 2006; Eliasson *et al.*, 2008) and that the treatment of LBP utilizing rehabilitation therapy reduced the symptoms of the UI (Ghaderi *et al.*, 2016), only one veterinary publication has found a correlation between reduced mobility of lumbar vertebrae L3–L5 and the existence of urethral sphincter mechanism incompetency (USMI) (Thude, 2015). One recent publication has examined whether treatment of LBP could improve symptoms of acquired, non-neurologic urinary incontinence in dogs (Lane & Hill, 2022). USMI is the most common acquired non-neurogenic cause of urinary incontinence in dogs (Chew *et al.*, 2011; Byron *et al.*, 2017) and Lane and Hill reported on therapeutic outcomes in 39 patients with LBP treated over a 6-year period using combined manual therapy and acupuncture (with 33 of these patients also having been treated concurrently with PBM). Treated patients had significantly reduced frequency ($p < 0.01$) and volume ($p < 0.01$) of UI episodes. Responses to treatment ranged from no improvement to complete resolution of clinical signs. Hill and Lane logically concluded that this decrease in USMI clinical symptoms following treatment for LBP suggested a relationship between the two conditions, and that combined treatment using manual therapy and acupuncture with or without PBM was effective for USMI. PBM parameters reported to be utilized in the treatment of these patients were varied and were not described in detail in the publication. USMI incontinence should be considered a potential pain symptom, and dogs presenting with UI should be examined carefully for LBP. For laser operators who wish to treat UI patients with back pain, further details on appropriate dosimetry and technique for treating the spine are described in Chapters 11, 16, and 23.

Treating the Veterinary Patient with Lower Urinary Tract Disease

In any scenarios involving chronic lower urinary tract disease or urethral obstruction, it is recommended to apply PBMT to all applicable areas of the urinary bladder (Figure 15.1a and b, as well as to the perineum (and the penis in male patients) to target the urethra. Additionally, treating the lumbar and sacral spine could be of added benefit, targeting the sensory neurons innervating the bladder via the pelvic and hypogastric nerves originating from the dorsal horn of the sacral and lumbar spinal cord, respectively. A deep-tissue dosage of 6–10 J/cm^2 for the caudal abdomen is recommended (scaling up with the size of the patient and the depth of the target tissues), treating on-contact to minimize loss of light from reflection (Lavallee and Olson, 2017). When treating transabdominally, irradiance at the level of the urinary bladder is determined by irradiance at the skin surface, determined in turn by both spot size of the laser beam (choice of treatment handpiece) and the treatment power (watts). The author and colleagues have previously used an on-contact

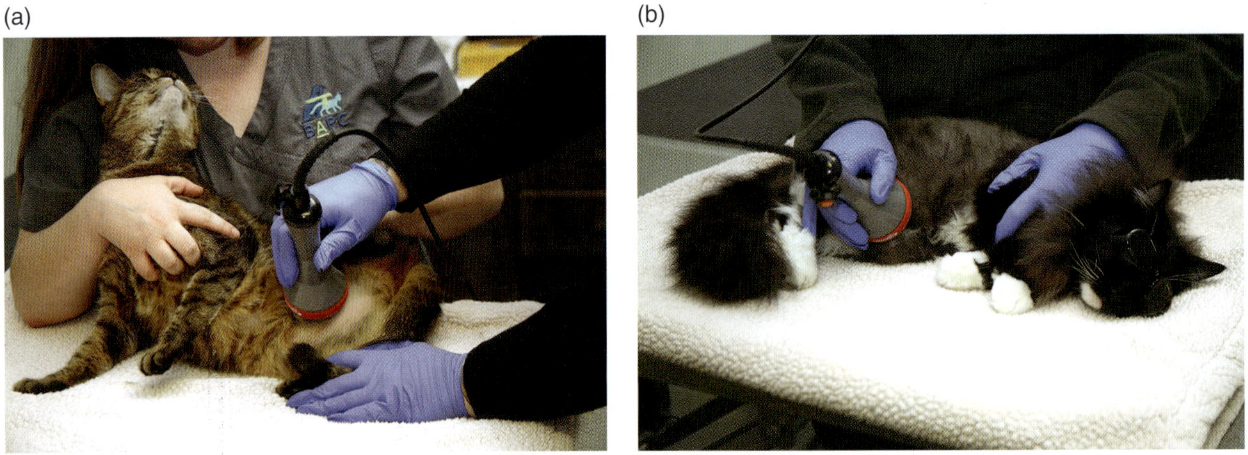

Figure 15.1 (a) and (b) Treating the urinary bladder in feline patients with handheld device.

treatment head with a spot size of 5 cm^2 and power settings in the 4–8 W range (0.8–1.6 W/cm^2) at the skin surface (again, scaling up with the size of patient and depth of target tissue). Extrapolating from computational modeling and previous cadaver work in dogs (Piao *et al.*, 2018), treatment using these irradiances at the target tissue should be approximately 155–250 mW/cm^2. The author recommends scanning the entire caudal abdomen to treat the urinary bladder, aiming for all aspects of the bladder where it is positioned in the abdomen and utilizing a technique similar to scanning the area for a diagnostic ultrasound. The perineum should be treated with an off-contact technique, due to often being contaminated with urine or already having been prepped for catheterization. Since the target tissues in question are usually more superficial in this area, the operator may turn the power setting (W) down when treating the perineal area, using a target fluence similar to a wound setting (3–5 J/cm^2). Care should be exerted to treat the entire perineal area without hovering over sensitive areas, such as inflamed or swollen tissues where urethral catheterization has been attempted or a catheter has been placed. Allow sufficient time for such tissues to thermally relax appropriately before returning to the same area with the treatment beam.

The same technique of treating the urinary bladder may also be applied to canine or feline patients experiencing discomfort from cystitis, or for patients that have had a cystotomy performed for urolithiasis. For acute situations or hospitalized patients, PBMT sessions may be performed daily for pain management until resolution, weaning the frequency of treatment sessions as the patient improves. In mild cases, one to three treatment sessions is often sufficient in combination with other appropriate treatments for a urinary tract infection (UTI). Techniques for intraoperative treatment of the urinary bladder during or immediately post-cystotomy while the abdomen is still open, are described in Chapter 7.

For more chronic situations (FLUTD/FIC or chronic UTIs), weaning to a maintenance schedule of treatments (typically once every 2–4 weeks) is recommended after initial improvement is clinically noted to aid in keeping a patient's symptoms to a minimum. Many colleagues have reported anecdotal success in maintaining patients on a chronic treatment schedule with regards to subjectively reducing the number of overall occurrences of acute presentation for lower urinary tract "flare ups" in chronically affected patients.

Acute and Chronic Kidney Disease

Dense with mitochondria, the kidney is a metabolically active organ and is hemodynamically dependent on adenosine triphosphate (ATP) in order to regulate solute and water balance. Processes that stress or disrupt mitochondrial function, reduce the production of ATP, and create oxidative stress subsequently lead to cellular injury, harming kidney function. Mitochondrial dysfunction has been associated with acute kidney injury (AKI) in different disease states, including in ischemia reperfusion injury (Clark & Parikh, 2020; Hall *et al.*, 2013; Szeto *et al.*, 2017) and mitochondria-targeted antioxidants have been investigated for their protective effects on kidney tissues especially from ischemic injury, and in reducing AKI (Jankauskas *et al.*, 2016; Szeto *et al.*, 2017). Similarly (depending on etiology), mitochondrial dysfunction, reactive oxidative stress, inflammation, and renal tissue fibrosis are inherent components in chronic kidney disease (CKD). Studies have investigated PBMT for its potential to aid in the treatment of these conditions due to its ability to reduce superoxide radicals, reduce mitochondrial dysfunction in ATP production, the potential to decrease apoptosis, to stimulate repair and attenuate the sequelae of inflammation and fibrosis, and potentially for its ability to mitigate gut microbiota dysbiosis. It should be noted here that the author is not advocating that PBMT be used in place of traditional CKD management, including nutritional modifications, renoprotective treatments, phosphorus reduction, or the identification and correction of any existing prerenal or postrenal disorders and/or primary disease processes or complicating disorders. As with most complex disease management, a multimodal approach is best, taking therapeutic priorities into consideration based on the patient's presentation and stage of CKD.

A study in diabetic rats on IR-induced kidney damage showed that PBM attenuated kidney injuries caused by this pathology, which was associated with reduced lipid peroxidation, an enhanced antioxidant defense system, and polymorphonuclear leukocyte (PMN) infiltration (Asghari *et al.*, 2016). Another recent study further verified that the protective effect of PBM was mediated through the modulation of oxidative stress in kidney damage induced by γ-radiation. PBM significantly attenuated oxidative stress in this same model while also enhancing the activity of enzymes involved in detoxification, leading to tubular and corpuscular improvement in the kidney (Abdel-Magied *et al.*, 2020).

Another recent publication examined the effects of PBM and caffeine on AKI in rodents. Rat pups were subjected to the Modified Rice–Vannucci model (a hypoxic ischemic encephalopathy (HIE) intervention) replicating pathology in humans. Either PBM or caffeine was administered for a few days following the HIE. Urine biomarkers and weights were analyzed, as well as histologic changes in the kidney. Both treatments individually resulted in decreased kidney injury seen on electron microscopy, but not when treatments were combined. HIE elevated urinary albumin, neutrophil gelatinase-associated lipocalin (NGAL), and kidney injury molecule (KIM-1) but these elevations were significantly reduced by either treatment. Individual treatments, but not combination of caffeine + PBM, improved the reductions noted in the enzymatic activity of mitochondrial complexes II-III following kidney injury and also improved weight gain. Ultimately, both caffeine and PBM were found to reduce AKI in this model (Groves *et al.*, 2023).

Numerous PBM application studies have indicated positive outcomes on CKD and have described beneficial findings with regards to decreasing inflammatory cytokines, decreasing renal hypertension, preserving glomerular filtration rate, and decreasing renal fibrosis particularly through affecting TGFβ1 signaling (Yamato *et al.*, 2013; Ucero *et al.*, 2013; Bian *et al.*, 2022). As one example, the PBM was shown to be renoprotective in a model of metabolic syndrome-induced CKD in rats, which was associated with increased glomerular filtration rate, reduced blood pressure, and decreased tubulointerstitial fibrosis (Ucero *et al.*, 2013). In another study, PBM using 670 nm light and a fluence of around 10 J/cm^2 contributed to improved renal function and lowered azotemia as well as the blood urea nitrogen (BUN)/creatinine ratio in streptozotocin-induced type-1 diabetic rats (Lim *et al.*, 2010). In a model of ureteral obstruction (UO), PBM decreased several inflammatory markers as well as Smad3 and TGF-β1, demonstrating that PBM mitigated inflammation and provided protection against interstitial fibrosis induced by UO (Oliveira *et al.*, 2012). These anti-inflammatory effects were also verified in a crescentic glomerulonephritis rodent model. PBM significantly reduced pro-inflammatory cytokines (TNF-α and IL-1β) in the renal cortex as well as inhibiting crescent formation and accumulation of CD8+ lymphocytes and ED+ macrophages histologically in the glomeruli (Yamato *et al.*, 2013).

Attenuating Kidney Disease through the Gut–Kidney Axis

PBM may also exert effects on the gut-kidney axis, a factor increasingly considered a crucial contributor to CKD, at least in humans (Rukavina *et al.*, 2020). Disruptions in the GI microbiome worsen gut permeability in CKD patients, potentially leading bacterial translocation and endotoxin leakage through the gut barrier, increasing uremic toxins, and accelerating CKD progression (Chen *et al.*, 2021b; Stavropoulou *et al.*, 2021). Impaired kidney function subsequently leads to worsening retention of uremic toxins which are secreted into the lumen of the gastrointestinal tract, continuing to contribute to the severity of microbiota dysbiosis.

A growing body of evidence shows that PBM improves bacterial composition, function, and abundance, thus favorably restoring GI microbiota (Bicknell *et al.*, 2019; Chen *et al.*, 2021a, 2021b) contributing to increased production of short chained fatty acids and strengthening the gut barrier by decreasing endotoxins and uremic toxins.

Bicknell and colleagues researched gut microbiota modulation via PBM application. Findings in healthy Balb/c mice included that PBM using 660 and 808 nm light altered microbiome diversity increasing the abundance of certain bacterium associated with a healthy rodent microbiome (Bicknell *et al.*, 2019). Furthermore, these gut microflora-regulating effects of PBM may be of benefit in various neurodegenerative diseases as well (Chen *et al.*, 2021a; Wang *et al.*, 2021). Strategies to possibly attenuate some of the symptoms of kidney disease by improving the gut microbiota through the use of PBMT have been suggested in human publications (Bian *et al.*, 2022).

Treating the Veterinary Patient with Kidney Disease

Veterinary colleagues as well as the author have noted anecdotal subjective improvements in their own CKD-patients treated with PBM with regards to decreasing azotemia and stimulating appetite and overall well-being (Godine, 2017).

To attempt to treat the kidneys themselves, the recommendation is to use a deep tissue dose of 6–10 J/cm^2 on-contact (scaling up with the size of the patient and the depth of the target tissues) with a focus on the cranial abdomen, including the area of the kidneys (as though performing a diagnostic ultrasound scan of that area). Approaching from both the ventral aspect and the lateral walls of the abdomen, the left kidney is often palpable and usually easier to localize than the right kidney due to its lateral location along the mid-abdomen. The right kidney, located more craniodorsally, may have to be treated based on aiming the beam in that orientation under the rib cage on that side of the abdomen (Figure 15.2), or even utilizing a lateral approach in large deep-chested dogs through the 11th or 12th intercostal space. The laser operator should utilize good technique, making sure to keep the beam scanning and moving at all times.

If the laser operator wishes to include the intestines in the treatment field, to help with any GI symptoms from uremia or for the potential benefits of improving gut microbiota as previously described, the author would recommend expanding the field of treatment to include the remainder of the abdomen, utilizing the same dosimetry described above, and continuing to treat on contact over the abdominal wall. Similar doses and techniques have been applied in veterinary patients suffering from chronic idiopathic large bowel diarrhea and resulted in decreased frequency of diarrhea episodes, increased body weight, and improved body condition scores (Alves *et al.*, 2022).

For CKD, this author and other veterinary colleagues recommend an initial treatment session frequency of two to three times per week, weaning the frequency of treatment sessions after 2 weeks, until a maintenance phase treatment session of typically once every 2–3 weeks is established based on the patient's response (keeping clinical symptoms to a minimum), and any improvements noted in labwork. For AKI, hospitalized patients could certainly be treated daily to help reduce inflammation or pain associated with pyelonephritis or to potentially help reduce oxidative stress and overall kidney injury.

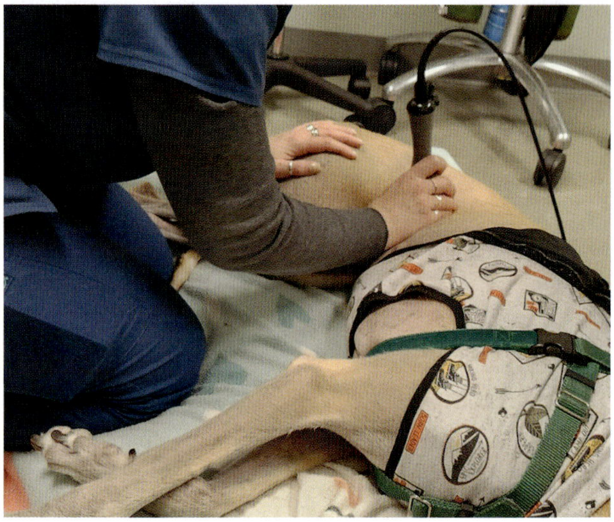

Figure 15.2 Treating the kidney in a canine patient.

Conclusion

A large amount of research has been done over the last 60 years to elucidate the mechanisms behind PBM. Ongoing research is exploring additional cellular mechanisms and optimal dosing parameters for various conditions; however, research and clinical progress has been made. While further veterinary-specific studies are needed, photobiomodulation could be very impactful for many veterinary patients being treated for renal and lower urinary tract disease. This modality should be strongly considered for these patients, both as part of the overall strategy to reduce their pain and hasten recovery wherever possible and also to ameliorate other long-term consequences of their chronic conditions.

References

Abdel-Magied, N. *et al.* (2020). Effect of low-level laser on some metals related to redox state and histological alterations in the liver and kidney of irradiated rats. *Biol Trace Elem Res.* 194:410–422.

Alves, J.C. *et al.* (2022). The effect of photobiomodulation therapy on the management of chronic idiopathic large-bowel diarrhea in dogs. *Lasers Med Sci.* 37(3):2045–2051.

Asghari, A. *et al.* (2016). Effect of photobiomodulation on ischemia/reperfusion-induced renal damage in diabetic rats. *Lasers Med Sci.* 31:1943–1948.

Bian, J. *et al.* (2022). Therapeutic potential of Photobiomodulation for chronic kidney disease. *Int J Mol Sci.* 23(14):8043.

Bicknell, B. *et al.* (2019). Photobiomodulation of the microbiome: implications for metabolic and inflammatory diseases. *Lasers Med Sci.* 34:317–327.

Butrick, C.W. and Lamvu, G. (2022). Transvaginal Photobiomodulation improves pain in women with pelvic muscle tenderness and interstitial cystitis/bladder pain syndrome: a preliminary observational study. *Urology.* 170:14–20.

Byron, J.K. *et al.* (2017). Urethral sphincter mechanism incompetence in 163 neutered female dogs: diagnosis, treatment, and relationship of weight and age at neuter to development of disease. *J Vet Intern Med.* 31:442–448.

Chen, Q. *et al.* (2021a). Gut flora-targeted photobiomodulation therapy improves senile dementia in an Aβ-induced Alzheimer's disease animal model. *J Photochem Photobiol.* 216:112152.

Chen, T.H. *et al.* (2021b). Gut microbiota composition and its metabolites in different stages of chronic kidney disease. *J Clin Med.* 10:3881.

Chew, D.J. *et al.* (2011). *Disorders of micturition and urinary incontinence.* In: *Canine and Feline Nephrology and Urology.* (eds. D.J. Chew *et al.*), 2 edn, pp. 409–433. W.B. Saunders, Saint Louis, MI.

Clark, A.J. and Parikh, S.M. (2020). Mitochondrial metabolism in acute kidney injury. *Semin Nephrol.* 40:101–113.

Cotler, H.B. *et al.* (2015). The use of low level laser therapy (LLLT) for musculoskeletal pain. *MOJ Orthop Rheumatol.* 2(5):1–7.

de la Torre, S. and Miller, L.E. (2017). Multimodal vaginal toning for bladder symptoms and quality of life in stress urinary incontinence. *Int Urogynecol J.* 28:1201–1207.

Eliasson, K. *et al.* (2008). Urinary incontinence in women with low back pain. *Man Ther.* 13:206–212.

Forrester, S.D. and Towell, T.L. (2015). Feline idiopathic cystitis. *Vet Clin Small Anim.* 45(4):783–806.

Freitas and Hamblin (2016). Proposed mechanisms of photobiomodulation or low-level light therapy. *IEEE J Sel Top Quantum Electron.* 22(3):1–22.

Gao, Y. *et al.* (2018). The role of C-fibers in the development of chronic psychological stress induced enhanced bladder sensations and nociceptive responses: a multidisciplinary approach to the study of urologic chronic pelvic pain syndrome (MAPP) research network study. *Neurourol Urodyn.* 37(2):673–680.

Gaspar, A. and Leibaschoff, G. (2018). Preliminary study using a device for photobiomodulation and controlled exercises in the perineum floor. In: *World Society of Cosmetic Gynecology Congress.* ISAPS, Cartagena.

Ghaderi, F. *et al.* (2016). Effects of stabilization exercises focusing on pelvic floor muscles on low back pain and urinary incontinence in women. *Urology.* 93:50–54.

Godine, R. (2017). *Abdominal conditions.* In: *Laser Therapy in Veterinary Medicine: Photobiomodulation.* (eds. R.J. Riegel and J.C. Godbold), pp. 169–178. John Wiley and Sons, West Sussex, UK.

Groves, A.M. *et al.* (2023). Effects of photobiomodulation and caffeine treatment on acute kidney injury in a hypoxic ischemic neonatal rat model. *Physiol Rep.* 11:15.

Hall, A.M. *et al.* (2013). In vivo multiphoton imaging of mitochondrial structure and function during acute kidney injury. *Kidney Int.* 83:72–83.

Houston, D.M. *et al.* (2003). Feline urethral plugs and bladder uroliths: a review of 5484 submissions 1998–2003. *Can Vet J.* 44(12):974–977.

Jankauskas, S. *et al.* (2016). Dysfunction of kidney endothelium after ischemia/reperfusion and its prevention by mitochondria-targeted antioxidant. *Biochem Mosc.* 81:1538–1548.

Kohli, N. *et al.* (2021). An observational cohort study of pelvic floor photobiomodulation for treatment of chronic pelvic pain. *J Comp Eff Res.* 10(17):1291–1299.

Lane, D. and Hill, S. (2022). The relationship between urethral sphincter mechanism incompetency and lower back pain: positing a novel treatment for urinary incontinence in dogs. *Open Vet J.* 12(1):105–113.

Lanzafame, R.J. (2019). The rationale for Photobiomodulation therapy of vaginal tissue for treatment of genitourinary syndrome of menopause: an analysis of its mechanism of action, and current clinical outcomes. *Photobiomodulation, Photomed and Laser Surg.* 37(7):395–407.

Lavallee, J. and Olson, J. (2017). Feline-specific conditions. In: *Laser Therapy in Veterinary Medicine: Photobiomodulation.* (eds. R.J. Riegel and J.C. Godbold), pp. 198–211. John Wiley and Sons, West Sussex, UK.

Lavelle, J. *et al.* (2000). Urothelial pathophysiological changes in feline interstitial cystitis: a human model. *Am J Physiol Renal Physiol.* 278:540–553.

Lev-Sagie, A. *et al.* (2017). Low-level laser therapy for the treatment of provoked vestibulodynia – a randomized, placebo-controlled pilot trial. *J Sex Med.* 14(11):1403–1411.

Lim, J. *et al.* (2010). Effects of low-level light therapy on streptozotocin-induced diabetic kidney. *J Photochem Photobiol B.* 99(2):105–110.

Oliveira, F.A. *et al.* (2012). Low-level laser therapy decreases renal interstitial fibrosis. *Photomed Laser Surg.* 30(12):705–713.

Parsons, C.L. (2007). The role of the urinary epithelium in the pathogenesis of interstitial cystitis/prostatitis/urethritis. *Urology.* 69:9–16.

Piao, D. *et al.* (2018). Flexible nine-channel photodetector probe facilitated intraspinal multisite transcutaneous photobiomodulation therapy dosimetry in cadaver dogs. *J Biomed Opt.* 23(1):010503.

Rukavina, M. *et al.* (2020). Gut microbiota and chronic kidney disease: evidences and mechanisms that mediate a new communication in the gastrointestinal-renal axis. *Pflugers Arch.* 472:303–320.

Sculptoreanu, A. *et al.* (2005). Protein kinase C contributes to abnormal capsaicin responses in DRG neurons from cats with feline interstitial cystitis. *Neurosci Lett.* 381(1–2):42–46.

Stavropoulou, E. *et al.* (2021). Microbiome, Immunosenescence, and chronic kidney disease. *Front Med.* 8:661203.

Szeto, H.H. *et al.* (2017). Mitochondria protection after acute ischemia prevents prolonged upregulation of IL-1β and IL-18 and arrests CKD. *J Am Soc Nephrol.* 28:1437–1449.

Thude, T.R. (2015). Chiropractic abnormalities of the lumbar spine significantly associated with urinary incontinence and retention in dogs: chiropractic associated with incontinence. *J Small Anim Pract.* 56:693–697.

Ucero, A.C. *et al.* (2013). Laser therapy in metabolic syndrome-related kidney injury. *Photochem Photobiol.* 89:953–960.

Wang, Y. *et al.* (2021). Oral berberine improves brain dopa/dopamine levels to ameliorate Parkinson's disease by regulating gut microbiota. *Signal Transduct Target Ther.* 6:77.

Westropp, J.L. *et al.* (2006). Evaluation of the effects of stress in cats with idiopathic cystitis. *Am J Vet Res.* 67(4):731–736.

Yamato, M. *et al.* (2013). Low-level laser therapy improves crescentic glomerulonephritis in rats. *Lasers Med Sci.* 28(4):1189–1196.

Zhang, J. *et al.* (2006). A case series of reduced urinary incontinence in elderly patients following chiropractic manipulation. *J Chiropr Med.* 5:88–91.

Zipper, R. *et al.* (2021). Transvaginal photobiomodulation for the treatment of chronic pelvic pain: a pilot study. *Womens Health Rep.* 2(1):518–527.

16

Neurological Conditions

Lisa A. Miller[1], *Juanita J. Anders*[2], *and Ann K. Ketz*[3]

[1] *Companion Animal Health, New Castle, DE, USA*
[2] *Uniformed Services University of the Health Sciences, Bethesda, MD, USA*
[3] *Recovery Sciences, Enovis, Lewisville, TX, USA*

1st Edition Contributor:

Richard L. Godine

North American Association for Light Therapy, Ruckersville Animal Hospital and Veterinary Laser Therapy Center, Ruckersville, VA, USA

Introduction

Photobiomodulation therapy (PBMT) offers an effective, nonpharmacological approach for treating the nervous system. *In vitro* and *in vivo* preclinical studies indicate that PBMT promotes cellular regeneration, reduces neuronal oxidative stress and neuroinflammation, and modulates pain while increasing mitochondrial function, oxygen consumption, and blood flow in many traumatic injuries and diseases of the peripheral and central nervous systems (CNSs). The principal chromophores for absorption of red and near-infrared light are located within the mitochondria. Therefore, it is not surprising that tissues rich in mitochondria, such as brain, spinal cord, and neurons in peripheral nerve ganglia respond readily to PBMT, resulting in repair and regeneration (Hamblin, 2024). In this chapter, we will review the science supporting the use of PBMT for peripheral nerve conditions, neuropathic pain, spinal cord injury (SCI), and injury and diseases of the brain.

Peripheral Nerve Injury

Injury to a peripheral nerve results in loss of associated motor and sensory function. In an extremity, such a loss results in severe impact on quality of life. Peripheral nerve injury (PNI) results in degeneration of the axons and retrograde degeneration of the corresponding neurons of the spinal cord, followed by a very slow regeneration. Total nerve regeneration of the peripheral nerve does not occur, which leads to muscle atrophy. Therefore, of major research interest are developing methods to enhance/accelerate regrowth of injured peripheral nerves and decrease or prevent atrophy of the corresponding muscles (Fellin *et al.*, 2024). Surgery is the preferred method for complete or severe PNI. However, recovery of the repaired nerve's function almost never occurs. Improving posttraumatic peripheral nerve regeneration, especially when nerve surgery has been carried out, still represents a major challenge of restorative medicine (Evans, 2000; Lundborg, 2002). One method proposed to enhance peripheral nerve repair is PBMT. Although the first pioneering report on the use of light for peripheral nerve repair was published by Rochkind (1978), it has been in the last 20 years that many PBMT papers have reported positive effects on peripheral nerve regeneration (Rochkind, 2023). In the Anders' laboratory, we investigated the effects of PBMT on incomplete PNI (crush injury, facial nerve) (Anders *et al.*, 1993; Alcântara *et al.*, 2013) and on complete transection without repair (facial nerve) (Anders *et al.*, 2004), with autograph repair of the rat median nerve (Moges *et al.*, 2011) and with end-to-end epineural suture of transected peroneal nerves in New Zealand white rabbits (Anders *et al.*, 2014). In these studies, 632.8 nm light was used to treat the facial nerve, which is located sub dermally in the rat face, and either 810 or 980 nm light for the median and peroneal nerves. In all cases the laser and treatment parameters were optimized, and axonal regrowth and functional improvements occurred. Here are some of our findings:

- The rate of regeneration was increased in crush-injured rat facial nerve as measured by retrograde transport of horseradish peroxidase to neuronal cell bodies in facial motor neurons.
- There was an accelerated return of choline acetyltransferase (ChAT) immunoreactivity in the facial nerve crush injury model.
- mRNA for cr-calcitonin gene-related peptide (cr-CGRP) increased by 10-fold ($p < 0.0001$) at 11 days post-transection using an axotomy facial nerve injury model.
- Neuronal survival in the facial motor nucleus increased threefold ($p < 0.0001$) at 6–9 months post-transection.

With PBMT of the transected rat median nerve repaired with an autograph, there was faster functional recovery of grip strength ($p < 0.05$), shorter compound motor action potential (CMAP) latency ($p < 0.05$), and higher S-100 immunoreactivity, indicating increased Schwann cells in the nerve trunks when compared to the autograph repaired nerves (Moges *et al.*, 2011). These results demonstrate that PBMT can accelerate functional recovery and improve the quality of nerve regeneration after autograft repair of severely injured peripheral nerves.

In the study on the effects of the transected and end-to-end sutured peroneal nerve, it was demonstrated that treatment parameters can be determined initially using *in vitro* models and then translated to *in vivo* research and clinical practice. *In vitro*, 980 nm light at 10 mW/cm^2 significantly improved neurite elongation at energy densities between 2 and 200 mJ/cm^2. *In vivo* transmission of the near infrared light measured in anesthetized rabbits showed that on average, 2.45% of the light applied to the skin reached the depth of the peroneal nerve. An *in vivo* pilot study revealed that an output power of 4 W applied to the skin over the injury/repair site inhibited nerve regeneration while an output power of 2 W significantly improved axonal regrowth. For the definitive study, the irradiated group performed significantly better in the toe spread reflex test compared to the control group from week 7 post-injury, and the average length of motor endplates returned to uninjured levels, indicating a reinnervation of the involved muscles (Anders *et al.*, 2014).

These studies and those of many other investigators demonstrate that PBMT at various wavelengths with optimized parameters accelerates nerve regeneration and improves functional recovery. The wavelength selection should be based on the depth of the nerve to be treated. For nerves such as the median and sciatic, the near-infrared wavelengths were used because of their greater depth of penetration. Also, much higher output power is needed at the surface to deliver the appropriate therapeutic dose to the nerve. In summary, PBMT is one of the most promising adjunctive therapies to date for improved neuro-regeneration.

Peripheral Nerve Injuries in Veterinary Medicine

Peripheral nerve injuries in the dog and cat are usually the result of a traumatic incident. Brachial plexus avulsions are commonly seen in the dog, resulting in neurotmesis, axonotmesis, and neuropraxia (Inzana, 2000). Other peripheral nerve injuries can occur from fight wounds, ballistic injuries, and vehicular accidents (Welch, 1996; Mariani, 2010). Severe injuries are often permanent without proper surgical intervention, while neuropraxia will often resolve over 8 weeks (Rodkey and Sharp 2003). Inadequate peripheral nerve regeneration due to trauma can significantly contribute to the morbidity of surgical patients. Animals admitted in an emergency situation often have concurrent orthopedic injuries impairing mobility and potentially masking peripheral nerve dysfunction if a thorough neurological examination is not performed (Welch, 1996). The use of PBMT offers the clinician a way to increase the rate of peripheral nerve regeneration and motor neuron survival (Snyder *et al.*, 2002; Rochkind *et al.*, 2007; Anders *et al.*, 2014). PBMT has clinical evidence in cats, regarding analgesic effects on peripheral nerves (Kono *et al.*, 1993) via decrease of ascending signals from the spinal cord to the higher CNS. A study in dogs following severe SCI and implantation of a segment of the peripheral nerve into the injured area demonstrated diminished glial scar formation, induced axonal sprouting in the injured area, and restoration of locomotor function following laser irradiation of the spinal cord (Rochkind and Ouaknine, 1992). Other publications have also documented the use of PBMT for peripheral nerve injuries in veterinary patients (Gouveia *et al.*, 2024).

Recommended parameters for PBMT in peripheral nerve injuries are comparable to those recommended for deep-tissue musculoskeletal dosing (10–20 J/cm^2, scaling up with the size of the patient and depth of target tissues). Table 11.1 (Chapter 11) provides a range of recommended power settings for deep musculoskeletal conditions in veterinary patients of various sizes that is also appropriate for the application(s) described here. Treatment surface areas used for calculating dose should take into consideration an area encompassing the suspected site(s) of injury as well as the entire nerve tract(s) of the traumatized nerve(s), and any associated myofascial pain or spasms in adjacent muscles.

Ideally, the injury should be treated soon after it occurs (provided there is no remaining active hemorrhage in the area), as this will decrease the noxious cellular and biochemical environment, limit the extent of the damage, and increase the chances of success, while decreasing the time to healing. Treatment should be administered daily for 3 days and then every 2–3 days until resolution. Recovery of peripheral nerve injuries is a long, slow process, in which axonal growth rates may reach 1 mm/day in small nerves and 5 mm/day in large nerves (Recknor *et al.*, 2006). Thus, treatment with PBMT should continue for at least 8 weeks or until acceptable function has returned.

Neuropathic Pain

Both peripheral nerve and spinal cord injuries can result in neuropathic pain symptoms, which may become chronic. Neuropathic pain evolves through various fundamental mechanisms, including abnormal nerve activity, heightened sensitivity in peripheral nerves, increased sensitivity in the CNS, diminished inhibitory control, and abnormal activation of microglia (Moore, 2016). PBMT has been shown to have positive effects on several of these mechanisms.

As previously described, several labs have investigated the effect of different PBMT parameters on neuropathic pain-related behaviors in chronic constriction or spared nerve injury models of neuropathic pain. Hsieh et al. (2012) used a chronic constriction injury model and treated with CW 660 nm light, at an energy density of 9 J/cm^2, daily for 7 consecutive days. The PBM-treated animals demonstrated both decreased mechanical allodynia and improved indices of walking patterns of the injured nerves. Two other studies compared 660, 830, and 980 nm light with doses of 4 and 8 J/cm^2 and decreased mechanical allodynia as well as improved rat-knee incapacitation test (Bertolini *et al.*, 2011; Masoumipoor *et al.*, 2014). See Chapter 3 for further details.

In the rat-spared nerve injury model, both LED and diode laser light has been used to effectively mediate neuropathic pain mechanisms. Our laboratory used optimized laser parameters from *in vivo* and *in vitro* experiments using 980 nm light to characterize the activation of macrophages and microglia along ascending somatosensory pathways related to neuropathic pain. Light was applied to an affected hind paw (output power: 1 W; 20 seconds; 41 cm above skin; power density: 43.25 mW/cm^2; dose: 20 J), dorsal root ganglia (output power: 4.5 W; 19 seconds; on-contact with skin; power density: 43.25 mW/cm^2; dose: 85.5 J), and spinal cord (output power: 1.5 W; 19 seconds; on-contact with skin; power density: 43.25 mW/cm^2; dose: 28.5 J) regions every other day from day 7–30 postoperatively. Untreated animals demonstrated mechanical hypersensitivity 1–30 days postoperatively, though PBM-treated animals began to recover after two treatments, and reached baseline measurements at day 26 (Kobiela Ketz *et al.*, 2017). Additionally, immunohistochemical analysis of macrophage and microglial inflammatory markers showed a shift toward the M1 (pro-inflammatory) phenotype of microglia in injured spinal cord dorsal horn and dorsal column, though not in the injury + PBMT group. In dorsal root ganglion samples, macrophages expressing M2 markers (anti-inflammatory) were significantly increased in the PBMT group but not in the injury or sham groups, indicating that PBMT may contribute to resolution of inflammation (Kobiela Ketz *et al.*, 2017).

In another study, an LED array of 890 nm light was used following spared nerve injury in male Swiss mice. The LED pad was applied directly to the ventral side of the entire animal body and delivered 390 mW of power, with an energy density of 20.8 J/cm^2 and a power density of 17.4 mW/cm^2, 20 minutes per day for 21 days. The team showed that this treatment resulted in an analgesic effect in both mechanical hypersensitivity and cold allodynia measurements (Pigatto *et al.*, 2020).

Zhang and colleagues treated Sprague-Dawley rats with PBMT over the site of a crush SCI at the T10 vertebrae with 150 mW of CW 810 nm light for 60 minutes per day for 14 days following injury, for a total irradiation energy of 540 Joules per treatment. Unfortunately, full parameters were not reported. Treated animals demonstrated cellular responses to PBMT, including mediation of the NF-KB pathway, decreased expression of CXCL10 in glial cells, and microglial and astrocyte inhibition. Animals that received PBMT also had alleviation of neuropathic pain-related behaviors and improved motor function recovery (Zhang *et al.*, 2023).

Though treatment parameters and behavioral measurements differ between these studies, the findings suggest that PBMT can be effective in decreasing neuropathic pain behavior and altering the inflammatory process associated with peripheral nerve and spinal cord injuries in animals.

Spinal Cord Injury

The spinal cord lies within the spinal column and extends from the brainstem to the lumbar region. The spinal cord terminates in the lumbar region at L1–L2 level in adult humans. Below this, the vertebral canal contains the cauda equina, which consists of peripheral nerve roots (Standring, 2020).

The role of the spinal cord is to conduct information between the periphery and the brain via 31 pairs of segmentally organized spinal nerves and ascending and descending tracts within the spinal cord. SCI causes damage to the cells within the cord and severs the ascending and descending nerve tracts, disrupting the flow of sensory and motor information between the body and brain, resulting in loss of sensation, movement, and autonomic regulation (Bennett *et al.*, 2024). SCI can result in serious disabilities, including neurological deficits, loss of sphincter functions, and chronic pain.

Damaged axons fail to regenerate following SCI in adult mammals. After SCI, a secondary injury occurs that is mediated in part by the immune response (Popovich *et al.*, 2002) and causes further impairment (Dusart and Schwab, 1994; Fitch *et al.*, 1999). A number of therapeutic modalities have been tested including use of anti-inflammatory drugs, X-irradiation, elimination of inhibitory factors in the spinal cord, provision of neurotrophic factors, and cell transplantation (Byrnes *et al.*, 2005). Despite these efforts, there currently is no effective intervention for SCI. However, there is considerable research on the efficacy of PBMT for SCI.

Dr. Rochkind pioneered the use of light to treat SCI by combining PBMT with transplantation of embryonic cultured neurons in transected spinal cords. The result was an increase in axonal sprouting, decreased scar formation, and improved weight bearing and locomotion in dogs and rats in comparison to transplantation alone. Since these pioneering studies, several research groups demonstrated that transcutaneous PBMT improved locomotor function. These studies used near-infrared light. Three reports from Dr. Anders' laboratory looked at the use of transcutaneous 810 nm PBMT (150 mW output power, 0.3 cm^2 spot size, 1589 J/cm^2, 2997 sec daily for 14 days) to treat transected or contused rat spinal cords. PBMT using an 810 nm laser promoted regeneration and functional recovery of rats and suppressed immune cell activation and cytokine/chemokine expression (Wu *et al.*, 2009). Invasion/activation of immune cells has been implicated as a potential mediator of secondary injury. A variety of cell types invade or are activated within the first hours to days after SCI, including neutrophils, macrophages, microglia, astrocytes, and T and B lymphocytes. These cells are primarily activated or attracted to the lesion area by pro-inflammatory cytokines and chemokines, expressed within the first few hours after injury. Therefore, alteration of cell invasion/activation after SCI improves functional recovery. Von Leden and colleagues (Von Leden *et al.*, 2013) examined the effects of 808 nm irradiation on microglia, which are responsible for immune and inflammatory responses in the CNS. After exposure of microglia in culture to fluences of 0.2, 4, 10, or 30 J/cm^2, the phenotypic expression for pro- and anti-inflammatory markers were examined using immunocytochemistry, proteomic profiling, and reverse transcriptase-polymerase chain reaction. PBMT had a dose-dependent effect on the spectrum of microglia for M1 (pro-inflammatory) and M2 (anti-inflammatory). PBMT at energy densities between 4 J/cm^2 and 30 J/cm^2 induced expression of MI markers while lower fluences induced expression of M2 markers. When microglia were co-cultured with neurons, a dose-dependent effect was reported on microglial-induced neurite expression. These data are important in understanding the mechanistic basis for PBMT of the CNS as well as effects on signal transduction pathways (Von Leden *et al.*, 2013).

Intervertebral Disk Disease in Veterinary Medicine

One of the most common causes of neuropathic pain in veterinary medicine is intervertebral disk disease (IVDD). IVDD was first classified as type I or type II by Hansen (1951). Type I is commonly associated with chondroid disk degeneration and involves herniation of the nucleus pulposus through the annulus fibrosis, resulting in extrusion of disk material into the spinal canal and subsequent compression of the spinal cord to varying degrees.

Typically affecting younger, small-breed, chondrodystrophic dogs, though it may also occur in larger, non-chondrodystrophic breeds, Type I disk extrusion cases usually present as an acute-onset episode, and clinical signs vary depending on the severity of the resultant SCI and neuroanatomic localization. Clinical signs include varying degrees of spinal hyperesthesia and neurological deficits from paraparesis to paraplegia, with or without deep pain perception. Thoracolumbar disk herniation is reported in 66–87% of dogs with intervertebral disk herniation (Hansen, 1951; Gage, 1975). The disks located between T12 and L3 have been shown to be at higher risk of herniation (Brisson, 2010). IVDD with extrusion can also occur in the cervical spine, and many of these patients will present with varying degrees of lowered head and neck carriage, guarding, or cervical spinal muscle spasms. Root signature may be observed with impingement of C5–C8 nerve roots.

Type II IVDD is associated with fibroid degeneration and involves a shift of the nucleus pulposus secondary to weakening and partial rupture of the annulus, causing a focal protrusion into the spinal canal. Cases usually display a slow, progressive onset of clinical signs. Type II protrusions occur more commonly in older, non-chondrodystrophic breeds; chondrodystrophic breeds *can* develop them, but it is less common (Macias *et al.*, 2002).

Disk extrusion or protrusion causes SCI. The damage is usually most severe at the sites of occurrence, and the associated clinical signs are caused by concussion or compression. Pathologic changes progress, and the ensuing neurodegenerative process contributes to the development of inflammation, along with a complex cascade of vascular and biochemical events that contribute to secondary SCI and neuronal damage. Traumatic and biochemical injury to axons of the spinal cord can lead to demyelination, axonal degeneration, neuronal death, cavitation, and glial scarring. PBMT has been shown to be effective in reducing pro-inflammatory cytokines and reactive oxygen species (ROS) that infiltrate the spinal cord following injury (Byrnes *et al.,* 2005). Furthermore, laser light has been shown to stimulate neuronal sprouting and regrowth of severed axons (Rochkind, 2009). One *in vitro* study investigating the inflammation induced by the interaction between macrophages and human annulus fibrosus cells found that laser irradiation markedly suppressed IL6 and IL8 levels in a time-dependent manner (Hwang *et al.,* 2015).

An article titled "Rehabilitation and Physical Therapy for the Neurologic Patient" further explains:

> Even in the absence of persistent compression, ischemia, or decreased perfusion, local edema and secondary oxidative damage play a key role in the extent and severity of SCI. Of these, tissue perfusion may be the most responsive to physiotherapeutic intervention; thus, physiotherapy techniques and modalities that promote circulation are often central to the rehabilitation program for patients with SCI (Sims et al., 2015).

If for no other reason than its positive effects on tissue perfusion, PBMT is an excellent treatment modality in cases of IVDD regardless of other treatments employed, conservatively or surgically.

As detailed previously, PBMT has also been shown to promote axonal regeneration and functional recovery in cases of SCI as well. Another study investigating one of the major causes of pain in human degenerative lumbar spinal disease – chronic compression of the dorsal root ganglion (CCD) – examined the molecular-based irritation involving the localized release of inflammatory cytokines and the effects of laser irradiation on them. Two of the primary cytokines responsible for the hyperalgesia observed in lumbar spinal diseases are TNFα and IL1β. It has been demonstrated that herniated disk tissues release IL1β, which affects the somatosensory neural response at the dorsal root level. Previous studies have also shown that TNFα in the nucleus pulposus plays an important role in radicular pain (root signature or referred pain) and that sensory neurons display increased sensitivity to TNFα in a rat CCD model. This study demonstrated not only that the expression levels of both cytokines are reduced by the application of laser light but that it also promotes neural regeneration and significantly reduces CCD-mediated mechanical and thermal hyperalgesia (Chen *et al.,* 2014).

Canine models showed that PBMT improved neurologic function after experimentally-induced disc disease, with treated dogs being able to walk within 9–12 weeks after spinal cord transection and sciatic nerve autograft insertion, compared to a still-paralyzed untreated control group. Histologic analysis of treated dogs revealed that new axons and blood vessels had migrated into the graft (Millis *et al.,* 2005). An earlier study in dogs with disk disease examined the use of PBMT in non-ambulatory dogs with thoracolumbar IVDD following decompressive surgery compared to a control group that received hemilaminectomy alone. There was a significant difference between the two groups in the median time to ambulation (3.5 days in the PBMT-treated group versus 14 days in the control group), which was independent of age, weight, modified Frankel score, and duration of clinical signs on presentation (Draper *et al.,* 2012). Even though this study demonstrated a positive effect, more information needs to be gathered in order to optimize the parameters used to treat this condition. The irradiance in this study (25 000 mW/cm^2 applied "to the overlying skin of the spinal segment associated with the hemilaminectomy and the two adjacent ones (one cranial and one caudal)") is likely misreported, as this level would cause thermal damage to the tissue surface. Additionally, the calculations of irradiance and fluence "delivered to the spinal cord" were based on personal communications of unpublished data, emphasizing the need for more rigorous standards when conducting clinical laser research.

Two more recent studies showed contrasting results. One study found no difference in recovery-related variables among dogs that received PBMT and physical rehabilitation compared to those receiving physical rehabilitation with sham PBMT. The authors described treating the area over the affected spinal cord segment, one spinal segment cranial to, and one segment caudal to the injury site, using a wavelength of 810 nm, a power of 1 W, an irradiance of 5.5 W/cm^2, and a fluence of 329.7 J/cm^2 (Bennaim *et al.,* 2017). The second report described how including PBMT within the rehabilitation protocol during the postoperative period improved patients' neurological status, and there was a tendency for a shorter mean time to regain ambulatory ability. The reported parameters were 808 and 905 nm wavelengths, a power of 1.2–7.5 W, a fluence of 4 J/cm^2, and a total dose between 75.292 and 75.389 joules (Bruno *et al.,* 2020).

Based on the variety of treatment parameters reported in different studies, there is still a need to determine adequate laser device parameters prior to the beginning of a clinical study, and to ensure that those reported are correct for the condition being treated. There is also a need for further studies in veterinary patients, in both conservative-management and postsurgical-application models, and in dogs that have presented with and without deep pain perception. However, there is certainly enough evidence in the present body of literature to support the use of PBMT as an adjunct to current standard-of-care treatment regimens for patients with IVDD. It should be noted that, whether or not PBMT is available, current best practices and recommendations for both surgical and conservative management should be communicated to owners after examination of the patient.

Light Penetration to the Spinal Cord in Dogs

Historically, individuals have expressed polarizing viewpoints on the use of PBMT in treating spinal cord conditions in veterinary medicine. One end of the spectrum voiced concerns for the ability of a laser to penetrate transcutaneously through the relevant tissues and deliver a therapeutic dose of light to the spinal cord, while the other viewpoint(s) expressed concerns that photobiomodulatory irradiances could potentially cause collateral thermal damage to the spinal cord, especially in postsurgical situations in which a hemilaminectomy had been performed. Experimental dosimetric data has now reported the skin-to-spinal-cord light transmission in various species and enables some extrapolation of a photobiomodulatory dose that is translatable to veterinary patients.

As previously discussed in Chapters 2 and 4, only a small percentage of the dose applied to the skin penetrates to the spinal cord beneath the laser handpiece. In the study by Byrnes et al. (2005), only 6% of the 810 nm laser energy applied to the skin reached to spinal cord depth in rats. Though not specific to the spinal cord itself, a study by Anders et al. (2014) found that only 2.45% of 980 nm light applied to the skin reached the depth of the peroneal nerve in anesthetized rabbits. Work in cadaver dogs, using a single photodiode sensor placed in the spinal canal, showed that 0.00102% transcutaneous light transmission to the shallowest level of the spinal canal of the dog was comparable to the 0.00114% transcranial light transmission measured from the same subject (Piao *et al.,* 2017). The transcranial light transmission of 0.00114% in this dog cadaver also agreed with transcranial light transmission at 5 cm depth in human cadavers, demonstrating it was possible to deliver PBMT light to the spinal cord level in dogs at a dose that has shown the potential of improving human cerebral conditions (Tian *et al.,* 2016) at a clinically safe surface irradiation level. A later study by the same researchers attempted to improve upon the consistency of multisite measurements in the canine spinal cord and the reproducibility of inter-subject evaluation. In this study, Piao et al. (2017) reported on the development of a flexible multichannel probe that was deployed in the spinal canal of large cadaver dogs after hemilaminectomy, quantifying simultaneous intraspinal light irradiances at nine sites throughout the thoracolumbar spine during surface light irradiation (Piao *et al.,* 2018). The intraspinal light irradiances at these sites were measured both in the absence and presence of the skin, and with the laser handpiece held both on-contact and off-contact. The same surface continuous light illumination of 3.14 W/cm^2 was applied, and a peak light irradiance of 327.48 μW/cm^2 was recorded at approximately the L1–L2 area in the absence of the skin, while a peak light radiance of 5.68 μW/cm^2 was recorded in the presence of the skin. The difference of the light irradiances in the absence and presence of the skin and when held on- or off-contact indicated that the skin is the greatest barrier to light penetration and that treating in direct contact does make a significant difference in light penetration to deeper tissues. Though optimal power densities (at least for 980 nm wavelength light and for neurite elongation) at the level of target tissue are thought to be relatively low (Anders *et al.,* 2014), the therapeutic window is likely wider, and research should be continued to further define optimal parameters for various conditions, wavelengths, and depths of target tissues. Studies such as the aforementioned give us a reasonable place to start with some recommendations.

Treating the Spinal Cord in IVDD

Current deep-tissue musculoskeletal dosing (10–20 J/cm^2, scaling up with the size of the patient and depth of target tissues) is appropriate for treating the cervical, thoracic, lumbar, and sacral spine in most dogs and cats. Table 11.1 (Chapter 11) provides a range of recommended power settings for deep musculoskeletal conditions in veterinary patients of various sizes that is also appropriate for neurological applications in the spinal cord. These doses should be effective and safe for most commercially available laser units, but the practitioner should always confirm with the laser manufacturer regarding safety specifications. Treatment surface areas used for calculating dose should take into consideration a few spinal segments both cranial and caudal to the suspected area of intervertebral disk extrusion or protrusion. If any spasms in the paraspinal muscles are noted, these should be addressed concurrently, and if neurological deficits are present in the limbs, it is recommended to treat the remainder of the spine as well as descending nerve tracts. For thoracolumbar lesions, treatment should be applied directly over the spine (Figure 16.1) along with a few inches to either side, aiming toward the spine through the paraspinal musculature. In the neck area,

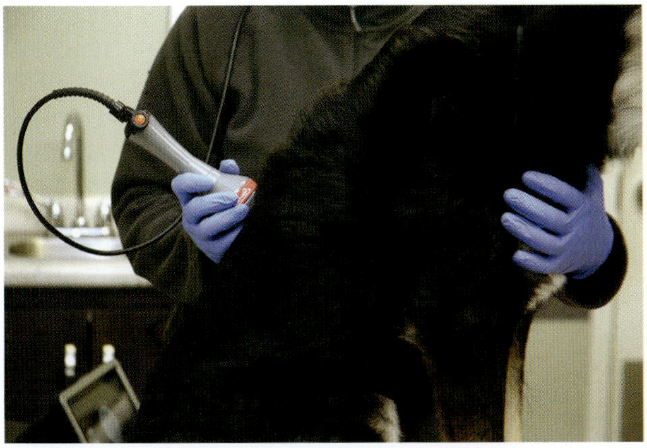

Figure 16.1 Treating the thoracic spine in a canine patient.

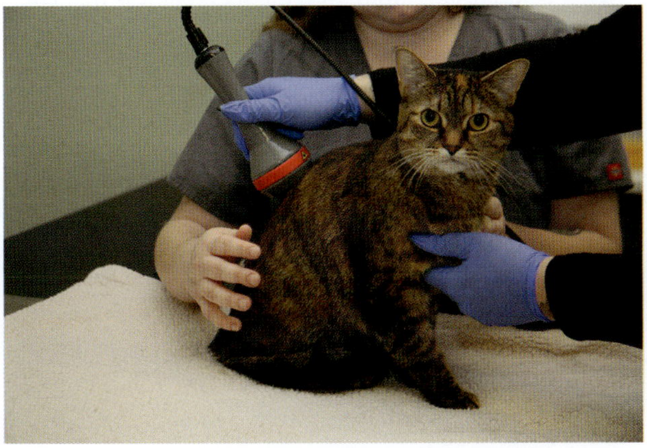

Figure 16.2 Treating the thoracic spine in a feline patient.

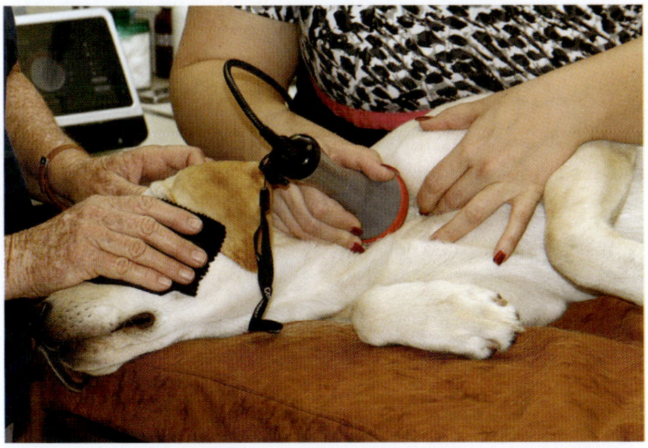

Figure 16.3 Treating the caudal cervical area.

a lateral and ventral approach is recommended, and the laser therapist is reminded that to effectively treat the caudal cervical area (Figures 16.2 and 16.3), manipulation of the front leg may be necessary, which is often painful for the patient due to radicular pain. This should be done with care, and a good knowledge of anatomy is critical to treating the correct areas in these patients. Patients with back and neck pain should be treated in the position that is most comfortable for them, which may involve standing, sitting, or lying down in various positions.

For patients prescribed conservative management, PBMT should begin immediately and continue daily, if possible, until significant improvement is seen. At this time, weaning to a transition phase of less-frequent treatments is possible, and continued until resolution of clinical signs. Some patients with chronic IVDD may benefit from continued maintenance-therapy treatment, as in patients with osteoarthritis (see Chapter 11 for further discussion).

For patients that have undergone surgical decompression, PBMT should be started immediately after surgery for the wound area, similar to recommendations for postoperative CCL patients. The paraspinal muscles in these patients should be treated in a similar manner to the techniques described above, aiming toward the spine and using deep-tissue dosing. Since the surgical incision often has staples or sutures in place, see the recommendations given in Chapter 11 regarding metal implants and suture material. Ideally, PBMT should be started daily for 3–5 days, if possible, and then continued at least three times weekly until significant improvement is seen, when the frequency of treatment can be weaned as described earlier. As always, results with PBMT are optimized when it is used in conjunction with an excellent physical rehabilitation program and other supportive care for neurologic patients.

Transcranial PBM

In 2004, following work by Oron on cardiac ischemia in a rodent model, PBMT was first applied to the human brain to treat acute ischemic stroke using noninvasively delivered (transcranial) near-infrared light (Oron *et al.*, 2006). Transcranial photobiomodulation (tPBM) of brain physiology is nonthermal and has been attributed to the absorption of red and/or near-infrared light by specific cellular chromophores (Karu, 1999). These chromophores include mitochondrial cytochrome C oxidase (CCO) and ion channels receptive to light (Karu, 1999). CCO-absorbed light energy is converted into ATP for cellular use, restoring or enhancing mitochondrial function, leading to gene transcription and then to cellular repair and healing. Additionally, the process creates mild oxidants (ROS), which further contribute to the healing process (Lubart and Breitbart, 2000; Alexandratou *et al.*, 2002). Notably, the effects of tPBM do not appear to be confined to specific near-infrared wavelengths (Hamblin, 2016).

Over the last two decades, tPBM has undergone extensive trials as a therapeutic intervention for various neurological conditions, consistent with findings from the NEST trials, which involved over 1400 patients (Lampl *et al.*, 2007). These trials found tPBM to be safe and have no serious side effects. However, the trials yielded varying results concerning treatment efficacy, a variability that can be attributed to the diverse range of diseases and disorders studied, as well as inconsistent tPBM dosing. Nonetheless, with an improved understanding of dosing, several recent tPBM trials have demonstrated both safety and efficacy in treating Alzheimer's (Iosifescu *et al.*, 2023b) and Parkinson's diseases (Mcgee *et al.*, 2023), traumatic brain injuries (Naeser *et al.*, 2016), major depressive disorders (Iosifescu *et al.*, 2022), and autism spectrum disorder (Ceranoglu *et al.*, 2022; Pallanti *et al.*, 2022) as well as improving cognitive performance in healthy young adults (Salehpour *et al.*, 2019).

The future of tPBM holds great promise, with ongoing well-funded trials like TRIADE (Iosifescu *et al.*, 2023a) and TRAP-AD (Iosifescu *et al.*, 2023b). There is a growing trend towards standardizing dosages, and researchers are exploring advanced PBM techniques that employ photosensitive nanoparticles to stimulate deeper brain activity. This approach has the potential to lead to significant advancements in the treatment of Parkinson's disease. Furthermore, due to its affordability, safety, and ease of self-administration, tPBM is likely to become a widely accessible neurologic therapy that individuals can use at home.

Cognitive Dysfunction Syndrome

Cognitive dysfunction syndrome (CDS) encompasses canine cognitive dysfunction and feline cognitive dysfunction. It is becoming more common in small-animal practice as veterinarians lengthen pets' lives through better nutrition and wellness care. Confusion, disorientation, excessive panting, nocturnal pacing, agitation, circling, separation anxiety, phobias, irritability, and vocalization often characterize canine CDS (CCDS). In the cat, one might see litterbox issues, wandering, increased vocalization, and nocturnal activity. CCDS is a naturally occurring degenerative brain disorder with a gradual onset and insidious progression (Landsberg *et al.*, 2012; Ozawa *et al.*, 2016) analogous to human Alzheimer's disease (AD) (Landsberg *et al.*, 2012; Dewey *et al.*, 2019).

The pathophysiology of AD and CCDS is multifactorial, involving vascular compromise, neuronal mitochondrial dysfunction, inflammation, oxidative brain damage, and deposition of β-amyloid (Aβ) around blood vessels and neurons. Over time, these factors lead to progressive loss of dendrites, synapses, and neurons, followed by cognitive decline (Landsberg *et al.*, 2012; Chapagain *et al.*, 2018; Dewey *et al.*, 2019). As for AD in humans, there is no cure, although a variety of supplements, pharmacological agents, and environmental strategies have been used to treat CCDS, including L-deprenyl, S-Adenosyl methionine, diets fortified with antioxidants, mitochondrial cofactors, and essential fatty acids (Landsberg *et al.*, 2011; Manteca, 2011). While these methods may be helpful, authors and colleagues have observed that the use of transcranial PBMT seems to be very effective in improving the symptoms of CCDS within 4–6 weeks in most cases.

What is interesting from a PBMT standpoint is that compromised blood flow, mitochondrial dysfunction, oxidative stress, and inflammation are at the core of this disease process, and these all happen to be where PBMT shines as a treatment modality, having been extensively discussed in this and other chapters. Vascular compromise and inflammation result in the accumulation of neurotoxic Aβ, generating the production of ROS and proinflammatory cytokines (e.g., IL-1β, IL-6, and TNF-α), stimulating premature neuronal apoptosis via various signalling pathways, and increasing formaldehyde levels (FA) in the brain, all of which can lead to cellular and neuronal damage (De Taboada *et al.*, 2011; Da Luz Eltchechem *et al.*, 2017; Hamblin, 2019). While neuronal mitochondria are the primary source of energy production in the brain, when functioning normally they can also mitigate the toxic effects of Aβ on neuronal cellular function. Compromised cerebral blood flow and the toxic effects of Aβ contribute to mitochondrial dysfunction (Landsberg *et al.*, 2012; Chapagain *et al.*, 2018; Dewey *et al.*, 2019), which subsequently worsens the adverse effects of Aβ on cellular and mitochondrial function in a vicious cycle (Gonzalez-Lima *et al.*, 2014; Da Luz Eltchechem *et al.*, 2017; De La Torre, 2017; Lu *et al.*, 2017).

Studies have demonstrated the ability of PBMT to cause disaggregation of Aβ via suppression of β-secretase activity and stimulation of enzymes responsible for degrading Aβ peptides (De Taboada *et al.*, 2011; Da Luz Eltchechem *et al.*, 2017; Yue *et al.*, 2019; Zhang *et al.*, 2020; Tao *et al.*, 2021). Microglia play a central role in the generation and dissolution of Aβ in rodent AD models. PBMT has been shown to favor a shift between the two main types of activated microglia to the neuroprotective and anti-inflammatory M2 phenotype (Hamblin, 2019; Tao *et al.*, 2021). Rodent studies have demonstrated that tPBMT application decreased brain levels of Aβ, improved cognitive test scores, increased cerebral vascular density, and decreased FA (Huang *et al.*, 2020; Tao *et al.*, 2021).

While there are no veterinary studies published regarding the efficacy of use of tPBMT for the treatment of CCDS, one publication has discussed the pathophysiology and previously mentioned mechanisms by which PBMT may be beneficial (Dewey *et al.,* 2022). The ideal parameters for use of tPBMT for CCDS are not well established. However, data extrapolated from rodent and human clinical trials involving AD (Barrett and Gonzalez-Lima, 2013; Naeser *et al.,* 2014; Saltmarche *et al.,* 2017; Chan *et al.,* 2019; Salehpour *et al.,* 2019; Spera *et al.,* 2021) may be used as a basis of where to start. Though numerous wavelengths within the therapeutic window have been investigated for this purpose, including 660, 810, 980, and 1064 nm, it is important to remember that the ability of each of these wavelengths to penetrate through the necessary tissues to reach the brain can vary, especially given differences in skin pigmentation and the depth of muscles overlying the calvarium in the dog (which is typically thicker than in rodents and humans). Dosimetry in published studies is varied and fluence has been reported sometimes at the level of the cortex and sometimes at the level of the skin, lending further complication. Authors of one study did report the beneficial effects of transcranial PBM on anxiety and depression in humans. Using an 810 nm LED array of 250 mW/cm^2 irradiance, they calculated that from the supplied dose of 60 J/cm^2 at the scalp, an effective dose of 2.1 J/cm^2 (3.7%) reached the dura of the brain (Schiffer *et al.,* 2009). This dose is within the ranges estimated by other light transmittance studies in human cadavers (Lychagov *et al.,* 2006; Tedford *et al.,* 2015). In the future, further tissue modelling studies and cadaver studies on light penetration to the canine brain could help guide dosing decisions. Different pulse structures have also been examined in some of these studies, though the most common wave forms investigated have been CW, 100 Hz, and 1000 Hz. The reasoning behind the use of pulsed delivery is because neural oscillations measured by electroencephalography recordings have been linked to different mental processes. Memory processes are most closely related to oscillations with theta (6Hz) and gamma frequencies (40 Hz), while attention seems closely associated with alpha and gamma oscillations (10 Hz and 40 Hz, respectively) (Ward, 2003). Pulsed light at alpha or gamma frequencies did elicit a positive effect on the brain in mouse models of AD (Iaccarino *et al.,* 2016). While it has been demonstrated that pulsing affects the biology of the brain differently than CW, true benefits remain to be elucidated and should be investigated further. Pulsing will also decrease the possibility of any thermal effect within the tissues, though using a reasonable surface irradiance and moving the laser handpiece over the scalp as described below would be safe.

In a recent literature review examining PBM to prevent and treat AD, authors Enengl, Hamblin, and Dunkl (Enengl *et al.,* 2020) suggested that based on the available body of research on PBM to the brain (which took into consideration both safety and efficacy), application should achieve a dose in the minimum effective range between 5 and 10 J/cm^2 at the level of the cortex. Based on the exponential energy decrease during transcranial application, energy densities of 20–60 J/cm^2 applied to the human scalp would be suggested and should be somewhat similar in large to very large dogs. The same authors suggest that pulsing with alpha or gamma frequencies might add additional benefit to tPBM against AD, and a 50% duty cycle would necessitate a doubling of the calculated treatment time to achieve the same dose as with CW light.

The authors recommend that the handpiece be held on-contact with the dorsal surface of the skull, treating both the right and left hemispheres (Figures 16.4, 16.5), when treating CCDS. Laser safe eyewear for the patient is recommended and is discussed further in Chapters 4 and 5. When treating with a higher power laser (or at the higher end of the irradiance range listed below), the laser operator is encouraged to keep the treatment head in continuous motion at all times. A handheld class 3b laser may be held in place and used to treat point-to-point as an alternative. An irradiance between 0.250 and 1.5 W/cm^2 at the skin surface is recommended. The resultant irradiances at the cortical surface in dogs should replicate dosing that was safe and effective in humans (Ilic *et al.,* 2006) and tested in other species. Therefore, the laser operator must know the spot area of their laser handpiece as well as the power setting and duty cycle (if pulsed) for their laser to adequately calculate dose. In a medium- to large-size dog, treating over the dorsal calvarium, the size area may be between 50 and 70 cm^2 which would result in a total dose of 1000–1400 total joules delivered over the entire area if using

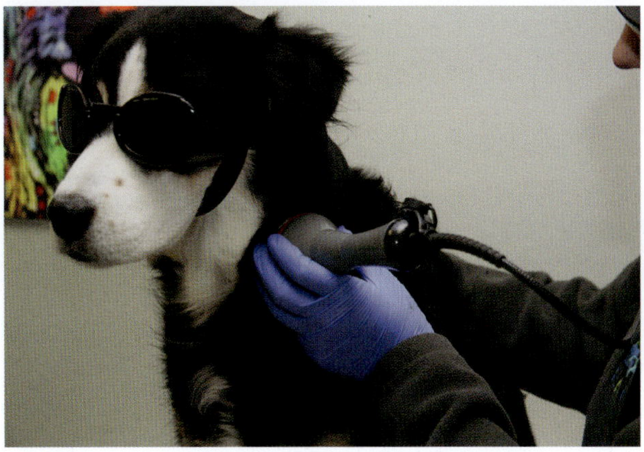

Figure 16.4 Treating the caudal cervical area.

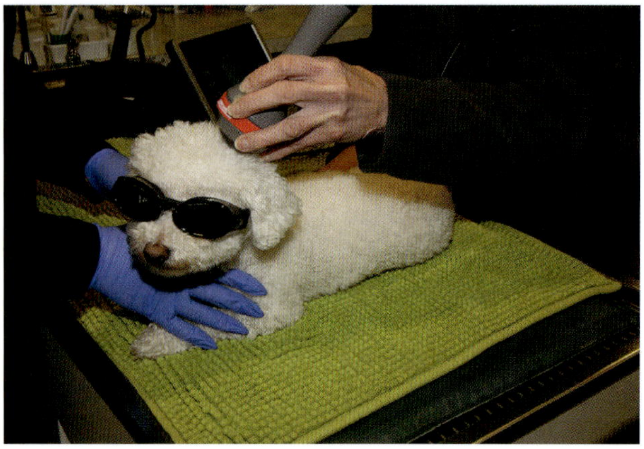

Figure 16.5 Canine patient receiving transcranial PBMT.

a fluence of 20 J/cm^2 (scale down for smaller patients and treatment size areas accordingly). As with most chronic, degenerative conditions, PBMT should be started with 2–3 sessions the first week, if possible, weaning to a transition phase of less-frequent treatments (twice weekly, then once weekly), and continued once every 2–3 weeks as needed, keeping clinical signs at a minimum. Treatments are painless and well tolerated. Some colleagues have noted that the patient may seem a little tired for the first 24 hours, but resolution of clinical signs usually begins within the first one or two treatments and gets progressively better in the first month (Godine, 2017). Bimonthly maintenance treatments offer the optimal chance for continued efficacy Figure 16.6.

Traumatic Brain Injuries

In the case of traumatic brain injuries, it has been shown that early intervention not only assists in early resolution of clinical signs, but also can be neuroprotective against lingering symptoms (Oron *et al.,* 2012).

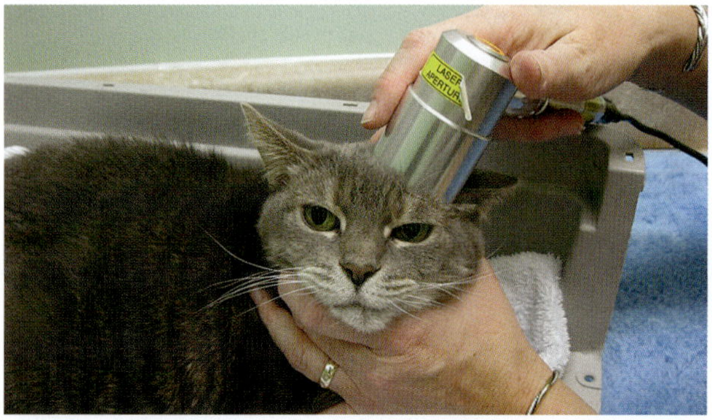

Figure 16.6 Feline patient with CDS receiving transcranial PBMT with a 500 mW, 810 nm multiprobe handpiece.

Animal-model studies using rats have demonstrated that transcranial near-infrared laser application may provide benefit in cases of acute traumatic brain injuries (Xuan *et al.,* 2013). The same parameters as used for treating CCDS can be used to treat traumatic brain injury. The frequency of treatment should be every 12–24 hours as needed for aiding in resolution of clinical signs. PBMT can decrease intracranial inflammation, decrease oxidative stress, and help stabilize damaged membranes. It is not recommended that subacute head trauma cases be treated with PBMT due to the possibility of intracranial hemorrhage; PBMT may cause a transient increase in blood flow. If there is any reason to suspect that intracranial bleeding is ongoing, PBMT should not be used.

Neurodegenerative Diseases and Degenerative Myelopathy

The body of evidence in the literature discussed above has shown that the application of PBMT can effectively modulate the inflammatory response following not only PNI but SCI as well. Statistically significant suppression of proinflammatory cytokine and chemokine gene expression, significant decreases in the invasion of cells involved in secondary damage (including macrophages, activated microglia, and T lymphocytes), a reduction in astrogliosis, and significantly improved axonal regrowth and function, are among the effects noted when PBMT is applied acutely after SCI. These studies provide evidence that light confers specific beneficial effects on the response of cells in the CNS to injury, leading to alteration of both the secondary injury response and the progression of the injury process.

Numerous studies have suggested that astrocytes and the astrocyte glutamate transporter (GLT-1; via deficiency of glial reuptake of excitatory amino acids) may play a role in modifying disease progression and motor neuron (MN) loss in neurodegenerative disease progression (Trotti *et al.,* 2001; Pardo *et al.,* 2006; Ogawa *et al.,* 2011; Lin *et al.,* 2012; Ogawa *et al.,* 2014). Astrocytes can induce MN degeneration through secretion of inflammatory mediators, including nitric oxide and prostaglandin E2 (Hensley *et al.,* 2006; Haidet-Phillips *et al.,* 2011). At least one study has demonstrated that neural progenitor cell-derived astrocytes from both familial amyotrophic lateral sclerosis (fALS) and sporadic ALS (sALS) patients were toxic to MNs *in vitro,* by co-culturing mouse embryonic stem-cell-derived MNs with the differentiated astrocytes from each patient (Haidet-Phillips *et al.,* 2011). Increased proliferation of glial fibrillary acidic protein (GFAP)-positive astrocytes has been observed in the presence of atrophied MNs in the spinal cords of human patients with both fALS and sALS, and has been correlated with the severity of the axonal loss and demyelination in the spinal cords of dogs with degenerative myelopathy (DM) (Ogawa *et al.,* 2011; Ogawa *et al.,* 2014). Ogawa and colleagues reported a significant and unique inducible nitric oxide synthase (iNOS) expression pattern in the gray matter of these same dogs, similar to that in SOD1 transgenic mice (Almer *et al.,* 1999; Lee *et al.,* 2009) and in ALS patients (Phul *et al.,* 2000; Sasaki *et al.,* 2000). The same authors concluded that there is likely an interaction between NO production and glutamate uptake occurring in DM. There are published studies reporting effects of PBMT on astrocytic activity. Yang *et al.* (2010) found that in astrocytes pretreated with PBMT, Ab-induced production of ROS and inflammatory response were eliminated in the cortical astrocytes of rats. PBMT has also demonstrated influence on the glial response, particularly that of the astrocytes, in a monkey model of Parkinson's disease (El Massri *et al.,* 2016). Sun *et al.* (2020) found that PBMT applied to the spinal cord of rats after SCI inhibited activation of GFAP-positive astrocytes, as well as inhibited astrocyte proliferation and the expression of astrocyte activation-related genes *in vitro*. Finally, one published study specifically examined the use of PBMT in an SOD1 transgenic mouse model of ALS (Moges *et al.,* 2009). This study reports that there was a statistically significant, yet short-lived, improvement in the group that received laser therapy. The data suggest that there was a delay in the onset of motor deficits, but this beneficial effect was only seen in the early stage of the disease. Furthermore, there was a statistically significant decrease in GFAP expression (an astrocyte marker) in the cervical and lumbar enlargements of the spinal cord in the laser-treated groups of mice compared with controls. The authors concluded that laser therapy may have suppressed astrocytes surrounding MNs in the spinal cord, possibly conferring a protective effect.

Canine DM is an adult-onset neurodegenerative disease characterized by progressive generalized proprioceptive ataxia of the pelvic limbs, asymmetric upper motor neuron (UMN) paraparesis, and a lack of paraspinal hyperesthesia, which progresses to lower motor neuron (LMN) paralysis of the pelvic limbs, and, eventually, the thoracic limbs (Averill Jr., 1973; Coates and Wininger, 2010). Sharing similarities in cause, clinical signs, and disease progression to some forms of ALS in humans, DM is a naturally occurring animal model for this disease. ALS and DM are progressive, incurable, fatal diseases. Clinicians thus look to available and novel therapies and clinical interventions to improve the overall quality of life and, hopefully, increase the life expectancy of affected patients. Dogs with DM are usually euthanized when they become nonambulatory and/or incontinent, both of which present challenges to at-home care by pet owners. Canine DM symptom progression is consistent across and within breeds, with distinct stages of disease progression, beginning with general proprioceptive ataxia with spastic UMN paraparesis (stage I) before progressing to nonambulatory paraparesis and paraplegia (stage II), followed ultimately in time by LMN tetraplegia and brain stem dysfunction (stage IV). Time of progression from stage I to stage II is generally 6–9 months (Coates and Wininger, 2010). Various therapeutic protocols have been attempted to slow DM's clinical symptom progression but none have been significantly successful (Clemmons, 1989; Polizopoulou *et al.,* 2008). Only daily intensive physiotherapy has demonstrated some benefit as a DM supportive therapy (Kathmann *et al.,* 2006).

Recently, a retrospective study was published examining the impact on the pathology of DM in canine patients by adding two different doses of PBMT to rehabilitation therapy (Miller *et al.,* 2020). The authors examined the records of dogs referred for presumed DM to a specialty rehabilitation facility and screened for patients meeting the study criteria. Qualifying patients were divided into two groups: a lower-dose group and a higher-dose group, based on the PBMT protocol used. Data related to demographics, diagnostics, rehabilitation protocols, and progression of clinical signs were collected and analyzed to determine differences in outcomes between the two treated groups and historical data expectations, as given by a previously published study. Authors reported that the time between symptom onset and euthanasia of dogs in the high-dose PBMT group was 38.2 $\pm$ 14.67 months (mean $\pm$ SD) and was significantly longer than that of dogs in the lower-dose group (11.09 $\pm$ 2.68 months). Similarly, the times between symptom onset and nonambulatory paresis or paralysis of dogs in the higher-dose group (31.76 $\pm$ 12.53 months), were significantly longer than those of dogs in the lower-dose group (8.79 $\pm$ 1.60 months). The data reviewed shows significantly slower disease progression – and longer survival times – for patients in the higher-dose group than those in the lower-dose group or published historical data. The authors suggested that potential mechanisms at play for the positive PBMT effects might include a protective effect on the MNs in the spinal cord of DM dogs through astrocyte-neuronal interactions suggested in the studies mentioned above, as well as PBMT acting as an ergogenic aid to therapeutic exercise and prevention of exercise-induced muscle fatigue or damage. Further details on these latter mechanisms are discussed in Chapter 23.

For optimal results in treating DM, the authors strongly recommend that all dogs should receive weekly to twice weekly in-clinic rehabilitation therapy, which includes PBMT as well as hydrotherapy exercise in an underwater treadmill and other therapeutic exercises as outlined by a rehabilitation therapist or practitioner. It is strongly recommended that the primary veterinarian consult with a rehabilitation-certified practitioner for therapeutic exercise recommendations, as DM dogs have a very finite exercise tolerance, and if exceeded, may take several days to recover and/or may become temporarily worse. Similarly, a rehabilitation practitioner may outline a suitable home exercise program for pet owners. Supportive care recommendations, including the use of assistive devices (such as slings for walking support and protective boots, socks, or bandages for the feet) are also strongly recommended. PBMT may be performed without the hair coat shaved, though of course, light penetration will be maximized in shaved areas. Treatment should be applied with the laser treatment head in direct contact with the dog's skin, directly over the spinal column, as well as several inches lateral to the right and left sides of the spinal column in the paraspinal musculature, treating the entire thoracic and lumbar spine. For dosimetry consistent with the aforementioned retrospective study, measure the area to be treated as described above in square centimeters, calculating a target energy density of 15–25 J/cm^2 to obtain the total joules desired (e.g., 700 $cm^2 \times 25\ J/cm^2 = 17\,500$ total joules). Once the total joules are calculated for the patient, select an appropriate treatment power in watts (W). Similar power ranges for use in intervertebral disc disease are recommended. Power should always be adjusted down if the patient is uncomfortable or if the laser operator feels any excessive thermal buildup in the haircoat or on the skin.

For any chronic degenerative condition such as DM, treatment sessions should begin with an "induction phase" of initial, more frequent treatment sessions (i.e., at least three times weekly if possible), until improvement is seen. With DM it is not unusual to be presented with patients that are in various stages of the disease progression. In the author's subjective experience and from personal communications with colleagues, better results are appreciated in dogs that are still in stage I of clinical progression. Each patient must be evaluated and treated as an individual; some take longer to respond than others. It is helpful for the practitioner to set expectations with pet owners to avoid their becoming discouraged when they do not see immediate results or to expect a "cure," as this is not possible. Once an improvement is noted in clinical signs, a "transition phase" of treatment sessions is begun. During transition, treatments are decreased to twice weekly, then once weekly, where this weekly "maintenance phase" of treatment sessions is maintained. These maintenance treatment sessions are more frequent than for pain-related chronic conditions such as osteoarthritis, likely due to the neurodegenerative nature of the disease.

Conclusions

PBMT is an innovative treatment strategy for a wide range of injures and diseases of the peripheral and CNSs. Its therapeutic effects have been demonstrated in numerous preclinical studies using animal models of neurological diseases, peripheral nerve injuries, pain relief, and brain and spinal cord injuries. These data, alongside that of the daily clinical experiences of colleagues utilizing this modality, provide strong evidence for the use of PBMT in veterinary practice for treatment of the nervous system. The benefits of PBMT for nervous system disorders include: a noninvasive, nonpharmacological treatment choice, a possible therapy for difficult clinical problems without proven and effective therapies, an adjunct alongside other best practices (including rehabilitation therapy), and lack of reported side effects in preclinical animal models. Without the limitations faced by the regulation of human medicine, veterinarians in clinical practice and academia can take the lead in using PBMT on nervous system disorders and demonstrating its potential as an effective treatment for difficult clinical problems with no current solutions.

References

Alcântara, C.C. *et al.* (2013). Effect of low-level laser therapy (LLLT) on acute neural recovery and inflammation-related gene expression after crush injury in rat sciatic nerve. *Lasers Surg Med.* 45:246–252.

Alexandratou, E. *et al.* (2002). Human fibroblast alterations induced by low power laser irradiation at the single cell level using confocal microscopy. *Photochem Photobiol Sci.* 1:547–552.

Almer, G. *et al.* (1999). Inducible nitric oxide synthase upregulation in a transgenic mouse model of familial amyotrophic lateral sclerosis. *J Neurochem.* 72:2415–2425.

Anders, J.J. *et al.* (1993). Low power laser irradiation alters the rate of regeneration of the rat facial nerve. *Lasers Surg Med.* 13:72–82.

Anders, J.J. *et al.* (2004). Phototherapy promotes regeneration and functional recovery of injured peripheral nerve. *Neurol Res.* 26:233–239.

Anders, J.J. *et al.* (2014). In vitro and in vivo optimization of infrared laser treatment for injured peripheral nerves. *Lasers Surg Med.* 46:34–45.

Averill, D.R. Jr. (1973). Degenerative myelopathy in the aging German Shepherd dog: clinical and pathologic findings. *J Am Vet Med Assoc.* 162:1045–1051.

Barrett, D.W. and Gonzalez-Lima, F. (2013). Transcranial infrared laser stimulation produces beneficial cognitive and emotional effects in humans. *Neuroscience.* 230:13–23.

Bennaim, M. *et al.* (2017). Preliminary evaluation of the effects of photobiomodulation therapy and physical rehabilitation on early postoperative recovery of dogs undergoing hemilaminectomy for treatment of thoracolumbar intervertebral disk disease. *Am J Vet Res.* 78:195–206.

Bennett, J., Das, J. M. & Emmady, P. D. (2024). *Spinal Cord Injuries.* Treasure Island, FL: StatPearls. Copyright © 2024, StatPearls Publishing LLC.

Bertolini, G.R. *et al.* (2011). Low-level laser therapy, at 830 nm, for pain reduction in experimental model of rats with sciatica. *Arquivos de Neuro-Psiquiatria.* 69:356–359.

Brisson, B.A. (2010). Intervertebral disc disease in dogs. *Vet Clin N Am: Small Anim Pract.* 40:829–858.

Bruno, E. *et al.* (2020). Perilesional photobiomodulation therapy and physical rehabilitation in post-operative recovery of dogs surgically treated for thoracolumbar disk extrusion. *BMC Vet Res.* 16:120.

Byrnes, K.R. *et al.* (2005). Light promotes regeneration and functional recovery and alters the immune response after spinal cord injury. *Lasers Surg Med.* 36:171–185.

Ceranoglu, T.A. *et al.* (2022). Transcranial photobiomodulation in adults with high-functioning autism spectrum disorder: positive findings from a Proof-of-Concept Study. *Photobiomodul Photomed Laser Surg.* 40:4–12.

Chan, A.S. *et al.* (2019). Photobiomodulation improves the frontal cognitive function of older adults. *Inter J Geriat Psychi.* 34:369–377.

Chapagain, D. *et al.* (2018). Cognitive aging in dogs. *Gerontology.* 64:165–171.

Chen, Y.-J. *et al.* (2014). Effect of low level laser therapy on chronic compression of the dorsal root ganglion. *PLoS One.* 9:e89894–undefined.

Clemmons, R.M. (1989). Degenerative myelopathy. In: *Current Veterinary Therapy X Small Animal Practice.* (ed. R.W. Kirk). W.B. Saunders Company, Philadelphia.

Coates, J.R. and Wininger, F.A. (2010). Canine degenerative myelopathy. *Vet Clin N Am: Small Anim Pract.* 40:929–950.

Da Luz Eltchechem, C. *et al.* (2017). Transcranial LED therapy on amyloid-β toxin 25-35 in the hippocampal region of rats. *Lasers Med Sci.* 32:749–756.

De La Torre, J.C. (2017). Treating cognitive impairment with transcranial low level laser therapy. *J Photochem Photobiol, B.* 168:149–155.

De Taboada, L. *et al.* (2011). Transcranial laser therapy attenuates amyloid-β peptide neuropathology in amyloid-β protein precursor transgenic mice. *J Alzheimers Dis.* 23:521–535.

Dewey, C.W. *et al.* (2022). Transcranial photobiomodulation (laser) therapy for cognitive impairment: a review of molecular mechanisms and potential application to canine cognitive dysfunction (CCD). *Open Vet J.* 12:256–263.

Dewey, C.W. *et al.* (2019). Canine cognitive dysfunction: pathophysiology, diagnosis, and treatment. *Vet Clin N Am: Small Anim Pract.* 49:477–499.

Draper, W.E. *et al.* (2012). Low-level laser therapy reduces time to ambulation in dogs after hemilaminectomy: a preliminary study. *J Small Anim Pract.* 53:465–469.

Dusart, I. and Schwab, M.E. (1994). Secondary cell death and the inflammatory reaction after dorsal hemisection of the rat spinal cord. *Eur J Neurosci.* 6:712–724.

El Massri, N. *et al.* (2016). Near-infrared light treatment reduces astrogliosis in MPTP-treated monkeys. *Exp Brain Res.* 234:3225–3232.

Enengl, J. *et al.* (2020). Photobiomodulation for Alzheimer's disease: translating basic research to clinical application. *J Alzheimers Dis.* 75:1073–1082.

Evans, G.R. (2000). Challenges to nerve regeneration. *Sem in Surg Oncol.* 19:312–318.

Fellin, C.R. *et al.* (2024). Photobiomodulation and vascularization in conduit-based peripheral nerve repair: a narrative review. *Photobiomodul Photomed Laser Surg.* 42:1–10.

Fitch, M.T. *et al.* (1999). Cellular and molecular mechanisms of glial scarring and progressive cavitation: in vivo and in vitro analysis of inflammation-induced secondary injury after CNS trauma. *J Neurosci.* 19:8182–8198.

Gage, E.D. (1975). Incidence of clinical disc disease in the dog. *J Am Anim Hosp Assoc.* 11:135–138.

Godine, R. (2017). Neurological Conditions. In: *Laser Therapy in Veterinary Medicine: Photobiomodulation.* (ed. R.J.R.A.J. C. Godbold). John Wiley and Sons Ltd, Chichester.

Gonzalez-Lima, F. *et al.* (2014). Mitochondrial respiration as a target for neuroprotection and cognitive enhancement. *Biochem Pharmacol.* 88:584–593.

Gouveia, D. *et al.* (2024). Early intensive neurorehabilitation in traumatic peripheral nerve injury-state of the art. *Animals (Basel).* 14(6):884.

Haidet-Phillips, A.M. *et al.* (2011). Astrocytes from familial and sporadic ALS patients are toxic to motor neurons. *Nat Biotechnol.* 29:824–828.

Hamblin, M.R. (2016). Shining light on the head: Photobiomodulation for brain disorders. *BBA Clin.* 6:113–124.

Hamblin, M.R. (2019). Photobiomodulation for Alzheimer's disease: has the light dawned? *Photonics.* 6.

Hamblin, M.R. (2024). Transcranial photobiomodulation for the brain: a wide range of clinical applications. *Neural Regener Res.* 19:483–484.

Hansen, H.J. (1951). A pathologic-anatomical interpretation of disc degeneration in dogs. *Acta Orthopaedica Scandinavica*. 20:280–293.

Hensley, K. *et al.* (2006). Primary glia expressing the G93A-SOD1 mutation present a neuroinflammatory phenotype and provide a cellular system for studies of glial inflammation. *J Neuroinflamm*. 3:2.

Hsieh, Y.L. *et al.* (2012). Low-level laser therapy alleviates neuropathic pain and promotes function recovery in rats with chronic constriction injury: possible involvements in hypoxia-inducible factor 1alpha (HIF-1alpha). *J Comp Neurol*. 520:2903–2916.

Huang, N. *et al.* (2020). Safety and efficacy of 630-nm red light on cognitive function in older adults with mild to moderate Alzheimer's disease: protocol for a randomized controlled study. *Front Aging Neurosci*. 12:143.

Hwang, M.H. *et al.* (2015). Low level light therapy modulates inflammatory mediators secreted by human annulus fibrosus cells during intervertebral disc degeneration in vitro. *Photochem Photobiol*. 91:403–410.

Iaccarino, H.F. *et al.* (2016). Gamma frequency entrainment attenuates amyloid load and modifies microglia. *Nature*. 540:230–235.

Ilic, S. *et al.* (2006). Effects of power densities, continuous and pulse frequencies, and number of sessions of low-level laser therapy on intact rat brain. *Photomed Laser Surg*. 24:458–466.

Inzana, K.D. (2000). Peripheral Nerve Disorders. In: *Textbook of Veterinary Internal Medicine*, 5 edn. Saunders, Philadelphia, PA.

Iosifescu, D.V. *et al.* (2023a). Grant report on the transcranial near infrared radiation and cerebral blood flow in depression (TRIADE) Study. *Photonics*. 10:90.

Iosifescu, D.V. *et al.* (2022). Very low-level transcranial photobiomodulation for major depressive disorder: the ELATED-3 multicenter, randomized, sham-controlled trial. *J Clin Psychia*. 83(5):21.

Iosifescu, D.V. *et al.* (2023b). Protocol report on the transcranial photobiomodulation for Alzheimer's disease (TRAP-AD) Study. *Healthcare (Basel)*. 11(14):2017.

Karu, T. (1999). Primary and secondary mechanisms of action of visible to near-IR radiation on cells. *J Photochem Photobiol, B*. 49:1–17.

Kathmann, I. *et al.* (2006). Daily controlled physiotherapy increases survival time in dogs with suspected degenerative myelopathy. *J Vet Intern Med*. 20:927–932.

Kobiela Ketz, A. *et al.* (2017). Characterization of macrophage/microglial activation and effect of photobiomodulation in the spared nerve injury model of neuropathic pain. *Pain Med*. 18:932–946.

Kono, T. *et al.* (1993). Cord dorsum potentials suppressed by low power laser irradiation on a peripheral nerve in the cat. *J Clin Laser Med and Surg*. 11:115–118.

Lampl, Y. *et al.* (2007). Infrared laser therapy for ischemic stroke: a new treatment strategy: results of the NeuroThera Effectiveness and Safety Trial-1 (NEST-1). *Stroke*. 38:1843–1849.

Landsberg, G.M. *et al.* (2011). Clinical signs and management of anxiety, sleeplessness, and cognitive dysfunction in the senior pet. *Vet Clin N Am: Small Anim Pract*. 41:565–590.

Landsberg, G.M. *et al.* (2012). Cognitive dysfunction syndrome: a disease of canine and feline brain aging. *Vet Clin N Am: Small Anim Pract*. 42(749-68):vii.

Lee, J. *et al.* (2009). Differential regulation of neuronal and inducible nitric oxide synthase (NOS) in the spinal cord of mutant SOD1 (G93A) ALS mice. *Biochem Biophys Res Commun*. 387:202–206.

Lin, C.L. *et al.* (2012). Glutamate transporter EAAT2: a new target for the treatment of neurodegenerative diseases. *Future Med Chem*. 4:1689–1700.

Lu, Y. *et al.* (2017). Low-level laser therapy for beta amyloid toxicity in rat hippocampus. *Neurobiol Aging*. 49:165–182.

Lubart, R. and Breitbart, H. (2000). Biostimulative effects of low-energy lasers and their implications for medicine. *Drug Dev Res*. 50:471–475.

Lundborg, G. (2002). Enhancing posttraumatic nerve regeneration. *J Periph Nerv Sys*. 7:139–140.

Lychagov, V.V. *et al.* (2006). Experimental study of NIR transmittance of the human skull. In: *Proceedings of SPIE - The International Society for Optical Engineering*, p. 6085. SPIE. doi:10.1117/12.650116.

Macias, C. *et al.* (2002). Thoracolumbar disc disease in large dogs: a study of 99 cases. *J Small Anim Pract*. 43:439–446.

Manteca, X. (2011). Nutrition and behavior in senior dogs. *Topics in Companion Animal Medicine*. 26(1):33–36. doi:10.1053/j.tcam.2011.01.003.

Mariani, C.L. (2010). Peripheral Nerve Disorders. In: *Textbook of Veterinary Internal Medicine*, 7 edn. Elsevier, St. Louis, MO.

Masoumipoor, M. *et al.* (2014). Effects of 660- and 980-nm low-level laser therapy on neuropathic pain relief following chronic constriction injury in rat sciatic nerve. *Lasers Med Sci*. 29:1593–1598.

Mcgee, C. *et al.* (2023). A randomized placebo-controlled study of a transcranial photobiomodulation helmet in Parkinson's Disease: post-hoc analysis of motor outcomes. *J Clin Med*. 12(8):2846.

Miller, L.A. *et al.* (2020). Retrospective observational study and analysis of two different photobiomodulation therapy protocols combined with rehabilitation therapy as therapeutic interventions for canine degenerative myelopathy. *Photobiomodul Photomed Laser Surg*. 38:195–205.

Millis, D.L. *et al.* (2005). Emerging modalities in veterinary rehabilitation. *Vet Clin N Am: Small Anim Pract*. 35:1335–1355, viii.

Moges, H. *et al.* (2009). Light therapy and supplementary Riboflavin in the SOD1 transgenic mouse model of familial amyotrophic lateral sclerosis (FALS). *Lasers Surg Med.* 41:52–59.

Moges, H. *et al.* (2011). Effect of 810 nm light on nerve regeneration after autograft repair of severely injured rat median nerve. *Lasers Surg Med.* 43:901–906.

Moore, S.A. (2016). Managing neuropathic pain in dogs. *Front Vet Sci.* 3:12.

Naeser, M.A. *et al.* (2016). Transcranial, red/near-infrared light-emitting diode therapy to improve cognition in chronic traumatic brain injury. *Photomed Laser Surg.* 34:610–626.

Naeser, M.A. *et al.* (2014). Significant improvements in cognitive performance post-transcranial, red/near-infrared light-emitting diode treatments in chronic, mild traumatic brain injury: open-protocol study. *J Neurotrauma.* 31:1008–1017.

Ogawa, M. *et al.* (2011). Immunohistochemical observation of canine degenerative myelopathy in two Pembroke Welsh Corgi dogs. *J Vet Med Sci.* 73:1275–1279.

Ogawa, M. *et al.* (2014). Neuronal loss and decreased GLT-1 expression observed in the spinal cord of Pembroke Welsh Corgi dogs with canine degenerative myelopathy. *Vet Pathol.* 51:591–602.

Oron, A. *et al.* (2006). Low-level laser therapy applied transcranially to rats after induction of stroke significantly reduces long-term neurological deficits. *Stroke.* 37:2620–2624.

Oron, A. *et al.* (2012). Near infrared transcranial laser therapy applied at various modes to mice following traumatic brain injury significantly reduces long-term neurological deficits. *J Neurotrauma.* 29:401–407.

Ozawa, M. *et al.* (2016). The Relation between canine cognitive dysfunction and age-related brain lesions. *J Vet Med Sci.* 78:997–1006.

Pallanti, S. *et al.* (2022). Transcranial photobiomodulation for the Treatment of Children with Autism Spectrum Disorder (ASD): a Retrospective Study. *Children (Basel).* 9.

Pardo, A.C. *et al.* (2006). Loss of the astrocyte glutamate transporter GLT1 modifies disease in SOD1(G93A) mice. *Exp Neurol.* 201:120–130.

Phul, R.K. *et al.* (2000). Expression of nitric oxide synthase isoforms in spinal cord in amyotrophic lateral sclerosis. *Amyotrop Lat Sclerosis and Other Motor Neuron Dis.* 1:259–267.

Piao, D. *et al.* (2017). Challenges of transcutaneous laser application for the potential of photobiomodulation of the spinal cord at the scale of a large companion animal. *Proc. SPIE, Mechanisms of Photobiomodulation Therapy XII.* 10048(17 February):10048M. doi:10.1117/12.2248164.

Piao, D. *et al.* (2018). Flexible nine-channel photodetector probe facilitated intraspinal multisite transcutaneous photobiomodulation therapy dosimetry in cadaver dogs. *J Biomed Opt.* 23:1–4.

Pigatto, G.R. *et al.* (2020). Low-intensity photobiomodulation decreases neuropathic pain in paw Ischemia-Reperfusion and spared nervus ischiadicus injury experimental models. *Pain Pract.* 20:371–386.

Polizopoulou, Z.S. *et al.* (2008). Evaluation of a proposed therapeutic protocol in 12 dogs with tentative degenerative myelopathy. *Acta Veterinaria Hungarica.* 56:293–301.

Popovich, P.G. *et al.* (2002). The neuropathological and behavioral consequences of intraspinal microglial/macrophage activation. *J Neuropathol Exp Neurol.* 61:623–633.

Recknor, J.B. *et al.* (2006). Nerve regeneration: tissue engineering strategies. In: *The Biomedical Engineering Handbook: Tissue Engineering and Artificial Organs.* Taylor & Francis, New York.

Rochkind, S. (1978). Stimulation effect of laser energy on the regeneration of traumatically injured peripheral nerves. *Morphogen Regen.* 83:25–27.

Rochkind, S. (2009). Phototherapy in peripheral nerve regeneration: from basic science to clinical study. *Neurosurgical Focus.* 26:E8.

Rochkind, S. (2023). Phototherapy (photobiomodulation) for peripheral nerve and muscle injury. *Laser Ther.* 30 (10):4081.

Rochkind, S. *et al.* (2007). Laser phototherapy (780 nm), a new modality in treatment of long-term incomplete peripheral nerve injury: a randomized double-blind placebo-controlled study. *Photomed Laser Surg.* 25:436–442.

Rochkind, S. and Ouaknine, G.E. (1992). New trend in neuroscience: low-power laser effect on peripheral and central nervous system (basic science, preclinical and clinical studies). *Neurol Res.* 14:2–11.

Rodkey, W.G. and Sharp, N.J.H. (2003). Surgery of the Peripheral Nervous Sytem. In: *Textbook of Small Animal Surgery*, 3 edn. Elsevier, Philadelphia, PA.

Salehpour, F. *et al.* (2019). Transcranial photobiomodulation improves cognitive performance in young healthy adults: a systematic review and meta-analysis. *Photobiomodul Photomed Laser Surg.* 37:635–643.

Saltmarche, A.E. *et al.* (2017). Significant improvement in cognition in mild to moderately severe dementia cases treated with transcranial plus intranasal photobiomodulation: case series report. *Photomed Laser Surg.* 35:432–441.

Sasaki, S. *et al.* (2000). iNOS and nitrotyrosine immunoreactivity in amyotrophic lateral sclerosis. *Neurosci Lett.* 291:44–48.

Schiffer, F. *et al.* (2009). Psychological benefits 2 and 4 weeks after a single treatment with near infrared light to the forehead: a pilot study of 10 patients with major depression and anxiety. *Behav Brain Funct.* 5:46.

Sims, C. *et al.* (2015). Rehabilitation and physical therapy for the neurologic veterinary patient. *Vet Clin N Am: Small Anim Pract.* 45:123–143.

Snyder, S.K. *et al.* (2002). Quantitation of calcitonin gene-related peptide mRNA and neuronal cell death in facial motor nuclei following axotomy and 633 nm low power laser treatment. *Lasers Surg Med.* 31:216–222.

Spera, V. *et al.* (2021). Pilot study on dose-dependent effects of transcranial photobiomodulation on brain electrical oscillations: a potential therapeutic target in Alzheimer's disease. *J Alzheimers Dis.* 83:1481–1498.

Standring, S. (2020). *Gray's Anatomy, 42nd Edition. The Anatomical Basis of Clinical Practice.* Elsevier, Amsterdam.

Sun, J. *et al.* (2020). Photobiomodulation therapy inhibit the activation and secretory of astrocytes by altering macrophage polarization. *Cell Mol Neurobiol.* 40:141–152.

Tao, L. *et al.* (2021). Microglia modulation with 1070-nm light attenuates Aβ burden and cognitive impairment in Alzheimer's disease mouse model. *Light Sci Appl.* 10:179.

Tedford, C.E. *et al.* (2015). Quantitative analysis of transcranial and intraparenchymal light penetration in human cadaver brain tissue. *Lasers Surg Med.* 47:312–322.

Tian, F. *et al.* (2016). Transcranial laser stimulation improves human cerebral oxygenation. *Lasers Surg Med.* 48:343–349.

Trotti, D. *et al.* (2001). Amyotrophic lateral sclerosis-linked glutamate transporter mutant has impaired glutamate clearance capacity. *J Biol Chem.* 276:576–582.

Von Leden, R.E. *et al.* (2013). 808 nm wavelength light induces a dose-dependent alteration in microglial polarization and resultant microglial induced neurite growth. *Lasers Surg Med.* 45:253–263.

Ward, L.M. (2003). Synchronous neural oscillations and cognitive processes. *Trends Cognit Sci.* 7:553–559.

Welch, J.A. (1996). Peripheral nerve injury. *Semin Vet Med Surg Small Anim.* 11:273–284.

Wu, X. *et al.* (2009). 810 nm Wavelength light: an effective therapy for transected or contused rat spinal cord. *Lasers Surg Med.* 41:36–41.

Xuan, W. *et al.* (2013). Transcranial low-level laser therapy improves neurological performance in traumatic brain injury in mice: effect of treatment repetition regimen. *PLoS One.* 8:e53454.

Yang, X. *et al.* (2010). Low energy laser light (632.8 nm) suppresses amyloid-β peptide-induced oxidative and inflammatory responses in astrocytes. *Neuroscience.* 171:859–868.

Yue, X. *et al.* (2019). New insight into Alzheimer's disease: light reverses Aβ-obstructed interstitial fluid flow and ameliorates memory decline in APP/PS1 mice. *Alzheimers Dement (N Y).* 5:671–684.

Zhang, Z. *et al.* (2020). Activation of PKA/SIRT1 signaling pathway by photobiomodulation therapy reduces Aβ levels in Alzheimer's disease models. *Aging Cell.* 19:e13054.

Zhang, Z. *et al.* (2023). Photobiomodulation reduces neuropathic pain after spinal cord injury by downregulating CXCL10 expression. *CNS Neurosci Ther.* 29:3995–4017.

17

Laser Therapy for the Geriatric Patient

Erin O'Leary

HEAL Mobile Veterinary Laser Therapy, Cary, NC, USA

1st Edition Contributor:

Dianne Adjan Logan

Wilmington Animal Fitness & Rehabilitation Center at Needham Animal Hospital, Wilmington, NC, USA

Introduction

Geriatric pets make up a steadily growing population in veterinary medicine due to improved veterinary care, innovations in technology, and our ability as practitioners to catch diseases earlier in their progression. A growing population of older pets means more companion animals are suffering from age-related conditions, including organ failure, malignancies, joint disease, and cognitive deterioration. In the United States, nearly 45% of dog owners and 46% of cat owners have a pet of age 7 years or older (PR Newswire, 2016).

It is imperative that we offer the most comprehensive treatment and maintenance options for this expanding population of patients as they age. Though we cannot prevent the process of aging, we are responsible for recognizing and minimizing its effects (both physical and cognitive) on our patients' quality of life and their relationships with their families (AVMA, 2016). The purpose of this chapter is to illustrate the use and benefits of laser therapy in senior geriatric pets and offer tools to deal with this very specific and unique subset of patients. We will discuss why the introduction of laser therapy into senior protocols can be particularly rewarding and look at some special approaches that should be taken with aging patients (Rodier, 2016).

Laser therapy, now called photobiomodulation therapy (PBMT), is one tool in a growing arsenal of methods for providing the best care for our patients. This mode of therapy, along with a focused and appropriate pain medication regimen, utilization of physical and alternative therapy options, and, most importantly, a thorough evaluation of each individual patient, allows us to provide an optimal strategy for meeting our patients' health needs. We will not go into detail in this chapter about other therapies available to treat chronic pain, skin, and inflammatory conditions, but it is important to note that any of them can be used in conjunction with laser therapy.

Geriatric animals are generally defined as 7 years old and above, though this varies according to breed and species. Most such pets have been in the home for a long time and have established a strong bond with their families. Though recent studies attempt to show that cats have less secure attachment bonds (Potter and Mills, 2015) than are reported for dogs (Payne *et al.,* 2016), both species, as well as other companion animals, become well-loved family members. It therefore is crucial that you treat a senior pet with the same focus and attention that you do a new puppy whose owners are looking to you as the expert. The senior portion of life comes with a similar, if not increased, number of owner questions and concerns.

Utilizing PBMT not only provides a new option for concerned and invested pet owners but also allows them time during treatment sessions to discuss concerns, progress, and plans for their pet. The veterinarian's role in clients' decisions regarding their pets, particularly when those pets are geriatric or seriously ill, is dependent on open communication and good models of shared decision-making (Christiansen *et al.,* 2016). These sessions are optimal for the veterinarian as caregiver to see their patients on a regular basis and allow time for dialogue, questions, and observations of any new conditions that might arise.

Though many of the benefits of laser therapy can be applied to the general population, some are specific and

Laser Therapy in Veterinary Medicine: Photobiomodulation, Second Edition. Edited by Christopher J. Winkler and Lisa A. Miller.

advantageous to an aging population. These include maintaining mobility and a sense of security, preserving patients' status as family members, and managing and resolving long-term conditions (particularly those that can otherwise result in isolation for these pets).

As a mobile practitioner performing the majority of my patients' treatments in their own homes, I have some additional suggestions and insights, the details of which can also be of use in your practice location and applied to your laser protocols.

Important PBM Effects in Geriatric Patient Management

Before we begin discussing the specific approaches to treating senior pets with laser therapy, it is worth mentioning the cellular effects of PBM that can help counteract some of the natural degeneration of physiological processes within geriatric patients' bodies.

Application of PBMT to impaired tissue results in a number of complex and well-documented effects. The mechanisms of PBM are detailed in Chapter 3, as well as in other publications (Pryor and Millis, 2015). When considering the application of laser therapy to the specific needs of geriatric patients, a number of those mechanisms are important.

Increased Cellular Energy

PBM stimulates the production of adenosine triphosphate (ATP) in damaged and impaired cells (Hamblin and Demidova, 2006). In aging patients, this interaction can lead to healthier, more normalized cells and tissue via increased growth factor production and cellular metabolism.

Increased Blood Flow and Circulation

Vasodilation and improved circulation result in increased oxygenation of tissues, decreased effects of exposure to environmental and physical stressors, and improved response to chronic inflammation (Maegawa *et al.*, 2000).

Improved Neural Tissue Effects

As animals age, nerve cells die and are not replaced. In some cases, nerve cells malfunction or their nerve potentials or communication capabilities are altered. PBM can affect the conduction of neurotransmitters, assist in the repair of damaged nerves, and aid in the normalization of nerve potentials, leading to decreased pain sensitivity (Cambier *et al.*, 2000; Chow *et al.*, 2011; Farivar *et al.*, 2014).

Decreased Inflammation

Many geriatric patients have diseases associated with the aging process that involves chronic inflammatory changes. Dental disease, arthritis, neurological deterioration, and chronic skin inflammation are common. Prolonged inflammation can lead to a progressive destruction of the affected tissue and incite further inflammatory activity. PBM has a direct effect on the reduction of negative inflammatory processes (Cotler *et al.*, 2015; Huang *et al.*, 2015).

Improved Healing

Healing tissue fibers align themselves in a more linear and uniform direction when exposed to therapy laser light. Scarring is reduced and tissue strength improves. As aging progresses, tissues lose elasticity and become more prone to injury. PBM contributes to normal healing and can help prevent injuries by improving tissue flexibility and elasticity (Medrado *et al.*, 2003; Peplow *et al.*, 2010; Tabakoglu *et al.*, 2015; Kuffler, 2016).

Improved Serotonin and Endorphin Release

Older pets have a decreased ability to cope with stress and can experience behavioral changes, including aggression, noise phobias, and increased anxiety. PBM can help support the natural secretion of serotonin and endorphins, which can make pets feel better, happier, and less anxious (Labajos, 1988; Montesinos, 1988; Ceylan *et al.*, 2004; Hagiwara *et al.*, 2007, 2008).

Utilization of Laser Therapy in Geriatric Patients

As they have earned their place in our homes and hearts, geriatric patients come with years of ingrained desires, needs, and peculiarities that we as practitioners need to take into consideration when we initiate a laser therapy session with them. This section details some of those considerations, provides tools to deal with them, and assists in creating an ideal environment for treatment.

Communication

Learn Who Is Under the Handpiece

First, get to know your patient. Who is this creature that will be under your handpiece? Often, you are starting a new relationship, and it helps to know a bit about your new partner. Have a thorough conversation with the pet's owner to get a good understanding of who it is. What are its idiosyncrasies, preferences, or special needs? Administering laser therapy treatments to geriatric patients is unique for most veterinarians, technicians, and nurses, since it involves a relatively long one-on-one contact time with patients who are not sedated or under anesthesia. Taking special care to learn all you can about the patient and the owner will contribute significantly toward a successful (and peaceful) treatment. Learn from the owner and from personal observation what the patient might take as an act of aggression. Note the patient's level of sensitivity to loud noises. Confirm with the owner whether the patient's shaking is typical or if it demonstrates a high degree of nervousness. All are valuable pieces of information that can help make everyone involved more comfortable and avoid patient aggression as the laser therapy treatment session begins.

Make the Owner a Partner in the Initial Treatment

I recommend allowing the pet owner to be present for at least the first treatment session so they can apprise you of the aforementioned information and learn exactly what takes place during a session, which will increase their own (and their pet's) comfort level. In addition, this is a wonderful opportunity for you to discuss senior care, any issues they have noted, and any concerns they have. It also gives you a chance to talk with the pet owner about their bond with their pet. This will give you a very good idea of what they are looking for in terms of care and guidance, and may even open the door to future discussion of their inevitable loss as their pet continues to age.

It is rare for veterinarians to have such uninterrupted quiet time in person with clients in such a positive and relaxing environment. Collaborating with the client and your technician or nurse in the first treatment session can ensure all members of the pet care team are on the same page. As further treatments sessions ensue, I recommend maintaining a progress log, noting the observations of the therapist as well as the pet owner. This will help you catch any subtle changes, positive results, or new concerns. I often find that we get one geriatric problem under control when another starts to develop. Consistent monitoring and follow-up are beneficial to all involved. Maintaining a log ensures that with each visit you are getting a true update.

The time during a laser treatment is ideal for discussions about geriatric health care topics like nutrition, weight, activity level, home environment, and supplementation. You have a captive audience and the focus is on you and the patient, your senior health care management plan, and your recommendations for the patient and owner. This is a time for delivering care, for strengthening the veterinarian-client-patient relationship, and for marketing to your current and future geriatric pet owners.

Communicate Clear Expectations

When working with geriatric patients, it is critical to discuss with the owners what their expectations are for their pet. While their pet ages, we can give them the tools they need to measure the aging process and help them take appropriate actions to improve their pet's quality of life. Laser therapy can help geriatric pets be more mobile and get them moving more comfortably. This is an incredibly beneficial element, both psychologically and physically. Exercising, walking, running, and playing are among the biggest connections pets have with their owners, and increased function and mobility will help maintain their emotional bond. In addition, laser therapy will help decrease the frequency of other unpleasant events like bed sores, accidents in the house, and skin issues, all of which can put a distance between a pet and its owners.

It is important to communicate that laser therapy is not a magic wand, however. Owner expectations should be reasonable. Laser therapists need to be clear about what this technology can and cannot achieve: age-related bone changes will not be reversed, but the associated pain and inflammation can be reduced. Managing expectations for owners is important when working with geriatric patients, because their conditions will often have been ongoing for long periods of time. Clients need to understand that changes may be slow and subtle. They need to understand when results take longer to appear and may not as dramatic as they might have hoped. The measure of success with geriatric patients is any improvement, any increase in mobility, function, and quality of life.

Understand the Obstacles Geriatric Pets Experience at Home

As a mobile laser therapy practitioner, I have the fortune of assessing each patient's home environment and having conversations about its bedding, the obstacles to its getting around the house, its traction on hardwood floors, why area rugs may be an issue, and so on. It is important for you to have these same discussions with your geriatric pet owners so that what you accomplish with laser therapy is not reversed by the home environment.

Discuss with owners where problems occur at home. Does the pet avoid parts of the house? Does it have problems making it outside for eliminations? Does it hesitate to use the litter box? Does it no longer get on the bed or sofa? Can it no longer comfortably bend over to eat and drink? Do the owners and the pet spend a lot of time in the car? Where, when, and how do they ride? How do they get in and out? These questions help to identify what the patient's quality of life is like.

Your recommendations concerning options like booties, ramps, orthopedic bedding, lowered litterboxes, harnesses, bed stairs, and raised bowls will assist in improving your patients' quality of life, and demonstrate your partnership in ensuring their success.

Remember, Your Geriatric Pet Owners Are Invested

People who are interested in laser therapy for their geriatric pets will likely be your most engaged and informed clients. In addition to being the most familiar with their particular pet, they will also likely do a lot of investigation and have lots of propositions for alternatives to try. There are many ideas, theories, and products that promise to be the magic solution to a dog's aging problem. Do not disregard their suggestions and thoughts; be their educator, and be open to things they may come up with, while giving them good information about things that may or may not be a waste of their time and money. A large number of my clients report that they asked their primary veterinarians about laser therapy for their pet's arthritis and were dismissed or redirected. You have the opportunity to debunk, inform, and perhaps even learn something new from them.

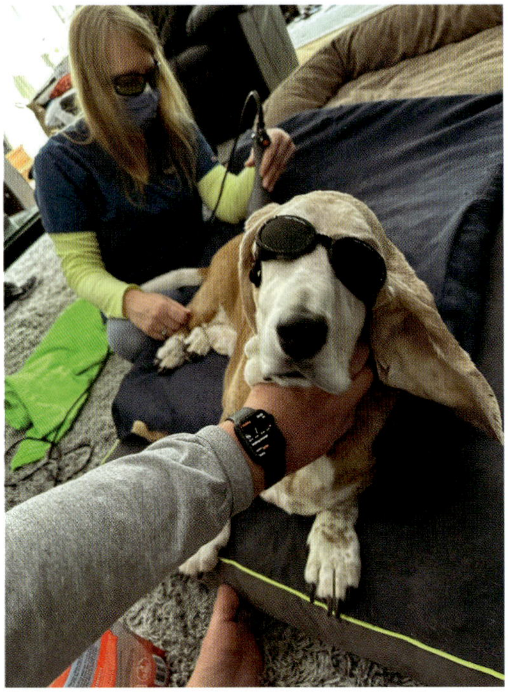

Figure 17.1 Ensure that patients are in a comfortable position during treatment. Smaller patients are frequently more comfortable in your lap rather than on the floor or a table.

Treating Geriatric Patients

Before Treatment Begins

As pets age, they are more likely to have impaired vision and hearing, so it is important to slow your approach, make sure they know you are coming, allow them to acclimate to the sounds the laser might make, and get used to having the handpiece in contact with their body. If pets are noise-sensitive (particularly common in cats), ask the manufacturer if your laser's audio may be reduced or muted, or how best to reduce its noise with some type of cover that still allows normal function of its cooling system. It is ideal to provide comfortable bedding or seating, a pillow for their head, or a tilted back that they can lean on. Ensure that they are in a comfortable position (according to their individual preference) during treatment.

Positioning for Laser Therapy

Laser therapy is generally easier to administer with the pet standing, giving the therapist access to all body surfaces and areas that may need to be treated. In an elderly patient, standing for a prolonged period of time may be uncomfortable or impossible. Create a pleasant, comfortable environment for geriatric patients so that they have an enjoyable experience and a complete treatment can take place. Smaller patients are frequently more comfortable in your lap, rather than on the floor or a table (Figure 17.1). Also, understand that you will likely have multiple areas to treat in an elderly animal. The patient may need to take a break and walk around rather than remain stationary for a long period of time. This applies to lying in one position for a prolonged period also. I find that older pets often have a preferred side that they tend to lie on, often their weaker side. Though getting access to this side can be tricky, it is important to do so. Do not be above using treats and bribery. As a last resort, use gentle repositioning.

Along with positioning, the therapist should also consider the pros and cons of manipulating and putting a joint through its range of motion in pets that are severely arthritic or have pain from chronic conditions. Though it is ideal to treat joints through a passive range of motion when applying laser therapy, a geriatric patient with chronic pain may not allow manipulation of joints. After multiple treatments, pain will reduce and flexibility will increase, and movement through range of motion may be allowed. You will want to monitor and measure these changes in range of motion and flexibility of the joint in order to have an objective measure of the progress you are making. In addition, you want to be very careful when repositioning patients during a treatment session, as they may have become protective of certain areas and they may not be used to being moved. Be gentle, be aware of the patient's responses as you move them, and protect yourself and your assistants from a patient's possible reprisal.

Cats may require more creativity to find a good compromise between position and accessibility, since their body areas are much smaller and more difficult to effectively reach with a laser handpiece. With large animals, unless they are lying down or have placed themselves in a corner or against a wall, accessibility is not typically an issue.

Having an experienced handler present is the general solution, but again, watch for sudden reprisal if positioning upsets the patient.

Adjusting Treatment Protocols

As pets age, they are less able to thermoregulate and may become more temperature-sensitive. This may require you to adjust your treatment protocols for these patients. Discuss with the pet owner whether their pet is heat-seeking or tends to prefer bathroom tiles over their bed. Many pets are sensitive to heat, and you may observe increased panting or a desire to move away from the laser during treatment. Ensure that you are moving the handpiece in an appropriately consistent manner, at the correct speed. Understand that some pets will need to have the power decreased (and time increased) during their treatment. Adapt to what patients will tolerate and make appropriate changes in the therapy laser protocol to ensure that the appropriate dose is being delivered to the tissues.

Also, adjust your protocol depending on whether there has been significant muscle atrophy or a decrease in fat stores. You are more likely to have prominent bony structures in pets with these structural changes, and any contact between the head of the handpiece and bone might be unpleasant and uncomfortable. Measure the areas that you will be treating with a cloth tape and ensure that if you are treating a 40 kg dog, the area you are treating is representative of a 40 kg dog.

Physical Barriers

As pets age and clients become more and more conscientious of their needs, you may have to deal with physical barriers that can cause difficulty during laser therapy treatment sessions. Anxiety-reducing shirts, diapers, walking harnesses, braces, booties, and a variety of bandaging and cast options can be barriers to administering laser therapy. Since our goal is to provide the most comfortable and least stressful environment for treatment, learn to navigate around these barriers.

As mentioned previously, sometimes even the position of the pet can provide an obstacle – particularly if you have a determined patient that is not going to budge from one side or a corner of a room or stall. Be prepared for these situations, work with the owner to have acceptable treats available, and have the owner prepare their pet prior to treatment when possible. Try to avoid spending valuable time having to remove a recently placed bandage or a harness. If it is possible to perform a complete treatment with dog-appeasing pheromone collars, anxiety-reducing shirts, or anxiety wraps in place, then do so.

Incontinence

Many older pets experience urinary or fecal incontinence or both, and this must be taken into account during your treatment session. Often, the treatment itself will cause them to relax (gas is a very common part of my treatment sessions, particularly when I treat the back). Make sure that you are prepared for an accident or the potential need to get up and go outside during treatment. If possible, have the owner take their pet outside prior to the visit so they can relieve themselves. This is especially important for pets that are unable to walk or require assistance to eliminate.

Balancing Concurrent Conditions

By virtue of their age, older patients will likely have been diagnosed with multiple conditions that need to be taken into consideration while treating with laser. Ensure that you have a full understanding of the medications prescribed, the supplements being used, and the medical conditions that have been diagnosed. Knowing whether a patient is on medications or has an underlying condition such as cancer or a bleeding disorder will allow you to ensure that your protocol is well calculated and appropriate. As your treatment progresses, it is also useful to begin eliminating or titrating down pain medications. Having a good method for charting progress allows you to monitor these changes, have a clear idea of what is working, and stay updated on anything else that may be affecting your progress (e.g., a change in medication could cause a backslide that appears to be orthopedic but is in fact weakness secondary to a change in blood pressure medication). It is also imperative to understand previous surgeries that have been performed and any hardware that may still be present.

For a full discussion of the special considerations required when considering PBMT in a patient with a malignancy, see Chapters 5 and 19. When treating an elderly patient, you will need to weigh the benefits it could derive from the laser treatment with the concern of potentially worsening a present neoplastic condition. As 50% of dogs over the age of 10 are diagnosed with cancer, it is common to encounter this dilemma in senior pets. Ensure full disclosure of the risks to the owner and document the conversations you have about the decision to treat. I personally have not observed a perceptible increase in the rate of growth of a known cancer after PBMT. For osteosarcoma in particular, I have found laser therapy to be an invaluable tool in managing pain, but I always ensure that the owners are making an informed decision to proceed with treatment.

Cats, and Other Animals for Which We Have Limited Options

As a population, cats have benefited immensely from laser therapy in the veterinary world. Historically, we either did not identify that cats were in pain or had to accept that if they were in pain, our options were limited. Available treatment options were often relatively difficult to administer to our patients. We are now able to increase their quality of life and avoid exacerbating some of the most common issues that we see in geriatric cats, including kidney disease and gastrointestinal upset. We can address some previously unmanageable conditions, such as stomatitis and nerve pain. As a bonus, we have also discovered a treatment that cats actually enjoy.

Usually no restraint or stressful positioning is required; most cats relax within minutes of initiating treatment, and are often noted to maintain a relaxed state (Figure 17.2). When utilizing laser therapy on cats, it is important to recognize that they are particularly good at masking pain and weakness, and that some of the clinical signs they demonstrate at home will respond to treatment. These include (but are not limited to) decreased activity, aggression, hiding, increased vocalization, pacing at night, changes in litterbox usage, decreased grooming, changes in sleep patterns, changes in eating habits, and self-mutilation. It is important to discuss any changes the owners are noting at home and to chart the cat's progress in these areas.

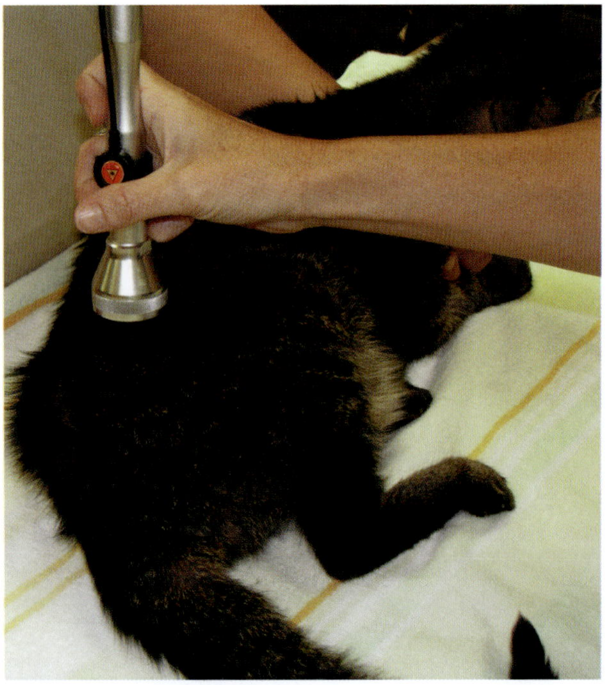

Figure 17.2 Always offer patients a comfortable surface during treatments. Cats usually require no restraint and relax within minutes of initiating treatment. Image courtesy of Dr. John C. Godbold Jr.

Senility

As pets age, they often suffer a decline in mental function. Their memory, their ability to learn, their awareness, and their senses of sight and hearing can all deteriorate. This deterioration can cause disturbances in their sleep–wake cycles, making them restless at night but sleepy during the day. It can make them forget previously learned cues (commands) or habits they once knew well. It can increase their anxiety and any tendency to react aggressively (Landsberg *et al.*, 2011, 2012). It can also change their social relationships with their owners, therapists, and other pets in their home. Some pets may become less interested in affection, petting, or social interaction, while others become more so. It is important to understand these changes as you approach any laser therapy management plan.

Treating senior patients increases the likelihood of dealing with senility or cognitive changes. Be aware that you may have to adjust your protocols accordingly. You may have to slowly familiarize the pet with PBMT, and you may have to do this repeatedly. You may have only short intervals of time during which the pet is accepting of laser therapy, and you may have to break up treatment times. Be watchful of erratic and unpredictable behavior and discuss the items mentioned in this section with the owners so you can educate them on changes in sleep cycles, appetite, self-care, activity levels, relationships, and reactions to strangers or to people and pets they know. (Will they feel better if their "person" is in sight or out of the room? Do they have a special blanket or toy that comforts them? Would an anxiety-reducing shirt or hormone diffuser help relax them during a treatment session?) Try to determine the ideal situation that will make the patient comfortable, both physically and emotionally.

Many of the medications that we use for pain management in aging pets can cause side effects that can be confused with senility. Utilizing laser therapy while minimizing or completely discontinuing the use of these medications can help you monitor the pet's "normal" cognitive state. Since cognitive function is one of the things veterinarians use to determine whether it may be time to recommend euthanasia, it is imperative that the signs are clear and are not based on muddled data and observations (Schütt *et al.*, 2015; Rodier, 2016).

Offering House Calls

As both pet and pet owner populations age, it may be beneficial to your practice to add house calls as an adjunct to your practice-based laser therapy. Transporting large arthritic dogs and uncooperative cats to your hospital for laser therapy may be difficult for a proportion of your clientele, and offering laser therapy at home may increase the number of senior pets being served who otherwise might not be able to utilize laser therapy as an option.

Case Studies

Unilateral Coxofemoral Joint Osteoarthritis in a Feline

Signalment
"Boomer," 12 years old, domestic short hair, MN, 5.5 kg.

Client Complaint
Decreased physical activity and social interaction with family.

History
Boomer had a chondrosarcoma and amputation of his right rear leg at 6 years of age. He was being treated with chemotherapy following surgery for a gastrointestinal adenocarcinoma.

Physical Examination
Physical examination confirmed pain in the left coxofemoral joint.

Laser Therapy Treatment
Boomer's left hip was treated every other day using contact delivery and laser settings that delivered a dosage of 5 J/cm^2. A total of seven treatments were administered.

Outcome
The owner reported in a follow-up email, "You know, one thing I just realized yesterday about Boomer that had not really struck me before is that since you treated him the second time, he's continuously hanging out with the family. For months and months he's gone and laid on our bed during the day, even if I'm at home. But he now just stays in the kitchen or family room with all the dogs all the time." Boomer is a great example of the opportunity for laser therapy and pain management to affect the human–animal bond and increase patient well-being.

Multiple-Joint Osteoarthritis in a Sheep

Signalment
"Angus," 14 years old, sheep, M.

Client Complaint
Increased difficulty in getting up and down and in moving about to graze.

History
Angus had previously been diagnosed with arthritis in the hocks and stifles. He also had chronic renal disease and was undergoing symptomatic treatment.

Physical Examination
A physical examination confirmed pain and reduced range of motion bilaterally in Angus's hocks and stifles.

Laser Therapy Treatment
A twice-weekly schedule of laser therapy treatments was initiated. The affected areas (bilateral hocks and stifles) were treated with a contact method and laser settings delivering a dosage of 20 J/cm^2 per area. Angus responded well to laser therapy, so treatments were continued long-term. At the time of writing, he has received 34 treatments. He also received acupuncture treatments.

Outcome
Angus showed increased mobility and the ability to get up on his own. Being able to stay mobile and graze was critical to his life on the farm. Angus was able to continue walking and to maintain muscle tone, and the potential for muscle atrophy and infections due to inactivity and pressure sores was decreased.

Though these changes can be dramatic in larger animals, this point is also very applicable to our smaller patients in terms of their ability to maintain muscle mass, mobility, and flexibility. Though we feel it is normal for our older patients to sleep more and be less active, keeping exercise (though perhaps shorter and less vigorous) as a mainstay of their daily schedule is crucial to their vitality and their ability to stay healthy and active for as long as possible.

Multiple-Joint Osteoarthritis in a Canine

Signalment
"Caleb," 10 years old, border collie mix, MN, 28 kg

Client Complaint
Caleb was previously an energetic dog who loved hiking, swimming, and outdoor activity. By 9 years of age, he had developed severe signs of arthritis and had slowed down substantially.

History
Caleb's regular veterinarian had diagnosed osteoarthritis of the stifles, hips, and lumbar spine.

Physical Examination
A physical examination confirmed pain and limited range of motion in both stifles and hips, and pain on deep palpation of Caleb's lumbar area.

Laser Therapy Treatment
Initial laser therapy treatments were administered every other day. Caleb was treated using on-contact delivery with

laser settings that delivered dosages of 20 J/cm^2 to his stifles, 23 J/cm^2 to his hips, and 25 J/cm^2 to his lumbar and sacral regions. After the fourth treatment, they were tapered to once a week, and then once every 2 weeks.

A total of seven treatments were administered, and then Caleb's family moved and laser therapy was continued at their new location.

Outcome

After treatments were initiated, Caleb quickly began to show an increase in activity levels, improved ability to walk up and down stairs, and renewed pleasure in playing with human and animal family members. His range of motion increased in both hips, and he demonstrated less pain on extension of his stifles.

Caleb had a very positive physical response to laser therapy. He also demonstrated an interesting psychological response to the treatment sessions. For the first two treatments, we moved Caleb's dog bed into the den to separate him from the other pets in the house during his treatment time. During both of these sessions, he displayed visible anxiety and paced around the room between treatments of each affected body area. When I arrived for the next treatment and began discussing his progress with his owner, we observed him pulling his bed into the den! We began treating him in the den, and from that point on, his anxiety level was decreased and he relaxed during his treatment sessions.

Multiple-Joint Osteoarthritis in a Canine with Chronic Renal Disease

Signalment

"Bitsy," 15 years old, cavalier King Charles spaniel, FS, 5.5 kg.

Client Complaint

Reduced activity and inability to move around comfortably.

History

Bitsy's regular veterinarian had identified severe osteoarthritis in her stifles, hips, shoulders, and spine. Bitsy had chronic renal disease, which was stable. She was unable to take any nonsteroidal anti-inflammatory drugs (NSAIDs). She did not tolerate other pain management options well, in terms of the effect on both her behavior and her gastrointestinal system.

Physical Examination

A physical examination confirmed pain and reduced range of motion in Bitsy's stifles, hips, and shoulders, and pain on deep palpation of her spine.

Laser Therapy Treatment

Laser therapy was initiated with every-other-day treatments. The treatments were administered using a contact delivery technique and dosages of 7 J/cm^2 to the stifles, 8 J/cm^2 to the shoulders and hips, and 10 J/cm^2 to the spine. After 2 weeks of every-other-day treatments, Bitsy was tapered to once-a-week treatments. Long-term, she received a total of 84 treatments.

Outcome

Bitsy showed improved mobility, a visible decrease in pain responses on palpation and manipulation of her joints, and increased barking when I came to the house.

Laser therapy substantially decreased her level of pain and gave her a reprieve from a decision to euthanize that her owners had been reluctantly considering. Due to the improvement in her ability to walk and function, Bitsy was afforded another year and a half with her family.

Multiple-Joint Osteoarthritis in an Aged Canine

Signalment

"Jelly," 17 years old, beagle, FS, 15.5 kg.

History

Jelly had a history of gradual reduction of musculoskeletal function and increased disability in getting about. Her regular veterinarian had diagnosed arthritis in the hips and shoulders, gall bladder disease, and an anal gland carcinoma.

Physical Examination

An initial physical examination verified pain and reduced range of motion in Jelly's shoulders and hips. During a treatment session several weeks later, an examination demonstrated that she was sensitive to touch in the lumbar area; this area was added to the areas initially being treated.

Laser Therapy Treatment

Laser therapy was initiated with two treatments the first week, two treatments the third week, followed by one treatment every other week. The treatments were administered using contact delivery and dosages of 10 J/cm^2 to the shoulders and 18 J/cm^2 to the hips.

One of the things we noted during Jelly's treatments was that she would often start panting and shift a lot during treatment sessions. After discussion with her owners, we noted that she opted not to take long walks on warmer days and chose to lie on cold tile or wood rather than the multitude of beds she had at her disposal. At that point, we adjusted the dosage to 9 J/cm^2 to the shoulders, 17 J/cm^2 to the hips, and, starting with the twelfth treatment, 20 J/cm^2 to the lumbosacral area. Jelly received a total of 68 treatments long-term.

Outcome

Jelly displayed an excellent response to laser therapy. Her activity increased, she was able to jump on and off the sofa, she was able to go for longer walks, and she generally showed an improvement of her overall demeanor.

Final Considerations

Working as I have in a mobile laser therapy practice, with a majority of senior patients, it has become clear that responses to laser therapy vary greatly. In most cases, the response is positive and observable. Our goal with senior patients is to create an opportunity for each to experience an optimal level of physical and mental well-being, while keeping the effects of aging at bay. There are several areas in our geriatric patients' lives that we can consistently improve with the addition of laser therapy to their overall management.

Mobility

Keeping older pets mobile through appropriate exercise helps keep them healthier and decreases the loss of muscle tone. Exercise is also important for the health of the heart, digestive system, and attitude, and can be an integral part of the human–animal bond. In addition to the benefit to the patient, pet mobility also contributes to the physical activity of the owner. A study exploring the associations between dog ownership, walking activity, and health outcomes in older adults demonstrated that the relationship with one's dog may be a positive influence on physical activity for older adults (Curl *et al.,* 2016).

Cognitive Function

Supporting serotonin and endorphin release helps geriatric patients cope with stress and anxiety and lowers requirements for behavior-altering medications. Future studies will advance our current knowledge of direct, transcranial PBM treatment of cognitive dysfunction (Barrett and Gonzalez-Lima, 2013; Naeser *et al.,* 2014).

Dental Disease

PBMT is ideal for addressing inflammation and pain associated with routine dental disease, dental procedures, and difficult-to-manage conditions such as stomatitis (Kathuria *et al.,* 2015).

Dermatologic Conditions

As pets age, their ability to heal becomes more and more diminished. A wound that might have taken days to heal when they were younger can now take weeks and may have many more complications associated with it. Along with the associated pain and discomfort, when pets are suffering from skin infections, they may find the level of interaction with their humans diminished. Wounds heal faster when laser therapy is part of their overall management (Kuffler, 2016). Speeding up the healing process returns the pet to its normal surroundings, sleeping with family members and being petted regularly once again.

Age Is Not a Disease

Age is not a disease, but with age comes disease. Laser therapy can and should be fully utilized when managing the diseases of geriatric patients. The mindset of accepting a pet's decline due to aging can be adjusted substantially by adding laser therapy to our senior management protocols and client conversations. Geriatric pets offer many benefits to humans. One of the advantages of being in the veterinary profession is that we can return the favor.

References

AVMA. (2016). Senior pet care (FAQ). Available from: https://www.avma.org/public/PetCare/Pages/Caring-for-an-Older-Pet-FAQs.aspx (accessed November 30, 2016).

Barrett, D.W. and Gonzalez-Lima, F. (2013). Transcranial infrared laser stimulation produces beneficial cognitive and emotional effects in humans. *Neuroscience.* 230:13–23.

Cambier, D. *et al.* (2000). The influence of low intensity infrared laser irradiation on conduction characteristics of peripheral nerve: a randomised, controlled, double blind study on the sural nerve. *Lasers Med Sci.* 15(3):195–200.

Ceylan, Y. *et al.* (2004). The effects of infrared laser and medical treatments on pain and serotonin degradation products in patients with myofascial pain syndrome. A controlled trial. *Rheumatol Int.* 24(5):260–263.

Chow, R.T. *et al.* (2011). Inhibitory effects of laser irradiation on peripheral mammalian nerves and relevance to analgesic effects: a systematic review. *Photomed Laser Surg.* 29 (6):365–381.

Christiansen, S.B. *et al.* (2016). Veterinarians' role in clients' decision-making regarding seriously ill companion animal patients. *Acta Vet Scand.* 58(1):30.

Cotler, H.B. *et al.* (2015). The use of low level laser therapy (LLLT) for musculoskeletal pain. *MOJ Orthop Rheumatol.* 2 (5) pii:00068.

Curl, A.L. *et al.* (2016). Dog walking, the human–animal bond and older adults' physical health. *Gerontologist* pii:gnw051.

Farivar, S. *et al.* (2014). Biological effects of low level laser therapy. *J Lasers Med Sci.* 5(2):58–62.

Hagiwara, S. *et al.* (2007). GaAlAs (830 nm) low-level laser enhances peripheral endogenous opioid analgesia in rats. *Lasers Surg Med.* 39(10):797–802.

Hagiwara, S. *et al.* (2008). Pre-irradiation of blood by gallium aluminum arsenide (830 nm) low-level laser enhances peripheral endogenous opioid analgesia in rats. *Anesth Analg.* 107(3):1058–1063.

Hamblin, M.R. and Demidova, T.N. (2006). Mechanisms of low level light therapy. *Proc of SPIE.* 6140(612001):1–12.

Huang, Z. *et al.* (2015). The effectiveness of low-level laser therapy for nonspecific chronic low back pain: a systematic review and meta-analysis. *Arthritis Res Ther.* 17:360.

Kathuria, V. *et al.* (2015). Low level laser therapy: a panacea for oral maladies. *Laser Ther.* 24(3):215–223.

Kuffler, D.P. (2016). Photobiomodulation in promoting wound healing: a review. *Regen Med.* 11(1):107–122.

Labajos, M. (1988). Beta-endorphin levels modification after GaAs and HeNe laser irradiation on the rabbit. Comparative study. *Invest Clin.* 1–2:6–8.

Landsberg, G.M. *et al.* (2011). Clinical signs and management of anxiety, sleeplessness, and cognitive dysfunction in the senior pet. *Vet Clin North Am Small Anim Pract.* 41(3):565–590.

Landsberg, G.M. *et al.* (2012). Cognitive dysfunction syndrome: a disease of canine and feline brain aging. *Vet Clin North Am Small Anim Pract.* 42(4):749–768.

Maegawa, Y. *et al.* (2000). Effects of near-infrared low-level laser irradiation on microcirculation. *Lasers Surg Med.* 27 (5):427–437.

Medrado, A.R. *et al.* (2003). Influence of low level laser therapy on wound healing and its biological action upon myofibroblasts. *Lasers Surg Med.* 32(3):239–244.

Montesinos, M. (1988). Experimental effects of low power laser in encephalin and endorphin synthesis. *J Eur Med Laser Assoc.* 1(3):2–7.

Naeser, M.A. *et al.* (2014). Significant improvements in cognitive performance post-transcranial, red/near-infrared light-emitting diode treatments in chronic, mild traumatic brain injury: open-protocol study. *J Neurotrauma.* 31 (11):1008–1017.

Payne, E. *et al.* (2016). Exploring the existence and potential underpinnings of dog-human and horse-human attachment bonds. *Behav Processes.* 125:114–121.

Peplow, P.V. *et al.* (2010). Laser photobiomodulation of wound healing: a review of experimental studies in mouse and rat animal models. *Photomed Laser Surg.* 28(3):291–325.

Potter, A. and Mills, D.S. (2015). Domestic cats (*Felis silvestris catus*) do not show signs of secure attachment to their owners. *PLoS One.* 10(9):e0135109.

PR Newswire. (2016). Packaged facts: key trends shaping the U.S. pet industry. Available from: http://www.prnewswire.com/news-releases/packaged-facts-key-trends-shaping-the-us-pet-industry-300028033.html (accessed November 30, 2016).

Pryor, B. and Millis, D.L. (2015). Therapeutic laser in veterinary medicine. *Vet Clin North Am Small Anim Pract.* 45(1):45–56.

Rodier, L. (2016). Caring for an elderly dog: what an owner thinks of as "just old age" is often a treatable illness. Available from: http://www.whole-dog-journal.com/issues/13_1/features/Diagnosing-Older-Dogs-Illnes_16189-1.html?zkPrintable=true (accessed November 30, 2016).

Schütt, T. *et al.* (2015). Cognitive function, progression of age-related behavioral changes, biomarkers, and survival in dogs more than 8 years old. *J Vet Intern Med.* 29 (6):1569–1577.

Tabakoglu, H.O. *et al.* (2015). Assessment of circular wound healing in rats after exposure to 808-nm laser pulses during specific healing phases. *Lasers Surg Med.* 48 (4):409–415.

18

Laser Therapy for Feline-Specific Conditions

Michael H. Jaffe

Mississippi State University College of Veterinary Medicine, Mississippi State, MS, USA

1st Edition Contributors:

Jennifer O. Lavallee and James Olson

Cat Specialist, Castle Rock, CO, USA

Introduction

Rehabilitation medicine in cats, a field that has long been overlooked, is now gaining the attention it deserves. Recent advancements in identifying and managing pain in cats have underscored the importance of a multimodal approach to pain management. In this context, rehabilitation therapy has emerged as a crucial component.

Alongside the need for a multimodal pain management approach, a similar approach to treating a range of conditions is also gaining recognition. Many cat owners are now embracing minimally or noninvasive approaches. Despite the limited research-backed data for many disease states, anecdotal evidence and findings from human medicine and translation studies support the use of photobiomodulation (PBM) for various conditions. Given its increasing prevalence in practice, laser therapy should be considered a potential adjunct or primary therapy for many disease states in cats.

Anal Sac Diseases, Non-Neoplastic

Anal sacculitis, impaction, and abscesses of the anal sacs are uncommon in cats (Bellah 2006). Anal sacculitis is an inflammatory condition that develops when material within the anal sac becomes impacted and the sac does not express well, eventually leading to inflammation. With time, a bacterial infection may develop into an abscess due to the lack of normal drainage. The distinction between these three conditions is not always initially apparent (Corbee *et al.,* 2022). Anal sacs have no apparent functional use in the cat.

- **Diagnosis:** Appearance on physical exam is typically diagnostic. Most anal sac abscesses are discovered by the owner when a large, painful swelling is found at 4 or 8 o'clock to the anus, or when the sac ruptures, draining purulent material. Cats may appear to excessively lick at the area of inflammation, which may cause a local alopecia.
- **Standard treatment:** Treatment of anal sacculitis and impaction involves a combination of anal sac expression, flushing the anal sacs, warm compresses, anti-inflammatory drugs, and systemic antibiotics. Surgical drainage may be necessary when an abscess forms or if it ruptures cutaneously.
- **Laser therapy:** A short series (one to three sessions) of laser therapy applications to help treat anal gland abscesses has demonstrated a good outcome. Photobiomodulation is effective in reducing pain and inflammation, decreasing pruritus, and promoting healing.
- **Prognosis:** Non-neoplastic anal gland diseases respond well to treatment, but recurrence is possible. Including a high-fiber diet and providing periodic anal gland expression may be indicated.
- **Dose:** 6–8 J/cm^2

Abscess, Cat-Bite

Cat-bite wounds are most common in young, male, feral, and free-roaming cats (O'Neill *et al.,* 2023). Abscesses secondary to a bite wound are acute to chronic infectious

Laser Therapy in Veterinary Medicine: Photobiomodulation, Second Edition. Edited by Christopher J. Winkler and Lisa A. Miller.

processes. Bites result in an area of cellulitis followed by formation of a pocket of purulent material in the subcutaneous tissue.

- **Diagnosis:** A painful, fluctuant to firm swelling palpated in a localized area of alopecia or (often) an open, draining wound. Cytology of the fluid reveals purulent material characterized by bacteria and neutrophils. Cats are commonly febrile, lethargic, anorexic, lame, and painful.
- **Standard treatment:** Closed abscesses should be surgically lanced, drained, and lavaged. Systemic antibiotics based on culture results should be administered (usually in the penicillin or cephalosporin groups) to combat *Pasturella* spp., *Staphylococcus* spp., and *Streptococcus* spp. Open, draining abscesses should be clipped and the skin surrounding the bite wound cleaned with an antiseptic. The draining tract may need to be opened wider to facilitate drainage and to prevent premature healing. Warm compresses and pain medication typically accompany antibiotic therapy.
- **Laser therapy:** Treatment of small to medium-sized puncture wounds or cellulitis swellings with only laser therapy treatment has demonstrated some degree of effectiveness in preventing abscess formation in patients. Cats with an active abscess may receive one to three laser treatment sessions in addition to antibiotic therapy. Continued observation for abscess formation should be monitored, and if this occurs, more aggressive conventional therapy should be initiated.
- **Prognosis:** Cat-bite abscesses are expected to be responsive to treatment. Including laser therapy in the conventional treatment plan will assist in reducing inflammation, reduce pain, and promote healing.
- **Dose:** 6–8 J/cm^2

Allergic Dermatitis

Allergic dermatitis is a type 1 hypersensitivity reaction that erupts with miliary lesions, causing pruritus, inflammation, destructive scratching, and varying degrees of discomfort. Secondary cutaneous infection including pyoderma and *Malassezia* dermatitis is common (Bajwa 2018). Prevalence is higher than previously suggested, with young cats (<3 years of age) most often affected (Bajwa 2018). Breed predispositions (domestic mixed, Abyssinian, and Devon Rex) have been confirmed (Ravens *et al.*, 2014).

- **Diagnosis:** Physical exam reveals miliary dermatitis with patchy alopecia, crusting, erosions, and ulceration. Intradermal allergen testing is useful to confirm (Ravens *et al.*, 2014).
- **Standard treatment:** If an underlying allergic trigger can be identified and removed, this is the most definitive treatment. Symptomatic treatment of pruritis with glucocorticoids or cyclosporine (Atopica 7 mg/kg once daily) should help provide relief. Allergen specific immunotherapy is safe and effective for long-term treatment (Bajwa 2018)
- **Laser therapy:** Laser treatment protocols may decrease or remove dependence on medication. Laser therapy should be considered in patients with allergic dermatitis. Because it avoids the side effects of corticosteroids and immunosuppressive drugs, it may of great benefit for some cats. Maintenance therapy sessions can be spaced 7–60 days apart, depending on the condition and response. Use of photobiomodulation therapy for miliary dermatitis may provide relief from pruritis.
- **Prognosis:** Allergic skin disease has many causes and often needs life-long therapy. Laser therapy may reduce inflammation and pruritus and promote skin healing.
- **Dose:** 2–4 J/cm^2

Arthritis

Arthritis is defined as inflammation of a joint. Osteoarthritis is a chronic, progressive, degenerative condition resulting in cartilage destruction, joint capsule thickening, and periarticular muscle fibrosis. One study (Slingerland *et al.*, 2011) found the large majority (90%) of cats over 12 years of age have radiographic signs associated with osteoarthritis.

Feline arthritis has historically been underdiagnosed. Arthritis in cats manifests as behavioral changes as opposed to the more obvious gait changes noticeable in dogs. Cats do have stiffness and lameness as part of their arthritis but tend to hide these by appearing less active. Attention to owner-reported changes in mobility (particularly gait, jumping, and the use of stairs) is important (Klinck *et al.*, 2012).

- **Diagnosis:** Common signs include generalized decreased activity, increased weight gain, reluctance to jumping, limping, soreness around the affected joint(s), stiffness after rest, and possible changes in litter box usage. Physical exam may find muscle atrophy, limited and painful range-of-motion of joints, and crepitus on manipulation of joints (Bennett *et al.*, 2012). Good-quality orthogonal radiographs are helpful to confirm the diagnosis.
- **Standard treatment:** Multimodal management for treating arthritis in cats is recommended, with surgical options considered only for nonresponsive cases. Commonly used medications include those nonsteroidal anti-inflammatory drugs (NSAIDs) approved for cats (such as Robenacoxib), glucosamine and chondroitin sulfate joint supplements, glycosaminoglycan, and anti-NGF monoclonal antibodies. Weight management and

controlled exercise are vital for successful management. Acupuncture and physical therapy have also been applied. Supportive treatment can include modification of the environment: reducing joint stress by adding cat stairs to allow access to furniture; increasing traction on slippery floors with nonskid rugs; and putting food, water, and litter boxes in relatively close proximity in the house.

- **Laser therapy:** Photobiomodulation is one important component of a rehabilitation therapy plan to reduce inflammation and control chronic pain. The author has seen many patients show significant, rapid improvement in their mobility following this type of rehab plan.
- **Prognosis:** With a combined PBMT and multimodal therapy plan, the treatment of arthritis can be greatly improved. Many patients with chronic arthritis will benefit from life-long intermittent therapy to maintain good joint comfort.
- **Dose:** 6–10 J/cm^2

Asthma and Allergic Pulmonary Disease

Feline asthma is a chronic lower airway disease characterized by airway inflammation, airway hypersensitivity, and limitation of airflow (Trzil 2020). Treatment with glucocorticoids and bronchodilators has demonstrated mixed results, with some cats not responding to this therapy.

- **Diagnosis:** Cats with feline asthma may have the following clinical signs: cough, increased respiratory effort, open-mouth breathing, tachypnea, and vomiting. Upon physical exam, cats are noted to have an inducible cough on tracheal palpation and demonstrate an increased abdominal effort on expiration; an expiratory wheeze may also be heard on thoracic auscultation (Trzil 2020). Thoracic imaging demonstrates a characteristic radiographic appearance of bronchial lung pattern (Foster *et al.*, 2004). Bronchoscopy and bronchoalveolar lavage (BAL) may also be useful in making a diagnosis.
- **Standard treatment:** Severely dyspneic cats need oxygen therapy and cage rest to minimize stress. Corticosteroids are the mainstay of therapy for treating feline asthma to reduce inflammation. The route of administration can be oral, injectable, inhaled, or transdermal. Bronchodilators are used to reduce bronchoconstriction during acute attacks and in conjunction with corticosteroids. For asthmatic cats, it is important to consider the environment and look to minimize dust, perfumes, scents, second-hand smoke, and any other possible inhaled irritants.
- **Laser therapy:** Treatment of asthmatic cats with laser therapy at the thoracic inlet and both sides of the chest wall has been described. On-contact delivery over the chest wall is recommended if possible, though it is not necessary to attempt to treat between rib spaces on feline patients. Laser therapy inhibits bronchoconstriction, T-helper 2 inflammation, and airway remodeling in allergic asthma in mice (Silva *et al.*, 2014). Whether a similar effect occurs in cats has not been determined and no clinical reports document a positive effect.
- **Prognosis:** Feline asthma is often a chronic disease with acute flare-ups that requires ongoing treatment. The addition of laser therapy to reduce the inflammatory response in asthmatic patients could be beneficial in reducing lower airway inflammation, but further evaluation is needed.
- **Dose:** 6–8 J/cm^2

Myocardial Disease

Feline myocardial disease (cardiomyopathy) is the most common cardiac disease in cats, and of the classifications, hypertrophic cardiomyopathy accounts for roughly two-thirds of the cases (Ferasin 2009a,b).

Diagnosis: Definitive diagnosis of cardiac disease is based on echocardiographic criteria. Further classification of cardiomyopathy into hypertrophic (HCM), restrictive (RCM), dilated (DCM), arrhythmogenic right ventricular cardiomyopathy, and unclassified cardiomyopathy follows the World Health Organization definition and guidelines (Richardson *et al.*, 1996). Several clinical signs are described in cats with cardiomyopathy: presence of a heart murmur, dyspnea, tachycardia, paresis or paralysis of the hindlimbs (indicating an aortic thromboembolism), hypothermia, cardiac arrhythmias, hypotension, and ascites (Ferasin 2009a,b).

- **Standard treatment:** Treatment is focused on alleviating the underlying pathologic processes such as blood pressure changes, outflow obstructions, ischemia, arrhythmias, and hypercoagulable conditions (Ferasin 2009a,b). This may include diuretics, calcium channel blockers, beta-blockers, taurine supplementation, and inotropic drugs (Ferasin 2009a,b).
- **Laser therapy:** There are anecdotal reports of the use of laser therapy to reduce pain, increase muscle relaxation, and increase collateral circulation in the rear legs in cases of aortic thromboembolism; this seems a reasonable addition to treatment. For cardiac disease in general, the use of laser therapy over the chest wall appears to improve cardiac function when combined with standard medical therapy. In humans, cardiac disease has been treated via laser therapy delivered intravascularly (Derkacz *et al.*, 2014).
- **Prognosis:** Cardiac disease often needs lifelong treatment and serial re-evaluation. Further investigation into

the use of laser therapy as an adjunctive treatment for cardiac disease is warranted.

- **Dose:** 6–8 J/cm^2

Constipation and Obstipation

Constipation is characterized by incomplete, difficult, or infrequent passage of stool. Obstipation is a more severe form of constipation characterized by stool retention and the inability to pass stool. Idiopathic megacolon is the end-point presentation of prolonged constipation or obstipation due to colonic dilation and hypomotility in cats.

- **Diagnosis:** History of straining to defecate with little or no stool produced. Decreased appetite with possible vomiting. A large firm colon is palpable on abdominal palpation. Cats may also appear generalized cachectic.
- **Standard treatment:** Medical management is generally unrewarding in resolving obstipation. A combination of laxatives, prokinetic agents, dietary modifications, stool softeners, and enemas are often minimally successful in evacuating impacted stool from the colon. Subtotal colectomy is often considered the treatment of choice when medical management no longer helps.
- **Laser therapy:** Idiopathic megacolon, or megacolon secondary to pelvic stricture following trauma, typically results in poor colonic smooth muscle contractility. As such, administration of laser therapy before true megacolon develops may be helpful, but the window of opportunity for such treatment may be small. Lumbar and sacral neuromodulation in people with colonic dysmotility disorders using red LED light at 660 nm (10 min) and infrared LED light at 840 nm (10 min) has demonstrated changes in the autonomic nervous system, warranting further study into the effects of photobiomodulation for chronic colonic motility disorders (Ali *et al.,* 2022).
- **Prognosis:** Prognosis for megacolon is generally good following surgery. For constipation, medical management, including the possible use of laser therapy, is good if treatment is initiated prior to loss of colonic smooth muscle motility.
- **Dose:** 6–10 J/cm^2

Dental Extractions, Gingivitis, and Periodontal Disease

There are numerous dental conditions that may benefit from laser therapy in companion animal patients. Laser therapy is very commonly used in people and dogs for its anti-inflammatory effects as well as its analgesic and biostimulatory effects to aid in tissue healing (Bidar *et al.,* 2016) (Alves *et al.,* 2024).

- **Diagnosis:** Diagnosis is based on a thorough oral examination with dental radiographs performed.
- **Standard treatment:** Treatment is based on specific diagnosis of dental disease present.
- **Laser therapy:** Laser therapy is useful as an adjunct to dental prophylaxis to reduce inflammation of the gingiva. Cats with feline stomatitis benefit from treatment with laser therapy. One study demonstrated effective reduction in inflammation due to stomatitis when laser therapy was used (Squarzoni *et al.,* 2017).
- **Prognosis:** The prognosis depends on the specific dental condition. Consider laser therapy for inflammatory conditions such as feline chronic gingivostomatitis as well as periodontal and other gingival diseases. Laser therapy for pain management following dental prophylaxis and extractions should also be considered.
- **Dose:** 3–4 J/cm^2 if the mouth is open; 6–8 J/cm^2 if it is closed.

Eosinophilic Granuloma Complex

Eosinophilic granuloma complex (EGC) is not a specific dermatologic diagnosis; however, it is a manifestation of several etiologic factors presenting as cutaneous lesions. The most common etiology is due to a hypersensitivity reaction. Other causes include infectious agents, foreign body reaction, genetic predisposition, and idiopathic causes. Inflammatory lesions such as indolent (eosinophilic) ulcers, eosinophilic plaques, and eosinophilic granulomas are characterized by the presence of numerous leukocytes, with eosinophils present in large numbers.

- **Diagnosis:** Clinical signs of the characteristic lesions present on the lip of patients (confirmed by cytologic evaluation demonstrating numerous eosinophils) are suggestive of EGC. Histopathologic analysis following biopsy is necessary to rule out viral or neoplastic lesions (Buckley and Nuttall 2012).
- **Standard treatment:** EGC lesions respond well to treatment with glucocorticoid therapy. Immunomodulatory agents such as cyclosporine have also shown good efficacy. Chlorambucil may be used in nonresponsive cases. Other agents used include interferon omega and prostagens. Ruling out and eliminating causes of a hypersensitivity reaction such as food or environmental allergens may be necessary.
- **Laser therapy:** Photobiomodulation in conjunction with standard therapy may be effective in reducing the inflammatory response in cases of EGC and promoting

healing of tissue. Laser surgery has been used to excise lesions.

- **Prognosis:** Long-term medical management may be necessary in many cases. In general, medical management offers a good prognosis. Photobiomodulation therapy in conjunction with medical management may offer the possibility of lowering doses of drugs such as glucocorticoids and cyclosporine.
- **Dose:** Low dose: 3–4 J/cm^2 high dose: 20–30 J/cm^2. Though the lesions and tissues involved seem to indicate that a low dose would be appropriate, anecdotal reports from practitioners indicate better responses have been seen clinically when treating EGC with high doses (as are recommended for some granulomatous conditions in other species, such as lick granulomas in dogs). To avoid patient discomfort when using the high dose, a low power setting of 2–4 W delivered over a longer time is recommend (rather than a higher power setting over a shorter time) (Lavallee and Olson 2017).

Feline Acne

Feline acne is a dermatologic condition seen in feline practice that is believed to be an idiopathic disorder of follicular keratinization and glandular proliferation of the chin (Pieper 2018).

- **Diagnosis:** Comedones noted on the chin are early clinical signs that may progress to severe folliculitis and furunculosis. Histopathology of lesions may reveal lymphoplasmacytic periductal inflammation, sebaceous gland duct dilatation, folliculitis, pyogranulomatous adenitis, and furunculosis (Pieper 2018).
- **Standard treatment:** Systemic antibiotics are recommended to treat secondary bacterial infections. Chronic cases may include treatment with prednisolone once the infection is resolved. Topical therapy with salicylic acid, benzoyl peroxide, and other lotions are used to reduce infection, inflammation, and cutaneous reactions.
- **Laser therapy:** Feline acne appears to have an exaggerated inflammatory response, and PBMT removes the red, sore component of the disease, often within in the first 24 hours. A single session or a short series of laser therapy treatments for feline acne, especially if severe, may be beneficial to promote resolution of inflammation and promote healing.
- **Prognosis:** Prognosis for treatment is good, however, lifelong vigilance for recurrence is needed. Laser therapy has been remarkably helpful in severe or recurrent cases.
- **Dose:** 3–4 J/cm^2

Fracture Healing

- **Diagnosis:** A comprehensive orthopedic and physical exam in conjunction with diagnostic imaging to confirm the presence of a fracture.
- **Standard treatment:** Open reduction and internal fixation is needed with many fractures. However, external coaptation may be acceptable, depending on the fracture and anatomic location.
- **Laser therapy:** Photobiomodulation has been shown to help reduce pain, control inflammation, and accelerate bone healing in the presence of fractures by stimulating osteogenesis and reducing the time for fracture consolidation (Neto *et al.*, 2019) (Brassolatti *et al.*, 2018). Additionally, PBM enhances bone healing by promoting angiogenesis, which increases local blood flow and tissue oxygenation. Laser therapy stimulation of nonunion fractures can restart the healing process and may help to avoid more invasive techniques. The effect that laser therapy has on fracture healing in lab animals (improving bone healing by activating osteogenic factors and accelerating the development of newly formed bone) has been described (Jawad *et al.*, 2013; Son *et al.*, 2012; Tim *et al.*, 2014). Laser therapy has been demonstrated to be effective in treating experimentally induced chronic osteomyelitis in rats by methicillin-resistant *Staphylococcus aureus* (MRSA) (Kaya *et al.*, 2011).
- **Prognosis:** With adherence to appropriate fracture repair guidelines, laser therapy is an appropriate adjunct for the treatment of fractures.
- **Dose:** 6–10 J/cm^2

Hyperesthesia Syndrome

Feline hyperesthesia syndrome (FHS) is a condition where numerous behavioral changes are noted. Cats may exhibit signs of pain or frantic compulsive behavior such as tail twitching, chewing and self-barbering, vocalization, mydriasis, skin twitching, and others.

- **Diagnosis:** Diagnosis of this condition may be challenging as clinical signs are the only means of diagnosis. No laboratory testing is available to confirm this condition. However, ruling out dermatologic or other painful conditions is helpful.
- **Standard treatment:** Gabapentin and phenobarbital may be useful. Other treatments include clomipramine, fluoxetine, and acupuncture.
- **Laser therapy:** Anecdotal use of laser therapy in cats with hyperesthesia has shown mixed results. Localized areas of hyperesthesia characterized by licking and chewing are

targeted for treatment. Some clients report complete resolution of symptoms after a single treatment, while others had minimal response after a series of treatments.

- **Prognosis:** Prognosis for controlling the signs of FHS is generally good. Laser therapy as an adjunct to standard therapy may offer some improvement and should be considered.
- **Dose:** 5–10 J/cm^2

Inflammatory Bowel Disease

Inflammatory bowel disease (IBD) is a common immune-mediated and inflammatory disease of the small intestine. It is defined as chronic (>3 weeks), persistent, or recurrent gastrointestinal signs in which mucosal inflammation has been confirmed by histopathology (North 2018).

- **Diagnosis:** A thorough workup including CBC, serum biochemistry profile, and urinalysis should be performed. A total T4 is recommended in cats over 7 years of age. Abdominal ultrasound is often suggestive of IBD, although a normal ultrasound exam does not rule out the presence of disease. Full-thickness biopsies of multiple intestinal sites as well as lymph nodes is essential for diagnosis and helps to rule out other disease syndromes. Endoscopic biopsies may be limited to only the mucosa of intestine within reach of the endoscope.
- **Standard treatment:** A combination of treatment modalities includes dietary management, immunomodulatory therapy (typically with prednisolone, but may include budesonide, chlorambucil, or others), probiotics, omega-3 polyunsaturated fatty acids, antibiotics, cobalamin, and microbiome restorative therapy (North 2018).
- **Laser therapy:** Because of the inflammatory component of IBD, photobiomodulation appears to be a reasonable adjunct to standard therapy. Photobiomodulation included as an adjunct therapy for the treatment of large bowel diarrhea in dogs has demonstrated beneficial effects (Alves *et al.*, 2021). Anecdotal reports of use in cats have also shown positive results. Since PBM is a comparatively safe procedure, its use could be considered as a complementary form of therapy.
- **Prognosis:** Many cases of IBD can be successfully managed with standard therapy, although life-long care may be necessary.
- **Dose:** 6–8 J/cm^2

Chronic Renal Disease

Stage 4 of the International Renal Interest Society (IRIS) is the condition formerly known as chronic renal failure. It is characterized by severe renal azotemia, elevated creatinine, elevated symmetric dimethylarginine (SDMA), and systemic clinical signs of uremia. It commonly develops in geriatric cats but may begin in younger cats as earlier stages and progress throughout their life. Cats with IRIS Stages 1 and 2 may not present with any clinical signs. Cats with IRIS Stage 3 disease often show milder signs than Stage 4, but typically progressively worsen.

- **Diagnosis:** Clinical signs of uremia (such as weight loss, decreased appetite, polyuria, and polydipsia) coupled with elevated creatinine and SDMA are highly suggestive of IRIS Stage 4 disease. Further diagnostic findings may reveal decreased urine specific gravity, elevated urine protein: creatinine ratio, decreased hematocrit, microalbuminuria, and systemic hypertension. A complete urinalysis including a urine sediment exam will reveal similarly consistent changes. Diagnostic imaging modalities such as radiographs and ultrasound are helpful in ruling out other disorders as well as identifying comorbidities.
- **Standard treatment:** Depending on the stage of renal disease present, treatment is based on maintaining electrolyte balance, the use of phosphate binders, acid–base balance, maintaining weight and nutrition, preserving normal blood pressure, and mitigating the signs of azotemia. Hospitalization with IV fluid therapy may be needed in severely affected patients. Renal transplant may be indicated.
- **Laser therapy:** Laser therapy may be considered, though its use in clinical cases is anecdotal. However, beneficial effects of PBM use in mice with chronic kidney disease (CKD) are reported (Bian *et al.*, 2022).
- **Prognosis:** Prognosis is based on the IRIS Stage of disease and response to therapy. Cats with CKD will need life-long therapy and continued monitoring for progression of their disease.
- **Dose:** 4–6 J/cm^2

Hepatic Lipidosis

Hepatic lipidosis (also known as fatty liver syndrome) is the most common liver disease in cats and is characterized by the accumulation of triglycerides or neutral lipid in more than 80% of hepatocytes (Norsworthy and Romeo 2018). Cats with hepatic lipidosis are typically overweight and anorectic for 7 or more days. The cause of hepatic lipidosis is not fully known but is likely multifactorial. Primary diseases that precipitate the development of hepatic lipidosis may include cholangiohepatitis, biliary disease, and primary hepatic disease. Other factors may also play a role in the pathogenesis. Clinical signs include anorexia, weight loss, vomiting, and icterus.

- **Diagnosis:** Diagnosis is based on history of not eating and other clinical signs. Serum biochemical changes include elevated alkaline phosphatase, elevated ALT, hyperbilirubinemia, hypoalbuminemia, and increased AST. Bilirubinuria may be present on urinalysis. Ultrasound examination of the liver and biliary system may reveal a diffusely hyperechoic liver. Definitive diagnosis is confirmed by hepatic cytology or histopathology.
- **Standard treatment:** Treatment of hepatic lipidosis involves fluid therapy, anti-emetics, nutritional support (including appetite stimulants or feeding tubes if needed), maintenance of electrolyte balance, antibiotics (when an underlying suppurative process is suspected), and hepatic support supplements and vitamins.
- **Laser therapy:** The presence of an inflammatory disease such as cholangiohepatitis indicates that PBM may be considered an adjunctive modality to standard treatment. There are no veterinary reports of treating hepatic lipidosis or underlying disease with PBM.
- **Prognosis:** Prognosis is very good based on aggressive treatment and response to therapy.
- **Dose:** 6–8 J/cm^2

Musculoskeletal Acute Injury

Musculoskeletal injuries in cats tend to be due to trauma and may result in concurrent fractures. Muscle and tendon injuries (such as calcanean tendon ruptures) occur as well due to metabolic disease, high-rise syndrome, and low-impact injuries. Lameness is the most common presenting sign. Contusions and muscle strain/ruptures are the most common underlying mechanism of injury.

- **Diagnosis:** History of trauma and lameness on examination are the most common clinical findings. Fractures are usually detected with imaging such as radiographs or CT. Muscle and tendon injuries may be diagnosed with musculoskeletal ultrasound.
- **Standard treatment:** Fractures in conjunction with musculoskeletal trauma may need open reduction and internal fixation. Traumatic muscle strain injuries may be amenable to rest. Muscle/tendon injuries may require surgery. Regenerative therapy is commonly used in dogs with tendon strains, but reports are lacking for this form of therapy in cats. Physical therapy and rehabilitation (including photobiomodulation) are very helpful for recovery from many muscle injuries.
- **Laser therapy:** Photobiomodulation in conjunction with an aggressive rehabilitation therapy regimen is a mainstay of therapy for muscle injuries. Because muscle damage is amenable to treatment with laser therapy, healing of tissue using this modality adds great value to a treatment plan. Additionally, laser therapy provides pain relief and reduces inflammation associated with muscle and tendon injuries.
- **Prognosis:** The prognosis for recovery is generally good, depending on the nature of the injury. Laser therapy as part of the treatment plan in conjunction with surgery and a complete PT/Rehabilitation therapy regimen offer an improved chance of a successful outcome.
- **Dose:** 4–8 J/cm^2 (Pryor and Millis 2015)

Otitis Externa

Otitis externa is an inflammatory skin disease of the pinna and external ear canal. Although the primary cause of otitis externa may not be inflammatory in nature, the resultant inflammatory response produces a painful and chronic disorder. Chronic pruritis secondary to the underlying cause may result in development of external skin excoriations of the pinna and aural hematoma formation. Primary inciting causes of otitis externa include bacterial and fungal infections, external parasites such as ear mites, hypersensitivity reactions, tumors and polyps, and wax debris.

- **Diagnosis:** Cats with otitis externa are pruritic, shake their head frequently, and exhibit a malodorous discharge from their ears. Crusts and scabs frequently form due to pruritis. Otitis externa is diagnosed by physical exam findings, otoscopic exam, and cytology. Cultures of fluid and debris from the ears often are helpful in identifying the primary infectious pathogen.
- **Standard treatment:** A combination of topical and systemic antibiotics and antifungal agents are used for primary and secondarily infected ear canals. Ear cleansing agents are helpful to reduce the accumulation of debris and to soothe inflammation of the epithelium. When ear mites are present, topical and systemic parasiticides are available for treatment.
- **Laser therapy:** Laser therapy is very helpful in reducing the pain and inflammation associated with chronic otitis externa. In addition to treating the underlying primary cause, PBM may help relieve the inflammation and pruritis associated with otitis externa.
- **Prognosis:** Prognosis for cats with otitis externa is excellent when a comprehensive diagnostic and therapeutic plan is initiated. Recurrence of otitis externa is not uncommon when otitis media is also present, and this may precipitate more aggressive therapy. The presence of masses may require more aggressive therapy, especially when underlying malignancies are diagnosed.
- **Dose:** Superficial component: 3–4 J/cm^2; deep component: 8–10 J/cm^2. When treating otitis, two components, or anatomical areas, must be addressed. The first is the

affected portion of the pinna and the visible, more distal portion of the ear canal. These tissues should be treated with a laser setting that delivers 3–4 J/cm^2, usually with a noncontact delivery. The second component is the more proximal, deeper portion of the ear canal. This deeper tissue component requires a higher target dose of 8–10 J/cm^2 and is most commonly treated with on-contact delivery (Lavallee and Olson 2017).

Pancreatitis

Acute and chronic pancreatitis is an idiopathic inflammatory disorder with several notable risk factors, such as trauma, infectious disease, hypotension, hypertriglyceridemia, and secondary to pharmacologics. Nonspecific signs observed (anorexia, lethargy, dehydration, weight loss, hypothermia or fever, abdominal pain, vomiting, icterus, and diarrhea) may be noted in both acute and chronic cases. Chronic cases are characterized by the presence of fibrotic changes or atrophy of the pancreas. Cats with concurrent pancreatitis, inflammatory bowel disease, and cholangitis are referred to as having "triaditis" or triad disease (Steiner 2018).

- **Diagnosis:** Diagnostic testing includes serum feline pancreatic lipase immunoreactivity concentration (fPLI), the presence of a hyperechoic pancreas on ultrasound (in chronic cases), and cytology or histopathology. Concurrent small intestinal disease must also be ruled out, and serum cobalamin and folate concentrations should be evaluated, as are serum feline trypsin-like immunoreactivity concentration (fTLI), fasting serum triglyceride concentrations, and serum calcium concentrations.
- **Standard treatment:** Aggressive supportive care is mandatory for cats with pancreatitis, in the form of fluid therapy, nutritional management, antiemetics, and analgesics. Any comorbidities will also need to be treated. Corticosteroids may be used in cases related to autoimmune pancreatitis.
- **Laser therapy:** Laser therapy may be helpful in reducing inflammation of the pancreas. Transcutaneous application of light over the pancreas at a dose of 8–10 J/cm^2 is reported in an attempt to reduce inflammation of the pancreas and assist in healing (Lavallee and Olson 2017). It is unproven whether this facilitates healing, but appears to be well-tolerated by patients.
- **Prognosis:** Prognosis is guarded for cats with pancreatitis depending on their response to conventional therapy. Treatment with laser therapy is well-tolerated and may help reduce inflammation.
- **Dose:** 8–10 J/cm^2

Feline Chronic Rhinosinusitis

Chronic rhinitis is an inflammatory condition of the nasal cavity due to infection from feline herpesvirus 1, bacterial and fungal infection, neoplasia, and foreign bodies. Secondary bacterial infections may develop, and the subsequent rhinitis may ascend into the frontal sinus resulting in concurrent sinusitis (Reed 2020).

- **Diagnosis:** History of sneezing, nasal discharge, and increased upper airway sounds are presumptive of nasal disease. Computed Tomography (CT) is more likely to confirm nasal and frontal sinus involvement than radiographs. Rhinoscopy is difficult in cats due to their small nares, but nasal lavage may provide samples for culture and cytology. Biopsies may be performed but are blind as to the tissue collected. Polymerase chain reaction testing (PCR) for several likely pathogens may provide useful results.
- **Standard treatment:** Treatment is based on the underlying cause. Antibiotics are effective for bacterial infections of the nasal cavity and frontal sinus. Rhinotomy may be performed when there is the presence of a foreign body or a mass, or to lavage the nasal cavity in the presence of inflammatory material (Norsworthy and Restine 2018).
- **Laser therapy:** Laser therapy has given the practitioner the advantage of treating both infectious and inflammatory triggers in nasal disease, and may be a good adjunct to standard treatments. If there is any question whether a neoplasia is present, do not use laser therapy. A recent study with human cadaver skulls demonstrated that photons of near-infrared laser therapy wavelengths do penetrate through bone (Tedford *et al.*, 2015). Protective eyewear goggles (rated for laser therapy wavelengths) must be worn by the patient for treatments around the eyes (Figure 18.1).
- **Prognosis:** The prognosis depends on the underlying cause and the extent of the disease into the frontal sinus. Most infections are amenable to treatment, whereas neoplasia such as lymphoma is initially responsive to chemotherapy.
- **Dose:** 8–10 J/cm^2

Surgery, Treating Incisions Postoperatively

Post-op incision laser treatment has become commonplace in veterinary practice. Treatment of incisions postoperatively with laser therapy has been shown to speed up wound healing and result in a more cosmetic healed

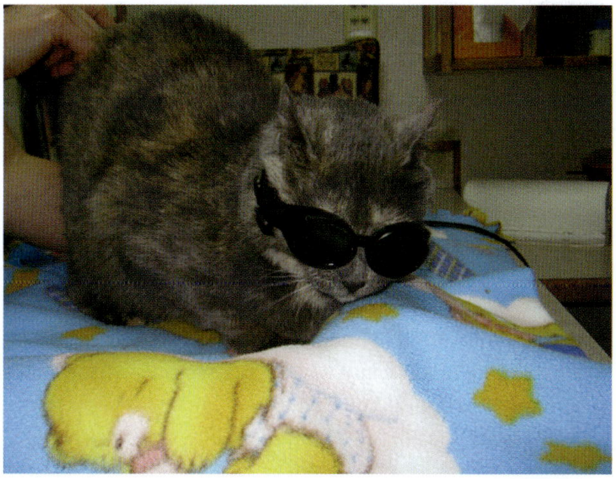

Figure 18.1 Protective eyewear goggles (rated for laser therapy wavelengths) must be worn by the patient during treatments around the eyes.

incision (Wardlaw *et al.*, 2019). Photobiomodulation has been shown to have a positive influence on the inflammatory, proliferative and maturation phases of wound healing. The overall result is improvement of the wound's tensile strength. Additionally, laser therapy provides some degree of analgesia to post-op incisions through a reduction in local inflammation.

- **Standard treatment:** Basic post-op incision management involves vigilance for any signs of infection and dehiscence. Treating incisions with cold compresses in the first 48 hours, followed by warm compresses, also provides analgesia and reduces inflammation.
- **Laser therapy:** PBM is safe for use after most surgeries. As detailed in Chapter 5, care should be exercised during use around eyes, thyroid glands, tumors, or testicles in breeding cats (Lavallee and Olson 2017). Post-op laser therapy of incisions can encourage more rapid healing with less scar tissue, and a reduction in post-surgical pain.
- **Dose:** 2–4 J/cm^2 (Pryor and Millis 2015).

Urethral Obstruction

Feline lower urinary tract conditions are amenable to laser therapy included with the treatment protocol. Less resistance to urethral catheterization in cats with FLUTD (feline lower urinary tract disease) due to urethral calculi is reported (Buijs and Godbold Jr. 2017). It is suspected that this may be due to decreased local edema and swelling as well as relaxation of muscle spasms in the urethra. Additionally, following perineal urethrostomy (PU) surgery, noncontact laser delivery will reduce inflammation around the stoma site and reduce patient discomfort.

- **Diagnosis:** Urethral obstruction is characterized by lower urinary tract signs such as dysuria, stranguria, pollakiuria, or hematuria. Typically, the urinary bladder will be large, firm, and painful upon abdominal palpation; such examination should be performed gently so as not to compromise the bladder, which could rupture. Other systemic signs noted may include lethargy, dehydration, anorexia, and vomiting. In long-standing cases cats may be recumbent or comatose. Diagnostic imaging with radiographs and ultrasound is useful for confirming the diagnosis. If urine can be obtained safely, it should be analyzed along with a serum biochemistry profile and a CBC.
- **Standard treatment:** Cat with urinary tract obstruction should have a urinary catheter placed to relieve the obstruction and allow emptying of the bladder. PU surgery is considered in recurrent cases and for some cats following their first obstruction.
- **Laser therapy:** PBM is an adjunct to treatment in cases where the cat has first been stabilized. Urinary catheterization is often an emergency procedure to empty an overdistended bladder. Laser therapy is helpful to reduce urethral smooth muscle spasms, reduce inflammation around the urethra, and promote healing around a PU site without directly contacting the incision.
- **Prognosis:** The prognosis is guarded for chronic urinary obstructions, but much better for stabilized and post-op PU patients.
- **Dose:** 6–8 J/cm^2

Vestibular Disease, Peripheral

Feline idiopathic vestibular syndrome may affect cats of any age, but is most commonly seen in middle-aged adult cats. It is a condition where the vestibular receptors of the middle ear (or the vestibulochoclear nerve) are affected, resulting in clinical signs of acute falling, rolling, ataxia, circling, or head tilt (Wexler-Mitchell 2018).

- **Diagnosis:** Clinical signs are strongly suggestive, but rule outs include inner ear disease, trauma, and access to potential neurotoxins. A thorough neurological examination must be performed to identify any other neurological abnormalities. Standard radiographic imaging, computed tomography (CT), or MRI should be performed to rule out neoplasia or disease of the inner ear.
- **Standard treatment:** Supportive care for cats with vestibular disease includes nutritional and fluid support,

antiemetics when necessary, and antibiotics for concurrent otitis interna. Sedatives may be helpful to ease anxiety.

- **Laser therapy:** Use of PBM in rats with peripheral vestibular dysfunction is described. PBM treatments of cochlear damage related to gentamicin therapy is observed to have a regenerative effect (Lee *et al.*, 2017). There are no reports of treatment of cats with vestibular dysfunction with this therapy. Anecdotal reports exist as to the efficacy of PBM in cats with vestibular dysfunction (Lavallee and Olson 2017).
- **Prognosis:** Prognosis is guarded. However, laser therapy appears to be safe for cats with vestibular dysfunction, and its use should be considered as an adjunctive therapy.
- **Dose:** 4–6 J/cm^2

Wound Healing

Adjunctive management of chronic wounds is a well-described use for photobiomodulation therapy. PBM has a positive influence on the inflammatory, proliferative, and maturation phases of wound healing. The effect of laser therapy, in conjunction with standard wound management techniques, is development of greater wound tensile strength.

- **Diagnosis:** Open wound management and visual inspection of wounds.
- **Standard treatment:** There are a variety of techniques available for open wound management. The goal of wound management is to create an environment that promotes vascular ingrowth of tissue in a clean, sterile environment while enhancing epithelialization and contraction of tissue.
- **Laser therapy:** Laser therapy is used as part of basic wound management. Wounds that are treated with bandage changes, debridement, tissue lavage, and topical therapy can be easily treated with noncontact laser therapy.
- **Prognosis:** There are multiple factors that contribute to prognosis for wound management cases. The local wound environment, vascular supply of the wound, location and size of the wound, presence of infection, and many other factors contribute to the healing process. Laser therapy has a role in promoting tissue healing and decreasing inflammation and edema at the wound surface.
- **Dose:** Superficial wound 3–4 J/cm^2; deep wounds 6–8 J/cm^2

Case Studies

Calcanean Tendon Injury

The author has treated several cats with calcanean tendon injuries with a combination of surgery and photobiomodulation therapy. Calcanean tendon injuries are notoriously slow to heal and rarely achieve 100% of their original strength following repair. Cats are typically maintained in a rigid splint following surgery to support the repair. During sedated splint changes, PBM therapy is easily performed at the incision site and across the repaired tendons to facilitate healing. Bandage changes and laser therapy are performed once weekly for 6 weeks.

Perineal Urethrostomy

The author has performed laser therapy on multiple cats following PU surgery. Because the tissue handled during a PU procedure is generally very sensitive and prone to developing some swelling and edema, it is felt that PBMT is a great modality to reduce inflammation and encourage healing in these cases. Cats were treated postop and for the next 2 days following surgery as well as 1 week and 2 weeks postop.

Idiopathic Cystitis

Idiopathic cystitis is a common, painful, and often recurrent disease of the lower urinary tract that can make management frustrating. The ultrasound images in Figure 18.2 show the urinary bladder of a cat with significant irregular bladder thickening on initial exam. The cat was treated with six sessions of laser therapy over 1–2 weeks, and the repeat ultrasound showed a normal thin bladder wall. Laser therapy has proven to be a valuable addition to the treatment of these cats.

Overgrown Nails

Nails that overgrow and puncture the digital pad can cause a persistent infection because of the structural fat in the pad. Cats' nails grow in a curve, and if they are not worn down or trimmed they can take on a ram's horn-type curl and puncture the digital paw pad (Figure 18.3). Laser therapy can minimize the chances of infection and promote quicker healing. The authors always recommend laser therapy when paw-pad injuries are identified.

Otitis Media and Peripheral Vestibular Disease

The combination of otitis media and peripheral vestibular disease is an uncommon diagnosis, but is one that requires

(a) (b)

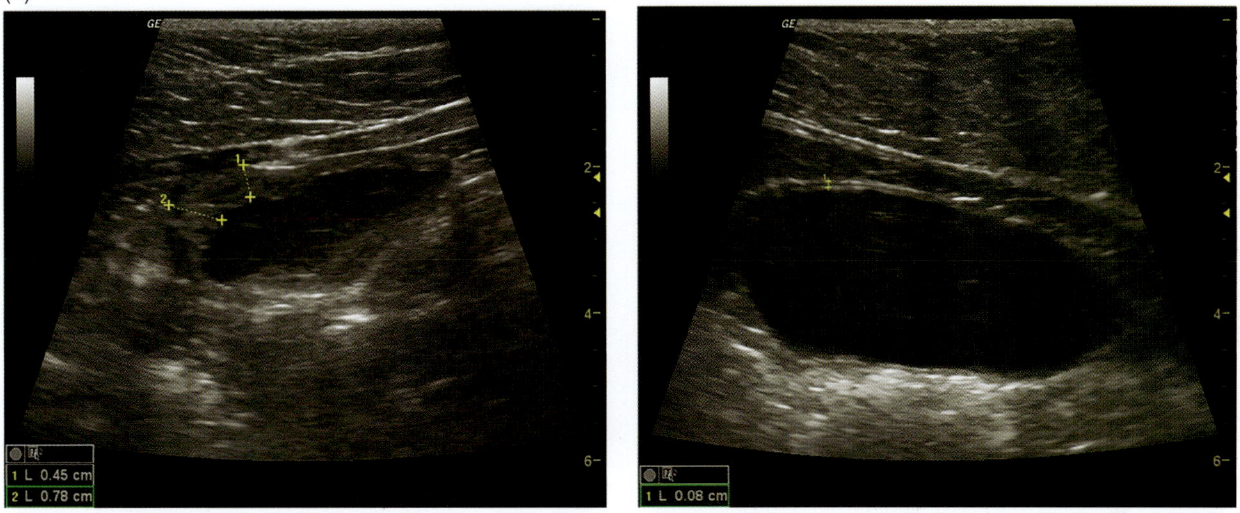

Figure 18.2 (a) Ultrasound image showing the urinary bladder of a cat with significant irregular bladder thickening on initial exam. Idiopathic cystitis was diagnosed. (b) Ultrasound image showing the urinary bladder of the same cat after six laser therapy treatments.

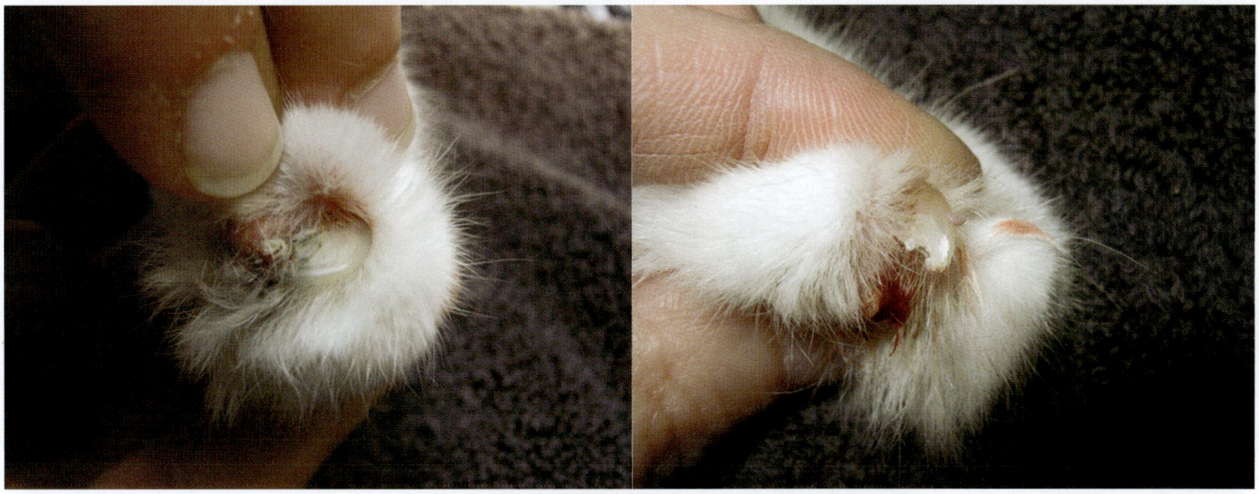

Figure 18.3 Curled nail appearance and the resulting paw-pad wound.

rapid appropriate treatment if there is to be a chance of restoring normal function of the affected vestibular nerve where it courses through the middle ear. This case (Figure 18.4) shows a kitten with a left-sided head tilt that was acute in onset. Physical exam found a bulging discolored tympanum on the left side. The cat was treated with oral broad-spectrum antibiotics, corticosteroids, and a series of six laser therapy sessions over 2 weeks. Figure 18.4 shows the head tilt on initial presentation and the marked improvement and resolution after laser therapy treatment sessions. The authors have found laser therapy to be a great asset in difficult cases of bacterial or yeast otitis with or without secondary vestibular disease.

Feline Acne

When the authors are presented with moderate to severe cases of feline acne, they routinely add a series of three laser therapy sessions on three consecutive days to help speed recovery. Figure 18.5 shows a case (a) upon presentation, (b) during a laser treatment session (wearing goggles), and (c) on a recheck visit 2 weeks later. This cat is a great example of the rapid positive responses seen.

Allergic Dermatitis

Allergic dermatitis can be an uncomfortable disease for the patient, and therefore one where any aid in speeding

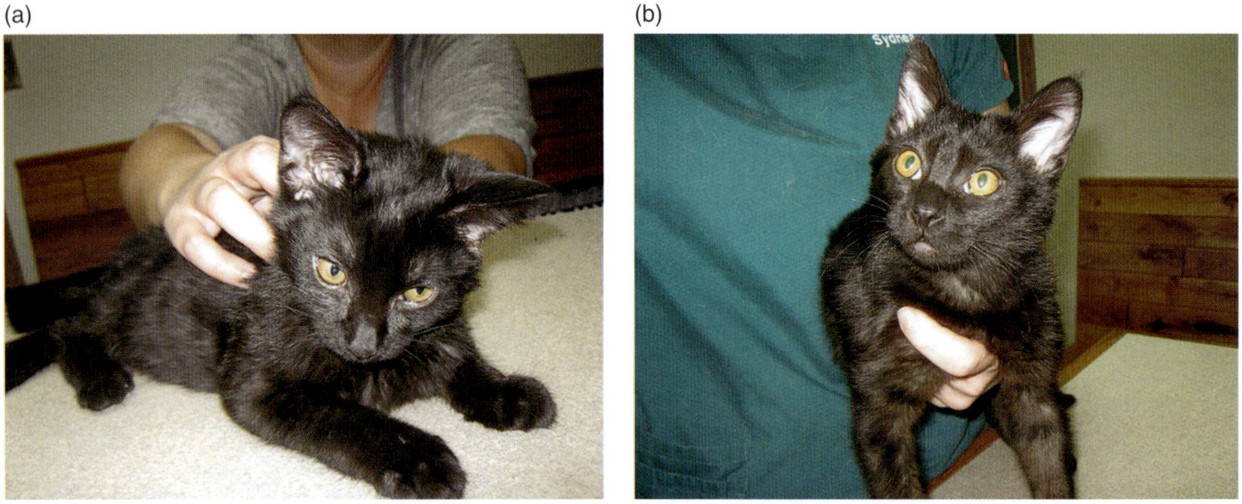

Figure 18.4 (a) Patient with head tilt from acute vestibular disease. (b) Resolution of head tilt from acute vestibular disease after six laser therapy sessions over 2 weeks.

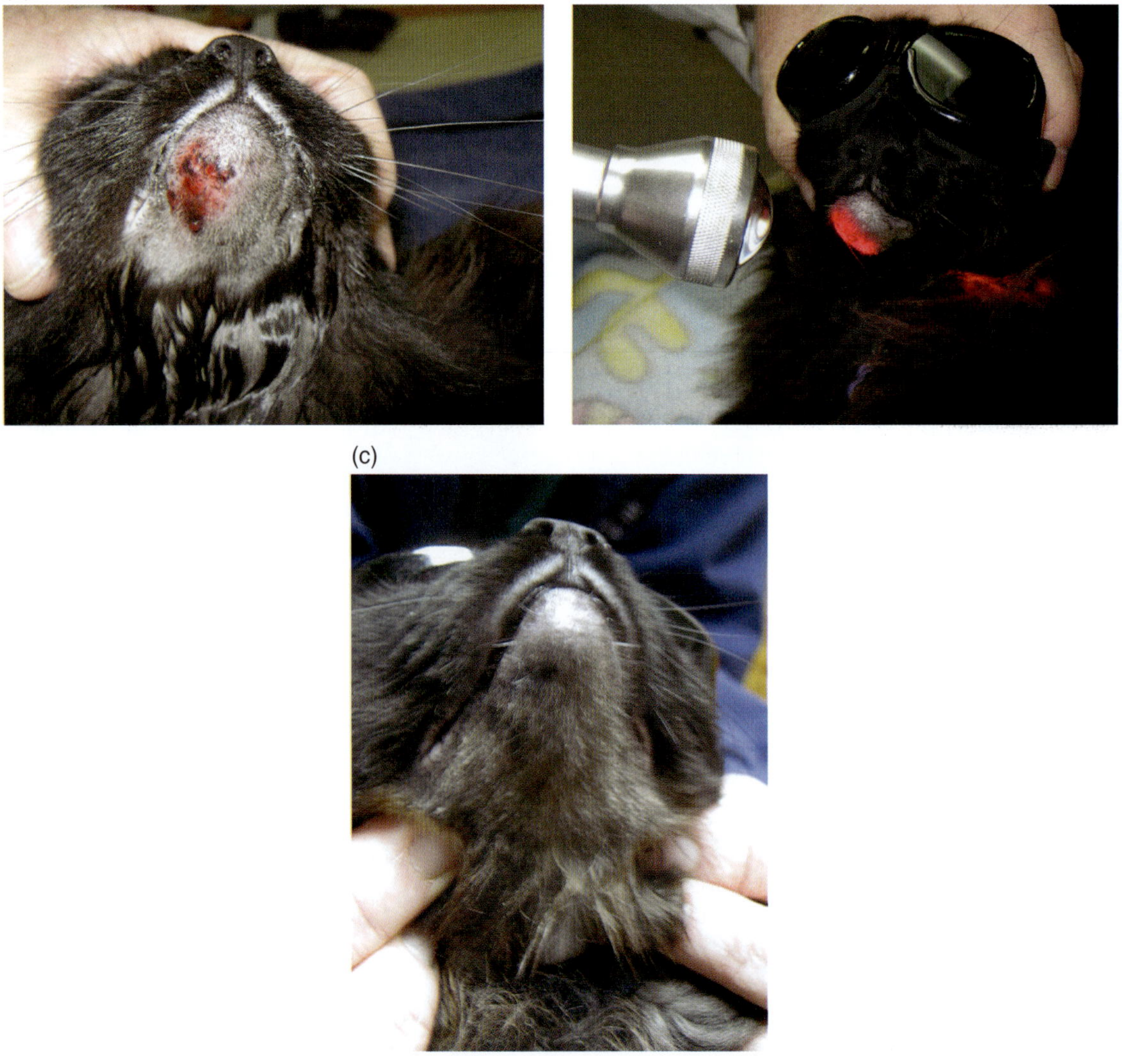

Figure 18.5 (a) Patient with feline acne lesions on presentation. (b) Laser therapy treatment of the same patient. (c) Resolution of the feline acne lesions 2 weeks after presentation, following three laser therapy sessions on three consecutive days.

(a) (b)

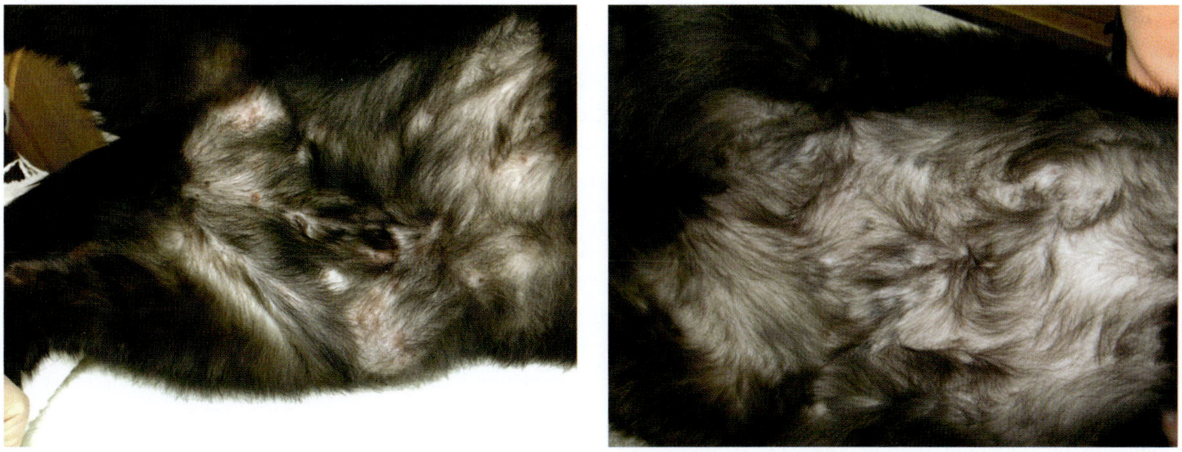

Figure 18.6 (a) Self-inflicted excoriation and dermal lesions due to allergic dermatitis on presentation. (b) The same patient without erythema and with significant hair regrowth 3 weeks later, following three laser therapy treatments.

relief is important. The authors routinely use laser therapy on these cases. Figure 18.6a shows a cat with self-inflicted excoriation and dermal lesions on the belly due to allergic dermatitis. This seasonal flare-up was worse than typical; laser therapy was added as a series of three treatments over 1 week. The owner noted immediate relief of pruritus after the first treatment, and healing of skin lesions was 50% faster than expected. Figure 18.6b shows the skin without erythema and with significant hair regrowth 3 weeks later.

References

Ali, M.K. *et al.* (2022). Modulation of the autonomic nervous system by one session of spinal low-level laser therapy in patients with chronic colonic motility dysfunction. *Front Neurosci.* 16:882602.

Alves, J. C., Jorge, P. & Santos, A. (2021). The effect of photobiomodulation therapy on the management of chronic idiopathic large-bowel diarrhea in dogs. Available at: 10.1007/s10103-021-03469-w [Accessed 8 March 2024].

Alves, J.C. *et al.* (2024). The effect of photobiomodulation therapy on inflammation following dental prophylaxis. *J Vet Dent.* 41(1):26–30.

Bajwa, J. (2018). Atopic dermatitis in cats. *The Canad Vet J.* 59(3):311–313.

Bellah, J.R. (2006). Tail and perineal wounds. *Vet Clini Small Anim Pract.* 36:913–929.

Bennett, D. *et al.* (2012). Osteoarthritis in the cat: 1. how common is it and how easy to recognise? *Journal of Feline Medicine and Surgery.* 14(1):65–75.

Bian, J. et al. (2022). Therapeutic potential of photobiomodulation for chronic kidney disease. Available at: 10.3390/ijms23148043 [Accessed 8 March 2024].

Bidar, M. *et al.* (2016). The effect of low level laser therapy on direct pulp capping in dogs. *J Laser Med Sci.* 7(3):177–183.

Brassolatti, P. *et al.* (2018). Photobiomodulation on critical bone defects of rat calvaria: a systematic review. *Lasers Med Sci.* 33:1841–1848.

Buckley, L. and Nuttall, T. (2012). Feline eosinophilic complex(ities) some clinical clarification. *J Feline Med Surg.* 14:471–481.

Buijs, S. and Godbold, J.C. Jr. (2017). Intra- and postoperative laser therapy. In: *Laser Therapy in Veterinary Medicine Photobiomodulation.* (eds. R.J. Riegel and J.C. Godbold Jr.), pp. 95–96. John Wiley and Sons, Inc., Chichester, West Sussex.

Corbee, R.J. *et al.* (2022). A cross-sectional study on canine and feline anal sac disease. *Animals.* 12:95.

Derkacz, A. *et al.* (2014). Effects of intravascular low-level laser therapy during coronary intervention on selected growth factors levels. *Photomedicine and Laser Surgery.* 32(10):582–587.

Ferasin, L. (2009a). Feline myocardial disease 1: classification, pathophysiology and clinical presentation. *J Feline Med Surg.* 11:3–13.

Ferasin, L. (2009b). Feline myocardial disease 2: diagnosis, prognosis and clinical management. *J Feline Med Surg.* 11:183–194.

Foster, S.F. *et al.* (2004). Twenty-five cases of feline bronchial disease (1995–2000). *J Feline Med Surg.* 6:181–188.

Jawad, M.M. *et al.* (2013). Effect of 940 nm low-level laser therapy on osteogenesis in vitro. *Journal of Biomedical Optics.* 18(12):128001.

Kaya, G.Ş. *et al.* (2011). The use of 808-nm light therapy to treat experimental chronic osteomyelitis induced in rats by methicillin-resistant *Staphylococcus aureus. Photomedicine and Laser Surgery.* 29(6):405–412.

Klinck, M.P. *et al.* (2012). Owner-perceived signs and veterinary diagnosis in 50 cases of feline osteoarthritis. *The Canadian Veterinary Journal.* 53(11):1181.

Lavallee, J.O. and Olson, J. (2017). Feline-specific conditions. In: *Laser Therapy in Veterinary Medicine.* (eds. R.J. Riegel and J.C. Godbold Jr.), pp. 198–211. Wiley Blackwell, s.l.

Lee, M.Y. *et al.* (2017). Treatment of peripheral vestibular dysfunction using photobiomodulation. *J Biomed Opt.* 22(8):1–7.

Neto, F. C. J. *et al.*, (2019). Effects of photobiomodulation in the treatment of fractures: a systematic review and meta-analysis of randomized clinical trials. Available at: 10.1007/s10103-019-02779-4 [Accessed 2019].

Norsworthy, G.D. and Restine, L.M. (2018). Nasal and frontal sinus disease, chronic. In: *The Feline Patient.* (ed. G.D. Norsworthy), 5 edn, pp. 420–421. John Wiley & Sons, Inc., Hoboken, NJ.

Norsworthy, G.D. and Romeo, A. (2018). Hepatic lipidosis. In: *The Feline Patient.* (ed. G.D. Norsworthy), 5 edn, pp. 258–261. John Wiley and Sons, Inc, Hoboken, NJ.

North, C. (2018). Inflammatory bowel disease. In: *The Feline Patient.* (ed. G.D. Norsworthy), 5 edn, pp. 349–351. John Wiley & Sons, Inc., Hoboken, NJ.

O'Neill, D.G. *et al.* (2023). Commonly diagnosed disorders in domestic cats in the UK and their associations with sex and age. *J Feline Med Surg.* 25(2):1–9.

Pieper, J.B. (2018). Acne. In: *The Feline Patient.* (ed. G.D. Norsworthy), 5 edn, pp. 5–6. John Wiley & Sons, Inc., Hoboken, NJ.

Pryor, B. and Millis, D.L. (2015). Therapeutic laser in veterinary medicine. *Vete Clini Small Anim Pract.* 45:45–56.

Ravens, P.A. *et al.* (2014). Feline atopic dermatitis: a retrospective study of 45 cases (2001–2012). *Vet Dermatol.* 25:95–e28.

Reed, N. (2020). Chronic rhinitis in the cat. *Vet Clin: Small Anim Pract.* 50(2):311–329.

Richardson, P. *et al.* (1996). Report of the 1995 World Health Organization/international society and Federation of Cardiology Task Force on the definition and classification of cardiomyopathies. *Circulation.* 93(5):841–842.

Silva, V.R. *et al.* (2014). Low-level laser therapy inhibits bronchoconstriction, Th2 inflammation and airway remodeling in allergic asthma. *Respiratory Physiology & Neurobiology.* 194:37–48.

Son, J. *et al.* (2012). Bone healing effects of diode laser (808 nm) on a rat tibial fracture model. *in vivo.* 26(4):703–709.

Squarzoni, P. *et al.* (2017). NIR laser therapy in the management. *SM Dermatol J.* 3(3):1021–1031.

Steiner, J.M. (2018). Pancreatitis, chronic. In: *The Feline Patient.* (ed. G.D. Norsworthy), 5 edn, pp. 460–461. John Wiley & Sons, Inc., Hoboken, NJ.

Slingerland, L.I. *et al.* (2011). Cross-sectional study of the prevalence and clinical features of osteoarthritis in 100 cats. *The Veterinary Journal.* 187(3):304–309.

Tedford, C.E. *et al.* (2015). Quantitative analysis of transcranial and intraparenchymal light penetration in human cadaver brain tissue. *Lasers in Surgery and Medicine.* 47(4):312–322.

Tim, C.R. *et al.* (2014). Low-level laser therapy enhances the expression of osteogenic factors during bone repair in rats. *Lasers in Medical Science.* 29:147–156.

Trzil, J.E. (2020). Feline asthma: diagnostic and treatment update. *Vet Clin N Am: Small Anim Pract.* 50(2):375–391.

Wardlaw, J. L. *et al.*, (2019). Laser therapy for incision healing in 9 dogs. Available at: 10.3389/fvets.2018.00349

Wexler-Mitchell, E. (2018). Vestibular Syndrome. In: *The Feline Patient.* (ed. G.D. Norsworthy), 5 edn, pp. 673–674. John Wiley & Sons, Inc., Hoboken, NJ.

19

Laser Therapy in the Oncology Patient

Chelsea Tripp[1] *and Lisa A. Miller*[2]

[1] *Bridge Animal Referral Center, Edmonds, WA, USA*
[2] *Companion Animal Health, New Castle, DE, USA*

Challenges in the Geriatric Oncology Patient

In veterinary medicine, our goal is always to do no harm. When we have to treat cancer, this becomes more challenging as many of the therapies needed to help target cancer have serious and sometimes deleterious side effects. We tend to focus on smaller doses and less-intense protocols to minimize the side effects in our patients, but in turn likely sacrifice efficacy for these patients. We need to balance treatment for the patients to optimize efficacy, while still maintaining quality of life.

The majority of cancer patients are older and have other painful comorbidities. It is challenging to manage their dosing, the schedule of administration, and balance effectively treating the cancer with a complex medical presentation as well as background pain. Older dogs notoriously also have cognitive decline, health conditions such as heart disease and renal disease, and a general decrease in physiologic reserve. It is likely that we grossly underestimate the amount of pain in our patients and need to balance these other physiologic processes to obtain multimodal control. Many of our therapies also cause discomfort with side effects for rapidly dividing tissues such as the gastrointestinal tract and bone marrow. Diarrhea is a common side effect of IV chemotherapy agents. Many veterinarians prescribe metronidazole, a nitroimidazole antibiotic, for acute diarrhea. The commonplace usage of antibiotics for treating a self-limiting condition raises concerns regarding appropriate antimicrobial stewardship. Alternative approaches to address the diarrhea and inflammation would be a better approach.

For any patient with cancer, a geriatric assessment is another tool and an important part of treatment planning. In a study in humans, patients who had undergone this assessment were much less likely to experience serious side effects of their chemotherapy (Mohile *et al.*, 2021). The assessment includes evaluations in physical performance, functional status, comorbidities, cognition, nutrition, social support, polypharmacy. These principles also apply in veterinary oncology (Box 19.1).

Pain is another factor that markedly affects quality of life in the cancer patient. The source of cancer pain is variable, complicated and intertwined with other physiologic processes. Pain is related to a variety of host-related factors, processes and tumor-related factors that generally include direct tumor effects such as tissue damage, compression, or invasion by neoplastic growth; and indirect effects caused by unknown paraneoplastic mediators (such as hypertrophic osteopathy). Opioids are the mainstay approach and remain the most effective intervention to sharp C-fiber pain. However, the evolving landscape of chronic opioid abuse and misuse has changed accessibility and limited the long-term use for cancer patients. The need for other options is clear; despite research, no other class of equivalent analgesics has been discovered. This research has actually determined additional therapeutic targets to hone drug development to establish new pharmaceuticals to help pain.

Recently, the monoclonal antibodies bedvintanab (Librela® – Zoetis, USA) and frunevetmab (Solensia® – Zoetis, USA) have become possible and attractive alternatives to help manage osteoarthritis in these patients. These monoclonal antibodies target nerve growth factor (NGF), the main neurotransmitter in nociception. While preliminary work is ongoing, NGF is upregulated in cancer pain. For example, squamous cell cancers of many locations secrete high levels of NGF. Most cancer cells produce chemical mediators and modulators that interact with their microenvironment. These mediators help to sensitize or deactivate nociceptors associated with pain and include prostaglandins, NGF, bradykinin, and endothelin (Falk & Dickenson, 2014; Mantyh, 2014). NGF is recognized by tyrosine kinase-based pain nociceptors as a substrate and can play a crucial role in modulating pain. This binding can further crosstalk, leading

Laser Therapy in Veterinary Medicine: Photobiomodulation, Second Edition. Edited by Christopher J. Winkler and Lisa A. Miller.

Box 19.1 Components of a Geriatric Assessment

• Physical performance	Assess balance, gait, and strength.
• Functional status	Assess difficulties with eating, urination, defecation.
• Comorbidities	Assess the presence of other illnesses.
• Cognition	Assess orientation, sleep habits, and ability to concentrate on tasks.
• Nutrition	Assess body weight and change over last 6 months.
• Polypharmacy	Assess the number of regular medications and any high-risk medications.
• Support	Assess support for daily activities when needed (e.g. mobility, eating, etc.).

to the upregulation of other receptors and increasing the binding affinity of other partner kinases, magnifying the signal. It has also been documented that NGF has been associated with neuronal sprouting, activating the neural inflammatory cascade causing additional neuroma formation within bone and disorganized arborization of axons causing extreme, neuropathic pain. These monoclonal Ab that block NGF are another potential to add to our cancer patients for their pain-relief regime (Williams & MacDonald-Dickinson, 2023).

With the complex interplay between the availability of drugs and their use, additional approaches will have to focus on non-pharmacologic options. Given that up to one-third of human cancer patients remain in uncontrolled pain (Greco *et al.*, 2014), this is likely to be higher in our veterinary companion patients who are unable to verbalize their level of pain. It is important for us to remember to be continually vigilant in our evaluation for pain. Other modalities that also help with pain relief in cancer patients should be considered: injectable agents such as ketamine, acupuncture, and photobiomodulation.

Growing evidence on the human side supports the use of injectable or intranasal ketamine in human cancer patients as an intermittent, nonopioid approach for treatment for patients with intractable pain. Ketamine inhibits the inflammatory signaling pathway of certain glial cell types, thereby modulating and inhibiting neuropathic pain (Culp *et al.*, 2020). Ketamine is also reported to reduce pain behaviors in an arthritis model, distal tibial fractures, ischemia, and perfusion injury.

Evidence has mounted that suggests intractable pain decreases both the quality of life and survival of patients. In a recent rodent model, researchers created persistent pain signaling via electrocautery or sciatic nerve ligation thereby increasing the expression of sensory-located growth factors and peptides and promoting tumor growth. Tumor volume in the mice receiving electrocautery was significantly higher than in patients with no stimulus (sham) (Tanaka *et al.*, 2023). Thus, with intractable pain, the tumors grew faster and were more likely to metastasize.

We need to remember that the unique treatments (such as photobiomodulation) that we currently do have at our disposal are effective against cancer pain in the majority of patients. Also, as these patients have side effects from surgery (swelling from facial and airway surgery, open wounds or draining tracts), have potential unique toxicities from a chemotherapy (sterile hemorrhagic cystitis (SHC) from cyclophosphamide, compartment syndrome from Stelfonta®, pulmonary fibrosis from Bleomycin), and contract secondary conditions/infections from myelosuppression (pneumonia, diarrhea, cystitis, pancreatitis), we should remember the goal of addressing the inflammatory process and breaking the cancer pain cycle. It will likely take multiple modalities of pain relief to achieve this in our cancer patients.

Introduction to the Use of PBM in the Oncology Patient

Historically, there have been mixed recommendations about the use of photobiomodulation therapy (PBMT) in oncology patients. These recommendations have ranged from cautions to not using the modality at all in patients that were currently or previously being treated for neoplastic disease, or in those that could have unknown neoplasia, to using it only in patients so long as photobiomodulation (PBM) was not applied directly over the area of known tumor tissue. Early recommendations, as covered extensively in this first edition's chapter, "Contraindications, Special Considerations, and Precautions," were originally made out of an abundance of caution. This was largely based on a few early studies that showed PBM stimulated the growth of cancer cells in cell culture (Sroka *et al.*, 1999, Al Ghamdi *et al.*, 2012). Not all experimental studies produced the same results, however, and not only does a growing body of research show that PBM can be very beneficial in mitigating numerous side effects that occur as a result of cancer therapies (Zecha *et al.*, 2016a, 2016b; Baxter *et al.*, 2017; Paglioni *et al.*, 2019) but also other research shows that there may even be some potential mechanisms by which PBM can actually be applied against cancer (Hamblin *et al.*, 2017).

Cancer Stimulation *In Vivo*

Taking a deeper dive into the initial concerns of PBM potentially increasing the growth *in vitro* of cancer cells, there are only a few studies that suggest that PBM can actually stimulate cancer growth *in vivo* in animal tumor models. As an example, Rhee and colleagues investigated PBM delivered as a single dose (650 nm, 100 mW/cm^2) to an orthotopic mouse model of anaplastic thyroid cancer. For 4 weeks, tumor volume was measured and histopathological analysis was performed. Researchers reported that PBMT led to a decrease in TGF-β1 and increase of a signaling pathway that regulates certain cellular functions, resulting in proliferation and angiogenesis to the carcinoma. The authors suggested that this could influence cancer aggressiveness (Rhee *et al.*, 2016). A criticism that has been fairly leveled at this study was that it used an immunodeficient mouse model, failing to account for the protective role of the immune system (Hamblin *et al.*, 2017). Another study with a melanoma mouse model compared the effects of two different PBMT doses of 660 nm light – a lower dose (2500 mW/cm^2 and 105 J/cm^2) and a higher dose (2500 mW/cm^2, 1050 J/cm^2) delivered daily for three consecutive days. The researchers concluded that the lower dose PBMT did not influence tumor size; however, the higher dose did increase tumor volume, cell abnormalities, and the number of blood vessels. It is worth noting in this case that the "high" dose was several orders of magnitude above any typically recommended clinical recommendations, even for deeper tissue conditions in a small rodent. Myakishev-Rempel and colleagues examined the effect of PBMT on a standard non-melanoma rodent skin cancer model. They applied 670 nm PBMT (8 mW/cm^2, 5 J/cm^2) to the whole body twice daily for over 30 days. No significant changes in tumor growth were found (Myakishev-Rempel *et al.*, 2012).

Ottaviani *et al.* looked at the behavior of cancer cells both in cell culture and in animal models following PBM. Three PBM protocols using 660 nm, 880 nm, and 970 nm light, respectively, were applied once daily for 4 days: 50 mW/cm^2, 3 J/cm^2; 200 mW/cm^2, 6 J/cm^2; and 200 mW/cm^2, 6 J/cm^2. *In vitro*, PBMT significantly increased proliferation and cell metabolism of the mouse melanoma cells, but when the researchers further investigated the effect of the same PBM protocols *in vivo*, after melanoma cells were subcutaneously injected in syngeneic mice, PBMT application resulted in reduced invasiveness and tumor growth (Ottaviani *et al.*, 2016). The authors investigated further and showed that especially in the L3 group (970 nm, at 6 J/cm^2), alongside the changes noted above were the consistent upregulation of type I interferons (IFN) around the tumor mass and the presence of immune cells (T lymphocytes and dendritic cells [DC]). Type I IFN are known for their unique anti-angiogenic, pro-apoptotic, and anti-proliferative properties. Recently, it has been observed that PBM can be utilized to activate DCs in the dermis to migrate to draining lymph nodes and to induce CD8+/CD4+ T cell responses in melanoma models in mice (Terhorst *et al.*, 2015). These results may partially explain the mechanistic basis by which PBM could inhibit tumor growth *in vivo*. Interestingly, PBM treatment had no effect in IFNα receptor knockout mice, which have no IFNα/β activity, thus indicating that IFNα and IFNβ are the likely mediators of this anti-neoplastic activity of PBMT *in vivo*.

On the human side in the last 20 years, however, the use of PBM has been on the rise in the supportive care of cancer patients (Paglioni *et al.*, 2019). Its use to help manage the side effects of cancer therapies, including lymphedema, oral mucositis, neuropathy, radiodermatitis, and even extravasation injuries, is described in further detail below (Robijns *et al.*, 2017; Baxter *et al.*, 2017; Maria *et al.*, 2017; Argenta *et al.*, 2017; Hamblin, 2023). Two recent retrospective studies evaluating the safety of PBM in head and neck cancer patients did not show that PBM treatment favored the development of new primary tumors or tumor recurrences (Brandão *et al.*, 2018; Antunes *et al.*, 2017). The latter of these studies showed better disease-free survival and survival rates in the PBM-treated group compared to a placebo group. In 2019, a systematic review examined the safety of PBM for the management of cancer-related toxicities. The authors concluded that the majority of the 27 studies analyzed showed no observable side effects with the use of PBMT, and concluded that analysis of this current literature suggests that use of PBMT in the prevention and amelioration of treatment toxicities does not create tumor safety issues (Paglioni *et al.*, 2019). While the authors did mention that further prospective studies with long-term follow-up were needed, it should be noted that in their literature review, "longer term" follow-up periods were considered to be 24 months or more. Altogether, these studies seem to support that the effect of PBMT on *in vitro* cancer is not representative of *in vivo* settings. The majority of current literature suggests that PBMT using wavelengths and fluences typically recommended for clinical practice in veterinary medicine is likely well-tolerated and low-risk for application in cancer patients.

Evidence for PBM Mitigation of Cancer Treatment Side Effects in Humans

In humans, PBM has been shown to be effective for the treatment of several cancer-therapy side effects as described in a recent consensus review provided by World Association of Laser Therapy (WALT) "Guidelines for the Use of PBM to Mitigate Cancer Therapy Side Effects" (Robijns *et al.*, 2022). These side effects included radiodermatitis, oral mucositis, mucosal or bone necrosis, dysphagia, alopecia, chronic graft-versus-host disease, lymphedema, peripheral neuropathy, and other problems. Without treatment, some of these side effects may lead to the alteration or potential discontinuation of therap(ies) with consequential risk to patient(s). In this summary, we will cite the evidence for the use of PBM in three of the most common side effects in humans: radiodermatitis, lymphedema, and oral mucositis.

Acute radiodermatitis (ARD), an inflammatory skin reaction caused by radiotherapy, occurs in up to 95% of patients undergoing this treatment (Cox & Ang, 2010). Developing after 2–4 weeks following the first radiotherapy treatment, the progression and severity of skin reactions can vary and are graded based on the criteria of the Radiation Therapy Oncology Group on a scale of grade 1 (faint or dull erythema, epilation, dry desquamation) to grade 4 (ulceration, hemorrhage, necrosis). Grades 2–4 radiodermatitis can be very impactful to the patients' quality of life, causing severe discomfort (Cox *et al.*, 1995). In severe cases of ARD, premature interruption of radiotherapy might be necessary, which may impact treatment outcomes and overall patient survival. Radiodermatitis management strategies to reduce the risk of radiotherapy interruptions and morbidity have primarily utilized topical products for skin care, improved daily hygiene, and at times, the use of topically applied steroids (Wong *et al.*, 2013). However, due to limited scientific research, the effectiveness of these protocols remain unclear.

In-vitro and *in-vivo* studies previously described have demonstrated that PBMT affects all phases of wound healing. PBMT enhances angiogenesis, increases collagen synthesis, downregulates inflammatory mediators, and increases the proliferation and migration of fibroblasts and keratinocytes (Hawkins & Abrahamse, 2006a, 2006b; Chaves *et al.*, 2018; Lanzafame *et al.*, 2007; Pereira *et al.*, 2002). Moreover, PBMT increases the production of granulation tissue, causes faster reepithelization of wounds, and improves tensile strength (Stadler *et al.*, 2001; de Lima *et al.*, 2016; Lanzafame *et al.*, 2007; Chaves *et al.*, 2018) as well as modulating growth factor and cytokine production involved in ARD mechanisms (Peplow *et al.*, 2011; Peplow *et al.*, 2012).

There have been several human clinical trials examining the use of PBMT in the management of ARD (Robijns *et al.*, 2019a,b). Schindl and colleagues were the first to report a case series in which breast cancer patients experiencing ARD ulceration after mastectomy were treated with PBMT. PBMT was able to speed healing of the skin ulcers (Schindl *et al.*, 1999). Further breast cancer clinical trials have studied the use of PBMT in patients undergoing radiotherapy. Patients receiving a full course of radiotherapy were treated daily with PBMT. One trial demonstrated that PBMT reduced the incidence of grade 2 or higher radiodermatitis (Deland *et al.*, 2007) though these results could not be repeated in a later randomized controlled trial (Fife *et al.*, 2010). It is worth noting, that a possible explanation for the different outcomes was the use of different treatment and assessment parameters, emphasizing again the need for more consistent study design(s). Another prospective intervention trial in breast cancer patients demonstrated that the application of PBMT twice weekly (808–905 nm, 4 J/cm^2) prevented the aggravation of ARD and improved quality of life toward the end of radiotherapy (Censabella *et al.*, 2016). Two other studies investigated the prophylactic use of twice-weekly PBM in prospective trials with breast cancer patients. Both demonstrated that PBMT reduced the incidence of severe ARD (Strouthos *et al.*, 2017) and the latter also demonstrated that the use of PBMT improved patient quality of life scores (Robijns *et al.*, 2019b).

In humans, a common complication secondary to cancer treatments is breast cancer-related lymphedema (BCRL). BCRL significantly impacts the morbidity of breast cancer patients. Despite implementation of new surgical techniques like sentinel node biopsies instead of axillary dissection to try to reduce lymphedema rates, BCRL remains a common occurrence. One systematic review estimated that one out of every five women who survive breast cancer experience BCRL (DiSipio *et al.*, 2013). Previous and current mainstays of BCRL management approaches include physiotherapy, manual lymphatic drainage, and the use of compression garments. In the past 20 years, PBM has also been researched and promoted as a possible management tool for BCRL (Morrell *et al.*, 2005; Baxter *et al.*, 2017). In 2017, Baxter and colleagues performed a systematic review of studies involving the use of PBM in patients with BCRL. This review included an assessment of treatment adequacy in these trials to examine the clinical appropriateness of the PBM treatment regimen. Findings of this review supported the use of this modality for treating BCRL patients. There was strong evidence (three high-quality trials) favoring PBM over sham for reduction in limb edema, and moderate evidence favoring PBM for short-term pain relief.

Characterized by the ulceration of non-keratinized mucosa (such as on the buccal mucosa tongue, and the soft palate) oral mucositis (OM), is one of the most severe complications arising from certain cancer treatments in humans. Head and neck tumor patients that have undergone hematopoietic stem cell transplantation, or been diagnosed with other solid tumors, may experience severe pain, dysphasia, the need for parental feeding, or impaired speech and sometimes even psychological consequences from OM that severely impact quality of life and sometimes may even require further intensive interventions or hospitalization (Nascimento *et al.*, 2023).

The appearance of erythema and ulcers is preceded by cancer treatments causing tissue damage, thereby releasing reactive oxygen species, pro-inflammatory cytokines, and activating metalloproteinases and other substances which initiate inflammation and create widespread damage to the collagen connective tissues and accelerated cellular apoptosis in the basal layer of epithelium (Sonis, 2011; Pulito *et al.*, 2020). In 2020, guidelines of conduct and clinical practices for the prevention and management of OM were published (Elad *et al.*, 2020). Recommendations included the general promotion of oral health, the use of benzydamine or 0.2% morphine mouthwashes (for ongoing OM), the IV administration of keratinocyte growth factor, and cryotherapy for the prevention of OM. However, some of these methods may be difficult to access for patients or present other challenges, making their implementation difficult. One of the recommendations emphasized in the guidelines was PBMT, and there have been several studies confirming its effectiveness for this application (Zadik *et al.*, 2016; Cronshaw *et al.*, 2020; Lima *et al.*, 2010).

PBM's efficacy for pain management via its modulation of the inflammatory process, and selective inhibitory effects on axonal transmission of pain signals (amongst other mechanisms described extensively in Chapter 6) in addition to the promotion of collagen production and growth factors beneficial for healing tissues, favors the resolution of OM ulcers while also relieving pain for patients. A recent summary of the systematic reviews for oral mucositis was published, including outcomes from 16 clinical trials (Nascimento *et al.*, 2023). Most studies provided data on OM management in mixed cancer populations. Regarding the effectiveness of both prophylactic and therapeutic treatment, six studies indicated a statistical difference in favor of PBM therapy for the former and all studies reporting outcomes for the latter demonstrated statistical significance favoring PBM therapy for reducing the severity of OM. Most studies reported doses in the range of 1–6 J/cm^2 as effective for OM prevention across the different cancer treatments, which is consistent with the dosimetry for many veterinary oral conditions (see Chapter 13). The frequency of treatment sessions most recommended was daily to every other day throughout the entire cancer treatment, or until the resolution of OM lesions (Lai *et al.*, 2021; Anschau *et al.*, 2019; da Silva *et al.*, 2022). Overall, the summary authors concluded that OM prevention and treatment were favorable for PBMT in most studies, significantly reducing OM severity, with moderate confidence obtained in most studies.

The evidence summarized above for these three common conditions faced in oncology indicates that PBM represents an effective strategy in the management of ARD, BCRL, and oral mucositis, and this evidence is supported by numerous quality studies. It is important to note that Baxter and colleagues also identified that, much like many of the published PBM studies on other conditions, there were extensive study differences in treatment regimens and outcome measures used, and that a head-to-head comparison to determine optimal PBM dosing regimens (for lymphedema at least) was not possible (Baxter *et al.*, 2017). Future continued research into all these areas was a common suggestion by SR authors, which could further guide establishment of optimal PBM regimes for symptom management of cancer treatment side effects, both in human and veterinary medicine.

Anti-cancer Applications of PBM

We have discussed the possibilities of using PBMT to treat side effects associated with cancer treatment, but a more interesting possibility is whether it may also be possible to employ PBM as part of cancer treatment itself. Some recent studies seem to suggest that PBMT might have utility as a means of (in)directly attacking cancer via three varied mechanisms: utilizing high-dose PBMT to directly kill neoplastic cells, selectively destroying cancer based on inherent metabolic differences, and stimulating anti-tumor immunity (Hamblin *et al.*, 2017; Robijns *et al.*, 2019b).

So-called "overdosing" of cancer cells through application of high-dose PBM is achieved through the method of "high fluence, low-power laser irradiation" (HF-LPLI). This technique has been utilized in experiments both *in vitro* and *in vivo* primarily by researchers at a laboratory in China (Wu *et al.*, 2009). The fluence used in these studies has been reported at 1200 J/cm^2, approximately 20 times that of the upper end of energy densities typically recommended for even deep tissue conditions. In one study, a single dose using this fluence was delivered to mice bearing EMT6 breast tumors. The mice that were treated with this dose had complete regression which did not occur in rho-zero EMT6 tumors (without functional mitochondria) (Lu *et al.*, 2016).

PBM has a different effect on cancer cells compared to its effects on normal cells, which is likely related to a phenomenon known as the Warburg effect, in which cancer cells are able to convert their metabolism to promote growth, survival, and proliferation (Liberti & Locasale, 2016) by carrying out aerobic glycolysis rather than oxidative phosphorylation, even in the presence of completely functioning mitochondria. Normally, apoptotic programs require relatively large amounts of adenosine triphosphate (ATP) to execute in the cell (Eguchi *et al.*, 1997). As ATP supply is limited in neoplastic cells, the surge provided by the application of PBM may enable them to respond to pro-apoptotic stimuli more readily and execute apoptotic programs more efficiently (Hamblin *et al.*, 2018). In this strategy, cancer cells are selectively destroyed when PBM is applied in combination with additional cytotoxic therapies (photodynamic therapy and radiation therapy being two examples). The application of PBM releases reactive oxygen species that reduce the damaging effects these therapies have on healthy tissues, while potentiating the destruction of cancer cells (Tsai *et al.*, 2015; Djavid *et al.*, 2017). This differential effect could also be at play in certain veterinary oncology strategies that utilize the photothermal effects of laser combined with gold nanoparticles to selectively kill tumors but spare healthy surrounding tissues (Parshley *et al.*, 2022).

Lastly, PBM may be stimulating the immune system itself to fight against cancer. In the previously mentioned 2016 study by Ottaviani *et al.*, researchers showed that PBM increased the recruitment of T lymphocytes and dendritic cells secreting type I IFN while also reducing the quantity of highly angiogenic macrophages, thus promoting vessel normalization, and reduced tumor growth (Ottaviani *et al.*, 2016). In another study, researchers inoculated 72 Walker Tumor-induced Wistar rats, and after 2 weeks (allowing time for the development and assessment of the tumor mass), the animals were randomized and distributed in four groups: a control group (G1) or one of three treatment groups that received varying fluences (35–214 J/cm^2) of PBM using 660 nm and 100 mW three times on alternating days. The expression and regulation of certain inflammatory mediators were assessed and gene expression of iNOS, eNOS, COX-1, and COX-2 were also analyzed. The authors reported that the 35 J/cm^2 dose promoted a significant increase in the gene expression of COX-2, the levels IL-1β and iNOS, compared to the other treatment and control groups. They concluded that this fluence produced cytotoxic effects via generation of reactive oxygen species causing acute inflammation, though notably, they did not measure direct tumor effect (Petrellis *et al.*, 2017).

The research outlined here is exciting, but there are questions still to be answered. Optimal dosing parameters and timing of application(s), as well as the combined use of PBMT with other therapies, all need to be elucidated further. Nevertheless, the possibility to employ PBMT as a therapy, not only to benefit patients suffering side effects but also as part of their anti-cancer treatment strategy, is intriguing.

Conditions for Consideration in Veterinary Oncology

PBMT is becoming a well-established approach on the human side to help prevent or minimize the development of side effects associated with cancer therapies. As the authors here point out, veterinary patients, while experiencing many of the same side effects from cancer treatment that humans do, usually have a plethora of concomitant conditions common in geriatric patients that may also benefit from treatment with PBMT. This textbook goes into detail on a wide variety of various conditions by category that may benefit from PBMT in practice, but here the authors will focus on recommendations for a few common conditions seen in oncology practice that we have found to benefit from treating with PBMT.

Diarrhea and Digestive Changes

Gastrointestinal adverse effects (vomiting, diarrhea, nausea, and inappetence) are recognized in both dogs and humans after receiving chemotherapy (Mellanby *et al.*, 2002; Tomiyasu *et al.*, 2010; Mason et al., 2014). Toxicity may lead to increased patient morbidity, necessitating reduction in drug dosages or (in certain circumstances) withdrawal of treatment. Two retrospective publications reported on the gastrointestinal side effects of vincristine and cyclophosphamide in dogs. Though mild, GI side effects were reported in 20–50% of patients (Mellanby *et al.*, 2002; Tomiyasu *et al.*, 2010). Similarly, a retrospective analysis of nonradiation complications in dogs undergoing radiation therapy found that GI complications occurred in 37% of patients, though in that population, complications were usually mild or self-limiting (Farrelly & Shi, 2018). Inflammation associated with chronic diarrhea can alter the microbiome composition, affecting adequate digestion and the production of some metabolites (Redfern *et al.*, 2017; Whelan & Schneider, 2011). Combined with changes in how cancer patients metabolize nutrients and the altered permeability of their GI tract, this can further alter the normal microbiome as well. It has been established that the health and composition of the GI microbiome affects many diseases related to obesity, metabolism, autoimmunity, cardiovascular disorders, and others (Liebert *et al.*, 2019).

The potential for using PBMT as part of an overall strategy to reduce inflammation in the GI mucosa, decrease the frequency of episodes of diarrhea, reduce weight loss, and potentially reset the microbiome, is promising.

In a study in police working dogs that evaluated the effectiveness of PBMT in reducing the clinical signs of chronic inflammatory large bowel diarrhea, PBMT was compared to psyllium husk supplementation. The study utilized 980 nm and a fluence of 8.6 J/cm^2 (irradiance 2.4 W/cm^2) treating on-contact over the abdomen of large-breed dogs, initially starting with three sessions weekly and decreasing the frequency of treatment sessions over time. Patients treated with PBMT showed decreased frequency of diarrhea episodes, increased body weight, and better body condition scores (Alves *et al.*, 2022a).

Researchers have also shown that in healthy mice, PBM delivered to the abdomen produces significant changes in the GI microbiome. 808 nm near-infrared (NIR) light significantly altered the diversity of the microbiome, especially in mice treated multiple times per week, producing a 10 000-fold increase in the proportion of *Allobaculum* (a beneficial bacterium) in the microbiota of mice after 2 weeks of treatment (Liebert *et al.*, 2019). The same researchers that performed this original study reported that this same methodology has been repeated (though unpublished) with more mice in the experimental groups and that preliminary work (also unpublished) has been done involving the human (quasimetabolic syndrome) microbiome, and that preliminary results from both species showed the proportion of bacteria associated with a dysregulated microbiome generally decreased and the proportion of bacteria associated with a healthy microbiome generally increased (Liebert *et al.*, 2019). Proposed mechanisms behind how PBM may be impacting the microbiome in the reported experiments above have included that PBM is impacting the inflammatory response (via a reduction in proinflammatory cytokines and change in the activity of macrophages from a proinflammatory lineage to an anti-inflammatory M2 phenotype), and thus affecting the gut microbiota (Hamblin, 2017; Fukuda *et al.*, 2013; Fernandes *et al.*, 2015).

In another experimental series, researchers have shown a neuroprotective effect against an induced Parkinson's disease insult in mice with PBM delivered to other areas of the body distant to the brain (Ganeshan *et al.*, 2019; Johnstone *et al.*, 2014; Kim *et al.*, 2018). This "abscopal effect" of PBM is thought to be due to stem cells, immune cells, or another circulating mediator. Liebert and colleagues have proposed that this mediator may be associated to changes in the microbiome (Liebert *et al.*, 2019). Alongside other approaches to improve the microbiome (including dietary management, probiotics, and fecal transplantation), PBM may provide a means of beneficially altering the microbiome for numerous inflammatory diseases.

For treating diarrhea, a deep-tissue dosage of 6–10 J/cm^2 is recommended (scaling up with the size of the patient and depth of the target tissues), treating the entire abdomen as if performing a scanning abdominal ultrasound of the GI tract, continuously moving on-contact to minimize light loss(es) from reflection. The author and colleagues have previously used an on-contact treatment head with a spot size of 5 cm^2 and power settings in the 4–8 W range (0.8–1.6 W/cm^2) at the skin surface (again, scaling up with the size of the patient and the depth of the target tissue). For acute situations or hospitalized patients, PBMT sessions may be performed daily for pain management, weaning the frequency of treatment sessions as the patient improves, until resolution. For more chronic situations, after initial improvement(s) are clinically noted, weaning out to a maintenance schedule of treatments that aid in keeping a patient's symptoms to a minimum is recommended (typically once every 2–4 weeks).

The authors are not recommending that PBMT be used instead of appropriate nutritional management and pharmacological supplementation, but instead are advising that it should be used in conjunction with a comprehensive program of dietary management and administration of appropriate GI medications according to the clinician's judgment.

Urinary Tract Infections and Sterile Hemorrhagic Cystitis

Urinary tract infection (UTI) commonly affects patients in veterinary medicine and is characterized by the persistence of bacteria within the urinary tract, leading to inflammation and subsequent clinical signs (Smee *et al.*, 2013). Subclinical bacteriuria (SB) has a reported prevalence in healthy dogs between 2% and 9% (Wan *et al.*, 2014) and is defined by a positive urine culture (PUC) without clinical signs of actual urinary tract disease (Weese *et al.*, 2019). There is an increased prevalence of SB in dogs receiving immunosuppressive treatments reported in most studies (Peterson *et al.*, 2012), and treatment with antineoplastic chemotherapy or corticosteroids has been identified as the most common risk factor in dogs that have a PUC (Wong *et al.*, 2015; Seguin *et al.*, 2003). A study in 47 pyelonephritis dogs found non-urogenital neoplasia as the most common comorbidity (Bouillon *et al.*, 2018). The prevalence of PUC in dogs receiving chemotherapy has been reported for dogs with prostatic carcinoma (Ravicini *et al.*, 2018), transitional cell carcinoma (Budreckis *et al.*, 2015), and non-urogenital neoplasia (Harrer *et al.*, 2022) and indicates that (at least in these three studies) there is increased prevalence of PUC in dogs with urogenital tumors than in dogs with non-urogenital tumors (Harrer *et al.*, 2022).

SHC is a painful condition clinically characterized by lower urinary tract signs such as hematuria, stranguria, and pollakiuria, without evidence of a UTI. A well-documented adverse effect associated with cyclophosphamide administration in both humans and dogs, SHC can be debilitating and sometimes irreversible, and may necessitate discontinuation of the drug (Peterson *et al.*, 1992; Stillwell & Benson, 1988; Crow *et al.*, 1977; Gaeta *et al.*, 2014). The pathogenesis of SHC involves the formation and accumulation of byproducts of cyclophosphamide metabolism (acrolein and 4-hydroxymetabolites) in the urine, which cause submucosal edema, hemorrhage, necrosis, and fibrosis of the mucosal epithelium in the urinary bladder (Brock *et al.*, 1981) and may follow oral or IV administration of the drug. The risk of a patient developing SHC increases as the cumulative dose of administered cyclophosphamide increases. In dogs, the reported incidence of SHC ranges from 3.8% to 12.1% following administration of the maximum tolerated dose of cyclophosphamide, but is lower when cyclophosphamide is administered concurrently with IV or oral administration of furosemide, respectively (Charney *et al.*, 2003; Laberkey *et al.*, 2014; Chan *et al.*, 2016). Management strategies for SHC have included the discontinuation of the offending drug, managing secondary infections with appropriate antibiotics, and decreasing discomfort with pain medications (including NSAIDs if renal function is normal) (Kobayashi, 2015). Most cases resolve with time, but may take several weeks to months to reach resolution.

As immunosuppression (caused by both the cancer itself and chemotherapy) may predispose patients to be at increased risk for UTI, and antibiotic treatment of SB is only recommended in rare cases with particularly high risk of ascending or systemic infection, it may be helpful to have another modality which may help manage the symptoms of cancer patients with UTIs and/or cases of SHC. Both of these conditions are extremely painful, and current pain medication options may be insufficient and/or unable to be administered to the patient, depending on other factors including renal function. The benefits of PBM for treating the urinary tract are described in detail in Chapters 14 and 15. Briefly, PBMT results in analgesia through reducing inflammation and reducing C-fiber activation (a major contributor to the development of the allodynia responsible for the symptom of urinary frequency and bladder pain).

For treating the urinary bladder in the case of either UTI or SHC, a deep tissue dosage of 6–10 J/cm^2 is recommended (scaling up with the size of the patient and depth of the target tissues), treating the entire caudal abdomen on-contact utilizing the same power settings as described for diarrhea above, using a similar technique to scanning the area for a diagnostic ultrasound, aiming for all aspects of the bladder where it is positioned in the abdomen. In cases of mild UTIs, one to three treatment sessions may suffice. For more serious infections or SHC, begin with daily to every-other-day treatments, then wean the frequency of treatment sessions (twice weekly, then once weekly, and so forth) as the patient improves, until resolution may be needed.

PBM for Extravasation Injuries and Other Wound Management

While not a normal side effect of cancer treatment(s), some chemotherapeutics are classified as vesicants and may cause severe injury when accidently extravasated into tissue during an intravenous injection or infusion. Some cytotoxic drugs are worse than others when it comes to those causing extravasation injuries, and the anthracyclines (including doxorubicin, idarubicin, epirubicin, and some liposomal formulations) are amongst the most notorious. Less severe extravasation injuries can be caused by other chemotherapy drugs, such as vinca alkaloids, taxanes, and alkylating agents, amongst others. Acutely, these extravasations can cause swelling and pain at the infusion site, progressing to blistering or necrosis over the next few days (Kreidieh, 2016). Further damage to soft tissues in the area of injury can develop over weeks depending on the location of the infusion. Extensive wound care and sometimes surgical excision of necrotic tissue may be required in some cases. Traditional treatments in both human and veterinary medicine for extravasation injury have been extremely varied as well as variably successful, including saline dilution/lavage and needle aspiration to attempt removal of the offending chemotherapy agent, cold-packing the affected area(s), local injection of hyaluronidase, topical dimethyl sulfoxide (DMSO) application, local injection of corticosteroids, and/or systemic administration of antihistamines and anti-inflammatories, depending on the agent (Biller *et al.*, 2016; Hamblin, 2023).

Recently Freitas *et al.* reported on PBM's efficacy in minimizing anthracycline extravasation injury, both in both cancer patients and in animal models (Freitas *et al.*, 2022). In one study, 60 rats divided into four groups each received a subcutaneous doxorubicin injection. One group (G1) served as a control while groups 2–4 all received a different treatment (G2-topical hyaluronidase; G3-PBM; and G4-topical hyaluronidase and PBM combined). G3 and G4 PBM utilized 660 nm light at 1 J/cm^2, applied once daily until the lesion resolved. The patients in both PBM groups (alone or in combination) showed less hyperemia, bleeding, exudate, and necrosis, and better granulation tissue compared with the other two groups (G1 or G2). By 4 weeks, 40% of G3 patients and 13% of G4 patients showed complete healing. A retrospective study by the same group was also published where PBM was used in 15 cancer patients who had each experienced a chemotherapy extravasation event (Freitas *et al.*, 2020). Patients were treated daily with PBM in combination with topical hyaluronidase for two days and none of the patients developed any lesions or clinical signs upon evaluation following 48 hours of the extravasation event.

In a recent article on the use of PBM for extravasation injury, Hamblin points out that there are overlapping similarities between the use of PBM for this particular type of injury and its use in treating the localized effects of inflammation, pain, and necrosis seen in snake bite envenomation cases (Hamblin, 2023). The role of PBM in treating snake bites is discussed extensively in Chapter 10. Briefly, PBM has been shown to reduce pain and swelling, modulate the inflammatory response, and accelerate tissue healing in cases of certain types of snakebites (Silva *et al.*, 2018) as well as in wounds of other origins (see Chapter 8). Studies previously described have demonstrated that PBMT affects all phases of the wound healing process through enhancing angiogenesis, downregulating inflammatory mediators, favoring collagen deposition, and a more rapid reepithelization of wounds (Hawkins & Abrahamse, 2006a, 2006b (1&2); Chaves *et al.*, 2018; Lanzafame *et al.*, 2007; Pereira *et al.*, 2002; Stadler *et al.*, 2001; de Lima *et al.*, 2016; Lanzafame *et al.*, 2007; Chaves *et al.*, 2018). The use of photobiomodulation should especially be considered in patients with potential healing compromise from anticancer therapies that are undergoing surgery or have experienced wounds from other traumatic injuries.

Dosages listed and recommended in the literature for treating wounds are extensively discussed in Chapter 8, but usually range from 2–5 J/cm^2 for superficial wounds and 4–15 J/cm^2 (or higher), depending on the size and depth of the wound, the presence of any infection(s), and the chronicity (Al-Watban *et al.*, 2007; Hawkins and Abrahamse, 2007; Peplow *et al.*, 2012). Wounds should be treated in a noncontact manner to avoid contamination of either the wound or the treatment handpiece. The wound area should be measured, and a corresponding surrounding margin of 1–3 cm of healthy tissue should be added to this treatment area. Initial treatment may be daily to every other day for two to five sessions. If no improvement is noted within the two to five treatments, the dosage (total joules) should be increased by 25–50% per treatment until a positive response is being noted (Bradley, 2017). In larger or complicated wounds (including those created by extravasation injuries), following the more frequent initial treatments described above, treatment intervals should be weaned to twice weekly, then once weekly and so on, once the wound is showing a strong positive clinical response.

Osteoarthritis and Mobility Issues

Chronic pain is often underestimated in veterinary patients, and strategies should be integrative to help the patient's condition. Many cancer patients are geriatric and already experiencing some form of chronic pain, whether due to their neoplasia or other comorbidities (Withrow and Vail, 2020). Cancer can cause pain by several different mechanisms, including direct tumor effects such as invasion by tumor growth or tissue damage, compression, and indirect effects caused by paraneoplastic mediators (Willians and Macdonald-Dickinson, 2023). A recent meta-analysis in human oncology patients revealed that about one-third of patients experienced uncontrolled pain (Greco *et al.*, 2014). While it may be challenging to assess whether or not our patients have their pain adequately managed, it is likely that many of them do not (Withrow and Vail, 2020; Willians and Macdonald-Dickinson, 2023). In addition to the validated pain assessment and osteoarthritis tools discussed in Chapters 6 and 11, several validated quality-of-life and pain assessment scales have been published which are of particular use in oncology patients (Lynch *et al.*, 2011; Yazbek & Fantoni, 2005). In both human and veterinary medicine, the advantage of a multimodal analgesic plan over single-agent therapies has been demonstrated. The efficacy and use of pharmaceuticals for managing chronic pain in the veterinary oncology patient, while important, will not be discussed here in this textbook.

Accounting for the cause of at least 80% of lameness diagnoses and affecting around 20% of adult dogs in the United States, over 90% of elderly dogs show clinical signs of osteoarthritis (Anderson *et al.*, 2020; Johnston, 1997; Venable *et al.*, 2008). In cats, a similar scenario is observed. Osteoarthritis has a prevalence of over 90% in animals over 12 years (Lascelles, 2010; Lascelles *et al.*, 2012) and this prevalence is expected to increase due to increased life expectancy and obesity rates (Anderson *et al.*, 2020). While there are no published studies specifically looking at the prevalence of arthritis in veterinary oncology patients, with cancer affecting pets of all ages, it is safe to assume that the numbers are very similar. Keeping these patients moving with worsening arthritis and body condition changes is imperative.

Discussed in further detail in Chapter 11, current treatment strategies in veterinary medicine for arthritis are aimed primarily toward controlling pain, improving joint function, and minimizing functional incapacity in patients through pet owner education and home environmental management. Multimodal management of patients with osteoarthritis includes appropriate weight management, nutraceutical supplementation, pharmacological therapy, rehabilitation therapy, or regenerative medicine (including the use of platelet-rich plasma (PRP) or stem-cell therapy). PBMT may be utilized along with any or all of these therapies, and utilizing PBMT for its analgesic and anti-inflammatory effects is especially important, as it may reduce or eliminate the need for medications and the concomitant side effects that can come with their use. PBMT can be particularly effective in helping to control the degenerative disease-driving low-grade inflammation.

All veterinary oncology patients exhibiting signs of pain should undergo a thorough orthopedic and neurologic examination, as well as an investigation of their clinical history, prior to being prescribed PBMT for their osteoarthritis. In order to be effective, PBMT must be applied to the correct tissues. Many of these patients will, in addition to having joint pain from arthritis, also have other localized painful areas due to compensatory changes in biomechanics. Pain examinations should be repeated regularly on all patients, to evaluate for improvement after therapy has started, and to ensure there are no "new" issues that should be treated. In the case of a lack of improvement or a worsening, pain examinations can also help to determine whether further diagnostics are indicated. It is also important to remember that the degree of radiographic or pathologic change discovered may not necessarily be consistent with the amount of lameness displayed by the patient or the severity of their discomfort. Further details are provided in Chapters 11 and 23 on patient evaluation, validated pain questionnaires and other tools that may be used in diagnostics and outcome assessments, and on patient preparation and techniques. Prescribed treatment areas for PBMT should primarily be based on the orthopedic and pain-assessment examinations performed by the clinician.

For osteoarthritis and compensatory musculoskeletal pain, a general range of energy densities of 6–20 J/cm^2 is recommended (Looney *et al.*, 2018; Alves *et al.*, 2022b) scaling up with the size of the patient and the average thickness of soft tissues (including fat and muscle layers) in the treatment areas. Though the specifics are device- and design-dependent, the power used to achieve the desired fluence should be lower for smaller patients, areas with increased sensitivity, or areas with very little soft tissue present. Chapter 11 provides a range of recommended power settings for musculoskeletal conditions in veterinary patients of various sizes, but in general, settings from 2 to 15 W may be acceptable (with the appropriate treatment head and spot size), again scaling up with patient size, size of treatment area(s) and depth of tissues. For any acute or chronic painful condition such as osteoarthritis, an "induction phase" of initial, more frequent treatment sessions are recommended (i.e. every-other-day treatments until a significant effect is seen). Though significant improvement may be appreciated sooner for some patients with osteoarthritis, it is usually noted between four and six treatment sessions. However, for those with severe osteoarthritis or multiple joint involvements, improvement may not be noted for 7–10 sessions. It is helpful for the practitioner to set expectations with pet owners, to avoid their becoming discouraged when they do not see immediate results. Once a significant improvement is noted in clinical signs, a "transition phase" of treatment sessions is begun. During transition, treatments are decreased to twice weekly, then once weekly, and so on as the patient improves, until a "maintenance phase" of treatment is established (typically once every 2–4 weeks) such that a patient's symptoms are kept to a minimum.

PBM Cases in an Oncology Clinical Practice

Postsurgical Pain Relief

Signalment: 9 years, M/N French Bulldog; "Smudge."

History: Presented in February of 2022 for CT scan and biopsy of lytic oral mass found during dental radiography for routine dental prophylaxis.

Diagnostics: Histopathology of oral mass revealed squamous cell carcinoma; CT scan showed no evidence of lymph node involvement or metastasis.

Surgery: mandibulectomy

Laser therapy: PBM utilizing a dose of 5 J/cm^2 was applied in a noncontact manner to the surgical site and ventral neck area in post-op recovery and twice daily for the first 48 hours following surgery for pain relief, with decreasing frequency of treatment sessions over the next 14 days as the patient became more comfortable.

Results: The patient recovered from surgery without complications and went on to receive further treatment including IV chemotherapy and maintenance metronomic chemotherapy (satraplatin) and immunotherapy (vorinostat). Patient remains in complete remission at 25 months (Figures 19.1 and 19.2).

Chronic Diarrhea and Inappetence

Signalment: 14.5 years, M/N Doberman Pinscher; "Balboa."

History: Chronic hepatopathy and a nasal carcinoma with pulmonary metastasis treated with satraplatin and palliative radiation for control of nasal tumor more than 6 months prior. Patient had chronic intermittent diarrhea, nausea, and reduced appetite despite discontinuation of

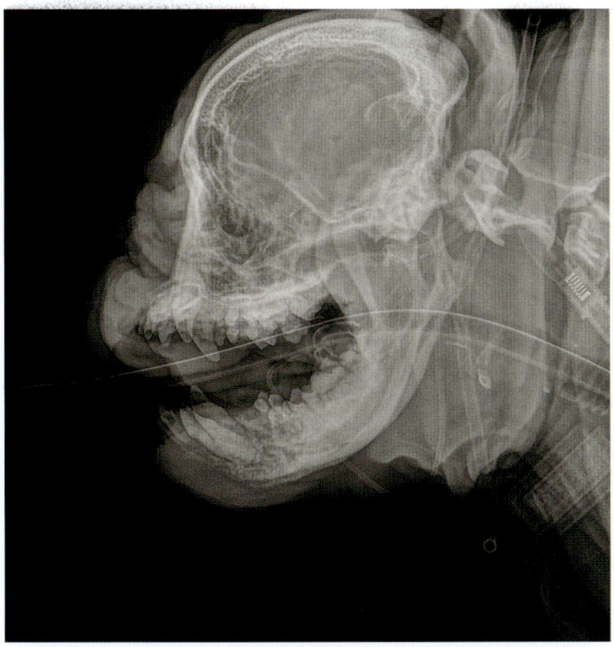

Figure 19.1 Radiographs of patient mandible prior to surgery.

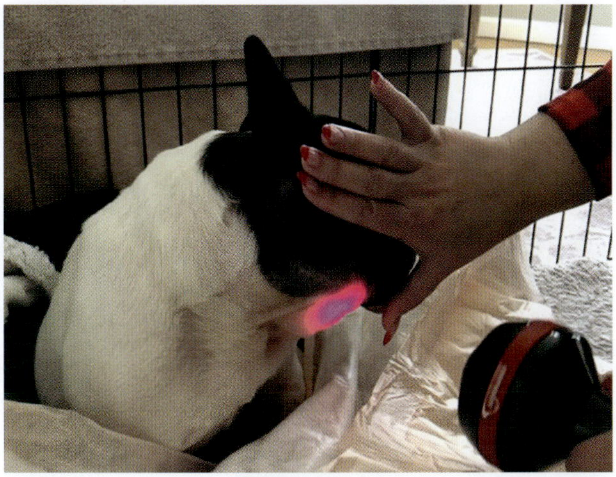

Figure 19.2 Patient receiving PBM treatment for post-op pain.

chemotherapy and use of multiple gastrointestinal support medications over the past several months.

Diagnostics: Abdominal palpation revealed no pain, mass effect, organomegaly, or distension. Mild elevations to ALP and ALT were noted on serum chemistry panel. Abdominal ultrasound with fine needle aspirates of the liver and spleen revealed no evidence of neoplasia on cytology.

Laser Treatment: PBM using an abdominal disorders protocol setting (10 J/cm^2) at 15 W power was applied on-contact to the entire abdomen initially twice weekly, then

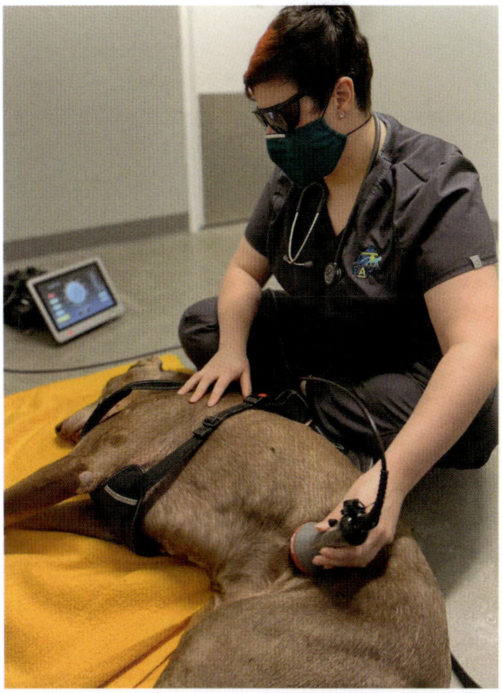

Figure 19.3 Patient receiving PBM treatment for diarrhea.

weaned to once weekly as the patient improved over a 6-week period.

Other Treatments: Denamarin®, ursodiol, gabapentin, yunnan baiyao, Ellevet®, doxycycline, omeprazole, Visbiome®, Entyce®, and ondansetron were initially all being administered. Ondansetron and Entyce were able to be ultimately discontinued as the patient's symptoms resolved.

Results: After a single PBM treatment, liquid stools became soft-formed stools, and following two sessions, soft-formed stools became solid stools. Gastrointestinal support medications were weaned with no nausea or vomiting noted despite discontinuing some of these medications. Ultimately, the patient also received laser therapy for chronic osteoarthritis due to improved quality-of-life noted by the pet owners after resolution of the dog's chronic diarrhea (Figure 19.3).

Compartment Syndrome Wounds

Signalment: 6 years, M/N Pit Bull; "Bentley."

History: Recurrent mast cell tumor (dimensions 2.0 cm × 1.2 cm × 2.4 cm) along dorsal carpus. Patient was treated with intra-tumoral injection of 1.44 ml tigilanol tiglate (Stelfonta).

Exam findings: 48 hours post-injection, patient presented with lethargy and decreased appetite. Significant swelling was present both proximal and distal to the injection site. The patient was significantly painful and toe-touching lame on the forelimb, even with oral pain medications (gabapentin, prednisone, and codeine).

Laser treatment: PBM using an edema/swelling protocol (8 J/cm^2) at 7–9 W was applied on-contact over areas of closed skin and off-contact over any area(s) that were open/draining throughout the carpal, elbow, and shoulder areas (approximately 540 cm^2). The patient was initially treated daily for 3 days in a row; treatment session frequency was weaned as the lesions improved. Five total treatment sessions were applied in a 10-day period.

Results: Swelling decreased significantly and the patient was much more comfortable following the first laser treatment. By the third treatment session, devitalized tissue had sloughed but only in limited areas, and a good granulation tissue bed(s) were noted. One week following the first treatment session, the wounds were contracting and healed without further sequelae (Figures 19.4–19.6).

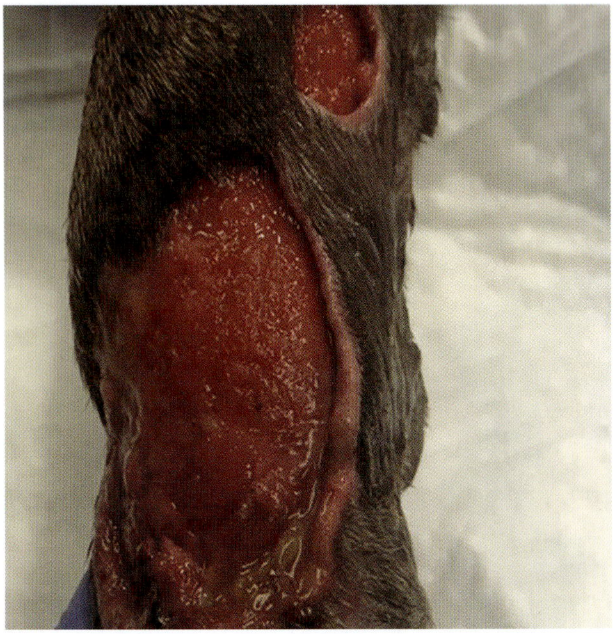

Figure 19.5 Day 7 tissue sloughing and granulation bed following 3 PBM treatments.

Sterile Hemorrhagic Cystitis

Signalment: 11.5 years., MN Cockapoo; "Henry."

History: 6 months history of duodenal soft tissue sarcoma treated with surgical resection followed by metronomic cyclophosphamide. During the course of treatment, the patient presented with paraphimosis, urinary incontinence, polyuria, and polydipsia.

Diagnostics: Urinalysis and culture results were consistent with SHC.

Initial treatments and response: Cyclophosphamide was discontinued and patient was tapered off prednisone. Two weeks later, upon recheck examination, urinary

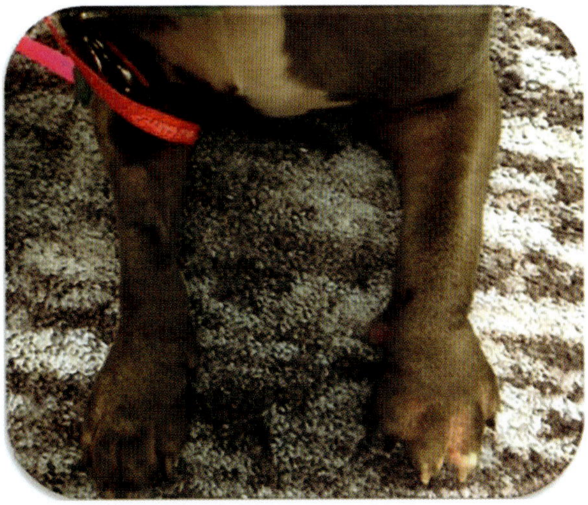

Figure 19.4 Close up photo showing left forelimb edematous with draining tract(s) from compartment syndrome 48 hours post tigilanol tiglate injection.

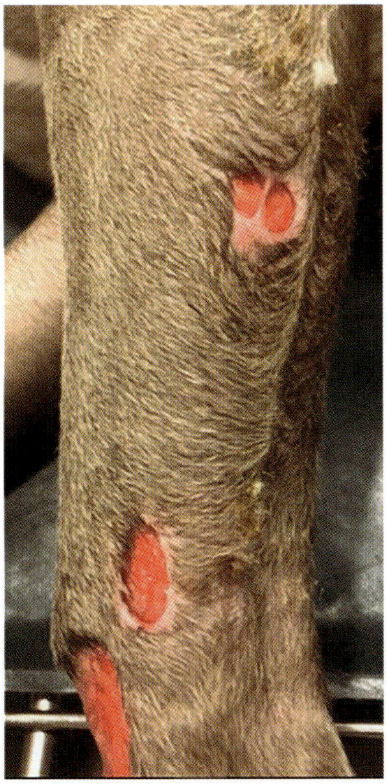

Figure 19.6 Day 9 wound contracture following 4 PBM treatments.

incontinence was only slightly improved and the patient still had paraphimosis.

Further diagnostics: Ultrasound of urinary bladder showed thickened ventral bladder wall (diameter 0.59 cm).

Laser Treatment: PBM using a urinary disorders protocol (7 J/cm^2 at 9 W power) on-contact over the caudal abdomen. The patient initially received three treatment sessions over a 2-week period, weaning the frequency of treatments as symptoms improved.

Results: Within three treatments, the paraphimosis resolved, symptoms drastically improved, and the ventral bladder wall decreased in thickness by half on bladder ultrasound (Figures 19.7 and 19.8).

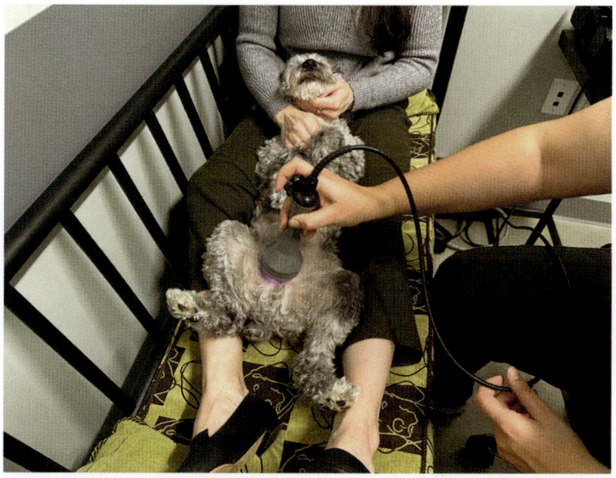

Figure 19.7 Patient receiving PBM treatment for sterile hemorrhagic cystitis.

Deciding to Treat an Oncology Patient with PBM

Balancing all the factors of geriatric cancer patients is important to maintaining their quality of life. Actually, standard of care options are often the concern for causing side effects in the cancer patient, and we need to keep this in mind with our conversations. Alternative options to help support these patients should be considered. Many clients have concerns about their pets with cancer and are interested in trying anything that may help them, including complementary and alternative supportive treatments. The majority of clients would welcome any suggestion to help their pet. Always remember these options are available and can help support the patient in their end-of-life journey. These patients are terminal, and the more we can do to help support them in maintaining their quality of life, the better.

Our historic understanding of photobiomodulation suggested to many not to use it at all in a cancer patient. Just as medications have multiple uses at different doses, PBM can be used successfully in cancer patients. Judicious evaluation of the location of active cancer is still prudent. Off-label prescribing of any drug or therapy is uncharted territory where we lack the usual level of evidence. This was done in the last 10 years, and now the evidence exists that inflammation propagates cancer. The more we can control inflammation and support the immune system in the right direction, the better for these patients. As we improve our understanding of the GI microbiome, this will continue to help our decision making as well. Recent evidence suggests the gut microbiome and the metabolites can act as promotors or inhibitors to cancer development. The relationship

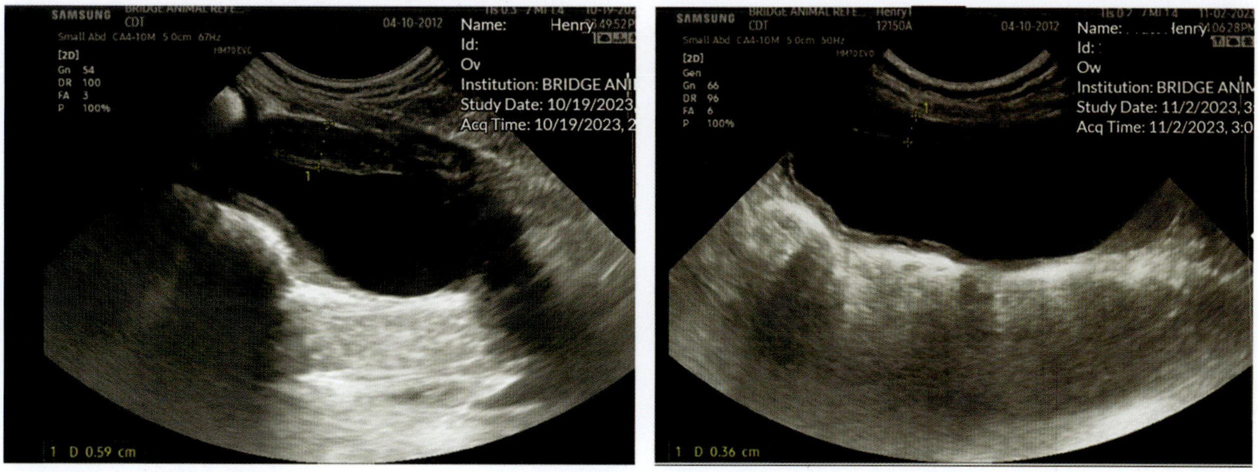

Figure 19.8 Initial bladder ultrasound (left) showing thickened ventral bladder wall. Follow up bladder ultrasound (right) showing significantly improved bladder wall.

between the gut microbiota and the efficacy of radiation therapy, chemotherapy and immunotherapy is starting to take shape with the move toward precision medicine. Tumors and other causes of the disruption of the intestinal mucosal barrier may provide access for these gut microbes, resulting in their switching to intra-tumoral microbes directly involved in the development of cancer. Therefore, it is not surprising that both gut and intratumoral microbes can exert cancer-promoting effects. Controlling this inflammatory state in cancer patients through PBM is an exciting new arena to help slow this impact on tumorigenesis and improve therapeutic efficacy in our patients (Zhao *et al.*, 2023).

Ultimately, the veterinarian with laser therapy at their disposal is encouraged to use their own best clinical judgment when taking into account all the evidence presented here, as well as considering the oncology patient's quality of life and unique challenges that may benefit by treatment with photobiomodulation. An informed consent discussion with the pet owner is encouraged if any concerns are expressed or if palliative treatment for pain directly over a tumor site is being considered.

References

Al Ghamdi, K. *et al.* (2012). Low-level laser therapy: a useful technique for enhancing the proliferation of various cultured cells. *Lasers Med Sci.* 27:237–249.

Alves, J.C. *et al.* (2022a). The effect of photobiomodulation therapy on the management of chronic idiopathic large-bowel diarrhea in dogs. *Lasers Med Sci.* 37(3):2045–2051.

Alves, J.C. *et al.* (2022b). A randomized double-blinded controlled trial on the effects of photobiomodulation therapy in dogs with osteoarthritis. *Am J Vet Res.* 83(8).

Al-Watban, F.A.H. *et al.* (2007). Low-level laser therapy enhances wound healing in diabetic rats: a comparison of different lasers. *Photmed Laser Surg.* 25(2):72–77.

Anderson, K.L. *et al.* (2020). Risk factors for canine osteoarthritis and its predisposing Arthropathies: a systematic review. *Frontiers in Vet Sci.* 7.

Anschau, F. *et al.* (2019). Efficacy of low-level laser for treatment of cancer oral mucositis: a systematic review and meta-analysis. *Lasers Med Sci.* 34(6):1053–1062.

Antunes, H.S. *et al.* (2017). Long-term survival of arandomized phase III trial of head and neck cancer patients receiving concurrent chemoradiation therapy with or without low-level laser therapy(LLLT) to prevent oral mucositis. *Oral Oncol.* 71:11–15.

Argenta, P.A. *et al.* (2017). The effect of photobiomodulation on chemotherapy-induced peripheral neuropathy: a randomized, sham-controlled clinical trial. *Gynecol Oncol.* 144(1):159–166.

Baxter, G.D. *et al.* (2017). Low level laser therapy (Photobiomodulation therapy) for breast cancer-related lymphedema: a systematic review. *BMC Cancer.* 17(1):833.

Biller, B. *et al.* (2016). 2016 AAHA oncology guidelines for dogs and cats. *J Am Anim Hosp Assoc.* 52:181–204.

Bouillon, J. *et al.* (2018). Pyelonephritis in dogs: retrospective study of 47 histologically diagnosed cases (2005–2015). *J Vet Intern Med.* 32:249–259.

Bradley, D. (2017). Wounds. In: *Laser Therapy in Veterinary Medicine: Photobiomodulation*. (ed. J. Ronald), pp. 100–113. Riegel and John C Godbold, John Wiley and Sons, West Sussex, UK.

Brandão, T.B. *et al.* (2018). Locally advanced oral squamous cell carcinoma patients treated with photobiomodulation for prevention of oral mucositis: retrospective outcomes and safety analyses. *Support Care Cancer.* 26(7):2417–2423.

Brock, N. *et al.* (1981). Detoxification of urotoxic oxazaphosphorines by sulfhydryl compounds. *J Cancer Res Clin Oncol.* 100:311–320.

Budreckis, D.M. *et al.* (2015). Bacterial urinary tract infections associated with transitional cell carcinoma in dogs. *J Vet Intern Med.* 29:828–833.

Censabella, S. *et al.* (2016). Photobiomodulation for the management of radiation dermatitis: the DERMIS trial, a pilot study of MLS([R]) laser therapy in breast cancer patients. *Support Care Cancer.* 24:3925–3933.

Chan, C.M. *et al.* (2016). Incidence of sterile hemorrhagic cystitis in tumor-bearing dogs concurrently treated with oral metronomic cyclophosphamide chemotherapy and furosemide: 55 cases (2009–2015). *J Am Vet Med Assoc.* 249(12):1408–1414.

Charney, S.C. *et al.* (2003). Risk factors for sterile hemorrhagic cystitis in dogs with lymphoma receiving cyclophosphamide with or without concurrent administration of furosemide: 216 cases (1990–1996). *J Am Vet Med Assoc.* 222:1388–1393.

Chaves, M.E. *et al.* (2018). Effects of low-power light therapy on wound healing: LASER x LED. *An Bras Dermatol.* 89:616–623.

Cox, J. and Ang, K. (2010). Radiation oncology: rationale, technique. In: *Results*, 9 edn. Mosby Elsevier.

Cox, J.D. *et al.* (1995). Toxicity criteria of the radiation therapy oncology group (RTOG) and the European Organization for Research and Treatment of Cancer (EORTC). *Int J Radiat Oncol Biol Phys.* 31:1341–1346.

Cronshaw, M. *et al.* (2020). Photobiomodulation and oral mucositis: a systematic review. *Dent J (Basel).* 8(3):87.

Crow, S.E. *et al.* (1977). Cyclophosphamide-induced cystitis in the dog and cat. *J Am Vet Med Assoc.* 171:259–262.

Culp, C. *et al.* (2020). Ketamine use for cancer and chronic pain management. *Front Pharmacol.* 11:599721.

DeLand, M. *et al.* (2007). Treatment of radiation-induced dermatitis with light-emitting diode (LED) photomodulation. *Lasers Surg Med.* 39:164–168.

DiSipio, T. *et al.* (2013). Incidence of unilateral arm lymphoedema after breast cancer: a systematic review and meta-analysis. *Lancet Oncol.* 14(6):500–515.

Djavid, G.E. *et al.* (2017). Photobiomodulation leads to enhanced radiosensitivity through induction of apoptosis and autophagy in human cervical cancer cells. *J Biophotonics.* 10(12):1732–1742.

Eguchi, Y. *et al.* (1997). Intracellular ATP levels determine cell death fate by apoptosis or necrosis. *Cancer Res.* 57:1835–1840.

Elad, S. *et al.* (2020). MASCC/ISOO clinical practice guidelines for the management of mucositis secondary to cancer therapy. *Cancer.* 126(19):4423–4431.

Falk, S. and Dickenson, A.H. (2014). Pain and nociception: mechanisms of cancer-induced bone pain. *J Clin Oncol.* 32(16):1647–1654.

Farrelly, J. and Shi, Q. (2018). Retrospective analysis of nonradiation complications in dogs undergoing radiation therapy. *Vet Radiol Ultrasound.* 59(1):116–123.

Fernandes, K.P. *et al.* (2015). Photobiomodulation with 660-nm and 780-nm laser on activated J774 macrophage-like cells: effect on M1 inflammatory markers. *J Photochem Photobiol B.* 153:344–351.

Fife, D. *et al.* (2010). A randomized, controlled, double-blind study of light emitting diode photomodulation for the prevention of radiation dermatitis in patients with breast cancer. *Dermatologic Surg.* 36:1921–1927.

Freitas, K.A. *et al.* (2020). Association of photobiomodulation and topical hyaluronidase in extravasation and infiltration of antineoplastics. Retrospective study. *Rev Nurs (Sao Paulo).* 23(271):4971–4978.

Freitas, K. *et al.* (2022). Effects of photobiomodulation (laser 660nm) on anthracycline extravasation: an experimental study. *Rev Lat Am Enfermagem.* 30:e3693.

Fukuda, T.Y. *et al.* (2013). Infrared low-level diode laser on inflammatory process modulation in mice: pro-and anti-inflammatory cytokines. *Lasers Med Sci.* 28:1305–1313.

Gaeta, R. *et al.* (2014). Risk factors for development of sterile haemorrhagic cystitis in canine lymphoma patients receiving oral cyclophosphamide: a case-control study. *Vet Comp Oncol.* 12:277–286.

Ganeshan, V. *et al.* (2019). Pre-conditioning with remote photobiomodulation modulates the brain transcriptome and protects against MPTP insult in mice. *Neuroscience.* 400:85–97.

Greco, M.T. *et al.* (2014). Quality of cancer pain management: an update of a systematic review of undertreatment of patients with cancer. *J Clin Oncol.* 36:49–54.

Hamblin, M.R. (2017). Mechanisms and applications of the anti-inflammatory effects of photobiomodulation. *AIMS Biophys.* 4(3):337–361.

Hamblin, M.R. (2023). Photobiomodulation therapy for treatment of extravasation injuries in Cancer chemotherapy. *Photobiomodul Photomed Laser Surg.* 41(1):1–2.

Hamblin, M.R. *et al.* (2017). Photobiomodulation and cancer: what is the truth? *Photomed Laser Surg.* 36(5):241–245.

Harrer, J. *et al.* (2022). Bacterial urinary tract infection and subclinical bacteriuria in dogs receiving antineoplastic chemotherapy. *J Vet Intern Med.* 36(3):1005–1015.

Hawkins, D.H. and Abrahamse, H. (2006b). The role of laser fluence in cell viability, proliferation, and membrane integrity of wounded human skin fibroblasts following helium-neon laser irradiation. *Lasers Surg Med.* 38:74–83.

Hawkins, D. and Abrahamse, H. (2006a). Effect of multiple exposures of low-level laser therapy on the cellular responses of wounded human skin fibroblasts. *Photomed Laser Surg.* 24:705–714.

Hawkins, D. and Abrahamse, H. (2007). Phototherapy – a treatment modality for wound healing and pain relief. *Afr J Biomed Res.* 10:99–109.

Johnston, S.A. (1997). Osteoarthritis. Joint anatomy, physiology, and pathobiology. *Vet Clin North Am Small Anim Pract.* 27(4):699–723.

Johnstone, D.M. *et al.* (2014). Indirect application of near infrared light induces neuroprotection in a mouse model of Parkinsonism – an abscopal neuroprotective effect. *Neuroscience.* 274:93–101.

Kim, B. *et al.* (2018). Remote tissue conditioning is neuroprotective against MPTP insult in mice. *IBRO Reports.* 4:14–17. doi:10.1016/j.ibror.2018.01.001.

Kobayashi, T. (2015). Management of Chemotherapy Side Effects. World Small Animal Veterinary Association World Congress Proceedings (2015)

Kreidieh, F.Y. (2016). Overview, prevention and management of chemotherapy extravasation. *World J Clin Oncol.* 7(1):87–97.

Lai, C.C. *et al.* (2021). Effectiveness of low levellaser therapy versus cryotherapy in cancer patients withoral mucositis: systematic review and network meta-analysis. *Crit Rev Oncol Hematol.* 160:103276.

Lanzafame, R.J. *et al.* (2007). Reciprocity of exposure time and irradiance on energy density during photoradiation on wound healing in a murine pressure ulcer model. *Lasers Surg Med.* 39:534–542.

Lascelles, B.D.X. (2010). Feline degenerative joint disease. *Vet Surg*. 39(1):2–13.

Lascelles, B.D.X. *et al*. (2012). Relationship of orthopedic examination, goniometric measurements, and radiographic signs of degenerative joint disease in cats. *BMC Vet Res*. 8:10.

Liberti, M.V. and Locasale, J.W. (2016). The Warburg effect: how does it benefit cancer cells? *Trends Biochem Sci*. 41(3):211–218.

Liebert, A. *et al*. (2019). "Photobiomics": can light, including photobiomodulation, alter the microbiome? *Photobiomodul Photomed Laser Surg*. 37(11):681–693.

Lima, A.G. *et al*. (2010). Efficacy low-level laser therapy and aluminum hydroxide in patients with chemotherapy and radiotherapy-induced oral mucositis. *Braz Dent J*. 21(3):186–192.

de Lima, F.J. *et al*. (2016). Is there a protocol in experimental skin wounds in rats using low-level diode laser therapy (LLDLT) combining or not red and infrared wavelengths? Systematic review. *Lasers Med Sci*. 31:779–787.

Looney, A.L. *et al*. (2018). A randomized blind placebo-controlled trial investigating the effects of photobiomodulation therapy (PBMT) on canine elbow osteoarthritis. *Can Vet J*. 59(9):959–966.

Lu, C. *et al*. (2016). Phototherapy-induced antitumor immunity: long-term tumor suppression effects via photoinactivation of respiratory chain oxidase-triggered superoxide anion burst. *Antioxid Redox Signal*. 24:249–262.

Lynch, S. *et al*. (2011). Development of a questionnaire assessing health-related quality-of-life in dogs and cats with cancer. *Vet Comp Oncol*. 9:172–182.

Mantyh, P.W. (2014). Bone cancer pain: from mechanism to therapy. *Curr Opin Support Palliat Care*. 8(2):83–90.

Maria, O.M. *et al*. (2017). Radiation-induced oral mucositis. *FrontOncol*. 7:89.

Mason, S. *et al*. (2014). Gastrointestinal toxicity after vincristine or cyclophosphamide administered with or without maropitant in dogs: a prospective randomised controlled study. *J Small Anim Pract*. 55:10.

Mellanby, R.J. *et al*. (2002). Treatment of canine lymphoma by veterinarians in first opinion practice in England. *J Small Anim Pract*. 43(5):198–202.

Mohile, S.G. *et al*. (2021). Evaluation of geriatric assessment and management on the toxic effects of cancer treatment (GAP70+): a cluster-randomised study. *Lancet*. 398 (10314):1894–1904. doi:10.1016/S0140-6736(21)01789-X.

Morrell, R.M. *et al*. (2005). Breast cancer-related lymphedema. *Mayo Clin Proc*. 80(11):1480–1484.

Myakishev-Rempel, M. *et al*. (2012). A preliminary study of the safety of red light phototherapy of tissues harboring cancer. *Photomed Laser Surg*. 30:551–558.

Nascimento, M. *et al*. (2023). Management of cancer therapy-induced oral mucositis using photobiomodulation therapy: an overview of systematic reviews. *Photobiomodul Photomed Laser Surg*. 41(10):513–538. doi:10.1089/photob.2023.0091.

Ottaviani, G. *et al*. (2016). Laser therapy inhibits tumor growth in mice by promoting immune surveillance and vessel normalization. *E Bio Medicine*. 11:165–172.

Paglioni, M. *et al*. (2019). Tumor safety and side effects of photobiomodulation therapy used for prevention and management of cancer treatment toxicities. A systematic review. *Oral Oncol*. 93:21–28.

Parshley, L. *et al*. (2022). Using nanoparticles and laser induced photo thermal ablation to treat low grade canine mast cell tumors: evaluation of efficacy and safety. *J Nanotechnol Res*. 4(2):45–58.

Peplow, P.V. *et al*. (2011). Laser photobiomodulation of gene expression and release of growth factors and cytokines from cells in culture: a review of human and animal studies. *Photomed Laser Surg*. 29:285–304.

Peplow, P. *et al*. (2012). Photodynamic modulation of wound healing: a review of human and animal studies. *Photomed Laser Surg*. 30:118–148.

Pereira, A.N. *et al*. (2002). Effect of low-power laser irradiation on cell growth and procollagen synthesis of cultured fibroblasts. *Lasers Surg Med*. 31:263–267.

Peterson, J.L. *et al*. (1992). Acute sterile hemorrhagic cystitis after a single intravenous administration of cyclophosphamide in three dogs. *J Am Vet Med Assoc*. 201(10):1572–1574.

Peterson, A.L. *et al*. (2012). Frequency of urinary tract infection in dogs with inflammatory skin disorders treated with ciclosporin alone or in combination with glucocorticoid therapy: a retrospective study. *Vet Dermatol*. 23:201–205.

Petrellis, M.C. *et al*. (2017). Laser photobiomodulation of pro-inflammatory mediators on Walker tumor 256 induced rats. *J Photochem Photobiol B*. 177:69–75.

Pulito, C. *et al*. (2020). Oral mucositis: The hidden side of cancer therapy. *J Exp Clin Cancer Res*. 39(1):210.

Ravicini, S. *et al*. (2018). Outcome and prognostic factors in medically treated canine prostatic carcinomas: a multi-institutional study. *Vet Comp Oncol*. 16:450–458.

Redfern, A. *et al*. (2017). Role of the gastrointestinal microbiota in small animal health and disease. *Vet Rec*. 181(14):370–370.

Rhee, Y.H. *et al*. (2016). Low-level laser therapy promoted aggressive proliferation and angiogenesis through decreasing of transforming growth factor-beta1 and increasing of Akt/hypoxia inducible factor-1alpha in anaplastic thyroid cancer. *Photomed Laser Surg*. 34:229–235.

Robijns, J. *et al*. (2017). The use of low-level light therapy in supportive care for patients with breast cancer: review of the literature. *Lasers Med Sci*. 32(1):229–242.

Robijns, J. *et al*. (2019a). Biophysical skin measurements to evaluate the effectiveness of photobiomodulation therapy in the prevention of acute radiation dermatitis in breast cancer patients. *Support Care Cancer*. 27:1245–1254.

Robijns, J. *et al.* (2019b). Photobiomodulation therapy for acute radiodermatitis. *Curr Opin Oncol.* 31(4):291–298.

Robijns, J. *et al.* (2022). Photobiomodulation therapy in management of cancer therapy-induced side effects: WALT position paper. *Front Oncol.* 2022:12.

Schindl, M. *et al.* (1999). Induction of complete wound healing in recalcitrant ulcers by low-intensity laser irradiation depends on ulcer cause and size. *Photodermatol Photoimmunol Photomed.* 15:18–21.

Seguin, M.A. *et al.* (2003). Persistent urinary tract infections and reinfections in 100 dogs (1989–1999). *J Vet Intern Med.* 17:622–631.

Silva, L. *et al.* (2018). Photobiomodulation therapy on bothrops snake venom-induced local pathological effects: A systematic review. *Toxicon.* 152:23–29. doi:10.1016/j.toxicon.2018.07.006.

da Silva, B.M. *et al.* (2022). Most used photobiomodulation dosimetry parameters to treat oral mucositis after preconditioning for hematopoietic stem cell transplantation: systematic review and metaanalysis. *Support Care Cancer.* 30(5):3721–3732.

Smee, N. *et al.* (2013). UTIs in small animal patients: part 1: etiology and pathogenesis. *J Am Anim Hosp Assoc.* 49:1–7.

Sonis, S.T. (2011). Oral mucositis. *Anti-Cancer Drugs.* 22(7):607–612.

Sroka, R. *et al.* (1999). Effects on the mitosis of normal and tumor cells induced by light treatment of different wavelengths. *Lasers Surg Med.* 25:263–271.

Stadler, I. *et al.* (2001). 830-nm irradiation increases the wound tensile strength in a diabetic murine model. *Lasers Surg Med.* 28:220–226.

Stillwell, T.J. and Benson, R.C. (1988). Cyclophosphamide-induced hemorrhagic cystitis. A review of 100 patients. *Cancer.* 61:451–457.

Strouthos, I. *et al.* (2017). Photobiomodulation therapy for the management of radiation-induced dermatitis: a single-institution experience of adjuvant radiotherapy in breast cancer patients after breast conserving surgery. *Strahlenther Onkol.* 193:491–498.

Tanaka, K. *et al.* (2023). Cancer aggravation due to persistent pain signals with the increased expression of pain-related mediators in sensory neurons of tumor-bearing mice. *Mol Brain.* 16:19. doi:10.1186/s13041-023-01001-5.

Terhorst, D. *et al.* (2015). Laser-assisted intradermal delivery of adjuvant-free vaccines targeting XCR1+ dendritic cells induces potent antitumoral responses. *J Immunol.* 194(12):5895–5902. doi:10.4049/jimmunol.1500564.

Tomiyasu, H. *et al.* (2010). Gastrointestinal and hematologic adverse events after administration of vincristine, cyclophosphamide, and doxorubicin in dogs with lymphoma that underwent a combination multidrug chemotherapy protocol. *J Vet Med Sci.* 72(11):1391–1397.

Tsai, S.R. *et al.* (2015). Low-level light therapy potentiates npe6-mediated photodynamic therapy in a human osteosarcoma cell line via increased ATP. *Photodiagn Photodyn Ther.* 12:123–130.

Venable, R.O. *et al.* (2008). Examination of synovial fluid hyaluronan quantity and quality in stifle joints of dogs with osteoarthritis. *Am J Vet Res.* 69(12):1569–1573.

Wan, S.Y. *et al.* (2014). Prevalence and clinical outcome of subclinical bacteriuria in female dogs. *J Am Vet Med Assoc.* 245:106–112.

Weese, J.S. *et al.* (2019). International Society for Companion Animal Infectious Diseases (ISCAID) guidelines for the diagnosis and management of bacterial urinary tract infections in dogs and cats. *Vet J.* 247:8–25.

Whelan, K. and Schneider, S.M. (2011). Mechanisms, prevention, and management of diarrhea in enteral nutrition. *Curr Opin Gastroenterol.* 27(2):152–159.

Williams, K. and MacDonald-Dickinson, V. (2023). Progress in palliation: managing pain caused by cancer in veterinary medicine. *Can Vet J.* 64(8):789–791.

Withrow, S.J. and Vail, D.M. (2020). *Withrow and MacEwen's Small Animal Clinical Oncology*, 6 edn, pp. 286–297. Elsevier, St. Louis, Missouri.

Wong, R.K. *et al.* (2013). Clinical practice guidelines for the prevention and treatment of acute and late radiation reactions from the MASCC skin toxicity study group. *Support Care Cancer.* 21:2933–2948.

Wong, C. *et al.* (2015). Antimicrobial susceptibility patterns in urinary tract infections in dogs (2010–2013). *J Vet Intern Med.* 29:1045–1052.

Wu, S. *et al.* (2009). High fluence low-power laser irradiation induces mitochondrial permeability transition mediated by reactive oxygen species. *J Cell Physiol.* 218:603–611.

Yazbek, K.V.B. and Fantoni, D.T. (2005). Validity of a health-related quality-of-life scale for dogs with signs of pain secondary to cancer. *J Am Vet Med Assoc.* 226:1354–1358.

Zadik, Y. *et al.* (2016). Systematic review of photobiomodulation for the management of oral muco-sitis in cancer patients and clinical practice guidelines. *Support Care Cancer.* 27(10):3969–3983.

Zecha, J.A. *et al.* (2016a). Low level laser therapy/ photobiomodulation in the management of side effects of chemoradiation therapy in head and neck cancer: part 1: mechanisms of action, dosimetric, and safety considerations. *Support Care Cancer.* 24:2781–2792.

Zecha, J.A. *et al.* (2016b). Low-level laser therapy/ photobiomodulation in the management of side effects of chemoradiation therapy in head and neck cancer: part 2: proposed applications and treatment protocols. *Support Care Cancer.* 24:2793–2805.

Zhao, L.Y. *et al.* (2023). Role of the gut microbiota in anticancer therapy: from molecular mechanisms to clinical applications. *Signal Transduct Target Ther.* 8:201.

20

Laser Therapy in Critical Care Patients

Michael H. Jaffe

Mississippi State University College of Veterinary Medicine, Mississippi State, MS, USA

Introduction

Rehabilitation therapy has historically been considered a modality limited to patients who have undergone orthopedic or neurologic injury. Whereas rehabilitation therapy aids these patients in their return to function and has demonstrated the ability to enhance recovery, patients with chronic and critical systemic illnesses can also benefit from a rehabilitation recovery program. Patients with long-term systemic medical issues that require hospitalization or limited activity can significantly improve following a recovery program that includes photobiomodulation (PBM).

Patients with chronic and critical illnesses undergo many physiologic changes directly and indirectly associated with their condition. Some of these changes are due to the underlying disease, while others may be secondary to co-morbidities and changes related to long-term hospitalization. Cancer patients are especially prone to numerous physiologic changes from their neoplasia and secondary to the effects of surgery, chemotherapy, and radiation treatments.

Patients treated in hospitals for chronic illnesses may be unable to leave their kennels for extended periods and are prone to cachexia and developing muscle atrophy. In these patients, clinicians should direct a dedicated rehabilitation therapeutic regimen. PBM can be vital in treating many of these patients. In some cases, PBM may directly affect tissue healing and recovery from the primary disorder and should be considered part of the patient's treatment plan.

There needs to be more published information regarding the clinical use of PBM in veterinary patients with chronic or critical illnesses. There is also a need for more knowledge about its use in chronically ill people. Clinicians can extrapolate research in people with chronic disease to promote its clinical benefits in companion animals. A few isolated veterinary case series exist, which indicate its potential. This chapter attempts to offer some evidence for incorporating its use into a rehabilitation therapeutic regimen for chronically ill small animal patients.

Physiologic Changes Associated with Chronic Disease

Musculoskeletal Changes

Cachexia in patients with chronic illness can accelerate rapidly due to a negative energy balance (Remillard, 2002). Evans *et al.* (2008) define cachexia as "a complex metabolic syndrome associated with underlying illness and characterized by loss of muscle with or without loss of fat mass." Insufficient intake of calories to meet nutritional demands causes the weight loss that accompanies cachexia (Freeman, 2012). Muscle is broken down during acute and chronic illness, as amino acids are catabolized as a source of energy instead of fat (Evans *et al.*, 2008). Body fat is also depleted during the cachectic state, but this is to a lesser degree than the concurrent muscle loss. Altered concentrations of chemical mediators in the disease state (inflammatory cytokines, catecholamines, cortisol, insulin, glucagon) impact the metabolic processes necessary for fat to be utilized as an energy source, resulting in the depletion of lean body mass (Freeman, 2012). In septic dogs, activating the inflammatory response and release of stress hormones promotes a hypermetabolic state, resulting in even worsening protein catabolism (Liu *et al.*, 2012).

Cachexia and chronic illness may also be associated with decreased appetite, thus further worsening the negative energy balance of these patients. Reduced consumption of calories by a sick animal may be due to the primary disease or changes in diet and feeding routine during hospitalization (Corbee & Van Kerkhoven, 2014).

Laser Therapy in Veterinary Medicine: Photobiomodulation, Second Edition. Edited by Christopher J. Winkler and Lisa A. Miller.

Hyporexia (decreased appetite) and anorexia (total loss of appetite) must be corrected to return the patient to a metabolic state where the caloric intake meets caloric needs providing the animal with sufficient energy.

Certain conditions may preclude the animal from eating, such as gastrointestinal disease. For these animals, maintenance of caloric needs is even more critical since they frequently have anorexia. Animals become weak and fatigued, resulting in reduced muscle strength, decreased VO_2 max to muscles, and diminished physical activity to conserve energy for bodily functions (Evans *et al.*, 2008). Nutritional support for these patients is vital for their recovery. Proper dietary support allows tissue healing, recovery, and improved immune response (Corbee & Van Kerkhoven, 2014).

Patients in the catabolic state caused by a chronic illness can benefit significantly from concurrent physical rehabilitation. Many animals are reluctant to rise independently and may be recumbent for extended periods. In humans, prolonged inactivity results in rapid muscle atrophy and exercise intolerance resulting from changes in the myocytes, myosin filaments, and increases in proteolytic enzymes (Cirio *et al.*, 2003) (Winkelman, 2004).

Mitochondrial Dysfunction Secondary to Chronic Disease

Physiologic changes associated with mitochondrial dysfunction in animals with chronic disease can precipitate changes that may worsen ongoing muscle atrophy and cachexia. In people with chronic illnesses, such as cancer and sepsis, cachexia associated with skeletal muscle mass deterioration is highly correlated with increased morbidity and mortality (Srikanthan & Karlamangla, 2014). Protein synthesis and breakdown of protein balance homeostasis is needed to maintain muscle mass. Various signaling pathways to which mitochondrial dysfunction contributes trigger skeletal muscle wasting (Hyatt & Powers, 2021). Muscle wasting because of mitochondrial dysfunction occurs by three mechanisms: (i) increased production of reactive oxygen species (ROS); (ii) pro-apoptosis-inducing factors release; and (iii) decreased production of ATP (Hyatt & Powers, 2021).

ROS is produced by the mitochondria promote muscle wasting by inhibiting protein synthesis and accelerating proteolysis (Hyatt & Powers, 2021). There are four mechanisms by which proteolysis occurs, resulting in protein degradation: (i) autophagy through lysosomal pathways, resulting in cellular organelle degradation and cell lysis; (ii) ubiquitin-proteasome system, which is an enzymatic pathway causing proteolysis; (iii) calpain 1 and calpain 2, which are calcium-activated proteins that cleave cytoskeletal proteins; and (iv) caspase-3, which acts similarly to the calpains to cleave actin and myosin complexes as well as other muscle proteins and is activated by oxidative stress (Powers *et al.*, 2016; Powell, 2006; Goll *et al.*, 2003; Whidden *et al.*, 2010).

Increased ROS production causing muscle wasting is also seen in recumbent patients for prolonged periods (Talbert *et al.*, 2013). Oxidative stress occurs when elevated intracellular levels of ROS are present and contribute to depressed protein synthesis in skeletal muscle, which is another means by which muscle atrophy occurs secondary to increased mitochondrial production of ROS (Scheiber & Chandel, 2014).

Chronic illness may produce systemic factors that result in mitochondrial dysfunction, leading to changes in the mitochondrial membrane permeability. These changes initiate intracellular processes that lead to the activation of caspases. Caspases are enzymes that execute apoptosis by cleaving proteins that contribute to the disassembly of the cell (Bloemberg & Quadrilatero, 2019). The permeability of the mitochondrial membrane occurs through the formation of mitochondrial permeability transition pores (mPTP). The appearance of mPTPs develops through several mechanisms initiated by cellular oxidative stress (Bernardi, 2013). These changes within the cell promote apoptosis, furthering skeletal muscle atrophy.

Synthesis of ATP for cellular energy may also be depressed due to mitochondrial dysfunction. Oxidative phosphorylation is the final step in cellular respiration and is associated with the electron transport chain, which passes electrons through a series of carriers within the inner mitochondrial membrane. A terminal carrier links electron transport reactions to ATP production (Cooper & Adams, 2000). Muscle cells use the ATP synthesized within the mitochondria to power muscle contraction. For normal muscle function, ATP must continue to be resynthesized since the muscle's ability to store ATP is minimal. Depressed ATP production leads to cellular energy production by the less efficient anaerobic glycolysis process, which also builds up lactic acid within the muscle (Hultman & Greenhaff, 1991). The inability of the body to process lactic acid fast enough may lead to lactic acidosis. Lactic acidosis occurs when high levels of lactic acid are produced, and this buildup may result in organ and tissue damage. Hyperlactatemia indicates a hypoxic condition in septic patients and occurs when oxygen consumption becomes dependent on oxygen delivery during anaerobic metabolism (DeBacker, 2003). Hyperlactatemia may be caused by increased lactate production and/or decreased hepatic clearance (DeBacker, 2003).

Sarcopenia

Sarcopenia is the loss of lean body mass associated with aging (Freeman, 2012). Many animals maintain normal body weight with sarcopenia due to increased fat mass despite losing muscle. Aging in dogs is associated with sarcopenia (Freeman, 2012). The cause of sarcopenia is multifactorial. Factors implicated in the resultant loss of muscle mass associated with aging include physical inactivity, increased cytokine production, decreases in growth hormone and testosterone concentrations, insulin resistance, reduced protein synthesis, and changes in type II muscle fibers (Lang *et al.,* 2010). Mitochondria in muscle cells produce a large amount of ATP as an energy source for the muscle. Decreased mitochondrial function due to the accumulation of ROS in animals with sarcopenia is one of the mechanisms by which muscle mass is lost in sarcopenia (Lang *et al.,* 2010).

Photobiomodulation and the Mitochondria

For cells to respond to light therapy, they must first be able to absorb the light. *Chromophores* are molecules that can absorb photons of light. PBM uses light in the near-infrared (NIR) spectrum (780–980 nm). Light absorption in this spectrum is made possible by chromophores in the mitochondria of cells. Cytochrome c oxidase (CCO) is a subunit of the mitochondrial respiratory chain along the inner mitochondrial membrane that is part of the oxidative phosphorylation electron transport chain, which produces ATP. CCO is an enzyme activated *in vitro* by red light in the 670 nm range (Pastore *et al.,* 2000). When activated by red or NIR light photons, photodissociation of nitric oxide within the mitochondria causes CCO to increase its activity, leading to increased cellular respiration and ATP production (Hamblin, 2018). It is believed that PBM may have a more dramatic effect on injured or diseased tissue while generally sparing its effects on normal healthy tissue because damaged cells have a higher concentration of nitric oxide producing this effect (Lane, 2006).

Cells that contain many mitochondria (skeletal and cardiac muscle cells and neurons) and those with high metabolic activity are particularly responsive to light therapy (Hamblin, 2018). This effect is due to the primary chromophores that PBM acts on within their mitochondria. Due to their location within tissue, these chromophores are not naturally exposed to light (Hamblin, 2018). When chromophores absorb light and activate the cell, the mitochondria of these cells have the capacity to produce a large amount of ATP to power these cells, which can aid in their recovery when there is tissue or cellular insult due to injury.

Challenges in an ICU Setting

The challenge of treating patients with critical illnesses is that many are cage-bound due to various medications, injuries, catheters, and monitoring devices. Some patients may be capable of traveling to an area where laser therapy is performed via walking, by gurney, or carried. For more critical patients, or when transporting a patient is not feasible, the laser must travel to the patient.

Great care to shield and protect the eyes of personnel and other patients when treating a patient with laser therapy in a busy ICU setting is imperative. The author has used a combination of towels and shields when working in a cage with patients receiving laser therapy. Portable rolling screens are commercially available to protect ICU personnel and other patients. Of course, the patient and personnel performing the treatment must wear appropriate eye protection. Proper eye protection and signage must be accounted for when a patient is in an area with other patients and personnel. Stray laser light is less of a concern if the cage is isolated, such as a large run.

Rehabilitation Therapy for Chronic Disease

Many of the changes that develop in the muscles and joints that are associated with cachexia are reversible. Muscle atrophy is typically characterized as disuse atrophy when seen in hospitalized patients and those immobilized long-term. Once these patients recover and remobilize, their muscle mass often dramatically increases. During remobilization, therapeutic exercises emphasizing movement and reloading promote improved muscle oxidative capacity (Millis & Levine, 2014). Muscle regeneration occurs following the mechanical reloading of postural muscles; however, this is a slow process. PBM increases the activity of mitochondrial respiratory chain complexes, resulting in increased ATP synthesis, which may accelerate muscle healing (Silveira *et al.,* 2009). Information extrapolated from *in vitro* work shows that patients with chronic disease resulting in a cachectic state and older patients with changes consistent with sarcopenia would benefit from a physical rehabilitation regimen that includes PBM therapy. Chronic diseases such as neoplasia and chronic renal disease are more frequently seen in older patients. These patients may have more profound muscle loss due to concurrent cachexia and sarcopenia.

Treating animals with chronic disease needs to take a multimodal approach. In addition to the therapeutic regimen for the patient's primary condition, physical rehabilitation should be an essential adjunct to therapy. Due to their primary illness, disuse atrophy may occur in nonambulatory or cage-bound patients. When generalized atrophy occurs, the most dramatic changes are typically in the postural extremity muscles and the epaxial muscles along the spine. PBM therapy should focus on treating these large muscle groups for these patients.

Decubitus Ulcers in Recumbent Patients

Small animal patients hospitalized for extended periods risk developing decubital ulcers unless they are on a well-padded surface. Even then, if they are not allowed to move around or if not turned when recumbent for long periods, ulcers over pressure areas may form. Treatment is initiated at the first sign of a possible ulcer developing to prevent it from worsening and allow it to heal. Clinicians can use appropriate padding and pressure-relieving bandages to relieve pressure from the ulcer. A well-padded roll of cotton shaped into a circle (like a doughnut) and placed around the ulcer, or pressure point, will distribute pressure from the ulcer. However, PBM therapy to heal the skin should be considered.

Decubitus ulcers are areas where the skin or soft tissue over a bone surface may suffer ischemia, leading to cellular necrosis (Ruh, 2017). The most common sites we see these ulcers form in recumbent small animals are over the ischial tuberosity, skin of the elbow at either the humeral epicondyle or olecranon, skin over the hip joint at the greater trochanter, and skin over the lateral stifle at the fibular head. Patients with lean body mass and those with certain endocrine disorders are especially prone to developing these. Hyperadrenocorticism (Cushing's disease) and diabetes mellitus are endocrine disorders most associated with these lesions in recumbent animals.

Patients may be unable to sense cutaneous pressure in these areas secondary to neuropathies. Secondary ischemia develops when vascular impairment exists, leading to delayed healing, decreased wound oxygen, and poor tissue nutrition. Patients with diabetes mellitus are especially prone to developing infections when decubital ulcers exist (Ruh, 2017). Treating these lesions with PBM enhances wound healing by increasing vascular endothelial growth factor (VEGF) and TGF-β while reducing TNF-α (Ruh, 2017).

Fibroblasts are one of the critical cells in the wound-healing process. During the inflammatory phase of wound healing, fibroblasts modulate the recruitment of immune cells and regulate the synthesis of extracellular matrix and collagen during the wound proliferative phase (Solmaz *et al.*, 2017). Following stimulation, fibroblasts differentiate into myofibroblasts, which contract the wound, reducing its size (Li and Wang, 2011). Solmaz *et al.* (2017) demonstrated a positive effect of laser irradiation *in vitro* at 635 nm at 1 J/cm^2 *in vivo* 5 and 7 days following wound creation concerning fibroblast proliferation, collagen formation, and healing tissue tensile strength.

Chronic Gastrointestinal Disease

PBM therapy has demonstrated efficacy in a study of dogs with chronic idiopathic large-bowel diarrhea. Dogs with chronic idiopathic large-bowel diarrhea received PBM treatments for 1 month compared to controls. At the end of 30 days, those dogs treated with PBM showed improved clinical signs, body weight, and body condition scores (Alves, 2022). Although there is little evidence in treating chronic gastrointestinal disorders with PBM, this study offers promise for future exploration. For patients with chronic gastrointestinal diseases, this may provide relief.

Dose: 6–10 J/cm^2

PBM therapy may benefit cats with chronic inflammatory bowel (IBD) disease treated over a short term. Treatment with 20–25 J (Godine, 2017) per point or 6–10 J/cm^2 (Lavallee & Olson, 2017) across the abdomen provides doses of light that stimulate the intestine and relieve clinical signs of diarrhea. Depending on their size and skin pigment, larger doses in dogs may be necessary. Including mesenteric and sublumbar lymph nodes in the treatment field is recommended (Godine, 2017).

IBD disease is a complex process resulting in generalized inflammation. Proinflammatory cytokines, including TNF-α, IL-6, and TGF-β, have been associated with the pathogenesis and progression of IBD (Laakso, 2023) (Lee, 2018). Bicknell (2022) observed that PBM alters the gut microbiome diversity, increasing bacteria associated with a healthy gastrointestinal microbiome. Although this provides the further belief that PBM may be beneficial in treating chronic IBD in small animal patients, it has not been confirmed in clinical veterinary patients.

Alebastrov and Butov (2005) reported that gastric ulcer healing may be improved experimentally by transcutaneous PBM. Compared to patients treated by direct endoscopic treatment with laser therapy, transcutaneous PBM also proved beneficial in gastric ulcer healing (Godine, 2017).

Dose: 6–10 J/cm^2

Pancreatitis

Conventional therapy – involving fluid therapy, enteral nutrition, antiemetics, etc., – is the mainstay of treatment for pancreatitis. Transcutaneous application of light over the pancreas at a dose of 8–10 J/cm^2 is reported in the treatment of the pancreas to reduce pancreatic inflammation and assist in healing (Lavallee & Olson, 2017). Whether this facilitates recovery is unproven, but it appears well-tolerated by patients.

Dose: 8–10 J/cm^2

Chronic Pain Management

PBM should be considered a part of the multimodal analgesia plan for patients with chronic pain. Many patients with chronic disease have longstanding, underlying pain that needs to be addressed. Management of patients with chronic pain with PBM has several distinct advantages. The greatest of which is the fact that it is a noninvasive form of therapy with good efficacy. Treatment of chronic pain with PBM is accomplished by activation of endogenous antioxidant enzymes that have the effect of reducing chronic inflammation. Increasing antioxidant nitric oxide (NO) levels results in vasodilation and removal of pro-inflammatory mediators such as Interleukin-1 and pro-inflammatory prostaglandins (Hochman, 2018).

PBM decreases transmission of pain along afferent nerves by inhibiting action potentials of neurons and blocking depolarization of C fibers of nerve cells (De Oliveira *et al.,* 2022). The effect of PBM is rapid onset in as little as 10–20 minutes, but of short duration and must be repeated every 24 hours. It is indicated for relief of minor muscle and joint pain, arthritis, and muscle spasms. Pain relief also occurs by the relief of muscle stiffness while promoting muscle relaxation. For many patients, a decrease in the use and need for nonsteroidal anti-inflammatory drugs (NSAIDs) and opioids is observed. Few side effects of PBM therapy are noted except where chronic pain secondary to neoplasia or active infection are present. Caution should also be observed for use in pregnant patients (De Oliveira *et al.,* 2022).

Dose: varies based on the level and underlying cause of pain

Neoplasia

Treatment of neoplasia with PBM is highly controversial. Based on the known mechanism of PBM to stimulate cellular activity, it is intuitive that clinicians should not perform PBM in these cases for fear of further growth and metastasis of the cancer. However, it is not known whether this is true for all cancer cell types. There exist conflicting studies regarding PBM-induced cellular proliferation of neoplastic cells. Until more is known about PBM's effects on all neoplasms, PBM therapy should be considered carefully for patients with cancer. Please see Chapter 19 for a more in-depth discussion.

Renal and Lower Urinary Tract Disease

Chronic kidney disease (CKD) is a progressive disease characterized by impaired function of one or both kidneys for over three months (Bartges, 2012). Renal tubular cells are metabolically active cells that maintain high levels of mitochondrial oxidative phosphorylation. As such, oxidative stress is a crucial aspect of CKD as these cells are prone to ROS formation, resulting in glomerulosclerosis and interstitial fibrosis (Brown, 2008). Oxidative stress may be decreased by lowering arterial hypertension, correcting chronic anemia, use of omega-3 fatty acids and ACE inhibitors (Brown, 2008). Tubulointerstitial nephritis is the most common histopathological diagnosis in cats with CKD; however, glomerular damage may also be present, resulting in inflammation and fibrosis of the nephron (Godine, 2017).

Treatment of CKD by PBM has generated significant interest in helping mitigate these inflammatory changes. Yamato et al. evaluated transcutaneous PBM of rats with experimentally induced glomerulonephritis and found that those treated with PBM had decreased levels of mRNA of pro-inflammatory mediators (IL-1β and TNF-α) in the renal cortex (Yamato *et al.,* 2013). Ucero *et al.* treated rats with experimentally induced CKD for 8 weeks with transcutaneous PBM. A significant dose-related decrease in tubulointerstitial fibrosis at high-dose PBM (12 J/cm^2, 5 mW, CW) was observed with a trend toward better-preserved GFR and lower systolic blood pressure in these rats (Ucero *et al.,* 2013). Ahrabi *et al.* (2020) reviewed differing low-power PBM settings and their effects on CKD. Reducing the inflammatory response decreases ROS with decreased fibrosis. Additionally, they showed that PBM enhances the anti-inflammatory response and glomerular cell proliferation.

Dose: 6–8 J/cm^2

Feline Lower Urinary Tract Disease

Feline lower urinary tract disease (FLUTD) may be amenable to PBM treatment. Cats who exhibit signs such as stranguiria, hematuria, pollakiuria, and inappropriate urination may have secondary inflammation of the urinary bladder and urethra. In addition to standard treatments such as fluid therapy, antibiotics, anti-inflammatory drugs, and urinary catheterization, PBM may be used as an adjunctive treatment to reduce inflammation. In addition to mitigating inflammation, PBM may provide some analgesia for these patients. Laser treatment of the caudal abdomen may be provided at a dose of 8–10 J/cm^2. Treatment should be safe even when an indwelling urinary catheter is in place (Lavallee & Olson, 2017).

Dose: 4–6 J/cm^2

Prostatitis

Prostatitis is amenable to PBM for its anti-inflammatory effects. Additionally, laser therapy may be used to reduce the size of the prostate as well as decrease inflammation for benign prostatic hypertrophy. Doses of 20–40 J per point focused on each prostatic lobe are reported to reduce prostatic inflammation and size. Focused NIR light at the superficial inguinal lymph node (10 J daily for 2–3 days, then twice weekly for 2 months following castration) is described to reduce prostatic size. A laser catheter is also described to reduce prostatic inflammation due to prostatitis when neoplasia has been ruled out (Godine, 2017).

Dose: 4–8 J/cm^2

Sepsis and Acute Respiratory Distress Syndrome

Septic patients have a high mortality rate due to several factors. In patients with early signs of sepsis, a marked inflammatory response releases numerous cytokines and pro-inflammatory mediators such as TNF-α, IL-2, IL-12, IFN-γ, and leukotrienes (Aziz, 2013). These mediators subsequently play a role in the defense response by the host, triggering numerous anti-inflammatory mediators such as TGF-β and IL-10 ((Yu, 1997; Aziz, 2013).

Immunosuppression during late sepsis is associated with lymphocyte ATP depletion and decreased proliferation. Early treatment of septic patients with ATP-$MgCl_2$ can improve lymphocyte ATP levels, which may reduce mortality from sepsis (Meldrum *et al.,* 1994). Open-abdomen PBM therapy of septic mice also had a stimulatory effect on ATP levels of lymphocytes (Argon Dye Laser at wavelength 630 nm, power 20 mW/cm^2, fluence 5 J/cm^2) (Yu *et al.,* 1997).

Acute respiratory distress syndrome (ARDS), also sometimes referred to as acute lung injury (ALI), is a systemic inflammatory condition resulting in acute hypoxemia and respiratory distress. These changes may progress to patients developing multiple organ dysfunction syndrome (MODS) (Balakrishnan *et al.,* 2017). PBM therapy in ARDS cases reduces inflammation by several mechanisms, including alteration of pro-inflammatory mRNA and DNA fragmentation of genes involved in inducing apoptosis in neutrophils and alveolar cells (Sergio *et al.,* 2018). Additionally, PBM increased the anti-inflammatory cytokine interleukin-10 expression in rats with sepsis-induced ALI (Alves *et al.,* 2020).

PBM therapy in mice with experimentally induced acute lung injury resulted in decreased inflammation with no adverse effects on the pulmonary tissue (transcutaneous at mid-axilla, 660 nm, 30 mW power continuous, fluence 10 J/cm^2) (Cury *et al.,* 2016). Acute lung injury induced by sepsis in mice treated with transcutaneous PBM was further evaluated. Results indicated decreased leukocytosis, decreased pro-inflammatory mediators in bronchoalveolar fluid, and increased anti-inflammatory cytokines in bronchoalveolar fluid (Costa *et al.,* 2017; da-Palma-Cruz *et al.,* 2019).

Dose: 6–8 J/cm^2

PBM was used in two clinical cases in people as adjunctive therapy for acute, infectious respiratory syndrome caused by the COVID-19 virus. In both cases, a treatment plan that included transcutaneous PBM therapy mitigated respiratory symptoms, pulmonary inflammation, and hypoxia. Patients in both cases were treated with 630 nm and 660 nm PBM with the transducer held 7 cm over the chest (irradiance 55 mW/cm^2, fluence 50 J/cm^2, three times daily for 10 days) (Pelletier-Aouizerate & Zivic, 2021).

Based on these and other studies, PBM may be a viable adjunctive therapy for patients with ARDS. Septic patients whose inflammatory syndrome progresses to include the respiratory tract may benefit from PBM. In addition to being minimally invasive, PBM therapy may be performed rapidly without causing further respiratory distress to these patients, even while receiving supplemental oxygen.

Thermal Burn Injuries

Thermal burn injuries in patients create a severe systemic inflammatory response. Treatment with PBM of third-degree burn injuries in patients has demonstrated success in facilitating the healing of tissue. Burn injuries that damage skin cause protein denaturation, tissue necrosis, and exudative wounds characterized by vascular leakage, edema, and venous congestion (Deana *et al.,* 2021). In addition to topical therapy with silver sulfadiazine and hydrogel dressings, PBM therapy provides anti-inflammatory and analgesic effects that promote wound healing. PBM promotes angiogenesis, fibroblast proliferation, and deposition of collagen, which provides an environment that facilitates epithelialization or early surgical closure of wounds (de Vasconcelos Catao *et al.,* 2015; Maligieri *et al.,* 2017; Fiorio *et al.,* 2014). PBM promotes activation of endogenous fibroblast and epithelial cell TGF-β1 in mice. Transforming growth factor-beta one is a cytokine that promotes cell growth and differentiation, immunosuppression, angiogenesis, and wound healing (Khan *et al.,* 2021). By stimulating TGF-β1, the enhancement of wound healing is believed to be a factor.

In contrast, some studies demonstrate no effect on healing with PBM use. One such study in rats found that PBM had no beneficial effect on wound healing following a burn (Schlager *et al.,* 2000). However, a nonthermal wound study in rabbits demonstrated a decreased inflammatory phase of healing with increased epithelialization of skin wounds, indicating PBM's beneficial effect on wound healing (Hodjati *et al.*, 2014).

Treatment for thermal burns by PBM recommendations (Bradley, 2017) includes starting initially with a low power setting of 2 J/cm^2. Treatment should be performed daily for 2–3 days, followed by every other day treatment. This protocol may continue if the treatment is successful. However, if the response is unsatisfactory after the first two to four treatments, the dosage may be increased by 25–50% Joules per treatment by increasing treatment duration or power settings. More extensive wounds that respond well may require twice-per-week treatments.

As Gal et al. demonstrated, histologic evaluation of skin showed that thermal burn wound healing in rats treated with PBM at 670 nm can shorten the inflammatory phase of wound healing. Additionally, treatment with PBM accelerated the proliferative and maturation phases of healing. Damaged epidermis and underlying striated muscle regeneration were enhanced in these subjects (Gal *et al.*, 2006).

Dose: 4–6 J/cm^2

Case Examples

Pancreatitis

The author has treated patients with severe pancreatitis hospitalized long-term with a combination of adjunctive laser therapy directed over the abdomen and physical therapy to maintain muscle mass. The belief holds that PBM may contribute to decreased pancreatic inflammation. Patients may be in pain when using the laser during the acute phases of their disease due to the pressure placed on the abdomen, although they tolerate the laser well. We have found that it is helpful to perform these treatments shortly after analgesic administration.

Polytrauma Cases

Patients who have undergone significant injuries following severe trauma, such as being hit by a motor vehicle, will benefit significantly from laser therapy. Blunt force trauma will result in multiple, often whole-body, muscle contusions, subcutaneous hemorrhage, fractures, neurologic damage, and potentially internal injuries to the chest and abdomen. Many patients hit by a car will have whole-body contusions to both sides of their body, as well as road-rash superficial injuries and deep lacerations. Treating whole-body muscle contusions with laser therapy will promote healing of muscle damage, decreased edema and inflammation, and analgesia. The author finds that treatment of fractures is beneficial only when the patient is either heavily sedated or under general anesthesia at the time of surgical repair. We have treated other soft tissue injuries after analgesia administration. We are careful not to apply too much pressure since the structures treated are often relatively superficial and subcutaneous.

Care must be taken when treating anesthetized patients or in patients with decreased sensation due to trauma. These patients may have a limited ability to feel and respond appropriately to discomfort. Avoiding thermal build-up by the operator of the laser is important to prevent untoward injury to these patients who may not be able to respond to potential tissue damage.

Thermal Burn Injuries

Patients who have undergone severe third-degree burns benefit greatly from PBM. The author has treated several patients undergoing sedated bandage changes, tissue debridement and lavage, and wound management with adjunctive laser therapy. With the treatment head cone positioned 1–2 in. over the lesion, the laser does not contact the affected tissue in these cases. We always wipe the laser head with alcohol and allow it to dry thoroughly before treatments to prevent introducing new bacteria to the wound. The laser promotes healing and decreases pain in these patients; patients tolerate this well since there is no contact with the wound. We routinely sedate patients for more extensive wound management and have found that this is the optimal time to perform laser treatments. Laser treatments may occur at each bandage change without detrimental effects on the wound bed. Some burn wounds can be quite extensive, so in these cases, breaking the treatments up into sections may be advised.

References

Ahrabi, B. *et al.* (2020). The effect of low-power laser therapy on the TGF/Beta signaling pathway in chronic kidney disease: a review. *J Lasers in Med Sci.* 11(2):220–225.

Alebastrov, A.P. and Butov, M.A. (2005). Potentialities of alternative non-drug therapy of gastric ulcer. *Klinicheskaia Meditsina.* 83(11):69–71.

Alves, J. (2022). The effect of photobiomodulation therapy on the management of chronic idiopathic large-bowel diarrhea in dogs. *Lasers Med Sci*. 37:2045–2051.

Alves, W.E. *et al.* (2020). *Verification of the Effects of Red Light-Emitting Diode Therapy on Acute Lung Injury in a Sepsis Model in Rats*, p. 63. Brazilian Archives of Biology and Technology.

Aziz, M. (2013). Current trends in inflammatory and immunomodulatory mediators in sepsis. *J Leukocyte Biol*. 93(3):329–342.

Balakrishnan, A. *et al.* (2017). Retrospective evaluation of the prevalence, risk factors, management, outcome, and necropsy findings of acute lung injury and acute respiratory distress syndrome in dogs and cats: 29. *J Vet Emerg Crit Care*. 27(6):662–673.

Bartges, J.W. (2012). Chronic kidney disease in dogs and cats. *Vet Clin N Am: Small Anim Pract*. 42(4):669–692.

Bernardi, P. (2013). The mitochondrial permeability transition pore: a mystery solved? *Front Physiol*. 4:95.

Bicknell, B. (2022). Microbiome changes in humans with Parkinson's disease after photobiomodulation therapy: a retrospective study. *J Personal Med*. 12(1):49.

Bloemberg, D. and Quadrilatero, J. (2019). Autophagy, apoptosis, and mitochondria: molecular integration and physiological relevance in skeletal muscle. *Am J Physiol Cell Physiol*. 317:C111–C130.

Bradley, D.S. (2017). Wounds. In: *Laser Therapy in Veterinary Medicine Photobiomodulation*. s.l.:. (eds. R.J. Riegel and J.C. Gobold Jr.), pp. 100–113. John Wiley and Sons, Inc.

Brown, S.A. (2008). Oxidative stress and chronic kidney disease. *Vet Clin Small Anim Pract*. 38:157–166.

Cirio, S. *et al.* (2003). Muscle retraining in ICU patients. *Monaldi Arch Chest Dis*. 59(4):300–303.

Cooper, G. and Adams, K. (2000). *The Cell: A Molecular Approach*, 2 edn. Sinauer Associates, Sunderland (MA).

Corbee, R.J. and Van Kerkhoven, W.J. (2014). Nutritional support of dogs and cats after surgery or illness. *Open J Vet Med*. 4:44–57.

Costa, S.G. *et al.* (2017). Beneficial effects of red light-emitting diode treatment in experimental model of acute lung injury induced by sepsis. *Sci Rep*. 7:12670.

Cury, V. *et al.* (2016). Low level laser therapy reduces acute lung inflammation without impairing lung function. *J Biophotonics*. 9(11–12):1199–1207.

De Oliveira, M.F. *et al.* (2022). Low-intensity LASER and LED (photobiomodulation therapy) for pain control of the most common musculoskeletal conditions. *European J Phys Rehab Med*. 58(2):282–289.

Deana, N.F. *et al.* (2021). Photobiomodulation therapy in burn wound healing: systematic review and meta-analysis of preclinical studies. *Photobiomodulation Photomed Laser Surg*. 39(7):439–452.

DeBacker, D. (2003). Lactic acidosis. *Intensive Care Med*. 29:699–702.

Evans, W.J. *et al.* (2008). Cachexia: a new definition. *Clin Nutrit*. 27:793–799.

Fiorio, F. *et al.* (2014). Effect of low-level laser therapy on types I and III collagen and inflammatory cells in rats with induced third-degree burns. *Lasers Med Sci*. 29:313–339.

Freeman, L. (2012). Cachexia and sarcopenia: emerging syndromes of importance in dogs and cats. *J Vet Intern Med*. 26:3–17.

Gal, P. *et al.* (2006). Histological assessment of the effect of laser irradiation on skin wound healing in rats. *Photomed Laser Surg*. 24(4):480–488.

Godine, R. (2017). Abdominal conditions. In: *Laser Therapy in Veterinary Medicine*. s.l. (eds. J.C. Godbold Jr. and R.J. Riegel), pp. 169–178. John Wiley & Sons.

Goll, D.E. *et al.* (2003). The calpain system. *Physiol Rev*. 83:731–801.

Hamblin, M.R. (2018). Mechanisms and mitochondrial redox signaling in photobiomodulation. *Photochem Photobiol*. 94:199–212.

Hochman, L. (2018). Photobiomodulation therapy in veterinary medicine: a review. *Topics in Compan Anim Med*. 33:83–88.

Hodjati, H. *et al.* (2014). Low-level laser therapy: an experimental design for wound management: a case-controlled study in rabbit model. *J Cutaneous and Aesth Surg*. 7(1):14–17.

Hultman, E. and Greenhaff, P.L. (1991). Skeletal muscle energy metabolism and fatigue during intense exercise in man. *Sci Progress Edinburgh*. 75:361–370.

Hyatt, H.W. and Powers, S.K. (2021). Mitochondrial dysfunction is a common denominator linking skeletal muscle wasting due to disease, aging, and prolonged inactivity. *Antioxidants*. 10(4):588.

Khan, I. *et al.* (2021). Accelerated burn wound healing with photobiomodulation therapy involves activation of endogenous latent TGF-β1. *Sci Rep*. 11:13371.

Laakso, E.-L. (2023). A holistic perspective on how photobiomodulation may influence fatigue, pain, and depression in inflammatory bowel disease: beyond molecular mechanisms. *Biomedicines*. 11(5):1497–1510.

Lane, N. (2006). Cell biology: power games. *Nature*. 443:901–903.

Lang, T. *et al.* (2010). Sarcopenia: etiology, clinical consequences, intervention, and assessment. *Osteoporosis Internat*. 21:543–559.

Lavallee, J.O. and Olson, J. (2017). Feline-specific conditions. In: *Lasser Therapy in Veterinary Medicine*. s.l. (eds. R.J. Riegel and J.C. Godbold Jr.), pp. 198–211. John Wiley and Sons, Inc.

Lee, S.H. (2018). Immunological pathogenesis of inflammatory bowel disease. *Intest Res*. 16(1):26–42.

Li, B. and Wang, J.-C. (2011). Fibroblasts and myofibroblasts in wound healing: force generation and measurement. *J Tissue Viabil.* 20(4):108–120.

Liu, D.T. *et al.* (2012). Early nutritional support is associated with decreased length of hospitalization in dogs with septic peritonitis: a retrospective study of 45 cases (2000–2009). *J Vet Emerg Crit Care.* 22(4):453–459.

Maligieri, L. *et al.* (2017). Differing energy densities with laser 670nm InGaP controls inflammation and collagen reorganization in burns. *Burns.* 43(7):1524–1531.

Meldrum, D.R. *et al.* (1994). Energetics of lymphocyte "burnout" in late Sepsis: adjuvant treatment with ATP-MgCl2 improves energetics and decreases lethality. *J Surg Res.* 56:537–542.

Millis, D. and Levine, D. (2014). *Canine Rehabilitation and Physical Therapy*, 2 edn. Elsevier, Philadelphia.

Pastore, D. *et al.* (2000). Specific helium-neon laser sensitivity of the purified cytochrome c oxidase. *Int J Radiate Biol.* 76:863–870.

Pelletier-Aouizerate, M. and Zivic, Y. (2021). Early cases of acute infectious respiratory syndrome treated with photobiomodulation, diagnosis and intervention: two case reports. *Clin Case Rep.* 9:2429–2437.

Powell, S.R. (2006). The ubiquitin-proteasome system in cardiac physiology and pathology. *Am J Physiol Heart Circ Physiol.* 291:H1–H19.

Powers, S.K. *et al.* (2016). Redox control of skeletal muscle atrophy. *Free Radical Biol Med.* 98:208–217.

Remillard, R. (2002). Nutritional support in critical. *Vet Clin Small Anim.* 32:1145–1162.

Ruh, A. (2017). Laser photobiomodulation in pressure ulcer healing of human diabetic patients: gene expression analysis of inflammatory biochemical markers. *Lasers Med Sci.* 33:165–171.

Scheiber, M. and Chandel, N.S. (2014). ROS function in redox signaling and oxidative stress. *Curr Biol.* 24:R453–R462.

Schlager, A. *et al.* (2000). Healing of burns after treatment with 670-nanometer low-power laser light. *Plastic and Reconstruct Surg.* 105(5):1635–1639.

Sergio, L.P. *et al.* (2018). Photobiomodulation prevents DNA fragmentation of alveolar epithelial cells and alters the mRNA levels of caspase 3 and Bcl-2 genes in acute lung injury. *Photochem Photobiol Sci.* 17:975–983.

Silveira, P.C. *et al.* (2009). Evaluation of mitochondrial respiratory chain activity in muscle healing by low-level laser therapy. *J Photochem Photobiol B.* 95:89–92.

Solmaz, H. *et al.* (2017). Photobiomodulation of wound healing via visible and infrared laser irradiation. *Lasers Med Sci.* 32:903–910.

Srikanthan, P. and Karlamangla, A.S. (2014). Muscle mass index as a predictor of longevity in older adults. *The Am J Med.* 127(6):547–553.

Talbert, E.E. *et al.* (2013). Immobilization-induced activation of key proteolytic systems in skeletal muscles is prevented by a mitochondria-targeted antioxidant. *J Appl Physiol.* 115:529–538.

Ucero, A.C. *et al.* (2013). Laser therapy in metabolic syndrome-related kidney injury. *Photochem Photobiol.* 89:953–960.

de Vasconcelos Catao, M.H. *et al.* (2015). Effects of red laser, infrared, photodynamic therapy, and green LED on the healing process of third-degree burns: clinical and histological study in rats. *Lasers Med Sci.* 30:421–428.

Whidden, M.A. *et al.* (2010). Oxidative stress is required for mechanical ventilation-induced protease activation in the diaphragm. *J Appl Physiol.* 108:1376–1382.

Winkelman, C. (2004). Inactivity and inflammation: selected cytokines as biologic mediators in muscle dysfunction during critical illness. *AACN Clinical Issues.* 15(1):74–82.

Yamato, M. *et al.* (2013). Low-level laser therapy improves crescentic glomerulonephritis in rats. *Lasers Med Sci.* 28:1189–1196.

Yu, W. (1997). Improvement of host response to sepsis by photobiomodulation. *Lasers Surg Med.* 21:262–268.

Yu, W. *et al.* (1997). Improvement of host response to sepsis by photobiomodulation. *Lasers Surg Med.* 21:262–268.

da-Palma-Cruz, M. *et al.* (2019). Photobiomodulation modulates the resolution of inflammation during acute lung injury induced by sepsis. *Lasers Med Sci.* 34:191–199.

Part V

Clinical Applications of Laser Therapy in Canine Rehabilitation & Sports Medicine

21

Laser Therapy for the Canine Athlete: Performance Maintenance and Discipline-Specific Applications

Deborah Gross Torraca

Wizard of Paws Physical Rehabilitation for Animals, Colchester, CT, USA

1st Edition Contributor:

Debra Canapp

Veterinary Orthopedic and Sports Medicine Group, Orthobiologic Innovations, Annapolis Junction, MD, USA

Introduction

Sports medicine has become an integral component of all canine athletic activities. The principles of sports medicine are routinely applied during conditioning, rehabilitation protocols, surgical and nonsurgical treatments, and in all stages of training. Sports medicine skills are used to maintain canine athletes at their individual peak performance levels. Research in humans and other species are being applied to canine athletes. The quantity of studies using dogs and photobiomodulation (PBM) continues to grow.

Canine athletes perform in athletic endeavors that range from professional racing to recreational agility events on the weekends. Each athletic discipline is divided into amateur and professional levels, each with unique training and preparation methodology. With the increasing popularity and demand of canine sports, the rate of injuries is also increasing. Stretch-induced and acute muscle and tendon injuries are estimated to account for greater than 30% of the injuries seen in a human sports medicine practice. Acute muscle and tendon injuries are slowly being recognized and detected with various diagnostic techniques.

Irrespective of the athletic discipline, a great amount of time, effort, and attention is spent on training, trialing, and preparation. This involves a diverse range of activities, including events focused on agility, obedience, racing, flyball, water work, rally, hunting, field trialing, sledding, scent work, and conformation. It also encompasses all working endeavors, including drug and bomb detectors, protection and guard dogs, guide dogs, service dogs, and therapy dogs.

Each sporting and working dog is a unique individual in the eyes of the owner, trainer, and handler, and in its ability to excel in its distinctive task. Each discipline demands specific actions of the body relative to physiology, strength, and performance. Laser therapy, also known as photobiomodulation therapy (PBMT), provides these individuals with the best probability of preventing injuries, enjoying an extended career, and experiencing a good quality of life.

The rapidly expanding number of canine athletic competitions demands canine sports medicine applications of both a proactive and a reactive nature. Proactively, PBMT is an essential component in the effort to prevent injuries (Ribeiro *et al.*, 2015), maintain the highest level of performance possible (Levine *et al.*, 2015), and provide a higher quality of life. Reactively, it is an important part of the treatment and accelerated healing of all musculoskeletal injuries (Ferraresi *et al.*, 2012). PBMT provides a higher level of available energy, accelerated gains in strength and conditioning, and a faster recovery period after each athletic endeavor. Therefore, when PBMT is integrated into strength, conditioning, and training programs, it results in a more comfortable athlete that is easier to train and can compete at a high level.

Injuries sustained in canine sports may cause damage to the soft tissues: muscles, tendons and ligaments. The initial injury may cause inflammation, pain, and dysfunction. If the problem persists, the chronic inflammation, pain and dysfunction may cause premature osteoarthritis. The chronicity

Laser Therapy in Veterinary Medicine: Photobiomodulation, Second Edition. Edited by Christopher J. Winkler and Lisa A. Miller.

of the soft tissue injury has the potential to prolong a return to sporting activities, or prevent a canine athlete from returning to sports. PBMT has been demonstrated to reduce tissue inflammation and pain. (Soriano *et al.*, 2006). PBMT is used in human sports medicine to treat the problems, and minimize athletes' down time. The treatment of canine athletes with PBMT is an area requiring additional research. However, the expansion and utilization of PBM in human sports has assisted in the support of research and clinical application in sporting and working dogs.

Types of Canine Sports

Most of the canine sports involve a combination of endurance, speed, power, obedience, and explosive activities. Knowledge of balance, proprioception, and normal physiologic parameters, as well as familiarity with the sport and common sense, are needed to evaluate and support these athletes. Some of the popular sports seen in a canine sports medicine environment are listed in Box 21.1.

Additional activities many dogs perform with their owners include hiking, walking, running, guard work, and, of course, counter surfing! All these activities are important to each individual dog, trainer, handler, and owner. Our goals as professional practitioners include injury prevention, appropriate treatment, and rehabilitation. Accomplishing these goals culminates in the dog maintaining the highest level of function and performance.

Each of the common sports can be broken down into individual components. As we split them into endurance, power, speed, and strength, we can determine what is needed for preventative activities, training, rehabilitation, and a return to activity (function). Common endurance sports and activities include hunting, field trials, sledding, skijoring, and detection work. Explosive activities include flyball, protection work, agility, and dock diving. Activities requiring speed include racing, agility, lure coursing, protection work, flyball, and water work. Power and obedience are fundamental to all the athletic disciplines.

Many events involve a combination of traits. For example, a dog may participate in one agility run of approximately 40 seconds that involves explosive running, turning, ascending and descending frames and obstacles, and jumping. Though the event may last only 40 seconds, the dog might participate in three to six of these runs in one day, or 15–18 runs over the course of a long weekend. Therefore, endurance also plays a significant role in participation in this explosive event.

Box 21.1 Popular Canine Sports

Agility	Herding
Barn hunts	Hunting
Canicross	Lure coursing Nosework
Conformation	Obedience
Disk dog	Protection work
Dock diving	Racing
Earthdog	Rally
Field trial	Schutzhund Skijoring
Freestyle dancing	Sledding
Flyball	Tracking Trick dog Treibball

Understanding of Individual Sports and Breeds

To provide optimal care, it is essential to have a thorough understanding of the individual sport and the unique breed-specific athletic ability to perform that sport. For example, sight hounds are very different from many working breeds in their composition of body fat and muscle. Jeusette *et al.* (2010) examined the different body compositions of greyhounds, rottweilers, standard poodles, Siberian huskies, dachshunds, and golden retrievers and found greyhounds had significantly lower levels of body fat and higher levels of muscle compared to other breeds. Golden retrievers have the distinction of having the highest percentage of body fat among all dog breeds (Raffan, 2013).

Certain sports have a much higher participation among particular breeds compared to others. For example, Sighthounds commonly participate in racing events, such as straight and oval racing. Herding dogs include a predominance of Border Collies, German Shepherd dogs, Shetland Sheepdogs, and Australian Shepherds. Protection dogs normally include German Shepherd dogs, Belgian Malinois, Doberman Pinchers, and Russian Terriers. Any dog may participate in agility, but Border Collies, Shetland Sheepdogs, Papillion, Australian Shepherds, and Portuguese Water Dogs excel due to their natural speed and accuracy. Dogs involved in flyball are typically fast and are very ball-motivated. Water work is typically performed by breeds that can swim, including Labrador Retrievers, Portuguese Water Dogs, Newfoundlands, and other type of retriever.

Breed clubs have specific types of activity, as well. For example, Bernese Mountain Dogs are common drafters and Portuguese Water Dogs perform water sports specific to their breeds. Newfoundlands compete in draft and water rescue. Parson Terriers and Jack Russell Terriers compete in barn hunts and racing.

Since each breed has a propensity to perform different athletic activities, as the practitioner, it is important to factor breed propensity into specific considerations about treatment and preventative care in different disciplines. Our goal is to assist with the prevention of injuries while maintaining a high level of performance. If an injury occurs, knowledge about breed propensity helps individualize the rehabilitation program to accelerate the patient's return to its previous level of competition.

General Principles of PBMT in Canine Sports Medicine

In the human field, athletic trainers and physical therapists utilize various physical, therapeutic, and electrophysical techniques and modalities as additions to the manual care of patients. They share the same goals as practitioners in the canine sports medicine field: optimum athletic performance, prevention of injuries, and accelerated recovery. Skeletal muscles utilized in high-intensity repetitive muscle activities eventually show fatigue, resulting in a direct decrease in performance of the core strength and the corresponding peripheral musculature. Whether it is a person running a 5 km race or a dog running an agility course, decrease in performance is caused by fatigue.

Many factors contribute to fatigue, including nutrition, age, training, conditioning, specific exercise conditions, and the environmental temperature. Ultimately, the depletion of energy sources within the cells results in fatigue. Proper nutrition, conditioning, and exercises specifically tailored to a discipline assist the canine athlete in avoiding fatigue.

Muscle contractions are either aerobic or anaerobic in nature. Aerobic muscle contractions are oxidative and more associated with endurance events. Anaerobic muscle contractions are lactic and alactic and are associated with short bursts of energy and strength training. High-intensity and strength training exercise creates a metabolic change in the musculature from the anaerobic metabolic pathways. Low-intensity and endurance exercise promotes a change in the energy recruitment from the aerobic metabolism (Billat *et al.*, 2009; Sundberg and Bundle, 2015).

Successful applications and approaches in the human field can be applied in the canine world. Common techniques and protocols have included cryotherapy, moist heat, massage, hot–cold contrast baths, stretching, low-intensity exercises, neuromuscular electrical stimulation, and various combinations of the same. The results on effectiveness are varied (Barnett, 2006). The rationale behind the use of these techniques is an attempt to reduce inflammation within the tissues associated with exercise. They increase vascularization and circulation, which in turn reduce the pooling of fluids and metabolites resulting from exercises that cause muscle soreness. Though these techniques are commonly utilized, their effectiveness is limited, and there is a constant search for alternatives. PBMT has been proven effective in increasing the circulation and reducing inflammation following exercise (Antonialli *et al.*, 2014; Baroni *et al.*, 2015). These attributes make it an ideal modality for use in both the human and the canine physical therapy fields.

PBMT targets the mitochondria or "energy centers" of individual cells. Skeletal muscles are rich in mitochondria. When their photoacceptors are stimulated, there is an increase in metabolic rate. PBMT thus assists in athletic performance by facilitating muscle repair, decreasing muscle fatigue, and reducing oxidative stress, all of which reduces the incidence of injury (Avni *et al.*, 2005). It has been used to accelerate metabolic and structural changes within both the aerobic and the anaerobic metabolic cycles (Karu, 2010).

PBMT has been demonstrated to reduce inflammation on many levels (Bortone *et al.*, 2008). In addition, it increases mitochondrial function and adenosine triphosphate (ATP), ribonucleic acid (RNA), and protein synthesis (Karu, 2010). These actions assist in increasing the rate of cellular metabolism and the acceleration of the inflammatory process (Huang *et al.*, 2009; Pryor and Millis, 2015). The combination of these facts has led scientists and clinicians to study the effectiveness of laser therapy on humans and animals post-exercise and activity. Scientific studies have demonstrated conclusive evidence of laser therapy reducing inflammation and accelerating muscle repair when optimal parameters of treatment are applied (Assis, 2015; Levine *et al.*, 2015; Liu *et al.*, 2009). During the recovery stage post exercise, reduction of inflammation and acceleration of healing will accelerate the training process and maintain optimal performance levels in the canine athlete (de Marchi *et al.*, 2012).

Further studies support additional benefits of PMBT. It can improve mitochondrial function, which accelerates the healing process after exercise (Avni *et al.*, 2005). It can also decrease oxidative stress and reactive oxygen species (ROS) production (Bjordal *et al.*, 2001; Silveira *et al.*, 2009). Recent studies have provided scientific evidence that PBMT is effective in preventing the development of skeletal muscle fatigue and that it enhances recovery, and therefore helps to maintain performance (Ferraresi *et al.*, 2012; Ribeiro *et al.*, 2015).

Most injuries occur secondary to muscular and physiological fatigue (Allen *et al.*, 2008). Studies have examined whether PBMT could delay the development of skeletal muscle fatigue (Avni *et al.*, 2005; Leal Junior *et al.*, 2009a,b). With a delay of skeletal muscle fatigue, there should be an increase in the speed of muscle recovery, with a faster restoration and recovery to normal, and with a reduced possibility of injury (Lopes-Martins *et al.*, 2006). Leal Junior *et al.* (2009a) demonstrated a delay in skeletal muscle fatigue with laser therapy. In addition to the delay, improved biomechanical markers were noted in direct relationship with muscle recovery (Ferraresi *et al.*, 2011). While these were valuable initial studies, they were performed with single-diode laser therapy probes (handpieces), which irradiate only a very small area. Another study by the same group utilized a multi-diode cluster probe applied to the biceps brachii muscle (Leal Junior *et al.*, 2009b). This crossover, double-blind, placebo-controlled trial included healthy male volleyball players between the ages of 18 and 20. PBMT was administered utilizing a wavelength of 810 nm and a dosage of 6 J per point, applied to 10 treatment areas on the biceps brachii muscle. The laser-treated group demonstrated significantly delayed development of muscle fatigue while performing active exercise and repetitions to elbow fatigue. This study was also able to demonstrate a reduction in the blood lactate concentration level at 5 minutes postexercise. Blood lactate concentration is utilized to monitor recovery and serves as a marker postexercise. Historically, modalities used in human sports medicine and physical therapy to address recovery (cryotherapy, massage, and electrical stimulation) have failed to enhance blood lactate removal (Halson *et al.*, 2008; Jarvinen *et al.*, 2005). The ability of PBMT to reduce the blood lactate concentration alone makes this a valuable modality to facilitate recovery and healing.

Studies performed by Leal Junior *et al.* (2009a,b) targeted a specific muscle and demonstrated improvement within the specific movement of elbow flexion. In sports, a multitude of muscles work at the same time. To improve the performance level of our athletic patients, it is imperative to determine which muscles to specifically target, each of which will be unique to each sporting activity. This will be covered later in the chapter.

Endurance Exercises

Endurance or aerobic exercise is activity of low intensity lasting more than 30 minutes. Jogging and hiking are two examples. Since the oxidative capacity of muscle fibers is proportional to the density of the mitochondria (Coffey and Hawley, 2007), endurance exercise is a great way to promote mitochondrial growth, resulting in a decreased level of muscle fatigue. The addition of PBMT to muscle cells increases the cellular respiratory level, resulting in increased synthesis of ATP. This allows an increase in oxygen consumption and a reduction in the fatigue index (Silveira *et al.*, 2009). The addition of PBMT to an endurance-training program allows an increase in the ability of the muscle to function at an efficient level for long periods. A study performed in 2017 assessed the effects of PBMT applied before and/or after endurance training (Miranda *et al.*, 2017). It was determined that PBMT applied before and after endurance-training exercise sessions improved endurance three times faster than exercise alone, and increased the time to exhaustion and oxygen uptake while reducing body fat in healthy volunteers. In this study on healthy human volunteers, 17 sites had PBMT performed in the lower limb. A superpulsed or low-level laser therapy and light-emitting diode (LED) therapy was utilized in this study.

Strength Training

Strength or intensity training involves anaerobic metabolic pathways and commonly involves short exercises. Weightlifting, weight pulling, and bursts of activity are examples. PBMT increases mitochondrial activity, resulting in an increased production of ATP and a normalization of cellular respiration. Fiber recruitment occurs sequentially, first with type I fibers, then with type IIa, type IIb, and finally type IIx. Strength training involves type I fibers, and PBMT may have more of a direct effect on strengthening these fibers than endurance exercises.

PBMT applied directly to specific muscles before activity will enhance performance and decrease the rate of fatigue. Strength training demands a significant amount of ATP from the hydrolysis of phosphocreatine. The consumption of ATP is faster than the rate of phosphocreatine hydrolysis, and this produces an excessive amount of creatine. This excess of creatine is an additional cause of muscle fatigue. If ATP levels can be increased, creatine levels will ultimately be reduced; this diminishes the rate and level of muscle fatigue. PBMT will increase the production of ATP (Karu *et al.*, 1995). A study conducted in 2016 examined strength gains with an application of PBMT consisting of multi-wavelengths prior to exercise in peak torque reached in a maximum voluntary contraction, load in one-repetition maximum text and thigh circumference. Forty-eight male volunteers (ages 18–35 years old) completed all procedures in this study. Volunteers performed the strength training protocol where either a phototherapy and/or placebo before and/or after each training session was performed using cluster probes with four laser diodes of 905 nm, four LEDs of 875 nm, and four LEDs of 640 nm (manufactured by Multi Radiance Medical™) (Vanin *et al.*, 2017).

De Olivera *et al.* conducted a randomized, double blind control study on 28 high school football players. PBMT was applied prior to an eccentric contraction protocol with a cluster of five diodes at 810 nm and a 10 joule dose. There were three different output powers at 100, 200, and 400 mW per diode or a placebo at six different sites of the knee extensors or quadriceps. Voluntary maximal isometric contraction (MIVC), DOMS, CK, and lactate dehydrogenase, inflammation (IL-1β, IL-6, and TNF-α), and oxidative stress (catalase, superoxide dismutase, carbonylated proteins, and thiobarbituric acid) were evaluated before isokinetic exercise, as well as after 1 minute and 1 hour to 96 hours. PBMT increased MIVC and decreased DOMS and the biochemical marker levels with the best results for 100 mW output power per diode (500 mW in total) in improving performance and post-exercise restoration. This study is demonstrating a 500 mW treatment to the targeted muscle group will assist in performance and recovery after exercise. Understanding the target muscle group and the type of muscle contractions needed in an activity may improve performance with the recommended dosage.

Another study examined the influence of PBMT on the performance and recovery of top-tier rugby players during a high-intensity field test. A total of 12 elite male rugby players were involved in this randomized, double-blind control study. No treatments were administered before the initial Bangsbo Sprint Test (BST). In the subsequent weeks, either PBMT or a placebo was randomly assigned to each player. The therapy involved irradiating 17 points on each lower limb using a cluster of 12 diodes. Key metrics such as average sprint time, best sprint time, and fatigue index were gathered from the BST. Blood lactate levels were measured at various intervals before and after the test. Additionally, players' self-reported fatigue was evaluated via a questionnaire. The results indicated that PBMT significantly improved average sprint time and fatigue index during the BST. It also led to a significant reduction in blood lactate levels and perceived fatigue ($p \leq 0.05$). Pre-exercise PBMT using a combination of low-level laser, red LEDs, and infrared LEDs can boost performance and speed up recovery for high-level rugby players during field tests. This underscores the potential for extensive use of PBMT in real-world sports medicine (Pinto *et al.*, 2016; de Oliveira *et al.* 2017).

Athletic Injuries in the Canine Athlete

The treatment of any injury demands a systematic approach to determine the location of the lesion as well as the severity. In canine veterinary medicine, we examine the subject objectively to determine pain, loss of strength, loss of range of motion, specific location, and deficits in the body caused by the injury. Objective data will include a thorough hands-on examination, goniometric measurements of all joints, muscle-mass recordings, a dynamic gait analysis (if possible), radiographs, and other diagnostics (such as diagnostic ultrasound, MRI, and CT scan). In addition to the objective information, a thorough history of the injury, the activity, and the overall condition of the dog is essential. Factors to be considered when addressing a canine athlete are age, body mass, history of training, conditioning activities, and behavior.

Overview of Sports-Injury Rehabilitation

Injuries to the soft tissues may be broken down into four phases. Phase I is the acute phase and is typically one to three weeks from the injury. This phase is characterized by inflammation, pain, loss of range of motion, atrophy and loss of function and weight bearing. The goals of this phase are to reduce the time of immobilization, promote the healing of the injured area, minimize pain and inflammation, and make the patient more comfortable. PBMT is essential (indeed, game-changing) at this period to initiate a decrease in inflammation and begin healing. PBMT should be aimed at reducing pain and inflammation. The peripheral nerve endings of nociceptors, consisting of the thinly myelinated A∂ and unmyelinated, slow-conducting C fibers, lie within the epidermis. This complex network transduces noxious stimuli into action potentials. Moreover, these nerve endings are very superficial in nature and thus are easily within the penetration depths of the wavelengths used in PBMT. Laser therapy can assist in providing pain relief and can improve the clinical outcome in these instances. A recent study of frozen shoulder in human patients demonstrated that laser therapy provided significant pain relief through 8 weeks, allowing for appropriate manual therapy (Kim *et al.*, 2015). The initial phase of rehabilitation therapy should incorporate the application of PBMT. Laser therapy, a significant treatment method for shoulder injuries, is applied to the main joints, muscles, and tendons that are affected. The purpose of this therapy is to decrease inflammation, promote the synthesis of collagen, deactivate trigger points, and aid in the healing process (Lam *et al.*, 1986).

Phase II typically occurs 4–6 weeks after the initial injury and is marked by a restoration of normal range of motion for the animal, improvement of lameness, and improvement of pain and inflammation. Research supports utilizing PBMT during this phase of healing, and continuing into Phase III as well (Larkin-Kaiser *et al.*, 2015). One study looked at the impact of PBMT on the proliferation stage in the intermediate phase of healing and demonstrated better mechanical resistance of the injured area in the remodeling phase of healing (Amadio *et al.*, 2021).

Phase III, or the advanced strengthening phase, initiates where there is full or near-full nonpainful range of motion, and no pain or tenderness in the affected limb and area. The injury is approaching a healed status and we can expect to see the strength and muscle mass approaching the status of the contralateral limb with no pain or tenderness to the region. This is the stage in rehabilitation in which a return to a level of activity can be initiated. The plan should include activities that prepare the dog for a full return. It will require appropriate strength, range of motion, balance, proprioception, and endurance of the injured limb. PBMT plays a significant role in assisting the muscular activity with appropriate increases in blood flow, ATP activity and mitochondrial activity. In 25 studies, PBMT has proven to enhance performance and speed up recovery. This is also backed by 22 animal studies (Ailioaie & Litscher 2021).

Phase IV is the return to full activity and usually occurs 12 or more weeks after the injury and/or surgery. Of course, this interval is dependent upon complications and general health and recovery of the animal. The hallmarks of this phase include full and nonpainful range of motion, the absence of pain during and after exercise, symmetrical muscle mass, and normal gait pattern. The dog will also be able to return to sport-specific activity without pain during or after the activity.

Photobiomodulation Application in Musculoskeletal Injuries

Canine sports-related injuries are a common occurrence. They require a confirmed diagnosis, and this is often performed by a veterinary specialist. The injuries are accompanied by pain, inflammation, loss of range of motion, loss of strength, deficits in gait, deficits in lifestyle for both the owner and the dog, and inability to participate in canine sports. There are often multiple areas of involvement with a sports-related injury so it is judicious to treat the entire dog. Photobiomodulation is appropriate at all phases of healing, as well as the treatment of the secondary and tertiary areas of involvement.

Repair of Muscle Damage

Various levels of muscle damage and injuries are common in canine sports medicine. Whether it is a significant muscle tear with bleeding, sidelining the dog for a significant period, or a minor tear in a muscle resulting in just a slight decrease in athletic performance, application of PBMT will accelerate the healing process. The regeneration of muscle tissue takes place in six phases, and typically takes 21 days (Jarvinen *et al.*, 2005). Ultimately, the faster the tissue can move through these phases, the quicker the patient can return to their previous level of activity and training. Studies have demonstrated that PBMT can increase the formation of new myofibrils that assist in filling the gap created when a muscle is injured and decrease the formation of scar tissue (Roth and Oron, 1985). Bibikova and Oron (1994) demonstrated that PBMT promotes a greater maturation of younger myofibrils. Shefer *et al.* (2009) also demonstrated an improvement in the number of young myofibrils in a group that received PBMT compared to a group that did not. These are all promising studies, demonstrating that PBMT is beneficial in decreasing the deleterious effects of strenuous exercise and training.

Secondary and Tertiary Compensations

In many sports medicine scenarios, dogs perform an array of activities. Very often, the demands on one part of their body cause compensatory effects in other parts. For example, a dog with a straight shoulder set involved in a great deal of jumping activities might place a significant amount of stress on the thoracolumbar region. A significant component of treating the canine sports athlete is treating the entire dog. Understanding just where the compensatory issues lie is an important part of the successful management of the recovery of the canine athlete.

Palpation, range of motion tests, and digital thermal imaging are useful tools for determining whether any compensatory issues exist. Palpation is extremely useful but may not always be consistent. The results can vary between practitioners and breeds. Though palpation is one of the most accurate ways of determining pain and dysfunction, it is subject to variations in knowledge, sensory ability, the dog's coat, and the depth of the problem.

Both active and passive range of motion are useful for determining pain and dysfunction. Active range of motion assists with testing the contractile units of the joint and the dog's willingness to move. Passive range of motion assists with testing the inert units, such as bones, nerves, and ligaments.

Digital thermal imaging assists in the physiological examination of a patient. Thermal imaging creates a visual image of the temperatures of the body and allows for differentiation between normal areas and areas experiencing physiological differences (Figure 21.1). With this tool, the practitioner can determine where the primary problem is, as well as the location of any secondary or tertiary issues or conditions. Digital thermal imaging also allows a visualization of the extent of an issue. It answers these questions: "Is the problem within the joint or is it both in the joint and surrounding soft tissues?" and "Is there a problem in all the soft tissues supporting a joint or just one area?" These

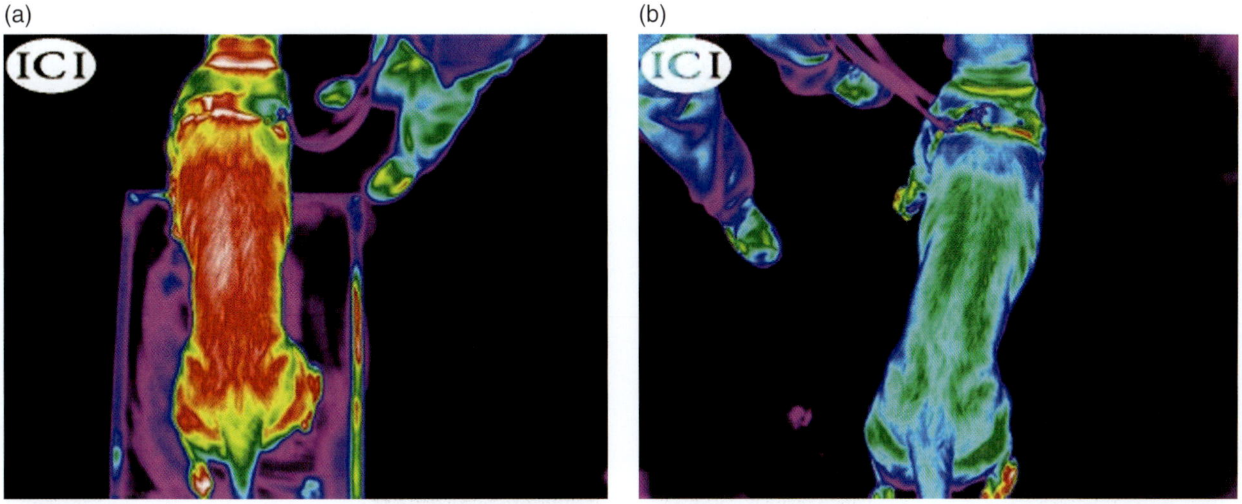

Figure 21.1 (a) Digital thermal image of a patient before PBMT. Increased thermal gradients are present throughout the thoracic and lumbar spinal musculature. Using this as a roadmap for PBMT, therapy was applied throughout all anatomical areas exhibiting an increase in thermal gradients. More energy was applied to the left side. (b) Digital thermal image taken 24 hours after PBMT of the same patient. All treated areas reveal a decrease in the thermal gradient. The patient was much more relaxed on palpation.

images serve as a very accurate roadmap for the application of PBMT to all primary, secondary, and tertiary areas of concern.

In addition, digital thermal imaging can assist in identifying problems before they become major issues. For example, detecting a minor iliopsoas problem is crucial in the canine athlete. Discovering issues before they become career ending is part of the practitioner's job. For more information on digital thermal imaging, please refer to Chapter 39.

Enhancement of Performance

Regardless of the athletic activity, the goal is always to safely maintain and maximize athletes' performance levels. In human sports medicine practice, numerous studies have demonstrated the efficacy of laser therapy in improving muscle performance. Ferraresi *et al.* (2011) examined 33 male athletes performing strength training with a load for 12 weeks. The athletes were divided into a control group, a training group, and a training group that received laser therapy. Immediately after training, the group receiving laser therapy to the quadriceps muscle had a 55% increase in muscle performance as measured by isokinetic dynamometry. This was the only group that demonstrated an increase in muscle performance, and the study concluded that PBMT can increase muscle performance compared with strength training alone. It is easy to extrapolate this study to the world of the canine athlete when the goal is to increase the level of performance and prevent injury. Strength training combined with laser therapy is more beneficial than strength training alone.

The wavelength plays a crucial role in shaping the spread, intensity, and distribution of photons in tissues exposed to light, in addition to determining the efficacy of noninvasive laser treatments. In the context of photobiomodulation, the chosen wavelength is a key factor influencing cell multiplication response, with the most effective noninvasive impact occurring within the range of 600–1070 nm (red/near-infrared) (Figure 21.1). It has been noted that shorter wavelengths are absorbed by hemoglobin or melanin, resulting in cellular changes, while longer wavelengths are absorbed by water, creating a sense of warmth and contributing to pain relief (Marshall & Vlkova 2020).

Other studies have also demonstrated the benefits of PBMT for athletic performance. One study concluded there was a greater endurance of rotator cuff muscles in a group that received PBMT before exercise than in a group that did not (Levine *et al.*, 2015). This was a double-blind crossover study, in which the infraspinatus and teres minor musculature was treated before the initiation of exercise.

Another study showed that PBMT applied immediately prior to injury had many positive effects during the muscle regeneration processes (Ribeiro *et al.*, 2015). This study has considerable application in canine sports medicine with regards to sports where there is a constant risk of injury.

While we do not have specific measuring systems such as isokinetic dynamometry, the understanding and expansion of applications continue to grow through the tested scientific technique of trial and error coupled with collaboration with colleagues. As we continue to see the benefits and possibilities of PBMT, the opportunities for its use will continue to expand. Success is measured in the performance of canine athletes and the extension of their individual sports activities.

Application Techniques

Practical applications of PBMT include performance enhancement, injury prevention, and preparation of canine athletes for their next activity. The goal is to assist with their quality of life and aid in their ability to compete safely to the best of their ability.

The first step is to understand and identify which muscles are important to an individual canine athlete's ability to perform at its maximum ability in a particular sport. The second step is to determine whether PBMT is intended for performance enhancement, injury prevention, recovery, or a combination of the three. The third step is to apply the appropriate dosage, utilizing the correct technique, at a frequency that optimizes athletic performance of the individual athlete.

Applying PBMT utilizing a contact method will help increase the blood flow, like a massage. This massage-like action potentiates the benefits of PBMT, since it puts the target tissue through a passive range of motion during administration. The soft tissue will be manipulated, which increases circulation. In addition, gently compressing the tissues forces the incidental absorbers, hemoglobin and oxyhemoglobin, away from the area. If this technique is performed properly, it is often very relaxing for the patient.

Before application of PBMT, make sure the area is clean. Clipping may not be feasible for performance dogs, so make sure the hair is clean and the laser equipment is adjusted appropriately for maximum penetration. In addition to preparing the skin, make sure the area is accessible.

Measure the treatment area to calculate the desired dose. Envisioning the area of a playing card is helpful in estimating the size of the treatment area. A single playing card is 57 cm^2; rounded up for ease of calculations, consider it 60 cm^2. Calculate the total number of playing cards needed to cover the intended area of treatment and then calculate the number of joules required to achieve the proper dosage. If a dosage of 10 J/cm^2 is desired, then administration of 600 J to an area equivalent in size to a single playing card would be correct. Always consider the patient's unique characteristics: hair color, hair length, skin color, and body mass. For example, a Border Collie will have pigmented and nonpigmented areas. The pigmented areas will absorb some of the photons being administered, so a higher dosage is warranted in these areas.

Superpulsed lasers are also being utilized and have a promising approach to improving endurance and strength.

In a study, participants underwent either active or placebo PBMT during the first session, and the alternative treatment in the second session. Each participant carried out a cardiopulmonary test on a treadmill post-treatment. For active PBMT, 17 specific areas on each lower limb were irradiated, including 9 on the quadriceps, 6 on the hamstrings, and 2 on the gastrocnemius muscles. The treatment was delivered using a cluster of 12 diodes, each with different wavelength and power and providing a total dose of 30 J per site. The conclusion determined the use of lasers and LEDs extended the duration, increased the distance, and enhanced pulmonary ventilation, while simultaneously reducing the dyspnea score in a cardiopulmonary examination (Miranda *et al.*, 2016).

Treatment time is directly correlated to the power of the laser equipment. Utilizing higher power will allow you to administer the required total dose in a shorter time, but safety is always a priority.

To maximize penetration, hold the laser handpiece perpendicular to the tissues receiving the energy. The dog may be in lateral recumbency or in a standing position. Prior to performance, a dog will very often be excited, and standing may be the optimal position, since lying in lateral recumbency may be difficult. Handle the dog with a minimum amount of restraint. This will allow you to determine whether the treatment or positioning is painful to them.

Apply the photonic energy in a direct-contact fashion, sweeping over and massaging the targeted muscle groups. Use an overlapping pattern of movement and repeat at right angles to ensure that all areas receive the same amount of treatment. The goal of the PBMT session is to increase blood flow, increase the flow of nutrients to the muscles and surrounding tissues, increase ATP levels, prepare the body for exercise, and decrease any inflammation present. This cascade of effects from PBMT essentially results in a pre-event warm-up.

Always follow all safety precautions unique to each piece of equipment. When using a high-power laser, keep the handpiece moving continuously. Drag a finger on the skin directly behind the handpiece to monitor the temperature of the treated area. Protective eyewear should be worn by the patient, the therapist, and anyone within the nominal hazard zone for the particular piece of equipment.

Dosages

There is always a question regarding the optimal dosage for the maximum consistent clinical response. Lopes-Martins *et al.* (2006) demonstrated a reduced fatigue in the tibialis anterior muscle in rats when a dosage of 0.5 J/cm^2 was applied, and decreased muscle damage at dosages of 1.0 and 2.5 J/cm^2. Another study examined the effects of different dosages of PBMT and found groups of rats receiving 1 and 3 J had a higher peak force compared to groups receiving 0.1 and 0.3 J (Leal Junior *et al.*, 2010). A third study reported doses of 1–3 J/cm^2 at 660 nm and 1, 3, and 10 J/cm^2 at 905 nm provided the best results (Santos, 2014). As these studies demonstrate, there are no universal dosages. Practitioners must dose each target and each muscle to effect. One successful way to do this is to palpate the target muscle manually while administering PBMT, and continue administration until you feel the target area relax and become free of any spastic areas.

Recommended doses for clinical use in canine sports medicine vary depending on the target area and the condition being treated. While there are no universal dosages, a range of 2–8 J/cm^2 will be very effective for most maladies (Saunders and Millis, 2014).

The physical characteristics of your patient also determine your dosage. Skin color, hair color, coat type, thick versus thin body conformation, and body mass should all be taken into consideration when calculating the initial dose. If the target area is deep on a heavily-muscled athlete, increase the dosage. If treating a dark-haired or dark-skinned patient with a long coat, increase the dosage. Fortunately, there are many laser units on the market with software that will do these calculations for you. The dosage can then be adjusted manually upon each reevaluation.

Clinical Applications

Agility and Flyball

Agility and flyball are two very popular sports. Both involve short bursts of activity with jumps, quick turns, and other movements dependent on terrain. The bursts may be anywhere from 30 to 90 seconds in length, but they can be repeated several times throughout the course of a day. Therefore, recovery and preparation for the next race are significant in these activities.

Agility and flyball participants require a significant amount of power and agility, and make a significant number of turns. Thus, these athletes utilize many different muscles during their events. Due to this high demand of muscle activity, it is often necessary to determine whether one muscle group needs therapy more than others do. Because of the time constraints between events, it is often difficult to treat all muscle groups, so a priority should be established.

The adductors and abductors of the shoulders and hips provide a significant amount of power, speed, and stability. They are often injured in agility and flyball. Medial shoulder injuries are also very common. The application of laser therapy to these areas before competitions and practice has a significant effect in reducing the incidence of injuries. To provide ideal access for the application of photonic energy to the medial shoulder, the patient should be positioned in lateral recumbency.

The iliopsoas is another area that is easily warmed up with PBMT. The dog should be placed in a lateral recumbent position with the hip in slight extension. The extended position will allow better access to the entire iliopsoas muscle from origin to insertion.

The canine athlete involved with flyball or agility should receive therapy approximately 20–30 minutes prior to their activity. The length of PBMT received will depend on the number of areas requiring treatment and the size of the dog. After the appropriate amount of PBMT has been delivered, the dog should be warmed up and stretched prior to the activity. If a muscle injury is suspected after an individual heat or sprint, additional PBMT should be applied to that specific region.

One PBMT session should be sufficient warm-up for the entire day. For example, a Border Collie involved with agility may receive PBMT to its shoulder adductors and hip adductors prior to a competition. A 22 kg Border Collie's shoulder adductors are approximately 120 cm^2 and its hip adductors approximately 240 cm^2. The dosage will range from 2–4 J/cm^2, or 240–480 J to the shoulder and 480–960 J to the hip. After the dog has received PBMT, a warm-up and dynamic stretching should be performed before it participates in its activity. If, after the activity, the dog is sore in its hip flexors, additional PBMT may be applied to the iliopsoas insertion, rectus femoris, and lumbar component from the second to the seventh lumbar vertebrae.

Jumping Activities

In jumping activities, the hip extensors, hip flexors, shoulder flexors, and spinal extensors are extremely active. The spinal extensors, specifically the lumbar and cervical muscles, are also very active during protection work. In these dogs, PBMT can be applied to a combination of muscles before their activities, as part of their warm-up routine. Treatment with PBMT should include the spinal extensors, hip flexors and extensors, and shoulder flexors and extensors. If there has been a previous injury, it is important to focus on the muscles in that area as well. This results in an increase in the blood flow and flexibility of these structures, with the goal of preventing re-injury. Stretches should be applied during therapy to any areas in which there is stiffness or reduced range of motion. After PBMT, warm-up with continued movement should be continued until the activity begins.

Power Events

In power events, such as Schutzhund, agility, and flyball, the muscles that are the most active include the hip and stifle extensors and the shoulder flexors. Of course, many other muscles are also very active, but a significant amount of the power will be generated by the hip and stifle extensors as the dog propels forward. The shoulder flexors will be involved, creating the power to propel forward from extension. Very often in power events, power with reach and extension is important.

In a fast-running dog, the shoulder flexors and elbow extensors will be very active during the stride, since they increase the forelimb extension.

PBMT should be applied to each of these muscles, from its origin to insertion:

- **Hip and stifle extensors:** The gluteal muscles originate from the posterior crest of the ilium and the posterior surface of the ilium. It then inserts into the gluteal tuberosity of the femur iliotibial band. The quadriceps are the main stifle extensors and comprise four separate muscles (vastus latus, vastus medialis, vastus intermedius, and the rectus femoris). They all insert into the patellar tendon.
- **Biceps femoris muscle:** Originates on the ischial tuberosity and sacrotuberous ligament, and inserts on the fascia lata, crural fascia, patellar ligament, and cranial border of the tibia.
- **Semitendinosus muscle:** Originates on the ischial tuberosity and inserts on the distocranial border of the tibia.
- **Semimembranosus muscle:** Originates from the ischial tuberosity and inserts into the aponeurosis of the origin of the gastrocnemius and on the medial condyle of the femur.
- **Shoulder extensors and elbow flexors:** The deltoid originates from the spine of the scapula and inserts into the deltoid tuberosity of the humerus. The brachialis is an elbow flexor and originates on the proximal portion of the brachial groove of the humerus. It then winds from the caudolateral to the cranial surface of the humerus as it travels distally and inserts on the ulnar tuberosity.
- **Triceps muscle:** Originates on the caudal border of the scapula and the tricipital crest and inserts on the olecranon.
- **Teres major muscle:** Originates on the caudal border of the scapula and inserts on the teres major tuberosity.
- **Supraspinatus muscle:** Originates on the Supraspinous fossa and inserts on the greater tubercle of the humerus.

To maintain or enhance performance, PBMT should be applied along the entire length, origin, and insertion of the three muscles of the hip and those involved with the extension of the stifle. Application to the hindlimb begins distal to the ischial tuberosity and proceeds distally to the cranial stifle. Repeat the same procedure for the three muscles of the forelimb. Photonic energy should be applied from the medial and distal shoulder down to the olecranon.

Protection Work

Protection work, such as Schutzhund, French ring, or guarding, often requires powerful bursts of energy. These activities involve a number of different types of muscle contraction, including isometric, concentric, eccentric, and plyometric. Dogs that engage in protection work are often jumping over objects or jumping up to perform bite work. Bite work involves running toward a decoy or a person, with the rear legs making powerful moves to propel the dog forward. The forelimb and spine complexes also extend and flex powerfully.

Figure 21.2 demonstrates the explosion onto the sleeve of a decoy. The hip extensors are very active as the dog explodes up to the sleeve. After the apprehension of the target, the dog requires a significant amount of control and focus to grip. The grip needs to be strong and powerful, requiring the dog to bound up in a powerful plyometric fashion and then, on release, slowly return to a guarding position. Figures 21.2 and 21.3 are from practice sessions, but in real-life situations, this is how a dog would apprehend a suspect. Police dogs, protection dogs, guard dogs, and other working dogs are familiar with this training. The combination of proper conditioning and pretreatment with PBMT has an important role in preventing injuries during this activity.

Speed Racing

Racing dogs, such as Sighthounds, need increased speed and distance. The hindlimb is responsible for propelling the body forward. The semitendinosus, semimembranosus, biceps femoris, and adductors also play a role in forward propulsion.

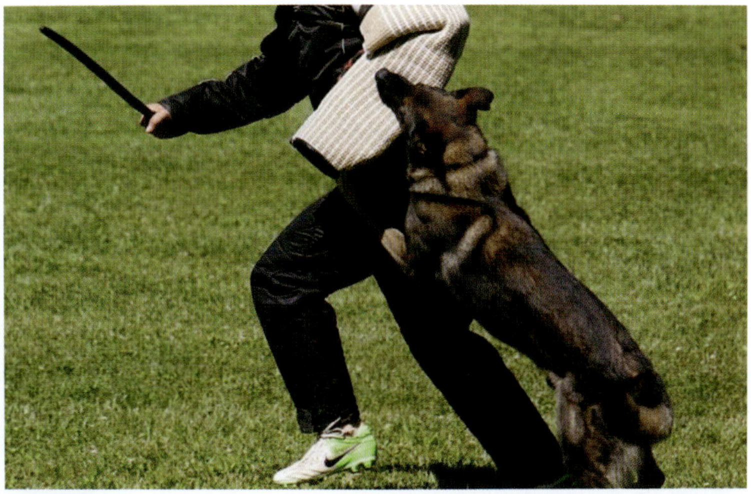

Figure 21.2 Explosion of a guard dog on to the sleeve of a decoy. The hip and spinal extensors are very active as the dog explodes up to the sleeve.

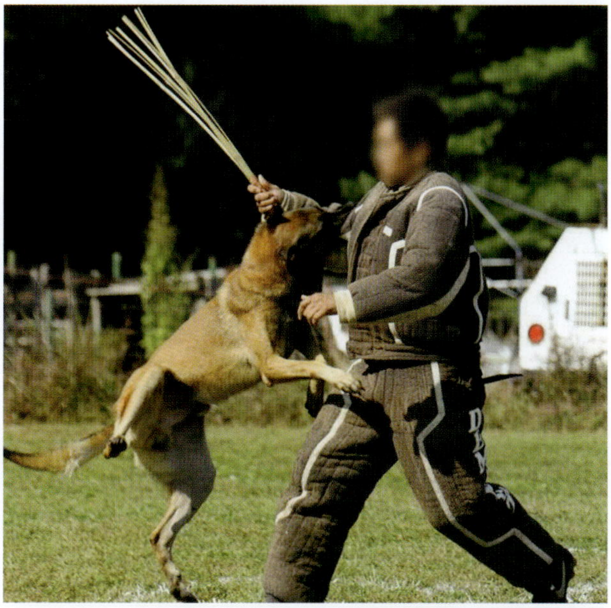

Figure 21.3 After apprehension of a target, a guard dog requires a significant amount of control and focus to maintain its grip.

The adductor group is often injured in Sighthounds, since it provides stabilization within the racing motion of these breeds. The shoulder extensors work to extend the forelimb and to widen the stride. The hip, stifle, and hock extensors are responsible for forward propulsion and increasing speed. Photonic energy should be applied to all these muscles (adductor groups, shoulder extensors, hip, stifle, and hock extensors, and hip and shoulder flexors) prior to an event. This general therapeutic protocol can be customized to an individual athlete's needs in order to maximize the clinical outcome.

Specific breeds involved in speed racing are primarily Whippets, greyhounds, Rhodesian Ridgebacks, and Borzois. Other breeds are involved in this event, but they are in a minority. The dogs may race in a straight line or in an oval. Dogs racing in an oval require particular attention to their medial musculature on both the fore and hind limbs, as they generate more power on these muscles when they navigate turns.

Racing Sighthounds are predisposed to soft-tissue injuries involving the adductor musculature in the hindlimbs. Individuals who have suffered previous injuries to the adductors should be examined closely before each event and should receive additional PBMT. In order to laser the adductor group, the dog must be in a lateral recumbent position or lying on its side, with the hip abducted. It is difficult to laser this group while the dog is standing.

Optimize the beneficial effects of PBMT by applying it approximately 30–60 minutes before the event. When there is a need to apply PBMT to a variety of muscle groups, treatment time for each patient can be 10–20 minutes, depending on the size of the dog and the areas in need of therapy. Utilize a contact method of application to impart the added benefit of a massage to the tissue. This results in a further increase in blood flow and maximizes the warm-up.

A case example is Weasel, a 4-year-old intact female Whippet. Figure 21.4 shows her receiving PBMT to the hip extensor muscles, utilizing the contact method. In Figure 21.5, she is receiving treatment to the biceps femoris muscle region. This dog prefers to be standing while receiving laser therapy, but appropriate therapy could also be performed in lateral recumbence or a lying-down posture. In Figure 21.6, an on-contact application of PBMT is being administered to Weasel's right shoulder and shoulder extensors. In Figure 21.7, PBMT is being administered to her right triceps region. Access to the triceps region can also be gained when in lateral recumbence. Apply gentle pressure along the triceps muscle and over the supraspinatus and teres major muscles.

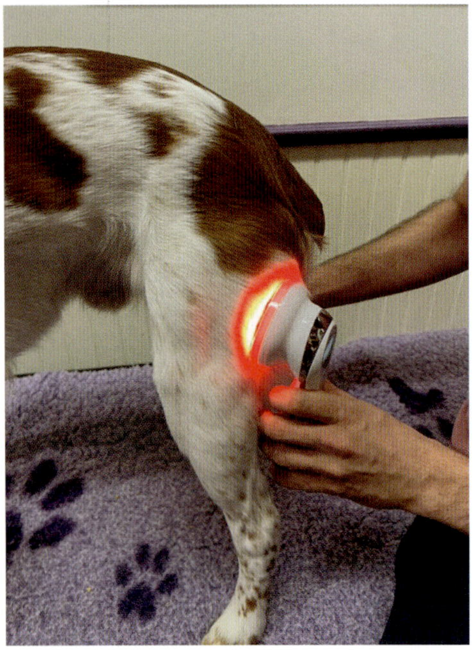

Figure 21.4 PBMT being administered to the hip extensor muscles, utilizing on-contact delivery with the handpiece in direct contact with the skin and hair coat.

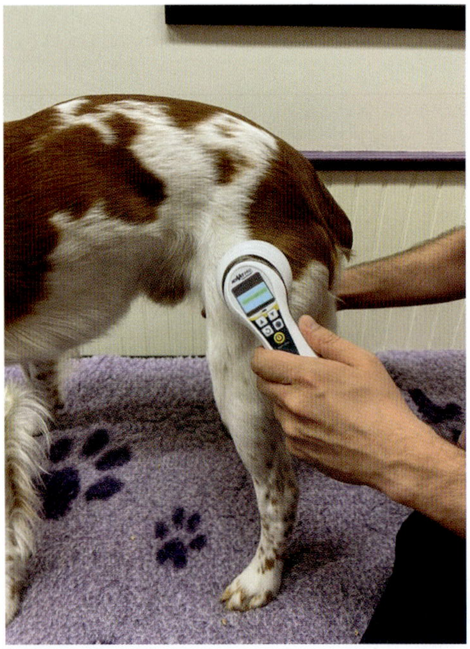

Figure 21.5 Administration of PBMT to the biceps femoris regions. To maximize photon penetration to the target tissues, the handpiece should be maintained perpendicular to the tissue and gentle pressure should be applied while moving it over the treatment area.

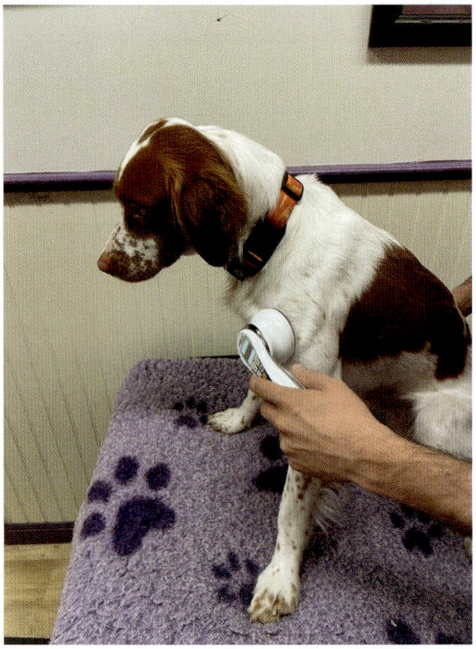

Figure 21.6 On-contact application of PBMT the right shoulder and shoulder extensors area. This treatment could also be administered with the patient in lateral recumbency or a lying-down posture.

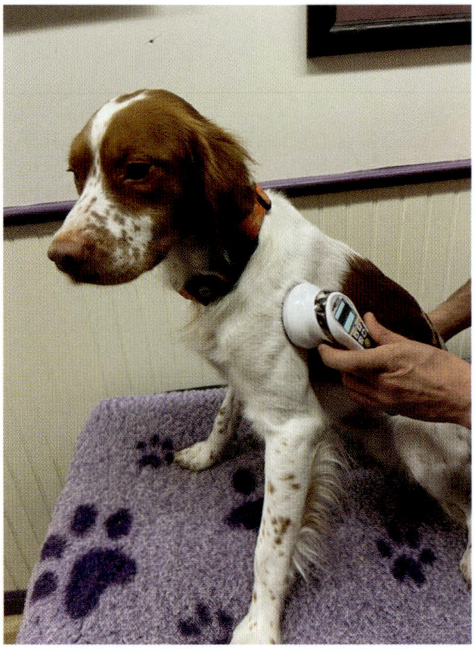

Figure 21.7 Administration of PBMT to the right triceps region. Access to the triceps region can also be gained with the patient in lateral recumbency. Gentle massage pressure should be applied along the triceps muscle and over the supraspinatus and teres major muscles.

Use the playing card system when calculating the total dose to these anatomical areas. In Figure 21.4, the area to be treated is roughly four playing cards. With each playing card measuring approximately 60 cm^2 and a dosage of 1–4 J/cm^2 required to achieve a clinical response, the total dose would be 60–240 J. The triceps area in Figure 21.7 is roughly the area of two playing cards, which is approximately 120 cm^2. Therefore, the correct dosage would be between 120 and 480 J. A larger area would require treatment at the same dosage but an increased total number of joules; the converse is applied for a smaller area.

In a racing dog, the goal of PBMT is to increase blood flow to the tissues. The vasodilation effects of PBMT allow additional nutrients to be provided to any cells that are going to be asked for an increase in their metabolic rate during the event. The application of PBMT to the racing dog should ideally be performed before the athlete stretches and warms up. The most beneficial time is approximately 30 minutes prior to any activity. This will facilitate an increased range of motion within the limbs and greater flexibility within the muscles. Utilization of this sequence of events maximizes performance.

In some smaller dogs, it is sometimes difficult to reach certain anatomical areas when attempting to massage or stretch before exercise. The application of PBMT will provide an increase in blood flow and an overall relaxation of the patient, which aids in this pre-event procedure. Particular attention should be paid to the hip region, the shoulder region, the medial muscle groups (such as the adductor and medial shoulder muscles), and the iliopsoas.

In Weasel's case, she had a previous injury to the rectus femoris and the iliopsoas muscles. She has been free of lameness for over 9 months at the time of writing, and has returned to both straight and oval racing at a very competitive level. She receives PBMT to the hip flexors, iliopsoas, and hip extensors 40 minutes prior to competition. After PBMT, she receives her warm-up, consisting of figure eights and dynamic hip extensor and flexor stretches. Movement is continued until the actual race time. The focus on the hip flexors and iliopsoas is secondary to the prior injury. An additional benefit of the application of PBMT to this area is the reduction of any preexisting inflammation. The result of all these efforts is a safe improvement in athletic performance.

Conclusion

PBMT has been demonstrated to have numerous benefits when applied to the canine athlete. If the practitioner is able to deliver the appropriate number of joules to the target tissues, positive results will be inevitable. This modality can be utilized for the treatment and prevention of injuries, pre-event preparation, and maintenance of the canine athlete at its highest performance level. Our ultimate goal when working with animals is to allow them to live the best life they can, for the longest time possible. This includes helping them safely work and compete to the best of their ability in their athletic endeavors. PBMT is an essential tool we can use to accomplish this.

References

Allen, D.G. *et al.* (2008). Skeletal muscle fatigue: cellular mechanisms. *Physiol Rev.* 88(1):287–332.

Ailioaie, L.M. and Litscher, G. (2021). Photobiomodulation and sports: results of a narrative review. *Life (Basel).* 11(12):1339.

Amadio, E.M. *et al.* (2021). Effect of photobiomodulation therapy on the proliferation phase and wound healing in rats fed with an experimental hypoproteic diet. *Lasers Med Sci.* 36(1):1427–1435.

Antonialli, F.C. *et al.* (2014). Phototherapy in skeletal muscle performance and recovery after exercise: effect of combination of super-pulsed laser and light-emitting diodes. *Lasers Med Sci.* 29(6):1967–1976.

Assis, L. (2015). Effect of low-level laser therapy (808 nm) on skeletal muscle after endurance exercise training in rats. *Braz J Phys Ther.* 19(6):457–465.

Avni, D. *et al.* (2005). Protection of skeletal muscles from ischemic injury: low-level laser therapy increases antioxidant activity. *Photomed Laser Surg.* 23(3):273–277.

Barnett, A. (2006). Using recovery modalities between training sessions in elite athletes: does it help? *Sports Med.* 36(9):781–796.

Baroni, B.M. *et al.* (2015). Effect of low-level laser therapy on muscle adaptation to knee extensor eccentric training. *Eur J Appl Physiol.* 115(3):639–647.

Bibikova, A. and Oron, U. (1994). Attenuation of the process of muscle degeneration in the toad gastrocnemius muscle by low energy laser irradiation. *Lasers Surg Med.* 14(4):355–361.

Billat, V. *et al.* (2009). Differential modeling of anaerobic and aerobic metabolism in the 800-m and 1,500-m run. *J Appl Physiol.* 17(2):478–487.

Bjordal, J.M. *et al.* (2001). Low level laser therapy for tendinopathy: evidence of a dose-response pattern. *Phys Ther Rev.* 6(2):91–99.

Bortone, F. *et al.* (2008). Low level laser therapy modulates kinin receptor expression in the subplantar muscle of rat paw subjected to carrageenan-induced inflammation. *Intss Immunopharm.* 8(2):206–210.

Coffey, V.G. and Hawley, J.A. (2007). The molecular bases of training adaptation. *Sports Med.* 34:663–679.

De Oliveira, A.R. *et al.* (2017). Pre-exercise infrared photobiomodulation therapy (810 nm) in skeletal muscle performance and postexercise recovery in humans: what is the optimal power output? *Photomed Laser Surg.* 35 (11):595–603.

de Marchi, T. *et al.* (2012). Low-level laser therapy (LLLT) in human progressive-intensity running: effects on exercise performance, skeletal muscle status, and oxidative stress. *Lasers Med Sci.* 27(1):231–236.

Ferraresi, C. *et al.* (2011). Effects of low level laser therapy (808 nm) on physical strength training in humans. *Lasers Med Sci.* 26(3):349–358.

Ferraresi, C. *et al.* (2012). Low-level laser (light) therapy (LLLT) on muscle tissue: performance, fatigue and repair benefited by the power of light. *Photonics Lasers Med.* 1(4):267–286.

Halson, S.L. *et al.* (2008). Physiological responses to cold water immersion following cycling in the heat. *Int J Sports Physiol Perform.* 3(3):331–346.

Huang, Y.Y. *et al.* (2009). Biphasic dose response in low level light therapy. *Dose-Response.* 7(4):358–383.

Jarvinen, T.A. *et al.* (2005). Muscle injuries: biology and treatment. *Am J Sports Med.* 33(5):745–764.

Jeusette *et al.* (2010). Effect of breed on body composition and comparison between various methods to estimate body composition in dogs. *Res Vet Sci.* 88(2):227–232.

Karu, T.I. *et al.* (1995). Irradiation with He-Ne laser increases ATP level in cells cultivated in vitro. *J Photochem Photobiol B.* 27(3):219–223.

Karu, T. (2010). Mitochondrial mechanisms of photobiomodulation in context of new data about multiple roles of ATP. *Photomed Laser Surg.* 28(2):159–160.

Kim, S.H. *et al.* (2015). Short-term effects of high-intensity laser therapy on frozen shoulder: a prospective randomized control study. *Man Ther.* 20(6):751–757.

Lam, T.S. *et al.* (1986). Laser stimulation of collagen synthesis in human skin fibroblast cultures. *Lasers Life Sci.* 1:61–77.

Larkin-Kaiser, K.A. *et al.* (2015). Near-infrared light therapy to attenuate strength loss after strenuous resistance exercise. *J Athl Train.* 50(1):45–50.

Leal Junior, E.C. *et al.* (2009a). Effect of 830 nm low level laser therapy in exercise induced skeletal muscle fatigue in humans. *Lasers Med Sci.* 24(3):425–431.

Leal Junior, E.C. *et al.* (2009b). Effect of cluster multi-diode light emitting diode therapy (LEDT) on exercise-induced skeletal muscle fatigue and skeletal muscle recovery in humans. *Lasers Surg Med.* 41(8):572–527.

Leal Junior, E.C. *et al.* (2010). Effect of low-level laser therapy (GaAs 904 nm) in skeletal muscle fatigue and biochemical markers of muscle damage in rats. *Eur J Appl Physiol.* 108(6):1083–1088.

Levine, D. *et al.* (2015). Effects of laser on endurance of the rotator cuff muscles. *Lasers Surg Med.* 47(s26):44–45.

Liu, X.G. *et al.* (2009). Effects of low-level laser irradiation on rat skeletal muscle injury after eccentric exercise. *Photomed Laser Surg.* 27(6):863–869.

Lopes-Martins, R.A. *et al.* (2006). Effect of low-level laser (Ga-Al-As 655 nm) on skeletal muscle fatigue induced by electrical stimulation in rats. *J Appl Physiol.* 101(1):283–282.

Marshall, R.P. and Vlkova, K. (2020). Spectral dependence on laser light on light tissue interactions and its influence on laser therapy: An experimental study. *Insights Biomed.* 5:1.

Miranda, E.F. *et al.* (2016). Using pre-exercise photobiomodulation therapy combining super-pulsed lasers and light-emitting diodes to improve performance in progressive cardiopulmonary exercise tests. *J Athl Train.* 51(2):129–135.

Miranda, D. *et al.* (2017). Multifunctional liposomes for image-guided intratumoral chemo-phototherapy. *Adv Healthc Mater.* 6(16). doi:10.1002/adhm.201700253.

Pinto, H.D. *et al.* (2016). Photobiomodulation therapy improves performance and accelerates recovery of high-level rugby players in field test: a randomized, crossover, double-blind, placebo-controlled clinical study. *J Strength Cond Res.* 30(12):3329–3338.

Pryor, B. and Millis, D.L. (2015). Therapeutic laser in veterinary medicine. *Vet Clin North Am Small Anim Pract.* 45(1):45–56.

Raffan, E. (2013). Obesity in labradors and golden retrievers. *Vet Rec.* 172(12):320.

Ribeiro, B.G. *et al.* (2015). The effect of low-level laser therapy (LLLT) applied prior to muscle injury. *Lasers Surg Med.* 47(7):571–578.

Roth, D. and Oron, U. (1985). Repair mechanisms involved in repair regeneration following partial excision of the rat gastrocnemius muscle. *Exp Cell Biol.* 53(2):107–114.

Santos, L.A. (2014). Effects of pre-irradiation of low-level laser therapy with different doses and wavelengths in skeletal muscle performance, fatigue, and skeletal muscle damage induced by tetanic contractions in rats. *Lasers Med Sci.* 29(5):1617–1626.

Saunders, D.G. and Millis, D. (2014). Laser therapy in canine rehabilitation. In: *Canine Rehabilitation and Physical Therapy*, 2 edn, pp. 359–380.

Shefer, G. *et al.* (2009). Low-energy laser irradiation promotes the recovery of atrophied gastrocnemius skeletal muscle in rats. *Exp Physilo.* 94(9):1005–1015.

Silveira, P.C. *et al.* (2009). Evaluation of mitochondrial respiratory chain activity in muscle healing by low level laser therapy. *J Photochem Photobiol B.* 95(2):89–92.

Soriano, F. *et al.* (2006). Photobiomodulation of pain and inflammation in microcrystalline arthropathies: experimental and clinical results. *Photomed Laser Surg.* 24(2):140–150.

Sundberg, C.W. and Bundle, M.W. (2015). Influence of duty cycle on the time course of muscle fatigue and the onset of neuromuscular compensation during exhaustive dynamic isolated limb exercise. *Am J Physiol Regul Integr Com.* 301(1): R51–R61.

Vanin, A.A. *et al.* (2017). What is the best moment to apply phototherapy when associated to a strength training program? A randomized, double-blinded, placebo-controlled trial: Phototherapy in association to strength training. *Lasers Med Sci.* 31(8):1555–1564. doi:10.1007/s10103-016-2015-7. Epub 2016 Jul 1. Erratum in: Lasers Med Sci. an;32(1):253.

22

Laser Therapy for the Working Dog

João C. Alves

Clinica Veterinária de Cães, Guarda Nacional Republicana, Lisbon, Portugal

Introduction

The evolution of dogs has occurred alongside human evolution, and dogs have historically been selected to perform multiple functions. They are employed worldwide in various task missions, serving as working, assistance, and therapy dogs. Even when considering only one of these fields, the employment range for dogs is quite wide. Considering working dogs alone, they are a part of many police and military forces worldwide, serving alongside their human counterparts in patrol, apprehension, search and rescue, product detection (including explosives, drugs, body fluids, poison, tobacco, guns, paper money, in ever-expanding possibilities), and others (McMichael & Singletary, 2021) (Figure 22.1).

Care for these special animals can be quite challenging as, independently of the specific task performed, working dogs must have adequate physical capability, mental aptitude, and proper cooperation with their handler. Only a balance between these factors will allow for adequate performance in challenging environmental conditions and situations (Hall *et al.*, 2021), which will ultimately translate into saved lives (McGraw & Thomas, 2021). There is increased interest worldwide in working dogs, recognizing their value and potential. Following this tendency, the field of working dogs' sports medicine will continue to grow in order to better care for these special animals, as working dogs should be considered and treated as performance athletes (Ramos *et al.*, 2021; Ridgway, 2021), and require a high standard of healthcare (Otto *et al.*, 2021).

As a part of this standard of care, photobiomodulation therapy (PBMT) plays a pivotal role as a solo treatment or as part of a treatment protocol, aiming to obtain better results and reduce recovery times. This chapter focuses on those specific uses.

Musculoskeletal Conditions

Working dogs are required to sprint, jump over obstacles, turn sharply, scale walls, overcome unstable surfaces, and bite, which adds physical and mental stress (Otto *et al.*, 2021). These activities may be required for short or very long periods in snow, desert, woods, or rubble (Toffoli & Rolfe, 2006; Zink & Schlehr, 2020) (Figure 22.2). As for sporting dogs, working dogs are at a higher risk of developing an orthopedic disease than companion dogs due to some breed predispositions and the increased stress related to the activities they are engaged in (Alves *et al.*, 2018). This may lead to injury, typically manifesting in musculoskeletal injury, altered mechanics, pain, and lameness (Hall *et al.*, 2021). Lameness is a common condition for early retirement in police working dogs. Depending on the report, lameness can add up to 69% of early retirement cases (Evans *et al.*, 2007; Worth *et al.*, 2013). Osteoarthritis (OA) (Alves *et al.*, 2020a,b) and degenerative lumbosacral disease (Alves *et al.*, 2018; Henderson, 2014) are the most commonly reported conditions in working dogs responsible for early retirement. They are also prone to developing cranial cruciate ligament injuries, tendinopathies, hyperextension lesions, and spinal trauma (McGraw & Thomas, 2021).

With musculoskeletal conditions having such a tool on working dogs' quality of life and work longevity, there is a need to detect early cases to improve early detection and disease prevention to maximize outcomes (Lafuente *et al.*, 2019). OA is a good example. In companion animals, it is diagnosed at a mean age of 8 years (Anderson *et al.*, 2018). In working dogs, OA is diagnosed at an earlier age of around 6 years (Alves *et al.*, 2020a,b). Still, a recent report looking at the prevalence of OA and associated clinical signs in young dogs (aged 8 months to 4 years old) found that 39.8% of animals had radiographic signs of OA in at

Laser Therapy in Veterinary Medicine: Photobiomodulation, Second Edition. Edited by Christopher J. Winkler and Lisa A. Miller.

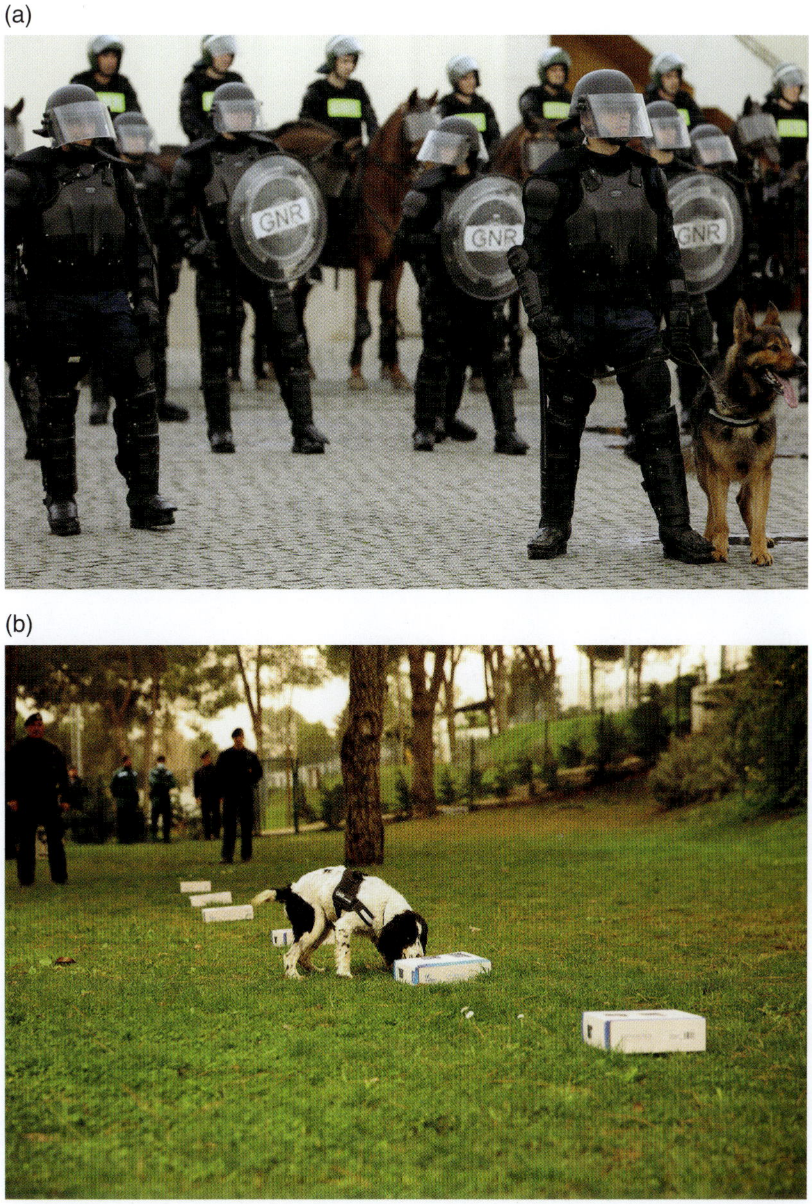

Figure 22.1 Example of two distinct tasks performed by working dogs – patrol (a) and product detection (b).

least one joint. Also, 23.6% of dogs had clinical signs of OA, corresponding to an overlap of radiographic OA and joint pain in the same joint (Enomoto *et al.*, 2022). This means that the actual prevalence of OA may be underrepresented in available reports. For that reason, a strong argument can be made for early treatment, particularly with treatment modalities aimed at changing disease progression that may have a regeneration effect (Alves *et al.*, 2021a,b). Available research shows that PBMT has a clinically significant improvement effect in working dogs with bilateral hip osteoarthritis, at a superior level than the nonsteroidal anti-inflammatory drug (NSAID) meloxicam.

In addition to providing greater pain control, a reduction in inflammation (as evaluated through infrared thermography), and an increased joint range of motion were also observed. The authors reported the use of 980 nm wavelength on hip osteoarthritis with a power of 6.5–8 W, an irradiance of 4.5–5.2 W/cm^2, and a fluence of 14.3–19.5 J/cm^2 over a 100 cm^2 area (Alves *et al.*, 2022a,b) (Figure 22.3). Despite having an effect by itself in the management of OA, PBMT is more commonly employed as a part of a multimodal approach. A recent study looked at the combined use of PBMT and platelet-rich plasma, compared to their isolated use, using the same parameters as above. The authors concluded that even though PBMT and platelet-rich plasma could improve objective outcomes and client-reported outcome measures in dogs with OA, their combined use leads to greater, longer-lasting, clinically significant improvements (Alves *et al.*, 2023).

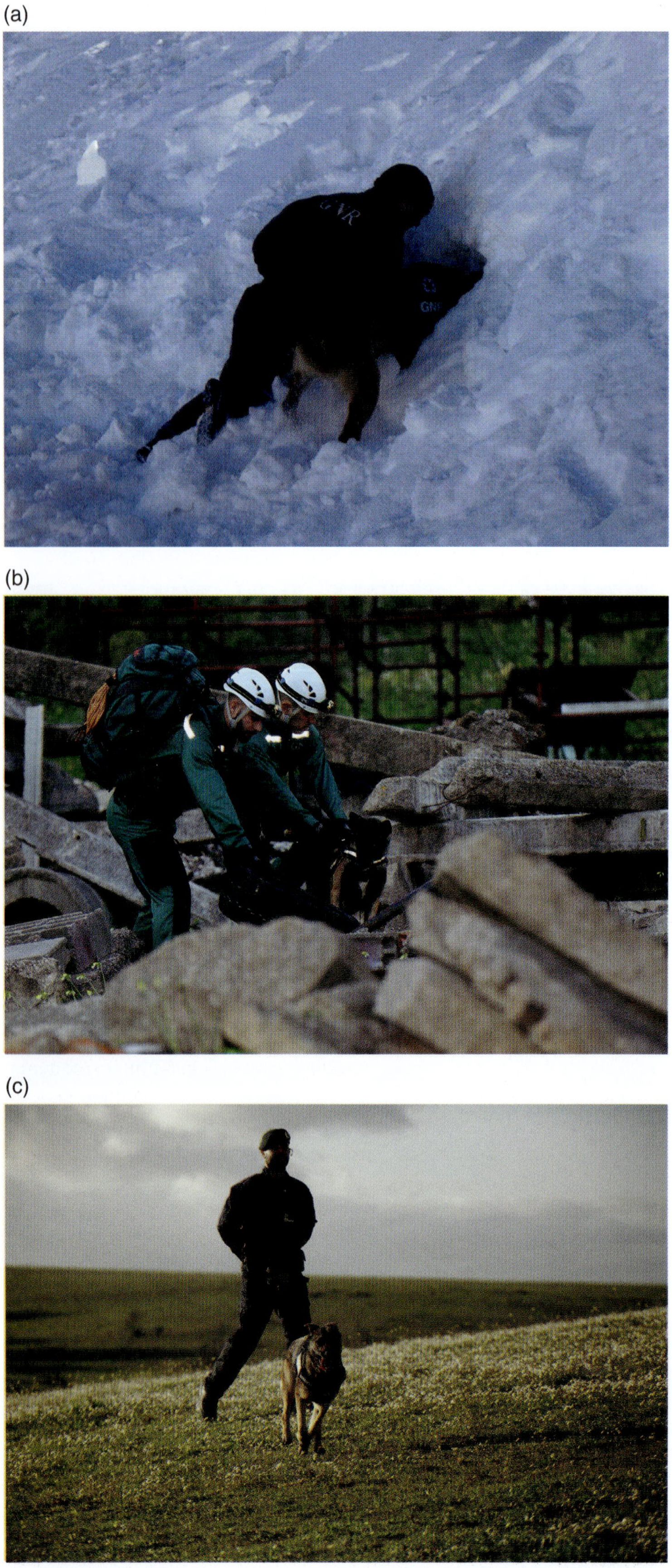

Figure 22.2 Even when performing the same task, a working dog can be called to work in distinct environments. Search and rescue dogs can be seen here working on (a) snow, (b) rubble, (c) and in an open field.

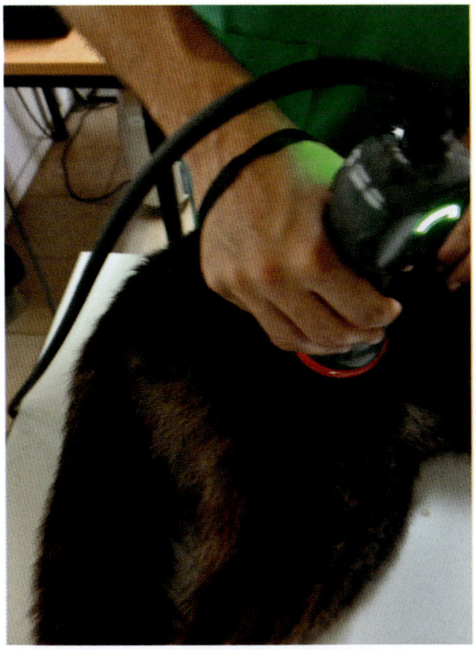

Figure 22.3 Photobiomodulation for the management of osteoarthritis is one of its common applications in working dogs.

It is also the author's experience that combining PBMT with other treatment modalities improves patient outcomes. For example, mesotherapy can effectively manage OA in dogs (Alves *et al.*, 2022a,b). Combining mesotherapy with PBMT increases the longevity of observed results.

Similar to joints, muscles are also subject to high demand in working dogs. Conditions affecting joints can either be primary or secondary to a different condition, such as due to a compensation mechanism. The treatment of muscle conditions is discussed in greater detail elsewhere in this book (please see Chapter 11). Still, one condition deserves a highlight in the present chapter, as it frequently affects working dogs. In working dogs, paraspinal soft tissue structures are under a great amount of repetitive stress, which leads to significant healing and remodeling, besides spondylosis deformans and facet joint osteoarthritis. These result in decreased spinal flexibility and range of motion, which leads to pain and stiffness and affects gait, posture, activity, and overall performance (Kinzel *et al.*, 2003; Kranenburg *et al.*, 2013; Steinberg & Coates, 2013). The PBMT protocols described for managing back pain are mainly related to intervertebral disk disease. In one study, an 810 nm wavelength, a power of 1 W, an irradiance of 5.5 W/cm^2, and a fluence of 329.7 J/cm^2 protocol has been described, using the affected spinal segment as a reference, and extended the treatment from one cranial to one caudal segment (Bennaim *et al.*, 2017). A second study reported different parameters, using 808 and 905 nm wavelengths, a power of 1.2–7.5 W, a fluence of 4 J/cm^2, and a total dose between 75.292 and 75.389 J (Bruno *et al.*, 2020).

In the author's experience, tendinopathies and conditions such as cranial cruciate ligament tears are not as common as OA and muscle conditions. This may be related to the nature of the work performed and the training environment, as the work performed can be of relatively low intensity but possibly for longer periods, and usually tends to be performed under controlled settings. The management of these conditions is discussed in greater detail in Chapter 11.

Gastrointestinal Conditions

Appropriate nutrition is paramount for a working dog. Feeding for optimal performance and health is quite demanding, as specific missions, work duration, environment, and individual needs can vary significantly (Zoran, 2021). Even when the best possible food is provided, many factors can influence a dog's ability to digest and absorb it adequately. Working and sporting dogs are at an increased risk of presenting with large bowel diarrhea due to the effects of prolonged exercise, their high drive, excitable (Simpson, 1998) and stressful nature (Leib, 2000), and competition events (McKenzie *et al.*, 2010). Many working dogs are identified as being nervous and excitable, and an association of the disease with some personality traits has been found (Simpson, 1998). The condition can be intermittent or persistent, with inflammatory enteropathies being the most common cause in dogs (Volkmann *et al.*, 2017). In working dogs, chronic large bowel disease is the most commonly diagnosed condition. Animals have a history of recurrent large-bowel diarrhea associated with increased fluidity, mucoid stools, and defecation frequency (Lecoindre & Gaschen, 2011). These dogs often present without other clinical findings, including negative fecal examination, no changes in blood counts and serum biochemistry, and a lack of histopathology abnormalities (Lecoindre & Gaschen, 2011). The underlying inflammation associated with chronic diarrhea can change the microbiome composition, affecting ingestion, nutrient extraction, and production of some metabolites (Redfern *et al.*, 2017; Whelan & Schneider, 2011). Different treatments have been described for this condition, but when dealing with working dogs, additional considerations exist. Many drugs are known to impact the dog's detection ability (Otto *et al.*, 2021), making their use undesirable. PBMT has been described as having a significant positive effect on disease progression in mice with induced colitis (Zigmond *et al.*, 2014). Besides having a possible effect on the underlying inflammation, PBMT can also stimulate analgesia and decrease other clinical signs such as flatulence, increasing patient comfort (Abreu Villela *et al.,* 2017; Anders *et al.,* 2017; Watson & Brundage, 2019; Zigmond *et al.,* 2014). In a study that evaluated the effectiveness of PBMT in reducing the clinical signs of chronic inflammatory large bowel diarrhea and frequency of diarrhea episodes in police working dogs, PBMT was compared to Psyllium husk. The authors reported using a 980 nm wavelength, with a power of 12 W, an irradiance of 2.4 W/cm^2, and a fluence of 8.6 J/cm^2 over a 500 cm^2 area (treating on-contact over the abdomen), for a total of 4320 J being delivered. A continuously moving grid pattern off-contact at a speed of 1–3 in./second was used. Patients treated with PBMT showed decreased diarrhea episodes frequency, increased body weight, and better body condition scores (Alves *et al.,* 2021a,b).

Oral Health

Proper oral health is a requisite for a working dog, as they will need to use their mouths to bite or play (Figure 22.4a and b).

Also, the oral cavity is juxtaposed with the nasal cavity, and oral disease can affect the animal's ability to perform as a detection dog (Juriga & Bilyard, 2021). Periodontal disease is a significant health problem in dogs; working dogs are no exception. It consists of the inflammation of the periodontium tissues (Bellows *et al.,* 2019; Harvey *et al.,* 2008; Reiter 2020) and progresses to the formation of plaque, followed by calculus accumulation and inflammation of the gingiva. Ultimately, it leads to tooth loss (Johnston *et al.,* 2011). The prevalence of periodontal disease varied according to reports, from 9.3% in England up to 80% in the United States and 90% in other regions (Marshall *et al.,* 2014; Niemiec & Stewart, 2020; Stella *et al.,* 2018), increasing with age (Harvey *et al.,* 1994). The treatment of canine gingivitis consists of professional dental prophylaxis (scaling and polishing) and tooth-brushing (Bonello & Squarzoni, 2008; Johnston *et al.,* 2011; Smith & Smithson, 2014). Even the dental prophylaxis procedure can influence inflammation due to the pressure applied to remove dental plaque and calculus from the teeth (Watson & Brundage, 2019). There is no ideal frequency of treatment, which is usually determined through signaling. There is a recommendation that working dogs should be assessed routinely twice a year (Otto *et al.,* 2021), and these moments can be used to evaluate the need for dental prophylaxis. Since gingivitis is the first stage of periodontal disease (Bellows *et al.,* 2019; Niemiec & Stewart, 2020), its control is paramount to maintaining good oral health. PBMT has been described in treating chronic gingivostomatitis and wound healing (Abreu Villela *et al.,* 2017; Arza, 2017; Wardlaw *et al.,* 2019), making it an interesting adjunct modality in dental prophylaxis. In a study to evaluate the effectiveness of PBMT in reducing gingivitis following professional dental prophylaxis in dogs, dental prophylaxis alone was compared to dental prophylaxis plus PBMT. The authors reported using a 980 nm wavelength, with a power of 3.5 W, an irradiance

(a) (b)

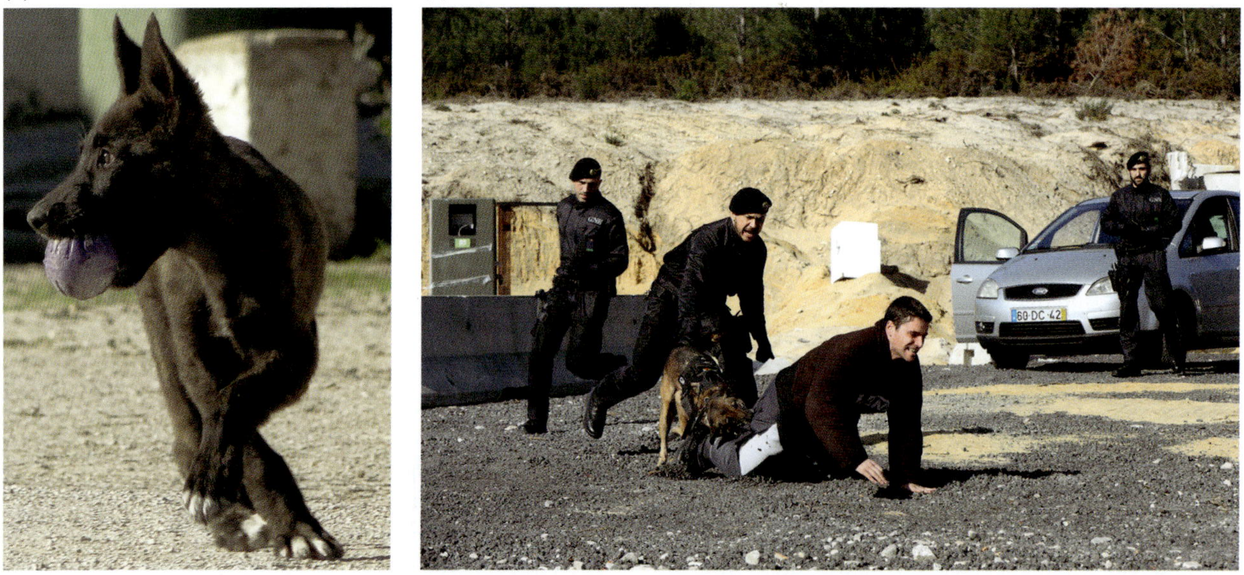

Figure 22.4 Good oral health is paramount for a working dog, from playing (a) to bite work (b). On the right (b), see also how musculoskeletal structures are challenged during work.

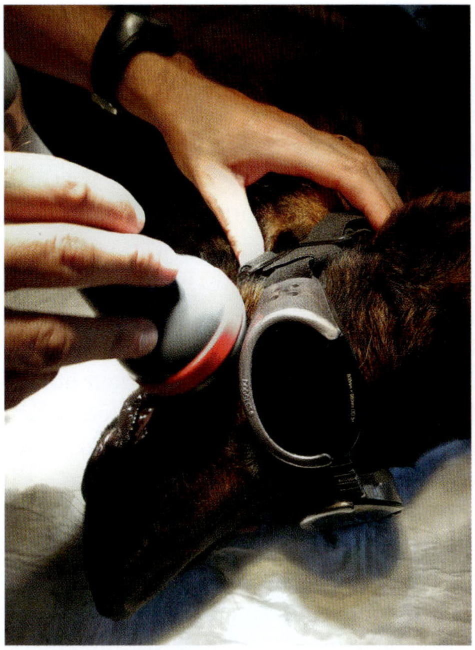

Figure 22.5 Photobiomodulation for the management of gingivitis following dental prophylaxis. Here the treatment is performed with the mouth closed.

of 2.3 W/cm^2, and a fluence of 6.2 J/cm^2 over a 35 cm^2 area, for a total of 217 J being delivered. In each patient, only one side received the combination of dental prophylaxis plus PBMT, while the other side was treated with dental prophylaxis alone. Overall, PBMT produced a significant decrease in grade of gingivitis and should be considered an adjuvant procedure following dental prophylaxis. While not evaluated, the authors also state that lower pain levels following the procedure could also be expected (Figure 22.5).

Other Conditions and Future Applications

Working dog sports medicine is a continuous process of optimizing performance, preventing injury, and mitigating performance-degradation factors (Ramos *et al.*, 2021; Ridgway, 2021). Working dogs also experience the same conditions as companion dogs, and situations must be addressed to achieve a fast and complete recovery, minimizing the time the dog is unavailable for service. One of the most common uses of PBMT to meet this goal is wound healing. It is not the goal of this chapter to discuss this topic in detail (more information can be found in Chapter 8). Another common use for PBMT is postsurgical recovery, with gastropexies being a relevant example. Many breeds used as working dogs are predisposed to gastric dilation and volvulus (GDV), making prophylactic gastropexy a common recommendation (McGraw & Thomas, 2021). In fact, some military forces perform prophylactic gastropexies for all their dogs, thus drastically reducing the number of dogs that die each year due to GDV (US Army Veterinary Services, 2019). In the author's experience, PBMT can be used immediately after surgery to increase patient comfort and decrease pain. One protocol includes 980 nm wavelength, with a power of 12 W, an irradiance of 2.4 W/cm^2, and a fluence of 8.6 J/cm^2 over a 500cm^2 area (treating on contact over the abdomen), for a total of 4320 J being delivered, with a continuously moving grid pattern off-contact at a speed of 1–3 in./second. While the impact on pain level is not as obvious, mostly due to using an effective multimodal analgesia protocol that leaves all dogs very comfortable, dogs treated with PBMT tend to start eating much sooner, a factor associated with a good prognosis, which may also reflect greater comfort.

Proper physical capacity is also paramount for working dogs to ensure success, longevity, and quality of life. The span for potential exercise-related applications for PBMT is enormous. However, little work has been done on dogs, and most available information is from human and animal model studies.

Research on muscle activity and recovery showed that a single PBMT treatment decreased delayed-onset muscle soreness, decreased creatine kinase activity, and enhanced maximal voluntary contraction, compared to placebo (Antonialli *et al.*, 2014). A different study, using 810 nm wavelength, a power of 200 mW applied in six sites on the quadriceps and delivering 50 J, had a remarkable effect on performance while reducing skeletal muscle's markers for damage and inflammation (Aver Vanin *et al.*, 2016).

Looking at aerobic capability, the effect of PBMT on high-level rugby players' performance and recovery was evaluated. Compared to placebo, PBMT improved average sprint time and reduced fatigue levels and blood lactate concentrations following exercise (Pinto *et al.*, 2016). PBMT can also increase muscle maximal isometric contraction while increasing the time to fatigue and improving recovery (de Oliveira *et al.*, 2017; Rossato *et al.*, 2018). Pre-exercise PBMT can also have positive effects. A study on high-level male soccer players evaluated the effect of pre-exercise PBMT to increase workout, speed up recovery, and attenuate oxidative stress, compared to a placebo. PBMT has several positive exercise-related effects, enhancing VO_2max, time to reach fatigue, exercise volume, and anaerobic and aerobic threshold appearance. At the same time, diminished CK and LDH activities were observed alongside lower pro-inflammatory activity (Tomazoni *et al.*, 2019). On the whole, positive effects of PBMT in physical activities and sports include protective and ergogenic effects, including but not restricted to a decrease in oxidative stress, muscle fatigue, blood lactate levels, and muscle injuries while increasing performance, muscle strength gain, speed of muscle adaptation, time to exhaustion, and recovery speed (Ailioaie & Litscher, 2021).

Studies in animals are scarcer and restricted to animal models. One study evaluated the effect of a 904 nm wavelength, a power of 15 mW, and a frequency of 700 Hz, delivering 1 J compared to a placebo in the progression of muscle dystrophy. The authors reported decreased morphological muscle changes, skeletal muscle damage, and inflammation (Leal-Junior *et al.*, 2014). In addition to working dogs, this finding may apply to managing sarcopenia in older animals. In a different study, an 808 nm wavelength, a power of 30 mW, and a density of 1071 W/cm^2 delivering 3 J over 100 s were evaluated in animals subjected to high-intensity forced exercise on an electric treadmill. Results showed that PBMT significantly reduced creatine kinase levels and oxidative stress compared to control (Silva *et al.*, 2015). When protecting muscle against damage and fatigue, 660 nm and 905 nm wavelengths delivering 1 to 10 J provided the best results (L. A. Santos *et al.*, 2014). Pre-exercise PBMT in animal models has also been conducted. The authors looked at different wavelengths (660, 830, and 905 nm) with a power of 50 mW and delivering doses of 1, 3, and 10 J. They observed an increase in cytochrome c oxidase expression and delayed onset of fatigue, in a dose- and wavelength-dependent manner, affecting muscle performance (Albuquerque-Pontes *et al.*, 2015). Based on currently available information from animal models, there is evidence to support the use of PBMT before and after exercise, having different effects, from improved performance in endurance training and aerobic metabolism while also showing a protective effect against muscle loss and a reduction in oxidative stress and inflammation (Ailioaie & Litscher 2021).

A growing field of interest is the promotion of welfare and well-being. Behavioral problems are the most common reason for the early release of working dogs, and they should be addressed from a very early age and with a comprehensive approach (Lazarowski *et al.*, 2021) to reduce stress and improve the quality of rest time and overall health. Stress can greatly impact a working dog's performance, and proper rest periods are essential for recovery and consolidation of the learning process (A. Santos *et al.*, 2015). Transcranial PBMT has been explored as a possible therapeutic route aiming at these exact goals. Several effects have been described with this approach justifying its use, including an increase in oxidized cytochrome-c-oxidase (CCO) and oxygenated hemoglobin, and a decrease in deoxygenated hemoglobin.

Interestingly, the effects on CCO were greater with increased age. Overall, PBMT alleviated age-related decline in mitochondrial respiration (Saucedo *et al.*, 2021). PBMT is also able to increase the mitochondrial respiratory chain, which in turn leads to ATP production, but also increases mitochondrial activity by promoting the dissociation of nitric oxide, restoring oxidative phosphorylation, and acting as a local vasodilator while increasing RNA and protein synthesis (Caldieraro & Cassano, 2019).

In human medicine and animal models, a growing number of possible PBMT applications have been described for behavioral and mood disorders, reporting promising results. An animal model study evaluating remote PBMT, directed at the abdomen or legs in mouse and non-human primate models of Parkinson's disease, concluded that PBMT parameters of 670 nm wavelength, an irradiance of 50 mW/cm^2 for 6 min/day covering the abdomen, was associated with a reduction of clinical signs and an increase in surviving midbrain dopaminergic cells compared to control. This effect was at least as pronounced as the one obtained with transcranial PBMT (Gordon *et al.*, 2023). In a human study looking at the effect of transcranial photobiomodulation in patients with generalized anxiety disorder, using an 830 nm wavelength, average irradiance of 30 mW/cm^2, a 36 J/cm^2 fluence, a power of 2.4 W, with 2.9 kJ being delivered per session, for 20 min over an 80 cm^2 area, the authors reported a decrease in different anxiety-related scores and an improvement in sleep quality associated with a lack of side effects. This effect could be of interest to working dogs, as many of the breeds commonly employed can be described as easily excitable or stressed, traits that also affect rest quality (Maiello *et al.*, 2019). Human reports on PBMT for traumatic brain injury, particularly for managing subsequent cognitive impairment and its impact on attention, motivation, and execution, show that PBMT can improve cognitive and emotional dimensions (Yao *et al.*, 2018). A different review on the application of transcranial PBMT for traumatic brain injury in an animal model also concluded that positive effects can be observed, but the results vary depending on the parameters used. Continuous wave appeared superior to pulsed wave. 660 and 880 nm wavelengths showed positive results when delivered from one to three times a day, leading to a neuroprotection effect, preventing the spread of brain cell death, linked to anti-inflammatory, anti-edema and proangiogenic effects (Huang *et al.*, 2012). As working dogs are also exposed to possible trauma episodes, this may certainly become a field for future applications of PBMT.

A recent review evaluated reports on the availability of evidence of effectiveness, useful parameters, and safety of PBMT in the management of four brain disorders: traumatic brain injury, stroke, Parkinson's, and Alzheimer's disease. Results of the review show mixed results in human studies, which the authors attribute to various outcome measures considered and PBMT parameters used. On the other hand, animal model studies seem to contribute to the standardization of PBMT parameters. Wavelengths varied from 610 to 950 nm, with an irradiance from 1.7–25 mW/cm^2 to 25–500 mW/cm^2, frequencies from 10–100 Hz, fluences from 1.2 to 60 J/cm^2, depending on the condition (Montazeri *et al.,* 2021). There are even reports on the effectiveness of PBMT in the management of different psychiatric diseases, such as bipolar disease (Mannu *et al.,* 2019).

A review of the potential application of PBMT in the management of canine cognitive dysfunction concluded that transcranial PBMT is a promising modality for patients exhibiting signs of cognitive decline. The available research still reports a variety of parameters, making an overall conclusion and recommendation of specific treatment parameters and protocols difficult (Dewey *et al.,* 2022). There are other conditions where PBMT can be helpful in working dogs. Working dogs with epilepsy can be challenging to manage, as the medication often prescribed can lead to what handlers and trainers describe as "sleepiness" or reduced levels of activity, leading to lower treatment compliance. Also, work anticipation or active work can lead to excitement, triggering further seizure episodes. In the author's experience, transcranial PBMT can reduce or even eliminate this reported "sleepiness" effect when using 810 and 980 nm wavelengths, a power of 5 W, for 3.5 min, with a frequency of 100 Hz, followed by the same treatment with a frequency of 10 Hz, for a total dose of 1050 J, over the entire cranium/calvarium and at the base of the skull and rostral portion of the neck, aiming toward the brainstem and spinal cord. For general well-being, a similar protocol can be used, with a power of 5 W and with a frequency of 100 Hz for 7 min, also aiming at the same anatomical areas. Treatment frequency usually starts at two to three treatments per week for 3–4 weeks. From this point, an adjustment can be made to meet individual needs.

Conclusion

Whatever the specific tasks they perform, caring for working dogs is challenging and demanding. Constant attention to the different dimensions of a well-balanced, fit, and happy working dog is paramount for success. There is ample information supporting the use of PBMT in caring for these dogs, addressing multiple areas of interest as applications of this therapy are constantly expanding. Still, much of our current knowledge is based on translational evidence-based medicine under a One Medicine/One Health approach. There is room and need for more research, on dogs as a whole and for working dogs in particular, in a promising field for future endeavors.

References

Abreu Villela, P. *et al.* (2017). Antimicrobial photodynamic therapy (aPDT) and photobiomodulation (PBM – 660 nm) in a dog with chronic gingivostomatitis. *Photodiagn Photodyn Ther.* 20:273–275. doi:10.1016/j.pdpdt.2017.10.012.

Ailioaie, L.M. and Litscher, G. (2021). Photobiomodulation and sports: results of a narrative review. *Life.* 11(12):1339. doi:10.3390/life11121339.

Albuquerque-Pontes, G.M. *et al.* (2015). Effect of pre-irradiation with different doses, wavelengths, and application intervals of low-level laser therapy on cytochrome c oxidase activity in intact skeletal muscle of rats. *Lasers Med Sci.* 30(1):59–66. doi:10.1007/s10103-014-1616-2.

Alves, J.C. *et al.* (2023). A preliminary report on the combined effect of intra-articular platelet-rich plasma injections and photobiomodulation in canine osteoarthritis. *Animals.* 13(20):3247. doi:10.3390/ani13203247.

Alves, J.C. *et al.* (2018). Evaluation of the effect of mesotherapy in the management of back pain in police working dogs. *Vet Anaesth Analg.* 45(1):123–128. doi:10.1016/j.vaa.2017.07.006.

Alves, J.C. *et al.* (2020a). Clinical and diagnostic imaging findings in police working dogs referred for hip osteoarthritis. *BMC Vet Res.* 16(1):425. doi:10.1186/s12917-020-02647-2.

Alves, J.C. *et al.* (2021a). The effect of photobiomodulation therapy on the management of chronic idiopathic large-bowel diarrhea in dogs. *Lasers Med Sci.* doi:10.1007/s10103-021-03469-w.

Alves, J.C. *et al.* (2021b). Platelet-rich plasma therapy in dogs with bilateral hip osteoarthritis. *BMC Vet Res.* 17(1):207. doi:10.1186/s12917-021-02913-x.

Alves, J.C. *et al.* (2022a). A randomized double-blinded controlled trial on the effects of photobiomodulation therapy in dogs with osteoarthritis. *Am J Vet Res.* 83(8). doi:10.2460/ajvr.22.03.0036.

Alves, J.C. *et al.* (2022b). A multiple-session mesotherapy protocol for the management of hip osteoarthritis in police working dogs. *Am J Vet Res*:1–8. doi:10.2460/ajvr.22.08.0132.

Alves, J.C. *et al.* (2020b). Clinical and diagnostic imaging findings in police working dogs referred for hip osteoarthritis. *BMC Vet Res.* 16(1):425. doi:10.1186/s12917-020-02647-2.

Anders, J. *et al.* (2017). Basic principles of photobiomodulation and its effects at the cellular, tissue, and system levels. In: *Laser Therapy in Veterinary Medicine: Photobiomodulation.* (eds. R.J. Riegel and J. Goldbold), pp. 36–52. Wiley Blackwell.

Anderson, K.L. *et al.* (2018). Prevalence, duration and risk factors for appendicular osteoarthritis in a UK dog population under primary veterinary care. *Sci Rep.* 8(1):5641. doi:10.1038/s41598-018-23940-z.

Antonialli, F.C. *et al.* (2014). Phototherapy in skeletal muscle performance and recovery after exercise: effect of combination of super-pulsed laser and light-emitting diodes. *Lasers Med Sci.* 29(6):1967–1976. doi:10.1007/s10103-014-1611-7.

Arza, R. (2017). Oral conditions. In: *Laser Therapy in Veterinary Medicine: Photobiomodulation.* (eds. R.J. Riegel and J.C. Godbold), 1 edn, pp. 161–168. John Wiley & Sons, Inc.

Aver Vanin, A. *et al.* (2016). Pre-exercise infrared low-level laser therapy (810 nm) in skeletal muscle performance and postexercise recovery in humans, what is the optimal dose? A randomized, double-blind, placebo-controlled clinical trial. *Photomed Laser Surg.* 34(10):473–482. doi:10.1089/pho.2015.3992.

Bellows, J. *et al.* (2019). 2019 AAHA dental care guidelines for dogs and cats∗. *J Am Anim Hospi Assoc.* 55(2):49–69. doi:10.5326/JAAHA-MS-6933.

Bennaim, M. *et al.* (2017). Preliminary evaluation of the effects of photobiomodulation therapy and physical rehabilitation on early postoperative recovery of dogs undergoing hemilaminectomy for treatment of thoracolumbar intervertebral disk disease. *Am J Vet Res.* 78(2):195–206. doi:10.2460/ajvr.78.2.195.

Bonello, D. and Squarzoni, P. (2008). Effect of a Mucoadhesive gel and dental scaling on gingivitis in dogs. *J Vet Dent.* 25(1):28–32. doi:10.1177/089875640802500108.

Bruno, E. *et al.* (2020). Perilesional photobiomodulation therapy and physical rehabilitation in post-operative recovery of dogs surgically treated for thoracolumbar disk extrusion. *BMC Vet Res.* 16(1):120. doi:10.1186/s12917-020-02333-3.

Caldieraro, M.A. and Cassano, P. (2019). Transcranial and systemic photobiomodulation for major depressive disorder: a systematic review of efficacy, tolerability and biological mechanisms. *J Affect Disord.* 243:262–273. doi:10.1016/j.jad.2018.09.048.

de Oliveira, A.R. *et al.* (2017). Pre-exercise infrared Photobiomodulation therapy (810 nm) in skeletal muscle performance and Postexercise recovery in humans: what is the optimal power output? *Photomed Laser Surg.* 35(11):595–603. doi:10.1089/pho.2017.4343.

Dewey, C. *et al.* (2022). Transcranial photobiomodulation (laser) therapy for cognitive impairment: a review of molecular mechanisms and potential application to canine cognitive dysfunction (CCD). *Open Vet J.* 12(2):256. doi:10.5455/OVJ.2022.v12.i2.14.

Enomoto, M., Castro, N., Hash, J., Nakanishi, A., Taylor, A., Snyder, A., Estrada, M., Ferris, K., Deresienski, D., Frey, E., Roe, S., Thompson, N., & Lascelles, B. D. (2022, April 1). Prevalence of radiographic osteoarthritis and associated clinical signs in young dogs. Poster presentation NC State College of Veterinary Medicine Research Forum (April 1, 2022).

Evans, R.I. *et al.* (2007). Causes for discharge of military working dogs from service: 268 cases (2000–2004). *J Am Vet Med Assoc.* 231(8):1215–1220. doi:10.2460/javma.231.8.1215.

Gordon, L.C. *et al.* (2023). Remote photobiomodulation targeted at the abdomen or legs provides effective neuroprotection against parkinsonian MPTP insult. *Eur J Neurosci.* 57(9):1611–1624. doi:10.1111/ejn.15973.

Hall, N.J. *et al.* (2021). Editorial: working dogs: form and function, volume II. *Front Vet Sci.* 8(July):8–11. doi:10.3389/fvets.2021.732304.

Harvey, C.E. *et al.* (2008). Scoring the full extent of periodontal disease in the dog: development of a Total mouth periodontal score (TMPS) system. *J Vet Dent.* 25(3):176–180. doi:10.1177/089875640802500303.

Harvey, C.E. *et al.* (1994). Association of age and Body Weight with periodontal disease in north American dogs. *J Vet Dent.* 11(3):94–105. doi:10.1177/089875649401100301.

Henderson, A.J. (2014). *Effect of a Core Conditioning Program on Lumbar Paraspinal Area, Asymmetry and Pain Score in Military Working Dogs with Lumbosacral Pain.* University of Tennessee.

Huang, Y. *et al.* (2012). Transcranial low level laser (light) therapy for traumatic brain injury. *J Biophotonics.* 5(11–12):827–837. doi:10.1002/jbio.201200077.

Johnston, T.P. *et al.* (2011). Canine periodontal disease control using a clindamycin hydrochloride gel. *J Vet Dent.* 28(4):224–229. doi:10.1177/089875641102800402.

Juriga, S. and Bilyard, K. (2021). Working Dog Dentistry. *Vet Clin N Am: Small Anim Pract.* 51(4):779–802. doi:10.1016/j.cvsm.2021.04.002.

Kinzel, S. *et al.* (2003). Diagnosis and treatment of arthrosis of cervical articular facet joints in Scottish deerhounds: 9 cases (1998–2002). *J Am Vet Med Assoc.* 223(9):1311–1315.

Kranenburg, H.C. *et al.* (2013). Spinal hyperostosis in humans and companion animals. *The Vet Quarter.* 33(1):30–42. doi:10.1080/01652176.2013.770181.

Lafuente, P. *et al.* (2019). Investigation into clients' perception of postoperative physiotherapy for dogs undergoing cranial cruciate ligament disease surgery. *Vet Rec.* 185(8):231–231. doi:10.1136/vr.105313.

Lazarowski, L. *et al.* (2021). Development and training for working dogs. *Vet Clin N Am: Small Anim Pract.* 51(4):921–931. doi:10.1016/j.cvsm.2021.04.009.

Leal-Junior, E.C.P. *et al.* (2014). Superpulsed low-level laser therapy protects skeletal muscle of mdx mice against damage, inflammation and morphological changes delaying dystrophy progression. *PLoS One.* 9(3):e89453. doi:10.1371/journal.pone.0089453.

Lecoindre, P. and Gaschen, F.P. (2011). Chronic idiopathic large bowel diarrhea in the dog. *Vet Clin N Am: Small Anim Pract.* 41(2):447–456. doi:10.1016/j.cvsm.2011.02.004.

Leib, M.S. (2000). Treatment of chronic idiopathic large-bowel diarrhea in dogs with a highly digestible diet and soluble Fiber. *J Vet Intern Med.* 14:27–32.

Maiello, M. *et al.* (2019). Transcranial Photobiomodulation with near-infrared light for generalized anxiety disorder: a pilot study. *Photobiomodulation Photomed Laser Surg.* 37(10):644–650. doi:10.1089/photob.2019.4677.

Mannu, P. *et al.* (2019). Transcranial photobiomodulation to augment Lithium in bipolar-I disorder. *Photobiomodulation Photomed Laser Surg.* 37(10):577–578. doi:10.1089/photob.2019.4674.

Marshall, M.D. *et al.* (2014). A longitudinal assessment of periodontal disease in 52 miniature schnauzers. *BMC Vet Res.* 10(1):166. doi:10.1186/1746-6148-10-166.

McGraw, A.L. and Thomas, T.M. (2021). Military working dogs: an overview of veterinary care of these formidable assets. *Vet Clin N Am: Small Anim Pract.* 51(4):933–944. doi:10.1016/j.cvsm.2021.04.010.

McKenzie, E. *et al.* (2010). Prevalence of diarrhea and enteropathogens in racing sled dogs. *J Vet Intern Med.* 24(1):97–103. doi:10.1111/j.1939-1676.2009.0418.x.

McMichael, M.A. and Singletary, M. (2021). The world of working dogs. *Vet Clin N Am: Small Anim Pract.* 51(4):xi–xii. doi:10.1016/j.cvsm.2021.04.016.

Montazeri, K. *et al.* (2021). Transcranial photobiomodulation in the management of brain disorders. *J Photochem Photobiol, B.* 221:112207. doi:10.1016/j.jphotobiol.2021.112207.

Niemiec, B.A. and Stewart, K. (2020). Current concepts in periodontal disease. *Today's Veterinary Practice.* (January/February):78–84.

Otto, C.M. *et al.* (2021). 2021 AAHA working, assistance, and therapy dog guidelines. *J Am Animl Hospi Assoc.* 57(6):253–277. doi:10.5326/JAAHA-MS-7250.

Pinto, H.D. *et al.* (2016). Photobiomodulation therapy improves performance and accelerates recovery of high-level rugby players in field test: a randomized, crossover, double-blind, placebo-controlled clinical study. *J Strength Cond Res.* 30(12):3329–3338. doi:10.1519/JSC.0000000000001439.

Ramos, M.T. *et al.* (2021). Sports medicine and rehabilitation in working dogs. *Vet Clin N Am: Small Anim Pract.* 51(4):859–876. doi:10.1016/j.cvsm.2021.04.005.

Redfern, A. *et al.* (2017). Role of the gastrointestinal microbiota in small animal health and disease. *Vet Rec.* 181 (14):370–370. doi:10.1136/vr.103826.

Reiter, A.M. (2020). Effects of diets, treats, and additives on periodontal disease. *Today's Veterinary Practice.* (January/February):23–26.

Ridgway, M. (2021). Preventive health care for working dogs. *Vet Clin N Am: Small Anim Pract.* 51(4):745–764. doi:10.1016/j.cvsm.2021.03.001.

Rossato, M. *et al.* (2018). Time response of photobiomodulation therapy on muscular fatigue in humans. *J Strength Cond Res.* 32(11):3285–3293. doi:10.1519/JSC.0000000000002339.

Santos, A. *et al.* (2015). Efeitos do enriquecimento ambiental e da coleira. *Vet Med*:30–36.

Santos, L.A. *et al.* (2014). Effects of pre-irradiation of low-level laser therapy with different doses and wavelengths in skeletal muscle performance, fatigue, and skeletal muscle damage induced by tetanic contractions in rats. *Lasers Med Sci.* 29(5):1617–1626. doi:10.1007/s10103-014-1560-1.

Saucedo, C.L. *et al.* (2021). Transcranial laser stimulation: mitochondrial and cerebrovascular effects in younger and older healthy adults. *Brain Stimul.* 14(2):440–449. doi:10.1016/j.brs.2021.02.011.

Silva, A.A. *et al.* (2015). Pre-exercise low-level laser therapy improves performance and levels of oxidative stress markers in mdx mice subjected to muscle fatigue by high-intensity exercise. *Lasers Med Sci.* 30(6):1719–1727. doi:10.1007/s10103-015-1777-7.

Simpson, J.W. (1998). Diet and large intestinal disease in dogs and cats. *J Nutrit.* 128(12):2717S–2722S. doi:10.1093/jn/128.12.2717S.

Smith, M.M. and Smithson, C.W. (2014). Dental wax decreases calculus accumulation in small dogs. *J Vet Dent.* 31(1):26–29. doi:10.1177/089875641403100103.

Steinberg, H. and Coates, J. (2013). Diagnosis of and treatment options for disorders of the spine. In: *Canine Sports Medicine and Rehabilitation*, 1 edn, pp. 311–337. John Wiley and Sons, Inc.

Stella, J.L. *et al.* (2018). A cross-sectional study to estimate prevalence of periodontal disease in a population of dogs (*Canis familiaris*) in commercial breeding facilities in Indiana and Illinois. *PLoS One.* 13(1):e0191395. doi:10.1371/journal.pone.0191395.

Toffoli, C.A. and Rolfe, D.S. (2006). Challenges to military working dog management and care in the Kuwait theater of operation. *Mil Med.* 171(10):1002–1005. doi:10.7205/MILMED.171.10.1002.

Tomazoni, S.S. *et al.* (2019). Infrared low-level laser therapy (Photobiomodulation therapy) before intense progressive running test of high-level soccer players: effects on functional, muscle damage, inflammatory, and oxidative stress markers—a randomized controlled trial. *Oxid Med Cell Longevity.* 2019:1–12. doi:10.1155/2019/6239058.

US Army Veterinary Services (2019). *Veterinary Care and Management of the Military Working Dog*: Vol. *TB MED 298.* U. S. Army.

Volkmann, M. *et al.* (2017). Chronic diarrhea in dogs – retrospective study in 136 cases. *J Vet Intern Med.* 31(4):1043–1055. doi:10.1111/jvim.14739.

Wardlaw, J.L. *et al.* (2019). Laser therapy for incision healing in 9 dogs. *Front Vet Sci.* 5. doi:10.3389/fvets.2018.00349.

Watson, A.H. and Brundage, C.M. (2019). Photobiomodulation as an inflammatory therapeutic following dental prophylaxis in canines. *Photobiomodulation Photomed Laser Surg.* 37(5):276–281. doi:10.1089/photob.2018.4614.

Whelan, K. and Schneider, S.M. (2011). Mechanisms, prevention, and management of diarrhea in enteral nutrition. *Curr Opin in Gastroenterol.* 27(2):152–159. doi:10.1097/MOG.0b013e32834353cb.

Worth, A. *et al.* (2013). Causes of loss or retirement from active duty for New Zealand police German shepherd dogs. *Anim Welfare.* 22(2):166–173. doi:10.7120/09627286.22.2.167.

Yao, X. *et al.* (2018). Transcranial near-infrared laser therapy in improving cognitive recovery of function following traumatic brain injury. *Curr Neuropharmacol.* 16(9):1320–1326. doi:10.2174/1570159X16666180321100439.

Zigmond, E. *et al.* (2014). Low-level light therapy induces mucosal healing in a murine model of dextran-sodium-sulfate induced colitis. *Photomed Laser Surg.* 32(8):450–457. doi:10.1089/pho.2013.3626.

Zink, C. and Schlehr, M.R. (2020). Working dog structure: evaluation and relationship to function. *Front Vet Sci.* 7(October):1–12. doi:10.3389/fvets.2020.559055.

Zoran, D.L. (2021). Nutrition of working dogs: feeding for optimal performance and health. *Vet Clin N Am: Small Anim Pract.* 51(4):803–819. doi:10.1016/j.cvsm.2021.04.014.

23

Laser Therapy in Postoperative and Injury Rehabilitation

Deborah Gross Torraca[1], *David Levine*[2,3], *and Matthew W. Brunke*[4]

[1] *Wizard of Paws Animal Rehabilitation for Animals, Colchester, CT, USA*
[2] *The University of Tennessee at Chattanooga, Chattanooga, TN, USA*
[3] *Veterinary Care and Specialty Group, Chattanooga, TN, USA*
[4] *Veterinary Referral Associates, Gaithersburg, MD, USA*

Introduction

Previous chapters have defined laser therapy principles, treatment regimens, and other dynamics. Before we can apply those concepts to injuries and postoperative rehabilitation, it is important to understand what can be treated with laser therapy.

In this chapter, we will focus on the musculoskeletal, neurological, and dermal systems. With insult (injury or recent pathology and necessary surgical intervention) to any of these systems, the veterinary practitioner must be cognizant of the phase of the injury (acute, subacute, chronic, or acute-on-chronic) and the phase of wound healing (inflammatory, reparative, remodeling, or maturation) of the tissue in question before planning treatment and rehabilitation. The effects of using laser therapy in injury rehabilitation are summarized in Box 23.1.

Box 23.1 The Effects of Using Laser Therapy in Injury Rehabilitation

Analgesia

Reduced pain in postoperative incisions

Decreased pain in meniscal tears

Reduced pain in arthritis

Dermatological Injuries

Wound healing	Capillary formation
Reduced tissue necrosis	Collagen formation
Increased angiogenesis	Vasodilation
Fibroblast stimulation	Lymphatic drainage

Musculoskeletal Injuries

Anti-inflammatory	Activation of osteogenic factors
Pain reduction in acute tendonitis	Improved cell proliferation and differentiation
Muscle recovery in athletes	Improved healing time
Promotion of oxygen uptake	Disruption of biofilm on implants
Promotion of exercise performance	Bactericidal effects
Faster return to function	Reduction of acute joint inflammation
Improved collagen organization	Improved tissue organization following cruciate ligament injury
Improved biomechanical properties	Inhibition of COX-2 enzyme and prostaglandins
Improved ligament healing	Fibrous healing of cartilaginous defects
Improved bone healing	

Neurological Injuries

Immunomodulation of brain damage	Increased axon numbers
Prevention of neuron death	Improved length of axonal regrowth
Better clinical outcome with cerebral ischemia	Improved motor function in peripheral nerve injury
Faster motor evolution following spinal cord injury	Regrowth of muscle fiber in brachial plexus injuries
Maintenance of the urinary system	Increased myelinization
Preservation of neural tissue	

Laser Therapy in Veterinary Medicine: Photobiomodulation, Second Edition. Edited by Christopher J. Winkler and Lisa A. Miller.

Wound Healing

Dermal System

Dermatological injuries can be associated with some of the causes of injuries to other parts of the body. Oftentimes, a crushing injury can affect multiple organ systems. Once the patient is properly stabilized, there is a need to address pain and inflammation from trauma to the skin, muscles, peripheral nerves, and spinal cord. Alternatively, dermal injuries can occur separately from other organ systems.

The dermal system benefits the most from the effects of photobiomodulation therapy (PBMT) to increase the speed of healing and the host response to bacteria and viruses. Examples of dermal injuries that can be independent of the musculoskeletal or neurological system include papillomas, lick granulomas, bacterial dermatitis, decubital ulcers, pressure sores, pododermatitis, nail and pad injuries, and otitis externa. Lacerations may be dermal only or may include muscle or nerve tissue. Patients that have been burned by chemicals or fire may have extensive injury to their skin. Patients with diabetes mellitus and hyperadrenocorticism may have delayed wound-healing potential and are prone to bacterial dermatitis. Cancer patients undergoing either chemotherapy or radiation are also at risk for dermatological injuries.

The inflammatory (lag) phase of dermatologic wound healing lasts approximately 5 days. It is characterized by increased vascular permeability, chemotaxis of circulatory cells, release of cytokines and growth factors, and cell activation.

The debridement phase is dominated by white blood cell action, recruitment of mesenchymal cells, stimulation of angiogenesis, and moderate matrix production in wounds, after preventing infection and debriding the area using phagocytosis. This phase can last another 4–5 days.

The repair phase usually begins 3–5 days after injury. Macrophages stimulate DNA and fibroblast production and collagen synthesis. The amount of collagen reaches a maximum within 2–3 weeks after injury. As collagen increases, the number of fibroblasts and the rate of collagen synthesis decrease; this marks the end of the repair stage.

Depending on the nature of the wound, the fibroblastic phase of healing lasts 2–4 weeks. Careful management of wounds during this time will avoid inappropriate epithelialization and poor wound healing.

The maturation phase begins once collagen has been adequately deposited in the wounds, 17–20 days after injury, and may continue for several years. Collagen fibers remodel with alteration of their orientation and increased cross-linking, which improves wound strength (Hedlund, 2002).

Patients with compromised wound-healing abilities (e.g., obesity, diabetes mellitus, malnourishment, hepatic disease, or hyperadrenocorticism) benefit from laser therapy in the early phases of wound healing, which helps minimize the risks, delays, or failures of the healing process (de Loura *et al.*, 2016). Additionally, those patients on corticosteroids, chemotherapeutic agents, or radiation therapy can have delayed wound healing. If the wound is over a neoplastic site, consultation with a veterinary oncologist is recommended prior to initiating laser therapy, to ensure that it will not promote proliferation of the neoplasia (Bensadoun & Nair, 2015).

Musculoskeletal System

The musculoskeletal system includes all bones, ligaments, tendons, cartilaginous joints, and muscles of the body. The potential for injury to these structures includes fractured bones and strained, sprained, or completely ruptured ligaments and tendons. Further, the muscle bodies themselves can be inflamed from trauma or infection. Even with optimal surgical technique, there is disruption of tissues. Autoimmune diseases can affect the joints or muscles and cause inflammation and pain. Articular cartilage injury can lead to osteoarthritis. Laser therapy can be beneficial at the time of injury, in preparation for surgical intervention, during postoperative pain management, and during rehabilitation.

Trauma (acute or chronic) to both the appendicular and the axial skeleton can lead to injury of the associated muscles, tendons, ligaments, bones, and cartilage. A working knowledge of normal anatomy and physiology is essential to understanding what is abnormal for a particular patient. A full physical examination, paying particular attention to the orthopedic and neurologic exam, should be completed prior to initiation of laser therapy for any injury.

Injuries to muscle occur as a result of ruptures, ischemia, strains, laceration, and contusions. A strain is described as any injury to a muscle and tendon unit. Strains have a tendency to occur near the myotendinous junction. They are described as grades I–IV, with grade I strains being disruption of a few muscle fibers and grade IV being complete rupture of the muscle belly. Damage to muscle includes tearing of the fibers and disruption of vascular and connective tissue support. Severity can range from mild injury to complete rupture. Complete rupture necessitates surgical correction. Lesser injuries can take 4–6 weeks to heal, during which time the patient should have protected activity (Williams, 2004).

Injuries to tendons can occur from similar causes as their companion muscles. A similar strain grading system is used. The goal of treatment is to minimize adhesion formation and return to full function. As with muscles, complete tendon rupture requires surgical stabilization and repair prior to rehabilitation. The size, location, and stress load on a particular tendon will dictate tensile strength and speed of return to function. Full healing is normally achieved in 6–10 weeks (Williams, 2004).

Ligamentous injuries can take up to 12 months to completely remodel and to complete the maturation phase of wound healing. At that point, ligament strength will only be 50–70% of the original tensile strength (Frank *et al.*, 1991). Factors that are important for ligament healing include apposition, nutritional status, endocrine imbalance, and severity of injury. Proper blood supply and load-bearing stress are also important. Complete tears will benefit from surgery first, then rehabilitation.

Cartilage healing is directly related to the type of trauma that caused the injury. Articular cartilage is avascular in nature, and this can be a limiting factor for repair. Partial-thickness injuries are dependent on the cartilage matrix for wound healing. Full-thickness injuries to the level of the subchondral bone can benefit from the available vascular supply in the bone. Cartilage healing can take 2–6 months, but often results in arthritis due to the poor repair potential of the tissue itself (Williams, 2004).

Bone is dynamic tissue composed of 35% organic and 65% mineral components. This complex nature dictates a prolonged healing time compared to soft tissues. Many factors can affect bone healing. Stress at the fracture site can cause micro-motion, which can disrupt tissue healing. Surgical stabilization is thus often indicated. The application of a splint or cast can be beneficial but does not allow for laser application unless a window is made in the material or the material is removed. Removal for laser therapy requires patient sedation to prevent the risk of motion and disruption of the healing bone.

Healing time will be dependent on fracture location, degree of trauma, and numerous other factors. A full return to normal lamellar bone structure accommodating normal weight-bearing forces can take 4 months or longer. Disturbances in bone healing can result in delayed unions, nonunions, and slowed healing (Williams, 2004).

In the postoperative period, care must be focused on a working knowledge of the surgery performed and awareness of the type of any implant(s). This is critical with laser therapy to prevent inadvertent heating of the implants, which can lead to postoperative complications (for more information, see Chapter 5).

All tissues of the musculoskeletal system will react differently to disuse and remobilization. After prolonged disuse, most tissues will atrophy and have decreased rates of new cell formation. The loss of tissue strength from atrophy can lead to further injury. Quick return to use and function through rehabilitation is almost always recommended.

Neurological System

Injuries to particular areas can result in injuries to the neurological system. The brain, spinal cord, and peripheral nerves can have different insulting injuries and different healing potentials.

The brain can be injured by trauma, infection, vascular events, inflammations, toxins, congenital defects, degenerative conditions, and neoplasia (Fenner, 2000). Laser therapy is normally not indicated for cancer, so proper diagnostic testing is essential before initiation of treatment. Additionally, the brain can be difficult to treat with laser therapy, since it is contained within the calvarium, though research is being done in this area with potentially promising results. Data indicate that photons can penetrate human cadaver skulls to a depth of 4 cm (Tedford *et al.*, 2015).

Causes of injuries to the spinal cord include those affecting the brain and herniated intervertebral disks. Common conditions affecting the spinal cord include trauma, intervertebral disk disease (IVDD), fibrocartilaginous emboli (FCE), vascular events, cervical spondylomyelopathy (Wobbler's disease), lumbosacral stenosis, discospondylitis, spondylosis deformans, syringomyelia, degenerative myelopathy, and trauma such as a spinal fracture and those resulting from being hit by a car. Trauma, IVDD, and FCE can have acute onset, where the spinal cord may have better healing potential than from more chronic conditions (e.g., lumbosacral stenosis, spondylosis deformans, and degenerative myelopathy). Proper diagnosis will aid in determining the prognosis and course of treatment (LeCouteur & Grandy, 2000).

Three basic categories of change occur after acute injury to the spinal cord: first, direct morphologic distortion of neuronal tissue, then vascular change, and finally biochemical and metabolic changes. Controversy exists regarding the relative importance of these closely related categories in the production of functional deficits.

Direct morphologic damage of the spinal cord (laceration, stretching, or compression) resulting in axonal interruption is thought to be irreversible and untreatable because central axons do not regenerate sufficiently to restore function. There may be some change in this theory with the advent of stem-cell and platelet-rich plasma therapy in both humans and animal models.

In the case of reversible spinal cord injury, a characteristic series of events occurs during the repair process. A heterogeneous population of small cells, including lymphocytes, macrophages, and plasma cells, invades the traumatized tissue 2 days after injury. This mimics the inflammatory phase, as shown in other organs. Within 7–20 days, fibroblasts appear and begin laying down scar tissue. A concurrent glial reaction consisting of astrocyte proliferation and expansion of axonal processes occurs. Depending on the extent of spinal cord injury, moderate to extensive fibrosis, nerve fiber degeneration, and multifocal malacia may be seen (Seim, 2002a).

Axons that have been severed, compressed, or stretched start to regrow, but growth will reach the edges of the scar mass and stop. Regeneration of spinal cord axons sufficient to restore function has not been achieved; however, if enough axons remain intact, return to clinically acceptable motor function may be expected.

The peripheral nervous system includes cranial nerves III–XII, the spinal nerves with their roots, peripheral nerves, and the peripheral components of the autonomic nervous system. These relay information to the central nervous system (CNS) and provide control of peripheral structures. They comprise the sole neural structure that controls skeletal muscle and are therefore essential for ambulation. A variety of diseases can affect this system, including congenital malformation, genetic diseases, metabolic conditions (diabetes mellitus, hypothyroidism), toxicities (botulism, tick paralysis), autoimmune and inflammatory diseases (acute polyradiculoneuritis, myasthenia gravis), neoplasia, trauma (brachial plexus avulsion), and vascular conditions (feline aortic thromboembolism) (Inzana, 2000).

Traumatic peripheral nerve injuries can be classified according to the degree of damage present. Class 1 is referred to as neurapraxia and includes mild or moderate focal compression. With class 2 injuries, complete recovery can occur within hours, or up to 6 weeks. Class 2 injury (axonotmesis) occurs with crushing injuries. The axons are interrupted, but the supporting connective tissue is intact and regeneration is usually effective. Axonal regeneration occurs at 1–2 mm/day, so the length of the injury will dictate the potential healing time. Classes 3–5 are varying degrees of neurotmesis. In Class 3 injuries, there is damage to the axons and endoneurium, but the perineurium is intact. Class 4 is similar but includes disruption of the perineurium. Class 5 is complete severing of the nerve (Inzana, 2000).

A peripheral nerve sustaining neurapraxia develops transient physiological dysfunction without anatomic disruption of the axons. The nerve regains normal function within 3 months, and regeneration occurs at 3 cm/month (1 mm/day). Peripheral nerves sustaining axonotmesis or neurotmesis will undergo immediate degeneration at the site of injury. This degeneration extends toward the cell body over a distance of two to three nodes of Ranvier, and regeneration begins from that site. Nerve processes distal to the injury degenerate completely (Wallerian degeneration), and after 1 week a connective-tissue framework called the "neurilemmal sheath" remains. Within 2 days, "sprouting" of the proximal end of the severed axon occurs.

Neuron regeneration and return of function depend on several factors. If continuity of the nerve is maintained (axonotmesis), the distance from the injury site to the end organ becomes the most important variable. Little function will be achieved if the distance is more than 30 cm. The best chance for functional regeneration is a distance of less than 10 cm. If anatomic nerve continuity is not maintained (neurotmesis), recovery depends on the distance from the injury to the end organ, the wounding mechanism, the time between injury and surgical repair, the patient's age and condition, and the surgical technique. The earlier a nerve is repaired, the better the chances of healing. Clean, sharp lacerations generally heal better than avulsion, crush, open, or chronic injuries (Seim, 2002b).

Proper diagnosis of injuries, involving consult with a veterinary neurologist and potentially an electromyography or advanced imaging techniques (or both) is important. Additionally, it is important to recognize that multiple types and classes of injury can occur along the same nerve.

How and Why Does Laser Therapy Work?

Studies of the successful use of laser therapy in promoting tissue repair and pain reduction are well established (Enwemeka *et al.,* 2004). Laser therapy is relatively new to our field of rehabilitation, and more studies are needed to evaluate and interpret its impact on our current treatment guidelines. Many have been done using *in vitro* models. While these are useful for establishing the fundamentals of laser treatment, they are rarely applicable in practice. As we continue to learn how to apply laser therapy in rehabilitation, it is essential that we pay proper attention to individual patient needs and responses to treatment. Precise medical records should include documentation of the areas treated, laser settings and parameters dates, and responses. Despite a lack of species-specific clinical studies, the foundation for the use of laser therapy in veterinary rehabilitation is established (Pryor and Millis, 2015).

Laser therapy works at a cellular level to activate cytokines and other mediators along various cascades in the tissue. Chromophores within the mitochondria and at the cell membrane absorb the photons. Oxygen and adenosine triphosphate (ATP) production can be enhanced. ATP may also act as a signaling molecule to enhance cell-to-cell communication (Karu, 2010). ATP may bind with a cell receptor to allow sodium and calcium to enter, resulting in cascades of intracellular activities. This increased intracellular calcium increases mitochondrial function. ATP is also thought to be a neurotransmitter, and this may explain some of the effects of laser therapy in pain management (Baxter & McDonough, 2007).

Laser therapy stimulates collagen synthesis (Abergel *et al.*, 1984), fibroblast development (Pourreau-Schneider *et al.*, 1990), and angiogenesis, allowing for repair of injured tissues (Corazza *et al.*, 2007). Additional studies have shown that laser therapy can lead to increased tensile strength (Vasilenko *et al.*, 2010) and faster closure of wounds (Hopkins *et al.*, 2004).

These cascades can enhance cellular growth and metabolism, and lasers therefore have the potential to accelerate tissue healing and cell growth in ligaments, tendons, skin, and muscles. Caution must be used, as excessively high doses of laser light may inhibit responses such as tissue healing (Huang *et al.*, 2009). Laser therapy has anti-inflammatory effects. Studies have indicated that inflammation can be reduced by using laser therapy to decrease prostaglandin E2 (PGE2) and cyclooxygenase 2 (COX-2) concentration (Honmura *et al.*, 1993; Sakarai *et al.*, 2000). This gives laser therapy the same potential treatment pathway as steroids and nonsteroidal anti-inflammatory drugs (NSAIDs). For those patients that cannot take these systemic medications, and for owners looking for alternative treatment, laser therapy has proven to be beneficial.

Reduction in inflammation and pain in both acute and chronic conditions will increase the patient's quality of life. By improving analgesia, laser therapy can be preemptive in the prevention or minimization of chronic pain or wind-up, and it can help reduce dependence on medications. If medications can be avoided, there is a benefit for the patient as a whole.

Evidence for Laser Therapy in Rehabilitation

Rehabilitation does not focus on one specific problem, but rather sees the patient as a whole and applies a multimodal approach. One of the main goals of rehabilitation is a return to normal or near-normal function (Millis & Ciuperca, 2015). The benefits of laser therapy for rehabilitation patients are focused in two main areas: the increase in healing times through faster, stronger tissue repair and the analgesic effect of the laser. These combine to allow the patient as a whole to feel better and to exercise efficiently (when indicated), gain strength, and return to function with an improved quality of life. Historically the research has focused on specific injuries, and we will review that first. Where possible, specific evidence for postoperative laser use will also be reviewed.

Tendon and Ligament Conditions

Most of the research on the effects of laser therapy on tendon and ligament conditions has been done either in experimental models in laboratory animals such as rats or in people. More evidence from studies in dogs, cats, and other animals is needed. Historically, laser therapy has been recommended for tendon and ligament conditions, but its clinical efficacy remained controversial. Recent research proves that laser therapy is appropriate for these types of injury (Tumilty & Baxter, 2015; Da Ré Guerra *et al.*, 2016).

A meta-analysis evaluated the use of laser in tendinopathies in people (Tumilty *et al.*, 2010). The 25 studies reviewed had conflicting results, half being inconclusive or demonstrating no effect and the other half showing a positive effect. Positive versus negative effects appear to be related to the dose applied. Those studies with positive results used doses similar to those recommended by the World Association for Laser Therapy (WALT): 1–8 J/cm^2 and $< 100\ mW/cm^2$ for superficial tendons and 3–9 J/cm^2 and 600 mW/cm^2 for deep tendons.

One study looked at seven people with bilateral Achilles tendinitis to see whether laser therapy has an anti-inflammatory effect (Bjordal *et al.*, 2006). In those treated with laser therapy the PGE2 levels were reduced for 75–105 minutes after laser therapy, and pain pressure threshold values increased. The authors concluded that laser therapy reduces pain and inflammation in people with acute Achilles tendinitis.

Another Achilles tendon study (de Jesus *et al.*, 2015) showed that laser therapy decreased Achilles tendon inflammation. The study evaluated interleukin 1 beta (IL1ß), COX-2, and PGE2 modulation in partially injured Achilles tendons of rats. The rats had a direct injury to the Achilles tendon and were placed in one of seven groups (negative control, three sham groups, and three treatment groups). The treatment groups received one, three, or seven treatments. A 780 nm laser was applied for 10 seconds once per day. The tendons were then surgically removed and assessed immunohistochemically for IL1ß, COX-2, and PGE2. In the group treated three times, all three inflammatory mediators were near-normal level. COX-2 and PGE2 were also near-normal in the group that had seven treatments.

A randomized blinded study looked at 74 people treated with laser therapy for tendinitis, along with 68 placebo patients (Lögdberg-Andersson *et al.*, 1997). Over 3–4 weeks, all patients received three to four treatments. Pain was measured using a pain threshold meter and a visual analog scale (VAS). Pain was measured prior to and at the end of treatment, and again 4 weeks later. Laser therapy had a positive effect on acute tendinitis throughout the study.

Laser therapy may also be of benefit to muscle recovery (Carvalho *et al.*, 2015). Assis *et al.* (2015) evaluated the effects of laser therapy on the biochemical markers and morphology of skeletal muscle in rats when applied after an endurance training protocol. They had a control group, a trained group, and a trained-and-laser-therapy group. The rats were walked on a treadmill for 1 hour per day, 5 days per week for 8 weeks, at 60% of maximal speed reached during a maximal-effort test. The trained-and-laser-therapy group showed significantly reduced lactate levels, increased tibialis anterior fiber cross-section area, and decreased fiber density. Myogenin expression was higher in both trained groups. Laser therapy produced myogenin down-regulation as well. This suggests that laser therapy could be an effective therapeutic approach for stimulating recovery in athletes.

Another treadmill study using rats showed that laser therapy promotes an increase in maximal oxygen uptake and exercise performance in a dose-dependent manner (Perini *et al.*, 2015). Laser therapy was applied in the treated (versus placebo) rats bilaterally to the biceps femoris, gluteus, lateral and medial gastrocnemius, iliopsoas, and adductor longus muscles once a day for 10 days. All animals performed the maximal-exercise test on a metabolic treadmill, with simultaneous gas analysis. The higher-dose (61.2 J/cm^2) laser therapy group showed increased VO_2 basal, VO_2 max, and VO_2 max levels and covered a longer distance compared to the other groups.

Conforti & Fachinetti (2013) showed that laser therapy is an effective treatment in humans with whiplash injury as compared to conventional simple segmental physical rehabilitation. They showed a reduction in VAS pain scores and a quicker recovery and return to work in the laser-treated group versus the non-laser-treated group.

Ligament healing may also benefit from laser therapy. Single-dose laser therapy has been shown to improve the healing of medial collateral ligaments in a rat model (Fung *et al.*, 2002). An earlier study demonstrated no improvement when patients were treated with suboptimal parameters (De Bie *et al.*, 1998). In a more recent animal-model study using rats, laser therapy was effective for the early improvement of the ultimate tensile strength of medial collateral ligament injuries (Bayat *et al.*, 2005). Further species-specific studies are warranted, and correct dose and treatment parameters are obviously important for successful results.

In human studies, laser therapy has been applied either before or during exercise to create an ergogenic effect and delay muscle fatigue (Borsa *et al.*, 2019, Crow *et al.*, 2023). In a triple-blind, repeated measures, placebo-controlled cross-over design, Borsa *et al.* (2019) applied laser therapy (10 J/cm^2) between bouts of isokinetic quadriceps exercise and found that subjects produced significantly more torque, total work output, and average power output during the active phototherapy condition compared to the sham phototherapy condition. In a recent human study (Crow *et al.*, 2023), laser therapy was found to be more effective than placebo for attenuating muscle fatigue of the external rotator muscle group of the shoulder in high-intensity and high-volume resistance exercise. In this case, laser therapy was utilized prior to a strenuous workout and between sets of exercise. While further studies are warranted, this could be a starting point to utilize laser therapy in a similar fashion for veterinary rehabilitation.

Bone and Cartilage Conditions

Bone and cartilage may also be affected by laser therapy. The focus within bone should be on healing following fracture and as an adjunct treatment for osteomyelitis.

Tim *et al.* (2014) looked at the effects of laser therapy on bone formation, immunoexpression of osteogenic factors, and biomechanical properties in a tibial bone defect model in rats. A total of 60 rats were distributed into a bone-defect control group and a laser-irradiated group. Rats were euthanized on days 15, 30, and 45 post-injury. Histological and morphometric analysis showed that the treated animals presented no inflammatory infiltrate and a better tissue organization at 15 and 30 days postsurgery. In addition, a higher amount of newly formed bone was observed at 15 days postsurgery. While this is a good reason to use laser therapy, the study also showed no statistically significant difference in COX-2 immunoexpression among the groups at 15, 30, and 45 days. Runt-related transcription factor 2 (RUNX2) was statistically higher in the treated group at 45 days. Bone morphogenetic protein (BMP-9) immunoexpression was higher in the treated group at day 30. However, there was no expressivity for this immunomarker in either group at 45 days. No statistically significant difference among the groups was observed in the maximal load at any time. This shows that laser therapy improved bone healing by accelerating the development of newly formed bone and activating osteogenic factors but did not improve the biomechanical properties of the bone.

Another study (Barbosa *et al.*, 2014) looked at 45 rats subjected to transverse osteotomy of the right femur and divided randomly into three experimental groups. One group did not receive laser therapy; one received therapy with a 660 nm laser; and one received therapy with an 830 nm laser. Animals were sacrificed after 7, 14, and 21 days. The bone calluses were evaluated by digital x-ray and submitted to variance analysis followed by the Tukey–Kramer test. The two laser-treated groups showed significant bone development at days 7 and 14. On day 21, a higher degree of bone repair was seen in the 830 nm group.

A 940 nm laser was used in an *in vitro* study on osteogenesis by Jawad *et al.* (2013). A human fetal osteoblast cell line was cultured and treated with laser therapy, and an assay was used to determine cell proliferation. Alkaline phosphatase and osteocalcin activity assays were used for cell differentiation. All treatment groups showed a significant increase in cell proliferation and differentiation compared to the control group.

A human *in vivo* study studied laser therapy on wrist and hand fractures and found positive results (Chang *et al.*, 2014). It evaluated the therapeutic outcomes of administering 830 nm laser therapy to closed bone fractures of 50 patients who had not had surgery. A control group was used, and the laser-treated group was treated five times per week for 2 weeks. The pain, functional disability, grip strength, and radiographic parameters of the participants were evaluated before and after treatment, and at a 2-week follow-up. The laser therapy group exhibited significant changes in all of the parameters compared with baseline. The results compared the two groups after treatment and at follow-up and indicated significant differences between them. The study concluded that laser therapy relieves pain and improves the healing process in these fractures.

Laser therapy has also been studied as a treatment for infections of the musculoskeletal system. Bacteria that surround medical devices, such as orthopedic implants, can create a bacterial coating (biofilm) that prevents penetration of antibiotics. Kizhner *et al.* (2011) used laser light to disrupt this biofilm and allow conventional treatment to reach the bacteria.

Kaya *et al.* (2011) examined rats with induced, chronic methicillin-resistant *Staphylococcus aureus* (MRSA) osteomyelitis of the tibia. The rats had either surgical debridement, surgical debridement with laser therapy, or no treatment. Treatment with an 808 nm laser for either 60, 120, or 180 seconds daily for five consecutive days decreased infection levels. The 180-second group had 93% less infection than the negative control, while the debridement-alone group had only 37% less. This study makes a good case for using laser therapy as an adjunct for osteomyelitis.

A recent review of 25 articles (13 *in vitro* and 12 animal studies) evaluated the influence of laser therapy on bone healing (Ebrahimi *et al.*, 2012). All animal studies showed improved bone healing in sites irradiated with laser. It was concluded that laser therapy could accelerate bone healing in extraction sites, bone fracture defects, and distraction osteogenesis.

While the majority of the benefits of laser therapy for cartilage involve arthritis, there is evidence for the use of laser therapy in nonarthritic cases.

Dos Santos *et al.* (2014) compared the effect of two laser therapy doses on the expression of inflammatory mediators on neutrophils and macrophages in acute joint inflammation. The synovial tissue of patients with initial osteoarthritis is characterized by mononuclear cell infiltration and the production of pre-inflammatory cytokines. In this study, rats were divided into a negative-control, an inflammatory injury positive-control, and two laser-treated groups (one at 2 J and one at 4 J), after being subjected to injury. On the day of euthanasia, articular lavage was collected and centrifuged. The supernatant was analyzed for tumor necrosis factor alpha (TNFα) protein expression by enzyme-linked immunosorbent assay (ELISA) and for IL1β, IL6, and IL10 mRNA by real-time polymerase chain reaction (RT-PCR). The joint tissue was also examined histologically. Analysis of variance with Tukey's post hoc test was used for comparisons. All data were expressed as means ±SD ($p < 0.05$). Both laser treatment modalities were efficient in reducing cellular inflammation and decreasing the expression of IL1ß and IL6. However, the 2 J treatments led to greater reduction in TNFα than the 4 J treatments. A single application of laser therapy with 2 J was more efficient in modulating inflammatory mediators and inflammatory cells. While this information proves the benefits of laser therapy, the dosing regimen reported in this study is not applicable in clinical practice. As with all such information, the practitioner must make informed decisions on how best to apply the concept to the reality.

Malliaropoulos *et al.* (2013) looked at meniscal pathology in a double-blind, placebo-controlled study. None of the patients in the study group underwent arthroscopy or new magnetic resonance imaging (MRI). The study included only symptomatic patients and showed that pain was significantly improved for the laser therapy group compared to the placebo group. Pain scores were also better after laser therapy. It was concluded that laser therapy should be considered in patients with meniscal tears who do not wish to undergo surgery.

Bublitz *et al.* (2014) analyzed the effects of laser therapy in the prevention of cartilage damage after transaction of the anterior (cranial) cruciate ligament in rats' knees. They divided 30 rats into three groups (10 each): a negative control, and two groups receiving laser therapy at different doses. An 808 nm laser was used immediately after surgery and was applied for 15 sessions. To evaluate the effects of the laser treatments, qualitative and semi-quantitative histological, morphometric, and immunohistochemistry analysis were performed. Initial signs of tissue degradation were observed in the control group. The laser-treated animals presented better tissue organization, especially at the lower (10 J/cm^2) settings. Laser therapy was capable of modulating some of the aspects related to the degenerative process, such as preventing loss of proteoglycans, and the increase in cartilage area. However, laser therapy was not capable of modulating chondrocyte proliferation and the immunoexpression of markers related to the inflammatory process (IL-1 and MMP-13).

In recent years a number of clinical studies have examined laser therapy for naturally occurring osteoarthritis in dogs. Looney *et al.* (2018) showed that increasing the dose of laser therapy to 20 J/cm^2 not only was safe but showed improvement when compared to control. This is helpful as historically arthritis was dosed at or around 8–10 J/cm^2. In a small study of 23 dogs (Barale *et al.*, 2023), the authors concluded that laser therapy may advance the management of arthritis by increasing the level of activity and subsequentially improving quality of life. Another group (Alves *et al.*, 2022) showed that laser therapy improved joint range of motion, as well as subjective outcome measures.

Numerous groups have investigated the use of laser therapy when evaluating postoperative conditions. Rogatko *et al.* (2017) compared laser therapy to placebo in 27 dogs undergoing tibial plateau leveling osteotomy (TPLO) and found that laser therapy may improve return to function following TPLO. However, Renwick *et al.* (2018) found only a mild improvement in gait function and no other improvements when comparing laser therapy to placebo in TPLO. In both studies there were no negative side effects reported, and this makes a case for laser therapy being safe in these patients. In 2023 a study comparing 24 dogs receiving laser therapy vs. 30 dogs in placebo (Chavez *et al.*, 2023) found that surgical site infections may be reduced in patients undergoing photobiomodulation.

While they are a common procedure and therefore helpful to utilize for study design, inherently a TPLO procedure has a low complication rate and a high degree of success for bone healing, so it may not be the ideal study model when looking for evidence to advocate use of laser therapy, especially at osteotomy healing. Hopefully with larger sample sizes and other study designs, a stronger case can be made for laser therapy in these scenarios.

Neurological System Conditions

Brain

A study by Morries *et al.* (2015) looked at using laser therapy to treat traumatic brain injuries. In 10 patients with chronic traumatic brain injury, given 10 treatments over the course of 2 months using an 810 or a 980 nm laser, symptoms of headache, sleep disturbance, cognition, mood dysregulation, anxiety, and irritability all improved. Depression scales and a novel patient diary system specifically designed for this study monitored symptoms. The authors concluded that laser therapy immunomodulates the response to brain damage.

A different study looked at the effect of laser therapy on wound healing following cerebral ischemia caused by cryogenic injury (Moreira *et al.*, 2011). This study used a 780 nm laser in rats following direct cortical cryogenic injury to look at the effects of laser treatment on inflammation and repair in the rat CNS. Wound healing in the CNS was monitored at 6 hours and 1, 7, and 14 days after laser treatment. The size of the lesions, the neuron cell viability percentages, and the distribution of lymphocytes, leukocytes, and macrophages were analyzed. Lasered lesions showed smaller tissue loss than control lesions after 6 hours. During the first 24 hours, the amount of viable neurons was significantly higher in the laser-treated group. The lesions of the laser-irradiated animals had fewer leukocytes and lymphocytes in the first 24 hours than those in the controls. The authors concluded that laser therapy exerts its effect in wound healing by controlling brain damage and preventing neuron death and severe astrogliosis and could indicate the possibility of a better clinical outcome.

Spinal Cord

Another rat study looked at the effect of a 780 nm laser on locomotor functional recovery and histomorphometric and histopathological changes of the spinal cord after moderate traumatic injury (Paula *et al.*, 2014). It divided 31 rats into seven groups: control without surgery, control surgery, laser therapy 6 hours after surgery, laser therapy 48 hours after surgery, medullar lesion without laser therapy, medullar lesion with laser therapy 6 hours after surgery, and medullar lesion with laser therapy 48 hours after surgery. Assessment of motor function and urinary dysfunction was performed. After 21 days, the animals were euthanized for analysis of the spinal cord. The results showed faster motor evolution in rats with spinal contusion treated with laser therapy, maintenance of the effectiveness of the urinary system, and preservation of nerve tissue in the lesion area with a notorious inflammation control and increased number of nerve cells and connections.

A 2015 study of human subjects with diskogenic back pain who failed to respond to a conventional physical therapy program examined the role of laser therapy in helping patients avoid operative intervention. The study concluded that laser therapy was a viable option in the conservative treatment of diskogenic back pain, with a positive clinical result of more than 90% efficacy, not only in the short term but also in the long term, with lasting benefits (Ip and Fu, 2015).

A 2012 publication (Draper *et al.*, 2012) showed laser therapy reduced the time to ambulation for dogs undergoing surgery for naturally occurring intervertebral disc disease (IVDD) when compared to a control group.

In another study looking at laser therapy for degenerative myelopathy, Miller *et al.* (2020) found that the group undergoing a 25-minute 14–21 J/cm^2 treatment of laser therapy and a rehabilitation program not only lived longer but had slower loss of function than the group with rehabilitation therapy coupled with a lower laser dose.

Peripheral Nerves

A pilot study investigated the effectiveness of 780 nm laser light in the treatment of patients suffering from incomplete peripheral nerve and brachial plexus injuries for 6 months to several years (Rochkind *et al.*, 2007). It was randomized, double-blind, and placebo-controlled and used 18 patients, applying 21 consecutive daily sessions of laser therapy or placebo transcutaneously for 3 hours to the injured peripheral nerve and for 2 hours to the corresponding segments of the spinal cord. Clinical and electrophysiological assessments were done at baseline, 21 days, and 3 and 6 months. The laser and placebo groups were in similar clinical conditions at the start of the study. Analysis of motor function during the 6-month follow-up period compared to baseline showed significant improvement in the laser-treated group compared to the placebo group. No significant difference was found in sensory function. Electrophysiological analysis showed statistically significant improvement in recruitment of voluntary muscle activity in the laser-treated group.

Another study reviewed the inhibitory effects of laser therapy on peripheral mammalian nerves and their relevance to analgesic effects (Chow *et al.*, 2011). It looked at 44 studies with variable laser settings. In 13 of 18 human studies, pulsed or continuous-wave (CW) visible and CW infrared laser application slowed conduction velocity or reduced the amplitude of compound action potentials, or both. In 26 animal experiments, infrared laser therapy suppressed electrically and noxiously evoked action potentials and pro-inflammatory mediators. Disruption of microtubule arrays and fast axonal flow may underpin neural inhibition. This could reduce acute pain through direct inhibition of peripheral nociceptors. In chronic pain, spinal cord changes induced by laser therapy may result in long-term depression of pain.

Rosso *et al.* (2018) showed in a systematic review that laser therapy has beneficial effects on peripheral nerve injuries when compared to not using it. This was despite the variances in settings over the 26 papers in this review.

Dermatological Conditions

Calisto *et al.* (2015) randomly distributed 24 rats into two groups, control and laser-treated, to look at laser therapy's effect in the healing of traumatic wounds. An induced surgical wound was made using a scalpel, and then the treated group received five sessions of laser therapy on consecutive days using the following laser parameters: 660 nm, 100 mW, 10 J/cm^2. The wounds were evaluated through measurement of the area and of the depth of the wound and histological analysis. The area and depth of the wounds treated with laser therapy were significantly less than those in the control group, and the laser group presented more epithelization than the control. This shows that the healing of wounds in rats was improved by the use of laser therapy.

Another study compared blue light (470 nm), red light (629 nm), and a negative control in induced ischemic abdominal flap wounds of rodents (Dungel *et al.*, 2014). Light from light-emitting diodes (LEDs) was applied for 10 minutes on five consecutive days. LED therapy of both wavelengths significantly increased angiogenesis in the subepidermal layer and intramuscularly, which was associated with improved tissue perfusion 7 days after ischemic insult. Accordingly, tissue necrosis was significantly reduced and shrinkage was less pronounced in the treated groups of both wavelengths. It should be noted that this study used LED and not laser therapy. LED may be efficacious when used for superficial applications; further study is needed (Opel *et al.*, 2015).

A rat study looking at induced wounds treated with 808 nm laser pulses showed good evidence for use of laser therapy (Tabakoglu *et al.*, 2015). In this study, a control group received no treatment, while three treatment groups received laser therapy immediately after wounding (inflammatory group), 24-hours post-wounding (proliferative group), or 72-hours post-wounding (remodeling group). Histological analyses were performed on days 3, 7, and 14 post-wounding. On day 7, wound diameters were smaller in all treated groups versus control, with the remodeling group having the smallest wound size. At 2 weeks, dermal tissue in the inflammatory and proliferative groups closed superficially, while control and remodeling groups were open. Mean wound-healing rates for all treatment groups were found to differ significantly from the control group. Comparing the proliferative group with the other treatment groups, a significant change was found, with the proliferative group being the most efficient at wound healing. Histological and morphometric results showed that laser application had the best effect when first applied 24 hours post-wounding (late inflammatory, early proliferative stage), as demonstrated by increases in granulation tissue, fibroblasts, and collagen deposition, which lead to faster rates of wound contraction and therefore accelerated healing.

In 2014 Andrade *et al.* did a review of laser therapy on wound healing. This paper reviewed studies between 2000 and 2011 in multiple languages. They found 14 papers and concluded that laser can be safely applied to the healing of wounds of the skin, with a dosing range of 3–6 J/cm^2. Wardlaw *et al.* (2019) showed that laser can improve incision healing in dogs undergoing hemilaminectomy for IVDD.

Role of Laser Therapy in Rehabilitation

Based on research, case reviews, and anecdotal reports, it can be concluded that the use of laser therapy is indicated in a clinical setting (Pryor and Millis, 2015). A practical approach is also needed, which can account for many factors, including patient need, patient cooperation, cost, efficacy, and frequency and duration of treatment. Some clients may allow their pet to be treated with the laser daily; some may only be able to do so two or three times a week. It is critically important for the veterinarian to prescribe a practical and realistic treatment plan for each individual patient. Laser therapy represents only one element of comprehensive rehabilitation (Figure 23.1). In 2020 Barger *et al.* discussed the economic impact of laser therapy for dogs in Missouri (Barger *et al.*, 2020). A survey of veterinary practices in that state showed that an average of patients with osteoarthritis were treated with laser therapy, with an average cost of treatment being US$28.00. The authors projects this to be an economic impact of 6.2 million USD per year just for the state of Missouri. This study shows the impact on the profession, but also highlights the need for more research in proper dosing, utilization, and frequency of laser use. While laser therapy can be safely and effectively combined with other modalities and integrated easily with other treatment approaches, it is important to prioritize the sequence of application with other modalities.

Laser Therapy as a Standalone Therapy

Examples of diagnoses that could benefit from laser therapy as a sole treatment modality include surgical incisions, wounds, lick granulomas, osteoarthritis, and tail-pull injuries.

The application of laser therapy to every surgical incision at the end of the anesthetic period can reduce postoperative pain and swelling. This can be provided either bundled or as an option for all appropriate surgeries in a practice.

Wounds can benefit from laser therapy in the late inflammatory or early proliferative phase, and laser therapy provides continued benefit in chronic or slow-healing wounds as healing progresses.

Lick granulomas can arise from many causes and can become cycles of healing and reoccurrence. Addressing pain relief, improved circulation, and antimicrobial pathways via laser therapy can provide improvement where other treatment modalities have either failed or only address a single potential cause.

Palliative management of chronic conditions can be achieved with the laser. End-stage otitis externa in cases that are not candidates for surgical resection will benefit from a reduction of bacterial load, inflammation, and pain.

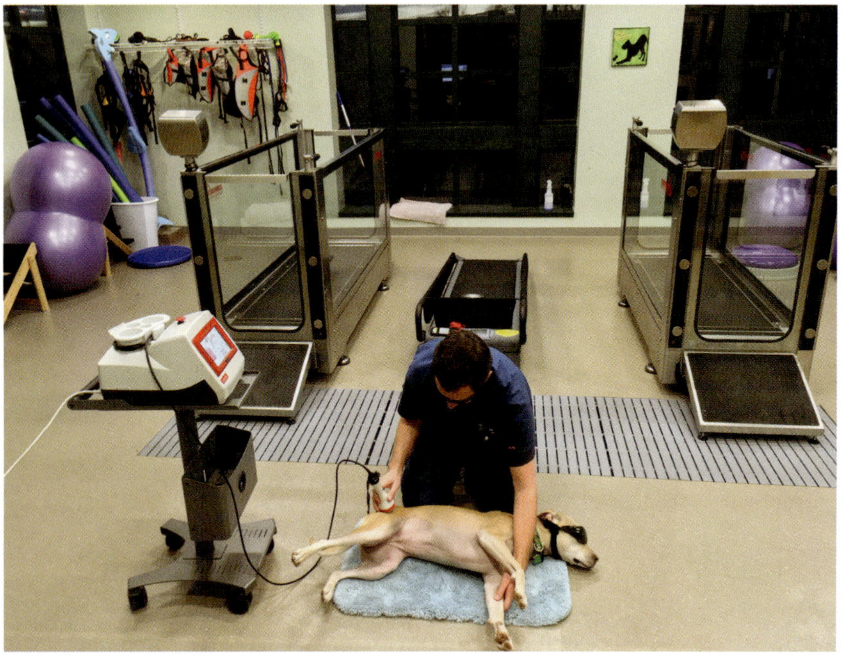

Figure 23.1 Laser therapy should be incorporated as one part of a complete rehabilitation program.

In some cases of osteoarthritis, the author has managed patients with standalone laser therapy. It is also a useful agent if other osteoarthritis management modalities need to be discontinued. An example is the severely arthritic patient on an NSAID that develops renal, hepatic, or gastrointestinal disease, meaning NSAID therapy has to be rapidly discontinued.

The therapeutic laser can be used to stimulate acupuncture points along meridians for those clinicians who practice traditional Chinese veterinary medicine (Lorenzini *et al.*, 2010; Law *et al.*, 2015). The author has found this helpful for anxious patients that may not sit for 20 minutes or more with acupuncture needles in place.

Neurological patients often need a comprehensive rehabilitation program (Sims *et al.*, 2015). Such a program should be multimodal and can include laser therapy to achieve favorable results. Tail-pull injuries provide a straightforward injury for which laser treatment may be the only modality that is available, practical, and easy to achieve. Additionally, patients suffering chronic pain from tail docking will also benefit from laser therapy.

Laser Therapy in Conjunction with a Rehabilitation Program

Proper rehabilitation starts with pain management. Regardless of the injury, no patient will be able to return to function through strength training, and maintain that outcome, if they are painful. Laser therapy is, in the author's opinion, an extremely valuable modality by which to achieve the goals of the clinician, the client, and the patient.

The release of endogenous opioids stimulated by laser therapy has applications throughout both acute and chronic conditions in injury rehabilitation (Labajos, 1988; Montesinos, 1988; Hagiwara *et al.*, 2008). The benefit of applying laser therapy to painful muscles, tendons, ligaments, or joints before (and sometimes after) having the patient do therapeutic exercises, such as underwater treadmill workouts, cavaletti rails, or other core exercises, makes sense and has been clearly demonstrated in human patients (Levine *et al.*, 2015).

Pain management is more effective and recovery is quicker after procedures when a multimodal postoperative protocol is used, because intervening in the pain and healing pathways at multiple points produces better outcomes than reliance on a single point. PBMT can be an important part of a multimodal postoperative plan for addressing pain (Enwemeka *et al.*, 2004; Fulop *et al.*, 2010; Sprouse-Blum *et al.*, 2010).

It is important for the clinician to incorporate PBMT as one part of a complete rehabilitation program. An example is incorporating laser therapy during the first few weeks of rehabilitation for a dog with biceps tendonitis. This aids in reducing pain and in stimulating cytokines and growth factors in order to achieve better tendon tissue healing. Laser therapy may be phased out of the rehabilitation program once the initial goals have been achieved and the patient has progressed to strength training and maintenance.

Osteoarthritis may initially require a high frequency of treatment (multiple times per week) through an induction phase. As pain and inflammation are reduced, the frequency can be reduced through a transition phase, until a maintenance-phase protocol is achieved. If an acute-on-chronic flare-up occurs, the induction phase can be easily repeated in order to keep the patient functional.

Neurological patients, such as those with brachial plexus avulsion or IVDD, may benefit from laser therapy throughout their entire rehabilitation process. It can be used early for management of pain at the insult site or in inflamed muscles. It can then be used to attempt a return of neurological function throughout recovery, and either to prevent or to manage the neuropathic pain that is a potential outcome in these cases.

Assessing Response to Laser Therapy

Based on the individual patient, diagnosis, prognosis, and plan, reassessments should be scheduled and documented appropriately by the clinician. The veterinary professionals delivering the treatment should be looking for both subjective and objective indicators of how the patient is doing.

Repeated physical examinations and photographs can be helpful in assessing patient function. The use of objective outcome measurements is important to track the progression (or potential regression) of cases. Simple outcome measures such as goniometry (Jaegger *et al.*, 2002) and limb circumference (Fox *et al.*, 2023) can be utilized in most clinics with minimal cost. Understanding the principles of musculoskeletal tissue healing and constructing the rehabilitation plan around them is vitally important. Kirkby Shaw *et al.* (2020) provided a specific review for postop cranial cruciate ligament surgery rehabilitation, and this can be applied to patients in general.

Case Studies

Cranial Cruciate Ligament Tear in a German Shepherd

Signalment

11-year-old German Shepherd, MN, 36.4 kg.

Client Complaint
Left hind limb lameness.

History
The patient had previously been diagnosed with bilateral anal sacculitis and spondylosis deformans. He had decreased mobility over the last 12 months and had become acutely lame in the left hind leg.

Current Medications
Cefpodoxime and cyclosporine were being given orally, along with topical Tacrolimus for anal sacculitis. Carprofen was being given for spondylosis.

Physical Examination
The patient was bright, alert, and responsive, with appropriate hydration and a body condition score (BCS) of 4/5. He displayed stiffness and discomfort in the lumbar muscles and was 3/5 lame in the left hind leg. There was moderate left stifle effusion, partial cranial drawer movement, cranial tibial thrust, and no meniscal click. Bilateral semilunar perianal fistulas measuring 2.5 × 5.0 cm were noted. All other systems were within normal limits.

Differential Diagnosis
Cranial cruciate injury.

Diagnostic Imaging
Lateral and anteroposterior radiographs of the stifles from the referring veterinarian showed disturbance of the infrapatellar fat pad and moderate osteoarthritic changes in the left stifle, with no significant findings in the right stifle. The pelvis was within normal limits in a ventrodorsal view. The lumbar spine showed a complete ventral fusion of all lumbar vertebrae. There was no evidence of lytic or proliferative lesions or any other indication for infection or neoplasia in any of the radiographs.

Laboratory Data
Complete blood count (CBC), chemistry panel, and urinalysis showed no significant findings.

Diagnosis
Bilateral anal fistulas, obesity, spondylosis deformans with muscle pain, and a partial tear of the left cranial cruciate ligament were diagnosed.

Treatment Plan
A weight-loss program with dietary restriction was implemented. Laser therapy was applied to the left stifle (6–10 J/cm^2 on-contact delivery) to aid in cruciate ligament healing. The laser was applied to the right hind leg and both thoracic limbs (6–10 J/cm^2, contact delivery), since increased weight bearing would occur on those limbs. The laser was also applied to the lumbar area (8–10 J/cm^2 on-contact delivery) and to the anal fistulas (6–8 J/cm^2 non-contact delivery).

Outcome
Laser therapy application was repeated twice per week for 4 weeks. During that time, the patient improved in ambulation, and lameness scores decreased. The fistulas decreased in size by 50%. The owner was then not able to bring the patient for treatment for 2 weeks, during which he became increasingly lame. Upon restarting laser therapy, the patient improved initially but then began stumbling at home, crying out, and limping more severely. Examination revealed a complete tear of the left cranial cruciate ligament. Surgery was not an option for this patient due to cost. The patient was fitted for a custom-made stifle brace and laser therapy was continued for another 4 weeks. During that time, the patient ambulated well and lameness scores returned to normal. The anal fistulas also resolved completely. Therapy was then discontinued due to cost and the patient was lost to follow-up.

Bicepital Tenosynovitis in a Standard Poodle

Signalment
8-year-old Standard Poodle, FS, 11.8 kg.

Client Complaint
Left foreleg lameness.

History
The owner had noted an on-and-off lameness for 4–6 weeks. It was worse after playing and running with other dogs in the household.

Current Medications
Heartworm, flea, and tick prevention medications were being given monthly.

Physical Examination
The patient was bright, alert, and responsive, with a BCS of 4/5. Moderate pain was elicited on left shoulder and biceps tendon palpation. Mild left-muscle atrophy was noted compared to the right. Mild pain was present in the right shoulder. No neck pain was noted. Neurological and other systems were within normal limits.

Differential Diagnosis
Shoulder osteoarthritis, biceps tendonitis.

Diagnostic Imaging

Lateral and anteroposterior radiographs of each shoulder were obtained. No abnormalities were found. While sedated, the patient underwent diagnostic musculoskeletal ultrasound of both shoulders, which showed inflammation and a grade I strain of both left and right biceps tendons.

Laboratory Data

CBC, chemistry panel, and urinalysis showed no significant findings.

Diagnosis

Bilateral biceps tendonitis.

Treatment Plan

While the patient was sedated, each tendon was injected with 10 mg of methylprednisolone acetate using ultrasound guidance. The patient was placed on restricted activity and was rechecked 7 days later. At that time, no lameness or discomfort was noted in either shoulder. An outpatient rehabilitation program was then instituted for further tissue healing and strength training. The patient was seen twice per week for 6 weeks and received laser therapy to both shoulders (8–10 J/cm^2 on-contact delivery, 12 treatments total) (Figure 23.2). The patient also did therapeutic exercises (cavaletti rails and core exercises on various devices) and walked on both land and underwater treadmills.

Outcome

The patient was sound within 2 weeks of beginning therapy and progressed to a return to full function.

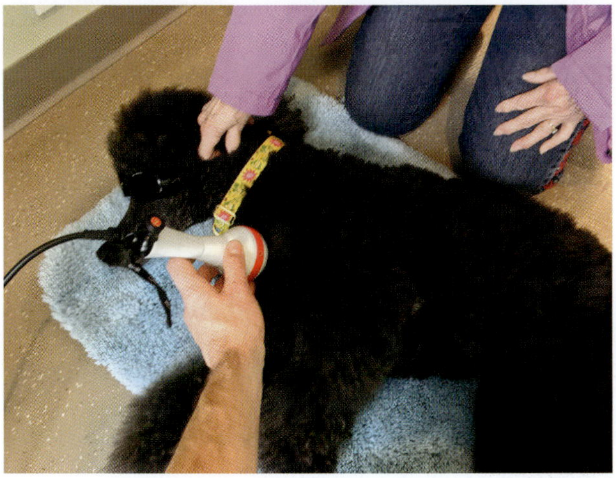

Figure 23.2 Laser therapy treatment of the shoulder for biceps tendonitis.

IVDD in a Dachshund

Signalment

7-year-old Dachshund, MN, 3.6 kg.

Client Complaint

Neurological deficits 2 weeks after T13–L1 right-sided hemilaminectomy.

History

This patient had experienced an acute disk herniation with loss of motor function and pain perception in the pelvic limbs. Within 12 hours, an MRI determined the diagnosis and surgery was performed to remove the herniated disk. The patient regained pain perception after surgery, but not motor function.

Current Medications

Gabapentin 100 mg BID.

Physical Examination

The thoracic limbs were within normal limits. Grade I motor function was present in the pelvic limbs. Pain and withdrawal reflexes were present in both hind legs. Upper motor neuron bladder function was noted, with the bladder requiring manual expression three times a day.

Treatment Plan

The patient received electroacupuncture treatments weekly for 6 weeks. He also had therapeutic laser, underwater treadmill, and other physical therapy modalities three times per week for 4 weeks, then twice per week for 6 weeks. Laser therapy was applied to the thoracic spine, lumbar spine, and pelvic limbs, delivering 8–10 J/cm^2 to each site. Treatments were delivered with a handpiece on-contact with the skin. When treating the pelvic limbs, the joints were taken through a passive range of motion to facilitate photonic penetration into the joint spaces.

Outcome

Over the course of 4 weeks, the patient regained all motor functions but was ataxic and had conscious proprioceptive deficits in both hind legs. In the following 6 weeks, the patient made a full recovery.

Presumed IVDD in a Jack Russell Terrier

Signalment

12-year-old canine Jack Russell terrier, MN, 8.2 kg.

Client Complaint

Acute nonambulatory paraplegia.

History
The patient was boarding, had been normal one evening, and in the morning could not use his hind legs. There was no evidence of trauma.

Current Medications
Famotidine 2.5 mg BID, prednisone 5 mg BID, gabapentin 100 mg BID.

Physical Examination
The thoracic limbs were within normal limits. Pain, withdrawal, and patellar reflexes were present in the hind legs. The patient had no motor function in either hind leg. His cutaneous trunci reflex stopped at approximately the second lumbar vertebrae. His bladder was large and turgid, but expressible.

Diagnostic Imaging
Survey radiographs did not show any fracture, lytic area, or other concerns.

Laboratory Data
CBC, chemistry panel, and urinalysis showed no significant findings.

Differential Diagnosis
IVDD was most likely. Fibrocartilagenous emboli and neoplasia were felt to be less likely.

Treatment Plan
The patient was treated as IVDD. Laser therapy was applied twice per week for 6 weeks as part of a full rehabilitation program. The patient also received transcutaneous electrical nerve stimulation, underwater treadmill therapy, massage, and range-of-motion and weight-bearing exercises. Laser settings delivered 8–10 J/cm^2 to the thoracic spine, lumbar spine, and pelvic limbs.

Outcome
Over the course of 4 weeks, the patient regained motor function in the pelvic limbs but was ataxic. This improved over the next 8 weeks.

Resultant Lumbosacral Issues and FHO in a Labrador Mix

Signalment
7-year-old Labrador Mix, FS, Hit by Car

Chief Complaint
Left hindlimb lameness due to FHO, right hindlimb distal paresthesia

History
The patient was hit by a car and referred to an emergency center. The patient underwent a left femoral head and neck osteotomy for a subluxation of the left coxofemoral joint. Four weeks into her recovery, she began to lick and mutilate the dorsum of the right hind foot.

Current Medications
Gabapentin 300 mg BID added after the mutilation began.

Physical Examination
Left hip extension limited to 134°, compared to right hip extension at 160°. Thigh circumference: left 31.3 cm, right 32.8 cm. Dorsum of right hind foot swollen, with an open wound. Conscious proprioception diminished, and flexor withdrawal limited to hip flexion. Pain on palpation of L6 to S1. Unable to actively flex the right hock and toes.

Diagnostic Imaging
Owner declined further diagnostic imaging secondary to cost. Dog was started on amoxicillin.

Treatment
The left hip was treated with photobiomodulation at wavelengths of 650 nm, 810 nm, 915 nm, 980 nm for blood flow and range-of-motion. Treatment began on the medial aspect of the coxofemoral joint with an on-contact method, and moved to the cranial, lateral and caudal aspect with a total of 450 joules. The right hindfoot was treated with blue light laser at 465 nm wavelength for infection control. This was followed by red light at 660 nm wavelength for the treatment of the wound. The lumbar region and sciatic nerve path was treated with laser therapy for a total of 500 joules at a variety of wavelengths for blood flow. Additional treatments included range-of-motion, balance and proprioception, wound wrapping, therapeutic exercise and a home laser for the treatment of the wound.

Conclusion

Rehabilitation in veterinary medicine is an expanding field that requires both a practical approach and a commitment to staying on the cutting edge of available treatment options. Laser therapy is a vital tool in the veterinary professional's armament. Its versatility, ease of administration, and proven benefits allow many types of patients to recover faster and more effectively. Further research is needed to identify other injuries that may benefit from laser therapy, as well as to further verify effective treatment settings and their time frames.

References

Abergel, R.P. *et al.* (1984). Control of connective tissue metabolism by lasers: recent developments and future prospects. *J Am Acad Dermatol.* 11(6):1142–1150.

Alves, J.C. *et al.* (2022). A randomized double-blinded controlled trial on the effects of photobiomodulation therapy in dogs with osteoarthritis. *Am J Vet Res.* 83(8): ajvr.22.03.0036. doi:10.2460/ajvr.22.03.0036.

Andrade, F.S. *et al.* (2014). Effects of low-level laser therapy on wound healing. *Rev Col Bras Cir.* 41(2):129–133. doi:10.1590/s0100-69912014000200010.

Assis, L. *et al.* (2015). Effect of low level laser therapy (808 nm) on skeletal muscle after endurance exercise training in rats. *Braz J Phys Ther.* 19(6):457–465.

Barale, L. *et al.* (2023). Effects of low-level laser therapy on impaired mobility in dogs with naturally occurring osteoarthritis. *Vet Med Sci.* 9(2):653–659. doi:10.1002/vms3.997.

Barbosa, D. *et al.* (2014). Laser therapy in bone repair in rats: analysis of bone optical density. *Acta Ortop Bras.* 22(2):71–74.

Barger, B.K. *et al.* (2020). Low-level laser therapy for osteoarthritis treatment in dogs at Missouri veterinary practice. *J Am Anim Hosp Assoc.* 56(3):139–145. doi:10.5326/JAAHA-MS-6851.

Baxter, G.D. and McDonough, S.M. (2007). Principles of electrotherapy in veterinary physiotherapy. In: *Animal Physiotherapy: Assessment, Treatment and Rehabilitation of Animals*, pp. 182–184. Blackwell, Oxford.

Bayat, M. *et al.* (2005). Low-level laser therapy improves early healing of medial collateral ligament injuries in rats. *Photomed Laser Surg.* 23(6):556–560.

Bensadoun, R.J. and Nair, R.G. (2015). Low-level laser therapy in the management of mucositis and dermatitis induced by cancer therapy. *Photomed Laser Surg.* 33(10):487–491.

Bjordal, J.M. *et al.* (2006). A randomized, placebo controlled trial of low level laser therapy for activated Achilles tendinitis with microdialysis measurements of peritendinous prostaglandin E2 concentrations. *Br J Sports Med.* 40(1):76–80.

Borsa, P. *et al.* (2019). Muscular preconditioning using phototherapy improves the physical work capacity of the quadriceps when applied between repeated bouts of resistance exercise. *J Athl Enhan.* 8(1):1–8. doi:10.4172/2324-9080.1000310.

Bublitz, C. *et al.* (2014). Low level laser therapy prevents degenerative morphological changes in an experimental model of anterior cruciate ligament transection in rats. *Lasers Med Sci.* 29(5):1669–1678.

Calisto, F.C. *et al.* (2015). Use of low-power laser to assist the healing of traumatic wounds. *Acta Cir Bras.* 30(3):204–208.

Carvalho, A.F. *et al.* (2015). The low-level laser on acute myositis in rats. *Acta Cir Bras.* 30(12):806–811.

Chang, W. *et al.* (2014). Therapeutic outcomes of low-level laser therapy for closed bone fracture in the human wrist and hand. *Photomed Laser Surg.* 32(4):212–218.

Chavez, O.A. *et al.* (2023). Photobiomodulation therapy in dogs undergoing TPLO after cranial cruciate ligament rupture shows promise but no statistically significant difference in a randomized trial. *Am J Vet Res.* 85(2):ajvr.23.06.0138. doi:10.2460/ajvr.23.06.0138.

Chow, R. *et al.* (2011). Inhibitory effects of laser irradiation on peripheral mammalian nerves and relevance to analgesic effects: a systematic review. *Photomed Laser Surg.* 29(6):365–381.

Conforti, M. and Fachinetti, G.P. (2013). High power laser therapy treatment compared to simple segmental physical rehabilitation in whiplash injuries (1 and 2 grade of the Quebec task force classification) involving muscles and ligaments. *Muscles Ligaments Tendons J.* 3(2):106–111.

Corazza, A.V. *et al.* (2007). Photobiomodulation of the angiogenesis of skin wounds in rats using different light sources. *Photomed Laser Surg.* 25(2):102–106.

Crow, J.A. *et al.* (2023). Therapeutic photobiomodulation before strenuous exercise attenuates shoulder muscle fatigue. *J Athl Train.* doi:10.4085/1062-6050-0171.23.

Da Ré Guerra, F. *et al.* (2016). Low-level PBMT modulates pro-inflammatory cytokines after partial tenotomy. *Lasers Med Sci.* 31(4):759–766.

De Bie, R.A. *et al.* (1998). Low-level laser therapy in ankle sprains: a randomized clinical trial. *Arch Phys Med Rehabil.* 79(11):1415–1420.

Draper, W.E. *et al.* (2012). Low-level laser therapy reduces time to ambulation in dogs after hemilaminectomy: a preliminary study. *J Small Anim Pract.* 53(8):465–469. doi:10.1111/j.1748-5827.2012.01242.x.

Dungel, P. *et al.* (2014). Low level light therapy by LED of different wavelength induces angiogenesis and improves ischemic wound healing. *Lasers Surg Med.* 46(10):773–780.

Ebrahimi, T. *et al.* (2012). The influence of low-intensity laser therapy on bone healing. *J Dent (Tehran).* 9(4):238–248.

Enwemeka, C.S. *et al.* (2004). The efficacy of low-power lasers in tissue repair and pain control: a meta-analysis study. *Photomed Laser Surg.* 22(4):323–329.

Fenner, W.R. (2000). Diseases of the brain. In: *Textbook of Veterinary Internal Medicine*, 5 edn, pp. 552–556. Saunders, Philadelphia, PA.

Fox, E.A. *et al.* (2023). Evaluation of a method to measure the ratio of pelvic limb to thoracic limb girth in dogs. *Vet Evid.* 8(4). doi:10.18849/ve.v8i4.667.

Frank, C. *et al.* (1991). Normal ligament: structure, function and composition. In: *Injury and Repair of the Musculoskeletal Soft Tissues. American Academy of Orthopedic Surgeons Symposium*. Park Ridge, IL.

Fulop, A. *et al.* (2010). A meta-analysis of the efficacy of laser phototherapy on pain relief. *Clin J Pain*. 26(8):729–736.

Fung, D.T. *et al.* (2002). Therapeutic low energy laser improves the mechanical strength of repairing medial collateral ligament. *Lasers Surg Med*. 31(2):91–96.

Hagiwara, S. *et al.* (2008). Pre-irradiation of blood by gallium aluminum arsenide (830 nm) low-level laser enhances peripheral endogenous opioid analgesia in rats. *Anesth Analg*. 107(3):1058–1063.

Hedlund, C.S. (2002). Surgery of the integumentary system. In: *Small Animal Surgery*, 2 edn, pp. 134–137. Mosby, St. Louis, MO.

Honmura, A. *et al.* (1993). Analgesic effect of GaA1As diode laser irradiation on hyperalgesia in carrageenin- induced inflammation. *Lasers Surg Med*. 13(4):463–469.

Hopkins, J.T. *et al.* (2004). Low-level laser therapy facilitates superficial wound healing in humans: a triple-blind, sham-controlled study. *J Athl Train*. 39(3):223–229.

Huang, Y.Y. *et al.* (2009). Biphasic dose response in low level light therapy. *Dose-Response*. 7(4):358–383.

Inzana, K.D. (2000). Peripheral nerve disorders. In: *Textbook of Veterinary Internal Medicine*, 5 edn, pp. 662–681. Saunders, Philadelphia, PA.

Ip, D. and Fu, N.Y. (2015). Can intractable discogenic back pain be managed by low-level PBMT without recourse to operative intervention? *J Pain Res*. 8:253–256.

Jaegger, G. *et al.* (2002). Reliability of goniometry in Labrador retrievers. *Am J Vet Res*. 63(7):979–986. doi:10.2460/ajvr.2002.63.979.

Jawad, M.M. *et al.* (2013). Effect of 940 nm low-level laser therapy on osteogenesis in vitro. *J Biomed Opt*. 18(12):128001.

de Jesus, J.F. *et al.* (2015). Low-level laser therapy in IL-1B, COX-2 and PGE2 modulation in partially injured Achilles tendon. *Lasers Med Sci*. 30(1):153–158.

Karu, T. (2010). Mitochondrial mechanisms of photobiomodulation in context of new data about multiple roles of ATP. *Photomed Laser Surg*. 28(2):159–160.

Kaya, G.S. *et al.* (2011). Use of 808-nm light therapy to treat experimental chronic osteomyelitis induced in rats by methicillin-resistant *Staphylococcus aureus*. *Photomed Laser Surg*. 29(6):405–412.

Kirkby Shaw, K. *et al.* (2020). Fundamental principles of rehabilitation and musculoskeletal tissue healing. *Vet Surg*. 49(1):22–32. doi:10.1111/vsu.13270.

Kizhner, V. *et al.* (2011). Laser-generated shockwave for clearing medical device biofilms. *Photomed Laser Surg*. 29(4):277–282.

Labajos, M. (1988). Beta-endorphin levels modification after GaAs and HeNe laser irradiation on the rabbit. Comparative Study. *Invest Clin*. 1–2:6–8.

Law, D. *et al.* (2015). Laser acupuncture for treating musculoskeletal pain: a systematic review with meta-analysis. *J Acupunct Meridian Stud*. 8(1):2–16.

LeCouteur, R.A. and Grandy, J.L. (2000). Diseases of the spinal cord. In: *Textbook of Veterinary Internal Medicine*, 5 edn, pp. 609–653. Saunders, Philadelphia, PA.

Levine, D. *et al.* (2015). Effects of laser on endurance of the rotator cuff muscles. *Lasers Surg Med*. 47(S26):44–45.

Lögdberg-Andersson, M. *et al.* (1997). Low level laser therapy (LLLT) of tendinitis and myofascial pains–a randomized, double-blind, controlled study. *Laser Ther*. 9:79–86.

Looney, A.L. *et al.* (2018). A randomized blind placebo-controlled trial investigating the effects of photobiomodulation therapy (PBMT) on canine elbow osteoarthritis. *Can Vet J*. 59(9):959–966.

Lorenzini, L. *et al.* (2010). Laser acupuncture for acute inflammatory, visceral and neuropathic pain relief: an experimental study in the laboratory rat. *Res Vet Sci*. 88(1):159–165.

de Loura, S.C. *et al.* (2016). Effect of laser therapy on immune cells infiltrate after excisional wounds in diabetic rats. *Lasers Surg Med*. 48(1):45–51.

Malliaropoulos, N. *et al.* (2013). Low-level laser therapy in meniscal pathology: a double-blinded placebo controlled study. *Lasers Med Sci*. 28(4):1183–1188.

Miller, L.A. *et al.* (2020). Retrospective observational study and analysis of two different photobiomodulation therapy protocols combined with rehabilitation therapy as therapeutic interventions for canine degenerative myelopathy. *Photobiomodul Photomed Laser Surg*. 38(4):195–205. doi:10.1089/photob.2019.4723.

Millis, D.L. and Ciuperca, I.A. (2015). Evidence for canine rehabilitation and physical therapy. *Vet Clin North Am Small Anim Pract*. 45(1):1–27.

Montesinos, M. (1988). Experimental effects of low power laser in encephalin and endorphin synthesis. *J Eur Med Laser Assoc*. 1(3):2–7.

Moreira, M.S. *et al.* (2011). Effect of laser phototherapy on wound healing following cerebral ischemia by cryogenic injury. *J Photochem Photobiol B*. 105(3):207–215.

Morries, L.D. *et al.* (2015). Treatments for traumatic brain injury with emphasis on transcranial near- infrared laser phototherapy. *Neuropsychiatr Dis Treat*. 11:2159–2175.

Opel, D.R. *et al.* (2015). Light-emitting diodes. A brief review of clinical experience. *J Clin Aesthet Dermatol*. 8(6):36–44.

Paula, A.A. *et al.* (2014). Low-intensity laser therapy effect on the recovery of traumatic spinal cord injury. *Lasers Med Sci*. 29(6):1849–1859.

Perini, J.L. *et al.* (2015). Long-term low-level laser therapy promotes an increase in maximal oxygen uptake and exercise performance in a dose-dependent manner in Wistar rats. *Lasers Med Sci.* 31(2):241–248.

Pourreau-Schneider, N. *et al.* (1990). Helium-neon laser treatment transforms fibroblasts into myofibroblasts. *Am J Pathol.* 137(1):171–178.

Pryor, B. and Millis, D.L. (2015). Therapeutic laser in veterinary medicine. *Vet Clin North Am Small Anim Pract.* 45(1):45–56.

Renwick, S.M. *et al.* (2018). Influence of class IV laser therapy on the outcomes of tibial plateau leveling osteotomy in dogs. *Vet Surg.* 47(4):507–515. doi:10.1111/vsu.12794.

Rochkind, S. *et al.* (2007). Laser phototherapy (780 nm), a new modality in treatment of long-term incomplete peripheral nerve injury: a randomized double-blind placebo-controlled study. *Photomed Laser Surg.* 25(5):436–442.

Rogatko, C.P. *et al.* (2017). Preoperative low level laser therapy in dogs undergoing tibial plateau levelling osteotomy: a blinded, prospective, randomized clinical trial. *Vet Comp Orthop Traumatol.* 30(1):46–53. doi:10.3415/VCOT-15-12-0198.

Rosso, M.P.O. *et al.* (2018). Photobiomodulation therapy (PBMT) in peripheral nerve regeneration: a systematic review. *Bioengineering (Basel).* 5(2):44. doi:10.3390/bioengineering5020044.

Sakarai, Y. *et al.* (2000). Inhibitory effect of low-level laser irradiation on LPS-stimulated prostaglandin E2 productions and cyclooxygenase-2 in human gingival fibroblasts. *Eur J Oral Sci.* 108(1):29–34.

dos Santos, S.A. *et al.* (2014). Comparative analysis of two low-level laser doses on the expression of inflammatory mediators and on neutrophils and macrophages in acute joint inflammation. *Lasers Med Sci.* 29(3):1051–1058.

Seim, H.B. (2002a). Surgery of cervical spine. In: *Small Animal Surgery*, 2., p.7 edn. Mosby, St. Louis, MO.

Seim, H.B. (2002b). Surgery of the lumbosacral spine. In: *Small Animal Surgery*, 2., pp.9 edn. Mosby, St. Louis, MO.

Sims, C. *et al.* (2015). Rehabilitation and physical therapy for the neurologic patient. *Vet Clin North Am Small Anim Pract.* 45(1):123–143.

Sprouse-Blum, A.S. *et al.* (2010). Understanding endorphins and their importance in pain management. *Hawaii Med J.* 69(3):70–71.

Tabakoglu, H.O. *et al.* (2015). Assessment of circular wound healing in rats after exposure to 808-nm laser pulses during specific healing phases. *Lasers Surg Med.* 48(4):409–415.

Tedford, C.E. *et al.* (2015). Quantitative analysis of transcranial and intraparenchymal light penetration in human cadaver brain tissue. *Lasers Surg Med.* 47(4):312–322.

Tim, C.R. *et al.* (2014). Low-level laser therapy enhances the expression of osteogenic factors during bone repair in rats. *Lasers Med Sci.* 29(1):147–156.

Tumilty, S. and Baxter, D. (2015). Effectiveness of class IV lasers for Achilles tendinopathy. *Lasers Surg Med.* 47(S26):38.

Tumilty, S. *et al.* (2010). Low level laser treatment of tendinopathy: a systematic review with meta-analysis. *Photomed Laser Surg.* 28(1):3–16.

Vasilenko, T. *et al.* (2010). The effect of equal daily dose achieved by different power densities of low-level laser therapy at 635 and 670 nm on wound tensile strength in rats: a short report. *Photomed Laser Surg.* 28(2):281–283.

Wardlaw, J.L. *et al.* (2019). Laser therapy for incision healing in 9 dogs. *Front Vet Sci.* 2019(5):349. doi:10.3389/fvets.2018.00349.

Williams, J. (2004). Wound healing: tendons, ligaments, bone, muscles and cartilage. In: *Canine Rehabilitation and Physical Therapy*, pp. 100–110. Saunders, St. Louis, MO.

Part VI

Clinical Applications of Laser Therapy in Exotic Animals

24

Photobiomodulation in Exotic Small Mammals

Jörg Mayer[1] and Robert D. Ness[2]

[1] Department of Small Animal Medicine and Surgery, University of Georgia, Athens, GA, USA
[2] Ness Exotic Wellness Center, Lisle, IL, USA

Introduction

The body of evidence regarding the efficacy of photobiomodulation (PBM) in small mammals is staggering as most of the research in this area usually includes at least one species of small mammal in the early stages of investigation. It is beyond the scope of this chapter to list all scientific publications that are currently available. The authors will focus on the most clinically applicable publications and applications of laser therapy commonly used in clinical daily practice. The body of knowledge will continue to grow in this area. The reader is encouraged to update their database frequently by searching for novel applications of PBM in small mammals.

Precautions

Safety precautions must be observed for all species when utilizing PBM, as with any form of medical therapy. Most of the precautions and contraindications discussed regarding exotic small mammals are extrapolated from recommendations for other species discussed in Chapter 5; see Box 24.1 for dose recommendations.

Due to the near-infrared (NIR) wavelength of therapeutic lasers, regulatory agencies require that protective eyewear be worn, which are calibrated to the proper laser light wavelength to prevent injury to the retina. Everyone in the room, including the patient, must have their eyes protected during laser therapy, since there is risk of retinal damage from direct exposure to the laser beam, as well as from reflection of the laser light. The patient's eyes are protected simply by covering the eyes with a dark cloth or towel.

Due to the inherent power of some therapy lasers in contrast to the small size of many of the exotic small mammal species, extra care should be exercised when using these devices in these patients. Smaller patients require a lower therapeutic dosing, which is accomplished by adjusting the laser settings. The adjustments can be made by modifying the delivery mode, power, or time. A pulsed delivery can be utilized instead of a continuous delivery, thereby reducing the rate of delivery 50% (assuming a 50% duty cycle). Similarly, a lower energy dose can be delivered by decreasing the treatment time or the laser power.

Overheating of the skin and fur is a potential risk of improper operator technique. Darkly pigmented skin or dark hair absorbs photons leading to greater ease of overheating, thereby requiring caution in dosing and administration of photobiomodulation. Running a finger behind the laser beam over the animal is encouraged, as the operator will immediately feel the temperature of the skin and hair as the laser handpiece is moved. If anything other than a pleasant and gentle warming is noted, then either reduce the power, enlarge the spot size, or move the handpiece more quickly.

It is recommended to avoid prolonged treatment over certain endocrine organs, such as the thyroid gland and gonads, even though there is minimal and contradictory data suggesting an adverse effect to these tissues.

Metal implants (such as bone plates and screws) do not absorb photons, but they do reflect them back into tissues that are more superficial, so decrease the dose of energy put into tissue directly over metallic implants.

Since photobiomodulation increases microcirculation in tissues, treatment of actively hemorrhaging tissue is discouraged.

The effect of PBM on a developing fetus or on parturition is unknown, thus prudent care suggests avoiding application of PBM directly over a gravid uterus. In one study,

Laser Therapy in Veterinary Medicine: Photobiomodulation, Second Edition. Edited by Christopher J. Winkler and Lisa A. Miller.

Box 24.1 Laser Therapy Dose Recommendations for Exotic Small Mammals

Integumentary disorders	
Abscesses	4–6 J/cm^2
Burn wounds	8–12 J/cm^2
Cuturebra larvae	2–4 J/cm^2
Deep wounds	8–10 J/cm^2
Edema	4–5 J/cm^2
Hair loss	8–10 J/cm^2
Lacerations	1–2 J/cm^2
Pododermatitis	2–6 J/cm^2
Superficial wounds	2–4 J/cm^2
Surgical incisions	1 J/cm^2 for skin, 2–3 J/cm^2 for deep
Musculoskeletal disorders	
Arthritis	8–10 J/cm^2
Fracture	8–10 J/cm^2
Muscular sprain and strain	2–4 J/cm^2
Scurvy	1–8 J/cm^2
Spondylosis	10 J/cm^2
Neurologic disorders	8–10 J/cm^2
Head and neck disorders	
Dental disease	2–4 J/cm^2
Otitis	10 J/cm^2
Otorhinolaryngological conditions	6–8 J/cm^2
Temporomandibular disorders	6–8 J/cm^2
Abdominal disorders	
Ascites	7–10 J/cm^2
Gastrointestinal disorders	7–10 J/cm^2
Urinary disorders	6–8 J/cm^2
Thoracic disorders	
Laryngitis	6–8 J/cm^2
Bronchitis & pneumonia	8 J/cm^2
Pulmonary congestion	6–8 J/cm^2
Pulmonary ischemia	6–8 J/cm^2

the hemodynamic changes and variations in liver and kidney function in pregnant rats with preeclampsia were observed after treatment with low-energy laser irradiation. In the treatment groups, laser irradiation of the chest was carried out after day 16 of gestation. Blood pressure, urine protein, liver and kidney function, and the hemodynamic changes in the rats were observed to assess systemic effects of the treatment and potential side effects. The study concluded that low-energy laser irradiation in the chest area may improve the hemodynamic indices, decrease blood pressure and urine protein, and ameliorate liver and kidney functions in pregnant rats with preeclampsia (Sun *et al.*, 2010). This suggests that the use of laser in pregnant rats with preeclampsia might be of benefit for the animal.

In human medicine, the CO_2 laser has the most evidence supporting its use during pregnancy. It is considered safe for the treatment of genital condylomas during pregnancy (Lee *et al.*, 2013). It has also been demonstrated that the use of laser therapy after a human cesarean section does not compromise blood prolactin levels and lactation status (Mokmeli *et al.*, 2009). This study concluded that photobiomodulation after cesarean section had no serious deleterious effects on lactation, and that it helped to modulate metabolic processes and promote wound healing postsurgery.

Contraindications to photobiomodulation are generally a result of prudence rather than clinical data. A current recommendation is that treatment over malignancy sites is usually contraindicated; however, some studies suggest photobiomodulation may have an inhibitory effect on some cancerous tissue in mammals (Myakishev-Rempel *et al.*, 2012; Santana-Blank *et al.*, 2012). The risk-to-benefit ratio has to be considered for each case, because the analgesic and anti-inflammatory effects of the treatment may be of greater benefit than the risk of stimulating a cancerous growth (e.g., the benefit of the analgesic property might outweigh the risk of complicating a case of osteosarcoma). Please see Chapter 19 for additional information.

Clinical Indications

Integumentary

Abscesses

Abscesses tend to heal more rapidly when treated with photobiomodulation. A deep wound setting of 4–6 J/cm^2 can expedite the recovery when used in conjunction with appropriate antimicrobial therapy. As expected, smaller and more superficial abscesses can be treated at lower therapeutic doses than deeper lesions penetrating beyond the skin and immediate superficial tissues.

Cuterebra Larvae

Cuterebra infestation in rabbits and other small mammals is a common example of a condition that responds well to photobiomodulation. The lesions are caused by the development of Cuterebra larvae under the skin after deposition of eggs by the Cuterebra fly. The treatment is careful removal of the infesting Cuturebra larvae and standard management of the resulting wound. Photobiomodulation at 2–4 J/cm^2 reduces the severe inflammation around the wound, reduces pain, accelerates the healing response, and accentuates resolution of tissue infection (Figure 24.1).

Deep Wounds

Deep wounds in exotic small mammals are treated similar to those treated in dogs and cats, at a starting dosage range of 8–10 J/cm^2. Minimal adjustment of treatment parameters is necessary for the size of the patients, since the therapeutic dosage is dependent on the size of the lesion, and is therefore lower in smaller patents with relatively smaller lesions. Higher dosages have been used in exotic small mammals without untoward effects.

Al-Watban and Zhang (1999) conducted a study to identify the ideal dose of laser light in the treatment of skin wounds on the backs of rats. In a comparison of fluency of 10, 20, and 30 J/cm^2 applied three times weekly, the best results were obtained with 20 J/cm^2. Another analysis showed that the combination of 685 and 830 nm wavelengths (10 J/cm^2 each; total 20 J/cm^2) promoted the best skin wound healing at the end of the experimental period (Mendez *et al.*, 2004). The importance of the application of the correct wavelength has also been documented in other wound healing studies (Hendler *et al.*, 2021). In their studies the authors have shown that when comparing photobiomodulation wavelengths, the 830-nm groups were more effective when compared with the naive and sham groups and those irradiated at 660 nm (Hendler *et al.*, 2021).

(a) (b) (c)

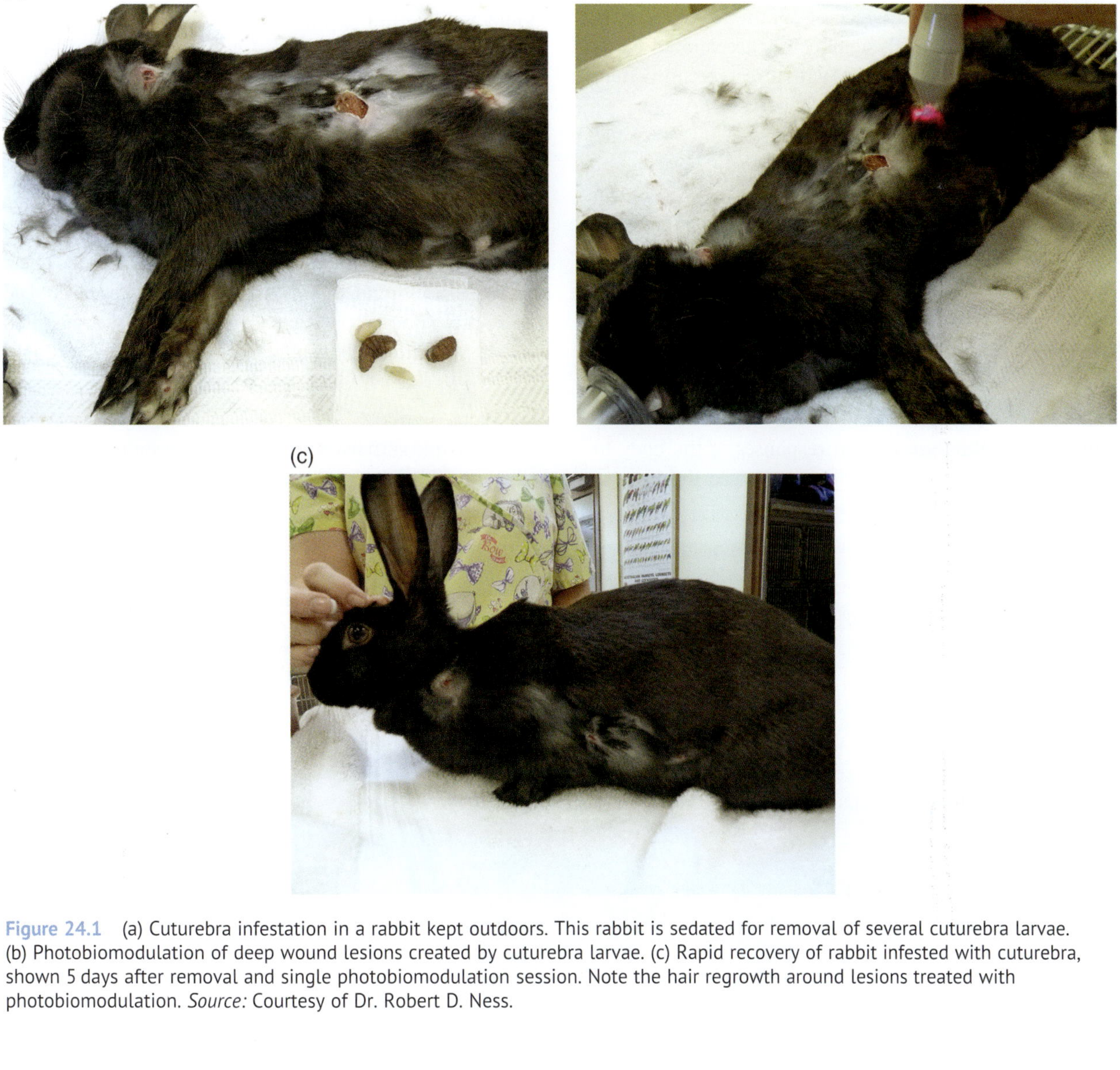

Figure 24.1 (a) Cuturebra infestation in a rabbit kept outdoors. This rabbit is sedated for removal of several cuturebra larvae. (b) Photobiomodulation of deep wound lesions created by cuturebra larvae. (c) Rapid recovery of rabbit infested with cuturebra, shown 5 days after removal and single photobiomodulation session. Note the hair regrowth around lesions treated with photobiomodulation. *Source:* Courtesy of Dr. Robert D. Ness.

However, a broader review of the literature focusing on wound healing indicated that daily laser exposure at a wavelength of a 600 or 800 nm range was the most beneficial across the rodent studies regardless of health status or wound type (Lopez & Brundage, 2019). The majority of the studies cited used an energy density of 1–5 J/cm^2, with the highest being 50 J/cm^2 for a single treatment (Demidova-Rice *et al.*, 2007; Lopez & Brundage, 2019). A study comparing different setting found a biphasic dose–response curve for fluence of 635 nm light with a maximum positive effect at 2 J/cm^2, and 820 nm was found to be the best wavelength tested compared to 635, 670, and 720 nm (Demidova-Rice *et al.*, 2007).

During the healing process of a wound, pericytes are relevant cells directly involved in wound healing, and they can be one of the main targets of photobiomodulation due to their plasticity and perivascular localization (do Valle *et al.*, 2020). Published data shows that photobiomodulation (at a wavelength of 660 nm, a power of 20 mW, an irradiance of 0.71 W/cm^2, a fluence of 5 J/cm^2, for 7 seconds, delivering a total of 0.14 J), significantly accelerated tissue repair through its vascular effects with direct recruitment of pericytes to the injury site (do Valle *et al.*, 2020).

Because of the large number of studies involving wound healing in small mammals in the laboratory that use widely varying parameters, there is no consensus about the ideal parameters for the application of photobiomodulation therapy (PBMT) for tissue repair and pain relief (Enwemeka, 2009). The parameters recommended in this chapter have produced positive clinical results; other parameters may do so as well.

Edema

Edema and swelling are normal responses of the body to inflammation and insult, leading to increased fluid in the tissues. Common causes include direct trauma, allergic response, circulatory compromise, cardiac disease, and metabolic disorders. Photobiomodulation relieves the swelling by improving local circulation and stimulation of the anti-inflammatory cascade. The higher end of the recommended superficial tissue target dosage (4–5 J/cm^2) is usually effective in a single or several laser therapy sessions (Figure 24.2).

Hair Loss

Hair loss in small mammals ranges from slight patchy thinning of the fur to complete alopecia. Many etiologies exist for each species, including ectoparasites, psychogenic barbering, endocrine disorders, metabolic diseases, chemical irritation, thermal burns, bite wounds, or other topical trauma. Regardless of the underlying cause, many of these patients will show hair coat improvement with PBM if the hair follicles are viable. Photobiomodulation addresses the outward clinical manifestation. The underlying etiology should be determined and treated appropriately as well. Initial target doses range from 8 to 10 J/cm^2, depending on the severity of the alopecia, with some recommendations as high as 20 J/cm^2. Superficial traumatic or direct physical insult cases may respond within one to two sessions of PBM, while systemic conditions may require multiple sessions with a plan for long-term maintenance treatments. It is interesting to note that the first report of what we now know of as photobiomodulation was its effect on hair follicles in mice (Mester *et al.*, 1968). Mester noticed a more rapid hair growth on shaven mice that were treated with therapeutic lasers versus nontreated control animals.

Lacerations

Laceration and skin tears are common in exotic small mammals due to their inquisitive nature getting them into

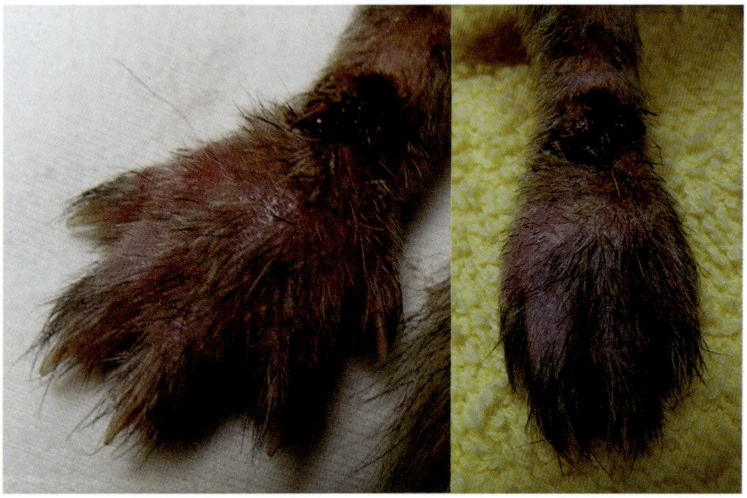

Figure 24.2 Cellulitis of the front paw of a ferret after surgical removal of mast cell tumor over carpus. Note the improvement seen 2 days later after a single photobiomodulation session. *Source:* Courtesy of Dr. Robert D. Ness.

trouble or from bite wounds among housemates. These types of injuries respond well to photobiomodulation and heal much more rapidly with fewer complications than with conventional therapy alone. The usual superficial photobiomodulation target dosing of 1–2 J/cm^2 is usually sufficient in only a few sessions repeated every few days until healed.

A study showing the benefits of photobiomodulation was conducted in rabbits where full thickness wounds (3 × 3 cm) were artificially created and then treated with laser exposure (4 J/cm^2) on days 0, 3, and 6 with a 808 nm diode laser. In the control group, a moist wound dressing was applied. The wound-healing process was evaluated by both gross and pathological assessment and demonstrated that PBM accelerates wound healing in some phases of healing process (Hodjati *et al.*, 2014) (Figure 24.3).

Pododermatitis

Pododermatitis is a common foot lesion encountered in clinical practice, resulting from improper cage flooring and substrate and complicated by obesity and improper hygiene. A recent publication noted that laser therapy has been used to encourage wound healing in a rabbit with pododermatitis (Blair, 2013). In the reported case, the treatments were performed twice weekly for six treatments in conjunction with topical medications, bandages, and improvements in the rabbit's husbandry. Because PBM is often used in conjunction with other therapies, the significance of its role in the resolution of these cases is difficult to determine, but clinicians often report positive results.

Osteoarthritis is a common sequela to pododermatitis, especially in guinea pigs and rabbits. A study in which osteoarthritis was induced in rabbits and then treated with PBM showed a significant improvement in the treated animals. In the study, two different lasers were used. One used 808 nm, with continuous delivery and an output of 1 W. The other used 904 nm, with an intermittent super-pulsed delivery and an average output of 1 W. The study concluded that photobiomodulation is effective in treating osteoarthritis based on superoxide dismutase activity, computed tomography (CT), gross observation, and histopathology, after induction of osteoarthritis. In addition, the study mentioned that no significant difference was seen between the two different laser irradiation methods, but a significant improvement was seen in both PBM groups compared to the osteoarthritis control group (Lee *et al.*, 2014) (Figure 24.4).

Superficial Wounds

In varying animal models, *in vitro* and clinically, wound healing is improved using a variety of different wavelengths and powers. As discussed above with lacerations, it was demonstrated that photobiomodulation accelerates wound healing in rabbits using a dose of 4 J/cm^2 (Hodjati *et al.*, 2014). This dose is representative of what is commonly used clinically. No optimal set of parameters has yet been identified (Kuffler, 2016) and in the literature evidence for both improved wound healing and no observed effect for wound healing is readily available.

In cases where the results of the study do not indicate a significant difference in wound healing when PBM is used, it is important to verify the methodology. In many wound healing studies, the same animal is used as the control. Multiple lesions are created on the same animal, and only

(a) (b)

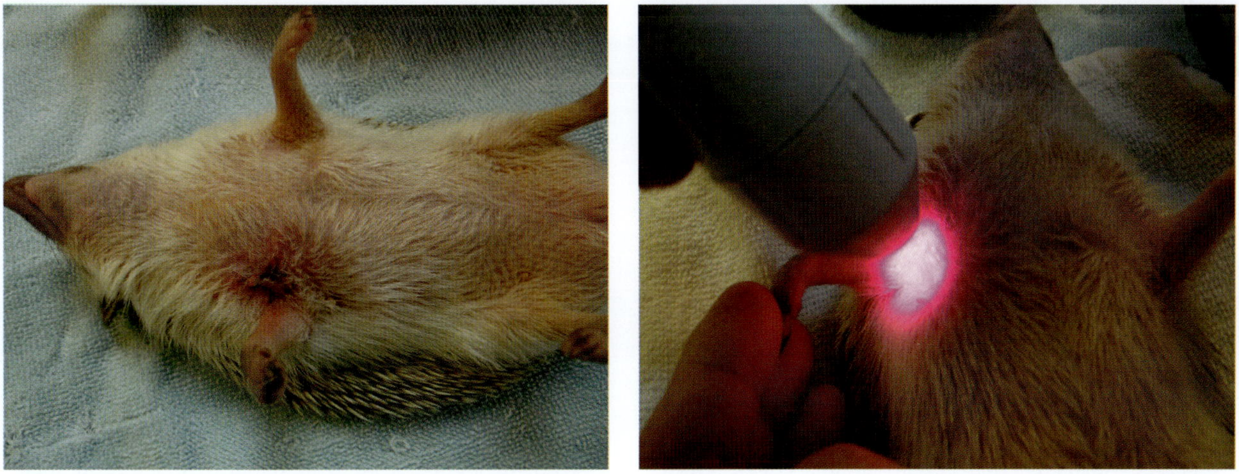

Figure 24.3 (a) Skin tear in the axilla of a hedgehog. (b) Photobiomodulation of skin tear in the axilla of a hedgehog using a superficial wound setting of 2 J/cm^2. *Source:* Courtesy of Dr. Robert D. Ness.

(a) (b)

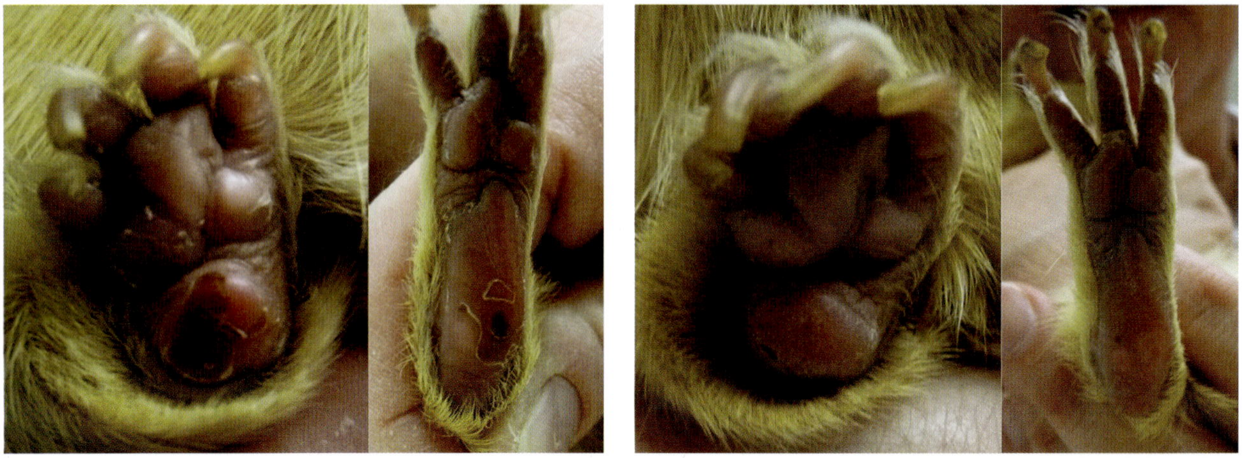

Figure 24.4 (a) Pododermatitis in a guinea pig, which presented with swelling and superficial abrasion of both front and hind foot pads. No significant ulcerations or bony involvment were detected in this case. (b) Full resolution of pododermatitis lesions on both front and hind feet within 1 week of single photobiomodulation session at a superficial lesion setting of 2 J/cm^2. *Source:* Courtesy of Dr. Robert D. Ness.

one lesion is treated with laser therapy while others serve as controls or receive other treatment modalities. Studies have clearly indicated that PBM has additional systemic effects besides the local effects on the treated tissues. Rodrigo *et al.* described a study in which rats were treated with PBM, and healing was more advanced in the wound located furthest from the point of laser application (Rodrigo *et al.*, 2009).

Another study evaluated the systemic effects of local PBM using rats with injuries in the peripheral and central nervous system, skin wounds, and burns. These animals were irradiated with a 632.8 nm laser at a power of 16 mW and different energy densities for 21 days (Gal *et al.*, 2006). In this study the laser was applied only to the right side of the animals after bilateral skin wounds were produced. At the end of the study, the authors observed superior healing of both wounds than in the control group, which did not receive any irradiation. Statistical analysis showed a significant difference between the group treated with PBMT and the control group. The authors concluded that the laser application had a marked systemic effect on the skin and adjacent tissues, as well as on the severely damaged peripheral nerves and the corresponding regions of the marrow. According to the authors, the effects persisted for a long time after laser irradiation. It is suggested that these systemic effects are relevant for the clinical application of laser therapy and for basic research about its possible mechanisms of action. Another study showed that PBMT accelerates the healing process of third-degree burns in rats (Ezzati *et al.*, 2009). These authors concluded that irradiation of a third-degree burn model with an 890 nm pulsed laser delivering 11.7 J/cm^2 in rats significantly increased wound-closure rate compared with control burns. In addition, the statistics also showed that the incidence of *Staphylococcus epidermidis*, *Lactobacillus*, and diphtheria decreased significantly in laser-treated groups compared with other groups.

Surgical Incisions

As with other superficial wounds, incisions treated with photobiomodulation at the conclusion of a surgical procedure appear to heal more rapidly with less inflammation and minimal scarring. Most elective surgery, minor wound closure, or basic dental procedure patients benefit from a single PBMT treatment at 1 J/cm^2 immediately after the procedure. Surgical patients with procedures causing more extensive tissue disruption, such as orthopedic or laparotomy cases, should receive additional treatments at 2–3 J/cm^2, administered every second to third day until healed.

Musculoskeletal

Arthritis

Arthritis is a common consequence of aging in all species. In human medicine, photobiomodulation has been evaluated in the conservative care of knee arthritis and been found to successfully postpone the need for joint replacement (Ip, 2015). In this longitudinal study, which included follow-ups after 6 years, it was concluded that photobiomodulation should be incorporated into standard conservative treatment protocol for symptomatic knee arthritis.

Strong evidence from a systematic review and meta-analysis of the effectiveness of photobiomodulation for nonspecific chronic low back pain in humans indicated that photobiomodulation is an effective method for relieving pain (Huang *et al.*, 2015). Similarly to humans, it has been demonstrated in a comparative evaluation of laser and systemic steroid therapy in adjuvant-enhanced arthritis of rat temperomandibular joints, that photobiomodulation has a long-term promising effect on reducing inflammation severity of temperomandibular joint syndrome, similar to betamethasone in earlier stages (Khozeimeh *et al.*, 2015).

When rats were used as models to evaluate PBMT in different stages of rheumatoid arthritis (RA), photobiomodulation was shown to modulate inflammatory response in early and late progression stages of RA (Alves *et al.*, 2013). In rabbits, it was shown to have significant beneficial effects on joint pain, synovitis, anabolic, and catabolic factors in the progressive osteoarthritis rabbit model (Wang *et al.*, 2014). Similar effects have been shown in osteoarthropathy induced in the rabbit (Cho *et al.*, 2004).

In the clinical setting, PBMT is used to control pain and reduce inflammation of this degenerative condition in exotic small mammals. The initial starting dosage in most cases is about 8–10 J/cm^2, depending on severity and chronicity.

Fractures

Fracture healing is stimulated with the use of photobiomodulation at deep tissue settings of 8–20 J/cm^2. Patients have healed in 25–50% less time compared to those without photobiomodulation. However, the laser light is scattered by bandage material, so fractures cannot be treated through splint or casting material. To overcome this obstacle, practitioners can design the splint or cast with a small window or fenestration over the fracture site that can be accessed during photobiomodulation.

It is interesting to note that in the research setting much higher doses have been used with good success. A study showed that the 830 nm wavelength, at 120 J/cm^2, was able to increase the biomechanical properties and bone mineral density of osteopenic rats without causing side effects (Renno *et al.*, 2006). Thus, current dose recommendations may continue to be adjusted over time.

The reported effects of PBMT on bone regeneration depend not only on the total dose of irradiation but also on the irradiation time, and the irradiation model (Saito & Shimizu, 1997). As early as 1987, evidence existed that the effect of photobiomodulation on fractures produced increased osteoblastic activity, an increased number of blood vessels, and increases in the amount of mineralized bone, speeding up early bone repair (Trelles & Mayayo, 1987). Multiple scientific publications show significant benefits of using photobiomodulation on fracture healing. Studies demonstrate that a variety of wavelengths and doses provided a variety of beneficial effects so it is difficult to recommend the perfect dose.

One publication demonstrated a 10% increase in the amount of mineralized bone in animals irradiated with 790 nm laser light for 7 days (Silva Júnior *et al.*, 2002). The study reported a more positive effect of 830 nm laser light in comparison to lasers emitting 632.8 or 790 nm. This is most likely due to a higher penetration of laser light with a longer wavelength.

The energy delivered to the tissue is as important as the wavelength used when treating fractures. The influence of the power delivered to the area of interest has clearly been identified in a variety of studies (Silva Júnior *et al.*, 2002; Gomes *et al.*, 2015). In one experiment, rabbits received a dental implant and were treated with 5, 10, or 20 J/cm^2. The results clearly indicated a significant improvement in stability of the bone implant in the 20 J/cm^2 group (Gomes *et al.*, 2015).

In a similar study, when PBM at a wavelength of 808 nm was applied at different energy levels ranging from 5 to 25 J/cm^2 to determine the effect on bone regeneration, it was observed that there was significant increase in bone regeneration following the application of 15 J/cm^2 (Kuzu *et al.*, 2022).

High doses were used in another study, and it is interesting to note that there appears to be a ceiling effect: the healing benefits were not significantly different in another experiment where high doses (60 or 120 J/cm^2 at 830 nm) were used on rat fractures. While the results of this study support the notion that laser therapy improves bone repair in the tibia of osteoporotic rats by the stimulation of newly formed bone, fibrovascularization, and angiogenesis, no difference was found between these two doses (Bossini, 2012).

A study showed the benefit of using laser therapy as an adjuvant in combination with calcitonin (Ribeiro *et al.*, 2012). The results of the study showed that photobiomodulation (830 nm) combined with calcitonin improved bone repair and reduced the duration of the bone repair process.

Another study looked at the synergy of using laser therapy and an anti-COX-2 selective drug (celecoxib) on bone repair in the tibia of rats (Ribeiro & Matsumoto, 2008). The results showed that PBM improved bone repair as a result of upregulation of COX-2 expression in bone cells. In the study, the group that received celecoxib and photobiomodulation showed better results when compared to just celecoxib alone, which was better than the control group.

Muscular Sprain and Strain

Muscular sprains and strains in exotic small mammals are treated with photobiomodulation as they are treated in dogs and cats. A target dose of 2–4 J/cm^2 is typically sufficient with only a few sessions repeated over a couple weeks. The underlying causes of the lesions within the muscles and connective tissue are also similar to other companion animals and must be appropriately treated.

Scurvy

Scurvy in guinea pigs is caused by hypovitaminosis C and characterized by inflammation of the temperomandibular joints, limb joints, costochondral joints of the ribs, and the spine. Clinical signs include swelling of limbs, lameness, weakness, poor appetite, loose teeth, hemorrhage, and death. Treatment includes vitamin C supplementation and supportive therapy as indicated by presenting clinical signs. Photobiomodulation is useful in treating the resultant inflammation in the body presenting as swollen and painful joints. The dosage ranges from 1 J/cm^2 for the temperomandibular joint to 8 J/cm^2 in the spine or pelvis, repeated as needed relative to the severity of the inflammation.

Spondylosis

Spondylosis is common in rabbits due to their inherent biomechanics. The spinal arthritis is typically age related, but can also be initiated by spinal trauma or irritation. As with any case of arthritis, analgesia and anti-inflammation can be achieved with PBM. A higher therapeutic dosage of 10 J/cm^2 is often necessary to obtain a consistent therapeutic effect, especially in chronic or advanced cases.

Neurologic Disorders

Evidence of the beneficial effects of laser therapy for spinal cord injury (SCI) and other neurological conditions in small mammals are cumulating in the scientific literature. In one study, rat spinal cords were injured and the lesion sites were directly irradiated with an 808 nm diode laser positioned either perpendicular or parallel to the spine immediately after the injury and daily for 5 consecutive days. The authors found that regardless of the polarization direction, functional scores of SCI rats treated with 808 nm laser light were significantly higher than the untreated group from day 5 after injury. However, the locomotive function of SCI rats irradiated parallel to the spinal column was significantly improved from day 10 after injury, compared to SCI rats treated with the linear polarization perpendicular to the spinal column (Ando *et al.*, 2013).

Two rat models of SCI – one a hemisection SCI and the other a contusion SCI – were used in two studies. In both studies, the authors transcutaneously applied an 810 nm laser, which penetrated to the depth of the injured spinal cord and promoted axonal regeneration and functional recovery (Byrnes *et al.*, 2005; Wu *et al.*, 2009).

These studies demonstrated that laser irradiation significantly suppressed immune cell activation and cytokine and chemokine expression, suggesting that a decrease in the inflammatory response is one of the recovery mechanisms in photobiomodulation for spinal cord repair (Ando *et al.*, 2013).

Selecting the right wavelength and power setting is most likely of clinical importance when treating a small mammal for a neurological problem. A study specifically addressing this point measured the *in vivo* penetration of infrared light applied to the skin of anesthetized rabbits. An average of 2.45% of the light reached the depth of the peroneal nerve (Anders *et al.*, 2014). This *in vivo* pilot study data revealed that the 4 W treatment inhibited nerve regeneration while the 2 W treatment significantly improved axonal regrowth, despite the fact that both groups received a total energy dose of 65 J. Overall the irradiated group performed significantly better in the toe spread reflex test compared to the control group from week seven post-injury.

A recent study on neurogenic pain in mice demonstrated that 808 nm wavelength PBM at a higher energy density of 20 and 40 J/cm^2 was more effective in the control of neuropathic pain (de Andrade *et al.*, 2017). Regarding the management of pain with PBM, the wavelength of the treatment protocol also appears to be significantly important. It has been demonstrated that the effect of PBM depends on the wavelength used, with 800 nm light mainly acting on mitochondrial metabolism, and 970 nm light acting on nociceptive signal transmission (Zupin *et al.*, 2019).

Head and Neck Disorders

Dental Disease

Photobiomodulation has been shown to enhance tissue regeneration and tissue growth, including effects on fibroblastic (Almeida-Lopes *et al.*, 2001) and chondral proliferation (Schultz *et al.*, 1985), collagen synthesis (Majaron *et al.*, 2000), wound healing (Lowe *et al.*, 1998), bone regeneration (Saito & Shimizu, 1997; Ekizer *et al.*, 2015), and nerve regeneration (Anders *et al.*, 2004). These effects mean that photobiomodulation can be used to treat a variety of dental diseases in the exotic small mammal patient. A systematic literature review regarding the effects of PBM on dental surgery patients has shown that a higher concentration of osteogenesis markers was consistently reported across studies and across species (man, rodent, rabbit), as well as a higher percentage of bony trabeculae and bone density. Improvement in bone repair can also be found when photobiomodulation is used on extraction sockets (Kulkarni et *al.*, 2019).

Dental malocclusion is common in rabbit and rodents, ranging from incisor malocclusion with elongation to molar root deviation and abscessation. This disorder results in oral lesions and anorexia in these species. Photobiomodulation is beneficial in controlling pain and inflammation associated with trimming and extraction of the affected teeth, as well as healing of the oral soft tissues and subsequent jaw and temporomandibular lesions. A single photobiomodulation session administered at a setting of 2 J/cm^2 can facilitate healing of the mouth following incisor extraction in rabbits and rodents. Therapeutic dosages for molar malocclusion with jaw lesions are 2–4 J/cm^2 and should be administered at least two to three times weekly until appetite returns. Higher photobiomodulation dosages and increased intervals may be indicated in chronic or more severe cases.

Otitis

Otitis and torticollis respond to photobiomodulation when treated at higher therapeutic dosages of at least 10 J/cm^2. The clinical improvement is thought to be the result of reduced inflammation within the vestibular apparatus and healing of deeper tissues within the ear canal. Although the benefit of photobiomodulation on otitis has been demonstrated in humans and companion animals, further evaluation is warranted to assess its clinical effects on torticollis, since current information is based on only a few clinical cases.

Otorhinolaryngol Disorders

The positive effect of photobiomodulation for a variety of otorhinolaryngol problems has been documented in human medicine. Treatment of pollinosis, adenoiditis and rhino-sinusitis, tonsillitis, and otitis with red and infrared laser irradiation led to positive results in 85% of patients (Gogeliia *et al.*, 2006; Nikitin *et al.*, 2008). Data from these studies suggests that similar effects would be expected with photobiomodulation used for comparable otorhinolaryngol disorders in exotic small mammals.

Temporomandibular Disorder

Temporomandibular disorder (TMD) is characterized by pain. It is sometimes a sequela to primary dental disease in small mammals such as guinea pigs. In rats, TMD was experimentally induced and then photobiomodulation applied for 10 minutes daily, starting the day after the confirmation of osteoarthritis. Treatment was at the right side of the temporomandibular joint with an 880 nm laser at 100 mW (Peimani & Sardary, 2014). After 7 days of therapy, the grade of cartilage defects, number of inflammatory cells, number of cell layers, and degree of arthritis improved compared to controls.

Abdominal Disorders

Ascites

Ascites is the resultant accumulation of fluid in the abdominal cavity from a metabolic imbalance causing changes in osmotic pressure and hemodynamic permeability. Classic etiologies in exotic small mammals include hepatic disorders, cardiovascular disease, and cancer. Photobiomodulation is appropriate for treating ascites resulting from hepatic and cardiac diseases. It should be avoided in cases of suspected neoplasia.

A study showed that 904 nm laser irradiation of an induced peritonitis at fluences of 1 and 5 J/cm^2 reversed signs of inflammation indicated by neutrophil infiltration and oxidative stress (de Souza Costa *et al.*, 2018).

Photobiomodulation has the potential effect of decreasing fluid accumulation by improving the cellular integrity of vessels and lymphatics, affecting the cell membrane potential and sodium ion exchange in the abdomen, and reducing inflammation of the tissues. A dose of 7–10 J/cm^2 is recommended.

Gastrointestinal Disorders

Gastrointestinal disorders are common in many exotic small mammals kept as pets. Conditions ranging from gastrointestinal stasis to gastritis, and inflammatory bowel disease are commonly seen. Malnutrition, gastrointestinal foreign bodies, and trichobezoars can all lead to slowing of gastrointestinal transit and ultimately stasis. Photobiomodulation should be included with other appropriate medical therapies in the management of these cases. In one study using rats with experimental chronic atrophic gastritis, laser treatment showed a good adjuvant therapeutic effect on the rat's gastric mucosa (Yang *et al.*, 2005).

In practice, utilizing photobiomodulation in cases with gastrointestinal disorders at around 7–10 J/cm^2 has greatly improved the recovery of these patients by reducing inflammation and providing abdominal pain relief similar to other deep conditions in companion small animals (Ness, 2016).

Urinary Disorders

Urinary disorders of exotic small mammals include cystitis and cystic calculi. They can be positively affected with photobiomodulation by reducing inflammation of the bladder and managing pain experienced by the patient. The target dosage is calculated from approximating the entire three-dimensional area that the bladder and other affected tissues occupy in the abdomen. Certain laser therapy units have specific preset parameters intended for treating the urinary tract, while others may have abdominal settings that are typically calculated for the entire abdominal cavity.

Therefore, it is prudent to integrate one's own starting target dose of approximately 6–8 J/cm^2, until confident with the laser device and its software. Depending on the degree of inflammation, the effective dose may be significantly higher or lower than the device's proposed dosage or preset. In addition, the frequency of photobiomodulation treatments will depend on the case, ranging from daily in severe acute cases to possibly weekly in chronic low-grade conditions.

Older rats often suffer from glomerulonephritis, and photobiomodulation has the potential to be used for its direct treatment. It has been demonstrated that externally-directed photobiomodulation suppresses the activity of rat anti-GBM crescentic glomerulonephritis (Yamato *et al.*, 2013).

Thoracic Disorders

Laryngitis

Intubation can be challenging in some exotic small mammal patients. Blind intubation is often performed, which carries an inadvertent risk of laryngeal damage and inflammation. The placement of a nasogastric tube is often associated with laryngitis in humans (Lima-Rodrigues *et al.*, 2008). Multiple studies in rats with experimentally induced laryngitis followed by laser therapy treatment have demonstrated that photobiomodulation is potentially useful to control reflux laryngitis secondary to nasogastric intubation. Photobiomodulation reduces the influx of neutrophils to the injured area and improves the reparative collagenization of the laryngeal tissues (Marinho *et al.*, 2013a, 2013b).

Bronchitis and Pneumonia

Bronchitis and pneumonia cases can benefit from PBM through reduced inflammation, increased leukocyte activity, and improved fluid resorption in any species. Rats with mycoplasma pneumonia develop poor compliance to the chest from dramatically increased inflammation and congestion in their lungs. Investigating the use of PBM regarding the resolution of inflammation during acute lung injury (ALI) induced by sepsis showed that treatment (660 nm, 100 mW of power, a fluence of 5 J/cm^2, and an Irradiance of 33.3 mW/cm^2), attenuated ALI by modulating the cell mobilization from their reserve compartments (da- Palma-Cruz *et al.*, 2019). While this treatment mentioned above appears to be very low energy when compared to other treatments, another study using a similarly low energy density showed similar results (Brochetti et *al.*, 2017).

PBM applied to the thorax once a day for 8 days (wavelength 660 ± 20 nm, power 100 mW, fluence 5 J/cm^2, irradiance 33.3 mW/cm^2) showed that PBM significantly reduced the number of inflammatory cells in the alveolar space, collagen production, interstitial thickening, and static and dynamic pulmonary elastance (Brochetti et *al.*, 2017).

Patients who are difficult to manage with standard treatments alone can show clinical improvement with the addition of photobiomodulation at approximately 8 J/cm^2. The same results are seen in rabbits with *Pasteurella multocida* or guinea pigs with *Bordetella bronchiseptica*.

Pulmonary Congestion and Pleural Edema

Pulmonary congestion and pleural effusion occur in respiratory cases involving excess fluid accumulation within (pulmonary congestion) or around (pleural effusion) the lungs. Photobiomodulation assists with the resorption of excess fluid through improved circulation and osmotic pressure changes. Target dosing for pulmonary congestion starts at 6–8 J/cm^2, while pleural effusion requires a higher target dose of at least 10 J/cm^2 to show clinical improvement.

Pulmonary Ischemia

A study evaluated the effect of PBM on remote organ injury of the lung induced by skeletal muscle ischemia and reperfusion. The animals' hindlimbs were subjected to ischemia induced by femoral artery occlusion followed by reperfusion. They were then treated with laser therapy applied to the skin over the right upper bronchus at varying intervals afterward. The study found that PBM alleviated the lung tissue injuries following skeletal muscle ischemia and reperfusion in this experimental model (Ashrafzadeh Takhtfooladi *et al.*, 2015).

Summary

A wealth of information is available about the use of photobiomodulation in mammals. Knowledge continues to grow as practitioners in both human and veterinary fields realize the potential of this phenomenal modality. Much of the information available in the literature regarding photobiomodulation in the exotic small mammal species is from research for human and companion animal applications. As with all other species, virtually any condition affecting an exotic small mammal that benefits from analgesia, anti-inflammation, and increased rate of healing can improve with PBMT.

The information provided here is intended as a starting point from which to expand the use of photobiomodulation in exotic small mammals. Although many of the common disorders treated in exotic pet practice have been presented, this is not an exhaustive list. The authors hope the information provided here will encourage and stimulate the use of this treatment modality in exotic pet practice.

Practitioners are also encouraged to add to this practical knowledge base by documenting and reporting their own PBM applications, the use of which is constrained only by one's imagination and ingenuity.

When applying this modality, the authors encourage documentation of treatment parameters as detailed as possible, including but not limited to wavelength and dose (J/cm^2), in order to standardize the treatment and to facilitate communication with other clinicians.

References

da- Palma-Cruz, M. *et al.* (2019). Photobiomodulation modulates the resolution of inflammation during acute lung injury induced by sepsis. *Lasers Med Sci.* 34(1):191–199.

Almeida-Lopes, L. *et al.* (2001). Comparison of the low level laser therapy effects on cultured human gingival fibroblasts proliferation using different irradiance and same fluence. *Lasers Surg Med.* 29(2):179–184.

Alves, A.C. *et al.* (2013). Low-level laser therapy in different stages of rheumatoid arthritis: a histological study. *Lasers Med Sci.* 28(2):529–536.

Al-Watban, F.A.H. and Zhang, X.Y. (1999). The acceleration of wound healing is not attributed to laser skin transmission. *Laser Ther.* 11(1):6–10.

Anders, J.J. *et al.* (2004). Phototherapy promotes regeneration and functional recovery of injured peripheral nerve. *Neurol Res.* 26(2):233–239.

Anders, J.J. *et al.* (2014). In vitro and in vivo optimization of infrared laser treatment for injured peripheral nerves. *Lasers Surg Med.* 46(1):34–45.

Ando, T. *et al.* (2013). Low-level laser therapy for spinal cord injury in rats: effects of polarization. *J Biomed Opt.* 18(9):098002.

de Andrade, A.L.M. *et al.* (2017). Effect of photobiomodulation therapy (808 nm) in the control of neuropathic pain in mice. *Lasers Med Sci.* 32(4):865–872.

Ashrafzadeh Takhtfooladi, M. *et al.* (2015). Effect of low-level laser therapy on lung injury induced by hindlimb ischemia/reperfusion in rats. *Lasers Med Sci.* 30(6):1757–1762.

Blair, J. (2013). Bumblefoot: a comparison of clinical presentation and treatment of pododermatitis in rabbits, rodents, and birds. *Vet Clin North Am Exot Anim Pract.* 16(3):715–735.

Bossini, P.S. (2012). Low level laser therapy (830 nm) improves bone repair in osteoporotic rats: similar outcomes at two different dosages. *Exp Gerontol.* 47(2):136–142.

Brochetti, R.A. *et al.* (2017). Photobiomodulation therapy improves both inflammatory and fibrotic parameters in experimental model of lung fibrosis in mice. *Lasers Med Sci.* 32(8):1825–1834.

Byrnes, K.R. *et al.* (2005). Light promotes regeneration and functional recovery and alters the immune response after spinal cord injury. *Lasers Surg Med.* 36(3):171–185.

Cho, H.J. *et al.* (2004). Effect of low-level laser therapy on osteoarthropathy in rabbit. *In Vivo.* 18(5):585–591.

Demidova-Rice, T.N. *et al.* (2007). Low-level light stimulates excisional wound healing in mice. *Lasers Surg Med.* 39(9):706–715.

Ekizer, A. *et al.* (2015). Effect of LED-mediated-photobiomodulation therapy on orthodontic tooth movement and root resorption in rats. *Lasers Med Sci.* 30(2):779–785.

Enwemeka, C.S. (2009). Intricacies of dose in laser phototherapy for tissue repair and pain relief. *Photomed Laser Surg.* 3:387–393.

Ezzati, A. *et al.* (2009). Low-level laser therapy with pulsed infrared laser accelerates third-degree burn healing process in rats. *J Rehabil Res Dev.* 46(4):543.

Gal, P. *et al.* (2006). Histological assessment of the effect of laser irradiation on skin wound healing in rats. *Photomed Laser Surg.* 24(4):480–488.

Gogeliia, A. *et al.* (2006). Experience on treatment of children with otorhinolaryngological diseases by low intensity laser irradiation. *Georgian Med News.* 130:84–86.

Gomes, F.V. *et al.* (2015). Low-level laser therapy improves peri-implant bone formation: resonance frequency, electron microscopy, and stereology findings in a rabbit model. *Int J Oral Maxillofac Surg.* 44(2):245–251.

Hendler, K.G. *et al.* (2021). Comparison of photobiomodulation in the treatment of skin injury with an open wound in mice. *Lasers Med Sci.* 36(9):1845–1854.

Hodjati, H. *et al.* (2014). Low-level laser therapy: an experimental design for wound management: a case-controlled study in rabbit model. *J Cutan Aesthet Surg.* 7(1):14–17.

Huang, Z. *et al.* (2015). The effectiveness of low-level laser therapy for nonspecific chronic low back pain: a systematic review and meta-analysis. *Arthritis Res Ther.* 17:360.

Ip, D. (2015). Does addition of low-level laser therapy (LLLT) in conservative care of knee arthritis successfully postpone the need for joint replacement? *Lasers Med Sci.* 30(9):2335–2339.

Khozeimeh, F. *et al.* (2015). Comparative evaluation of low-level laser and systemic steroid therapy in adjuvant-enhanced arthritis of rat temporomandibular joint: a histological study. *Dent Res J.* 12(3):215–223.

Kuffler, D.P. (2016). Photobiomodulation in promoting wound healing: a review. *Regen Med.* 11(1):107–122.

Kulkarni, S. *et al.* (2019). Efficacy of photobiomodulation on accelerating bone healing after tooth extraction: a systematic review. *Lasers Med Sci.* 34(4):685–692.

Kuzu, T.E. *et al.* (2022). Effect of photobiomodulation therapy on peri-implant bone healing in extra-short implants in a rabbit model: a pilot study. *Photobiomodulation Photomed Laser Surg.* 40(6):402–409.

Lee, K.C. *et al.* (2013). Safety of cosmetic dermatologic procedures during pregnancy. *Dermatologic Surg.* 39(11):1573–1586.

Lee, J.Y. *et al.* (2014). Healing effects and superoxide dismutase activity of diode/Ga-As lasers in a rabbit model of osteoarthritis. *In Vivo.* 28(6):1101–1106.

Lima-Rodrigues, M. *et al.* (2008). A new model of laryngitis: neuropeptide, cyclooxygenase, and cytokine profile. *Laryngoscope.* 118(1):78–86.

Lopez, A. and Brundage, C. (2019). Wound photobiomodulation treatment outcomes in animal models. *J Vet Med.* 2019:6320515.

Lowe, A.S. *et al.* (1998). Effect of low intensity monochromatic light therapy (890 nm) on a radiation-impaired, wound-healing model in murine skin. *Lasers Surg Med.* 23(5):291–298.

Majaron, B. *et al.* (2000). Deep coagulation of dermal collagen with repetitive Er:YAG laser irradiation. *Lasers Surg Med.* 26(2):215–222.

Marinho, R.R. *et al.* (2013a). Potentiated anti-inflammatory effect of combined 780 nm and 660 nm low level laser therapy on the experimental laryngitis. *J Photochem Photobiol B.* 121:86–93.

Marinho, R.R. *et al.* (2013b). Potential anti-inflammatory effect of low-level laser therapy on the experimental reflux laryngitis: a preliminary study. *Lasers Med Sci.* 29(1):239–243.

Mendez, T.M. *et al.* (2004). Dose and wavelength of laser light have influence on the repair of cutaneous wounds. *J Clin Laser Med Surg.* 22(1):19–25.

Mester, E. *et al.* (1968). The effect of laser beams on the growth of hair in mice. *Radiobiol Radiother.* 9(5):621–626.

Mokmeli, S. *et al.* (2009). The application of low-level laser therapy after cesarean section does not compromise blood prolactin levels and lactation status. *Photomed Laser Surg.* 27(3):509–512.

Myakishev-Rempel, M. *et al.* (2012). A preliminary study of the safety of red light phototherapy of tissues harboring cancer. *Photomed Laser Surg.* 30(9):551–558.

Ness, R.D. (2016). Photobiomodulation in exotic pet practice. In: *Proceedings CE at SEA: Raising the Standard of Veterinary Care with Laser Therapy.* The American Institute of Medical Laser Applications. 22–26 February 2016, Fort Lauderdale.

Nikitin, A.V. *et al.* (2008). Effectiveness of laser puncture in elderly patients with bronchial asthma accompanied by chronic rhinosinusitis. *Adv Gerontol.* 21(3):424–426.

Peimani, A. and Sardary, F. (2014). Effect of low-level laser on healing of temporomandibular joint osteoarthritis in rats. *J Dent.* 11(3):319–327.

Renno, A.C. *et al.* (2006). Effects of 830-nm laser, used in two doses, on biomechanical properties of osteopenic rat femora. *Photomed Laser Surg.* 24(2):202–206.

Ribeiro, D.A. and Matsumoto, M.A. (2008). Low-level laser therapy improves bone repair in rats treated with anti-inflammatory drugs. *J Oral Rehabil.* 35(12):925–933.

Ribeiro, T.P. *et al.* (2012). Low-level laser therapy and calcitonin in bone repair: densitometric analysis. *Int J Photoenergy.* 2012:829587.

Rodrigo, S.M. *et al.* (2009). Analysis of the systemic effect of red and infrared laser therapy on wound repair. *Photomed Laser Surg.* 27(6):929–935.

Saito, S. and Shimizu, N. (1997). Stimulatory effects of low-power laser irradiation on bone regeneration in midpalatal suture during expansion in the rat. *Am J Orthod Dentofacial Orthop.* 111(5):525–532.

Santana-Blank, L. *et al.* (2012). Concurrence of emerging developments in photobiomodulation and cancer. *Photomed Laser Surg.* 30(11):615–616.

Schultz, R.J. *et al.* (1985). Effects of varying intensities of laser energy on articular cartilage: a preliminary study. *Lasers Surg Med.* 5(6):577–588.

Silva Júnior, A.N. *et al.* (2002). Computerized morphometric assessment of the effect of low-level laser therapy on bone repair: an experimental animal study. *J Clin Laser Med Surg.* 20(2):83–87.

de Souza Costa, M. *et al.* (2018). Photobiomodulation reduces neutrophil migration and oxidative stress in mice with carrageenan-induced peritonitis. *Lasers Med Sci.* 33(9):1983–1990.

Sun, L. *et al.* (2010). Hemodynamic changes of pregnant rats with pre-eclampsia after treatment with low-energy laser irradiation of the chest. *Nan Fang Yi Ke Da Xue Xue Bao.* 30(10):2259–2262.

Trelles, M.A. and Mayayo, E. (1987). Bone fracture consolidates faster with low-power laser. *Lasers Surg Med.* 7(1):36–45.

do Valle, I.B. *et al.* (2020). Photobiomodulation drives pericyte mobilization towards skin regeneration. *Sci Rep.* 10(1):19257.

Wang, P. *et al.* (2014). Effects of low-level laser therapy on joint pain, synovitis, anabolic, and catabolic factors in a progressive osteoarthritis rabbit model. *Lasers Med Sci.* 29(6):1875–1885.

Wu, X. *et al.* (2009). 810 nm wavelength light: an effective therapy for transected or contused rat spinal cord. *Lasers Surg Med.* 41(1):36–41.

Yamato, M. *et al.* (2013). Low-level laser therapy improves crescentic glomerulonephritis in rats. *Lasers Med Sci.* 28(4):1189–1196.

Yang, Y. *et al.* (2005). Effects of He-Ne laser on gastric mucosa in rat with chronic atrophic gastritis. *Sheng Wu Yi Xue Gong Cheng Xue Za Zhi.* 22(5):926–929.

Zupin, L. *et al.* (2019). Analgesic effect of photobiomodulation therapy: an in vitro and in vivo study. *J Biophotonics.* 12(10): e201900043.

25

Laser Therapy for Birds

Robert D. Ness[1] *and Jörg Mayer*[2]

[1] *Ness Exotic Wellness Center, Lisle, IL, USA*
[2] *Department of Small Animal Medicine and Surgery, University of Georgia, Athens, GA, USA*

Introduction

To date, very little scientific information is available on the effect of laser therapy on the avian patient in the clinical setting. This chapter accumulates the information currently available from a variety of experimental studies and looks at how it might apply in the clinical setting. In addition, the authors share their clinical experience on the use of laser therapy. A 2015 publication of a round-table discussion shared the clinical experience of the authors and other practitioners using laser therapy in exotic patients (Ritzman *et al.*, 2015). Undoubtedly, the knowledge of how this treatment modality can affect the avian patient will continue to grow. While the general effects of photobiomodulation (PBM) on the avian system will be the same as for other species, anatomical and physiological differences in the avian patient dictate certain adjustments, as outlined in this chapter.

Photobiomodulation therapy (PBMT) has shown well-documented benefits in many species. The purpose of this chapter is to define the science behind this new treatment modality in avian medicine, and to elucidate its practical uses and applications in the clinical setting.

Precautions and Contraindications

Certain safety precautions must be observed for all species when utilizing PBMT, as with any form of medical therapy. This is especially true with birds, due to their high metabolism and thin skin. Most of the precautions and contraindications discussed regarding the avian species are extrapolated from recommendations for other species.

Due to the near-infrared (NIR) wavelength of therapeutic lasers, regulatory agencies require that protective eyewear be worn, appropriate to the laser light wavelengths in use. Everyone in the room, including the patient, must have their eyes protected when the laser is in use, since there is risk of retinal damage from direct exposure to the laser beam, as well as from reflective scatter of the laser light. The bird's eyes can be protected by covering them with a dark cloth or towel. Raptor hoods can be effective eye shields for patients that tolerate them.

Due to the inherent power of some therapy lasers and the relatively thin skin of birds, special considerations should be taken when treating avian species. Adjustments can be made to lower the power density and dose by modifying the delivery mode, power, or time. A pulsed delivery can be utilized to modify the delivery rate instead of a continuous delivery (assuming a 50% duty cycle, the rate of delivery would be thus reduced 50%). Similarly, a lower energy dose can be delivered by decreasing the treatment time or the laser power. Overheating of the skin and feathers is a potential risk from improper operator technique. The pigments in darkly pigmented skin or dark feathers absorb NIR photons and thus overheat easily, requiring caution and adjustment in dosing and administration of laser therapy. Running a finger over the animal behind the laser beam is encouraged, as the temperature of the skin and feathers will immediately be felt as the laser handpiece is moved. If anything other than a pleasant, gentle warming is noted, the handpiece should be moved more quickly, the power reduced, or the spot size enlarged.

Contraindications to PBMT are generally a result of prudence rather than clinical data. A current recommendation is that treatment over malignancy sites is usually considered contraindicated, though some studies suggest PBMT may have an inhibitory effect on some cancerous tissue. A number of published studies confirm that, under certain parameters, PBMT might indeed be safe for use in cancer patients, despite decades of controversy (Myakishev-Rempel *et al.*, 2012; Santana-Blank *et al.*, 2012). The

Laser Therapy in Veterinary Medicine: Photobiomodulation, Second Edition. Edited by Christopher J. Winkler and Lisa A. Miller.

risk-to-benefit ratio should be considered on a case-by-case basis, such as when the analgesic and anti-inflammatory effects of the treatment may outweigh the risk of stimulating a cancerous growth.

It is recommended that prolonged treatment be avoided over certain endocrine organs, such as the thyroid gland and gonads, even though there is minimal suggestion of an adverse effect on these tissues, and the data that are available are contradictory. The effect of PBMT on a developing egg in the oviduct is unknown. Thus, one should avoid PBMT in the breeding hen while gravid. A study using different laser intensities on exposed embryos resulted in different responses in embryologic development (El-Hussein *et al.*, 2021). PBMT has been shown to decrease third-week mortality rates during the developmental phase when fertile chicken eggs are treated once per day on embryonic days 0–20 (Yeager *et al.*, 2006).

Metal implants do not absorb photons, but they do reflect them back into more superficial tissues. The dose of energy should therefore be decreased when delivered to tissue directly over metallic implants, such as bone plates or screws.

Since PBMT increases microcirculation in tissue, treatment of actively hemorrhaging tissue is discouraged.

Clinical Indications

Integumentary Disorders

The skin and feathers of birds are vastly different from the skin and fur of mammals, but many of the same conditions treated by laser therapy in companion mammals can also be treated in birds. In addition, several unique opportunities exist for PBMT of the integument of birds (see Figure 25.1).

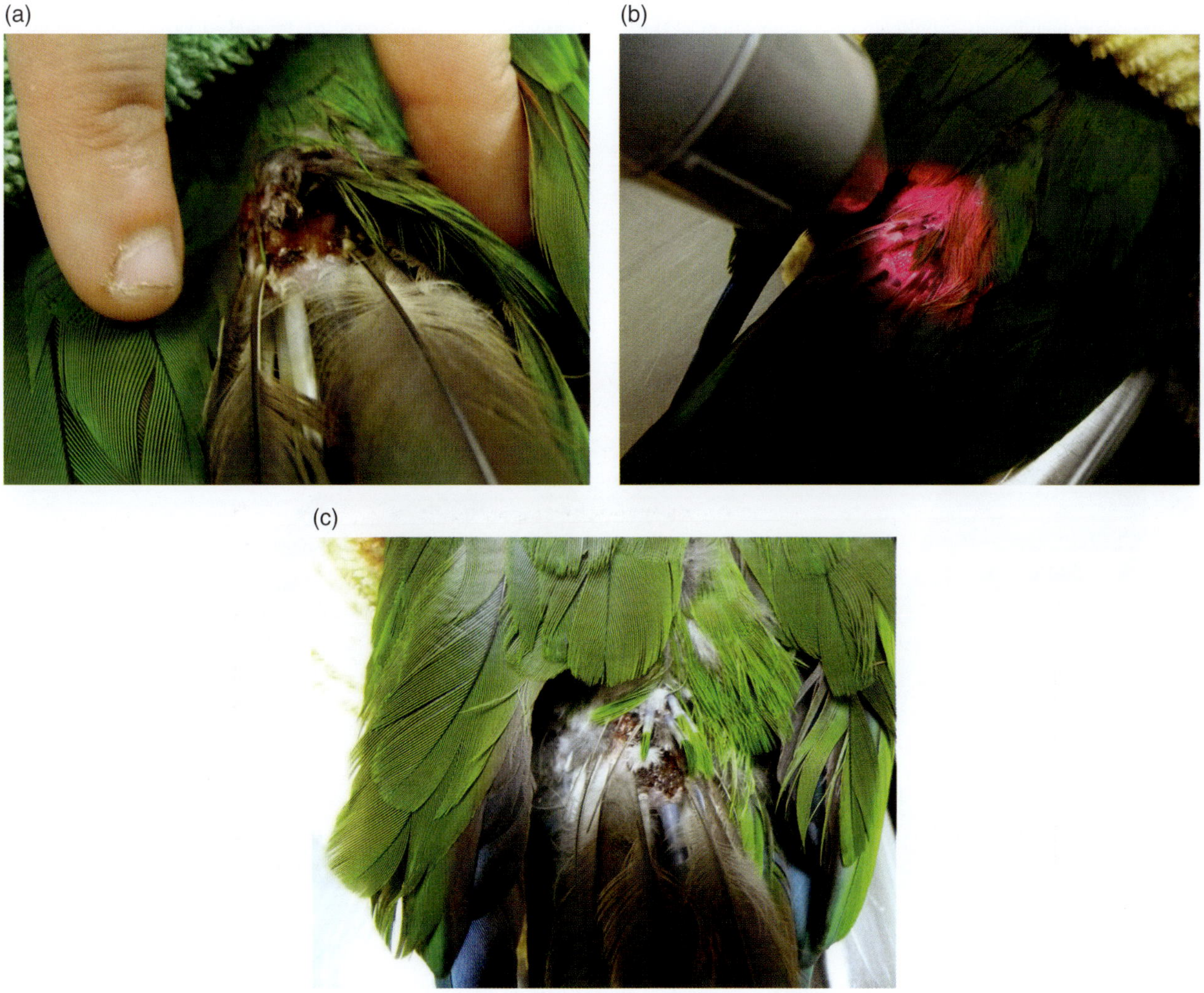

Figure 25.1 (a) Chronic self-mutilation of an impacted uropygial gland in a severe Macaw. (b) Application of laser therapy to the area of the traumatized, impacted uropygial gland. (c) Reduced inflammation and initial healing after laser therapy. Continued application of PBMT is indicated to further the healing process. Images courtesy of Dr. Robert D. Ness.

Deep Wounds

Deep wounds are treated with PBMT in the same manner as in mammals, but at relatively lower target dosages (Figure 25.2). A typical target dose of 4 J/cm^2 is often effective, rather than 6–8 J/cm^2 for a similar lesion in mammals (see Table 25.1). In addition, fewer treatment sessions are necessary to obtain a positive response. A case study involving PBMT as an adjunct therapy with conventional therapy and acupuncture demonstrated the effectiveness in treating a cervical injury with myopathy in an eclectus parrot (*Eclectus roratus*) (Hale-Mitchell *et al.*, 2023). The total energy delivered was 320 J at 2.5 W at both 980 and 810 nm wavelengths for 2 minutes 40 seconds.

Feather Disorders

Feather disorders are very common in birds, and the underlying causes are numerous and varied (Figure 25.3). This may range from snipped or chewed feathers due to overgrooming to complete feather loss due to psychotic feather plucking or underlying metabolic disease. Regardless of the underlying cause, PBMT can benefit patients that still possess some degree of follicular activity. PBM helps by reducing the inflammation of folliculitis and stimulating feather regrowth in quiescent follicles. As for most superficial conditions in birds, the target dose is generally between 2 and 3 J/cm^2 The frequency of treatment can vary greatly, from once every 1–2 days to as little as once a week, depending on the severity of the feather loss or damage and the level of inactivity of the feather follicles (Ness, 2015). Some clinical cases have shown limited response with sessions as infrequent as once a month.

Lacerations

Lacerations and skin tears in birds are treated with PBMT in a similar manner to how they are treated in mammals, except that the target dose is typically lower because of the thinner and more delicate skin (see Table 25.1). A superficial target dose of 2 J/cm^2 is typically sufficient, with only one to two sessions normally required.

Patagium Restriction

Patagium restriction is one of the unique conditions in birds for which PBMT is among the more promising therapies. The patagium often becomes limited in its range of motion due to fibrous tissue constriction following trauma to the tissue itself, or secondary to decreased range of motion of the wing due to arthritis or trauma. The authors' personal experience with clinical cases of patagium restriction indicates that PBMT can help reduce fibrous tissue and improve the elasticity of soft tissue, aiding in restoring a wider range of motion with treatment. We recommend a superficial target dose of 4–6 J/cm^2. This treatment appears to be effective in just a few sessions, scheduled at several-day intervals.

(a)

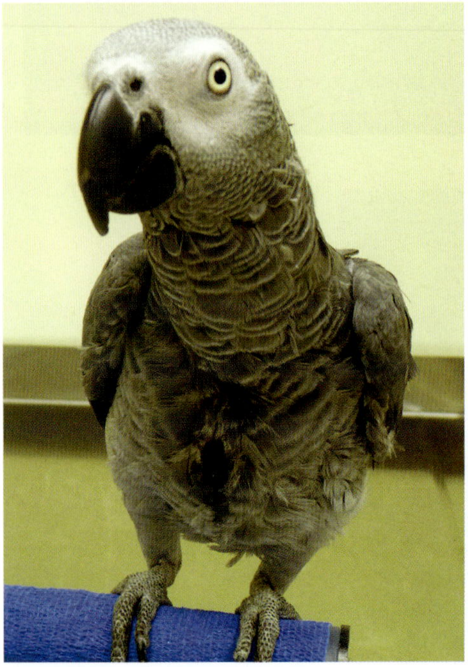

(b)

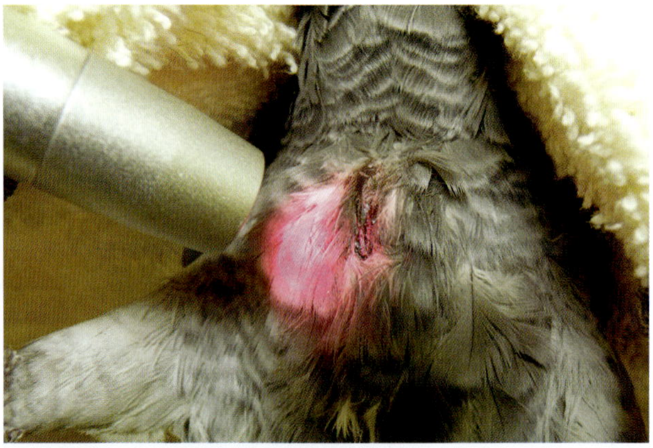

Figure 25.2 (a) African gray parrots are known for keel trauma from falling after over-trimming of their wings. (b) PBMT of the keel wound promotes healing of the lesion and helps minimize scar-tissue formation. Image courtesy of Dr. Robert D. Ness.

Table 25.1 Laser therapy dose recommendations for birds.

Disorders	Recommended dosage (J/cm^2)
Integumentary disorders	
Deep wounds	4
Feather disorders	2–3
Lacerations	2
Patagium restriction	4–6
Pododermatitis	3–4
Self-mutilation	2–4
Surgical incisions	1
Thermal burns	1
Musculoskeletal disorders	
Arthritis	4–8
Articular gout	6–8
Edema	1–3
Fractures	4–8
Muscular sprain and strain	4–8
Splayed legs	4–8
Wing-tip trauma	1–2
Coelomic cavity disorders	
Ascites	4–6
Gastrointestinal disorders	4–6
Renal disease	4
Miscellaneous	
Neuropathic pain	2

Though the response may be limited in severe cases, some birds can regain flight after successful therapy.

Pododermatitis

Pododermatitis is commonly referred to as "bumble foot" in birds, particularly in birds of prey. It can be quite severe and is often a challenge to treat, but typically responds favorably to PBMT as an adjunctive therapy. A case study of a northern bobwhite (*Colinus virginianus*) with bilateral pododermatitis demonstrated the effectiveness of PBMT by comparing the healing response between a laser-treated foot and the untreated (control) foot (Howard *et al.*, 2023). Comparable results have been documented in other avian species, including Megellanic penguins (*Spheniscus megellanicus*), ducks, and red-tailed hawks (*Buteo jamaicensis*). A dose of 3–4 J/cm^2 is usually sufficient in even the more complicated cases (Blair, 2013). Several laser therapy sessions may be necessary over a few weeks to elicit a successful outcome.

Self-Mutilation

Self-mutilation is a common condition in certain species of bird, and is usually related to underlying stress and other psychological issues. These cases are often aggravated by secondary infections and complications. PBMT can serve as an adjunctive therapy by reducing inflammation and pain at the trauma site, deterring the patient from further mutilation as well as reducing the healing time and minimizing scar-tissue formation. Depending on the depth of

(a)

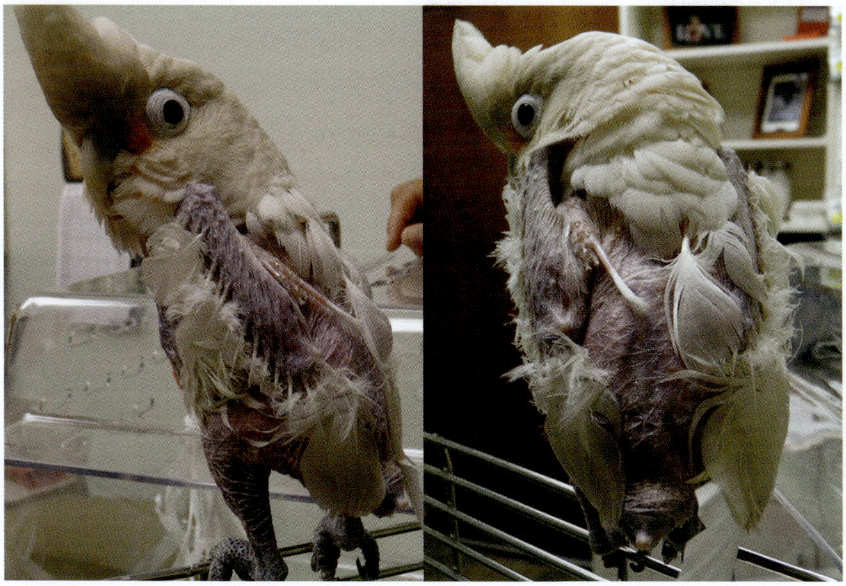

(b)

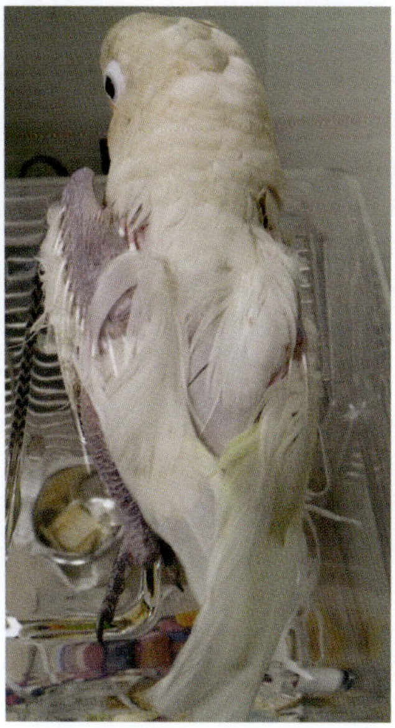

Figure 25.3 (a) Chronic feather plucking in a Goffins cockatoo. Self-induced feather trauma is common in many parrot species. Feather plucking stems from behavioral, hormonal, metabolic, and infectious etiologies, which must be addressed to enable a successful resolution. (b) Feather regrowth after several laser therapy sessions. PBMT stimulates feather growth by increasing follicular activity and reducing inflammation of feather follicles. Images courtesy of Dr. Robert D. Ness.

the lesions and the severity of mutilation, these cases typically require a moderate target dose of 2–4 J/cm^2 Self-mutilation cases usually require a minimum of twice-weekly treatment sessions until the healing is complete.

Surgical Incisions

As in other species, surgical incisions can be treated postoperatively in birds. A single brief PBMT session of approximately 1 J/cm^2 is usually effective in reducing postoperative pain and speeding the healing process of the surgical wound. Be cautious when hemorrhage is possible, since PBMT increases microcirculation in tissues, and do not treat over the surgical site from which a malignancy has been removed.

Thermal Burns

Though presentations of thermal burns in avian species will only rarely be seen, such injuries benefit from PBMT being a part of the overall management protocol. A case of extensive skin wound management from burn injuries was treated with 1 J/cm^2, and a dramatic improvement was noted in the first 48 hours (Zehnder *et al.*, 2007).

Musculoskeletal Disorders

Arthritis

Arthritis in avian species can result from age, metabolic dysfunction, or trauma. Regardless of the predisposing factors, the pain and inflammation associated with arthritic joints can be managed with appropriate use of laser therapy. A target dose of 4–8 J/cm^2 is administered as often as once a day in acute cases. Chronic cases may initially be treated several times a week, followed by long-term maintenance treatments every 10–14 days. Most avian cases of arthritis are treated on an as-needed basis once the initial pain and joint restriction is relieved. The ultimate therapeutic goal is management of the arthritic symptoms, but significant improvement in joint function and stability is possible with PBMT.

Articular Gout

Articular gout is a painful and debilitating condition associated with uric acid deposition in the joints of birds. PBMT reduces the pain and inflammation of affected joints, as in other arthritic conditions. In response to treatment, some cases can have a significant decrease in the swelling of joints from uric acid deposition. The target dose for articular gout is generally at the higher end of the recommended arthritic settings, typically around 6–8 J/cm^2.

Edema

Edematous swelling is a normal response of the body to injury or inflammation leading to increased fluid in the tissues. Common causes in birds, as in other species, include direct trauma, circulatory constriction, allergy, metabolic disease, and cardiac disease. PBMT relieves the swelling by improving circulation and stimulating anti-inflammatory cascades. Utilizing superficial target doses of 1–3 J/cm^2 is usually effective in a single or several PBMT sessions.

Fractures

Fractures in birds tend to heal more rapidly than comparable injuries in mammals, but they can heal quicker still, with less inflammation and pain, when PBMT is incorporated into their treatment (Figure 25.4). Avian practitioners have reported fractures healing in half the expected time when laser therapy was added to the overall fracture-management plan.

Tibia-tarsal fractures in cockatiels heal within 2–3 weeks when using a laser at 4–6 J/cm^2 twice weekly for 2 weeks, along with proper splinting of the fracture site. Lower target dosages can be administered more frequently to elicit similar results.

Fractures of the carpus or radius and ulna heal similarly in small to medium-sized birds, while larger parrots and raptors may take an additional week. Depending on the size of the patient and the bone that is fractured, a higher dose of 4–8 J/cm^2 may be required in some larger birds.

A bill fracture in a duck was managed with a dose of 1 J/cm^2 administered once daily for 4–5 days. The clinicians reported an increased rate of granulation and overall wound healing during the course of treatment (Zehnder *et al.*, 2007). A pilot study evaluating the addition of PBMT to other treatments of bone fractures in wild birds noted that preliminary observations suggested PBMT might be beneficial in promoting bone healing in birds (Desprez *et al.*, 2015).

Muscular Strain and Sprain

Muscular strains or sprains in birds are treated with PBMT as in other mammals, but at a lower target dose of 4–8 J/cm^2. Usually, a single PBMT session will result in significant improvement when administered acutely.

Splayed Legs

Splayed legs can appear in chicks as developmental tendon and ligament deformities from a number of underlying etiologies, including improper nesting material or nest box size, certain mineral deficiencies, and congenital deformities. Many cases also involve bowing and deformity of the long bones in the legs. The addition of PBMT to the treatment plan aids in tendon and ligament stability and function, which in turn aids in realignment of the deviated limbs.

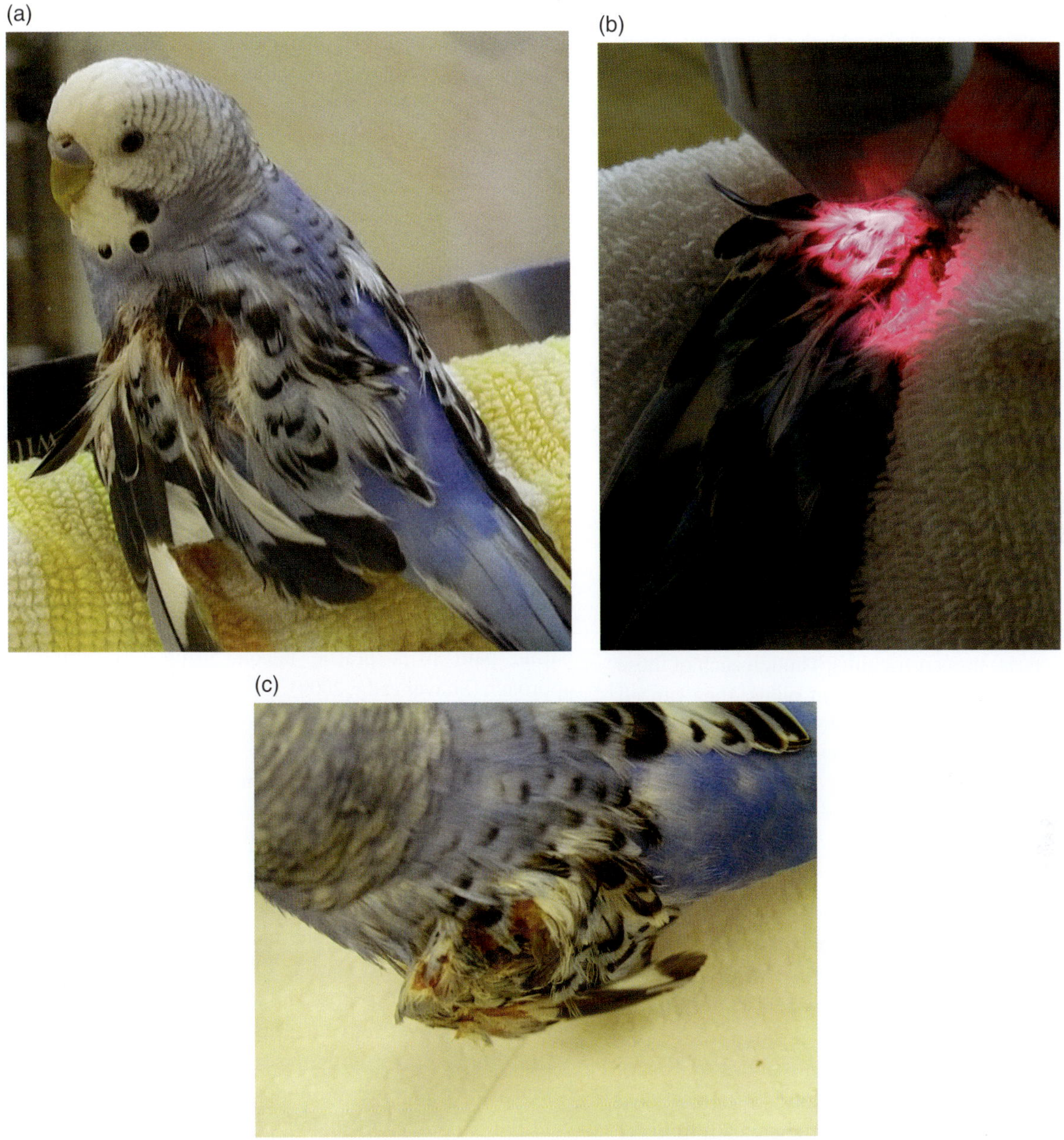

Figure 25.4 (a) Open-wing fracture in a budgerigar, caused by getting its wing caught in the cage bars. This client declined surgery to close the open fracture or amputate the wing. Instead, PBMT, bandaging, and oral medications were chosen for treatment. (b) Application of laser therapy to stimulate fracture repair and wound healing of the injured wing. The wing bandage was removed for laser therapy and reapplied after each session. Another option for bandaged or casted lesions is to leave access windows in the bandage, through which laser therapy can be applied. (c) Good healing response of the fractured wing was present after 1 week and three PBMT sessions. The injury was fully healed and the final bandage was removed in less than 3 weeks after the injury. Images courtesy of Dr. Robert D. Ness.

Wing-Tip Trauma

Wing-tip trauma and inflammation are often the result of a startled bird or the consequence of "night fright," when the bird traumatizes its wings by flapping against its cage's bars and accessories. The usual soft-tissue trauma of the carpus leads to swelling and inflammation, which benefit from PBMT. Many of these cases respond well to just one or two treatments at 1–2 J/cm^2.

Coelomic Cavity Disorders

Ascites

Ascites is the retention of fluid within the coelomic cavity of a bird when faced with a variety of metabolic conditions. The avian coelom is comparable to the abdomen in mammals, with the distinction that birds do not possess a diaphragm to separate the thorax from the abdomen.

Conditions that can lead to ascites in birds include hepatic disease, cardiac disease, and reproductive disorders. Reproductive disorders include egg binding, egg yolk peritonitis, cystic ovary, and ovarian or oviduct neoplasia. Neoplastic disease of any coelomic organ may lead to ascites within the coelom, in which case PBMT may be contraindicated. PBMT is an effective means of aiding fluid resorption in cases of non-neoplastic origin when dosed at 4–6 J/cm^2. The use of laser therapy on the coelomic cavity highlights the need to establish an appropriate diagnosis prior to treatment. The differentiation between an inflammatory, infectious, or neoplastic process should be established prior to treating coelomic pathology.

Gastrointestinal Disorders

Gastrointestinal disorders in birds often lead to inflammation and distention of digestive organs, particularly the proventriculus, intestines, and cloaca. Conditions that cause dilation of the proventriculus and intestine in birds include food or foreign-body impaction, heavy-metal toxicity, avian gastric yeast, avian bornavirus disease (Piepenbring *et al.*, 2012), and bacterial proven-triculitis. Though each of these has different etiologies and treatment plans, they can all potentially benefit from PBMT, especially if inflammation is part of the pathological process. The precise target dose varies, depending on severity and underlying etiology, but typically is 4–6 J/cm^2.

Renal Disease

Little is known about the use of PBMT in cases involving avian renal disease. However, in an experimental study in which chicken kidney tissue was insulted with the potent toxin 2,3,7,8-tetrachlorodibenzo-p-dioxin (TCDD), PBMT treatment with 670 nm light at 4 J/cm^2 resulted in a significant benefit to the renal tissue. The results of this study suggest that 670 nm PBMT may be useful as a noninvasive treatment for renal injury resulting from chemically induced cellular oxidative and energy stress (Lim *et al.*, 2008).

Similarly, in another toxicity (dioxin and TCDD) study conducted on developing chicks in the egg, it was shown that embryonic growth and hatching of the chicks was positively influenced in the 670 nm phototherapy treatment group. The therapy resulted in earlier pip times (a small hole created 12–24 hours prior to hatch) and an increased hatchling size and weight in the 200 parts-per-thousand dioxin dose group (Yeager *et al.*, 2006). While these studies explore the effects of PBMT in an experimental setting, knowledge of these data might be valuable when confronted with a clinical case of renal toxicity.

While the beneficial effect of PBMT is of value in the developing chick exposed to a variety of toxins, evidence also exists of its benefit in the normally developing avian embryo. Third-week mortality rates were decreased during the developmental phase when fertile chicken eggs were treated once a day from embryonic days 0–20 with 670 nm LED light at a fluence of 4 J/cm^2 (Yeager *et al.*, 2006). This study might be of interest to avian breeders, especially when dealing with endangered species. It found that there was a 41.5% decrease in mortality rate overall in the chickens treated with light. In addition, body weight, crown–rump length, and liver weight increased as a result of 670 nm phototherapy. Light-treated chickens pipped earlier and had a shorter time between pip and hatch (Yeager *et al.*, 2006).

Miscellaneous

Neuropathic Pain

The importance of appropriate dose and wavelength to the efficacy of treatment was recently demonstrated in a clinical case involving the management of suspected neuropathic pain in a prairie falcon, using a multimodal approach (Shaver *et al.*, 2009). Initially, the falcon was treated with a very low dose (<5 mW, 630–680 nm, 5-second application per site) directed to the skin wounds and healed metacarpus once daily. The falcon failed to improve, and changes to the overall management plan were made. One adjustment was to increase the PBM treatment parameters to a higher dose and longer wavelength (1040 mW, 830 nm, 2 J/cm^2). Clinical signs improved immediately. While in this case the changes in treatment were multimodal (medications were changed as well), the role of the increased and more appropriate laser dose and wavelength may have been part of the more effective treatment.

One author reported improvement in multiple avian patients affected with multiple inflammatory conditions (Gordon, 2011). Unfortunately, the specific settings of the treatment regimens were not provided. It is important to be precise when recording treatment settings in order to duplicate findings in future patients.

Conclusion

This chapter has summarized current knowledge on the use of PBMT in the avian patient. Many disorders common in avian medicine have been presented; however, this is not an exhaustive list of conditions that may benefit from PBMT. In fact, virtually any condition that benefits from analgesia, anti-inflammation, and accelerated rate of healing may show improvement with PBMT. The authors hope the information provided here will encourage and stimulate the use of PBMT in avian patients. When applying this modality, the authors encourage detailed documentation of treatment parameters, including spot-size, surface area, irradiance, power, and especially wavelength and fluence (J/cm^2), in order to standardize the treatment and facilitate communication between clinicians. With proper documentation, evaluation of effectiveness and meaningful recommendations can continue to be made.

References

Blair, J. (2013). Bumblefoot: a comparison of clinical presentation and treatment of pododermatitis in rabbits, rodents, and birds. *Vet Clin North Am Exot Anim Pract.* 16(3):715–735.

Desprez, I. *et al.* (2015). Potential benefit of low level laser in fracture healing in birds an initial assessment. In: *Proceedings of the I-CARE Conference.* I-CARE. April 18–23, Paris.

El-Hussein, A. *et al.* (2021). Photobiomodulation of avian embryos by red laser. *Lasers Med Sci.* 36(6):1177–1189.

Gordon, J. (2011). Cold laser therapy (3LT) in the management of avian inflammatory conditions. In: *Proceedings of the Association of Avian Veterinarians Conference.* Association of Avian Veterinarians. August 6–12, Seattle, WA.

Hale-Mitchell, L.K. *et al.* (2023). Successful treatment of a cervical injury and myopathy using integrative medicine techniques in an eclectus parrot (*Eclectus roratus*) following cervical entrapment. *J Avian Med Surg.* 37 (2):175–179.

Howard, L. *et al.* (2023). Effects of a therapeutic laser on pododermatitis: a case study in a Northern Bobwhite (*Colinus virginianus*). In: *Proceeding of 43rd Annual AZVT Conference*, p. 17. Corpus Christi, TX, October 7-11, 2023.

Lim, J. *et al.* (2008). Attenuation of TCDD-induced oxidative stress by 670 nm photobiomodulation in developmental chicken kidney. *J Biochem Mol Toxicol.* 22(4):230–239.

Myakishev-Rempel, M. *et al.* (2012). A preliminary study of the safety of red light phototherapy of tissues harboring cancer. *Photomed Laser Surg.* 30(9):551–558.

Ness, R.D. (2015). Laser therapy in avian patients. In: *Proceedings of the Association of Avian Veterinarians Conference.* Association of Avian Veterinarians. August 29–September 2, San Antonio, TX.

Piepenbring, A.K. *et al.* (2012). Pathogenesis of avian bornavirus in experimentally infected cockatiels. *Emerg Infect Dis.* 18(2):234–241.

Ritzman, T.K. *et al.* (2015). Therapeutic laser treatment for exotic animal patients. *J Avian Med Surg.* 29(1):69–73.

Santana-Blank, L. *et al.* (2012). Concurrence of emerging developments in photobiomodulation and cancer. *Photomed Laser Surg.* 30(11):615–616.

Shaver, S.L. *et al.* (2009). A multimodal approach to management of suspected neuropathic pain in a prairie falcon (*Falco mexicanus*). *J Avian Med Surg.* 23(3):209–213.

Yeager, R.L. *et al.* (2006). Brief report: embryonic growth and hatching implications of developmental 670-nm phototherapy and dioxin co-exposure. *Photomed Laser Surg.* 24(3):410–413.

Zehnder, A. *et al.* (2007). Physical rehabilitation in exotic species. In: *Proceedings of the Association of Avian Veterinarians Conference.* Association of Avian Veterinarians. August 5, Providence, RI.

26

Laser Therapy in Reptiles

Jörg Mayer[1] and Robert D. Ness[2]

[1] Department of Small Animal Medicine and Surgery, University of Georgia, Athens, GA, USA
[2] Ness Exotic Wellness Center, Lisle, IL, USA

Introduction

Very little is documented scientifically on the effect and efficacy of photobiomodulation in reptiles. Most of the evidence in this subset of the exotic patient population comes from personal experience, which is shared at conferences or in internet forums. At first glance, this may seem to devalue a clinician's expertise and reasoning, but "...evidence-based medicine (EBM) requires the integration of the best research evidence with our clinical expertise and our patient's unique values and circumstances" (Straus *et al.*, 2005).

Veterinarians have modified the definition slightly to describe evidence-based veterinary medicine (EBVM) since animal patients cannot communicate their values to us. "EBVM is a process of clinical decision-making that allows veterinarians to find, appraise, and integrate current best evidence with individual clinical expertise, clients' wishes, and patients' needs" (Schmidt, 2007). A good understanding of basic treatment principals and laser mechanics is very valuable when starting to treat reptiles, as very little scientific and peer reviewed material is currently available.

Nardini and Bielle point out that the wavelength used during the treatment has significant limitations. In their opinion, 685 nm light is very helpful to treat superficial and fresh wounds of the skin, exposed organs (such as those following carapacial fractures in Chelonians), and lesions on the oral and cloacal mucosa. By contrast, 830 nm light can be employed to reach deeper tissues, such as pericloacal tissues in Chelonians, to reduce swelling after bite trauma, or treatment of granuloma before surgery (Nardini & Bielli, 2011).

Photobiomodulation (PBM) is still in its infancy regarding scientific evidence. A few studies exist to document a potential benefit. However, the majority of data in this field originates from case reports in the clinical field. It is interesting to note that some of these case reports are using a fluence (J/cm^2) that is considered higher than usually recommended in reptiles. The authors recommend starting with lower fluences, and gradually increasing the energy if significant improvement of the condition is not observed. The chapter will highlight individual cases where higher than recommended doses were used with good results.

Precautions and Contraindications

Safety precautions must be observed for all species when utilizing photobiomodulation therapy (PBMT), as with any form of medical therapy. Most of the precautions and contraindications discussed regarding reptiles are extrapolated from dog and cat recommendations with modifications for skin characteristics and general metabolic differences. In general, the frequency of treatment in reptiles is less often then compared to similar conditions in mammals due to reptiles' relatively slower metabolic rate.

Due to the near-infrared (NIR) wavelength of therapeutic lasers, regulatory agencies require that protective eyewear appropriate to laser light wavelength be worn to prevent injury to the retina. Everyone in the room, including the patient, must have their eyes protected during laser therapy, since there is risk of retinal damage from direct exposure to the laser beam, as well as reflective scatter of the laser light. The patient's eyes may be protected simply by covering them with a dark cloth or towel.

Due to the inherent power of some therapy lasers in contrast to the small size of many reptile species, extra care should be exercised when using such devices in these patients. Smaller patients require a lower therapeutic dosing. The adjustments can be made by modifying the delivery mode, power, or time. A pulsed delivery can be utilized to modify the delivery rate instead of a continuous delivery

Laser Therapy in Veterinary Medicine: Photobiomodulation, Second Edition. Edited by Christopher J. Winkler and Lisa A. Miller.

(assuming a 50% duty cycle, the rate of delivery would thus be reduced 50%). Similarly, a lower energy dose can be delivered by decreasing the treatment time or the laser power.

Overheating of the skin is a potential risk of improper operator technique. Darkly pigmented skin or shells absorb photons, leading to overheating, thereby requiring caution in dosing and administration of photobiomodulation. Running a finger behind the laser beam over the animal is encouraged, as the operator will immediately feel the temperature of the skin and scales as the laser handpiece is moved. If any sensation other than a pleasant, gentle warming is noted, the therapist should either increase the handpiece speed, reduce the power, or enlarge the spot size.

Contraindications to photobiomodulation are generally a result of prudence rather than clinical data. A current recommendation is that treatment over malignancy sites is usually considered contraindicated, however some studies suggest photobiomodulation may have an inhibitory effect on some cancerous tissue in mammals (Myakishev-Rempel *et al.*, 2012; Santana-Blank *et al.*, 2012). The risk-to-benefit ratio should be considered for each case, because the analgesic and anti-inflammatory effects of the treatment may be of greater benefit than the risk of stimulating a cancerous growth, such as when the analgesic benefit of PBMT might outweigh the risk of complicating a case of osteosarcoma.

It is recommended to avoid prolonged treatment over certain endocrine organs, such as the thyroid gland and gonads, even though there is minimal and contradictory data suggesting an adverse effect to these tissues.

Metal implants do not absorb photons, but they do reflect them back into more superficial tissues. It is thus prudent to decrease the dose of energy applied directly over metallic implants such as bone plates or screws.

Since photobiomodulation increases microcirculation in tissues, treatment of actively hemorrhaging tissue is discouraged (Table 26.1).

Table 26.1 Laser therapy dose recommendations for reptiles.

Integumentary disorders	
Abscesses	6 J/cm^2
Blister disease	1–2 J/cm^2
Deep wounds	6–10 J/cm^2
Lacerations	5–10 J/cm^2
Rodent bites	10 J/cm^2
Pododermatitis	1–2 J/cm^2 for superficial
	4 J/cm^2 for deep
Surgical incisions	5–10 J/cm^2 for skin
Thermal burns	1–2 J/cm^2 for superficial
	4 J/cm^2 for deep
Oral disorders	
Stomatitis	0.5–1 J/cm^2
Musculoskeletal disorders	
Arthritis	6 J/cm^2
Fibrous osteodystrophy	8–10 J/cm^2
Fractures	8–10 J/cm^2
Muscular sprain and strain	4–6 J/cm^2
Spondylosis	7–10 J/cm^2
Coelomic cavity disorders	
Ascites	6–8 J/cm^2
Egg binding or retention	4–6 J/cm^2.
Constipation and regurgitation	4–10 J/cm^2
Inappetence	4–6 J/cm^2

Clinical Indications

Integumentary Disorders

Abscesses

Abscesses heal more rapidly when treated with photobiomodulation, a factor important in reptiles whose infections generally take longer to heal then in other species. A deep wound setting of approximately 6 J/cm^2 can expedite the recovery when used in conjunction with appropriate antimicrobial therapy. As expected, smaller and more superficial abscesses can be treated at lower therapeutic doses than deeper lesions that may penetrate beyond the skin and immediate superficial tissues.

Blister Disease

Blister disease is a form of dermatitis caused by poor hygiene and humidity. It is often complicated by secondary infection of the skin lesions if not addressed early. This condition can be resolved with photobiomodulation at superficial wound settings of 1–2 J/cm^2 if treated in the early stages, or as high as 6 J/cm^2 with complicated deep lesions. With correction of the environmental issues and prompt attention with photobiomodulation, these cases may resolve within three sessions.

Deep Wounds

Use of laser therapy was described on a soft-shelled tortoise with deep severe dermal ulcerations (Kraut *et al.*, 2013). Some of the cutaneous lesions were locally treated with laser therapy every fourth day (at a wavelength of 980 nm in continuous wave (CW), using a noncontact delivery with a power of 2–2.5 W). Laser therapy was performed beginning with three applications of 10 seconds per lesion, with a break of a few seconds to avoid heating the tissue, and a power of 2 W for the first three treatments. Laser therapy was continued with a power of 2.5 W and 40 seconds (two applications of 20 seconds each) per lesion. These high levels of power were delivered with a defocusing handpiece at a distance of 10 cm from the irradiated surface. The authors refrained from any topical treatment of the lesions to avoid falsification of the results from laser therapy. Comparing the healing process by inspection, the authors concluded that the irradiated lesions of the carapace, leg, and plastron showed a subjectively better and faster improvement than the untreated ones.

A case of ulcerative dermatitis in a turtle describes the use of a class IV laser at relatively high fluence rate (DiRuzzo *et al.*, 2022). Initially, a fluence range of 6–12 J/cm^2 was delivered to the wounds on the shell every 3 days for two treatments, but then the dose was increased to 15–22 J/cm^2. The authors report that after receiving a total of four PBM treatments over a 17-day period, visible improvement was noted in the treated lesions (DiRuzzo *et al.*, 2022). The energy dose used in this case was significantly higher than commonly recommended dosages for reptiles. No negative side effects of the therapy were observed.

The effects of photobiomodulation therapy on the healing of eastern box turtle shell fractures was investigated using a class 3B laser (Souza *et al.*, 2023). These animals were treated with 250 Hz red light (690 nm wavelength red light-emitting diodes – LEDs) every other day for a total of 2 months. The probe was held approximately 5–8 mm above the fracture site (noncontact delivery) and slowly moved back and forth, over the fracture for 3 minutes (Souza *et al.*, 2023). Unfortunately, fluence was not reported. The study concluded that the photobiomodulation group's fracture site width was significantly decreased between pretreatment and posttreatment measurements, showing that photobiomodulation could be a relatively easy and effective treatment to promote healing of fractured turtle shells (Souza *et al.*, 2023).

Lacerations

Skin lacerations from traumatic injuries can be effectively addressed with photobiomodulation. The successful treatment of two skin lacerations in turtles have been reported (Pelizzone *et al.*, 2014) where treatments were applied by means of a diode laser with a wavelength of 808 nm in CW mode. In both patients, the healing was complete, without any side effects. The authors summarized that, in their experience with PBMT on reptiles, its use has contributed to a 25% reduction in patients' recovery time.

Rodent Bites

Rodent bites are the result of clients feeding live prey to their snakes, and leads to severe damage of the skin and musculature. Considered deep wounds, these are treated with PBM at settings of up to 10 J/cm^2. Recovery is more rapid and complete with the use of photobiomodulation in conjunction with appropriate antibiotic therapy and wound dressing (Figure 26.1).

Pododermatitis

Pododermatitis in lizards and tortoises can be addressed with photobiomodulation as in other species. Superficial lesions can be treated with target doses of 1–2 J/cm^2, while deeper, contaminated wounds may require at least 4 J/cm^2 for effectiveness.

Surgical Incisions

A study was conducted on ball pythons (*Python regius*) to determine the effects of PBM on first-intention incisional wound healing (Cole *et al.*, 2015). The study examined if incisions treated with photobiomodulation would heal more rapidly with less histologic reaction (reduced inflammation, necrosis, and edema) than would untreated control incisions. The results showed no significant difference in wound healing between incisions treated with a therapeutic laser and the control group. However, there were lower

(a) (b)

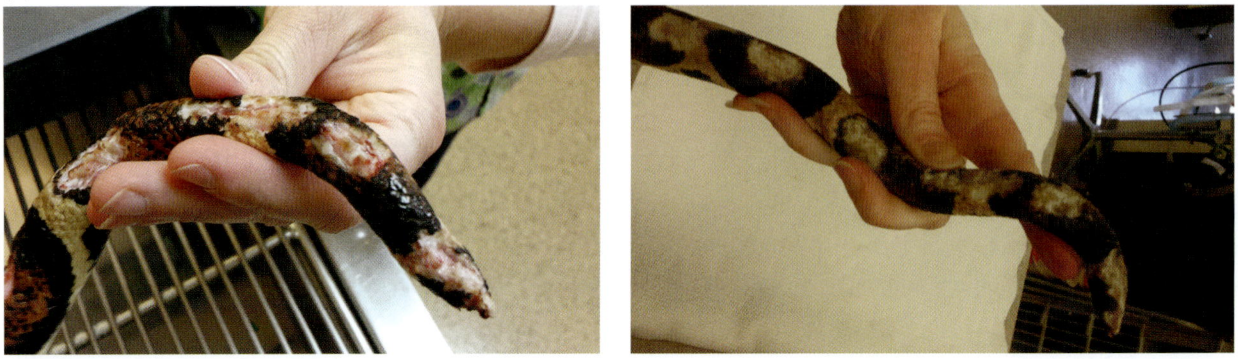

Figure 26.1 (a) Rat bite wounds on tail of boa constrictor caused by leaving live rat in snake's enclosure. (b) Relatively rapid healing of rat bite lesions after three sessions of photobiomodulation administered over 2 weeks.

gross wound scores and an increase in collagen deposition in the laser-treated incisions on day 14. In this study, treatment consisted of a power output of 0.5 W for 90 seconds once daily for 7 consecutive days. The dose delivered to each incision was 5 J/cm^2 with a wavelength of 980 nm emitted in CW. The authors acknowledge that it is possible that the protocols used in this study were insufficient, possibly due to greater reflection or absorption of photons by reptilian scales. A problem with this study is that each animal was treated and no true controls were used to assess the healing effects.

With laser treatment, it has been shown that if an area is treated locally, certain systemic effects can be observed in distant areas; this study in rats showed that the application of laser light directly to standardized skin wounds stimulated their healing, as well as the healing of wounds distant from the point of application (Rodrigo *et al.*, 2009). The authors noted that wounds located where the laser was applied had the worst mean ranks of healing while those in the intermediate position had the best. In conclusion, the study found that a systemic effect of PBMT was found in the wounds located most distally from the point of laser application on the third postoperative day. One of the authors (Mayer) of this chapter is currently conducting a study on wound healing in iguanas where a true control group is being used (and not each animal as its own control) because of the abovementioned systemic effects. At the end of the study, it was noted that wounds treated with PBMT at 10 J/cm^2 were significantly smaller than those treated with PBMT at 5 J/cm^2. On day 14, wounds treated with PBMT at 10 J/cm^2 were significantly smaller than those treated with a topical ointment. Based on these results, it might be suitable to treat skin wounds in iguanas with 10 J/cm^2.

Thermal Burns

Thermal burns are commonly encountered in reptile cases, particularly snakes, from direct contact with heating elements or uncovered flooring with under-tank heating. These lesions can vary from superficial discoloration to full-thickness third-degree burns. Photobiomodulation is quite useful in speeding the healing process and reducing inflammation when administered from 1–2 J/cm^2 for superficial lesions to 8–10 J/cm^2 for deep extensive wounds. Recovery of these cases can take months with standard treatment protocols, but may be resolve within several weeks when photobiomodulation is added to the regimen, with a typical 25–30% decrease in overall healing time (Figure 26.2).

Oral Disorders

Stomatitis

Stomatitis can be a symptom of a simple localized infection or indication of a much more serious systemic illness in reptiles. Therefore, proper diagnostics and systemic therapy are indicated in these cases. PBMT can positively affect most instances of stomatitis by reducing the inflammation and relieving the painful effects of the gingival lesions, thus leading to a more rapid return to eating. A superficial therapeutic dose of 0.5–1 J/cm^2 is usually effective in reducing inflammation and healing the gingiva.

One case report of stomatitis in a ball python describes significant improvement using laser therapy, which was conducted for eight treatments over 23 days. Fluence was 2.28

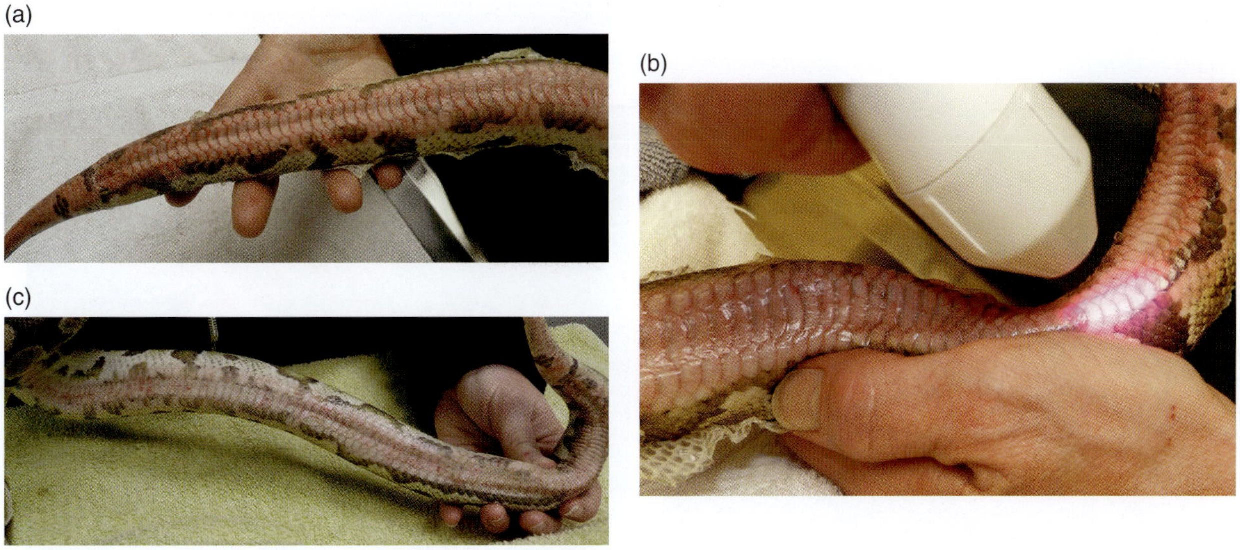

Figure 26.2 (a) Thermal burns on ventral aspect of ball python caused by contact to exposed healing element in cage. (b) Photobiomodulation at 2 J/cm^2 of thermal burns in snake. (c) Healing of thermal burns after two photobiomodulation sessions, administered 1 week apart.

and 4.04 J/cm^2 (Rungnirundorn *et al.*, 2021). The clinical signs significantly improved after three laser therapy sessions over 6 days. After eight laser sessions over 23 days, the inflammatory tissue was barely observed according to the authors. It is interesting to note that these laser dosages are higher than the commonly recommended doses for reptilian patients.

Musculoskeletal Disorders

Arthritis

Arthritis occurs in reptiles as experienced in other species, but often manifests itself more slowly and at a later stage in life. Photobiomodulation at around 6 J/cm^2 can reduce swelling and inflammation in the reptile's joints, thus increasing its mobility. Pain management in reptiles is difficult to assess and treat by conventional means, and research is lacking in analgesic effects of photobiomodulation in these species as well.

Fibrous Osteodystrophy

Fibrous osteodystrophy in reptiles is commonly referred to as metabolic bone disease. The typical causes are a deficiency of calcium, vitamin D3, or both in the diet, or due to the lack of proper UV-B lighting leading to nutritional secondary hyperparathyroidism. A related condition is renal secondary hyperparathyroidism caused by underlying renal disease, typically occurring in older reptiles. Common clinical signs include osteomalacia of the jaw and long bones, angular limb deformities, pathologic fractures, and seizures. The addition of photobiomodulation at fracture settings of at least 8–10 J/cm^2 can help strengthen bone integrity and speed recovery in these patients.

Fractures

As seen in other species, fracture repair in reptiles is augmented by photobiomodulation. Reptiles heal more slowly than their avian or mammalian counterparts, but their fractures typically heal 25–30% faster with photobiomodulation than without. A target dose of 8–10 J/cm^2 is a good starting point for fracture repair, but success depends on the general health status of the patient as well as the severity and characteristics of the fracture. Pathologic fractures should be treated with higher target doses then traumatic fractures, since the body must overcome the deficiency in integrity and bony foundation.

Muscular Strain or Sprain

Muscular sprains and tendon and ligament strains can be a challenge to diagnose effectively in reptiles. Since they are poikilothermic, they do not elicit the characteristic elevation in temperature with inflammation within the strained or sprained soft tissue. Photobiomodulation can be utilized at approximately 4 J/cm^2 in cases where the clinical manifestation suggests the sprain or strain.

A box turtle presented to one of the authors (Ness) with the inability to extend her left hind leg to ambulate (Figure 26.3). She was evaluated radiographically to rule out a fracture, a dislocation, or a mass. Since this appeared to be of soft tissue origin, a presumptive diagnosis of a sprain was made. The client declined photobiomodulation at initial evaluation. The patient was treated with an injection of buprenorphine for analgesia followed by daily administration of meloxicam as an anti-inflammatory for 10 days. Upon recheck examination, minimal improvement was seen in the use of the left hind leg. Photobiomodulation was permitted and administered at 8 J/cm^2.

(a) (b)

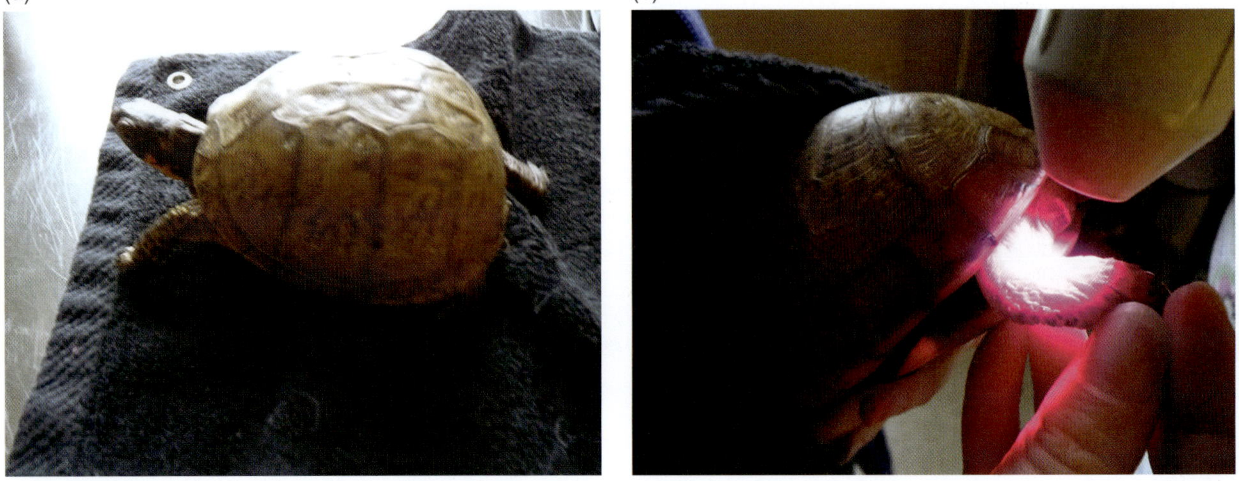

Figure 26.3 (a) Sprained leg in box turtle exhibiting lameness of unknown origin. (b) Photobiomodulation administered to lame leg in box turtle at 8 J/cm^2. Leg improved after treatment and resumed normal function within 1 week of laser session.

Significant improvement in the turtle's mobility was reported 3 days later, with normal extension of the hind limb and some persistent limping that resolved over the next few days.

Spondylosis

Spondylosis and spondylitis are described in reptiles as spinal arthritis caused by a number of contributing factors. Applying photobiomodulation at similar target dosages to other forms of arthritis can elicit clinical results. A case of a rainbow boa that had been diagnosed with spondylitis has been described. Treatment was started with meloxicam and tramadol, which had limited positive effects on the animal. The snake did not start to eat or move around normally, and it would strike when touched in the affected area. Laser therapy (1500 J) was applied to the affected area. It was noted that there was 80–90% improvement within just three treatments; the animal was eating normally and moving more normally the following week, and could be handled without striking or biting. Once the laser treatments were stopped, the patient relapsed to the original clinical signs. Medical therapy was started again, but it was noticed that the animal was only about 50% better. PBMT was initiated again, completely restoring the animal's behavior to normal and maintaining it for a longer time without any negative side effects (Stremme, 2012).

Coelomic Cavity Disorders

The coelom in reptiles, like birds, is equivalent to the combined thoracic and abdominal cavity of mammals in that reptiles lack a diaphragm to separate these two regions. In addition, the reptile's organs are modified to accommodate the longer and narrower body cavity. Therefore, photobiomodulation therapy of the body cavity of reptiles is different from that of mammals. Calculation of the therapeutic laser dosage for a general coelomic disorder would include measurement of the entire body cavity. Similarly, photobiomodulation of a gastrointestinal issue may include the entire coelom, whereas a specific lung or urinary bladder condition may only involve laser treatment of that particular portion of the coelom (Figure 26.4). This differentiation must be considered to accurately calculate therapy dosages when utilizing therapy laser software protocols designed to treat the entire coelomic cavity.

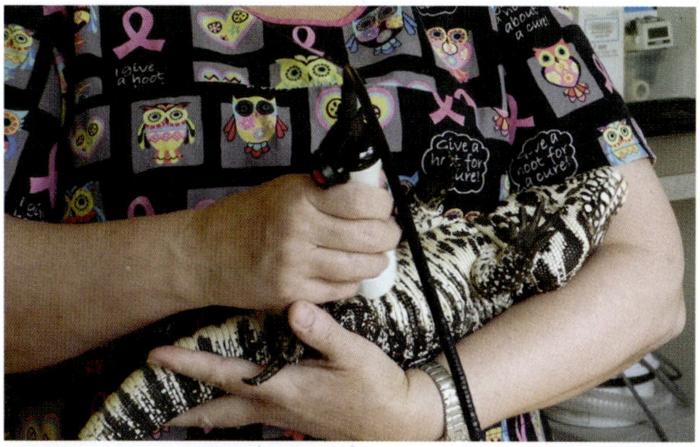

Figure 26.4 Calculation of the therapeutic laser dosage for a general coelomic disorder would include measurement of the entire body cavity. A lung or urinary bladder condition may only involve laser treatment of that particular portion of the coelom.

Ascites

Ascites is a consequence of osmotic difference caused by a circulatory disorder, hepatic disease, neoplasia, or other metabolic imbalance. Photobiomodulation can assist in dispersal of excess intracoelomic fluid in most of these disorders, except neoplasia. Therefore, if neoplasia has been ruled out, instituting a photobiomodulation protocol is indicated. Typical target dose settings of at least 6–8 J/cm^2 can facilitate the resorption of fluid. Further diagnostic and therapeutic regimens must be employed to address the etiologic component.

Egg Binding or Retention

Egg binding or retention is seen in certain reptile species, including various lizards, terrapins, and snakes. Extrapolating from studies of the effects of photobiomodulation on fertilized eggs of birds, there would appear to be no ill effect on the reptile egg when photobiomodulation is used on the gravid female. By reducing inflammation, the gravid patient may more successfully lay her eggs after a photobiomodulation session at 4–6 J/cm^2.

Gastrointestinal Disorders

Gastrointestinal disorders such as vomiting, maldigestion and constipation may improve with photobiomodulation, depending on the underlying cause. If inflammation is a factor in the clinical presentation, then photobiomodulation is likely to be beneficial. Target dosages of 4–10 J/cm^2 have been implemented with positive results in patients with constipation and regurgitation. In addition, snakes and lizards with inappetence have shown increased appetite after a single session of photobiomodulation of 4–6 J/cm^2, whereas other cases showed no response. Of course, identification and treatment of the underlying medical factors and environmental issues are vital in eliciting a positive outcome.

Miscellaneous

In the scientific literature, multiple studies have reported the use of PBMT for the treatment of a variety of inflammatory responses including snake venom (Nadur-Andrade *et al.*, 2012; Aranha de Sousa *et al.*, 2013). A study has shown that laser therapy was effective in the reduction of myonecrosis after injection of *Bothrops moojeni* snake venom (Dourado *et al.*, 2003). Another study reported that laser therapy significantly reduced the edema and leukocyte influx induced by *B. jararacussu* snake venom when the muscle was treated with a dose of 4.2 J/cm^2 from a semiconductor laser operating at 685 nm. This antiedematogenic action is magnified when laser and antivenin therapies are used together (Barbosa *et al.*, 2008).

Conclusion

As with all other species, virtually any reptile condition that benefits from analgesia, anti-inflammation, and increased rate of healing can improve with photobiomodulation. The information provided here is intended as a starting point from which to expand the use of photobiomodulation in reptilian patients. When applying this modality, the authors encourage detailed documentation of treatment parameters, including spot-size, surface area, irradiance, power, and especially wavelength and fluence (J/cm^2), in order to standardize the treatment and facilitate communication between clinicians. As with much of reptile medicine, further research on the use of photobiomodulation in reptiles and clinical documentation of results is needed to serve these patients better in the future.

References

Aranha de Sousa, E. *et al.* (2013). Effects of a low-level semiconductor gallium arsenide laser on local pathological alterations induced by *Bothrops moojeni* snake venom. *Photochem Photobiol Sci.* 12(10):1895–1902.

Barbosa, A.M. *et al.* (2008). Effect of low-level laser therapy in the inflammatory response induced by *Bothrops jararacussu* snake venom. *Toxicon.* 51(7):1236–1244.

Cole, G.L. *et al.* (2015). Effect of laser treatment on first-intention incisional wound healing in ball pythons (*Python regius*). *Am J Vet Res.* 76(10):904–912.

DiRuzzo, S. *et al.* (2022). Successful treatment of severe ulcerative dermatitis in an Aubry's Flapshell turtle (*Cycloderma aubryi*). *J Herpetol Med Surg.* 32(4):262–270.

Dourado, D.M. *et al.* (2003). Effects of the Ga-As laser irradiation on myonecrosis caused by *Bothrops Moojeni* snake venom. *Lasers Surg Med.* 33(5):352–357.

Kraut, S. *et al.* (2013). Laser therapy in a soft-shelled turtle (*Pelodiscus sinensis*) for the treatment of skin and shell ulceration. A case report. *Tierarztl Prax Ausg K Kleintiere Heimtiere.* 41(4):261–266.

Myakishev-Rempel, M. *et al.* (2012). A preliminary study of the safety of red light phototherapy of tissues harboring cancer. *Photomed Laser Surg.* 30(9):551–558.

Nadur-Andrade, N. *et al.* (2012). Effects of photobiostimulation on edema and hemorrhage induced by *Bothrops moojeni* venom. *Lasers Med Sci.* 27(1):65–70.

Nardini, G. and Bielli, M. (2011). *Low Level Laser Therapy (LLLT) in Reptile Medicine.* Association of Reptilian and Amphibian Veterinarians, Seattle.

Pelizzone, I. *et al.* (2014). Laser therapy for wound healing in chelonians: two case reports. *Veterinaria (Cremona).* 28 (5):33–38.

Rodrigo, S.M. *et al.* (2009). Analysis of the systemic effect of red and infrared laser therapy on wound repair. *Photomed Laser Surg.* 27(6):929–935.

Rungnirundorn, T. *et al.* (2021). Alternative treatment of stomatitis in ball python (*Python regius*) with class IV laser therapy: a clinical case. *Energy Health.* 21:16–18.

Santana-Blank, L. *et al.* (2012). Concurrence of emerging developments in photobiomodulation and cancer. *Photomed Laser Surg.* 30(11):615–616.

Schmidt, P.L. (2007). Preface. *Vet Clin North Am Small Anim Pract.* 37(3):xi–xii.

Souza, A.R. *et al.* (2023). The effects of photobiomodulation therapy on the healing of eastern box turtle (*Terrapene carolina*) shells. *J Zool Bot Gard.* 4:578–586. doi:10.3390/jzbg4030041.

Straus, S.E. *et al.* (2005). *Evidence-Based Medicine: How to Practice and Teach EBM*, 3 edn. Elsevier, Philadelphia.

Stremme, D.W. (2012). Confessions of a therapy laser neophyte. *Vet Pract News.* 24(3):20.

27

Laser Therapy for Aquatic Species

Micah C. Brodsky

Pono Scientific, Kaneohe, Hawaii, USA

1st Edition Contributor:

Donald W. Stremme

Academy of Natural Sciences of Drexel University and AQUAVET & Cornell University College of Veterinary Medicine, Cape May Beach, NJ, USA

Introduction

Aquatic animal species represent an extraordinary range of organisms, from microscopic invertebrates to gigantothermic reptiles (the Leatherback sea turtle) and facultative symbionts (such as corals) to the largest animal ever to have existed on planet Earth, the blue whale. By definition, the roughly 335,000 documented aquatic animal species (125,530 freshwater and 209,462 marine) representing 32 phyla are linked by the fact that they live all (or nearly all) of their lives in the water (Balian *et al.*, 2008; World Register of Marine Species Statistics, 2024). Over the past few decades there has been a significant increase in the number and range of aquatic animals maintained in collections at zoological and aquarium facilities, private aquariums, conservation breeding centers, wildlife rehabilitation centers, and in the aquaculture industry for both food production and the ornamental aquarium market. Veterinarians providing services for aquatic animals may encounter invertebrates (cephalopods, sea stars, jellyfish, corals, and snails), amphibians (frogs, salamanders, and axolotl), fish (Koi, fresh- and saltwater ornamentals, sharks, rays, and eels), reptiles (turtles, sea turtles, crocodilians, sea snakes, even marine iguanas), aquatic birds (penguins, flamingos, seabirds, ducks, geese, and other anseriformes), and aquatic mammals (cetaceans, pinnipeds, sirenians, hippopotamus, otters, and beavers).

The tiny fraction of extant aquatic species that veterinarians are likely to encounter in a clinical or research setting may still include a broad range of species from across multiple phyla; each with different physiologies, immunological systems, healing mechanisms, and husbandry considerations. While the practice of aquatic animal medicine has some inherent challenges (e.g., working in and around water, reduced physical access to patients, limited availability of validated diagnostic and therapeutic options, and a paucity of species-specific reference information) it also provides many opportunities for innovation (too often driven by necessity). Incorporating photobiomodulation therapy (PBMT) into aquatic animal practice represents one such opportunity. Photobiomodulation (PBM) has enormous potential in aquatic animal medicine because it is generally safe, noninvasive, has few known contraindications or side effects, can be applied to a broad range of disease processes, and has been shown to have analgesic effects for multiple types of pain (Bjordal *et al.*, 2003; Chow *et al.*, 2011). There are huge knowledge gaps in the basic anatomy, physiology, and pathophysiology of disease in most of the aquatic species maintained in collections today. As a result, much of aquatic animal medicine is the practice of applied comparative medicine, with clinicians adapting diagnostic and therapeutic tools from human and domestic animal medicine.

Laser therapy is a tool that can be applied with a wide safety margin in most species and we, as a profession, have just begun to scratch the surface of possible clinical applications for PBM in aquatic animals. A mounting body of scientific evidence spanning half a century of basic biological research across all kingdoms and phyla suggest that all living organisms have a biological response to near-infrared

Laser Therapy in Veterinary Medicine: Photobiomodulation, Second Edition. Edited by Christopher J. Winkler and Lisa A. Miller.

light (Hamblin *et al.*, 2019). The paucity of published information on clinical PBMT in aquatic animals means that there are few established treatment protocols or dosing references available. In the published literature that is available, there does not appear to be a conventionally accepted standard for reporting the different parameters associated with dosing and measurement of near-infrared light administration. This lack of conventional standardization can add an additional layer of confusion to the task of developing a treatment plan and manually calculating a therapeutic dose for PBMT.

Laser Safety

The general principles of laser safety and special considerations for administration are covered in detail in Chapters 4 and 5. The safety and treatment considerations for utilizing PBM with aquatic animals are fundamentally the same as with any domestic or zoological species. The two primary safety considerations when using laser therapy are providing effective eye protection for all people and animals present in the treatment area and avoiding thermal injury to the patient. Working around water adds additional safety consideration because of water's ability to reflect and refract light. When treating aquatic animals, the laser equipment will often need to be taken to the patient, and treatment administered poolside or tank-side, with the patient partially (or entirely) submerged in water. Regardless of location, when treating patients in the water it is important to consider reflection and refraction at the water surface, and from the sides and the bottom of the enclosure. Every person in the treatment area needs to wear laser-safe eyewear with the correct optical density to protect against the specific wavelengths of light produced by the laser equipment being used. The manufacturer of the therapeutic laser being used should be able (and willing) to provide guidance for determining the nominal ocular hazard distance (NOHD), establishing a nominal hazard zone (NHZ), and operational protocols to ensure the safety of people and animals in the laser treatment area (just as they would for a companion animal practice).

Where you conduct laser treatments will dictate the safety measures that need to be implemented.

Securing the Laser Treatment Area

The first order of business is to secure the laser treatment area to prevent facility staff or members of the public from accidentally entering the NHZ without appropriate eye protection. This can be accomplished by locking all access doors (if inside a facility) or establishing a perimeter using physical barriers, chain, rope, or even caution tape. If physical exclusion from the NHZ is not logistically possible, an alternative is to set up privacy screens around the treatment area (screens of nearly any configuration can be quickly and inexpensively constructed out of PVC pipe and a black painter's tarp or similar dark colored material).

Patient and Animal Safety

Aquatic species are often housed in multispecies or multi-animal enclosures. If it is not feasible to isolate the patient for laser treatment, preventive measures should be taken to minimize ocular exposure risk to other animals in the enclosure or nearby in the treatment area.

For the aquatic animal PBMT patient, it is important to protect both eyes, especially when treating in a tank or pool with reflective bottom and sides. This is partially to protect the patients' eyes from reflected light, but also because you may want to treat the same target from both sides of the animal. For species with eyelids, a wet towel, soft cloth, or other mechanical barrier (preferably black or dark) works well if the patient will tolerate it. In some species covering both eyes may help to calm the patient or reduce movement, and therefore reduce the level of restraint needed (chemical, manual, or both). It can be challenging to keep a cloth in place over a patients' eyes while in the water. A long, narrow piece of soft material draped over the head and eyes, then gathered underneath the jaw and held (not too tightly) by an assistant, can be an effective solution for maintaining eye protection.

Species without eyelids, and patients that will not tolerate (or are otherwise not good candidates for) a cloth eye covering, require a bit more creativity. Opaque plastic containers, plastic sheets, cones, paddles, or scoops can be used to provide effective eye protection. More rigid plastic can be cut and heated to form shapes such as paddles, cones, cylinders, or semi-circles. In situations where a smaller curved or hemispherical shape may be needed (such as treating close to the eye on a fish with Head and Lateral Line Erosion [HLLE]), black plastic spoons and scoops are readily available, cheap, and already have handles. Regardless of the item used, it is important to carefully check for and remove any sharp or rough edges (such as manufacturing seams) that could injure the patient's eye or skin if they were to struggle or move suddenly.

Thermal injury is the other major patient concern with PBMT, and the presence of water does not necessarily reduce the risk of thermal injury. Water has a relatively low absorption coefficient for electromagnetic energy within the wavelength range used for PBMT (the "therapeutic window" ranges from approximately 600–1100 nm). However, water is one of the main constituents of biological tissue associated with absorption of laser light energy (the other two being hemoglobin and melanin) (Palmer & Williams, 1974; Scholle *et al.*, 2010; Santana-Blank *et al.*, 2015). Melanin and hemoglobin have significantly higher absorption coefficients within that therapeutic window, but are present in much smaller quantities than water (mammalian skeletal muscle, for example, is about 76% water). Within an applied clinical standpoint, this author considers water to absorb laser energy, and heat up, at roughly the same rate as mammalian soft tissues.

As is the case with terrestrial animals, pigmentation significantly affects energy absorption and the heating rate of tissues, with darker pigments absorbing more energy and heating up faster than less pigmented or lighter colored tissues. In contrast to the two primary pigments that absorb light energy in terrestrial animals (melanin and hemoglobin), there are dozens of pigments (that we know of) in marine animals and likely many pigments from the aquatic environment that have yet to be identified (Bandaranayake, 2006; Muñoz-Miranda *et al.*, 2023). Even if the pigments present in an aquatic animal patient have been identified, the absorption spectra of those pigments may not be known.

Neoplasia and the Gonads

The safety considerations related to PBM of gonadal and neoplastic tissues are covered in detail in Chapters 5 and 19, respectively. While consideration should be given to treating over gonads and around neoplastic tissue, an increasing body of evidence suggests that there is less risk associated with PBM of these tissues than previously thought. In some aquatic species, the gonads extend nearly the entire length of the coelomic cavity and may occupy much of the coelom in reproductively active animals. At clinically relevant doses, PBM has not been shown to negatively impact gametogenesis in aquatic species. However, both fish and sea urchin sperm have been shown experimentally to exhibit dose-dependent motility increases that shift to decreased motility at high doses. Experiments with laserpuncture (using PBM to trigger acupuncture points) suggest that PBM may accelerate gonadal maturity and increased fecundity in male and female catfish, and sea urchin sperm irradiated at 192 J/cm^2 resulted in faster development of early-stage zygotes (Amaroli *et al.*, 2017; Mukti *et al.*, 2020; Plavskii *et al.*, 2021; Patmadevi *et al.*, 2022; Astuti *et al.*, 2023).

Equipment Safety

Therapeutic laser equipment is expensive, complex, and sensitive electronic equipment that is easily damaged by exposure to water (especially salt water) and moisture. The risk of damage is one reason practitioners may be hesitant to take their laser poolside to treat aquatic species, but there are ways to protect your equipment. I find that inexpensive, lightweight, disposable methods are more likely to be used consistently than big, expensive, fancy cases. Although I have invested in expensive waterproof cases to protect equipment during transport, I prefer either a plastic tote turned on its side or a cardboard box covered with a trashbag that can be turned away from the possible source of splashing when poolside or tank side (Figure 27.1). Regardless of the approach used, it is important to provide enough space around the back and sides of the machine to allow air circulation, so that heat generated by the base unit can be dissipated. Methods for protecting the handpiece will depend on the size and shape of handpiece and if it has interchangeable heads. A rubber exam glove can be trimmed and stretched over the handpiece, or a plastic bag with one corner cut off can be stretched over the handpiece and taped into place (Figure 27.2). To my knowledge, there is no therapeutic laser currently on the market with a submersible or waterproof handpiece. The handpiece of your laser should be thoroughly disassembled and carefully cleaned and dried

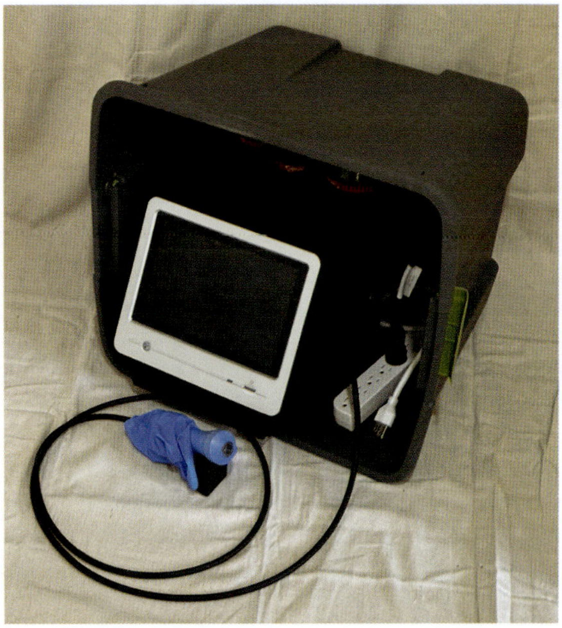

Figure 27.1 A plastic tote used to the protect the laser from being splashed. Note the surge protector inside the tote; for lasers that need to be plugged in, the extension cord plug can also be placed inside the tote.

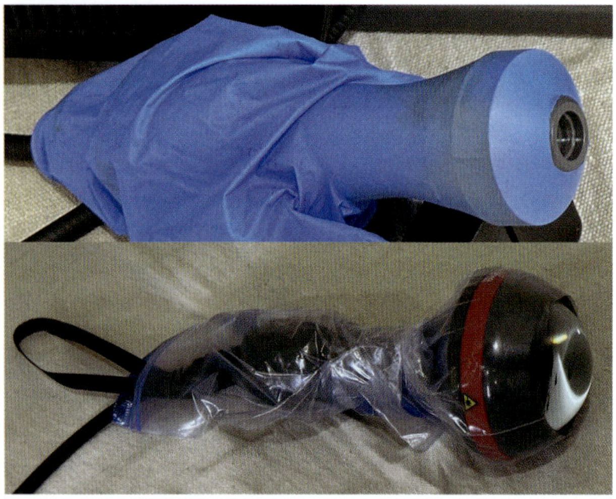

Figure 27.2 Laser handpiece with a small off-contact treatment head protected using an exam glove that has had the fingertip cut off (top) and a large on-contact head protected with a plastic bag with the corner cut off (bottom).

after each use (even if it did not get splashed). If you anticipate using electronic equipment around water frequently, consider pricing an insurance policy that will cover accidental damage (including water damage) to medical equipment.

General Approach to Treatment and Dosing

Utilizing PBMT in aquatic species is fundamentally the same as treating a patient with any other medical therapy, including keeping detailed medical records. There are few established protocols for aquatic animals and there will generally not be an option for selecting automatically calculated doses for aquatic species from the software in your therapy laser. This leaves the practitioner with two options; either extrapolate the disease process and the size, location, and type of target tissue from the aquatic patient to a comparable situation in a cat, dog, or horse (species commonly available in the laser's software), or calculate doses and plan treatment protocols manually.

Manually calculating the dose and treatment protocol is reasonably straightforward but does require consideration of numerous variables. The concepts of fluence (measured in J/cm^2) and irradiance (measured in W/cm^2) are critically important to understand for making manual calculations. Fluence represents energy density, the amount of energy delivered per unit area (in J/cm^2). Irradiance is the power density, which is arrived at by dividing the power delivered by the area of the laser beam (aka spot size) (in W/cm^2). Historically, fluence was accepted as the primary dosing consideration for PBMT. However, both fluence and irradiance have been determined to affect the clinical efficacy of PBMT (Zein *et al.*, 2018). These concepts and manual dose calculation are covered in detail in Chapter 4.

It is critically important that detailed records are kept of the initial calculations and treatment parameters used, in case the treatment protocol needs to be modified for any reason. Your own medical records will likely serve as your primary resource for specific protocols and dosing for future cases (at least until the volume of peer-reviewed literature has increased significantly). Dose and protocol changes are common when treating nondomestic animals with PBMT, and if no response is observed after three to four treatments, it is recommended that the dose be increased or the treatment protocol otherwise modified to increase the amount of energy reaching the target tissues. Even when using computer-calculated protocols and doses, it is good practice to double check the calculations manually and to record all parameters shown in the laser's software.

The parameters I recommend recording when manually calculating dosing and planning PBMT protocols are:

1) Indication for treatment (either the confirmed or suspected disease process, or a differential list).
2) Estimated size and anatomical location of the target tissue (in cm^2, including the surrounding margin).
3) Brand and model of laser equipment being used.
4) Treatment head of the handpiece (if interchangeable).
5) Spot size at the exit aperture of the handpiece/treatment head (cm^2), and the divergence angle of the beam (degrees).
6) Wavelength(s) of laser light (nm).
7) Treatment method (on-contact vs. off-contact; scanning or point-to-point).
8) Continuous wave or pulsed wave. If using pulsed wave, dose calculation will require knowing the duty cycle (% time the laser is actively emitting) and the average power (in W); average power is calculated from the peak power (W), pulse frequency (Hz), and pulse width (seconds). Refer to Chapter 4 for detailed guidance on these calculations.
9) Fluence (J/cm^2).
10) Irradiance (W/cm^2).
11) Power setting of the laser (W).
12) Duration of treatment (in Minutes:Seconds).
13) Total dose to be delivered (J).
14) Prescribed frequency of administration (q24h, q2day, 3×/week, etc.) and duration of therapy.

Each time PBMT is administered:

1) Date, time, and location of administration.

2) Patient identification.
3) Name of the person administering treatment.
4) Reference to the detailed PBMT protocol being used (above).
5) Power setting of the laser (W).
6) Duration of treatment (in Minutes:Seconds).
7) Total dose delivered (J).
8) Notes:
    a) The appearance of any visible lesions or changes in lesion appearance since initiating treatment.
    b) Any response observed during treatment (signs of discomfort, avoidance or attempts to withdraw, flushing of the skin, changes in posture, etc.).
    c) Any behavioral or kinematic changes observed since the previous treatment by the owner, aquarist, or person administering PBMT (swimming, coordination, buoyancy, feeding, hiding, etc.).

It can be challenging to gauge response to therapy, especially in nondomestic animals and in slow-healing species such as reptiles. Prospectively identifying clear metrics for assessing response to therapy will make it much easier to determine if treatment is working, and guide decisions to modify dose and/or administration protocols if the criteria for treatment success have not been met. For visible lesions, serial photographs at standard intervals (weekly or every other week) that include a scale (ruler) in the photograph can be very helpful in determining response to therapy. For nonvisible targets affecting movement or buoyancy, serial video can serve the same purpose. The owner, aquarist, or keeper is probably the best-available source of information on patient progress, as they know the individual animal and spend far more time observing and tending to the husbandry needs of the patient than the clinician or laser technician in most cases.

Dose Calculation and Treatment Considerations

The fundamentals of PBMT and detailed discussions of dosing, manual dose calculations, application methods, and other considerations (such as treating around neoplasia and gonadal tissues) are covered in Chapters 4, 5, and 19. The first step in dose calculation is estimating the size and location of the tissues targeted for treatment, which includes the lesion plus a 2–5 cm margin of "normal" tissue surrounding the lesion (the larger the lesion, the larger the margin should be). Current dosing recommendations in terrestrial animals are based on delivering a cumulative amount of energy to specific target tissues. It should be noted that while PBMT has a wide safety margin, dose response studies on clinical diseases have not been carried out in aquatic species. Dermal wound healing studies in rats showed the best results at 20 J/cm^2 and delayed wound healing at 50 J/cm^2 (Mendez *et al.*, 2004; Al-Watban *et al.*, 2007). Unless there is a specific indication to do otherwise (such as species-specific doses from successfully treated cases reported in the literature or provided by colleagues), I start with the recommended dose ranges used in terrestrial animals, which are:

1) 1–5 J/cm^2 for superficial tissues (those visible to the eye) (Peplow *et al.*, 2010).
2) 8–20 J/cm^2 for deep tissue targets, scaled up based on patient size and target tissue location and depth (Bjordal *et al.*, 2003; Roberts *et al.*, 2013; Looney *et al.*, 2018).

Deciding where in the dose range to start depends on multiple variables, but do not hesitate to modify the treatment approach to best meet the needs of the patient based on the available resources and limitations in that specific situation.

One of the primary considerations when selecting a dose is treatment method (on-contact vs. off-contact). Off-contact administration may be the only option for many aquatic animal patients. This could be due to restraint requirements, patient reactivity, facility or operational constraints, or because the patient has rough skin or scales (such as sharks, filefish, triggerfish, etc.), which could damage the surface of an on-contact treatment head and negatively affect the functioning of the laser unit. When treating off-contact in aquatic animals, I calculate starting doses at:

1) 5 J/cm^2 for superficial tissues.
2) 12 J/cm^2 for target tissues less than 5 cm deep.
3) 15 J/cm^2 for target tissues more than 5 cm deep.

Much of the benefit from on-contact administration is derived from not losing light energy to reflection, and to compression of soft tissues resulting in dispersion of blood and extracellular fluid that would otherwise absorb photons before they reach deeper target tissues. A study comparing on-contact to off-contact treatment at the same dose reported 70% more light delivered into the spinal canal of large dogs using the on-contact treatment method (Piao *et al.*, 2018). While wet skin or hair has no clinically relevant impact with on-contact administration in companion animals, a thin layer of water or shiny epidermal mucus (slime layer) on an aquatic animal will reflect a lot of light when treating off-contact. As a result, the amount of energy actually delivered into the target tissues may be significantly lower than that emitted from the handpiece (the calculated dose).

Point-to-point and scanning treatment methods (covered in detail in Chapter 4) each have their place and are useful for different applications. The primary consideration to remember about point-to-point administration is that it is limited to treating with relatively low irradiance (low power delivery). If treating with higher irradiance (as would be required to deliver the dose ranges described above in a reasonable amount of time) the handpiece must be kept in constant motion (the scanning method). Consistent movement of the handpiece reduces the risk of thermal injury by minimizing focal tissue heating while effectively saturating the target tissues with photons from multiple directions. It is standard practice in companion animals for the operator to monitor temperature in the treatment area by keeping their pinky finger in constant contact with the skin and hair while treating. This may not be feasible with many aquatic patients, but it is good practice where applicable.

Minimizing the risk of thermal injury is a primary component of creating a PBMT plan for any patient. The skin of aquatic animals differs significantly from that of terrestrial animals, and there is remarkable variation across aquatic species (consider the differences between jellyfish, cephalopods, crustaceans, finfish, sharks, and marine mammals). Pigmentation plays a central role in tissue heating with aquatic animals, just as it does in terrestrial animals. Many aquatic species, such as fish and sharks, exhibit countershading (light on the bottom transitioning to dark on the top) or have multi-colored ornate patterns. Cephalopods (octopus, squid, and cuttlefish) are famous for exhibiting metachrosis (the ability to change color and pattern) and many fish species change coloration based on behavioral or environmental factors, such as feeding or exhibiting territorial aggression. When treating a new species (or color morph) for the first time, if there are no references describing an irradiance (W/cm^2) that has been safely delivered in the past, the risk of thermal injury can be reduced by starting at 50% of what you think a conservative "safe" irradiance would be (based on a similar species or similarly colored animal from the same genus) and increasing the irradiance by 25% with the two subsequent administrations. One simple way to accomplish this is to first program all the settings on the laser for the planned treatment. Then without changing any other parameters (including the handpiece and treatment head so that a fixed spot size is maintained), reduce the power setting by 50% for the first treatment. If no signs of discomfort or thermal injury are observed, increase the power setting by 25% for each of the next two treatments. This approach will result in a reduced dose for the first two treatments, which should be accounted for before increasing the dose if no therapeutic response is observed after three to four treatments. Hypopigmentation following PBMT has been observed in fish (Johnson & Saint-Erne, 2022) and other species. Hypopigmentation is more likely to occur in darkly pigmented patients, and pigment loss may be temporary or permanent. It is important to communicate the potential for transient or permanent loss of pigment and discoloration to clients and aquarists before initiating PBMT.

In species with an epidermal mucus layer (or slime layer), the capture, handling, on-contact laser administration, and drying of an area to treat with topical medication and/or laser can all disrupt or remove that slime layer. Epidermal mucus is immunologically active and serves as an important environmental barrier. Disrupting the mucus layer (especially repeatedly) has the potential to exacerbate a primary condition and open the patient up to secondary infections. In those species with a mucus layer, the benefits of handling and restraint, on-contact administration, and drying or not drying the treatment area, must all be weighed against the potential risks associated with disrupting the mucus layer. For superficial and dermatological lesions, the mucus layer may already be disrupted and/or dysbiotic, in which case the risks associated with drying the treatment area to facilitate PBMT combined with topical and/or systemic therapy (as indicated) may be reduced relative to the benefits.

In contrast to companion animals, safely accessing the aquatic animal patient for therapeutic or diagnostic purposes can be one of the more challenging aspects of practicing aquatic animal medicine. Human and animal safety should be the primary concern for every procedure with every patient. It is critically important to have trained, capable personnel manage patient collection and handling (especially with large, venomous, or otherwise potentially dangerous animals) in order to minimize stress on the patient and allow the person administering PBMT to focus exclusively on safe laser operation. Capture, handling, and restraint of nondomestic animals can trigger profound stress responses. Stress-induced elevations of cortisol and glucocorticoids have been shown to negatively impact immune function and delay wound healing in humans and animals (Gouin *et al.*, 2011). The benefit of any therapy or treatment (even noninvasive procedures such as PBMT) must be weighed against the potential risks and stress induced by repeated capture and handling of the patient. In some situations, aquarists, curatorial staff, or owners may strongly oppose any capture, restraint, or handling of nondomestic patients for even a single diagnostic or therapeutic procedure, which presents a serious impediment to providing medical care that could improve the patients' health, well-being, and quality of life.

Decision-making around the risks and benefits of repeated handling of aquatic animals for medical procedures can be stressful for all involved parties, not just the patient. Because PBMT is noninvasive, provides pain relief, and is often perceived by owners or facility staff as having "no downside," this challenging situation can sometimes present an opportunity to generate buy-in for training husbandry and medical behaviors. A few basic behaviors, such as targeting, feeding at station, and hand-feeding (with tongs) can be accomplished with just about any aquatic animal patient and will significantly reduce the handling stress and risk of injury for patients and people alike. Over the past few decades, training medical and husbandry behaviors to minimize or eliminate the need for capture and physical restraint of collection animals has gained in popularity and become synonymous with best practices in the zoo and aquarium industry (Ramirez, 1999). More recently, incorporating Cooperative Veterinary Care and behavioral approaches to reducing fear and stress in patients (and owners) has also become more mainstream in companion animal practice (Feyrecilde, 2024).

Yes, training takes time and skill, and yes, there may be scoffing, laughter, and downright incredulity when you suggest training a fish to target and hold at station so that it can be treated with PBMT or have topical medications applied. No one would bat an eyelash if you were talking about a dolphin or sea lion, because they have seen shows while visiting an aquarium or watched videos of trained behaviors. Rays, eels, fish, turtles, crocodiles, alligators, and other aquatic species are being trained at facilities all over the world; and it improves the health, well-being, and quality of life of those animals and the people who work with them. I have been pleasantly surprised by how many aquarists and hobbyist owners get super excited about training their fish to target or to hand feed at station, so they can be calmy netted without being chased around the enclosure, which stresses the patient and every other animal in the system. Laser therapy represents an outstanding opportunity to open these discussions because the modality is (accurately) perceived as being safe, noninvasive, and effective for treating chronic wounds with a history of treatment failure.

Training and husbandry may be viewed by some as being outside the purview of the veterinary team, and you are likely to encounter resistance. In my experience, providing support to the people responsible for day-to-day husbandry and operations can help to build trust between individuals and across teams, and may well mean the difference between having zero patient access (not even being told about a health problem) and having some opportunity to diagnose and treat the aquatic animal patient, even if the situation is suboptimal.

Determining and prescribing the number and frequency of PBM treatments is covered in detail in Chapter 4. In companion animals, the approach is based largely on what PBM is being used to treat and the chronicity of that process. The generalized approach is to treat acute conditions more frequently (daily or every other day) for a short time, and chronic conditions frequently at first (an "induction phase" conceptually similar to a loading dose with systemic medication) followed by progressively less frequent applications until reaching the longest duration between treatments that will maintain the desired effect. In practice, the aquatic animal practitioner is more likely to be presented with chronic or non-healing lesions because aquarists and owners rarely seek veterinary support prior to multiple treatment failures or for self-limiting conditions.

If access to the aquatic animal patient is limited, it may be necessary to deviate significantly from the recommended number or frequency of administrations. While it is generally preferred to administer serial treatments with PBMT, sometimes a single treatment is all that is logistically possible. A study on dermal wound healing in rats showed no difference between nontreatment controls and single dose PBM at 14-days post injury. However, that study was conducted on acute injuries (Rezende *et al.*, 2007). Conversely, a chronic, nonhealing skin wound of 2-month duration in a freshwater stingray (*Potamotrygon motoro*) was described as completely healed 4 weeks after a single laser treatment and concurrent administration of becaplermin (Figure 27.3). The PBM dose delivered in that case was reported as "similar" to the protocol used by the same clinician to treat HLLE in Purple Tang (which was 4 W, off-contact, continuous wave, for 180 seconds = 720 J for the entire treatment area over the head and lateral line of a 12 cm long fish) (Stremme, 2017). Estimating a treatment area of approximately 40 cm^2, a delivered dose of 720 J translates to a fluence of 18 J/cm^2. This is more than three times higher than the 5 J/cm^2 upper limit of the range for superficial tissue targets that is carried over from terrestrial dosing recommendations, but it is also difficult to quantify how much of that energy might have been lost to reflection with off-contact administration on wet skin. A similarly high fluence (15–22 J/cm^2) was reported as part of successful multimodal treatment for delayed wound healing in a softshell turtle with septicemic ulcerative dermatitis (shell rot) that received a total of nine PBM treatments (DiRuzzzo *et al.*, 2023). While shell rot generally presents as a dermatological condition, deep tissue involvement and osteomyelitis are almost always present, so this higher fluence is more congruent with the recommendations for treating deep tissues (Figure 27.6). Anecdotal experience and these few reported cases suggest that a single or limited number of PBMT treatments at a fluence of between 15 and 20 J/cm^2 as part of multimodal therapy (wound debridement, antimicrobials if indicated, becaplermin, topical wound

(a) (b) (c)

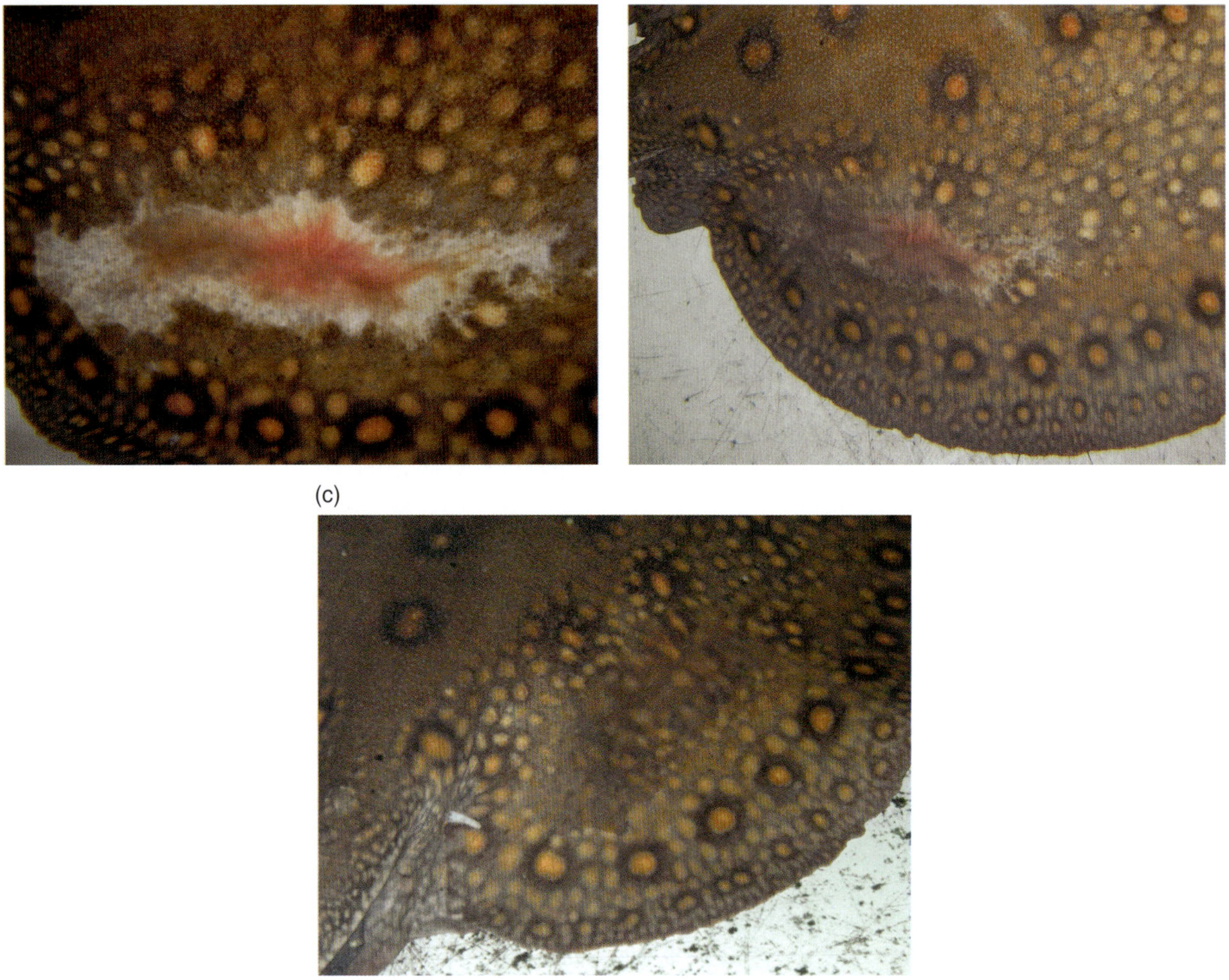

Figure 27.3 Chronic, nonhealing wound in a stingray. Clockwise from upper left: (a) before laser treatment, (b) after 5 days, (c) after 1 month.

dressings, etc.) *may* help to stimulate healing in chronic or nonhealing wounds. Additional research is clearly needed to understand the clinical efficacy of a single or limited number of PBMT treatments in these cases.

Laser therapy is most efficacious when utilized as part of a multimodal treatment approach. If any type of topical medication or wound dressing is used in the treatment area, the skin should be thoroughly cleaned and dried before laser administration, and the topical agent applied after PBMT has been completed. Any time PBMT is used in conjunction with a medication with the potential to cause photosensitization, irradiance and/or fluence reductions may be indicated and extra care should be taken to monitor for any signs of discomfort or thermal injury. Photosensitization can also be leveraged to clinical benefit in a modality called photodynamic therapy (PDT), which consists of intentionally administering an exogenous photosensitizing agent in conjunction with laser light to target specific cells, tissues, or microorganisms. Laser-driven PDT has been used to treat cancer in experimental animal models since the 1960s and was first utilized in human medicine in 1976 to treat bladder cancer (Ackroyd *et al.*, 2001; Hamblin *et al.*, 2017). There are multiple current routes of exploration and clinical trials for PDT in human and animal medicine, largely focused on treating cancer and developing effective treatment options for multi-drug-resistant microbes (Correia *et al.*, 2021; Sabino *et al.*, 2023; Zdubek *et al.*, 2024). In aquatic animals, PDT has been used experimentally to treat cutaneous fibropapillomatosis in green sea turtles (*Chelonia mydras*), as an antimicrobial treatment for a contaminated carapace (shell) fracture in a green sea turtle, and to treat chronic pododermatitis in penguins (Nascimento *et al.*, 2015; Filho *et al.*, 2021; Sellera *et al.*, 2014a, 2014b, 2017). PDT has significant unexplored potential for use in aquatic animal medicine, especially in situations where other treatment modalities or surgical intervention may not be good options.

Cases, Case Reports, and Publications

The current literature describing clinical applications of PBM in aquatic animals is limited largely to case reports. Basic research utilizing zebrafish as an animal model provides some valuable insight into the mechanisms of PBM that happens to be carried out in a fish model, and there are some interesting applications of PBM being explored for theriogenology in commercial aquaculture. In general, there is quite a bit of inconsistency in how doses are reported in the literature, but the fluence and/or irradiance can be calculated in many instances, which provides a useful starting point for identifying a fluence or irradiance that has been safely administered to a specific aquatic species.

Head and lateral line erosion (HLLE, aka "Hole in the Head") is a multifactorial condition of fish characterized by chronic erosive or ulcerative dermatopathy on the head and along the lateral lines. A range of environmental, nutritional, and infectious etiologies have been explored but the exact etiology of HLLE remains unidentified and effective treatment continues to be challenging in most situations. As is the case with all aquatic animals, water quality is an important component of preventing, managing, and treating HLLE. Multimodal therapy utilizing PBMT and becaplermin has been effective in some cases and has been anecdotally reported to be more effective than treatment with becaplermin alone (Adams & Michalkiewiz, 2005; Fleming *et al.*, 2008; Roberts, 2009; Stremme, 2017). In an informal experiment comparing PBMT to sham laser treatment for chronic HLLE lesions in two purple tang (*Zebrasoma xanthurum*), the fish treated with laser therapy showed visible signs of healing (lesions shrinking and repigmentation) after four treatments, while no change was observed in the control animal (Figure 27.4). The initial dose was reported as 4 W, continuous wave, for 90 seconds, total energy delivered 360 J (180 J per side), administered twice per week. Conservatively estimating a treatment area of 40 cm^2, this would calculate out to a fluence of 9 J/cm^2. The dose was increased by increasing the duration of treatment to 180 seconds at 4 W, resulting in the delivery of 720 J (fluence = 18 J/cm^2) for multiple treatments before logistical constraints necessitated discontinuing PBMT (Stremme, 2017).

PBM has been used to treat ulcerative dermatitis in Koi (caused by infection with *Dermocystidium* sp.). The authors reported improved healing in 9 out of 10 fish with chronic ulcerative lesions and a history of antimicrobial treatment failure. Dosing was reported as 9 J/cm^2 with a 980 nm diode laser (Pees *et al.*, 2011).

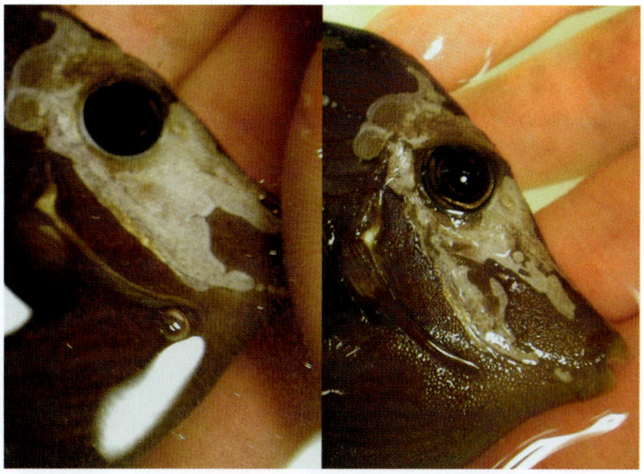

Figure 27.4 HLLE lesions in a purple tang before and after multiple laser treatments.

An adult *Plecostomus* presented with an approximately 3.0 cm, nonhealing deep ulcerative lesion on the head which had been present for 2 years. Minimal improvement was observed after 2 weeks of injectable antimicrobial therapy (guided by histopathology and microbial culture and sensitivity) and an additional 2 months in an isolation tank in water treated with Melafix. Seven days after PBMT was initiated (at a reported dose of "0.5 W and a pulse rate of 20hz for 2 minutes and 8 seconds each session") the lesion appeared significantly improved, and after 1 month the lesion was mostly healed. Twice weekly PBMT was continued until a total of 40 treatments had been administered over approximately 5 months, and the lesion appeared fully healed. One month after discontinuing PBMT the treatment area became markedly hypopigmented, but the pigmentation returned approximately 3 months later (Figure 27.5) (Johnson & Saint-Erne, 2022).

A 15-year-old green moray eel (*Gymnothorax funebris*) that presented with inappetence, reduced mobility, and positive buoyancy received PBMT as part of a multimodal treatment plan after diagnostic imaging revealed spondylosis, multifocal spinal cord compression, and a distended swim bladder. The authors reported observing "normal anguilliform motion" after the first PBM treatment and "markedly improved" feeding and swimming after five treatments. The dose was reported as "1616 joules, applied with a noncontact head, 8 watt, cold laser (Companion therapy lasers) along the vertebrae on each side for 2–3 min." Administration frequency was three PBM treatments/week for the first month, then one to two per week for 1 year. Buoyancy issues continued and were addressed through multiple other therapeutic approaches (Boylan *et al.*, 2017).

(a) (b) (c) (e) (d)

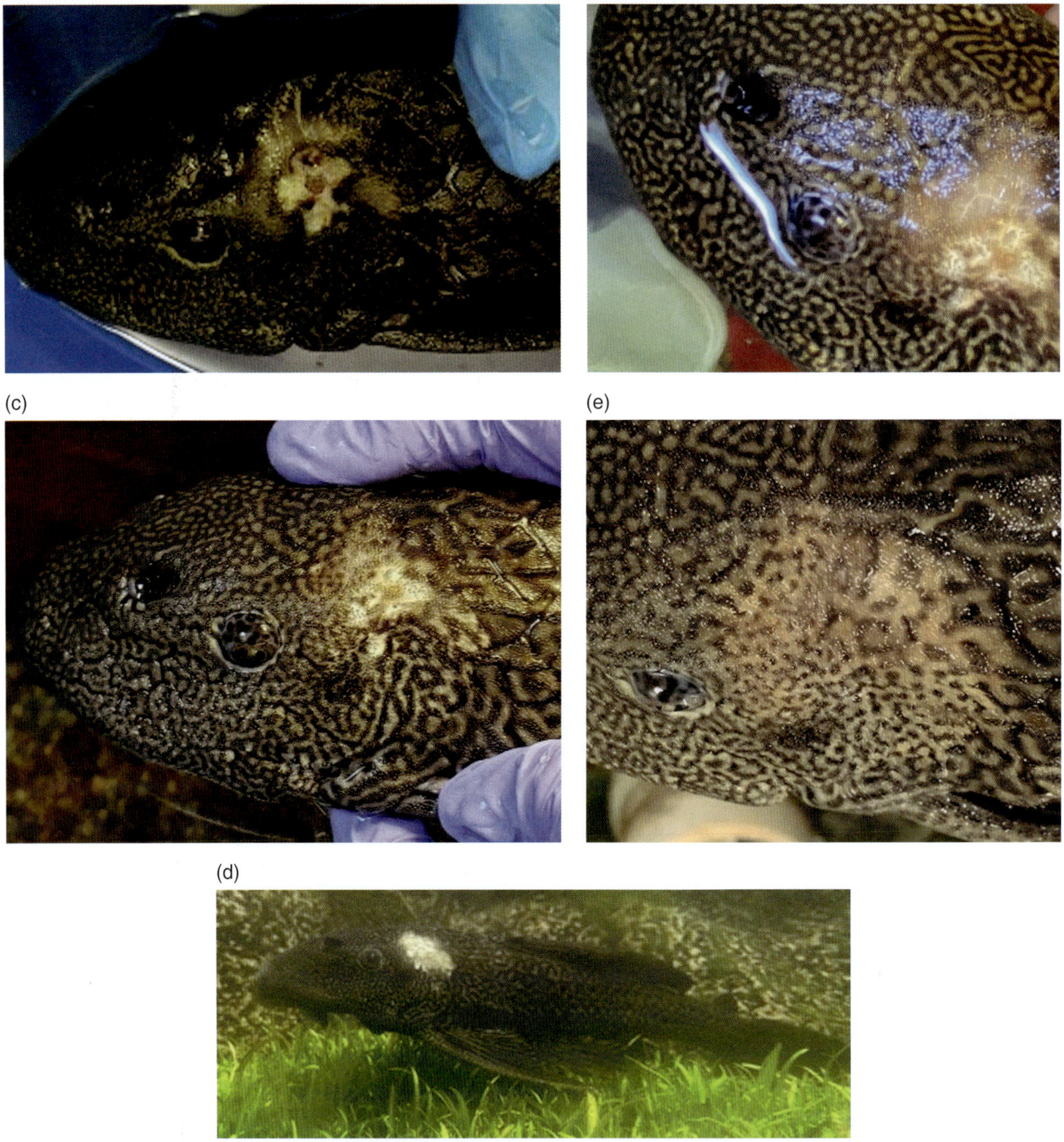

Figure 27.5 Adult *Plecostomus* with a chronic ulcerative lesion on the head: (a) original presentation; (b) 1 week after initiating PBMT; (c) one month after initiating PBMT; (d) 1 month after completing PBMT; (e) 4 months after completing PBMT. Images courtesy of the Arizona-Sonora Desert Museum, Tucson, AZ, USA.

A recently published study assessing the effects of PBMT on dermal abrasions in cownose rays (*Rhinoptera bonasus*) reported no visually appreciable difference between the non-PBMT control group ($N = 5$) and the PBMT treatment group ($N = 5$) at a dose of 5 J/cm^2 delivered off-contact at 2 W (irradiance = 0.28 W/cm^2 at the exit aperture). The authors suggest that incrementally higher dosing should be explored if no response is observed after three to four treatments (Gilewski *et al*., 2024). This recommendation is congruent with the higher fluence delivered as a single administration for a persistent dermal lesion in the freshwater stingray case described earlier (Stremme, 2017).

PBM has been utilized as a component of multimodal treatment for septicemic ulcerative dermatitis (shell rot) in softshell turtles, including a Chinese softshell turtle (*Pelodiscus sinensis*) and an Aubry's flapshell turtle (*Cycloderma aubryi*) (Kraut *et al.*, 2013; DiRuzzo *et al.*, 2022). In the case of the Aubry's flapshell turtle, PBMT was initiated to address delayed healing of surgical sites approximately 2 months after surgical debridement and ostectomy. Dosing was as follows (DiRuzzo *et al.*, 2022):

Anatomic treatment area: Multiple select ostectomy and debridement sites on the carapace and plastron, including 2–3 cm margin of normal tissue.
Dose (J): Not reported
Fluence (first three treatments): 6–12 J/cm^2 depending on lesion size (including margin)
Fluence (treatments four to nine): 15–22 J/cm^2 depending on lesion size (including margin)
Irradiance: 1.3 W/cm^2 (radiant power was set to 2.0 W using a small off-contact head with a 1.54 cm^2 aperture)
Method of treatment: off-contact scanning (2.5 cm from the treatment surface)
Notes: 980 nm wavelength, continuous wave, treatment frequency every 3 days.

After the first three treatments, the dose was increased to a fluence of 15–22 J/cm^2 by increasing the duration of treatment, with all other parameters unchanged. After the fourth treatment, visible indications of healing were observed in the treated sites and the decision was made to treat all lesions on the patient. PBM was discontinued after a total of nine treatments for logistical reasons. The patient made a full recovery over the next 5 months, with varying degrees of permanent depigmentation present on the treatment areas of the carapace (Figure 27.6) (DiRuzzo *et al.*, 2022).

PBM has been used to treat a broad range of soft tissue, shell, and osteological injuries and disease processes in sea turtles, primarily in the rehabilitation setting. The earliest report in the literature is a conference proceedings abstract describing the use of low-level laser therapy (LLLT) to treat traumatic head and carapace (shell) injuries in stranded loggerhead sea turtles (*Caretta caretta*) during rehabilitation (Vignoli *et al.*, 2007). Despite a relative paucity of published literature (considering nearly two decades of use), many sea turtle rehabilitation facilities that have access to laser equipment use PBMT to promote healing of acute and chronic injuries and wounds in soft tissues, shells, and bones. Multimodal treatment incorporating PBMT has been used with head and spinal cord injuries, osteomyelitis (including shell infections), septic arthritis, swelling and edema, and to address the sequelae of strangulating flipper entanglements (such as ischemia, reperfusion, and necrosis) (Figure 27.7) (Vignoli *et al.*, 2007; Nardini *et al.*, 2011; Levine *et al.*, 2022; Dr. G. Levine, personal communication; Dr. P. McCurdy, personal communication; Dr. T. Norton, personal communication; The Turtle Hospital, 2011; New England Aquarium, 2012).

PDT has been used in green sea turtles (*Chelonia mydas*) to treat a chronic, infected, nonhealing shell fracture and as an experimental treatment for fibropapillomatosis (FP). A green turtle with a chronic, nonhealing carapace fracture of 6-month duration was treated using topically-applied methylene blue as the photosensitizing agent (60 μM concentration solution with 5-minutes contact time) to target microorganisms, followed by irradiation with 660 nm red laser administered on-contact, point-to-point, at 100 mW (0.1 W) and an energy density of 180 J/cm^2. (*Note:* The duration of treatment application, irradiance, number of points treated, and total delivered energy [J] were not reported. The same author reported a spot size of 0.02 cm^2 in a different publication describing PDT using the same laser equipment (Sellera *et al.*, 2014a, 2014b). With a 0.2 cm^2 spot size, the delivered dose calculates out to 3.6 J of energy per point [$180\ J/cm^2 \times 0.02\ cm^2 = 3.6\ J$ per point]). In this case, PDT was used primarily for antimicrobial activity, or antimicrobial photodynamic therapy (aPDT), with the stimulation of wound healing considered an added benefit. PDT was applied once per week for 4 weeks. Re-epithelialization and keratinization at the fracture site were observed after 30 days (four treatments) and the aPDT was discontinued (Sellera *et al.*, 2017).

PDT has also been used as an experimental treatment for FP in green sea turtles (*Chelonia mydas*). Fibropapillomatosis is a multifactorial disease affecting marine turtles, characterized by the development of external and/or visceral (internal) epithelial tumors. Though classified as benign, tumors may become life-threatening as a result of mechanical obstructions and impingement that impair normal functioning such as sight, swimming, and feeding. All current evidence points toward a multifactorial etiology that includes infection with an alpha herpes virus (Chelonid alphaherpesvirus 5) and some combination of pathogen-host-environment interactions that have yet to definitively elucidated. Treatment options for FP are limited and have historically focused on surgical tumor debulking and supportive care. However, tumor recurrence is not uncommon. Five green turtles with multiple external tumors received two treatments with PDT, 15-days apart. Intralesional injection of methylene blue was used to photosensitize select tumors on each turtle, followed by irradiation with 660 nm red laser. Laser dosing was reported as on-contact, point-to-point, at 100 mW (0.1 W) for 160 seconds at each point, with a reported fluence of 560 J/cm^2 and total delivered dose of 16 J per point. Seven days after the first treatment all PDT treated lesions were reported to be dark blue, swollen, and firm. 30 days after

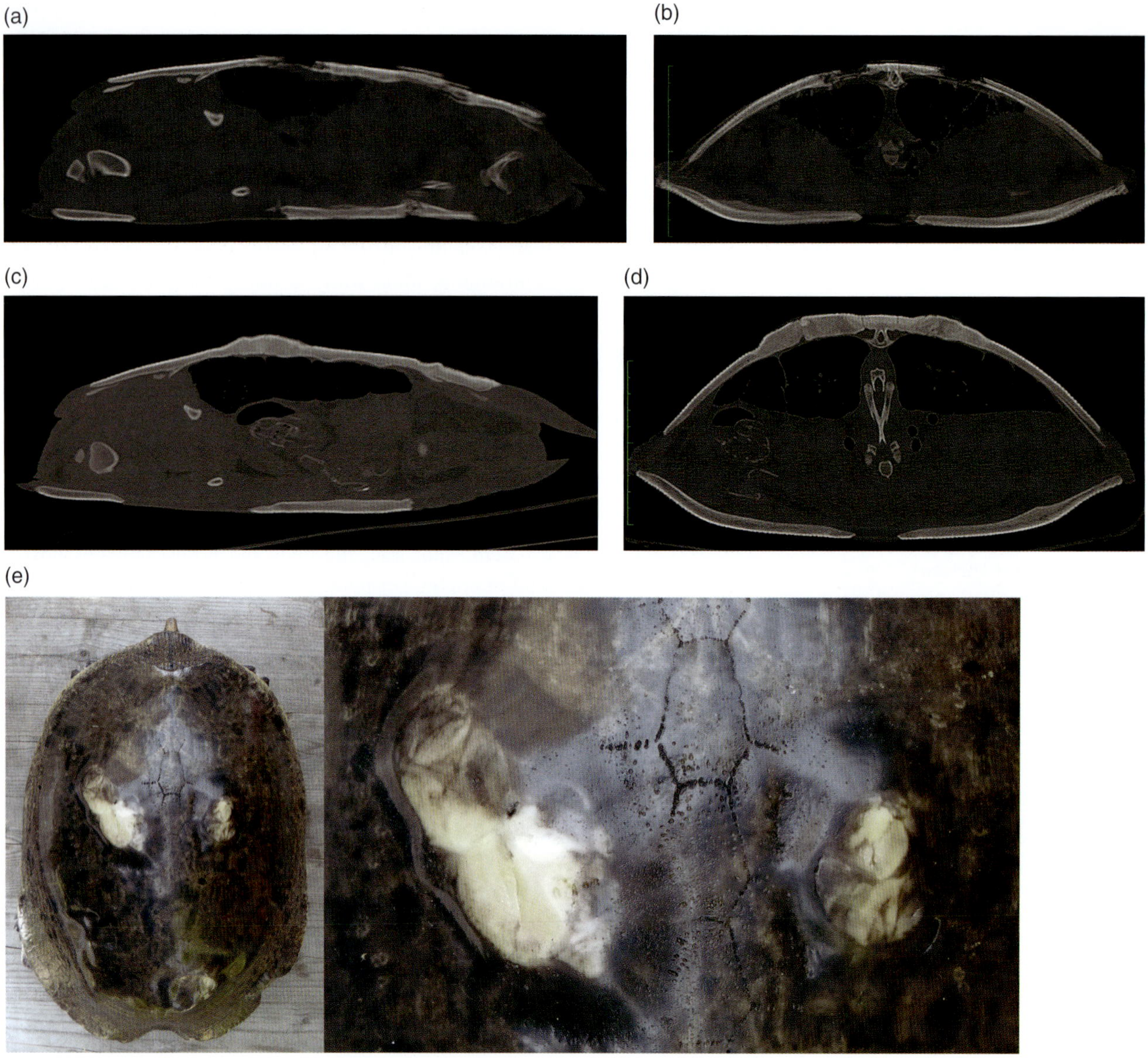

Figure 27.6 An Aubry's flapshell turtle (*Cycloderma aubryi*) with penetrating lesions to the shell. Sagittal (a) and transverse (b) computed tomography images of penetrating lesions and bone lysis 11 weeks after initial presentation. Sagittal (c) and transverse (d) computed tomography images of the same penetrating lesions shown in Figure 27.6 (a, b) from follow-up, 29 months after discontinuing medical treatment, showing healed shell lesions with bone regrowth. (e) Carapace lesions in the same patient more than 2 years after discontinuing medical treatment. The image on the right shows a close-up of the same lesions. Images courtesy of Turtle Island, Austria, EU.

the first treatment, all PDT-treated lesions had necrosed and were sufficiently detached from the epidermis to be removed using tweezers. Tumors treated with laser alone, methylene blue injection alone, or receiving no treatment, exhibited no macroscopic signs of changes (Herbst, 1994; Sellera *et al.*, 2014a; Jones *et al.*, 2016; Morrison *et al.*, 2018).

aPDT was used to treat chronic, moderate (Class III) pododermatitis in five Magellanic penguins (*Spheniscus magellanicus*) in an aquarium collection. Following surgical debridement, methylene blue was used as a photosensitizing agent to target microorganisms, and 660 nm laser light was delivered on-contact, point-to-point, to five points over each foot. The dose was reported as "100 mW at 660 nm of wavelength (λ), distributed in five equidistant points of 0.02 cm^2 ... that received 140 J/cm^2 each." This calculates out to 2.8 J of energy delivered per point (140 $J/cm^2 \times 0.02\ cm^2 = 2.8$), times 5 points, for a total delivered dose of 14 J (2.8 J/point × 5 points = 14 J). After irradiation, 10% urea cream was applied and the foot bandaged and covered with a rubber glove. Treatment and bandaging were repeated weekly until lesions were completely resolved (average = 8 weeks; range = 5–16 weeks); no

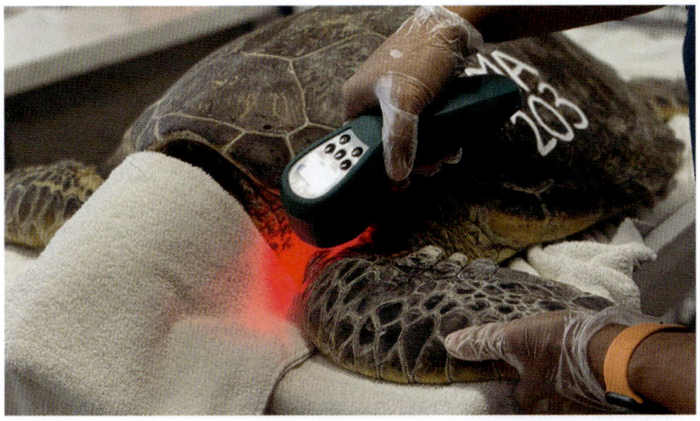

Figure 27.7 A green sea turtle in rehabilitation being treated with PBMT for a strangulating flipper entanglement. Photo courtesy of the Maui Ocean Center Marine Institute, Maui, HI, USA, and NOAA. Photo taken under USFWS Permit #TE-72088A-3.

recurrence was observed after 6 months of monitoring (Sellera *et al.*, 2014b).

After a limp of 1-year duration was diagnosed as DJD of the stifle via radiography and CT, an 18-year-old female African penguin (*Spheniscus demersus*) was treated with PBMT. The stifle joint and margins proximal and distal to the joint were treated twice per week (the dose was reported as 5 W, continuous wave, for 240 seconds; total energy delivery of 1200 J). The limp resolved after 2 weeks of PBMT (four treatments), and the patient was tapered to once-monthly treatments. All other medications (NSAIDs, opioids, and supplements) were gradually reduced, and ultimately discontinued. The patient was maintained long term on PBMT alone, administered once every 1–2 months (Figure 27.8) (Stremme, 2017).

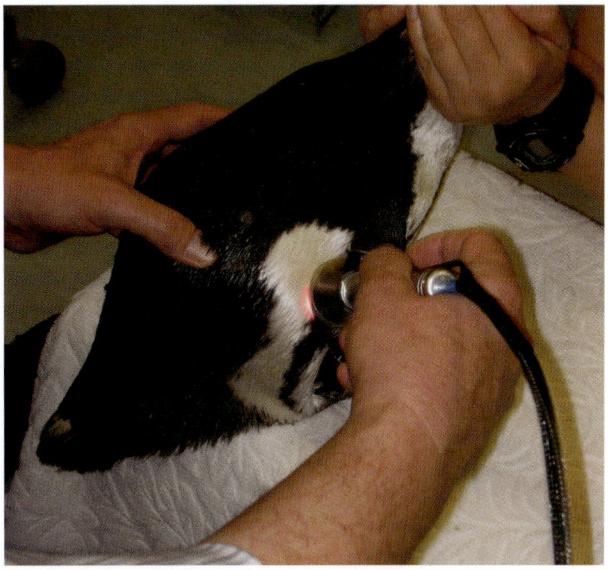

Figure 27.8 Administration of laser therapy to a penguin.

Research with Information Translatable into Clinical Practice

In the research arena, zebrafish are used as animal models for disease and have been used to investigate the cellular mechanisms of PBMT. While this research is not directly focused on clinical applications of PBMT, it is scientifically rigorous fish-specific information that can help to inform clinical application of this modality.

A zebrafish model used to investigate the potential of PBM to mitigate the inflammatory cytokine storm associated with SARS-CoV-2 (COVID-19) in humans showed decreases in pro-inflammatory markers across a broad range of tissues. Adult male zebrafish were inoculated with recombinant SARS-CoV-2 spike protein, and the treatment group received a single, whole-body administration of PBM (reported as 2 J/cm^2 of 660 nm laser light delivered at 100 mW) 5 hours post-inoculation. Specimens were euthanized for analysis at 6 and 24 hours. The PBM-treated group showed downregulation of the inflammatory response across multiple inflammatory markers measured via gene expression (qPCR), *Danio rerio* predicted protein–protein interactions, and metabolomic analysis (Rosa *et al.*, 2023).

Wound closure and neutrophil migration into fin tissue injuries were measured via real-time in-vivo imaging in transgenic zebrafish larva using a fluorescing neutrophil marker. Control and experimental groups were treated 30 minutes post-injury with 635 nm continuous wave Helium:Neon laser delivering 5 mW for a total fluence of 0 J/cm^2, 3 J/cm^2, or 18 J/cm^2. Cell migration was tracked using fluorescing light microscopy and three-dimensional time-lapse images taken every 60–75 seconds for 120 minutes. Wound healing was assessed at 24 hours. The 3 J/cm^2 treatment group had significantly reduced neutrophil migration into the wound area and more rapid wound closure than the control or 18 J/cm^2 treatment groups (Paredes *et al.*, 2022). The same research group assessed oxidative stress, macrophage migration, and wound closure in larval zebrafish utilizing similar equipment and methods described above. Control and experimental PBM treatment groups consisted of 0 J/cm^2, 3 J/cm^2, 9 J/cm^2, or 18 J/cm^2. The 3 J/cm^2 treatment group showed significantly reduced reactive oxygen species and increased macrophage migration into the wound during the first 120 minutes. At 24 hours, both the 3 and 9 J/cm^2 groups showed significantly accelerated wound closure (Paredes *et al.*, 2019).

In both studies described above, the zebrafish larvae used were 0.4 cm (4 mm) long and were treated using a laser with a 0.4 cm × 0.2 cm spot size, which effectively resulted in full thickness, whole body saturation with photons. It is possible (if not likely) that higher doses might be required to achieve similar physiological responses in the clinical setting with animals that are many orders of magnitude larger.

Recent research in the aquaculture arena has focused on utilizing PBM to increase reproductive output and productivity in catfish and sturgeon. In three catfish studies, once-weekly laserpuncture (laser stimulation of acupuncture points) for 4 weeks has been reported to accelerate gonadal development and to improve sperm quality and fecundity in male and female fish, respectively. All three studies used standardized, reasonably objective methods for evaluating gonadal development and the quantity and/or quality of sperm or eggs. All studies included a control group (no treatment), a comparative treatment group treated with Ovaprim (Salmon gonadotropin releasing hormone analog [sGnRHa] + domperidone, which is used to induce spawning in finfish) or with Ovaprim and human chorionic gonadotropin (hCG), and multiple laserpuncture treatment groups treated at different fluence. While some critical dosing information is not provided, the authors report accelerated gonadal development and increased sperm quality and fecundity at 0.4 J/cm^2 with a 975.2 nm, 20 mW laser; 0.4 J/cm^2 and 0.5 J/cm^2 with a 650 nm, 20 mW laser; and 0.4 J/cm^2, 20 mW laser (frequency not provided), respectively (Mukti *et al.*, 2020; Plavskii *et al.*, 2021; Patmadevi *et al.*, 2022; Astuti *et al.*, 2023; Mukti *et al.*, 2023).

Conclusion

The potential applications for PBM as a therapeutic modality in aquatic animal medicine have only begun to be explored. Modalities such as PDT open an entirely new set of opportunities for early intervention in chronic diseases processes that are not amenable to surgical intervention or have been minimally responsive to other treatment modalities, such as oral and genital papillomas in marine mammals (which can undergo malignant transformation into aggressive forms of neoplasia) and Fibropapillomatosis in sea turtles. Perhaps aPDT or PBMT could provide additional options for treating those chronic lesions that are too frequently unresponsive to antimicrobials and husbandry changes in aquatic animals. Clearly, there is a significant need for clinically focused research and case-based reporting to enhance our understanding of safety, efficacy, and possible uses for PBM in aquatic animals. I am optimistic that PBM can increase future therapeutic options and thereby increase our collective capacity to effectively meet the needs of so many aquatic animal patients.

Acknowledgments

The author would like to acknowledge and thank Donald W. Stremme, for his support and for contributions to this chapter, which have been conserved from the first edition of *Laser Therapy in Veterinary Medicine*.

References

Ackroyd, R. *et al.* (2001). The history of photodetection and photodynamic therapy. *Photochem Photobiol.* 74:656. doi:10.1562/0031-8655(2001)074<0656:THOPAP>2.0.CO;2.

Adams, L. Michalkiewiz J *et al.*(2005). Effect of Regranex Gel concentration or post application contact time on the healing rate of head and lateral line erosions in marine tropical fish. *IAAAM 36th Annual Conference Proceedings*. International Association for Aquatic Animal Medicine. May 14–18. Seward, AK.

Al-Watban, F.A.H. *et al.* (2007). Low-level laser therapy enhances wound healing in diabetic rats: a comparison of different lasers. *Photomed Laser Surg*. 25(2):72–77.

Amaroli, A. *et al.* (2017). The effect of photobiomodulation on the sea urchin *Paracentrotus lividus* (Echinodermata) using higher-Fluence on fertilization, embryogenesis, and larval development: an *in vitro* study. *Photomed Laser Surg*. 35(3):127–135. doi:10.1089/pho.2016.4136.

Astuti, S.D. *et al.* (2023). Photobiomodulation effect of infra-red laser on the level of gonad maturity in the Simese catfish (*Pangasianodon hypophthalmus*). *Heliyon*. 9(12):e23253. doi:10.1016/j.heliyon.2023.e23253.

Balian, E.V. *et al.* (2008). The freshwater animal diversity assessment: an overview of the results. *Hydrobiologia*. 595(1):627–637. doi:10.1007/s10750-007-9246-3.

Bandaranayake, W.M. (2006). The nature and role of pigments of marine invertebrates. *Nat Prod Rep*. 23(2):223–255. doi:10.1039/b307612c.

Bjordal, J. *et al.* (2003). A systematic review of low level laser therapy with location specific doses for pain from chronic joint disorders. *Aust J Physiother*. 49(2):107–116.

Boylan, S.M. *et al.* (2017). Spondylosis in a green moray eel, *Gymnothorax funebris* (Ranzani 1839), with swim bladder hyperinflation. *J Fish Dis*. 40(7):963–969. doi:10.1111/jfd.12563.

Chow, R. *et al.* (2011). Inhibitory effects of laser irradiation on peripheral mammalian nerves and relevance to analgesic effects: a systematic review. *Photomed Laser Surg*. 29(6):365–381.

Correia, J.H. *et al.* (2021). Photodynamic therapy review: principles, photosensitizers, applications, and future directions. *Pharmaceutics.* 13(9):1332. doi:10.3390/pharmaceutics13091332.

DiRuzzo, S. *et al.* (2022). Successful treatment of severe ulcerative dermatitis in an Aubry's Flapshell turtle (*Cycloderma aubryi*). *J Herpetol Med Surg.* 32(4). doi:10.5818/JHMS-D-22-00002.

Feyrecilde, M. (2024). *Cooperative Veterinary Care.* Wiley, Hoboken, NJ.

Filho, F.A. *et al.* (2021). Antimicrobial photodinamic therapy combined with laser photobiomodulation in the treatment of skin wounds in a dog (*Canis lupus familiaris*). *Acta Sci Vet.* 49. doi:10.22456/1679-9216.116169.

Fleming, G. *et al.* (2008). Treatment factors influencing the use of recombinant platelet-derived growth factor (Regranex®) for head and lateral line erosion syndrome in ocean surgeon fish (*Acanthurus bahianus*). *J Zoo Wildl Med.* 39(2):155–160.

Gilewski, A.L. *et al.* (2024). Effect of photobiomodulation therapy as a multimodal approach to treatment of dermal abrasions in cownose rays (*Rhinoptera bonasus*). *Zoo Biol*:1–7. doi:10.1002/zoo.21832.

Gouin, J.P. *et al.* (2011). The impact of psychological stress on wound healing: methods and mechanisms. *Immunol Allergy Clin N Am.* 31(1):81–93. doi:10.1016/j.iac.2010.09.010.

Hamblin, M.R. *et al.* (2017). *Imaging in Photodynamic Therapy.* Taylor & Francis Group, Boca Raton, FL, USA.

Hamblin, M.R. *et al.* (2019). Non-mammalian hosts and photobiomodulation: do all life-forms respond to light? *Photochem Photobiol.* 95(1):126–139. doi:10.1111/php.12951.

Herbst, L.H. (1994). Fibropapillomatosis of marine turtles. *Annu Rev Fish Dis.* 4:389–425.

Johnson, E. and Saint-Erne (2022). Utilization of photobiomodulation to heal a chronic wound in a Plecostomus (Hypostomus Plecostomus). *Aquat Vet.* 16(1):28–29.

Jones, K. *et al.* (2016). A review of fibropapillomatosis in green turtles (*Chelonia mydas*). *Vet J.* 212:48–57. doi:10.1016/j.tvjl.2015.10.041.

Kraut, S. *et al.* (2013). Laser therapy in a soft-shelled turtle (*Pelodiscus sinensis*) for the treatment of skin and shell ulceration: a case report. *Tierarztl Prax Ausg K Klientiere Heimtiere.* 41(04):261–266. doi:10.1055/s-0038-1623709.

Levine, G. *et al.*, (2022). A Noninvasive Integrative Multimodal Approach to Treating Flipper Strangulation Injuries Caused by Fishing Gear Entanglements in the Hawaiian Green Sea Turtle (*Chelonia mydas*). 53rd Annual IAAAM Conference Proceedings. International Association for Aquatic Animal Medicine. May 16 – 26. Virtual

Looney, A.L. *et al.* (2018). A randomized blind placebo-controlled trial investigating the effects of photobiomodulation therapy (PBMT) on canine elbow osteoarthritis. *The Canadian Veterinary Journal.* 59 (9):959–966.

Mendez, T.M. *et al.* (2004). Dose and wavelength of laser light have influence on the repair of cutaneous wounds. *J Clin Laser Med Surg.* 22(1):19–25. doi:10.1089/104454704773660930.

Morrison, C.L. *et al.* (2018). Genomic evolution, recombination, and inter-strain diversity of chelonid alphaherpesvirus 5 from Florida and Hawaii green sea turtles with fibropapillomatosis. *PeerJ.* 6:e4386. doi:10.7717/peerj.4386.

Mukti, A.T. *et al.* (2020). The effects of laserpuncture on gonadal maturity and sperm quality of male striped catfish (*Pangasianodon hypophthalmus*). *Theriogenology.* 147:102–107. doi:10.1016/j.theriogenology.2020.02.030.

Mukti, A.T. *et al.* (2023). Acceleration of gonadal maturity of female striped catfish, *Pangasianodon hypophthalmus* (*Pisces, Pangasiidae*) by irradiation to low-power soft-laser. *Anim Reprod Sci.* 258:107332. doi:10.1016/j.anireprosci.2023.107332.

Muñoz-Miranda, L.A. *et al.* (2023). An extensive review of marine pigments: sources, biotechnological applications, and sustainability. *Aquat Sci.* 85:68. doi:10.1007/s00027-023-00966-8.

The Turtle Hospital (2011). https://www.turtlehospital.org/past-patients/cold-laser-physical-therapy/ (accessed 4/15/24)

The New England Aquarium (2012). http://rescue.neaq.org/2012/09/laser-turtle.html (accessed 4/15/24)

Nardini G. *et al.*, (2011). Low level laser therapy (LLLT) in reptile medicine. *Proceedings Association of Reptilian and Amphibian Veterinarians.* 171. August 6–12. Seattle, Washington

Nascimento, C.L. *et al.* (2015). Comparative study between photodynamic and antibiotic therapies for treatment of footpad dermatitis (bumblefoot) in Magellanic penguins (*Spheniscus magellanicus*). *Photodiagn Photodyn Ther.* 12(1):36–44. doi:10.1016/j.pdpdt.2014.12.012.

Palmer, K.F. and Williams, D. (1974). Optical properties of water in the near infrared*. *J Opt Soc Am.* 64(8):1107. doi:10.1364/JOSA.64.001107.

Paredes, A.D. *et al.* (2019). The effect of fluence on macrophage kinetics, oxidative stress, and wound closure using real-time *in vivo* imaging. *Photobiomodulation Photomed Laser Surg.* 37(1):45–52. doi:10.1089/photob.2018.4494.

Paredes, A. *et al.* (2022). The effect of fluence on neutrophil kinetics in zebrafish wounds using real-time in vivo imaging. *Med Res Arch.* 10(12). doi:10.18103/mra.v10i12.3238.

Patmadevi, M. *et al.* (2022). The effect of laserpuncture on accelerate gonadal maturity of female striped catfish (*Pangasianodon hypophthalmus*). *IOP Conf Ser Earth*

Environ Sci. 1036(1):012036. doi:10.1088/1755-1315/1036/1/012036.

Pees, M. *et al.* (2011). Pilotstudie zum Einsatz der Diodenlasertherapie zur Behandlung von Dermatitiden bei Koi-Karpfen (*Cyprinus carpio*) [Pilot study on the use of diode laser therapy for treatment of dermatitis in koi carp (*Cyprinus carpio*)]. *Tierarztl Prax Ausg K, Kleintiere/ Heimtiere.* 39(2):89–96.

Peplow, P.V. *et al.* (2010). Laser photobiomodulation of wound healing: a review of experimental studies in mouse and rat animal models. *Photomed Laser Surg.* 28(3):291–325. doi:10.1089/pho.2008.2446.

Piao, D. *et al.* (2018). Flexible nine-channel photodetector probe facilitated intraspinal multisite transcutaneous photobiomodulation therapy dosimetry in cadaver dogs. *J Biomed Opt.* 23(1):1–4. doi:10.1117/1.JBO.23.1.010503.

Plavskii, V.Y. *et al.* (2021). Effect of continuous wave, quasi-continuous wave and pulsed laser radiation on functional characteristics of fish spermatozoa. *J Photochem Photobiol B Biol.* 216:112112. doi:10.1016/j.jphotobiol.2020.112112.

Ramirez, K. (1999). *Animal Training: Successful Animal Management through Positive Reinforcement.* Shedd Aquarium, Chicago, IL.

Rezende, S.B. *et al.* (2007). Effects of a single near-infrared laser treatment on cutaneous wound healing: biometrical and histological study in rats. *J Photochem Photobiol B.* 87 (3):145–153. doi:10.1016/j.jphotobiol.2007.02.005.

Roberts, H. (2009). *Fundamentals of Ornamental Fish Health.* John Wiley and Sons, New York.

Roberts, D.B. *et al.* (2013). The effectiveness of therapeutic class IV (10 W) laser treatment for epicondylitis. *Lasers Surg Med.* 45(5):311–317.

Rosa, I.F. *et al.* (2023). Photobiomodulation reduces the cytokine storm syndrome associated with COVID-19 in the zebrafish model. *Int J Mol Sci.* 24(7):6104. doi:10.3390/ijms24076104.

Sabino, C.P. *et al.* (2023). The biochemical mechanisms of antimicrobial photodynamic therapy[†]. *Photochem Photobiol.* 99:742–750. doi:10.1111 php.13685.

Santana-Blank, L. *et al.* (2015). Water's many roles in laser photobiomodulation. *J Cancer Res Treat.* 3(1):1–5. doi:10.12691/jcrt-3-1-1.

Sellera, F. *et al.* (2014a). Green turtle (*Chelonia mydas*) cutaneous fibropapillomatosis treatment by photodynamic therapy. *Mar Turt Newsl.* 142:6–10.

Sellera, F.P. *et al.* (2014b). Photodynamic therapy for pododermatitis in penguins. *Zoo Biol.* 33(4):353–356. doi:10.1002/zoo.21135.

Sellera, F. *et al.* (2017). Photodynamic therapy in consolidation of carapace fracture in green turtles (*Chelonia mydas*). *Nat Res Forum.* 5(1):50–55. doi:10.6008/SPC2237-9290.2015.001.0005.

Scholle, K. *et al.* (2010). 2 μm Laser Sources and Their Possible Applications. In: *Frontiers in Guided Wave Optics and Optoelectronics.* (ed. B. Pal). InTech. doi:10.5772/39538.

Stremme, D.W. (2017). Laser Therapy for Aquatic Species. In: *Laser therapy in veterinary medicine: Photobiomodulation.* (eds. R.J. Reigel and J.C. Godbold), pp. 313–319. John Wiley & Sons, Ltd, Ames, Iowa.

Vignoli, M. *et al.* (2007). Imaging of two trauma cases in loggerhead sea turtles (*Caretta caretta*). In: *Proceedings European College of Veterinary Diagnostic Imaging.*, p. 107.

World Register of Marine Species Statistics. 2024 https://www.marinespecies.org/aphia.php?p=stats (accessed March 10, 2024)

Zdubek, A. *et al.* (2024). On the possibility of using 5-aminolevulinic acid in the light-induced destruction of microorganisms. *Int J Mol Sci.* 25(7):3590. doi:10.3390/ijms25073590.

Zein, R. *et al.* (2018). *Review of light parameters and photobiomodulation efficacy: dive into complexity. J Biomed Opt.* 23(12):1. doi:10.1117/1.JBO.23.12. 120901.

28

Zoological Applications of Laser Therapy

Liza Dadone[1] *and Tara Harrison*[2]

[1] *Giraffe Veterinary Services, Colorado Springs, CO, USA*
[2] *North Carolina State College of Veterinary Medicine, Raleigh, NC, USA*

Introduction

Photobiomodulation therapy (PBMT) is used in zoos as part of a multimodal approach to case management. It is a noninvasive and generally safe treatment modality that can help manage medical conditions, including wound management, neurologic injuries, and age-related degenerative conditions.

PBMT, colloquially known as cold laser therapy, is a photochemical process that utilizes red and infrared light to reduce inflammation and pain and promote healing (González and Mayer, 2019). This has been studied in a range of species including humans (Pryor, 2009; Dompe *et al.*, 2020), laboratory animals, and other domestic species (Draper *et al.*, 2012; Pryor and Millis, 2015; Pluim *et al.*, 2020; Rico-Holgado *et al.*, 2021). In humans, PBMT is used for conditions including wound healing and burn management, brain injuries and spinal cord damage, dentistry, and diabetes (Dompe *et al.*, 2020). There are a growing number of peer-reviewed studies on the efficacy of laser therapy in nondomestic species (Archibald *et al.*, 2020; Comunian *et al.*, 2017; Cusack *et al.*, 2018).

While still an area of active research for zoo species, PBMT may help reduce pain and improve healing time, and ultimately may help reduce patient mortality. This benefits animal welfare and could also help reduce treatment costs and staff time.

Background

Class 3B and Class 4 lasers are used in zoo medicine. Class 3B lasers are those with power not exceeding 500 mW, while Class 4 lasers emit at a power greater than 500 mW. While 3B lasers can be used for a wide variety of patients depending on the condition being treated, Class 4 lasers may be more effective and practical in larger patients, including megavertebrates. Some zoos partner with local veterinary clinics for access to their equipment and expertise.

Variability in patient size, skin thickness, coloration, pelage, and depth of target tissues means an effective treatment in one species might not be universally therapeutic, and that additional studies could help to develop species-appropriate protocols. When developing protocols for zoo species (pending further studies), in general longer wavelengths will be needed to reach deeper tissues. Notably in human patients, up to 66% of percutaneous laser light energy is absorbed or scattered in the first 2 mm of skin (Esnouf *et al.*, 2007). For a mid-sized dog, the therapeutic window of wavelengths is generally from 600 to 1100 nm; a wavelength of 635 nm might be appropriate for treating superficial wounds, and a longer wavelength of 800 nm would reach most musculoskeletal conditions (Pryor and Millis, 2015). Above a certain wavelength, treatments will not be therapeutic and may inhibit the desired tissue response (Sims *et al.*, 2015). The safety and penetration of laser light through the epidermis of reptiles and fish is currently unknown (Rychel *et al.*, 2011), as is the ability of the therapy laser to penetrate the thick skin of megavertebrates such as elephants.

An additional consideration is how to access the patient for laser treatment in a way that is both safe and minimally stressful for patient and staff. Positive reinforcement training can make laser treatment sessions safer, less stressful, and less time-consuming for zoo staff compared with other ways of accessing the patient such as general anesthesia. This training is especially helpful for patients that are too large or dangerous to restrain manually. It is strongly recommended that zoos invest in staff time to train the animals under their care for stationing or holding near where laser therapy could be used prior to a medical

Laser Therapy in Veterinary Medicine: Photobiomodulation, Second Edition. Edited by Christopher J. Winkler and Lisa A. Miller.

condition developing, as ill patients and patients in pain may be slower to learn trained behaviors (Dadone *et al.*, 2016).

As in any species and with any treatment, clinicians should use equipment appropriately and should adjust treatments as warranted for the case. Safety precautions include always wearing appropriate eye protection when operating the laser and taking care around reflective surfaces. Additional safety measures may be needed to work in close proximity with some zoo species, particularly venomous snakes, primates, carnivores, and megavertebrates. Therapy lasers should be used according to manufacturer instructions and treatments should not be directed at eyes and are generally not recommended for use in pregnant or neonatal animals. For additional information on safety, see Chapter 5.

Evaluating Treatment Efficacy

The wide range of anatomic differences in zoo species makes it challenging to determine appropriate laser therapy settings for effective tissue penetration. To evaluate this, Burgos *et al.* (in review) measured PBMT tissue penetration with cadaver skin samples from birds, reptiles, amphibians, and small mammals. Opportunistic samples for study included skin from a red-tailed hawk, a box turtle, a guinea pig, a rabbit, a green iguana, a bullfrog, and a Kemp's Ridley sea turtle. The results suggest that feathers may inhibit the passage of light through the tissue to the photometer. Additionally, lighter-colored and less-pigmented skin had higher power readings and thus higher tissue penetration when compared with darker colored or pigmented samples. While this postmortem study did not measure tissue response to treatment, it does suggest that feathers and darker skin pigmentation may reduce tissue penetration with photobiomodulation treatments.

For most clinical cases, the effectiveness of PBMT is based on an individual patient receiving multiple concurrent therapies, and if the case does well, histopathology will not be available. For this reason, it is important to have clear metrics of whether patient therapies are effective. Monitoring should include periodic visual assessments, behavioral assessments, physical exams, physiological assessments such as bloodwork, and imaging, such that adjustments can be made as appropriate to the case and help ensure best possible outcome for the patient (Table 28.1).

Wound Management

Superficial wounds are relatively accessible for laser therapy treatments and are not limited by challenges related to deep-tissue penetration. In a small study of the effects of laser therapy in multiple cases at one zoo, it was found to be helpful in wound management more consistently than in the management of lameness or joint pain (Howard *et al.*, 2014). In human medicine, PBMT has helped in the healing of chronic wounds (Dompe *et al.*, 2020). While there are few systematic studies verifying the effectiveness of laser therapy, wound management is likely one of the better clinical applications.

Based on a study in rabbits, PBMT accelerates wound healing in some phases of the healing process (Hodjati *et al.*, 2014). In this study, wounds were treated with PBMT (4 J/cm^2, 808 nm, day 0, 3, and 6) and histopathology then confirmed a significant increase in epithelialization and reduced wound diameter when compared with the control group, but no significant difference in fibrin levels or wound inflammation. The histology results suggest PBMT activates primary photoreceptors as well as NADH-dehydrogenase. PBMT also initiates phagocytic cells' nonmitochondrial respiratory burst as well as

Table 28.1 As species-specific optimal dosing of photobiomodulation therapy is generally not available for zoo species, patient monitoring and adjustments to the treatment plan should be based on periodic monitoring of multiple metrics.

Monitoring modality	Examples (may vary by species and case)
Visual assessment	Activity level, lameness score, posture, wound appearance, proprioception, evaluation of body positioning when sleeping (i.e., laying down at night in a normal position)
Behavioral assessment	Willingness to participate in training session or to shift between enclosures
Physical exam	Baseline heart rate, wound size, and granulation
Physiological measures	Measures of inflammation (i.e., fibrinogen, serum amyloid A/SSA), muscle injury (i.e., creatinine kinase/CK, lactic acid), histology (i.e., granulation tissue)
Imaging	Photographs, radiographs, ultrasound, thermography, computed tomography (CT)

activating NADPH-oxidase. A similar study (Karu, 2003) reports that PBMT indirectly activates cells by activating secondary messengers released by those cells activated by PBMT, such as phagocytes, lymphokines, and cytokines that are produced by lymphocytes, macrophages that produce nitric oxide, or blood cells with nitric oxide hemoglobin photolysis.

Based on findings in humans and companion and laboratory animals (Kuffler, 2016), it is strongly recommended that surgical wounds in any species be treated with a single laser treatment after they have been closed, both to promote wound healing and to minimize postoperative pain (for safety reasons, this is not recommended for ocular or skin cancer surgeries). In general, PBMT for traumatic open wounds should be treated with a noncontact head and is usually dosed between 2 and 8 J/cm^2 (Fessehav, 2020). One of the authors (Harrison) has instituted the use of laser therapy postoperatively for every surgical procedure in exotic pet species, including rabbits, guinea pigs, and birds. The therapy seems to have subjectively improved healing in these species. Similarly, accelerated wound healing and analgesic benefits have been appreciated when managing a range of trauma cases in zoo patients (E. Lipanovich, personal communication).

Birds

In Magellanic penguins (*Spheniscus magellanicus*), pododermatitis (bumblefoot) showed clinical improvement with multimodal treatments that included photodynamic therapy (PDT). Magellanic penguins with preexisting advanced pododermatitis underwent surgical debridement of the lesions and were then treated either medically (topical and systemic antibiotics, plus anti-inflammatory medications) or with PDT without other medications (Nascimento *et al.*, 2015). For the PDT group, the wound was first instilled with an aqueous solution of methylene blue (the photosensitizer) for 5 minutes, then irradiated every 1 cm, with the number of treatment sites varying based on wound size. The wound was treated using a wavelength of 660 nm at a dosage of 133.3 J/cm^2 every 3 days for 84 days. Using this protocol, healing rates and average healing times were significantly better for penguins treated with PDT than for those solely receiving medical management. In another study, five Magellanic penguins with pododermatitis lesions on their foot pads were treated with PDT (Sellera *et al.*, 2014). All the treated lesions regressed and no recurrence was noted during a 6-month follow-up.

Pododermatitis lesions in an American flamingo (*Phoenicopterus ruber*) clinically improved with laser therapy (Harrison, unpublished results). The flamingo had a history of chronic, recurrent pododermatitis. Once per week photobiomodulation and acupuncture was added to the medical management (Ceftiofur CFFA 10 mg/kg; and meloxicam 0.5 mg/kg) and the foot lesions then showed clinical improvement (Figure 28.1) (5 Hz, 1 SPL 8.14 J/cm^2 @ 905 nm, 3 IRD [80 mW each] 153.4 J/cm^2 [total] @ 850 nm, 3 LED [64 mW each] = 122.7 J/cm^2 [total] @ 630 nm).

Chronic pododermatitis cases in other bird species have also improved when treated with laser therapy. In a multiple bird species including fulvous tree ducks (*Dendrocygna*

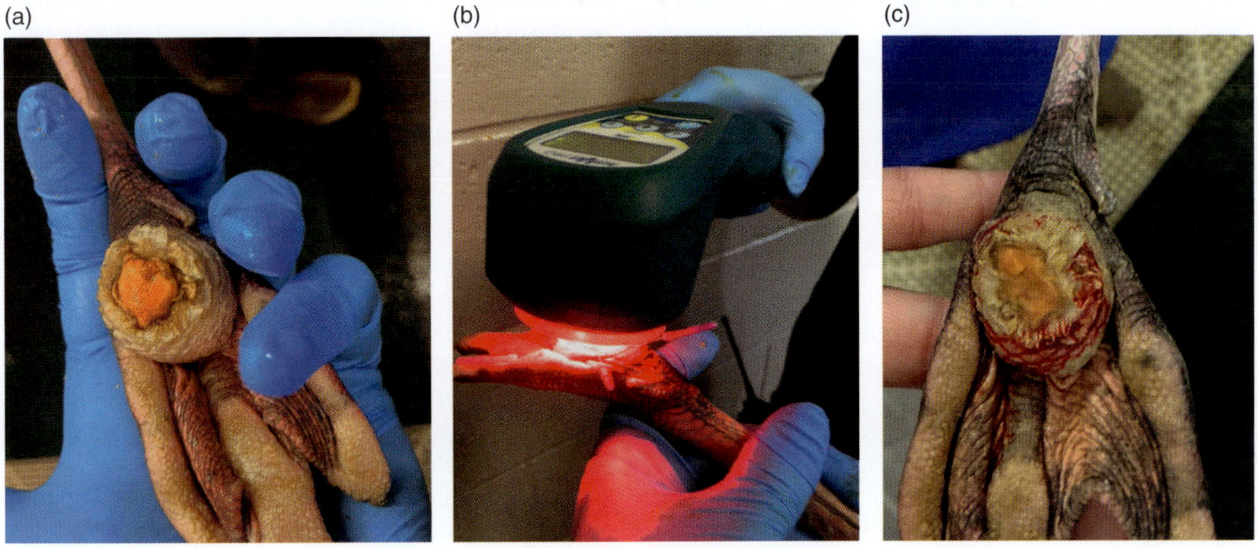

Figure 28.1 Chronic pododermatitis lesions in an American flamingo were managed with laser therapy. (a) Before starting treatment. (b) Positioning for treatment. (c) After 2 weeks of one time weekly treatments, and immediately post-acupuncture treatment (source of blood in photo), the chronic nonhealing pododermatitis lesion was smaller than prior to starting laser therapy treatments.

bicolor), lesions were treated with PBMT at 5 Hz (1 SPL 8.14 J/cm^2 @ 905 nm, 3 IRD [80 mW each] 153.4 J/cm^2 [total] @ 850 nm, 3 LED [64 mW each] = 122.7 J/cm^2 [total] @ 630 nm) for 3–5 minutes, once per week for 4 weeks (Harrison, unpublished results). The wounds showed clinical improvement, though the calluses appeared to progress more slowly. Similarly, chronic pododermatitis in a red-tailed hawk (*Buteo jamaicensis*) improved with laser therapy (L. Wright, personal communication). After managing chronic nonhealing foot-pad scabs for over 6 months, laser therapy was started. Within several months, the wounds had healed enough that the hawk no longer needed bandages on its feet.

Wing-tip lesions may show improved healing with laser therapy treatment, depending on the severity of the injury. In some raptors with wing-tip lesions associated with edema, avascular necrosis, and dry gangrene, laser therapy may assist in tissue recovery (Lacasse, 2015). A distal wing-tip fracture in a rock dove (*Columba livia domestica*) was initially treated with laser therapy but ultimately required amputation (Harrison, unpublished results). Initially, the dove's fracture site was treated twice weekly with laser therapy for 3 weeks at 250 Hz (1 SPL 8.14 J/cm^2 @ 905 nm, 3 IRD [80 mW each] 153.4 J/cm^2 [total] @ 850 nm, 3 LED [64 mW each] = 122.7 J/cm^2 [total] @ 630 nm) and then once-per-week thereafter. The fracture site ultimately still required surgical debridement, after which laser therapy treatments were continued, and the wound appeared nearly healed within a week.

A keel wound in a bald eagle (*Haliaeetus leucocephalus*) showed clinical improvement when management included laser therapy (Cushing *et al*., 2013). A healing time faster-than-expected was seen when laser therapy treatments were incorporated.

Mammals

Pododermatitis in rabbits has been managed with multimodal therapies, which can include medical and surgical management, bandaging, correction of underlying causes, and laser therapy (Blair, 2013). In one case, a rabbit was dosed with 150 J/cm^2 for each foot lesion. Laser treatments were carried out twice weekly for six doses, in conjunction with topical medications, bandages, and husbandry changes (Figure 28.2).

Pododermatitis has also been treated with laser therapy in a rat, *Rattus norvegicus* (Harrison, unpublished results). Lesions were treated with PBMT with 5 Hz (1 SPL 8.14 J/cm^2 @ 905 nm, 3 IRD [80 mW each] 153.4 J/cm^2 [total] @ 850 nm, 3 LED [64 mW each] = 122.7 J/cm^2 [total] @ 630 nm) for 3 minutes one time weekly. Although the pododermatitis never fully resolved, the lesions showed improvement and the rat had an improved quality of life.

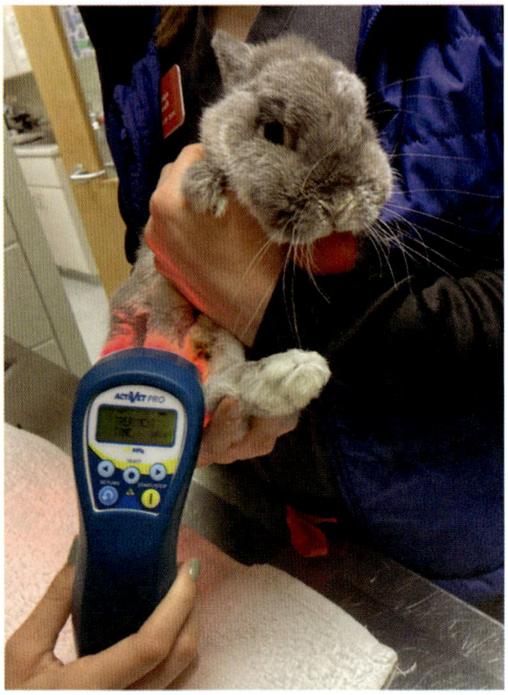

Figure 28.2 Pododermatitis in a domestic rabbit was treated with PBMT and resulted in improved wound healing.

Thermal burns in two domestic ferrets (*Mustela putorius furo*) healed well when treated with medical management and laser therapy (Harrison, unpublished results). Burns occurred accidentally from supplemental heat during a surgical procedure. The ferrets were treated three times a week for 4 weeks with 5 Hz (1 SPL 8.14 J/cm^2 @ 905 nm, 3 IRD [80 mW each] 153.4 J/cm^2 [total] @ 850 nm, 3 LED [64 mW each] = 122.7 J/cm^2 [total] @ 630 nm) for 5 minutes per treatment to assist in wound healing. Blue light laser therapy was also added to assist in managing infection (Figure 28.3).

A nonresolving scab on the front leg of a hedgehog became markedly worse after a single PBMT and was later diagnosed as a squamous cell carcinoma (L. Wright, personal communication). This case highlights the potential risks of treating a chronic wound prior to biopsy. Further details on treating patients with cancer or potential cancer are discussed in Chapter 19.

Complications from declaw surgeries in both a caracal (*Caracal caracal*) and a serval (*Leptailurus serval*) healed well when management included laser therapy (E. Lipanovich, personal communication). Both cats were housed at a sanctuary and had chronic complications and granulomas at the declaw sites. While declaws of large cats is strongly not recommended, in this case surgical removal of third phalangeal bone remnants combined with medical management and laser therapy helped both cats heal superficial wounds and have improved long-term comfort.

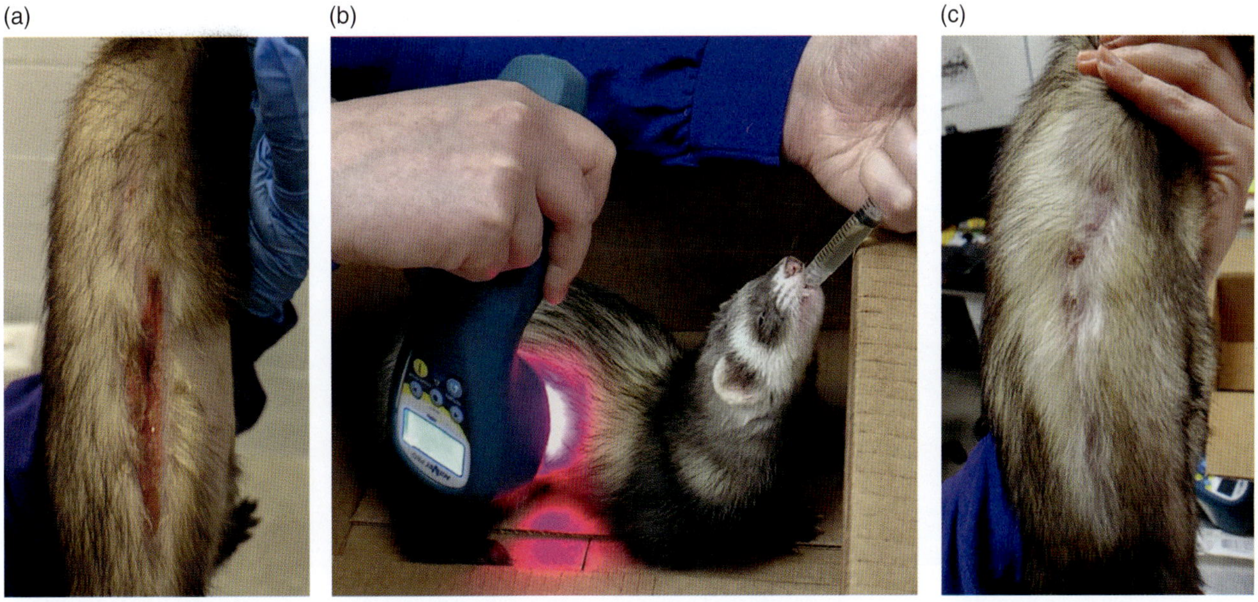

Figure 28.3 Thermal burns in a domestic ferret managed with laser therapy. The burns were from a heating bag placed next to the patient during an otherwise routine anesthetic procedure. (a) Three weeks after initial injury, the wound remained ulcerated. (b) Photobiomodulation therapy was administered three times weekly for 1 month while the ferret was slowly syringe-fed. (c) Six weeks after starting laser treatments the wound was no-longer ulcerative and most of the fur had regrown (Photo by L. Walosin, S. Kniseley).

Hygromas in three 2-year-old Amur tigers (*Panthera tigris altaica*) were successfully managed using laser therapy (Harrison, unpublished results). All hygromas were present to varying degrees on the elbows bilaterally for each animal (Figure 30.1a). When the hygromas were first seen, husbandry changes were made, but there was no obvious clinical improvement after 1 month. The tigers were target-trained to station in a squeeze chute for PBMT. They would position themselves between 2 and 4 in. from the side of the squeeze chute and the laser was placed outside of the chute. PBMT was administered twice a week for 2 months at 5 Hz (1 SPL 8.14 J/cm^2 @ 905 nm, 3 IRD [80 mW each] 153.4 J/cm^2 [total] @ 850 nm, 3 LED [64 mW each] = 122.7 J/cm^2 [total] @ 630 nm). Application was centered on the hygromas, as well as acupuncture points LI-11 and SI-9. After starting laser therapy, the hygromas noticeably decreased in size, and resolved within 2 months.

An okapi with fly strike skin lesions showed good wound healing when treatment included laser therapy. The lesion was treated with a PBMT treatment of 5 Hz (1 SPL 8.14 J/cm^2 @ 905 nm, 3 IRD [80 mW each] 153.4 J/cm^2 [total] @ 850 nm, 3 LED [64 mw each] = 122.7 J/cm^2 [total] @ 630 nm) for 5 minutes three times per week for 2 weeks. The wound was also regularly cleaned with chlorhexidine and additional fly control was used in the barn. Once laser therapy was included, the wounds rapidly resolved (Figure 28.4).

Elephants

There have been a number of attempts to facilitate wound healing in elephants by using PBMT. In several cases, PBMT has assisted in and resulted in faster wound healing than expected. At other times, no clinical improvement has been seen. To avoid damaging the optics of the laser unit and maximize the chances for treatment success, it is strongly recommended to avoid using a contact handpiece in a scanning application on elephants (R.J. Riegel, personal communication).

Before the increased availability of Class 3b and 4 lasers, pressure sores on the hips of a 58-year-old female Asian elephant (*Elaphas maximus*) were managed using direct-contact infrared irradiation, which was associated with clinical improvement (Gage *et al.*, 1997). Initially, the wounds appeared in areas of devitalized tissue near the ischial tuberosity. Prior to each treatment, the wounds were debrided and gently cleaned. They were treated for 30–45 minutes daily for 60 days, then every other day until the end of the experimental period. Infrared light-therapy pads were applied over cleaned wounds at each treatment and kept moist between treatments using isotonic saline gel. In this case, irradiation of pressure sores seemed to result in faster wound healing than expected, and the clinicians reported that the treatment was notably associated with no wound infections and with a good bed of granulation tissue.

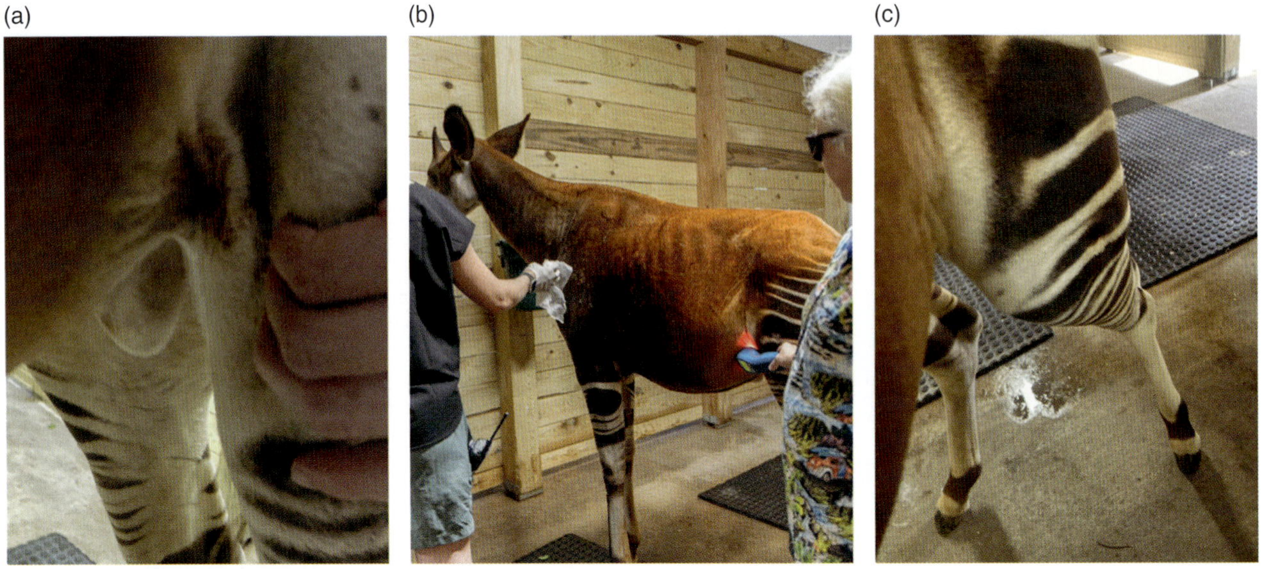

Figure 28.4 Fly strike dermatitis in an okapi was managed with daily cleanings, fly repellant, and laser therapy. (a) Before starting laser treatment, the wound was ulcerative and was not showing clinical improvement. (b) The laser was positioned on the lesion while the okapi received neck and chin scratches and browse from his trainer. (c) One month after starting laser therapy, the skin lesion had resolved (Photo by T. Harrison (Chapter Contributor) and B. Robinson).

Cheek-patch dermatitis in an Asian elephant (*Elaphas maximus*) improved with therapy laser treatments (Cushing *et al*., 2013). A schedule of three treatments in the first week, two in the second week, and one weekly thereafter was used in this case. The clinicians reported that this treatment was associated with reduced healing time and inflammation compared with clinical expectations. When a similar protocol was attempted for an African elephant (*Loxodonta Africana*) with cheek-pad dermatitis, no clinical improvement was appreciated (Dadone, unpublished results).

Pressure sores and superficial wounds in multiple elephants were successfully managed with treatment that included PBMT (L. Young, personal communication). Treatment with PBMT seemed to be well tolerated by the elephants and was associated with rapid healing, although all animals were generally treated so no control cases could be assessed.

A trunk laceration in an elephant healed rapidly when treated with laser therapy (E. Lipanovich, personal communication). A 31-year-old female Asian elephant (*Elaphus maximus*) presented with a large laceration to the distal third of her trunk, possibly caused by another elephant (Figure 28.5). Under a standing sedation, the wound was debrided and sutured closed twice in the first week but dehisced each time and showed signs of infection despite routine wound care and antibiotics. The elephant was sedated again 10 days after the initial injury, the wound was debrided, and laser therapy was started. Bandages were not tolerated by the patient. The laceration was dosed with mixed wavelengths of 808 and 905 nm at 1.2 J/cm^2. Treatments were carried out three times the first week, then twice weekly for 3 weeks, then once weekly for 3 weeks. During the first 3 weeks of treatment, the elephant was also sedated weekly for wound debridement. Within 2 weeks of starting the laser therapy, the wound had excellent granulation and reduced infection and seemed less sensitive during wound care. About 7 weeks after starting treatment, the laceration had healed and medical management was discontinued. The site of the wound appeared to be slightly lighter in coloration than the other side and had no obvious nerve damage.

Reptiles

PBMT has had variable results when used for reptile wound management. While laser treatments were generally associated with improvements in some aspects of wound healing, the most consistent benefits have been anecdotally reported in severe cutaneous wounds including degloving injuries, thermal burns, and contaminated ulcerative dermatitis lesions. Notable differences between clinical outcomes include that the wounds with the best outcomes were often more severe or chronic, were treated and monitored for several weeks or months, and were managed with multiple therapies concurrently.

The effects of PBMT on first intention, or primary, incisional wound healing was evaluated in ball pythons

(a) (b) (c) (d)

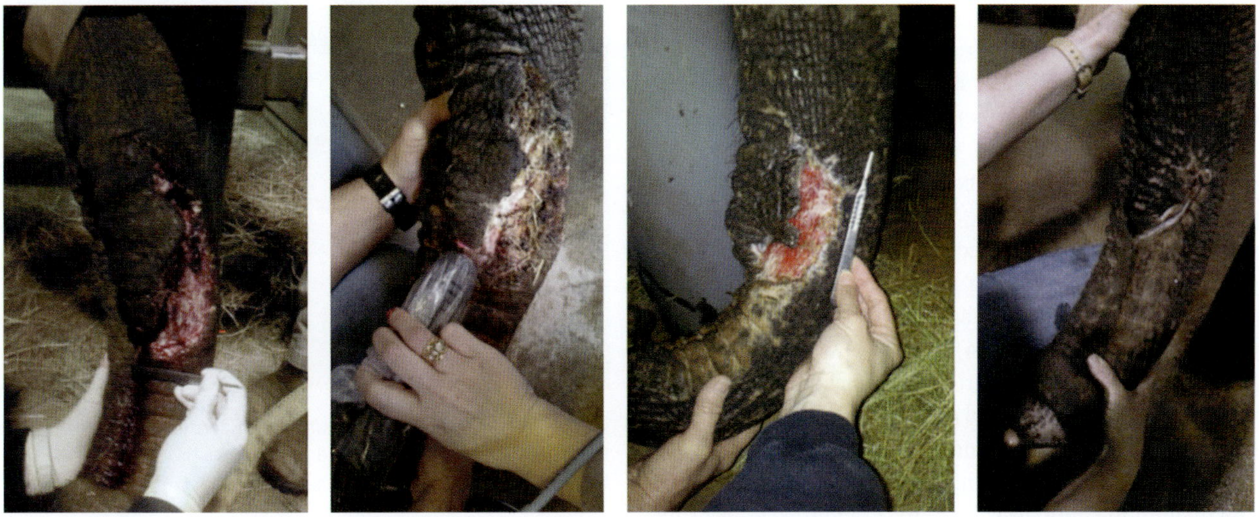

Figure 28.5 Laser therapy helped with wound healing and analgesia in an elephant with a trunk laceration. The wound was surgically repaired twice in the first week but dehisced both times and became infected. Laser therapy began 10 days after initial injury and resulted in complete wound closure within about 6 weeks. (a) Trunk laceration before wound debridement on day 10 when laser therapy treatments began. (b) Laser therapy treatment of the contaminated trunk wound on day 19 after injury. Despite contamination, the wound shows some contraction. (c) Wound healing of the laceration on day 26 after injury. (d) Trunk laceration on the final day of laser therapy treatment, 54 days after initial injury (Photo by Dr. Erica Lipanovich).

(*Python regius*) and resulted in significant improvement in collagen maturity for the laser-treated wounds 14 days after initial injury, but no improvement in other metrics of wound healing (Cole *et al.*, 2015). In this study, six healthy adult pythons were sedated and eight 2 cm skin incisions were made on each snake, then closed with surgical staples. Four incisions on each snake were treated daily for seven consecutive days (at 5 J/cm^2, 980 nm, continuous wave) then excisional biopsies were collected of control and laser-treated wounds over the subsequent weeks. While PBMT resulted in a significant increase in collagen maturity at day 14, it did not otherwise significantly improve necrosis, fibroplasia, inflammation, granuloma formation, or bacterial contamination between the laser treatment and the control incisions. The authors noted that dosing at 5 J/cm^2, a dosing protocol often used with mammal wound healing, may have been too low as the snakes' scales may have theoretically absorbed or reflected photons.

In a similar study, the effects of PBMT on incisional wound healing was evaluated in green iguanas (*Iguana iguana*) and showed laser-treated wounds were significantly smaller 14 days after the initial injury, but there was no difference on histopathology based on treatment protocols (Cusack *et al.*, 2018). For this study, 16 healthy subadult iguanas were anesthetized, three 5 mm skin biopsy samples were collected from each animal, and lesion healing was monitored for 14 days. Wounds were treated with either laser therapy, topical antimicrobial products daily, or no treatments. Laser therapy treatments were 980 nm continuous wave, direct contact daily for 14 days, at either 0.5 W for 60 seconds at 5 J/cm^2, or 1.0 W for 60 seconds at 10 J/cm^2. After 14 days, wounds treated with 10 J/cm^2 laser therapy were significantly smaller than those treated with the silver sulfadiazine, but there were no other differences (including histologically) between the treatment groups. Based on this study, treatment with 10 J/cm^2 appears to be a safe and well tolerated dosage for green iguana skin incisions and was not associated with delayed wound healing. The authors noted that future studies should evaluate wound healing for an extended study period (longer than 14 days).

Wound healing in bearded dragons (*Pogona vitticeps*) did not show histologic evidence of epithelialization after a single laser therapy treatment (Gustavsen *et al.*, 2013). Two full-thickness 4 mm-diameter punch biopsies were created on the dorsum of each dragon and splinted open to minimize dermal contact. In the study group ($n = 5$), one wound in each dragon received a single treatment of 4 J of 670 nm light. The wounds from all the study animals were resected en bloc for histologic evaluation 4 days after the initial biopsy. Compared with the control group ($n = 4$), the wound margins were not correlated with epithelialization. While lack of histologic evidence of wound healing may suggest that laser therapy is not a useful treatment modality in bearded dragons, further study could help determine whether faster wound healing occurs closer to the time of a normal shed or with repeat applications of laser therapy.

A severe degloving injury in a green tree python (*Morelia viridis*) was successfully managed with multimodal therapy that included PBMT (Vetere *et al.*, 2021). The snake presented with a full-thickness skin wound (16 × 2.5 cm) with exposed epaxial muscles along dorsal midline. The patient was stabilized, the wound was surgically debrided, the wound was treated with PBMT and irrigated with autologous thrombocyte-leukocyte rich plasma (TLRP), and the surgical site was then closed. The snake was not treated with antibiotics. Following surgery, the snake received PBMT every 4 days for five additional treatments (8 J/cm^2 of 808 nm, 3 minutes/session). Four weeks later, the wound had fully healed without further complications.

Extensive thermal burns in a savannah monitor (*Varanus exanthematicus*) were treated with laser therapy and showed clinical improvement (Cushing *et al.*, 2013). Minimal wound healing was seen in 11 months of routine wound care. The monitor was then treated with PBMT three times in week 1, twice in week 2, and weekly thereafter. The wound showed considerable improvement to full healing over the next 4 months. No adverse effects were reported.

Ulcerative dermatitis in multiple turtle species has been successfully managed with laser therapy. An Aubry's flapshell turtle (*Cycloderma aubryi*) with severe ulcerative dermatitis and delayed wound healing was initially managed with antibiotics and then surgical debridement and ostectomy, but 2 months later still had delayed wound healing (DiRuzzo *et al.*, 2022). Some of the lesions were then treated with photobiomodulation and showed improvement within 17 days, so the remaining lesions were then treated, resulting in a full recovery. Similarly, a soft-shelled turtle (*Pelodiscus sinensis*) with a septicemic ulcerative dermatitis was effectively treated using laser therapy and medical management (Kraut *et al.*, 2013). In this turtle, the laser therapy treatments were associated with good clinical outcomes for both the skin and the shell lesions. A western pond turtle (*Actinemys marmorata*) with chronic shell lesions associated with excessive algae growth was managed with laser therapy treatment (Harrison, unpublished results). PBMT was performed twice a week with 5 Hz (1 SPL 8.14 J/cm^2 @ 905 nm, 3 IRD [80 mW each] 153.4 J/cm^2 [total] @ 850 nm, 3 LED [64 mW each] = 122.7 J/cm^2 [total] @ 630 nm) for 2 months and then once a week for 2 months. Improvements were noticed in the shell within 1 month and continued over the 4 months of treatment.

Amphibians

A study on marine toads (*Rhinella marina*) evaluated wound healing when comparing PBMT with sulversulfadiazine wound treatment and showed less scar tissue formation in the PBMT group (Figure 28.6). A 6 mm skin biopsy was collected from the mid dorsum of their abdomen, and animals were then randomly assigned to a PBMT group, silversulfadiazine group, and control groups. The toads were placed in a container and covered with a plastic covering the cranial portion of the amphibian and with the laser pointing toward their caudal abdomen through the opening in the plastic. Each toad was treated with 5 Hz (1 SPL 8.14 J/cm^2 @ 905 nm, 3 IRD [80 mW each] 153.4 J/cm^2 [total] @ 850 nm, 3 LED [64 mW each] = 122.7 J/cm^2 [total] @ 630 nm). Doses at the skin level could not be estimated. There were no issues with ocular exposure in this study. Lower levels of fibrosis were noted in PBMT-treated amphibians, but differences in the other outcomes were not noticed in this study. Some of these results may have been attributed to the sample size (Archibald *et al.*, 2020).

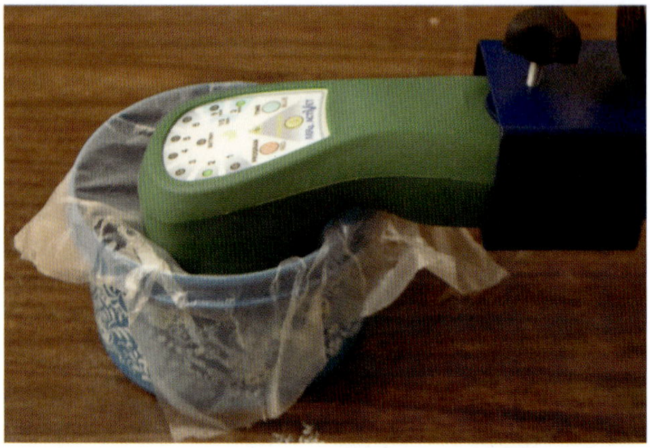

Figure 28.6 Laser therapy treatment of dermal wounds in marine toads (*Rhinella marina*) resulted in less scar tissue formation than for control groups.

Neurologic Injuries

Neurologic injuries may show clinical improvement with photobiomodulation associated with pain relief, improved healing, and improvements in mentation and proprioception.

Birds

Trauma-induced torticollis in raptors was more likely to resolve in birds treated with physical therapy, sometimes including laser therapy, than with medical management alone (Nevitt *et al.*, 2015). In three cases, laser therapy (1–2 J/cm^2) was applied to the soft-tissue restrictions to promote muscle relation and improve circulation. The beam of the laser was also focused on the caudal calvarium overlying the cerebellar and vestibular regions of the nervous system. This was done in conjunction with passive range of motion, soft-tissue therapy, and sometimes acupuncture. In this study, all five raptors treated with physical therapy improved clinically to the point that they could be released to the wild, while none of the birds that were not treated with physical therapy were releasable.

An eclectus parrot (*Eclectus roratus*) with a cervical injury and myopathy from cervical entrapment was effectively managed with integrative therapies that included photobiomodulation (Mitchell *et al.*, 2023). The parrot presented with severe ventroflexion of the cervical spine and had a dull mentation. Management included analgesics, steroids, subcutaneous fluids, vitamins, gavage feedings, photobiomodulation, acupuncture, massage, and rehabilitation exercises. Photobiomodulation was dosed at 320 J total (2.5 W, 980/810 nm wavelengths) and used for the neck region using a scanning technique (Mitchell *et al.*, 2023). Acupuncture points used consisted of GV-21, GV-20, GV-17, GV-12-14, Ah-shi, and Jing-jia-ji. Within 3 days of starting treatment, mentation was improved and was holding its head nearly 80% of expected normal positioning with no signs of ongoing cervical pain based on palpation.

Lameness in an ostrich (*Struthio camelus*) was not successfully managed with laser therapy (Harrison unpublished results). Acupuncture and laser therapy 250 Hz (1 SPL 8.14 J/cm^2 @ 905 nm, 3 IRD [80 mW each] 153.4 J/cm^2 [total] @ 850 nm, 3 LED [64 mw each] = 122.7 J/cm^2 [total] @ 630 nm) were used at Bai hui, BL-40, GB-21, BL-23, and BL-10. The ostrich tolerated the laser therapy well, and no adverse effects were seen. However, it did not show improvement and was euthanized. Postmortem, a femoral fracture was diagnosed.

Mammals

Acute-onset torticollis in a 2-year-old male reticulated giraffe (*Giraffa camelopardalis reticulata*) showed marked clinical improvement using a combination of medical management, chiropractic adjustments, laser therapy, and range-of-motion exercises (Dadone *et al.*, 2013). During transport between zoos, the giraffe developed a severe mid-cervical segmental torticollis that progressed to focal muscle spasms of the neck, marked neck sensitivity, and decreased range of motion. With positive reinforcement training, PBMT was used to manage soft-tissue pain and hypertonicity (Figure 28.7b). Laser therapy was applied twice weekly for 4 weeks, with treatments focused over sites of muscle contracture. Sites were treated with a blended wavelength of both 810 and 980 nm, and each treatment site received a total dose of 4800 J. The cervical range of

(a) (b)

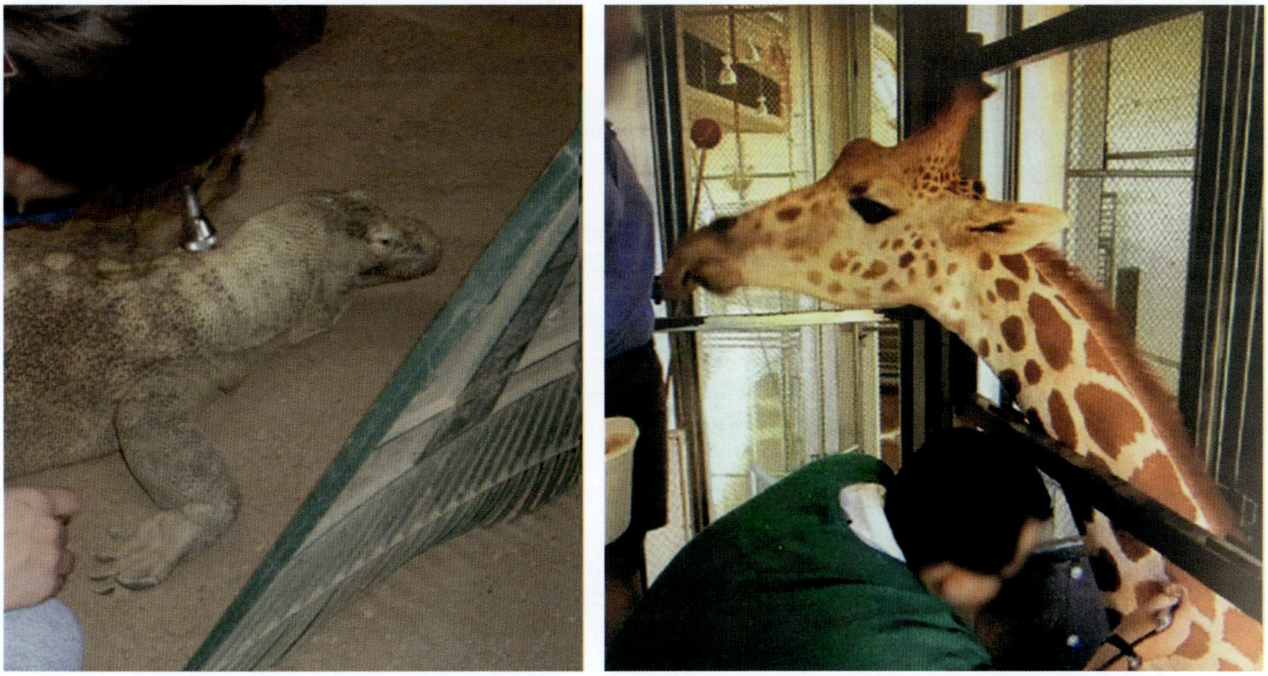

Figure 28.7 Photobiomodulation therapy to help manage neurologic injuries. (a) A 17-year-old female Komodo dragon with acute onset proprioceptive deficits, a lateral bend in the neck, and neck pain was treated with laser therapy and showed marked clinical improvement within 1 week of starting treatment. During treatments, a rake was brought into the enclosure for human safety. (b) A 3-year-old male reticulated giraffe with acute onset torticollis was treated with laser therapy targeted to sites of muscle contracture and sensitivity on the neck. In combination with medical management, chiropractic adjustment, and range-of-motion exercises, this giraffe made a full clinical recovery (Photo by R. Romero (28.7a), Liza Dadone, Cheyenne Mountain Zoo (Chapter Contributor) (28.7b)).

motion was significantly improved in left lateral bending, muscle hypertonicity and contracture were reduced, and the left side of the neck was less sensitive to palpation 1 month after initiation of laser therapy. Therapy was continued weekly for 9 months. The giraffe continued to be maintained with regular range-of-motion exercises more than 12 years later and has sired multiple calves.

Nutritional metabolic bone disease and subsequent fractures in a 5-year-old spayed striped skunk (*Mephitis mephitis*) were effectively managed with laser therapy (Dadone and Marsden, unpublished results). This former pet presented with hind-leg paresis associated with bilateral femoral fractures and suspected microfractures around the spine. Management included analgesics, laser therapy of the lumbar spine region, diet change, and supplemental vitamin D3. The skunk was treated with a blended wavelength of 810 and 980 nm and was dosed with 8–10 J/cm^2 administered to the lower back, the hips, and the left rear leg. Over several months, the skunk showed marked improvement in her gait and radiographic evidence of both fracture healing and improved bone density.

Reptiles

Acute-onset paresis in a Komodo dragon (*Varanus komodoensis*) showed short-term marked clinical improvement with laser therapy treatments to the cervical spine when used with medical management (Dadone, Marsden, and Johnston, unpublished results). A 17-year-old female Komodo dragon presented with mild dragging of a front leg. Within 1 week, she was severely ataxic on all four legs, had difficulty eating, had a visible bend in the proximal neck (Figure 28.7a), and had a distended gullar pouch area. Management included broad-spectrum antibiotics, anti-inflammatories, analgesics, heat therapy to the neck, and laser therapy to the neck. PBMT was dosed at 25 J/cm^2. Within about 1 week of starting laser therapy, the dragon showed marked improvement in strength, coordination, and ability to eat, and reduced neck-guarding behaviors. She was found dead 54 days after presentation. Histopathology indicated the cause of death was an egg yolk embolus, potentially unrelated to the suspect spinal cord injury. This case resembles past reports of cervical subluxation and compressive myelopathy in Komodo dragons, which thus far have not been successfully managed with either supportive care or surgical decompression (Zimmerman *et al.*, 2009). The clinical improvement suggests that laser therapy may help manage pain and reduce inflammation in other cases of suspected compressive myelopathy in Komodo dragons.

Musculoskeletal Injuries

Animals with bone fractures can be treated with laser therapy to assist in bone healing, as part of a multimodal treatment regimen. Similarly, animals with muscles sprains, strains or other injuries can benefit from treatments of LLLT and have improved healing times.

Mammals

Laser therapy has provided inconsistent but sometimes marked clinical benefits when managing lameness and soft-tissue injuries in giraffe. Dosing may vary but is generally extrapolated from equine settings for chronic inflammation and acute/chronic pain. Marked clinical improvement was observed in a geriatric giraffe with a pressure sore and suspect cellulitis of a hock joint (lateral hock treated off-contact using with 980/810 nm, 10 W, total dose 8000 J at 10–20 J/cm^2, twice weekly for 1 month); in this case marked improvement in posture and willingness to participate in hoof trim training sessions was noted within 2 days of the first laser therapy treatment (Figure 28.10b, Dadone, unpublished results). For a different adult giraffe with front-hoof overgrowth, suspect laminitis, and partial tears of the deep digital flexor tendons, a laser treatment was administered one time to the swollen region below the fetlock during general anesthesia, in conjunction with a corrective hoof trim and digital perfusion of medications. That giraffe had an excellent anesthetic recovery and lameness resolved within days of the anesthesia. During the same anesthesia, the giraffe developed muscle inflammation in one region of the neck. This was resolved during anesthesia after repositioning the neck, doing focal tissue massage, administering laser therapy to the site, applying ice, and NSAIDs.

A closed distal metacarpal fracture in an orphaned newborn mountain bongo (antelope, *Tragelaphus eurycerus isaaci*) was successfully managed with stall rest and laser therapy (Reillo and Clubb, 2015). About 1 week after presentation, laser therapy was applied circumferentially to the fracture site using a wavelength of 635 nm at a dosage of 0.68 J/cm^2 daily for 3 weeks. Follow-up radiographs at about 6 weeks and 6 months showed excellent remodeling and lengthening of the metacarpus. Normal walking was observed by day 65, and the calf continued to have no long-term health issues about 1 year later. The authors concluded that these noninvasive management techniques were warranted and effective for this antelope with such high conservation value.

Reptiles

Eastern box turtles (*Terrapene carolina*) with traumatic shell fractures from injuries incurred in the wild had significantly faster healing when treated with photobiomodulation (Souza *et al.*, 2023). In this study of 20 turtles, all received similar treatments but 10 animals also then were treated with PBMT (red light laser at a frequency of 250 Hz (1 SPL 8.14 J/cm^2 @ 905 nm, 3 IRD (80 mW each) 153.4 J/cm^2 (total) @ 850 nm, 3 LED (64 mW each) = 122.7 J/cm^2 (total) @ 630 nm), 3 minutes/session, 3 times weekly, 8 weeks duration). Computed tomography imaging was done to evaluate bony healing. The greatest healing was found in the width of the fracture and it was found to be significantly different between the treatment and control groups. However, the scans also showed there was no significant difference in shell density measurements at the wound healing sites between the study groups. This study suggests there may be benefits in wildlife rehabilitation cases for including photobiomodulation in the treatment plans (Figure 28.8).

Orofacial Diseases

While laser therapy is increasingly utilized to accelerate healing in human dentistry and is frequently applied in laboratory animal studies (Aoki *et al.*, 2015; Massotti *et al.*, 2015; Matos *et al.*, 2016; Tang and Arany, 2013), it is uncommonly used to help manage dental diseases or other orofacial conditions in zoos. A study in humans validated a significant reduction in pain, trismus, and swelling in patients receiving PBMT immediately following mandibular third molar-removal surgery and on the third postoperative day (Abdel-Alim *et al.*, 2015).

Mammals

Necrobacillosis (lumpy jaw) in a Parma wallaby (*Macropus parma*) was effectively treated using a combination of comprehensive endodontic therapy, apicoectomy, and laser therapy (Kilgallon *et al.*, 2010). In this case, an apicoectomy was performed on the mandibular incisor, and laser

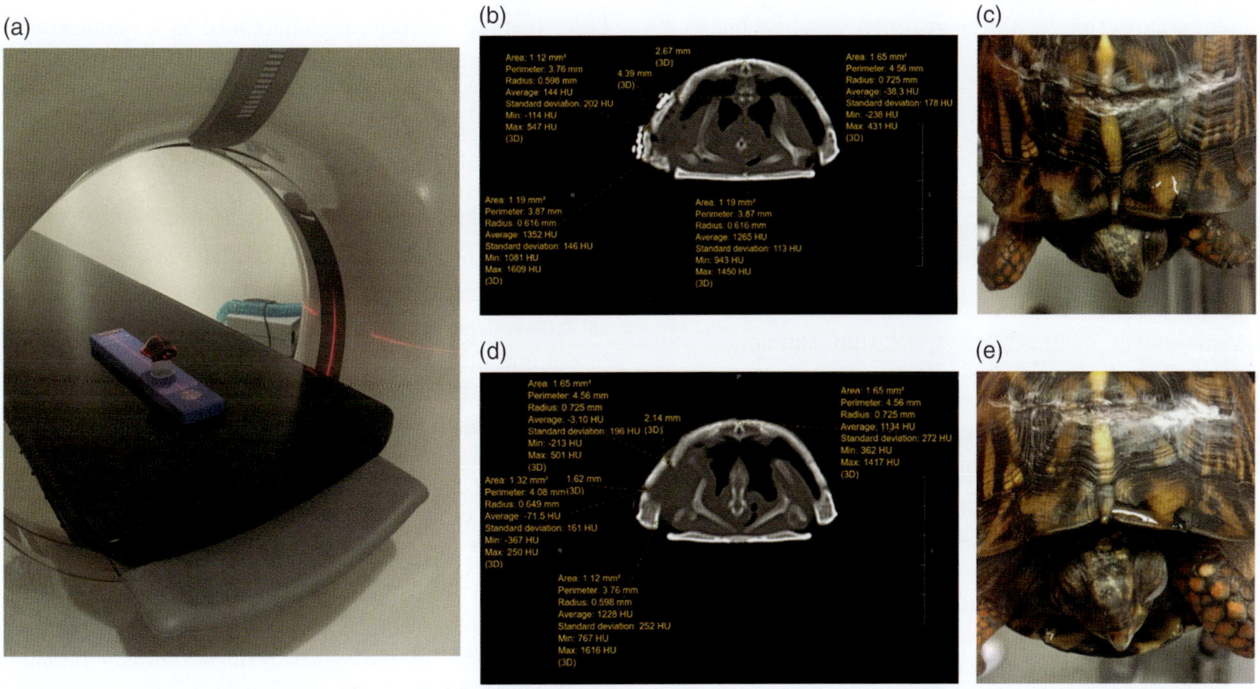

Figure 28.8 Shell fractures in box turtles at a rehabilitation center healed more quickly when management included laser therapy. (a, b, d) Turtles in the study had computerized tomography (CT) imaging to evaluate fracture width and bone density by the fracture sites at the start of the study and after 8 weeks of treatment. The turtles treated with laser therapy had significantly smaller fracture width than the control group but CT evaluation showed no significant difference in bone density by the fracture sites between the laser and control groups. (c, e) Turtle shell wounds at the start of LLLT treatment and 2 weeks later showed visible improvement in the lesion (Photo by T. Harrison (Chapter Contributor) and A. Souza).

treatment was applied to the site to decontaminate the pulp cavity and provide anti-inflammatory and biostimulatory effects. Using a wavelength of 810 nm and 2.0 W, the pulp cavity and alveolar bone defect were treated in pulsed mode with three passes of 5-second duration each for a total of with 15 J before starting dental restoration.

In rabbits, photobiostimulation at a site of incisor extraction and dental implant placement promoted new bone formation around the implant (Massotti *et al.*, 2015). In this study, 24 male New Zealand rabbits were randomly divided into four groups, then each had a mandibular incisor extracted and a titanium dental implant immediately inserted. Except for the control group, all rabbits were treated with laser therapy every 48 hours for seven treatments, and then the mandibles were evaluated histologically. Significantly more collagen fibers and bone-to-implant contact were seen in the treatment group that received 20 J/cm^2 each treatment. This helps validate the potential accelerated wound healing but does not quantify any possible analgesic benefits from this treatment.

A study in female New Zealand white rabbits with experimentally induced maxillary rhinosinusitis showed significant improvement with PBMT based on computed tomography, inflammatory cytokine levels, and histopathology (Park *et al.*, 2023). The treatment group rabbits were anesthetized daily for 7 days for PBMT treatments with laser probes inserted into the nares using multi-wavelength and multi-power treatments (20 minutes total per treatment using 670 nm with 3 mW and then 830 nm with 20 mW). This suggests PBMT applied inside the nares could have clinical benefits in the management of rabbit rhinosinusitis but warrants further study in naturally infected patients.

Chronic Degenerative Diseases

As zoo animals develop age-related degenerative conditions such as osteoarthritis, multimodal therapies including photobiomodulation can help patients maintain good comfort and welfare (Robinson, 2019). As the pharmacokinetics and pharmacodynamics of analgesics vary widely across species (Balko and Chinnadurai, 2017), treatments with photobiomodulation can provide neuromodulation in a noninvasive way and help counter spinal cord wind-up pain (Robinson, 2019).

Birds

A military macaw (*Ara militaris*) with flexor tendon mineralization showed clinical improvement when managed long-term with photobiomodulation (Sparrow, 2020). The bird presented with intermittent lameness, soft tissue swelling, and reduced range of motion. Medical management included analgesics and joint supplements. PBMT was administered off-contact with a five diode 820 nm wavelength 200 mW probe, 8 J/cm^2, with between 1 and 5 kHz of treatment over 2–5 minutes per session (variability based on how willing parrot was to participate in training each session). The parrot was initially treated three times weekly for a month, then reduced to two times weekly then one time weekly, but it showed signs of deterioration again when only treated weekly so was maintained long-term on two times weekly PBMT.

Chronic leg swelling and fusion ("peg leg") in a Victoria crowned pigeon (*Goura victoria*) improved when treated with laser therapy (L. Wright, personal communication). The pigeon had a chronic nonunion fracture above the foot with a large fibrous callous and severe osteomyelitis involving the joint. The fracture was over a year old when laser therapy was tried. Laser therapy was associated with reduced swelling of the foot and a return of some range of motion that had not been seen in over a year, but the use of the foot remained limited.

Mammals

Laser therapy has been recommended as a management tool for chronic pain in geriatric mammals. In a small trial across multiple species at one zoo, managing lameness or joint pain had inconsistent and sometimes ineffective results (Howard *et al.*, 2014). This variability might be associated with limitations of PBMT penetration (especially given that the authors noted success in more superficial conditions, but challenges with deeper tissue conditions), excessive distance between the laser handpiece and the target tissue, degenerative changes being advanced and multifocal, or other factors. These variables highlight the importance of understanding dosimetry (especially in megavertebrates) and minimizing light losses from reflection via treating on contact to the degree that it is possible with the device(s) being used (Figures 28.9 and 28.10).

Osteoarthritis pain management with PBMT in a koala (*Phascolarctos cinereus*) resulted in marked clinical improvement (P. Bapodra/Columbus Zoo and Aquarium, personal communication). Using a contact handpiece with a large massage ball, the koala was treated both on the spine (10 W, 780 J, 1 : 18 minutes) and wrist/ankle region (5 W, 315 J, 1 : 03 minutes). In this case, medical management was subsequently reduced and laser therapy continued long-term.

A red panda (*Ailurus fulgens*) with intervertebral disc disease was managed with PBMT as part of a multimodal analgesia management plan (K. Leach, personal communication). The panda was on long-term meloxicam,

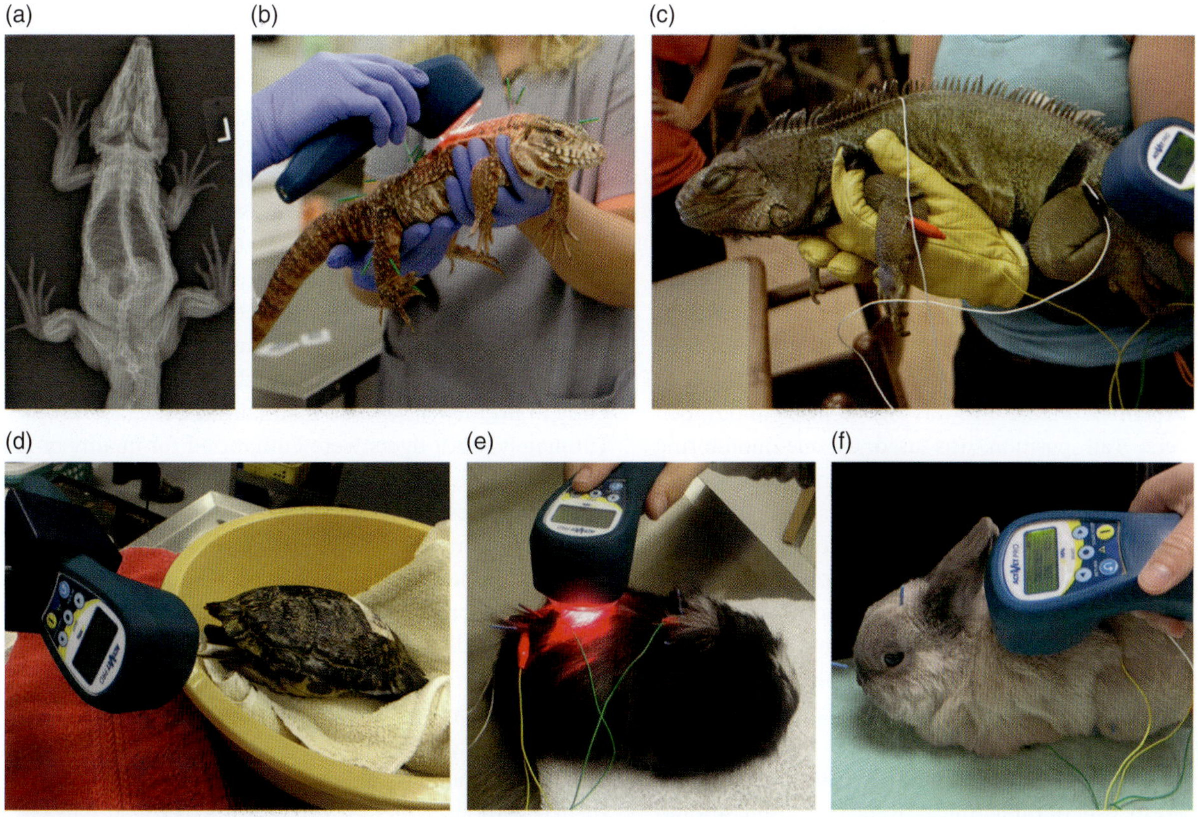

Figure 28.9 Photobiomodulation therapy can help manage osteoarthritis pain. Smaller and less dangerous patients can often be positioned using positive reinforcement or mild manual restraint. (a, b) A subadult tegu with nutritional secondary hyperparathyroidism was diagnosed from radiographs with severe kyphosis and scoliosis and showed clinical improvement with multimodal therapy that included laser treatments. Clinical improvements have also been observed in other species including (c) green iguana, (d) red eared slider turtles, (e) guinea pigs, and (f) domestic rabbits. In the above cases, the tegu, guinea pig, and rabbit concurrently also were treated with acupuncture needles in key meridian sites (Photo by T. Harrison (Chapter Contributor) and John Joyner, NC State Veterinary Medicine).

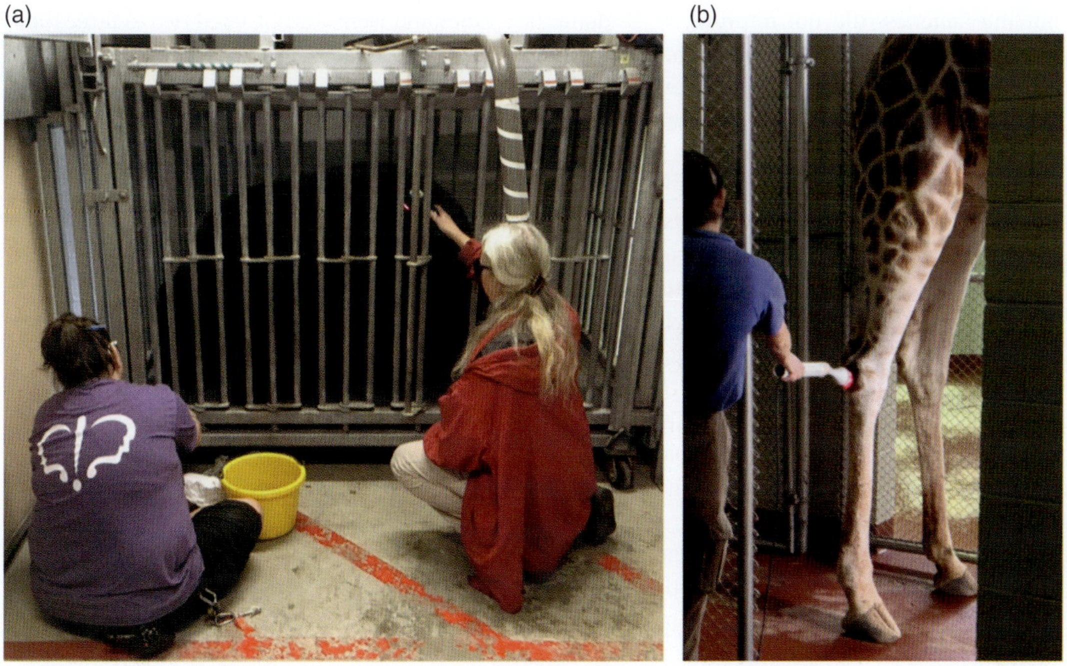

Figure 28.10 Photobiomodulation therapy for large and potentially dangerous patients in a restricted contact set-up with positive reinforcement training. (a) A North American black bear with osteoarthritis was trained to receive laser therapy treatments by lining up in a chute for food rewards. (b) A giraffe with osteoarthritis and a pressure sore was target trained and positively reinforced for laser therapy treatments. While the trainer remained in protected contact near the giraffe's head and provided food rewards, the giraffe was taught to stand with her hind leg positioned next to a doorway so laser treatments could be administered using an extension piece (a PVC pipe) (Photo by S. Samuels (28.10a), Liza Dadone, Cheyenne Mountain Zoo (Chapter Contributor) (28.10b)).

gabapentin, omega-3 fatty acid supplements, Adequan injections, and twice-weekly laser therapy. PBMT was administered using a domestic cat protocol for a patient with long hair and lumbar arthritis. The caudal lumbar, pelvic, and hip region of the panda were treated using 4.5–5 W, 720 J, using a large contact head. The panda had variable compliance with stationing for food rewards, and sometimes would walk away during treatments. A lightweight protective eye guard (modified cardboard box) was fabricated that also was a good place to put food reinforcers. Tail position was used as one monitoring parameter for the panda's overall comfort with the analgesia management plan.

PBMT helped manage degenerative joint disease (DJD) in small hoofstock species commonly housed in petting zoos. An 11-year-old domestic pygmy goat with healed fractures in both a front and hind limb and severe osteoarthritis was treated for chronic pain with red light therapy at 250 Hz frequency (1 SPL 8.14 J/cm^2 @ 905 nm, 3 IRD [80 mW each] 153.4 J/cm^2 [total] @ 850 nm, 3 LED [64 mw each] = 122.7 J/cm^2 [total] @ 630 nm) for 5 minutes PBM treatment three times a week (Harrison, unpublished). The goat tolerated the treatments well and showed clinical improvements following treatment. Similarly, a Sicilian burro with severe osteoarthritis of the coxofemoral joint and associated lameness showed dramatic improvement when treated with laser therapy (Harrison, unpublished results). Initially, the burro was treated medically for pain, including with gabapentin and firocoxib, but the lameness did not improve so laser therapy and acupuncture were added. The acupuncture points used were GB-21, BL-23, Bai-hui, Shen Shu, Shen Jiaco, BL-54, ST-31, and SP-11. The laser treatments were applied at Shen-jiao, BI-23, and BL-54, with aqua-acupuncture with vitamin B12 at Bai-hui, BL-23, BL-18, and BL-54. After two treatments, the burro's lameness was much less severe, so the firocoxib dose was decreased. Additional treatments included hyaluronic acid joint injection and a methylprednisolone acetate injection in the affected coxofemoral joint. With 1 month of all therapies, the burro was off all medications and the lameness had clinically resolved. Though laser therapy was one of multiple therapies, the use of nonsteroidal medication could be decreased after only two treatments.

Photobiomodulation has been used to help manage osteoarthritis lesions of zoo-housed giraffe as part of multimodal pain management plan. While clinical improvement varies by individual and diagnosis, osteoarthritis of the distal or proximal interphalangeal joint (DIP or PIP) of the front foot can be treated with 3000 J/digit (loading dose phase q72 hr for 1 month, maintenance phase with 1X weekly; Dadone, 2018).

Laser therapy was attempted for two geriatric tigers (*Panthera tigris altaica* and one hybrid tiger) at different zoos, with no obvious clinical benefits (Harrison & Dadone, unpublished results). One tiger was diagnosed radiographically with osteoarthritis of the lumbosacral spine and femoral heads, and the second tiger was diagnosed from MRI with intervertebral disc disease of the lumbar spine. Even with positive reinforcement training, access to the tigers was limited and laser therapy could not be applied consistently to priority sites while maintaining protected contact. Ultimately, both tigers were euthanized for quality-of-life concerns and necropsy confirmed severe degenerative lesions. In these two tigers, lack of clinical improvement with laser therapy may partly be attributable to the excessive distance between the laser handpiece and the target tissue, inappropriate settings, and/or the severity of the degenerative disease.

In geriatric primates, laser therapy has been recommended as a treatment option for pain management of osteoarthritis and degenerative disk disease (Boesch, 2012). At one zoo, four adult or geriatric gorillas (*Gorilla gorilla*) were treated with laser therapy for arthritis pain and flare-ups, but it was undetermined if the treatments were beneficial or appropriately dosed (Dave and Leach, 2014). Based on the individual case, treatments targeted arthritis of the hands, elbows, knees, feet, or hips. Treatments were voluntary and depended on trained behaviors to position the gorilla appropriately next to the mesh. Using a noncontact delivery, laser treatments were dosed by extrapolating from domestic species and were administered two to three times the first week, then one to two times weekly to biweekly, and then variably for maintenance (K. Leach, personal communication). Variation was seen, with females generally tolerating lower power (5–6 W) and one silverback comfortable with a higher power (8–9 W); this could be related to differences in patient size or sex, or to differences in skin color. Individual gorilla compliance was highly variable. For some individuals, limited mobility related to the targeted joint interfered with the ability to position themselves effectively for treatments.

Elephants

Multiple elephants at a sanctuary were treated for acute and chronic musculoskeletal diseases with PBMT, sometimes for years (L. Young, personal communication). Musculoskeletal diseases were identified from clinical lameness assessments and radiographic evidence of degenerative changes to joints. PBMT was administered as part of a multimodal approach to pain management, so the individual or synergistic effects of the treatments could not be determined. Dosing was extrapolated from equine settings for chronic inflammation and acute/chronic pain, generally increasing the power, which allowed for shorter treatment times, and with a noncontact laser head. For management of DJD, elephants were initially started with a daily loading dose phase, then maintained long term with weekly or biweekly treatments. For DJD cases that were only clinical during colder months, treatments were sometimes reduced to every other week during the spring/summer. Universally, laser therapy was well received and was performed in a positive reinforcement/protected contact setting. In multiple cases, elephants would visibly relax and lean into the treatment and would also move their bodies closer/into a different spot during treatment. Subjectively, there was variability in how well each individual elephant responded to long-term therapy, but even for some elephants that were treated daily for years, no negative side effects were ever noted.

Based on an analgesia survey in megavertebrates, a fair clinical response was reported in two Asian elephants (*Elephas maximus*) treated with laser therapy (Kottwitz *et al.*, 2016). The elephants were dosed at 80 J across four to eight points, administered three times weekly for 3 weeks, then weekly, then every 2 weeks. No additional details were recorded in the survey concerning anatomic location or possible diagnosis in each case.

Laser therapy for soft-tissue swelling and decreased joint mobility in the carpus of an Asian elephant seemed to help more with reducing soft-tissue swelling than with improving range of motion in the leg (L. Wright, personal communication). The geriatric elephant had decreased motion of the carpus and generalized swelling of the leg for several years. As part of multimodal treatment, the lower third of the leg was treated twice weekly until a marked decrease in swelling was seen; laser therapy was continued weekly thereafter.

Lameness associated with osteoarthritis of the stifle in an African elephant (*Loxodonta africana*) showed no clinical improvement with laser therapy (Dadone, unpublished results). This was likely due to both an insufficiently low dose and scuffing of the end of the massage ball-type handpiece, caused by the abrasive skin of the elephant. Because of the limited maximum power of the therapy laser used, each stifle treatment for an elephant took about 30 minutes, which could be time- limiting. With newer and more powerful units available, it is possible laser therapy could be an effective treatment for elephant osteoarthritis management, but for now results are inconsistent.

Reptiles

Limited mobility attributed to extensive spondylosis in a geriatric rosy boa (*Lichanura trivirgata*) was managed with laser therapy, which resulted in improved mobility (L. Wright, personal communication). Concurrently, the snake had an anal gland swelling. Laser therapy was targeted to the whole spine and the anal gland swelling. Following laser treatment, the snake resumed climbing and moved better, and the anal gland swelling resolved.

A 13-year-old male Komodo dragon with severe and progressive osteoarthritis was treated with PBMT for pain management and to slow disease progression (P. Bapodra/Columbus Zoo and Aquarium, pers. comm). The dragon was treated with a large ball/contact head to the elbow joint (12 W, 2712 J, for 3 : 46 minutes each treatment) and some clinical improvement was observed.

A subadult tegu was treated with acupuncture and cold laser therapy for relief of pain caused by nutritional secondary hyperparathyroidism (Harrison, unpublished data). This tegu had kyphosis as well as scoliosis and was treated weekly with both acupuncture and PBMT (1000 Hz, 1 SPL 8.14 J/cm^2 @ 905 nm, 3 IRD [80 mW each] 153.4 J/cm^2 [total] @ 850 nm, 3 LED [64 mW each] = 122.7 J/cm^2 [total] @ 630 nm for 5 minutes a treatment). The tegu's pain levels were well managed for months with this multimodal therapy, using activity and appetite levels as metrics of when PBMT and acupuncture should be repeated. Eventually, as the patient continued to grow, the kyphosis and scoliosis progressed and the patient was euthanized.

Fish

A green moray eel with spondylosis showed marked clinical improvement with laser therapy (Boylan *et al.*, 2016). The eel was at least 15 years old and presented for inappetence, abnormal buoyancy, and a 90° mid-body deviation. Spondylosis was diagnosed by radiographs and whole-body CT, and medical management was initiated including dexamethasone and glycosaminoglycans. PBMT was then applied with a noncontact head along the vertebrae on each side for 2–3 minutes (1616 J, 8 W for 2–3 minutes), from the spiracle to the caudal aspect of the swim bladder and was repeated three times weekly for the first month, then one to two times weekly for the next year. After the first laser therapy treatment, the eel was able to swim more normally again which had not been observed for the past year, and after its fifth laser treatment, the eel was able to achieve 180° turns in the water again.

Assisted Reproduction

While not yet widely studied in zoo medicine, laser therapy and laser acupuncture may have applications in assisted reproduction including in helping manage endangered species population. In humans this is an area of active research, including in the management of male infertility. In human males, PBMT can improve survival, motility, and speed of movement of spermatozoa, and can also help manage prostatitis and vesiculitis (Moskvin *et al.*, 2018).

Photobiomodulation for assisted reproduction requires further study across taxa. For example, farmed hybrid catfish treated with photobiomodulation had accelerated gonadotropin hormone formation which resulted in significantly improved fertilization rates, egg hatching rates, and larvae survival rates (Kusuma *et al.*, 2015). In a subsequent study on male striped catfish (*Pangasianodon hypophthalmus*), laserpuncture accelerated gonadal maturity and improved sperm quality (Mukti *et al.*, 2020). In comparison when PBMT was used in rams, it did not reverse signs of testicular degeneration and treatment instead induced sperm damage and did not improve testosterone levels (Alves *et al.*, 2016).

Laser Acupuncture

Laser therapy has been used as an acupuncture treatment with or without the use of needles. Most laser units have an acupuncture setting that helps to activate the nerves and the acupuncture points along the various meridians. Laser acupuncture (laserpuncture) has been especially useful for animals that are not yet trained to accept needles, are intolerant of needles, or it is helpful to treat more points than the animal will tolerate needles (Harrison and Brock, 2023). This has been an especially useful therapy and has been used by one of the authors (Harrison) to predominantly treat osteoarthritis in lions, tigers, bears, kudu, anteater, elephants, raptors, reptiles, and penguins among other animals. Laserpuncture has also been done with grizzly bear (*Ursus arctos*) trained to receive treatments through protected contact (Marziani *et al.*, 2017).

Future Role for Thermography-Assisted Laser Therapy

Ongoing challenges to validating the effectiveness of laser therapy in zoos include challenges with identifying pathologies premortem. Thermography aids in localizing surface temperature asymmetries which may be physiologically significant to the patient. These temperature asymmetries may be related to localized inflammation, poor perfusion, nerve injuries, or other potential abnormalities (Figure 28.11).

(a) (b) (c)

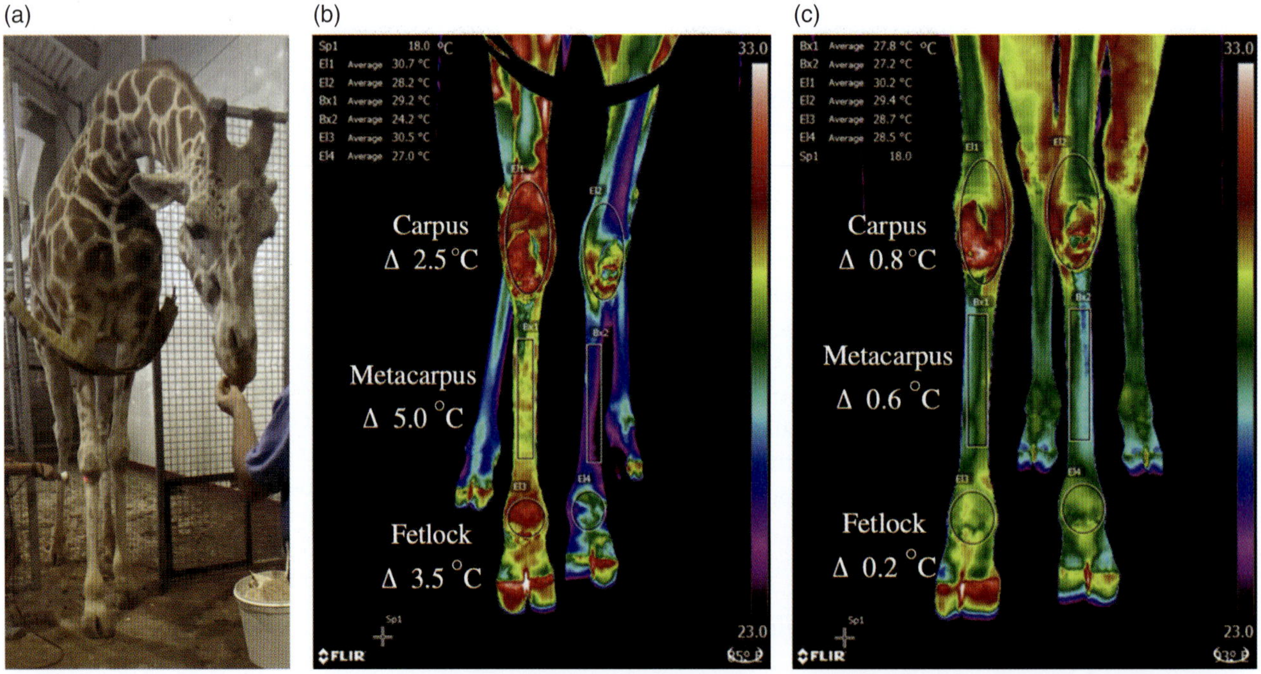

Figure 28.11 A geriatric giraffe with acute onset severe right front limb lameness was managed with stall rest, nonsteroidal anti-inflammatory medications, and laser therapy. (a) Laser therapy was started one day after presentation using positive reinforcement in a protected contact set-up with a noncontact laser. (b) Thermal imaging before the first laser therapy session helped identify priority areas for treatment by comparing surface temperature of different parts of the limb with the same anatomy on the clinically normal limb. The following day the giraffe showed moderate improvements in lameness and posture and (c) thermal imaging showed significant reduction in heat signatures of the right front leg including to the carpus, metacarpus, and fetlock (Photo by Liza Dadone, Cheyenne Mountain Zoo (Chapter Contributor).

Recent studies from equine sports medicine suggest PBMT can improve healing of suspensory branch ligament injuries (Pluim *et al.*, 2020). For zoo species like giraffe that may be prone to ligament and tendon injuries (Dadone *et al.*, 2020), further study is warranted to determine if PBMT could also help in management of similar injuries. In these cases, utilizing both thermal imaging and PBMT may help localize treatment priorities to improve healing success for some ligament and tendon injuries.

Conclusion

Laser therapy in zoo medicine can help improve clinical outcomes in some cases that are refractory to other types of medical management. To help improve the efficacy of laser therapy, more studies and widespread reporting of cases are needed. This ideally should include consistent reporting of doses (J/cm^2), techniques (on vs. off-contact, etc.), frequency of treatment(s), and other species-specific factors that would aid in more understanding and consistency through treating zoological patients. Thermography may also help localize abnormalities, especially in patients that cannot be readily handled or are too large for other types of imaging and could help quantify whether clinical improvements are observed with laser therapy and other treatments.

Acknowledgments

Thanks to our colleagues who shared cases and advice for this chapter, including Drs. Erica Lipanovich, Lydia Young, Lewis Wright, Kathryn Leach, Priya Bapodra/Columbus Zoo and Aquarium, Melanie Marsden, Matthew Johnston, Ron Riegel, and Kim Henneman, and Raymond Romano, CVT.

References

Abdel-Alim, H.M. *et al.* (2015). A comparative study of the effectiveness of immediate versus delayed photobiomodulation therapy in reducing the severity of postoperative inflammatory complications. *Photomed Laser Surg.* 33(9):447–451.

Alves, M.B.R. *et al.* (2016). Low-level laser therapy to recovery testicular degeneration in rams: effects on seminal characteristics, scrotal temperature, plasma testosterone concentration, and testes histopathology. *Lasers Med Sci.* 31 (4):695–704.

Aoki, A. *et al.* (2015). Periodontal and peri-implant wound healing following laser therapy. *Periodontol.* 68(1):217–269.

Archibald, K.E. *et al.* (2020). Effect of multiradiance low-level laser therapy and topical silver sulfadiazine on healing characteristics of dermal wounds in marine toads (*Rhinella marina*). *Vet Med Int*:8888328.

Balko, J.A. and Chinnadurai, S.K. (2017). Advancements in evidence-based analgesia in exotic animals. *Vet Clin North Am Exot Anim Pract.* 20(3):899–915.

Blair, J. (2013). Bumblefoot: a comparison of clinical presentation and treatment of pododermatitis in rabbits, rodents, and birds. *Vet Clin North Am Exot Anim Pract.* 16 (3):715–735.

Boesch, J.M. (2012). Update on primate analgesia. *Proceedings of the Annual Conference of the AAZV.* Oct 21–26. Oakland, CA.

Boylan, S.M. *et al.* (2016). Spondylosis in in a green moray eel, *Gymnothorax funebris* (Ranzani 1839), with swim bladder hyperinflation. *J Fish Dis.* 40:963–969.

Cole, G.L. *et al.* (2015). Effect of laser treatment on first-intention incisional wound healing in ball pythons (*Python regius*). *Am J Vet Res.* 76(10):904–912.

Comunian, C.R. *et al.* (2017). Photobiomodulation with LED and laser in repair of mandibular socket rabbit: clinical evaluation, histological, and histomorphometric. *Oral Maxillofac Surg.* 21:201–206.

Cusack, L.M. *et al.* (2018). Gross and histologic evaluation of effects of photobiomodulation, silver sulfadiazine, and a topical antimicrobial product on experimentally induced full-thickness skin wounds in green iguana (*Iguana iguana*). *Am J Vet Res.* 79(4):465–473.

Cushing, A.C. *et al.*, (2013). Abstract: The use of class IV laser therapy in zoo and wildlife medicine. *Proceedings of the Annual Conference of the AAZV.* September 28- October 4. Salt Lake City, UT.

Dadone, L. (2018). Lameness diagnosis & management in zoo giraffe. In: *Fowler's Zoo & Wild Animal Medicine, Current Therapy.* (eds. Miller *et al.*), Vol. 9, pp. 623–629. Elsevier.

Dadone, L.I. *et al.* (2013). Successful management of acute-onset torticollis in a giraffe (*Giraffa camelopardalis reticulata*). *J Zoo Wildl Med.* 44(1):181–185.

Dadone, L.I. *et al.* (2016). Training giraffe (*Giraffa camelopardalis reticulata*) for front foot radiographs and hoof care. *Zoo Biol.* 35(3):228–236.

Dadone, L.I. *et al.*, (2020). Computed tomography and pathology findings in the feet of zoo giraffe (*Giraffa camelopardalis reticulata*). *Proceedings of the Annual Conference of the AAZV.* Sept 20-24. Online conference.

Dave, M. and Leach, K. (2014). Poster: May the Force be With You: Laser Treatment in Gorillas. *2014 International Gorilla Workshop*. June 9–13. Atlanta, GA.

DiRuzzo, S. *et al.* (2022). Successful treatment of severe ulcerative dermatitis in an aubry's flapshell turtle (*Cycloderma aubryi*). *Journal of Herpetological Medicine and Surgery*. 32(4):262–270. doi:10.5818/JHMS-D-22-00002.

Dompe, C. *et al.* (2020). Photobiomodulation – underlying mechanism and clinical applications. *J Clin Med*. 9(6):1724. doi:10.3390/jcm9061724.

Draper, W.E. *et al.* (2012). Low-level laser therapy reduces time to ambulation in dogs after hemilaminectomy: a preliminary study. *J Small Anim Pract*. 53(8):465–469.

Esnouf, A. *et al.* (2007). Depth of penetration of an 850nm wave-length low level laser in human skin. *Acupunct Electrother Res*. 32(1–2):81–86.

Fessehav, H. (2020). Laser therapy and its potential application in veterinary practice – a review. *J Light Laser Curr Trends*. 3:007.

Gage, L.J. *et al.,* (1997). The use of direct contact infrared irradiation to aid the healing of pressure sores in elephants (*Elaphus maximus*). *Proceedings of the Annual Conference of the AAZV*. (October 26–30). Houston, TX.

González, M.S. and Mayer, J. (2019). Technological advances in wound treatment of exotic pets. *Vet Clin North Am Exot Anim Pract*. 22(3):451–470.

Gustavsen, K. *et al.,* (2013). Evaluation of low-level laser therapy in a model of cutaneous wound healing in bearded dragons (*Pogona vitticeps*). *Proceedings of the Annual Conference of the AAZV* (September 28–October 4). Salt Lake City, UT.

Harrison, T.A. and Brock, A.P. (2023). Integrative medicine in zoological species. In: *Fowler's Zoo and Wild Animal Medicine*. (eds. R. E. Miller *et al.*), Vol. 10, pp. 319–323. Saunders/El Sevier, St. Louis, MO.

Hodjati, H. *et al.* (2014). Low-level laser therapy: an experimental design for wound management: a case-controlled study in rabbit model. *J Cutan Aesthet Surg*. 7 (1):14–17.

Howard, L.L. *et al.,* (2014). Abstract: Functional assessment and multi-modal approach to pain management in zoo patients. *Proceedings of the Annual Conference of the AAZV*. (October 18–24). Orlando, FL.

Karu, T.I. (2003). Low-power laser therapy. In: *Biomedical Photonics Handbook*. (ed. T. Vo-Dinh), Vol. 48, pp. 7–20. CRC Press, London.

Kilgallon, C.P. *et al.* (2010). Successful treatment of chronic periapical osteomyelitis in a Parma wallaby (*Macropus parma*) using comprehensive endodontic therapy with apicoectomy. *J Zoo Wildl Med*. 41(4):703–709.

Kottwitz, J. *et al.* (2016). Results of the megavertebrate analgesia survey: elephants and rhino. *J Zoo Wildl Med*. 47 (1):301–310.

Kraut, S. *et al.* (2013). Laser therapy in a soft-shelled turtle (*Pelodiscus sinensis*) for the treatment of skin and shell ulceration. A case report. *Tierarztl Prax Ausg K Kleintiere Heimtiere*. 41(4):261–266.

Kuffler, D.P. (2016). Photobiomodulation in promoting wound healing: a review. *Regen Med*. 11(1):107–122.

Kusuma, P. *et al.* (2015). Utilization of laserpuncture induction as spawning stimulation in catfish (*Clarias* spp.) crossbreeding toward egg quality. *Egypt J Aquat Res* (2015) 41:353–335.

Lacasse, C. (2015). Falconiformes (falcons, hawks, eagles, kites, harriers, buzzards, ospreys, caracaras, secretary birds, old world and new world vultures). In: *Fowler's Zoo and Wild Animal Medicine*. (eds. R. E. Miller *et al.*), Vol. 8, pp. 127–142. Saunders/El Sevier, St. Louis, MO.

Marziani, J.A., *et al.,* (2017). Addition of complementary therapies in zoological medicine. *Proceedings of the Annual Conference of the AAZV* (September 23–29). Dallas, TX.

Massotti, F.P. *et al.* (2015). Histomorphometric assessment of the influence of low-level laser therapy on peri- implant tissue healing in the rabbit mandible. *Photomed Laser Surg*. 33(3):123–128.

Matos, F.S. *et al.* (2016). Effect of laser photobiomodulation on the periodontal repair process of replanted teeth. *Dent Traumatol*. 32(5):402–408.

Mitchell, L.K.H. *et al.* (2023). Successful treatment of a cervical injury and myopathy using integrative techniques in an eclectus parrot (*Eclectus roratus*) following cervical entrapment. *J Avian Med Surg*. 37(2):175–179.

Moskvin, S.V. *et al.* (2018). Effectiveness of low level laser therapy for treating male infertility. *Biomedicine (Taipei)*. 8(2):7.

Mukti, A.T. *et al.* (2020). The effects of laserpuncture on gonadal maturity and sperm quality of male striped catfish (*Pangasianodon hypophthalmus*). *Theriogenology*. 147:102–107.

Nascimento, C.L. *et al.* (2015). Comparative study between photodynamic and antibiotic therapies for treatment of footpad dermatitis (bumblefoot) in Magellanic penguins (*Spheniscus magellanicus*). *Photodiagn Photodyn Ther*. 12 (1):36–44.

Nevitt, B.N. *et al.* (2015). Effectiveness of physical therapy as an adjunctive treatment for trauma-induced chronic torticollis in a raptor. *J Avian Med Surg*. 29(1):30–39.

Park, S.R. *et al.* (2023). Efficacy of low-level laser therapy in a rabbit model of rhinosinusitis. *Int J Mol Sci*. 24(1):760. doi:10.3390/ijms24010760.

Pluim, M. *et al.* (2020). High-power laser therapy improves healing of the equine suspensory branch in a standardized lesion model. *Front Vet Sci*. 7:600. doi:10.3389/fvets.2020.00600.

Pryor, B. (2009). *Class IV Laser Therapy Interventional and Case Reports Confirm Positive Therapeutic Outcomes in Multiple Clinical Indications*. LiteCure, LLC, Newark, DE.

Pryor, B. and Millis, D.L. (2015). Therapeutic laser in veterinary medicine. *Vet Clin North Am Small Anim Pract.* 45(1):45–56.

Reillo, P.R. and Clubb, S.L. (2015). Natural metacarpus fracture remodeling in a bottle-reared mountain bongo antelope calf (*Tragelaphus eurycerus isaaci*) with presumed failure of passive transfer. *Int J Appl Res Vet Med.* 13 (2):89–92.

Rico-Holgado, S. *et al.* (2021). Effects of low-level laser therapy on bacterial counts of traumatic contaminated wounds in dogs. *J Lasers Med Sci.* 12:e78.

Robinson, N.G. (2019). Integrative medicine for geriatric zoo animals. *Proceedings of the Annual Conference of the AAZV* (September 28 October 4). Sr. Louis, MO.

Rychel, J.K. *et al.* (2011). Zoologic companion animal rehabilitation and physical medicine. *Vet Clin North Am Exot Anim Pract.* 14(1):131–140.

Sellera, F.P. *et al.* (2014). Photodynamic therapy for pododermatitis in penguins. *Zoo Biol.* 33(4):353–356.

Sims, C. *et al.* (2015). Rehabilitation and physical therapy for the neurologic veterinary patient. *Vet Clin North Am Small Anim Pract.* 45(1):123–143.

Souza, A.R. *et al.* (2023). The effects of photobiomodulation therapy on the healing of eastern box turtle (*Terrapene carolina*) shells. *J Zool Bot Gard.* 4:578–586.

Sparrow, S. (2020). Clinical applications of photobiomodulation therapy in a zoological setting. *Vet Nurs.* 11(10):2044–0065.

Tang, E. and Arany, P. (2013). Photobiomodulation and implants: implications for dentistry. *J Periodontal Implant Sci.* 43(6):262–268.

Vetere, A. *et al.* (2021). Treatment of a degloving lesion in a green tree python (*Morelia viridis*) with surgical approach adjuved by laser therapy and single application of thrombocyte-leukocyte rich plasma. *Veterinaria.* 35(5):257–263.

Zimmerman, D.M. *et al.* (2009). Compressive myelopathy of the cervical spine in Komodo dragons (*Varanus komodoensis*). *J Zoo Wildl Med.* 40(1):207–210.

Part VII

Clinical Applications of Laser Therapy in Large Animal Practice

29

Fundamentals of Equine Laser Therapy

Ronald J. Riegel

American Institute of Medical Laser Applications, Marysville, OH, USA

Introduction

Therapeutic lasers have been a mainstay in the equine industry for over three and a half decades. From the humble beginnings of a single milliwatt laser in the late 1970s, this technology has evolved to include lasers emitting over 60 W of power. Despite this evolution, new information emerges weekly, offering deeper insights into its broader clinical and regenerative medical applications. This chapter will delve into the specifics of dosages, general application techniques for localized treatment areas and their corresponding acupuncture points, and all associated compensatory areas. It will also cover the frequency of application and explore how this modality can be incorporated into a wholistic approach to achieve consistent clinical outcomes. For more fundamental information concerning the principles of physics and physiological and biochemical processes, readers are directed to the first few introductory chapters of this text.

Patient Preparation

Effective communication with both the owner and the trainer is crucial. It is important that they understand the rationale behind your recommendation for laser therapy and have realistic expectations regarding the clinical outcome. Key points to always discuss include: the absence of side effects, the fact that only dysfunctional cells are targeted, and the lack of a withdrawal period before competition. It is also important to establish realistic therapeutic goals and a detailed treatment plan. This approach not only promotes client compliance but also fosters a better understanding of your recommendations.

When administering laser treatment, it is crucial to ensure the patient's surroundings are calm, serene, and devoid of any distracting noise. An enclosed space that is impenetrable to light on all sides, such as a wash stall, is ideal. This completely adheres to laser safety standards and regulations. The patient should be held securely by someone familiar with their behavior and mannerisms. While it may not be the first choice, placing the animal in crossties is sometimes necessary when assistance is not readily available.

Photobiomodulation therapy (PBMT) uses light energy to modulate cellular functions. To ensure effective treatment, the animal's skin must be clean and free of any photo-absorbing materials. Microfiber cloths are particularly effective in removing dirt, sand, and dust. If the animal is particularly dirty or if leg paints, poultices, or ointments have been applied, washing may be necessary. Ideally, the animal should be dry when applying PBMT. However, even damp skin has little effect on photonic penetration. Wounds should be cleaned and debrided before applying PBMT. This allows better penetration of the photonic energy to the target cells, enhancing the effectiveness of the treatment.

Adherence to safety recommendations is crucial when operating any laser system. This is particularly significant when utilizing Class 3 or 4 therapeutic systems, which emit over 0.5 W. Before activating the laser, it is essential that the therapist, handlers, and patient wear appropriate eye protection. For the patient, a simple yet effective solution is to use a thick black towel or black felt, folded or doubled over several times. These material eye shields are not only easy to use but also comfortable and can be easily cleaned or replaced. It is also advisable to have assistance when applying laser therapy in areas near or directly to the head to minimize the risk of accidental eye exposure. Laser safety signage should be conspicuously displayed.

Laser Therapy in Veterinary Medicine: Photobiomodulation, Second Edition. Edited by Christopher J. Winkler and Lisa A. Miller.

Table 29.1 Calming and sedation acupuncture points.

Condition/disorder	Corresponding acupuncture points
Calming and sedation	Yin-Tang, GV 26, CV 24, KI 1, BL23, LV 3, BL 18, BL 19, SP 6, BL 20, LU 1, LU 11, BL 13

Calming and Sedation

Equines, being innately flight-response creatures, may exhibit nervousness and anxiety when introduced to new stimuli in their environment. Laser therapy, a relatively novel procedure, falls into this category. To mitigate any potential stress, it is recommended to apply an appropriate dosage of PBMT to the acupuncture relaxation points (Fuchtenbusch & Rosen, 2006). Over the past three decades, numerous studies have been conducted to understand the impact of laser therapy on nerves. It has been well-documented in several pieces of literature that one of the key mechanisms behind this analgesic effect is neural inhibition – meaning that laser therapy can slow down the speed of nerve impulses and reduce their intensity (Chow *et al.*, 2011).

An additional procedure to calm the patient, referred to as the "Unwind" protocol, is to apply laser therapy utilizing an on-contact scanning technique, emitting a blend of wavelengths of various power at 1000 Hz. Start at the base of the skull and closely following the bladder meridian, continuing the application to the base of the tail over a 10-minute period (Schoen *et al.*, 1994).

Patient responses to these techniques can vary significantly. While some individuals may experience a response after stimulation of the initial points, others may require higher doses. In some cases the techniques may not elicit a response at all. Despite these variations, the techniques do prove effective in approximately 80% of cases. It is important to note that good professional horsemanship is always expected (Table 29.1, Figure 29.1).

Therapeutic Dosage Considerations

Treatment of a Specific Localized Area

Proper dosing involves delivering a sufficient amount of energy (Joules) at a therapeutic wavelength over a specific anatomical area (cm^2). This results in enough energy reaching the target tissue to trigger a clinical response. In review, the formula used to calculate dosage is:

Table 29.2 Equine dosage guidelines.

Application	J/cm^2
Wounds and dermal lesions (lacerations, abrasions, post-operative incisions).	6 ± 4
Superficial structures (deep digital flexor, superficial digital flexor, suspensory tendons).	12 ± 5
Deep musculature (thoracolumbar spine, *gluteal m., cervical m.*).	25 ± 10
Distal joints (tarsal, carpal, metacarpal, metatarsal, phalangeal).	20 ± 5
Proximal joints (femoropatellar, femorotibial).	25 ± 5
Unique applications (lumbosacral area; L/S joint; SI joint and surrounding musculature).	30 ± 10
Trigger points	4 ± 2
Acupuncture points	**J/point**
Superficial	80–125
Deep	125–200

$$\text{Dose} = \text{Power (Watts)} \times \text{Time (seconds)}/\text{Area of treatment } (\text{cm}^2) = \text{Joules/cm}^2\,(\text{J/cm}^2)$$

As research continues to be published, recommended dosage levels have gradually increased. The following chart gives the recommended dosages currently being utilized when treating equines (Table 29.2).

Almost all therapeutic lasers on the market are equipped with sophisticated software designed to accurately calculate and administer the appropriate dosage for patients. Factors such as the patient's skin color, hair coat color, body weight, hair coat length, and the specific anatomical area being treated are considered. Some software even includes preset protocols for various specific conditions within each anatomical area.

This data is input into the program, which then calculates a dosage, determines how this dosage is to be emitted, sets the treatment time, and in some cases even recommends the appropriate handpiece to use. While these programs may not cover every disorder, they can easily be extrapolated to similar conditions to provide a suitable dosage.

These software programs provide a starting point for therapy, which can be adjusted according to the results of the patient's reevaluation examination conducted before each therapy session. This allows for personalized treatment plans, ensuring optimal results for each patient.

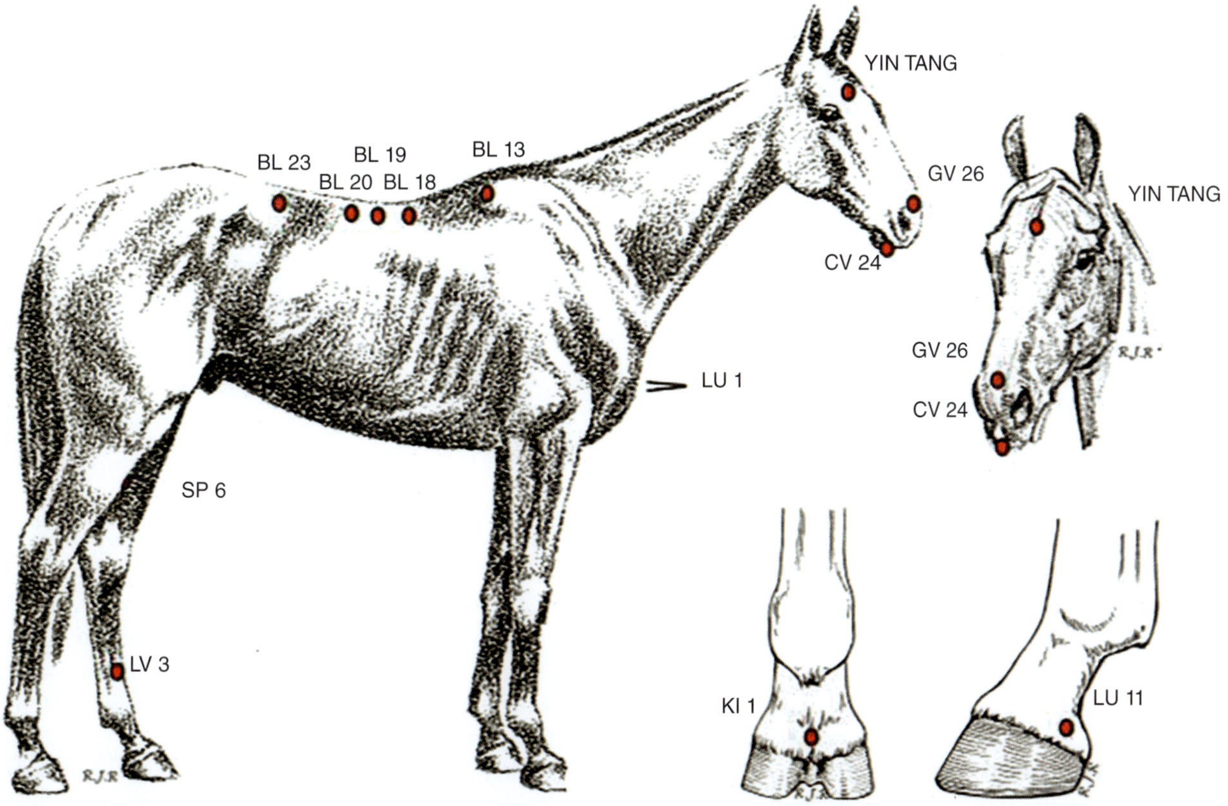

Figure 29.1 Acupuncture/laserpuncture points for calming and sedation.

Treatment of Trigger and Acupuncture Points

Acute myofascial trigger points are areas within the fascia surrounding muscle fibers that exhibit a painful response upon palpation. These points, which present as palpable nodules within taut bands of muscle fibers, are often the source of pain that radiates out in the direction of the surrounding muscle fibers (Travel & Simons, 1999).

The application of laser therapy to these points is very effective in relaxing spastic muscle fibers and relieving pain. Treat these points on-contact with sufficient pressure and photonic energy to release the muscle spasm and restore normal circulation. Applying 2–4 J/cm^2, using a pulsed or super-pulsed emission combined with a massage technique, will often cause the spastic nodule to disappear (Airaksinen *et al.,* 1989).

Performing acupuncture with the stimulatory power of photonic energy is a patient-friendly and painless alternative to the classic needle. The use of lasers to stimulate acupuncture points is termed "laserpuncture" or "laser acupuncture" (Lorenzini *et al.*, 2010). Laser acupuncture has several advantages when compared to classic needle acupuncture (Martin & Klide, 1987; Schoen & Wynn, 1998):

- Painless application
- Complication-free
- Short treatment time
- Noninvasive
- Minimal restraint

Acupuncture is a time-honored practice that has been used for centuries to alleviate pain and stimulate muscle circulation. Consider laserpuncture as another version of this practice. Recent studies have shown its broad range of effectiveness in various rehabilitation protocols (le Jeune, 2016), and even maintaining performance in the equine athlete (Pujalte *et al.*, 2023).

The dosage of photonic stimulation for each acupuncture point varies depending on the depth of that unique point and its relationship to the surrounding anatomical area. For average depth points, an irradiated dose of 125–200 J/point is recommended. However, deeper points, such as the Bai Hue point (which is surrounded by large muscle masses and bone) require a higher dose of 150–225 J/point (Fuchtenbusch & Rosin, 2006). These dosages should be administered slowly at a low wattage (0.5 W), using a super-pulsed or pulsed emission mode, emitting wavelengths within the therapeutic window.

The total treatment time per point also depends on the depth of the point and the average output power of the equipment. Therapy lasers that emit a higher-than-average power output require less treatment time than those with lower power outputs. Super-pulsed emissions are incorporated into specific treatment protocols for acupuncture point stimulation and are very effective in delivering photonic energy to these deep points.

When using laser acupuncture as the primary treatment, the frequency of treatment can vary. It is generally recommended to treat twice weekly until the therapeutic goal is reached. However, this can be adjusted based on the severity of the disorder and the compliance of the client. Laser therapy's results are cumulative in effect, and it is not unusual for it to be administered each or every other day when the patient would benefit.

A comprehensive meta-analysis of the human literature on laser acupuncture for treating musculoskeletal pain was conducted and published in the *Journal of Acupuncture and Meridian Studies* in 2015. The analysis found that two-thirds of the studies reported positive effects when dosages were properly reported, and the study was of methodological quality. However, the remaining studies, which were poorly designed and used lower dosages, did not show consistent positive clinical outcomes. Interestingly, consistent positive clinical outcomes were achieved after long-term follow-up rather than immediately after treatment (Law *et al.*, 2015).

Even though the beam's energy decreases as it penetrates deeper into the tissue, the stimulatory effect remains sufficient, even when the acupuncture point is difficult to locate. Ideally, a precise point location is desirable to ensure sufficient energy application. The ideal application technique involves on-contact administration with a circular massage motion and slight pressure for thorough penetration. A list of important equine acupuncture points, described using Western nomenclature, can be found in Chapter 31. However, more data is needed to refine these techniques. Parameters such as wavelength, type of emission, and frequency of treatment should be examined to optimize and refine results (Jagger, 1984).

Treatment of Secondary and Compensatory Areas

Laser therapy, when applied to the specific region affected by the diagnosed condition, will yield significant benefits. However, for even more impressive clinical outcomes, it is also advantageous to identify and treat all compensatory areas that would benefit from PBMT. This strategy, targeting both the primary area and any secondary compensatory regions, promotes a more comprehensive approach to treatment which can expedite the recovery process and potentially enhance the level of performance. Each secondary compensatory area must be identified and treated as a distinct entity, with its own suitable dosage, application technique, and frequency of sessions. This wholistic approach is beneficial when addressing and alleviating many lameness issues.

General Treatment Techniques

Diagnosis

An accurate diagnosis is essential before initiating PBMT. When treating lameness issues, this diagnosis should include all secondary and compensatory concerns and all corresponding acupuncture and trigger points involved. Utilizing this comprehensive approach to treatment will maximize the clinical response.

Similarly, when treating wounds, we must identify not only the area of injury but also the secondary and compensatory areas. These areas should also be included in the therapeutic protocol, along with generous margins surrounding the injury,

Infrared thermal imaging (IRTI), or infrared thermography (IR), identifies all areas that would benefit from further evaluation and possibly diagnostics. These images allow visualization of both the primary and secondary compensatory areas of stress. Infrared thermal images provide a "road map" for the application of laser therapy, allowing the therapist to target those anatomical areas that would benefit the most from treatment. The initial set of images taken prior to the commencement of therapy serves as a baseline to measure patient progress on subsequent reevaluations (Figures 29.2 and 29.3).

Before each subsequent therapeutic laser session, it is essential to conduct a reevaluation. This process allows the clinician to make necessary adjustments to the laser therapy parameters. Key clinical signs for which to observe include decreased swelling, reduced lameness, and other indicators of progress or regression.

Being not merely a subjective observation but an objective measurement, IRTI can be a valuable tool in tracking the progress of the case. By comparing temperature data from consecutive infrared thermal images, one can quantitatively assess the patient's progress and create a roadmap for each therapy session (Figure 29.3). This technology provides a visual representation of the progress to the owner

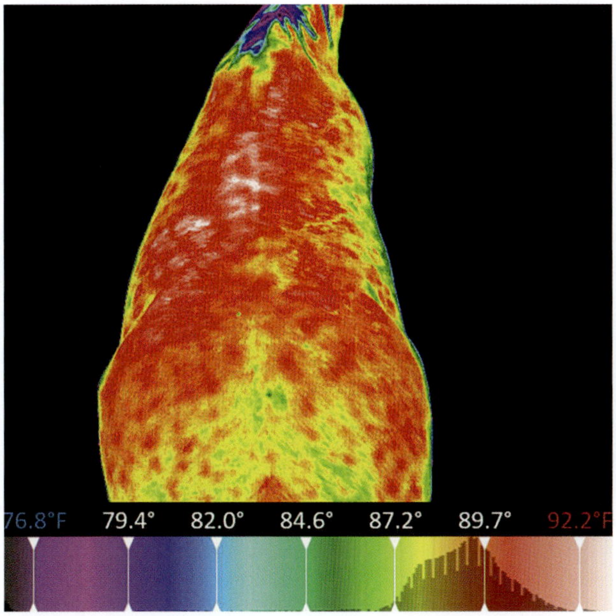

Figure 29.2 Dorsal infrared thermal image. There is an asymmetrical bilateral hyperthermia visualized in this infrared thermal image of the dorsal view of the spine. There are diffuse areas of increased circulation(red) and several focal areas of increased circulation and spastic muscle nodules (white) throughout. These focal areas (white), more numerous within the left paravertebral musculature, correspond to areas that present as painful and the muscle tissue in a state of spastic. This image is a visual representation of where the application of laser therapy is needed the most; throughout all reds areas with special attention to those areas that are white.

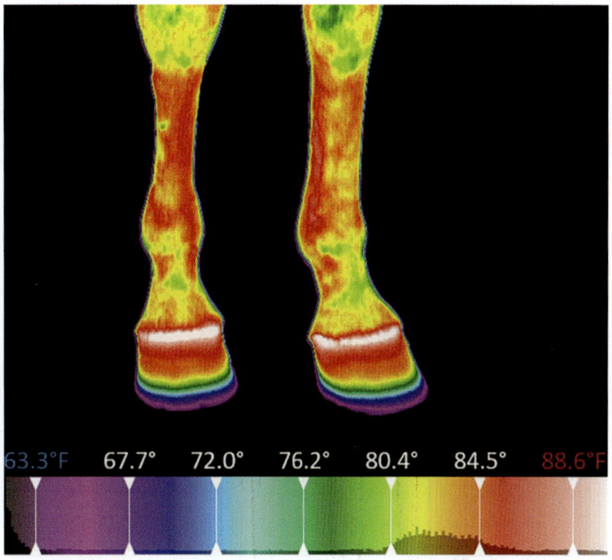

Figure 29.3 APLMO of distal forelimbs dorsal infrared thermal image. Asymmetrical bilateral hyperthermia exists between both forelimbs and within different areas on the same limb. The bilateral areas of increased circulation(red) correlate to inflammation, medially. The right forelimb depicts the extent of the inflammation in the extensor tendons. Laser therapy should be applied throughout both distal limbs, but higher dosages should be applied to those areas showing the highest increases in circulation.

and trainer, enhancing their understanding and promoting compliance with treatment recommendations. Therefore, it is recommended to utilize this technology until the issue is fully resolved (Figure 29.4).

General Application Techniques

When implementing PBMT on any part of an equine, it is crucial to consider the following guidelines:

- **Handpiece control:** Always maintain full control of the handpiece.
- **Beam orientation:** Ensure that the handpiece is always held perpendicular to the skin. Any deviation from this angle will increase the reflection of the energy, potentially reducing the therapy's effectiveness.
- **Treatment technique:** Regardless of whether the equipment uses a point-to-point or scanning treatment technique, it is essential to treat on-contact whenever possible if it is warranted by the condition and the patient permits. This approach minimizes reflective energy loss from the dermis, allowing more energy to penetrate the tissues. This technique also results in blanching of the tissue, reducing incidental energy absorption by the intervening blood supply. While the exact amount of this energy absorption is still under research, it is a crucial factor to consider.
- **Temperature monitoring:** When using either a point-to-point or scanning application, always place your finger next to the handpiece. This allows for easy temperature monitoring of the tissue, providing a more accurate assessment of the treatment's progress. There are therapeutic lasers on the market that do not produce thermal elements when emitting; placing a finger next to these units also aid in the orientation of the treatment beam angle.
- **Therapy angle:** Apply therapy at right angles to the target tissue in opposite directions. This ensures that the energy is applied evenly throughout the area, maximizing the therapy's benefits.
- **Medical recordkeeping:** Document the clinical progress of the case, recording the total number of joules administered to each anatomical area (J/cm^2), the specific application technique, infrared thermal images of the area, and the plan for the following therapy session in your medical records. This comprehensive recordkeeping aids in tracking the patient's response to therapy and adjusting the treatment plan as necessary.

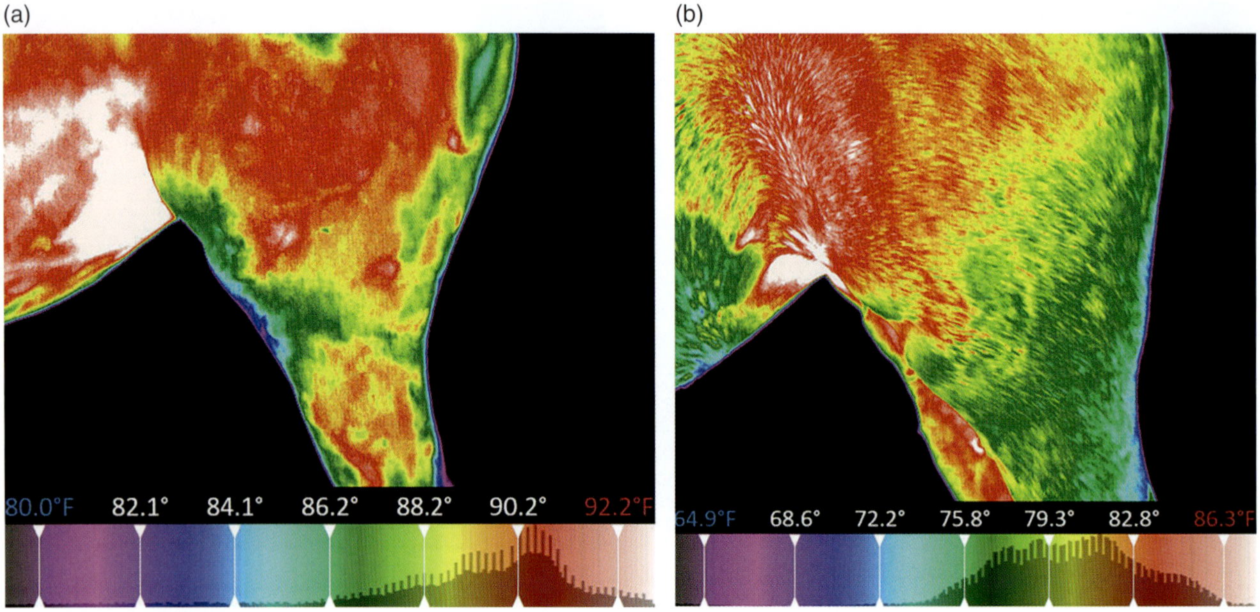

Figure 29.4 APLMO left stifle. (a) There are diffuse areas of increased circulation (red) radiating out from the stifle joint into areas of the quadriceps femoris, tensor facia latae, and superficial gluteal muscles. Note that the area of the femoropatellar and femorotibial joints are cooler (green and blue) due to the swelling just beneath the skin. (b) This image was taken 6 hours post-laser therapy. The circulation has normalized, with no distinct areas of increased thermal gradients in this area, and there is a reduction of the swelling within the stifle joint as indicated by the return of circulation.

Frequency of Administration

The frequency of laser therapy administration is tailored to each patient's unique needs. This frequency is influenced by several factors, including patient compliance, the patient's response to therapy, and the nature of the patient's condition. PBMT is typically applied across three distinct phases:

1) **Induction phase:** This is an aggressive phase where therapy is administered daily or every other day until a significant clinical response is observed. PBMT is cumulative in effect, and there are handheld units that can be prescribed to the owner for treatment more frequently and more economically.
2) **Transition phase:** During this phase, therapy applications are less frequent (usually twice a week) until the treatment goal is achieved. Utilization of a safe prescribed take-home laser provides more therapy sessions and an acceleration of clinical results.
3) **Maintenance phase:** In this final phase, therapy is administered as needed to maintain the treatment goal or to sustain the patient's quality of life over a prolonged period.

In summary, therapy is administered daily or twice a day to acute cases until a significant clinical response is noted. After this, therapy is administered less frequently until the condition is fully resolved.

Chronic cases may also initially receive therapy daily until a clinical response is noted; therapy is then administered less frequently until the therapeutic goal is reached. Subsequently, therapy is administered periodically to maintain the therapeutic goal of a level of performance or even quality of life.

Case Example: A Wholistic Approach to the Treatment of Cunean Tendonitis/Bursitis (Distal Tarsitis Syndrome)

Localized Treatment

The patient is diagnosed with cunean tendonitis/bursitis (distal tarsitis syndrome). The entire area around the tarsal bone is treated with appropriate dosages, wavelengths, and optimal emission. This includes the distal tarsal joint, the cunean tendon, and its corresponding bursa. Even though the hock is composed of soft tissue structures, joints, and bones, contact administration should be used when possible. This can be done using either a scanning or point-to-point treatment. If the area is extremely painful, start with off-contact treatment until immediate pain relief allows for on-contact administration.

In each laser therapy session, a focused application should be made over the primary area of concern. This treatment should also encompass all secondary and

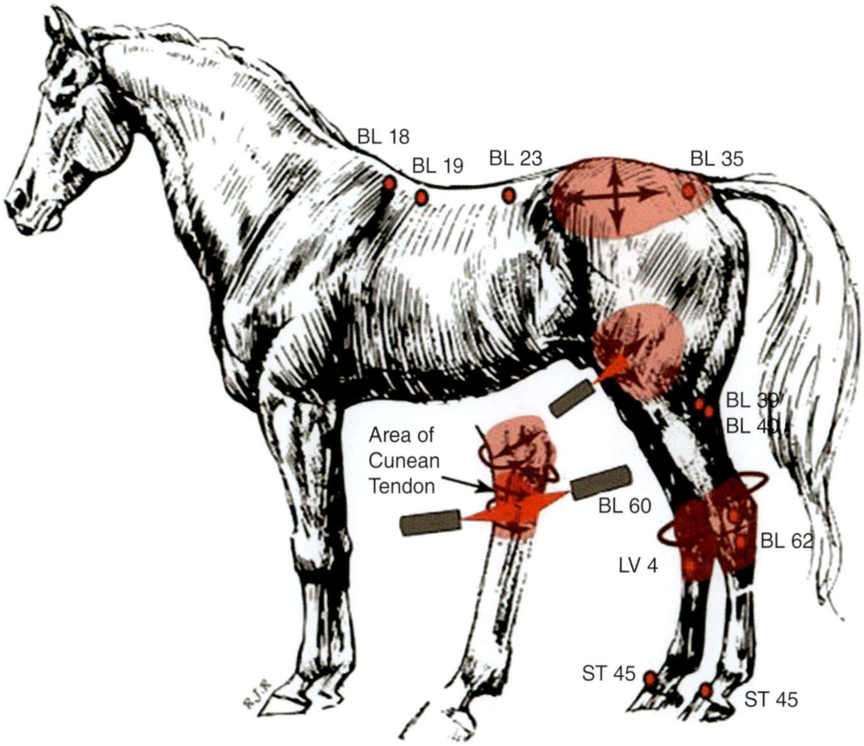

Figure 29.5 Administer PBMT circumferentially and at right angles on-contact throughout all the anatomical structures of the hock. Address every possible angle to saturate each soft-tissue structure and intraarticular surface. Administer a higher dosage to all the areas of both joints, the cunean tendon, and the cunean bursal lying beneath (darker shaded area on the insert). Treatment of all compensatory secondary areas of concern (the lumbosacral and sacroiliac areas, both hips and stifles, and the opposite hock) should be accomplished using appropriate dosages for each anatomical area. Lastly, apply photonic energy to stimulate all trigger and complementary acupuncture points.

compensatory anatomical involvements. Additionally, it should include the treatment of all associated trigger points and acupuncture points. Therapy should be administered from all angles on the medial side to ensure the distal tarsal joint and the length of the cunean tendon are saturated (see the darker shaded area on the illustration of the medial hock, Figure 29.5). It may be easier to administer this treatment from the opposite side of the horse, depending on the horse's temperament. Some patients may require lifting and holding one of the front legs off the ground to ensure the horse bears weight on the hind limb being treated.

Secondary and Compensatory Treatment

Issues with the cunean tendon place a biomechanical strain on at least the unilateral stifle structures. Both stifles should be examined by digital palpation to detect any soreness or swelling in the joints and surrounding soft tissue structures. Administer an appropriate dosage on-contact, utilizing ideal emissions and therapeutic wavelengths to all identified areas of soreness (Figure 29.5). This is an ideal time to utilize infrared thermal images to guide administration.

Consider treating both hips, gluteal areas, the lumbosacral area, and all other areas that palpate sore or show other clinical signs. These deeper target tissues require optimal parameters to reach and saturate them with a therapeutic dose. Attempt to administer to these tissues on-contact. When possible, utilize IRTI to identify all anatomical areas that would benefit from therapy and as a visual to monitor the patient's progress.

The ideal treatment would also include all tarsal structures on the opposite leg. These joint and soft tissue structures are under more weight-bearing stress as the patient compensates for the opposite limbs' painful cunean tendon, bursa, and other possible arthritic conditions.

Trigger Points and Laser Acupuncture

An appropriate dosage of photonic energy should be administered to all associated acupuncture and trigger points. Typically, these cases involve the points listed in Table 29.3 (Xie & Preast, 2007). Each individual case will be unique and must be assessed accordingly when choosing the proper points and areas to treat.

Table 29.3 Complementary trigger points and acupuncture points for the treatment of cunean tendonitis/bursitis – distal tarsitis.

Trigger points	BL 35 and BL 40
Acupuncture points	BL 18, BL 19, BL 23, BL35, BL 39, BL 60, BL 62, ST 45, LV 4

Conclusion

An inconsistent or unsuccessful clinical outcome can be attributed to several possible reasons. First, the diagnosis may have been incorrect. Second, all secondary and compensatory areas may not have been identified and included in the treatment. Third, the photonic energy may not have reached the target tissues with a significant therapeutic dose. Lastly, the therapy may not have been administered frequently enough.

Fundamental information and application techniques of laser therapy are crucial to achieving consistent clinical results. It is essential to consider factors such as dosages, application techniques, areas of treatment, and frequency of therapy administration on an individual basis. Each case should be treated uniquely, considering not just localized areas but all compensatory areas as well.

References

Airaksinen, O. *et al.* (1989). Effects of infra-red laser irradiation on the treated and non-treated trigger points. *Acupunct Electrother Res.* 14:9.

Chow, R. *et al.* (2011). Inhibitory effects of laser irradiation on peripheral mammalian nerves and relevance to analgesic effects: a systematic review. *Photomed Laser Surg.* 29(6):365–381.

Fuchtenbusch, A. & Rosin, P. (2006). *Laser Therapy and Acupuncture on Horses; Treatment Protocols.* pp. 102–105; 14–17.

Jagger, D.H. (1984). Alternative veterinary medicine. *Vet Rec.* 114(17):435.

le Jeune, S. (2016). Acupuncture and equine rehabilitation. *Vet Clin North Am Equine Pract.* 32(1):73–85.

Law, D. *et al.* (2015). Laser acupuncture for treating musculoskeletal pain: a systematic review with meta-analysis. *J Acupunct Meridian Stud.* 8(1):2–16.

Lorenzini, L. *et al.* (2010). Laser acupuncture for acute inflammatory, visceral and neuropathic pain relief: an experimental study in the laboratory rat. *Res Vet Sci.* 88(1):159–165.

Martin, B.B. and Klide, A.M. (1987). Treatment of chronic back pain in horses. Stimulation of acupuncture points with a low powered infrared laser. *Vet Surg.* 16(1): 106–110.

Pujalte, G. *et al.* (2023). Acupuncture in sports medicine. *J Acupunct Meridian Stud.* 16(6):239–247.

Schoen, A.M. and Wynn, S.G. (1998). Chapter 11). *Complementary and Alternative Veterinary Medicine Principles and Practice*, 1 edn, pp. 173–184. Mosby, USA.

Schoen, A.M. *et al.* (1994). *Veterinary Acupuncture: Ancient Art to Modern Medicine*, 1 edn. Mosby, USA pp. 425 and 559.

Travel, J.G. and Simons, L.S. (1999). Chapter 2). *Myofascial Pain and Dysfunction: The Trigger Point Manual*, 2 edn, pp. 11–93. Lippincott Williams and Williams, USA.

Xie, H. and Preast, V. (2007). Chapters 3 and 4). *Xie's Veterinary Acupuncture*, 1 edn, p. 260. Blackwell Publishing.

30

Administering Laser Therapy to the Equine Patient

Ronald J. Riegel

American Institute of Medical Laser Applications, Marysville, OH, USA

Introduction

Therapeutic lasers have been utilized in the equine industry for over 35 years. This modality has evolved from the first one milliwatt laser of the late 1970s to the 30–60+ W scientific and clinical evidence-based therapy equipment available today. The development of both new equipment and software has provided the therapist with the tools to achieve consistent and repeatable clinical results and expand the versatility of this modality.

This chapter will address general application techniques, dosages, and the frequency of application by anatomical area. The treatment protocols for several of the common disorders within each anatomical area will be presented with information for the treatment of the corresponding acupuncture points and associated compensatory areas. The goal is to provide basic guidance in treating the entire patient to maximize pain relief, modulation of inflammation, and acceleration of the healing processes. An understanding of how power, wavelength, mode of emission, current dosage recommendations, technique, and frequency of application is essential in obtaining consistent, efficacious clinical results. Laser therapy systems vary, but these fundamental elements must be addressed irrespective of the device to ensure maximum clinical success. In all cases, laser therapy should be used to supplement standard care procedures; not as a replacement.

The Head

The primary concern when implementing photobiomodulation therapy (PBMT) around the head is the protection of the patient's eyes. This can be achieved effectively using a thick, black cloth or felt. These materials can be folded to enhance protection while ensuring a high level of comfort for the horse. Even with such protective measures in place, it is crucial not to expose the eye to the direct beam of the therapy.

Lacerations in this region are managed as superficial wounds (see Chapter 32). The therapy should be administered off-contact with either a scanning or a point-to-point technique directly over the wound and to a margin of healthy tissue surrounding it. Dosages will vary depending on the exact anatomical location within the area, but most software will guide you to use a superficial range since the target tissues are on the skin's surface. A combination of red, infrared, and blue light will often be the treatment of choice after surgical closure.

Snakebites to the face and muzzle can be extremely traumatic injuries. Fortunately, laser therapy is an effective treatment for such (see Chapter 10). Once hemorrhaging is minimized and under control, maximize PBMT's benefits to the patient by administering as soon as possible. This condition would benefit from multiple treatments over several days, with the frequency governed by the clinical response. Some software will not have a preset protocol for the treatment of snakebite. The number one priority is to treat pain. If the therapy unit has a setting for pain, that will suffice; if not, use a dosage of 8 J/cm^2 and saturate not just the area encompassed by the fang marks but also a generous margin surrounding the bite. All initial administration will be off-contact utilizing a slow scanning technique.

Sinusitis responds well to laser therapy. Modulating the inflammatory response offers additional benefits when added to the traditional standard of care. As laser therapy is applied to the sinus cavity and adjacent structures, precautions must be taken to protect the eyes during the procedure. Drainage through the nostrils often occurs within the first 5 minutes of therapy. Use higher doses than usual to treat sinusitis, as the aim is to penetrate not only the skin and bone but also the photoabsorbing exudate within the

Laser Therapy in Veterinary Medicine: Photobiomodulation, Second Edition. Edited by Christopher J. Winkler and Lisa A. Miller.

sinus cavity. A starting dosage of 15–20 J/cm^2 is recommended, applied daily for three or four sessions, followed by every other day until the condition resolves.

In disciplines that demand natural balance and self-carriage, such as dressage, where the head and neck are positioned high to facilitate an upward movement as the center of gravity shifts backward, there is often stress on the anatomical area at the base of the skull and the first few cervical vertebrae. PBMT can achieve two objectives when applied to this region: it can alleviate any inflammation and soreness, and if applied before the event, it can enhance flexibility in the area. This results in increased comfort and suppleness within this area, resulting in better balance for both the horse and rider. This technique allows the patient to comfortably elevate the horse's front end, allowing for a more upward, airborne movement. The suggested dosage for this procedure is 8–12 J/cm^2, which should be applied directly on-contact around the base of the horse's skull and the adjacent muscles up to the C2–C3 vertebral level. Passive range of motion during the application (by an assistant gently flexing and extending the horse's head) will facilitate more saturation of the target tissues.

Numerous conditions within the oral cavity can benefit from the application of PBMT. This includes traumatized tissue of any kind, such as lesions caused by ill-fitting dental appliances, lacerations to the tongue, inflammation of the mucous membranes, periodontal disease, and bone fractures. Postoperative care following dental extraction should include PBMT. The target tissue in this area is often superficial, requiring only a dosage of 2–4 J/cm^2 to stimulate healing. Deeper target tissues may necessitate higher dosages. When applying PBMT, it is crucial to ensure that the oral cavity is adequately exposed using a full mouth speculum or mouth gag. The patient should always remain under control. These two pieces of equipment are essential for the safe and effective application of PBMT; caution should be exercised as these objects have reflective surfaces, necessitating protective eyewear be worn at all times. Sanitize the handpiece between application procedures.

Temporomandibular joint syndrome (TMJ), also referred to as TMJ dysfunction, has responded will to laser therapy in experimental settings (Lemos *et al.*, 2016) and clinically in human medicine (Ayyildiz *et al.*, 2015; Machado *et al.*, 2016). To administer the therapy, apply directly to the area highlighted in Figure 30.1. The therapy should be provided at a dosage of 8–12 J/cm^2 while the joint is undergoing a passive range of motion; this can be easily achieved by offering a treat (such as a carrot) to the patient and applying PBMT while the patient is chewing.

There are numerous superficial acupuncture points located on the head and ears that are complementary to the TMJ (Sutherland *et al.*, 1994). They include those listed in Table 30.1 and illustrated in Figure 30.1. Stimulate each point, dorsal to ventral, cranial to distal, after applying the localized therapy illustrated in Figure 30.1.

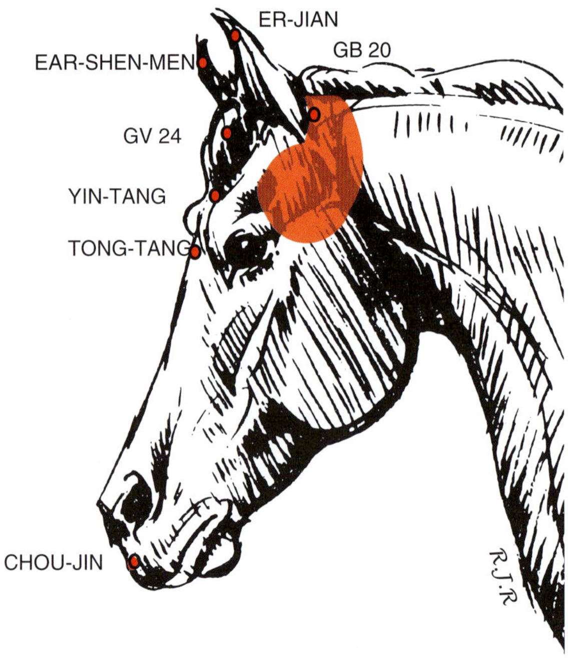

Figure 30.1 Acupuncture points for the temporomandibular joint.

Table 30.1 Acupuncture points for the temporomandibular joint.

Condition/disorder	Corresponding acupuncture points
Temporomandibular joint	Yin-Tang, Tong-Tang, Chou-Jin, ER-Jian, Ear Shen-Men, GB 20, and GV 24

The Throat

Laser therapy has proven effective in managing numerous disorders of the upper respiratory system in horses. Two key benefits of this therapy include the alleviation of pain and regulation of the inflammatory response. These benefits are universally applicable to all disorders within this anatomical region. The therapy is administered externally, directly to the skin of the horse. The handpiece should be in contact with the skin, applying a moderate amount of pressure. It is essential to apply the therapy bilaterally and semicircumferentially with enough energy to saturate all of the tissues in this area, as illustrated in Figure 30.2.

In this author's professional experience, pharyngeal lymphoid hyperplasia has shown a remarkable response to

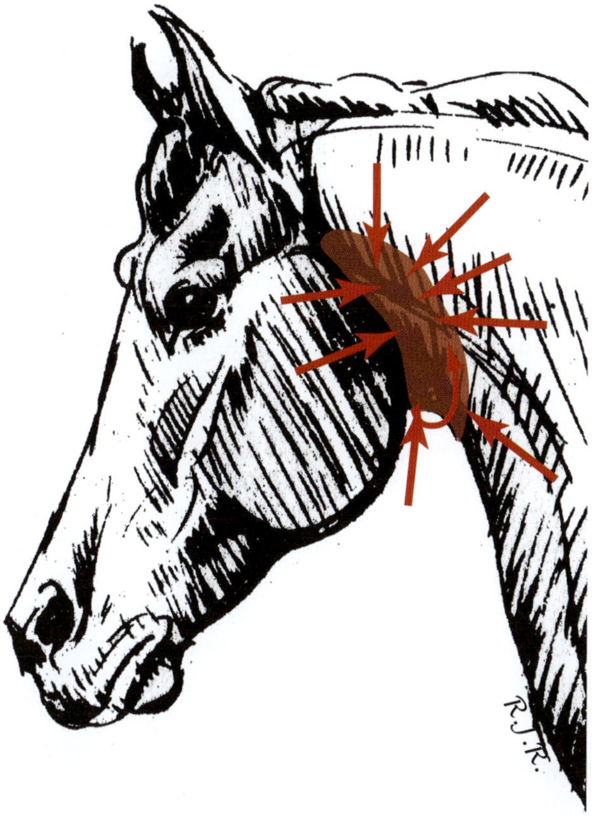

Figure 30.2 Application of PBMT to the throat: bilaterally and on-contact from all possible directions.

PBMT when used in conjunction with conventional standard-of-care treatments such as nebulization and systemic therapy. The therapy is administered to the skin at a dosage of 15–20 J/cm^2. If the therapy laser software is symptomatically based, initiate therapy with the anti-inflammatory preset protocols. Typically, within the first three therapy sessions, patients can expect to see a decrease in swelling and inflammation, as well as a reduction in the size and number of lymphoid follicles. After these initial sessions, a follow-up endoscopic examination is recommended. If the improvement is not as significant as expected, the dosage and frequency of treatments can be adjusted accordingly.

Guttural pouch disorders (tympany, mycosis, and emphysema) pose a unique challenge due to the difficulty in reaching these areas with sufficient photonic energy. While PBMT can be beneficial in the treatment of mycosis and emphysema when used as an adjunct to traditional methods, its effectiveness in treating tympany is quite limited.

There have been only anecdotal reports of the use of PBMT for the entrapment of epiglottis. While CO_2 lasers are efficient surgical tools for this condition, therapy lasers accelerate healing postoperatively. Standard postoperative PBMT protocols involve a dosage of 4–8 J/cm^2.

The cause of laryngeal hemiplegia is damage to the left recurrent laryngeal nerve. Theoretically, PBMT could re-establish this neural pathway (Anders *et al.*, 2004). However, there have been no consistent clinical successes using laser therapy alone. This could be attributed to the difficulty of reaching target tissues with the energy or improper dosing. Combining laser therapy on the surgical incision from a laryngoplasty with a ventriculectomy surgical correction can significantly speed up the healing process (Calisto *et al.*, 2015).

"Strangles," the bacterial infection caused by *Streptococcus equi*, is a highly contagious disease. PBMT, which could potentially reduce pain and inflammation associated with this disorder, should be considered as an adjunct to traditional care. However, before initiating treatment, one must consider the risk of spreading the disease. If PBMT is administered to a patient, it is crucial to follow strict sanitary procedures. This includes careful handling of the handpiece, the fiberoptic cable, the equipment, and the therapist. Simply placing the therapy unit inside a sealed plastic bag is not a guarantee of sterility. For instance, if the bag is punctured or if it encounters contaminated surfaces, the therapy unit could become contaminated. Consider the pros and cons of sterilization procedures before initiating therapy.

The Cervical Spine and Soft Tissues of the Neck

PBMT has proven effective in treating numerous disorders of the neck and cervical spine region, including injuries resulting from falls or injection site myositis, secondary or compensatory muscle soreness arising from distal primary lameness disorders, phlebitis, and transient neurological disorders. Large areas are typically treated with each disorder, with the administration of an on-contact dosage sufficient to saturate this large musculoskeletal region. The depth of the target tissue influences the dosage required to saturate it; thus, deeper tissues necessitate higher dosages. The frequency of treatment varies depending on the individual's condition, but aggressive treatment of acute cases is always recommended. While PBMT has shown some success in treating cervical vertebral compression and instability, its primary benefit is providing analgesia.

Combining PBMT and chiropractic adjustment will aid many equine athletes in maintaining their performance levels. These techniques are often used in conjunction to address muscle tension and misalignments.

Protocols for these treatments can vary, but a common approach involves giving a dosage of 5 J/cm^2, or a relaxing preset protocol, to all target muscles before any adjustments are made. This pre-adjustment treatment often results in a relaxed state in the horse, making the adjustments easier to perform.

Once all chiropractic corrections are made, PBMT is applied to any compensatory areas that may have been affected. In some cases, additional treatment of the target musculature within the neck can deliver another 10–15 J/cm^2 (or a pain and anti-inflammatory preset protocol) to provide further relief of pain and inflammation.

Stimulation of specific acupuncture points can also provide additional pain relief and increased circulation. The acupuncture points important for relieving cervical pain are listed and illustrated in Table 30.2 and Figure 30.3 (Fleming, 1998).

Table 30.2 Acupuncture points for cervical pain.

Condition/disorder	Corresponding acupuncture points
Cervical pain	GB 20, BL 10, TH 16, SI 16, LI 16, BL 11, GB 21

The Shoulder Region

This anatomical region includes the scapula, the scapulohumeral joint, and the muscles that make up the shoulder girdle. Several disorders in this area respond well when treated with laser therapy. These include bicipital bursitis, sweeny, myositis, some scapular fractures, and disorders within the scapulohumeral joint.

The bicipital bursa is a small sac found between the biceps brachii tendon and the bicipital groove of the humerus. This bursa can become inflamed and painful due to trauma or as a secondary compensatory lameness issue. Treating this area with laser therapy has been challenging because of its location, but the evolution of technology with the newer laser equipment has made it possible.

To treat this area, we apply laser therapy directly to the skin over the bursa at a dosage of 8–10 J/cm^2, or with an appropriate preset protocol that provides analgesia. This condition is acute, so we recommend treating it as frequently as possible. Daily treatment is ideal, but twice a day for a few days before administration every other day may provide more immediate clinical results. Laser therapy can be a valuable addition to other systemic treatments, such as anti-inflammatories and intrabursal injections. If an intrabursal injection is planned, administer laser therapy before the injection and then wait 24 hours post-injection before another therapy session.

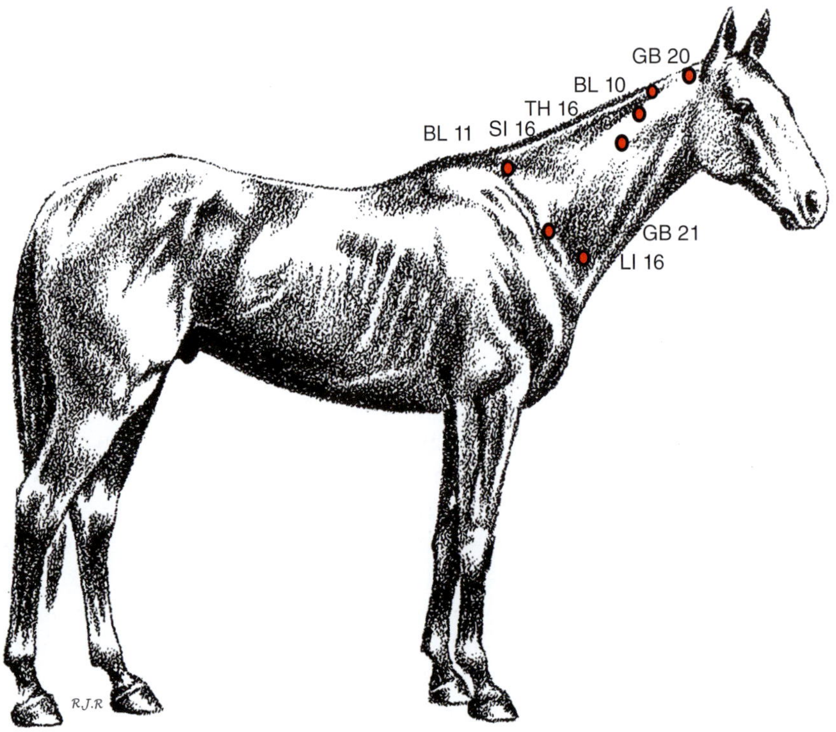

Figure 30.3 Acupuncture points for cervical pain.

Trauma to the suprascapular nerve can lead to atrophy of both the supraspinatus and infraspinatus muscles. PBMT has been observed to increase circulation within these muscles and therefore delay atrophy. There have been anecdotal reports of benefits to the damaged nerve.

PBMT should be administered on-contact at a dosage of about 8–10 J/cm^2 or with a preset protocol designed to address pain and inflammation. Concurrent physical therapy, including massage and stretching exercises, has yielded occasional resolution. While these treatments often result in immediate improvements, patients may still experience some long-term lameness due to the severity of the injury.

Laser therapy has been proven to accelerate the healing of fractures in numerous studies (Kazem *et al.*, 2010; Chang *et al.*, 2014). Most scapular fractures are accessible to photonic stimulation, which can relieve pain, modulate the inflammatory reaction, and accelerate the healing of these lesions. Administer the therapy on-contact, if possible, over an area encompassing all the anatomical structures, at dosages sufficient to saturate all the target tissues. It is important to note that the administration of laser therapy can do no harm in these cases, so its consideration is warranted when dealing with severe muscle atrophy or fractures.

The shoulder girdle muscles play a crucial role in the equine's locomotion. The unique anatomy of these muscles allows for a maximum range of motion, which is essential for the horse's ability to move efficiently and comfortably. However, this range of motion can also make the muscles susceptible to inflammation, strains, and injury.

When administering PBMT to this thick-muscled area, it is important to distribute the treatment throughout the entire muscle structure, from the origin to the insertion. This ensures that all areas of the muscle receive treatment, promoting overall healing and recovery. For larger muscle masses, use higher dosages to ensure complete saturation of the tissues. The dosage can range from 10 to 20 J/cm^2, administered on-contact in conjunction with massage. For more superficial muscle structures, use lower dosages.

Administration of PBMT to these structures before an event or after exercise can be beneficial in preventing injury and promoting recovery. Pre-event administration serves as a "warm-up" allowing for maximum flexibility and function (Levine *et al.*, 2015) aiding in ensuring the horse's comfort and performance.

In addition to the localized therapy applied to these muscles, it is beneficial to stimulate the corresponding acupuncture points, delivering a dosage sufficient to reach the depth of that individual point (Table 30.3) (Fleming, 1998).

Table 30.3 Acupuncture points for shoulder pain.

Condition/ disorder	Corresponding acupuncture points
Shoulder pain	SI 9, 10, TH 13, SI 3, LI 11, 4, 1, SI 1, LU 1

Case Study

History

A 4-year-old thoroughbred filly exhibited a left front limb lameness after a collision with another horse, which ran directly into its shoulder approximately 3 days before presentation.

Signalment

Short stride on left front. Grade 3/5 lame.

Work-up and Diagnostics

Manual palpation revealed only a slight tenderness within and around the origin of the supraspinatus muscles and along the anterior boarder of the scapula cartilage. Radiographs were negative for the scapulohumeral joint and all boney tissues of the shoulder. Ultrasound examination of soft tissues was within normal limits. Scintigraphic images were within normal limits. A complete series of nerve blocks to the limb did not alleviate the lameness.

Management

Initially, the animal rested in a stall for 30 days while administered a normal systemic regimen of analgesics and non-steroidal anti-inflammatories. This resulted in no change in the lameness status.

PBMT

PBMT was initiated 34 days after the onset of the lameness. The animal had been off all pharmaceuticals for the previous 72 hours. Laser therapy was applied to all the soft tissues surrounding the shoulder: both the trapezius cervicalis and thoracis muscles from the midline to their involvement with the scapula, the deltoideus, both the long and lateral head of the triceps brachii, and the brachiocephalicus. These were dosed at 30–40 J/cm^2 on-contact using a combination of scanning and point-to-point administration techniques. The goal of this high dosage was to allow sufficient photon penetration to the deeper musculature.

The scapulohumeral joint and surrounding soft tissues were treated in their entirety at a dosage of 25 J/cm^2.

Laserpuncture Administration

After treatment of all the localized tissues, a dose of 125 J/point was administered to the following acupuncture points in the following order: SI 9, 10, TH 13, SI 3, LI 11, 4, 1, SI 1, LU 1.

Frequency of Therapy

Three therapy sessions were conducted in the first week, each separated by 48 hours. Therapy was then administered twice a week for the next 3 weeks.

Rehabilitation

Following the first three treatments, the animal was massaged for 30 minutes over the shoulder musculature and then lightly across the whole body. The left front leg was brought forward in a controlled stretch, but only at about 30°. The animal was then hand-walked for at least 30 minutes under complete control.

As the therapy sessions progressed, the massage method remained the same, but the stretching of the limb became more aggressive. Hand-walking was increased to an hour twice per day. In the last week of treatment, the patient was placed on a walker for 1 hour thrice daily.

Resolution

A slight improvement in the walk was noticed after the first week of therapy. At the conclusion of the second week (five therapy sessions), the animal was only slightly off (grade 1/5 lame). Clinically, the patient was brighter and much more energetic. After the fourth week, the animal was completely sound and exhibited full range of motion of this front limb with no sign of lameness.

Recommendations and Conclusion

Light training was initiated and progressed normally over the next 5 weeks. When ready for competition, the animal proceeded to win over $3 000 000 in purse money before retiring. While this case is successful, no solid conclusions can be deducted from an N1. Further data should be collected to evaluate this therapy protocol versus others.

The scapulohumeral joint is a simple spheroidal joint with both extension and flexion as its major movements. Many disorders occur within the joint, including osteochondritis desscans and osteoarthritis. Applying PBMT to the structures within this joint is difficult. There are similar challenges when treating the same joint in a human patient. However, we can accomplish a thorough treatment in the human patient due to the ability to flex and extend this joint and perform abduction and adduction range-of-motion movements, allowing better access to the joint during administration. These movements cannot be accomplished in the equine species. Therefore, penetration is limited due to the accessibility of this joint, and often these disorders are clinically nonresponsive.

The Upper Arm and Forearm

The humerus, along with its associated structures, forms the anatomy of the upper arm. Concurrently, the radius and ulna, in conjunction with the humeroradial or elbow joint, create the forearm structure. Laser therapy can be a viable treatment option for several disorders found in this region, including fractures, radial nerve paralysis, hygroma of the elbow, superior check ligament strain, and epiphysitis.

Fractures in this region, typically caused by external trauma, respond well to PBMT. This includes stress fractures, fractures of the deltoid tuberosity, olecranon, and greater and lesser tubercles of the humerus.

In rare cases, fractures of the radius and ulna may occur. These usually require surgical intervention, and PBMT can be applied over surgical implants such as plates or screws without causing any harm. These implants merely reflect the laser light and do not heat up.

For postoperative cases, PBMT should be applied to the incision line and over the entire area of the fracture. In cases where fractures are treated conservatively, aggressive on-contact treatment, when possible, at a high dosage of, should be used.

However, it is important to note that diaphyseal fractures of the humerus often accompany radial nerve paralysis, and the prognosis is generally poor.

The radial nerve, the largest branch of the brachial plexus, is located along the humerus within the musculospiral groove. This area is particularly vulnerable to trauma. Therefore, when administering laser therapy, it should be applied not only perpendicularly but also in various directions to ensure complete saturation of the target tissues. Research has shown that nerve tissue responds well to laser therapy (Wang *et al.*, 2014a), with dosages as high as 25–30 J/cm^2 being effective.

A hygroma is a type of fluid-filled sac or cyst that forms over the point of the olecranon tuberosity. This condition typically results from trauma and is usually neither painful nor inflamed. However, if a hygroma becomes chronic or cosmetically offensive, surgical removal is often the best treatment. After surgery, treat the incision site using an off-contact technique with a dose of 2–5 J/cm^2, starting immediately after the procedure.

The radial head of the superficial digital flexor tendon is a vital component of the equine anatomy. It originates from the distal caudomedial surface of the radius and merges with the main tendon of the superficial digital flexor at the level of the carpus. This, by definition, is a ligament due to the absence of muscle tissue within its structure.

Injuries or strains to this ligament, often resulting from two distinct concurrent hyperextensions of the carpus and fetlock, result in significant pain and inflammation. These injuries are highly responsive to PBMT.

Traditional management of these injuries involved the injection of steroids into the ligament. While this method often provides immediate relief, it can significantly impede the healing process. A more effective approach involves the use of PBMT, physical therapy, and controlled exercises.

The application of laser therapy prior to physical therapy exercises (and ideally repeated several hours later) has proven to be particularly effective. This treatment is beneficial for only a few clinical conditions, this being one of them. Since the ligamentous tissue is quite dense, laser therapy should be applied at dosages of 10–15 J/cm^2 using an on-contact application technique, while placing the limb through a passive range of motion if possible.

Aggressive treatment is recommended initially until clinical results are observed. Without statistics to verify, acute cases responded well to treatment twice daily for the first few days. Gradually, the frequency of treatments can be reduced until the disorder is completely resolved.

Epiphysitis is a condition that affects yearlings and two-year-olds, characterized by swelling and pain. Lameness is uncommon, and the condition typically resolves itself with proper diet and rest. However, it can result in a blemish that impacts on the horse's market value.

There is a precautionary statement regarding the use of laser therapy due to theoretical concerns about abnormal bone growth, potentially leading to an angular limb deformity. However, it is important to note that such an outcome would be extremely difficult to achieve with PBMT.

Apply PBMT circumferentially to the growth plate in an even distribution. This approach can aid in alleviating pain and inflammation. Dosages of 10–12 J/cm^2 (or utilizing a preset protocol for inflammation) on-contact should be administered daily or every other day until resolution.

The Carpus

PBMT provides pain relief, modulation of inflammatory responses, and enhancement of blood circulation (Jang & Lee, 2012). These physiological changes make PBMT an excellent therapy for many carpal conditions, including degenerative joint disease, carpitis, synovitis, hygroma of the carpus, carpal tunnel syndrome, osteoarthritis, and postoperative care.

PBMT is particularly beneficial for animals such as jumpers, 3-day eventers, and thoroughbred racehorses. These animals often engage in strenuous activities that can lead to carpal stress and inflammation. Regular PBMT sessions can help maintain their performance levels by minimizing the inflammation that results from rigorous training.

Moreover, PBMT accelerates recovery time postexercise or event. This means that animals can quickly return to their training routine, minimizing downtime and maintaining their competitive edge. Thus, PBMT is not just a therapeutic tool, but also a performance maintenance tool for high-performance animals.

The application of PBMT to the three carpal joints is straightforward. Therapy should be administered in a circumferential manner, while the joints are in a flexed position and undergoing passive range of motion. It can also be administered at rest, while the limb is bearing weight. When administering PBMT, apply the laser handpiece perpendicular to the target tissues in a single direction, then repeat the process at a right angle to the initial direction (Figure 30.4). During passive range of motion exercises, the beam should be directed toward all parts of the joint capsule and every possible joint surface.

To ensure holistic treatment, consider starting with the entire carpal area, and then stimulate the corresponding acupuncture points (Table 30.4, Figure 30.5). The depth

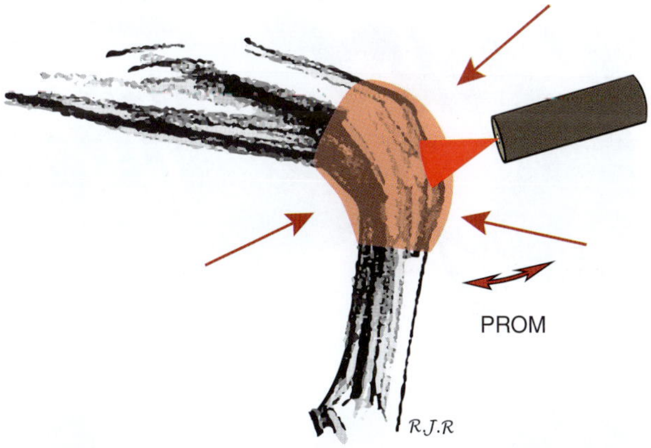

Figure 30.4 Application of PBMT for carpal pain. ~30% of the dose should be applied circumferentially at right angles while the animal is bearing weight on the limb. The remainder should be applied as illustrated while placing the joints and tissues through a passive range-of-motion (PROM) exercise. The handpiece should be kept perpendicular to the skin at all times. Note the margins receiving therapy above and below the carpus.

Table 30.4 Corresponding acupuncture points for the carpus.

Condition/disorder	Corresponding acupuncture points
Degenerative joint disease	LI 6, TH 5, LU 7, LI 4, SI 3
Carpal pain	LI 17, BL 13,BL14, BL 22, BL 25
Carpitis, synovitis, hygroma, carpal tunnel syndrome	BL 11, BL 23, SI 9, TH 5, PC 6, SI 3, TH 1, LI 1, LU 11
Performance maintenance	BL 11, TH 1, LI 1, LU 11

of the point will determine the dosage, which typically ranges from 80 to 200 J/point (Fleming, 1994; Xie & Preast, 2007).

When applying PBMT to the carpus, it is important to also apply treatment to all secondary and compensatory anatomical regions that are strained due to the malady within the carpus. These areas should be identified and addressed in each therapy session. One effective tool for identifying these areas is infrared thermal imaging (IRTI). IRTI provides a visual image of where to apply PBMT, which will provide better clinical results if it is applied where it is needed most. IRTI is a guide, providing a roadmap for therapy, and it will help identify all areas that would benefit from further investigation and possibly diagnostics (IRTI is also discussed in Chapter 39).

Figure 30.6 is a posterior to anterior infrared thermographic image of both carpi. Bilateral hyperthermia (red areas) is present medially. The medial areas on the left carpi are thermally asymmetrical when compared to the right, as there are more focal and diffuse areas of increased circulation present on the distal medial aspect of the radius and continue distally over the palmar areas of the radial, second, and third carpal bones.

PBMT should be applied to all areas of both carpi. The IRTI allows a visual guide to ensure those areas of hyperthermia are addressed. Application of the therapy to these anatomical areas on the IRTI is best accomplished by aiming the beam posteriorly to anteriorly while the joint is extended.

IRTI also identifies additional compensatory areas that would benefit from PBMT. Any anatomical structure that is under an unequal or undue strain will have more circulation present. This increased circulation pattern is easy to visualize when bilateral anatomic areas are compared.

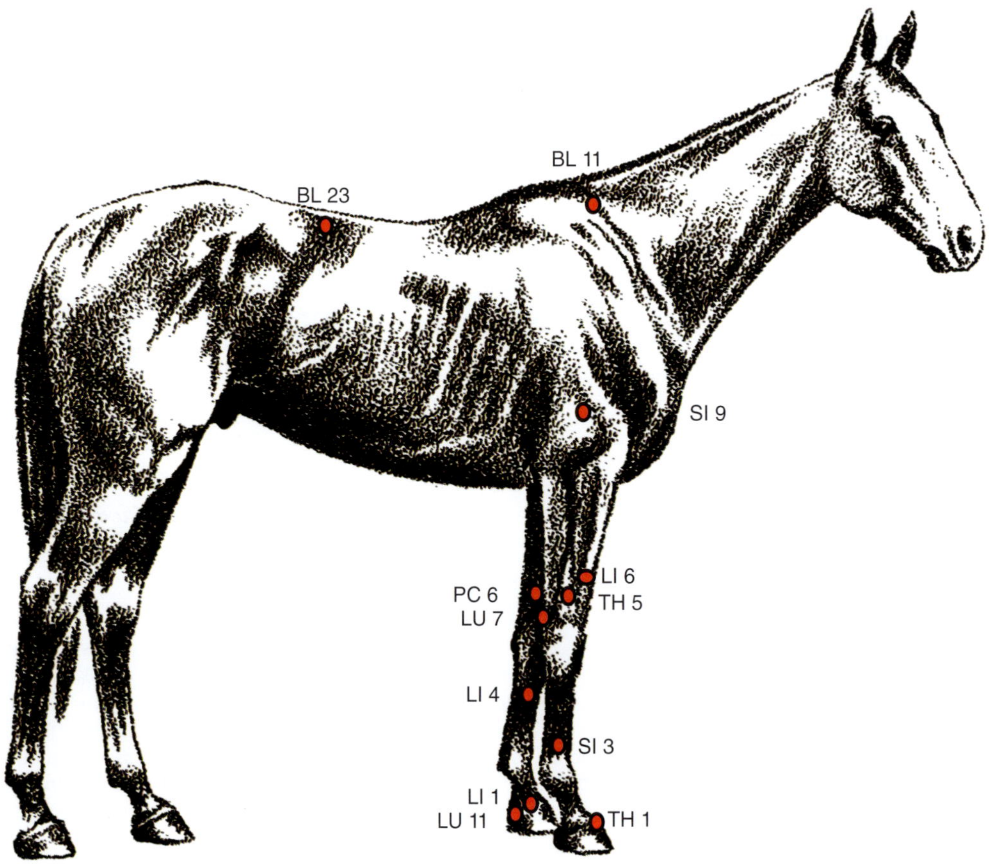

Figure 30.5 Acupuncture points for carpal pain.

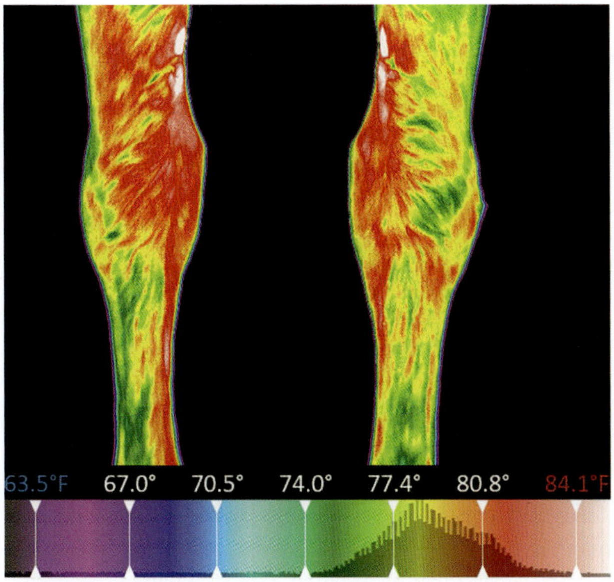

Figure 30.6 Posterior to anterior infrared thermograph image of both carpi. Hyperthermia present on both medially but the left has more focal and diffuse areas of increased circulation that begin on the distal medial aspect of the radius and continue distally over the radial, second, and third carpal bones.

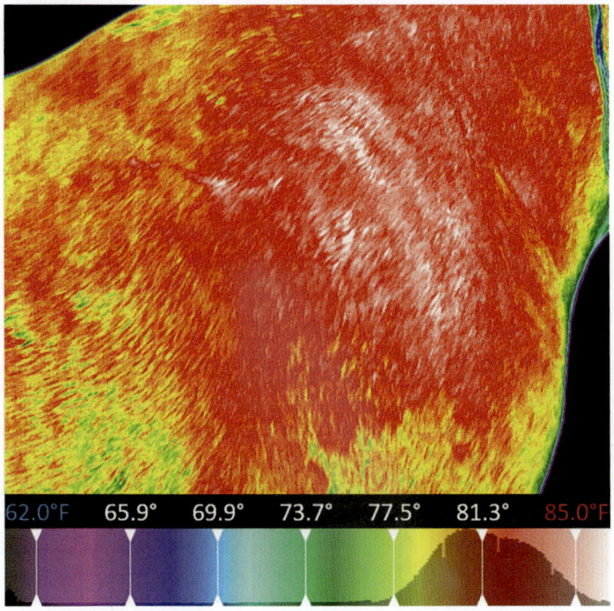

Figures 30.7 (a) and (b). There are increased thermal gradients, which directly correlate to an increased circulation, present in both these images. They are qualitatively visualized as red and white colors. These images provide a guide for the administration of PBMT. The reason for the increased circulation on the left side is a compensatory strain within these muscles because of a lesion distally within the left carpus.

When comparing the IRTI in Figure 30.7 a and b, there is more circulation within the structures of the left shoulder than the right. Both shoulders would benefit from PBMT, but in the areas that are qualitatively seen as white (more numerous on the left than the right), they should receive a higher dosage of photonic energy. All these areas would benefit from massage while the therapy is being administered.

The Metacarpus

The metacarpal region of the forelimb hosts a variety of conditions that respond well to PBMT. These conditions can arise from injuries to the soft tissues, the boney structures, or both. Common soft-tissue injuries include dorsal metacarpal disease, inflammation of the interosseous ligament, suspensory desmitis, tendonitis, tendosynovitis, bowed tendons, and inferior check ligament desmitis. PBMT is also beneficial when applied to hard tissues in the metacarpus, such as in the case of stress fractures and postoperative care after major orthopedic surgery.

The application of laser therapy to this specific anatomical area should not only stimulate the target cells but also the surrounding tissues. This stimulation is crucial for the effective treatment of soft-tissue disorders such as injuries to either the superficial or deep digital flexor tendons.

Treatment should include administering photonic energy along the entirety of these structures, starting from just distal to the carpus and concluding proximal to the metacarpophalangeal joint. This method ensures that the energy is delivered to the entire tendon structure. Administration should be delivered both at right angles and circumferentially while the animal is bearing weight and while the carpus and fetlock are flexed. This is to ensure that the tendons are in a relaxed posture, which allows the photonic energy to penetrate deeper into the tissues. A slight passive range of motion can be accomplished by manually flexing and extending the fetlock while the carpus is in a flexed posture. This technique aids in the overall treatment process by promoting blood flow and aiding in the healing process.

Metacarpal structures, despite appearing superficial, require a higher dosage than you would logically deduct due to their thickness and fibrous nature. The extensor, flexor, and suspensory tendons are extremely thick and fibrous and warrant higher dosages on the skin to achieve therapeutic levels of photonic energy deep into the target tissues. Many of the most recent laser therapy devices on the market have better optics and emit in a way that there is no thermal buildup in the target tissues. Dosages of 12–20 J/cm^2 are warranted for consistent clinical success. There also exists various new software that optimizes energy emissions and wavelengths with no thermal buildup in the tissue. Irrespective of the equipment, it is necessary to ensure that the photonic energy reaches the deeper layers of these thick fibrous and avascular tissues, providing the necessary stimulation for healing.

Stress fractures are common within the third metacarpal bone. Dosages of 10–12 J/cm^2 (administered on-contact and treated at every angle) are efficacious. Other fractures requiring surgery are treated postoperatively with similar doses. Laser therapy can be safely applied over any orthopedic implant, such as cortical bone screws.

Consider concurrent administration of PBMT to both the corresponding acupuncture points and any secondary or compensatory areas associated with the diagnosed disorder (Table 30.5, Figure 30.8) (Fleming, 1994; Xie & Preast, 2007). Even a case of inflammation within the interosseous ligament usually has a secondary inflamed area within the shoulder areas and possibly even the opposite front limb. Treat the entire patient for consistent and optimal clinical results.

Table 30.5 Corresponding acupuncture points for the metacarpus.

Condition/disorder	Corresponding acupuncture points
Dorsal metacarpal disease	TH 1 SI 1, SI 3, SI 4, SI 9, GB 21, BL 11, BL 23, HT 8,
Interosseous ligament tear, fracture of second & fourth metacarpal	TH 1, SI 1, SI 3, LU 1, LU 10, LU 11, LI 4, LI 11, LI 15, LU 1, PC 8, GB 21, BL 11, BL 23
Suspensory desmitis; superficial and deep flexor tendons, subacute, acute and chronic bowed tendons, inferior check ligament desmitis	BL 18, BL 19, GB 34, KI 3, LV, 3, LI 4, TH 1, PC 9

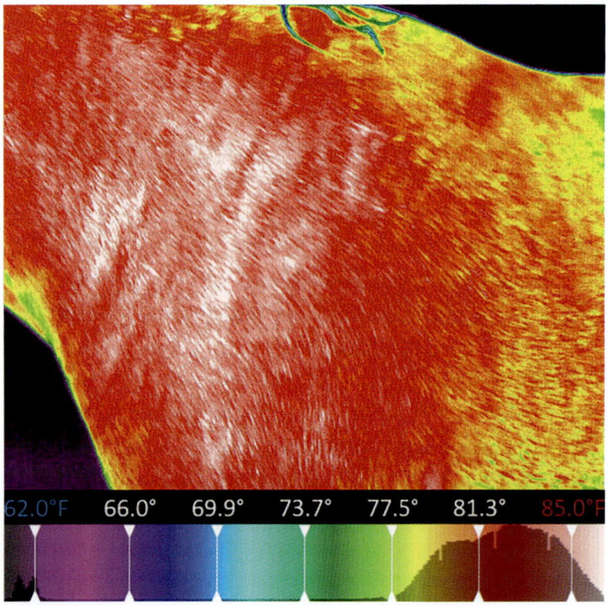

Figure 30.8 Acupuncture points and the recommended treatment area for painful disorders of the metacarpus.

The Fetlock and Pastern

The metacarpophalangeal joint, sesamoids, and the first and second distal phalanx areas are also susceptible to numerous lameness disorders that are very responsive to laser therapy. These include degenerative joint disease, sesamoiditis, fractures of the sesamoids, chronic proliferative synovitis, osslets, osteochrondosis, ringbone (all four classifications), and palmar annular ligament constriction.

Laser therapy should be administered in a circumferential manner across the entire anatomical area (Figure 30.9). The therapy session can be initiated while the patient is bearing full weight on the limb. As the patient becomes accustomed to the procedure, the foot should be lifted and the joint subjected to passive range-of-motion exercises during photonic energy administration.

The laser beam is directed internally, targeting the joint surfaces, the synovial membrane, and all areas surrounding the sesamoids. Dosages typically range from 8 to 12 J/cm^2. On-contact administration, using either a scanning method or a point-to-point method, is preferred over noncontact administration.

When treating degenerative joint disease (osteoarthritis) or osteochondrosis, the joint surfaces should be the primary target. Administer PBMT aggressively for several days and then every other day until a clinical response is observed. Laser therapy can be used as a complement to an intra-articular administration of platelet-rich plasma (PRP), hyaluronic acid (HA), or any other regenerative or anti-inflammatory intra-articular therapy. The general rule is to wait 3–7 days post-injection before initiating laser therapy. The decision on when to initiate PBMT should be made on an individual case basis.

Sesamoiditis, fractures of the sesamoid bones, and chronic proliferative synovitis, as well as most lameness disorders in this anatomical area, result from constant, repetitive, concussive force. These disorders start with an inflammatory response to this trauma. PBMT modulates this inflammatory reaction, slowing or stopping the detrimental process (Assis *et al.*, 2016). Direct the laser energy to encompass all the synovial membranes, joint capsules, surrounding ligaments, and sesamoid bones. Apply dosages of 10–12 J/cm^2 (or software with a preset protocol for inflammation) to penetrate and saturate these structures. In the acute phase, the therapy should be administered as often as possible, followed by a longer transitional phase between each therapy session

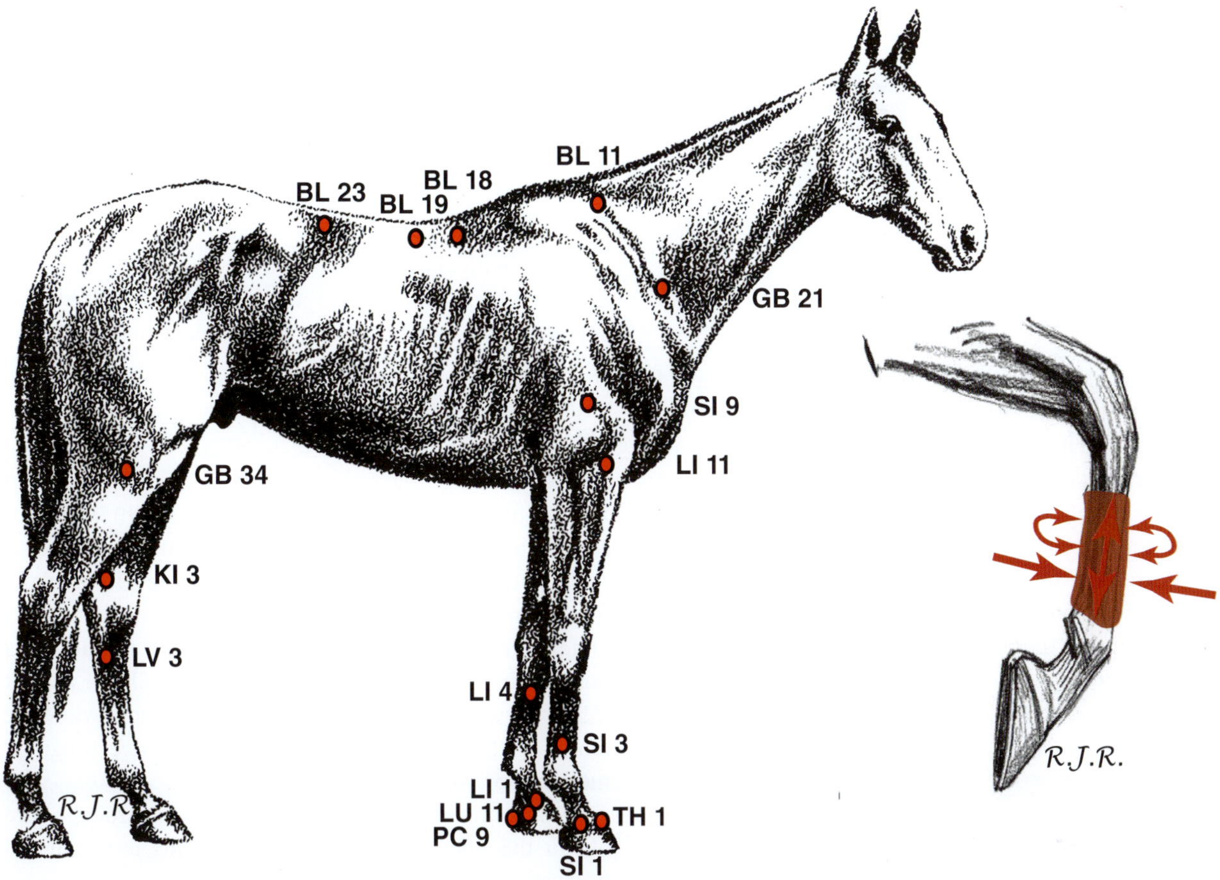

Figure 30.9 Recommended area and treatment technique for fetlock disorders.

based on the clinical response. Always ensure that the target structures are placed through passive range-of-motion during administration.

Osslets can form due to repeated impact on the metacarpophalangeal joint. This process is accompanied by joint inflammation and synovitis, leading to a condition comparable to arthritis. Over time, calcium deposits can form within the joint capsule, a condition known as ossification.

Ringbone is a similar condition where new bone growth occurs on the upper, upper-lateral, and upper-medial surfaces of the first and second phalanges and the extensor process of the third phalanx. This bone growth, like osslets, can be reduced (but will not be resolved) through PBMT.

While laser therapy can help reduce inflammation and pain associated with these conditions, it cannot halt the progression of the conditions. Therefore, it is crucial to treat these cases aggressively from the start. This includes daily administration of PBMT, followed by transitioning to a maintenance level of administration that is tailored to each patient's needs. Administer dosages directly on-contact while placing the area through passive range-of-motion exercises (Figure 30.10).

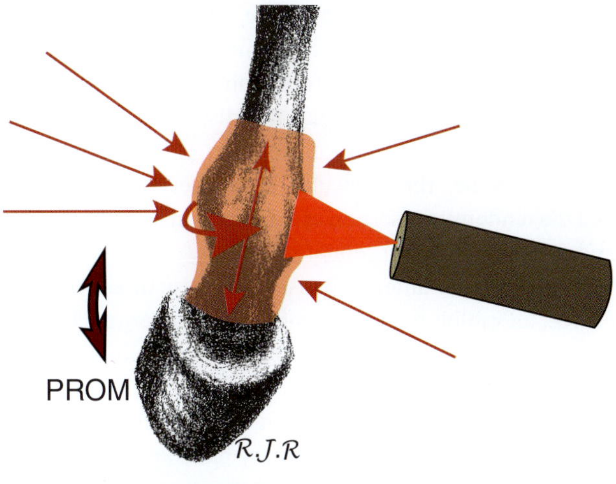

Figure 30.10 Acupuncture points for fetlock pain.

The synovial-lined joints are encircled by the strong, fibrous extensions of the fascial sheath, known as the annular ligaments. When these ligaments are strained or traumatized, they become inflamed, leading to a thickening

Table 30.6 Corresponding acupuncture points for the fetlock.

Condition/disorder	Corresponding acupuncture points
Degenerative joint disease, osslets, ringbone, sesamoinditis	BL 11, 23, 26, SI 9, LI 4, SI 3, TH 1, LI 1
Fetlock pain	LI 1, 16, BL 25, BL 23, LU 1, SI 9

and constriction of this structure. At the first clinical sign of this disorder, initiate PBMT. Once thickening occurs, PBMT can reduce inflammation and slow down this vicious cycle. It is important to provide performance-maintenance applications during both training and athletic endeavors.

After the localized treatment of the fetlock is completed, treat all corresponding acupuncture points (Table 30.6) and address any additional inflamed areas that may be compensatory arising from these fetlock disorders (Fleming, 1998; Xie & Preast, 2007).

The Hoof

The conformation or shape of the foot, with regards to the height of the heel, the length of the toe, and the overall angulation, determines which anatomical structures are accessible to the application of PBMT. The hoof is the interface between the musculoskeletal system and the ground. This structure is composed of the epidermal hoof itself (which is often pigmented), the connective tissue or dermal layer, the digital cushion, the distal phalanx, the lateral cartilages of the digital phalanx, the distal interphalangeal joint, the distal extremity of the short pastern bone, the navicular bone, the navicular bursa, several ligaments, and the tendons of insertion of the common digital extensor and deep digital flexor tendons.

All these parts differ in density and structure. To some degree, all inhibit the passage of photonic energy. The pigmented hoof wall inhibits almost 100% of the photonic energy. The efficacy of laser therapy is therefore limited to those structures that can be irradiated through the dermal areas surrounding the coronary band and throughout the heels. The higher the heel and the shorter the toe, the fewer are the targets that can receive PBMT. When considering the average foot, disorders of the following structures will respond to treatment:

- Attachment of the common digital extensor tendon.
- Insertion of the superficial digital flexor tendon.
- Portions of the deep digital flexor tendon.
- Portions of the lateral cartilage.
- Portions of the lateral and medial ligaments.
- Portions of the medial and lateral collateral ligaments.
- Portions of the "t" ligament.
- Portions of the navicular bursa.
- Portions of the navicular bone.
- Portions of the coffin joint.

Additionally, laser therapy applied to both the coronary band and corresponding acupuncture points will serve as a supplement to traditional care for both navicular syndrome and laminitis.

Techniques for the Application of Laser Therapy to the Foot

Localized treatment involves administering 8–10 J/cm^2, on-contact and using a point-to-point or scanning technique. Administer therapy from the middle of the first phalanx to the coronary band circumferentially, including the heels and pastern cavity (Figures 30.11 and 30.12). Administer a portion (approximately 30%) of the energy while the patient is bearing weight on the limb, and the remainder while the foot is picked up and placed through passive range-of-motion exercise.

PBMT influences both the vascular and neurologic supply to the hoof (Chow *et al.*, 2011). This is significant because a large number of equine foot disorders involve pain and inflammation and are accompanied by vasoconstriction. PBMT works by emitting specific wavelengths of light that interact with the cells in the hoof tissue, promoting healing, reducing inflammation, and causing vasodilation within the vasculature. Visualizing the location of these structures aids the therapist in guiding the application of PBMT, ensuring that the treatment is targeted and effective (Figure 30.13).

The neurovascular supply, which includes the digital artery, vein, and nerve, originates both medially and laterally. Specifically, arterial branches that emerge at the level of the coronet supply the perioplic and coronary dermis. Conversely, those that originate opposite the pastern joint supply branches to the digital cushion and the dermis of the caudal aspect of the hoof, including the frog. The third branch of the arterial supply arises from the dorsal and palmar terminal branches, providing blood flow to the laminella and sole. Interestingly, this is the only anatomical area where the venous supply does not correspond to the arterial supply. The venous system forms an extensive interlocking network in the dermis and underlying subcutis, continuous with the coronary band (Riegel & Hakola, 1996).

At the level of the fetlock, both the medial and lateral palmar nerves branch out in two directions, medially and laterally. These branches form the medial and lateral palmar

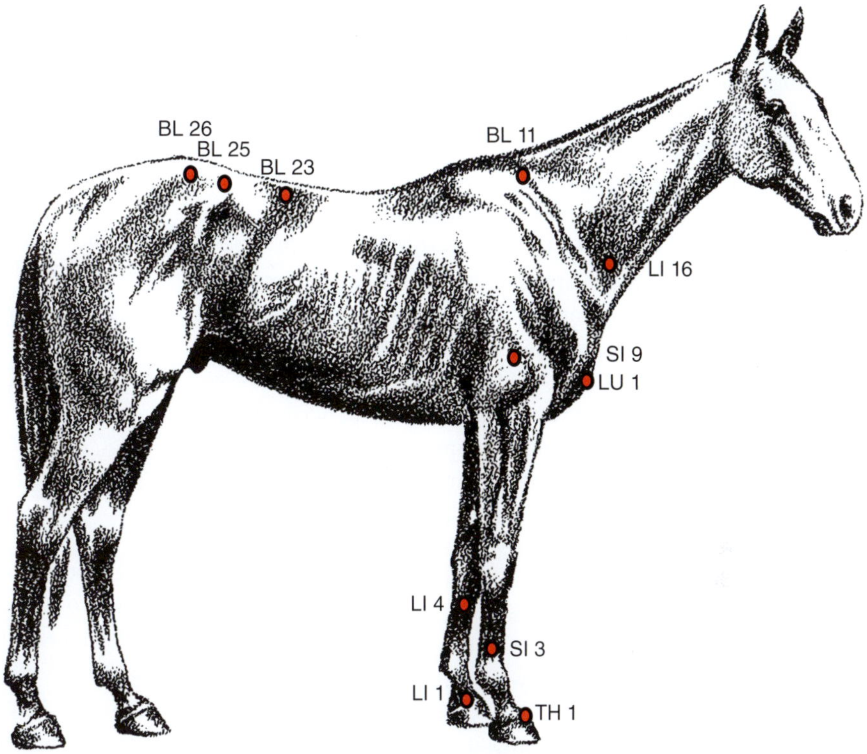

Figure 30.11 Application of PBMT to the hoof.

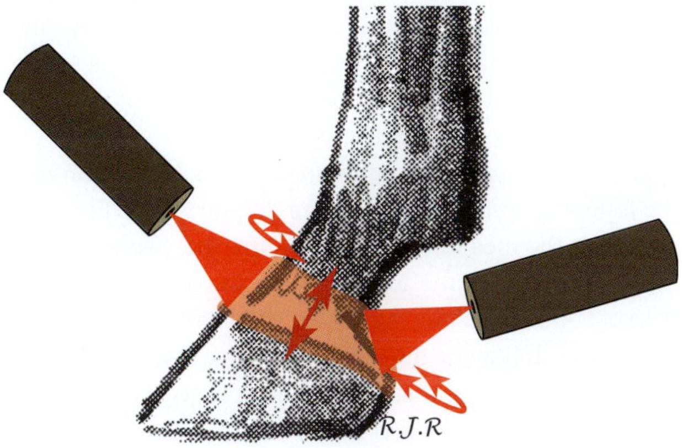

Figure 30.12 Application of PBMT to the heel.

digital nerves. As soon as these nerves form, they branch off into a dorsal division. These dorsal branches play a dual role, providing both sensory and vasomotor innervation to various structures. They innervate the skin over the fetlock, a part of the fetlock joint, the dorsal portions of the interphalangeal joints, the coronary corium, the dorsal parts of the laminar and solar coria, and the dorsal part of the cartilage of the distal phalanx.

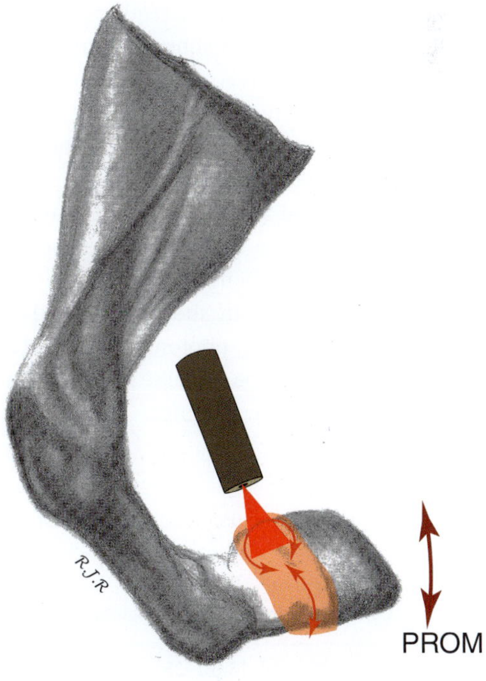

Figure 30.13 Application of PBMT throughout the coronary band.

As the palmar digital nerves continue their journey distally, they go on to innervate the palmar structures of the digit. These include the skin, the pastern joint capsule, the digital synovial sheath, the flexor tendons, the distal sesamoidean ligaments, the coffin joint capsule, the navicular bone (including its ligaments and bursa), the laminar corium, the coria of the sole and frog, and the digital cushion (Stashak, 1976). It is also worth noting that there are often branches of communication between the lateral and medial palmar nerves. These areas are crucial to consider when administering focused photonic energy.

Understanding the intricate structures of the foot, particularly its vascular and neurological components, is crucial when applying PBMT. Proper administration technique is vital for managing numerous foot disorders; laminitis, podotrochleosis, and degenerative joint conditions all benefit from the relief of pain and promotion of vasodilation (Maegawa *et al.*, 2000; Nakamura *et al.*, 2014). A therapeutic approach that utilizes these structures as a guide can therefore significantly enhance clinical outcomes. As illustrated in Figure 30.13, strategic administration of treatment can lead to improved patient care.

The use of photonic energy to stimulate acupuncture points in the foot has proven to be an effective treatment for various foot disorders. This technique offers several advantages: it is non-invasive, aseptic, requires minimal restraint, and can be completed in a short amount of time. The process involves a localized treatment where dosages of 150–200 J/point are administered on-contact (Xie & Preast, 2007). It is crucial to pay special attention to the Ting points, which are located on the coronary band (Table 30.7, Figures 30.14 and 30.15). These points are significant because they mark the beginning or end of the meridian, where energy is exchanged with the exterior (Rathgeber, 2001). Each Ting point should be stimulated separately with at least 50 J of photonic energy. This ensures that the energy exchange at these crucial points is effective and results in a clinical change.

Table 30.7 Corresponding acupuncture points for the foot.

Condition/ disorder	Corresponding acupuncture points
Hoof pain	LI 18, PC 1, BL 13, BL 25, BL 15, BL 27, BL 14, SI 9
Ting points forefoot	LI 1, HT 9, SI 1, LU 11, P 9, TH 1
Ting points hindfoot	LV 1, SP 1, BL 67, GB 44, ST 45, KI 1

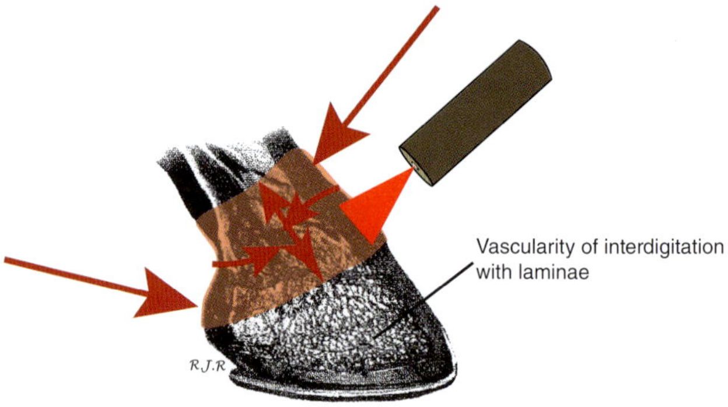

Figure 30.14 Ting points of the forefoot.

Treatment of Specific Disorders of the Foot

Foot Pain

The distal aspect of a horse's lower limb, specifically from the midpoint of the cannon bone to the sole of the foot, is characterized by a highly intricate anatomy. This complexity makes it susceptible to a wide range of injuries and disorders, ranging from prevalent conditions like laminitis and podotrochleosis to various disorders collectively referred to as "palmar foot pain." Regardless of the specific disorder, the two primary symptoms are pain and inflammation. The application of PBMT, which triggers a biochemical cascade leading to the relief of pain and modulation of inflammation in irradiated structures, therefore serves as an excellent supplemental therapy to traditional treatments for these disorders.

The relief of pain and inflammation is achieved through the following treatment technique (Figure 30.16). First palpate both the medial and lateral palmar nerves, which are located just above the fetlock. Then initiate therapy at a dose of 6–8 J/cm^2 along both the medial and the lateral palmar nerves, following the nerve pathway distally (including the dorsal branches of each) to the coronary band.

Next, treat the entire foot circumferentially along the coronary band, including the entire heel. This treatment should extend from the midpoint of the second phalanx to the coronary band. When applying the treatment, always ensure that the target tissues are anatomically considered, and focus the energy as perpendicularly as possible onto the target tissues. Finally, apply 150–180 J to each corresponding acupuncture point.

Laminitis

Despite our current advanced technology, laminitis remains something of a mystery. Regardless of the etiology, the horse's body undergoes a process known as lactic acidosis and systemic endotoxemia. This leads to an inflammatory response within the body, resulting in the release of

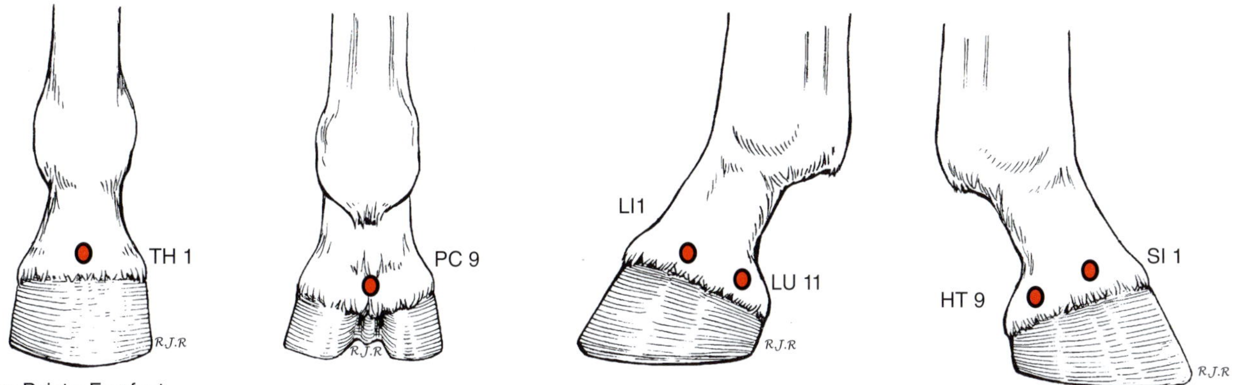

Ting Points: Forefoot

Figure 30.15 Ting points of the hindfoot.

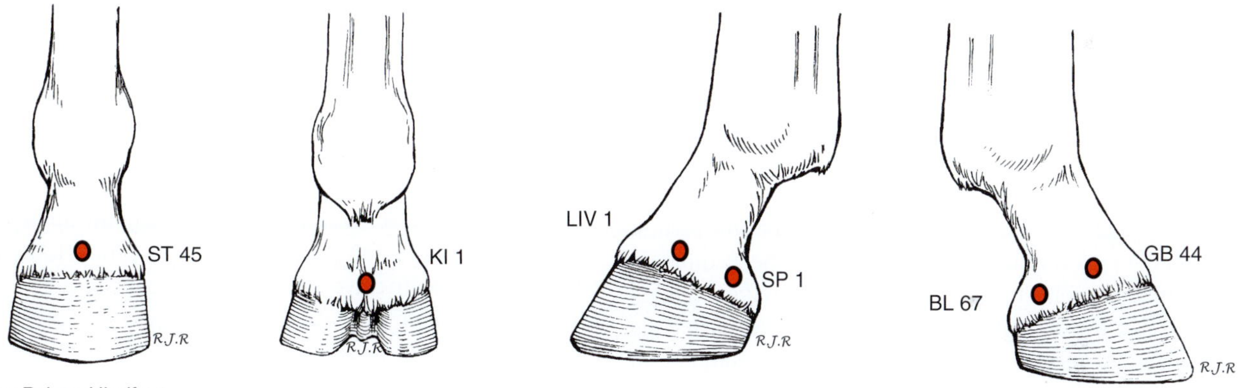

Ting Points: Hindfoot

Figure 30.16 Application of PBMT to relieve foot pain.

catecholamines, prostaglandins, histamine, serotonin, cachectin, and interleukin-1 (IL1). These inflammatory mediators have a significant impact on the foot. They initially cause an increase in arterial blood flow and systemic hypertension, which can lead to arteriovenous shunting within the microvasculature and decreased capillary perfusion within the laminae. Over time, this can result in ischemic necrosis at the laminar level (Riegel & Hakola, 1996).

Recent studies have suggested that inflammation may not be the only factor involved in the pathophysiology of laminitis. For instance, research using high-carbohydrate feeding to induce laminitis found that inflammation might not be the sole cause of the pathophysiologic change (Burns *et al.*, 2015).

Recent scientific research suggests that the lamellar attachment apparatus, a key component of the hoof structure, undergoes a deformation during the developmental phase of laminitis. This deformation begins with a compromise of the basement membrane zone, occurring when the production of certain enzymes, including metalloproteinase-9, membrane-type metalloproteinase, and aggrecanase, increases. These enzymes are responsible for breaking down key components of the lamellar suspensory apparatus (Coyne *et al.*, 2008; Loftus *et al.*, 2008; Budak *et al.*, 2009).

The level of pain experienced by laminitis patients is related to the amount of ischemic necrosis and deterioration of the lamellar attachment apparatus. This pain stimulus triggers a release of catecholamines from the adrenal glands, which in turn causes further vasoconstriction of the arteriovenous anastomoses within the laminae. This additional vasoconstriction leads to further ischemic necrosis of the laminar tissue, creating a perpetual vicious cycle that eventually allows the rotation of the distal phalanx. This is a severe complication of laminitis, which can lead to the horse's hoof becoming detached from the foot (Riegel and Hakola, 1996).

In brief, the underlying mechanism of laminitis involves inflammation, heightened production of lamellar enzymes, and pain. PBMT, serving as an adjunct to conventional

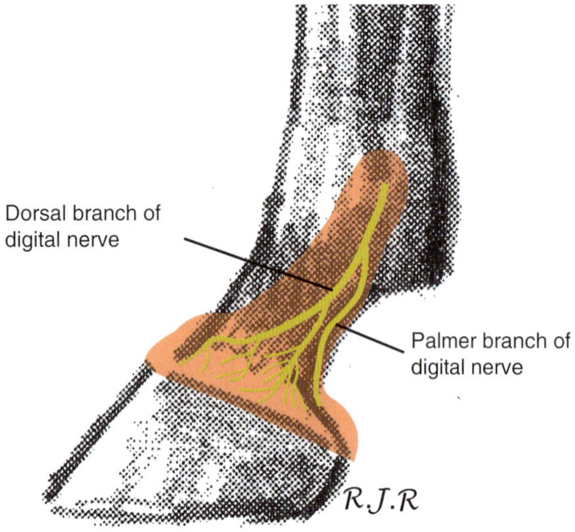

Figure 30.17 Application of PBMT to relieve laminitis pain.

treatment, offers pain relief (Enwemeka, 2009). More significantly, when applied to the coronary band, PBMT has a profound impact on the circulatory pattern of the entire foot (Maegawa *et al.*, 2000).

Administer PBMT on-contact if the patient will permit, across the region of the coronary band and heels utilizing a scanning or point-to-point technique. The recommended dose is 4–6 J/cm^2 (Figure 30.17). Concurrently, each Ting point should receive sufficient photonic stimulation. All corresponding acupuncture points should also receive laserpuncture stimulation in the range of 150–200 J (Xie & Preast, 2007). During the acute phase, this could initially be conducted twice a day, with the frequency gradually reduced as the laminitis condition improves.

Podotrochleosis

Podotrochleosis is a broad spectrum of conditions that affect the navicular bone, its bursa, and the flexor tendons. The navicular bone, also known as the distal sesamoid, is located palmar to the middle and distal phalanges and their corresponding joint space. It lies between the deep digital flexor tendon and is palmar to the distal interphalangeal joint. About 30% of its surface is covered in hyaline cartilage, forming the distal articular surface.

Early clinical signs of this disorder include an intermittent, progressive lameness that subsides with rest. Pressure applied to the middle of the frog will reveal pain in only 30–40% of the patients. Performing a phalangeal and fetlock flexion test for several minutes aggravates this condition in about 80% of the cases.

Due to the target tissues' anatomical location, it is often difficult to deliver sufficient photonic energy to elicit a clinical response. Access to these tissues is dependent on the conformation of the foot. Even with ideal conformation, only a portion of the deep digital flexor tendon, the navicular bursa, and the navicular bone will receive treatment.

In treating these cases, a multimodal approach is recommended, which includes proper shoeing, systemic medications, and PBMT. PBMT reduces local pain and inflammation commonly associated with the syndrome.

The protocol for the administration of PBMT is as follows (refer to Figure 30.18):

1) Apply 10–15 J/cm^2 on-contact in a safe manner to the entire area of the heel.
2) Place both the fetlock and the phalangeal joints through passive range of motion, while keeping the handpiece pointed perpendicular to the target tissues.
3) Treat all corresponding acupuncture points.
4) Treat aggressively for four to six therapy sessions, then reevaluate to determine when to transition to treatments spaced further apart.
5) If the treatment is successful, a program of less-frequent maintenance therapy can be initiated.

It is important to note that the response to PBMT can vary from case to case. Some cases may show a significant degree of response, while others may show very little. However, PBMT is a noninvasive procedure and can do no harm, and should therefore be considered on a case-by-case basis.

The Back (Thoracolumbar Spine)

Back disorders are one of the major causes of diminishing performance levels in equine athletes. Studies published in the United Kingdom indicate the incidence of thoracolumbar spine problems ranges from 0.9% in general practice to 94% in specialty referral practices (Anon, 1965; Jeffcoat, 1980a). The incidence of thoracolumbar problems is even higher in competitive jumpers, both show and eventing and dressage (Jeffcoat, 1980b). All these disorders manifest themselves as pain and a change in performance level.

The thoracolumbar spine is defined by those areas of the axial skeleton from the withers (T3-T7) to the lumbosacral joint (L6-S1), the bilateral sacroiliac joints, and the sacrum (S5). It includes the intervertebral disks, the overlying large thick muscles, fascia, ligamentous structures, and all their associated nervous and circulatory systems. All can cause a painful disorder (Dyce *et al.*, 2002). It is the complex nature of this large anatomical area, the variable clinical signs, and the distinctive, unique requirements for each discipline that often makes a definitive diagnosis difficult to obtain.

It is easy to visually identify and manually palpate those patients experiencing back pain and diminishing

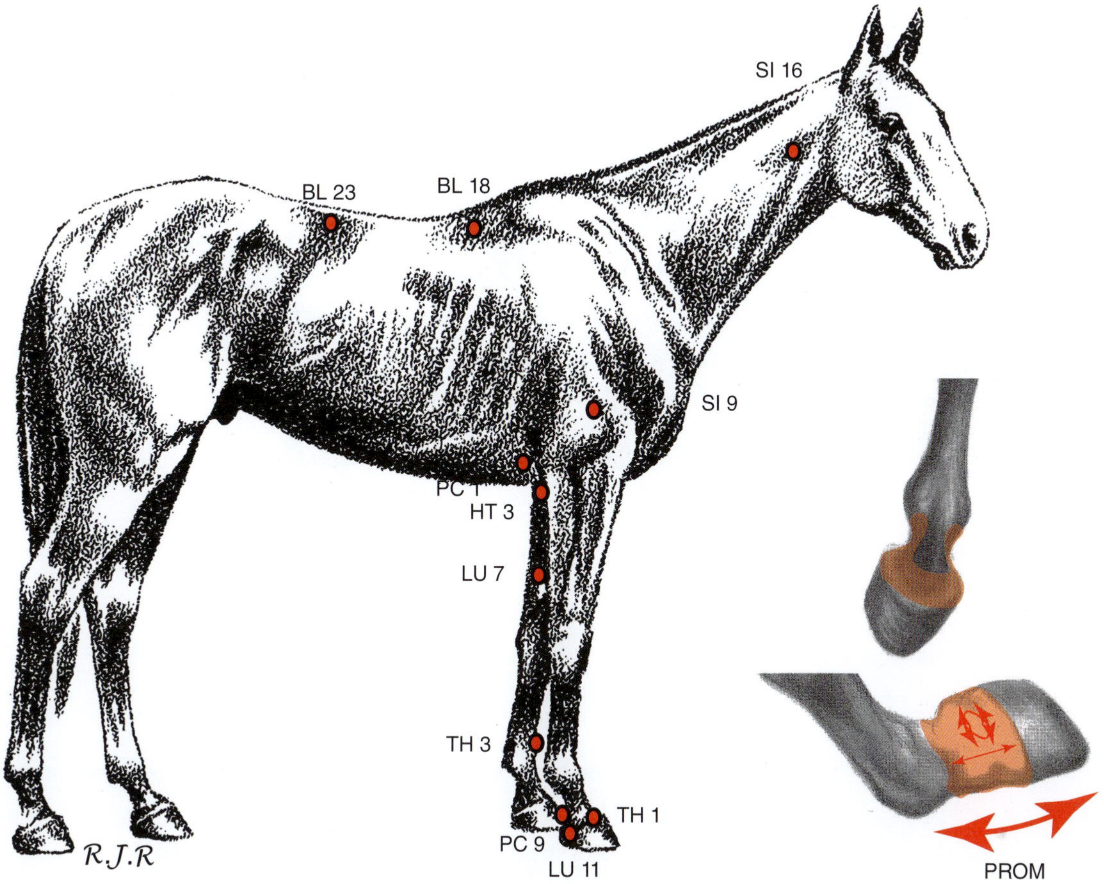

Figure 30.18 Application of PBMT to relieve pain in podotrochleosis.

performance, but exceedingly difficult to get a definitive diagnosis. Even with the use of the advanced diagnostic equipment at our disposal (digital radiography, sharper imaging ultrasounds, nuclear scintigraphy, and IRTI), it is difficult to identify and localize the exact problematic disorder or its origin. Consequently, large areas will require PBMT to achieve a clinical response.

Back pain is categorized as primary or secondary. Primary back pain is the clinical response to a direct insult to the anatomical structures, such as fractures, decompressions, subluxations, the sacroiliac joint, scoliosis, lordosis, arthritis, and myositis. There are many patients in which a combination of these etiologies occurs simultaneously. Secondary back pain is commonly a secondary or compensatory result of lower limb lameness, dental problems, poor-fitting saddles, and bits, and (more often than is admitted) poor riding technique and skill.

The goal is to identify all the areas that would benefit from therapy. Secondary back disorders will not be alleviated if the etiology is not identified and managed. Infrared thermal images can help identify all affected areas (Figure 30.19).

The crucial element in the application of PBMT to this anatomical area is the ability to deliver enough photonic energy to the skin safely to penetrate and saturate the target tissues, using a wavelength that the target chromophores can absorb. Correct dosages, the frequency of therapy, and the administration technique are all paramount to successful clinical outcomes.

Dosages of photonic energy administered to this area have increased from as low as 0.6 J/cm^2 in the late 1970s to 25–40 J/cm^2 today. Clinical results were realized when low dosages such as 5 J/cm^2 were administered. However, treatment outcomes in this anatomical area were very inconsistent. Logically, these results could have stemmed from the stimulation of the key acupuncture points that occur within this treatment area, or administration with wavelengths that did not penetrate very deeply. When laser therapy technology allowed a safe administration of higher dosages, treatment outcomes became more consistent and were achieved in less time.

PBMT should be administered to the entire thoracolumbar area from the withers to the last sacral vertebrae, including all paravertebral musculature (see Figure 30.20).

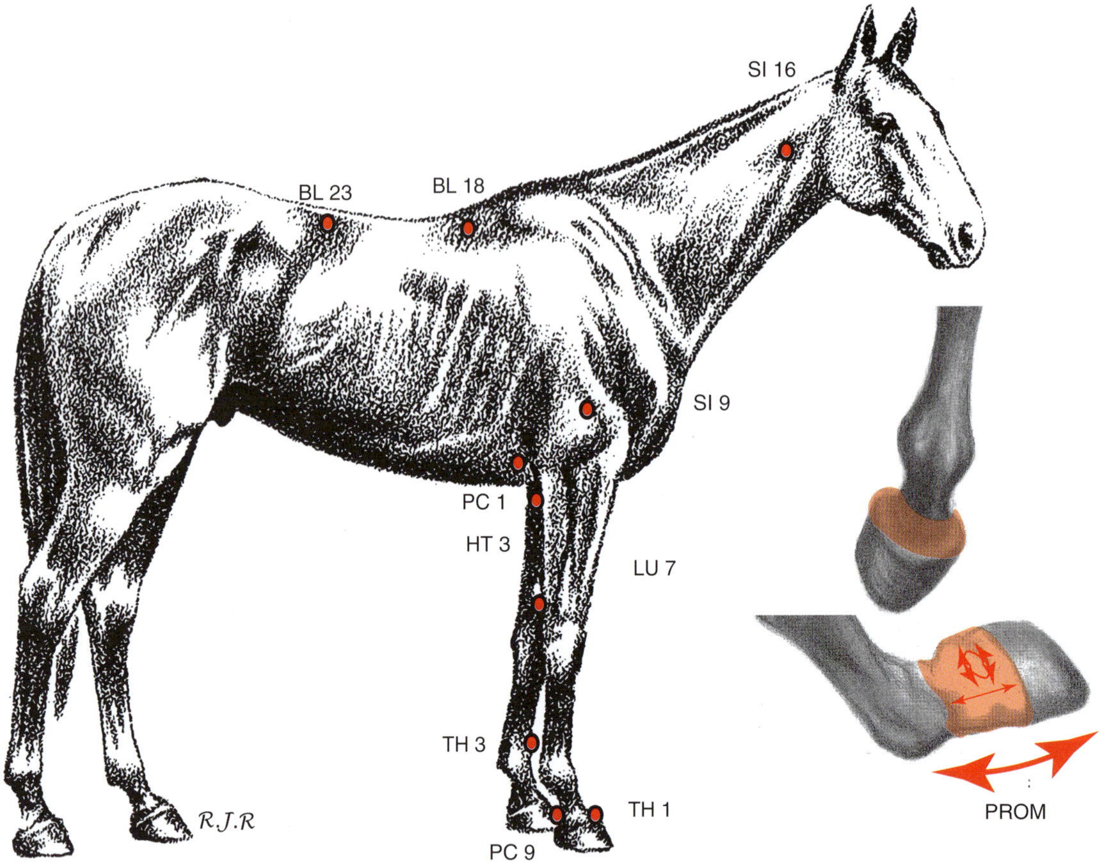

Figure 30.19 Infrared thermal image indicating areas of increased circulation on the patient's back. The areas of white and red within the ellipses. All areas of thermal asymmetry (red and white areas within the ellipses) warrant closer examination and thorough administration of PBMT.

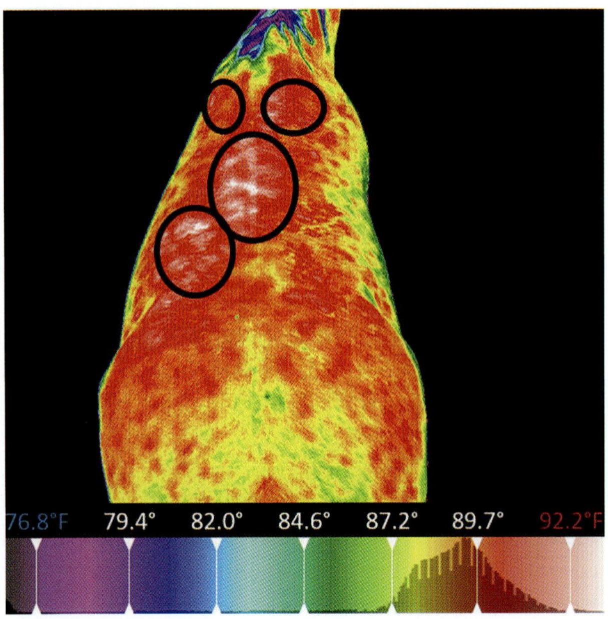

Figure 30.20 Acupuncture points and the recommended treatment area for the painful disorders of the thoracolumbar spine and surrounding musculature.

Administration of the energy should be done on-contact when possible and combined with therapeutic massage.

This combination of massage and PBMT allows a passive range of motion within the target tissues, (the muscle tissues) during administration. Additional benefits include an increase in circulation and a reduction in spasticity and tenderness within the muscles and trigger points.

Each patient should be treated to effect. Each is a unique individual and has specific physiology depending on the breed and discipline. The anatomy should be digitally palpated constantly during administration and treated until the tissues are as pain-free as possible. Frequency of administration will depend on the patient, the compliance of the client, and the amount of preparation time available before the next competitive event.

For simplicity, equine back cases are classified as either acute or chronic. When managing an acute case, administer treatment as aggressively as possible. Several daily treatment sessions are ideal, for two to four treatments, or at least every other day for the first week. When a significant clinical improvement is noted, a transition is made to less

Table 30.8 Corresponding acupuncture points for back pain.

Condition/ disorder	Corresponding acupuncture points
Back pain	Bai Hui, BL 18, BL 23, BL 25, BL 27, BL 28, BL 32, BL 40, BL 60, SI 3

frequent treatment by spacing more time between sessions. These cases are treated to resolution. Administer at least one additional treatment after the issue is resolved, and the patient should be rechecked periodically to see if a maintenance therapy regime is warranted.

Initially, chronic cases should also be managed aggressively, with therapy sessions at least every other day until clinical improvement is noted. Sessions can then be spaced further apart until the pre-established therapeutic goal is reached. The last stage is to determine a maintenance program to prevent reoccurrence or at least maintain as high a level of performance or quality of life as possible.

Acupuncture is well-established as an important part of the multimodal management of back pain in the equine (Xie *et al.*, 1997; Ridgway, 1999; Rogers, 1999). After applying therapy to all localized areas requiring it, stimulate the corresponding acupuncture points (Table 30.8, Figure 30.20) (Xie & Preast, 2007). Several of these points will be stimulated during the administration to the localized area. Check these points for sensitivity and retreat as necessary.

The Hip, Pelvis, and Upper Hind Limb

This anatomical area includes the pelvis (a part of the axial skeleton), the pelvic girdle, the coxofemoral joint, the sacroiliac joint, the femur, and all the sublumbar, cranial, lateral, and medial layers of musculature and their corresponding neurovascular supplies. It is the focal point for transferring supportive, locomotive, and propulsive forces from the hind limb to the trunk. PBMT is an excellent addendum to traditional standard-of-care treatment for many of the maladies originating here.

Historically, this area has been both a conundrum and an enigma. Injuries and lameness issues were thought to be a very uncommon finding and mostly the result of external trauma. Modern technologies in the development of digital radiography, nuclear scintigraphy, and diagnostic ultrasonography have expanded our ability to diagnose and appreciate the complexity of the disorders within this area. A prospective study, performed in Newmarket, England, over a period of 2 years, revealed 245 pelvic fractures in young racing thoroughbreds (Bathe, 1994).

The two universal clinical manifestations of all disorders within this area are pain and inflammation. Though there is still a great deal of research to be completed on the efficacy of PBMT in managing several of these disorders (e.g., sacroiliac joint injuries), there are numerous disorders that have a great deal of supportive clinical evidence for the use of PBMT. Those involving primary or secondary myositis, trochanteric bursitis, several tendon and ligament injuries, the coxofemoral joint, and fibrotic and ossifying myopathies all respond to PBMT. The technology will soon evolve to allow the safe penetration of photonic energy into deep tissue targets such as the structures surrounding the sacroiliac joint without a thermal buildup.

A physiological, biochemical cascade of events can only occur if photonic energy reaches the cellular photoreceptor cytochrome c oxidase (CCO) in the inner lining of the mitochondria (Poyton & Ball, 2011). Realization of the difficulty in efficiently delivering the energy required to produce effective photobiomodulation (PBM) within these cells requires an understanding of the light's loss of irradiance as it penetrates from the outer epidermis, through the epidermis, dermis, fat, and the very large muscle masses, to the target tissue (L. De Taboala, personal communication). Due to this loss, PBMT is commonly used in addition to both systemic and intra-articular pharmacological treatments. With a pharmacological or regenerative intra-articular administration to the coxofemoral joint, the cause of the disorder is then addressed, and PBMT can be administered to the inflamed, painful compensatory surrounding musculature and portions of the joint. The goal is always an accelerated recovery from the disorder. The stimulation of these structures will allow a holistic or multimodal approach by decreasing pain, increasing circulation, and modulating the inflammatory cycle (Bjordal *et al.*, 2006).

Dosages administered on-contact range from 20 to 40 J/cm^2. Higher doses, administered to all localized areas utilizing a massage technique, are required when treating any myositis. These areas include the psoas major and minor, the iliacus, the quadratus lumboram, the gluteals, the biceps femoris, and the semimembranosus and semitendinosus muscles.

When the patient suffers an acute injury, it should initially be treated as frequently as possible until a clinical response is recognized. Areas of inflammation within these muscles are present in all racing thoroughbreds and sport horses. A maintenance therapy program should be developed to minimize this and allow these athletes to compete pain-free at an elevated level.

Trochanteric bursitis is a localized inflammation of the bursa beneath the tendon of the middle gluteal muscle as it passes over the greater trochanter of the femur. This issue is usually a compensatory secondary result of a lameness issue within the tarsal structures. This is a common finding in standardbreds, who train many miles in the same direction on an inclined, hard-surfaced track. Administer therapy daily or at least every other day until this area is not painful upon palpation. The area can then usually be sustained pain-free with weekly maintenance therapy sessions.

The coxofemoral joint is a ball-and-socket joint capable of abduction, adduction, rotation, and circumduction movements. Even with a high dosage at an ideal wavelength, penetration to this joint is extremely limited. Doses of 35–40 J/cm^2 should be used, with the on-contact handpiece angled in all directions toward the target tissues. The benefit of PBMT in this disorder is the relief of pain and inflammation within the surrounding tissues and portions of the joint.

Fibrotic and ossifying myopathies are the result of traumatic insult to the semitendinosus, semimembranosus, biceps femoris, and gracilis muscles. These injuries are usually the result of an intramuscular injection or of the slide-to-a-stop movements frequently made in reining and rodeo events. They are very responsive to PBMT. The relief of pain and inflammation, coupled with increased circulation, allows an increased rate of cellular remodeling.

After administering localized treatment slowly at a high dose over the entire involved area, apply photonic stimulation to all complementary acupuncture points (Table 30.9, Figure 30.21) (Fleming, 1998).

Table 30.9 Corresponding acupuncture points for hip pain.

Condition/ disorder	Corresponding acupuncture points
Hip pain	Bai Hui, BL 27, BL 28, BL 35, BL 40, GB 28, GB 29, GB 30

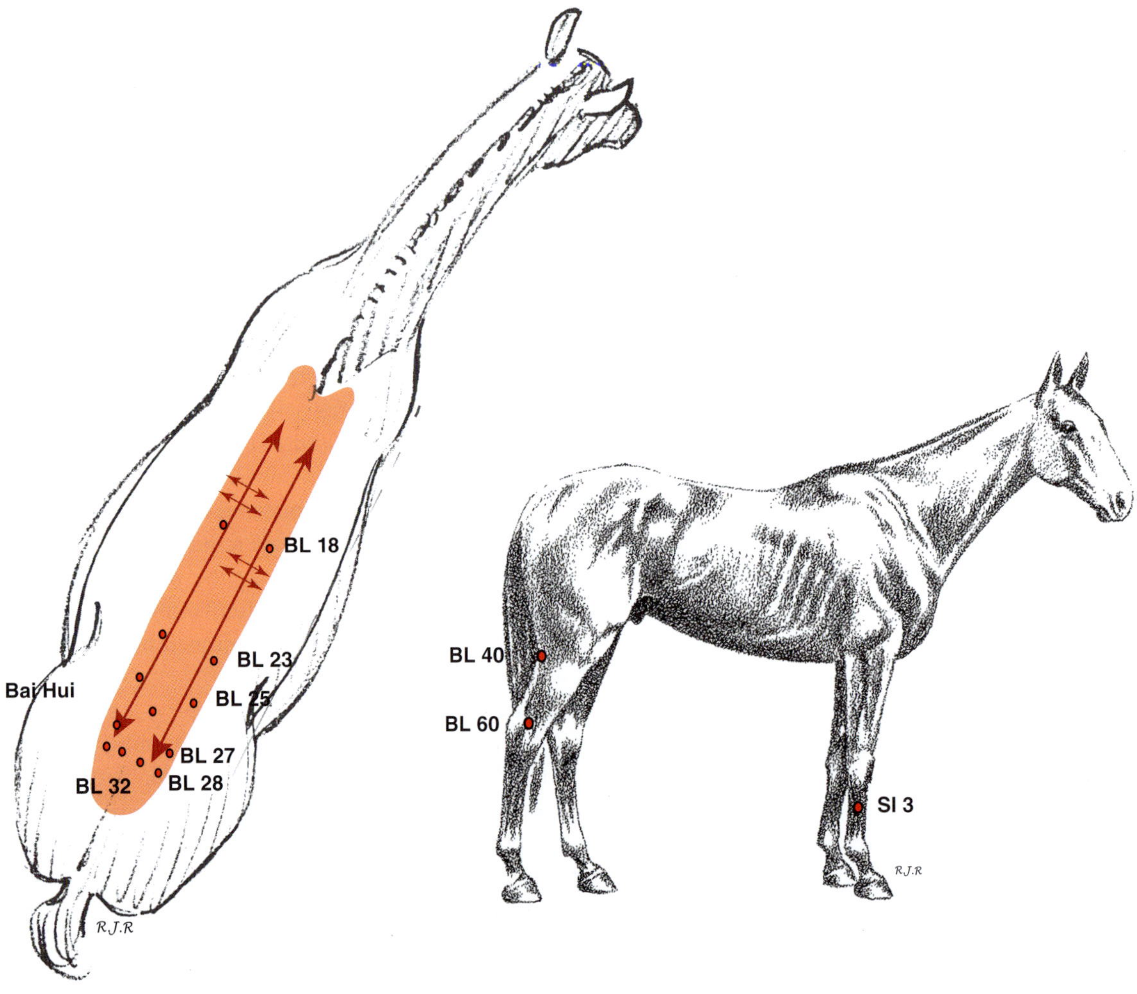

Figure 30.21 Acupuncture points and the recommended area of treatment for the painful disorders of the hip.

The Stifle

This is the largest and most intricate articulation in the equine. It consists of two joints, the femoropatellar and the femorotibial, which connect the femur, patella, and tibia, yet it contains three (sometimes communicating) synovial compartments. It is anatomically stabilized by numerous ligaments: lateral and medial femoropatellar ligaments; lateral, middle, and medial patellar ligaments; anterior and posterior cruciate ligaments; and medial and lateral collateral ligaments. The stifle joint extends through 150° range of motion, and it is often subjected to uneven stress loads during locomotion. In summary, this is the weakest joint in the horse. It is predisposed to numerous hard- and soft-tissue conditions, which result in a diminished level of performance or lameness.

Several of the lameness disorders of the stifle originate from the soft-tissue structures surrounding the joint. Numerous times, lameness is a combination of disorders within the joint itself and in the surrounding soft tissues. Both the joint and these adjacent ligaments are very responsive to PBMT. These structures are not obscured by massive amounts of muscle tissue and are therefore easier to saturate with photonic energy, but it is often not possible to reach some of the posterior anatomical areas. PBMT combined with traditional standard of care (e.g., intra-articular injection of an anti-inflammatory or regenerative substance) provides an accelerated route to recovery and return to competition.

There is a lack of double-blind scientific studies utilizing equines as the research model, yet there are an abundant number of documented clinical cases supporting a 90% efficacy rate. Scientific findings and techniques utilized in human medicine can be extrapolated to the equine athlete. An excellent example of this is a double-blind study by Ip and Fu (2015), in which they examined whether a combination of intra-articular HA injection and PBMT in addition to standard conventional physical therapy could successfully postpone the need for joint replacement surgery in elderly patients with bilateral symptomatic tricompartmental knee arthritis. They randomly divided 140 elderly patients into one of two treatment protocols. The first group received conventional physical therapy, a sham light source, and intra-articular saline. The second group received conventional physical therapy, PBMT (810 nm wavelength, 20 mW/cm^2 power density, therapy administered three times per week for 6 weeks), and an intra-articular injection of HA. Treatment failure was defined as breakthrough pain requiring joint replacement. Of the 70 subjects in the group receiving HA and PBMT, only 1 required joint replacement, compared to 15 of the 70 subjects in the control group.

One example alone is not the foundation of scientific evidence, but from January 2015 to June 2016, 16 papers were published using PBMT and the knee as the model, and all concluded efficacious results. During this time, one study was published that did not show efficacy, but it used exceptionally low dosages and the Achilles tendon as its model (de Jesus *et al.*, 2016).

Fekrazad *et al.* (2016) presented a paper on the effects of PBMT and mesenchymal stem cells on articular cartilage defects in rabbits. The results of this study showed the improvement of the control group was due to an increase in bone growth within the deficits. This study utilized 10 subjects with bone marrow-derived stem cells injected into both knees, with one knee receiving PBMT. PBMT was administered at a wavelength of 810 nm, at a dose of 4 J/cm^2, every other day for 3 weeks. Utilization of this dosage on the knee of the rabbit lends credibility to the much higher doses utilized on our equine patients since equine patients have significantly larger and more difficult-to-reach areas of target cells.

Visual identification of an upward fixation of the patella is a straightforward diagnosis. There is stress and insult to the medial patellar ligament, which results in inflammation and pain within this structure and all the surrounding tissues. Mild cases respond well to PBMT administered at 20–25 J/cm^2 on-contact for several consecutive days and then every other day as needed to re-establish normal function. If after three or four treatments there is still inflammation and pain within the medial patellar ligament, a medial patellar desmotomy should be considered. Post-procedure PBMT can then be delivered to the surgical site and surrounding tissues to accelerate healing and reduce scar formation.

Ligamentous strains and sprains of the structures surrounding the stifle joint are commonplace in competitive equine athletes. Uneven stress loads to these structures while training long and hard over unforgiving surfaces is universally unavoidable. These injuries can also result from biomechanical compensation from another primary lameness issue. Rarely do these injuries involve just one structure, so it is imperative to apply PBMT locally to the area of concern and to all adjacent structures. These are thick ligamentous bands of tissue requiring dosages of 20–30 J/cm^2, applied on-contact. It is impossible to place this area through a passive range of motion during treatment, so manual massage should be utilized during administration. Often, in the acute stage of these injuries, the patient will be experiencing enough pain to be uncooperative with on-contact treatment. This is easily resolved by treating off-contact for a period of time, or even for several treatment sessions until the analgesic effect has taken place and the patient allows contact administration. Acute cases benefit from daily or at least every-other-day therapy sessions. These are then spaced out until the case is resolved. Since the training surface seldom changes with these athletes, maintenance therapy sessions administered weekly after a hard workout will allow them to recover faster and perform at a higher level.

A considerable number of disorders occur within the stifle joint. These include capsulitis, synovitis, osteochondritis dessicans, subchondral bone cysts, and osteoarthritis. Due to the anatomical structure of this joint and its inaccessibility medially and posteriorly, it contains areas that are difficult to reach with photonic stimulation. The fluid within the joint is yet another incidental absorber for the light to penetrate. Dosages range from 20 to 40 J/cm^2 and are safely delivered on-contact, with particular attention being paid to applying them at all angles toward the target tissues. Therapy should be administered daily or at least every other day when an acute condition exists. This will continue until the resolution of the case. Chronic disorders benefit from establishing a maintenance program of at least one therapy session per week.

PBMT is a beneficial follow-up to post-intra-articular injection. Numerous combinations of intra-articular injection can be performed on this joint, so for simplicity, they will be categorized into non-regenerative (HA and cortisone) and regenerative (PRP and stem cells) types. The goal of treatment post intra-articular injection with a nonregenerative substance is to maintain the anti-inflammatory response. It is prudent to wait at least 3 days post injection before initiating a maintenance application of PBMT. This strategy allows for a greater time before repeating the injection. An added benefit is that, instead of a continuous cycle of "not-painful to painful" so that another intra-articular injection is needed, the patient is maintained with minimal pain and inflammation. This results in an animal that is more comfortable to train and a sounder competitor.

There is scientific evidence of the benefits of administering PBMT in conjunction with intra-articular regenerative therapies, but a controversy exists over when it is beneficial to apply PBMT post intra-articular injection of these regenerative substances (Ginani *et al.*, 2015). Initially, due to prudence caused by not knowing how PBMT works, it was advised that PBMT therapy not be applied for at least 90 days. The flaws with this advice are evident. There is absolutely a need for scientific studies on which to base sound recommendations for these cases, but through the time-

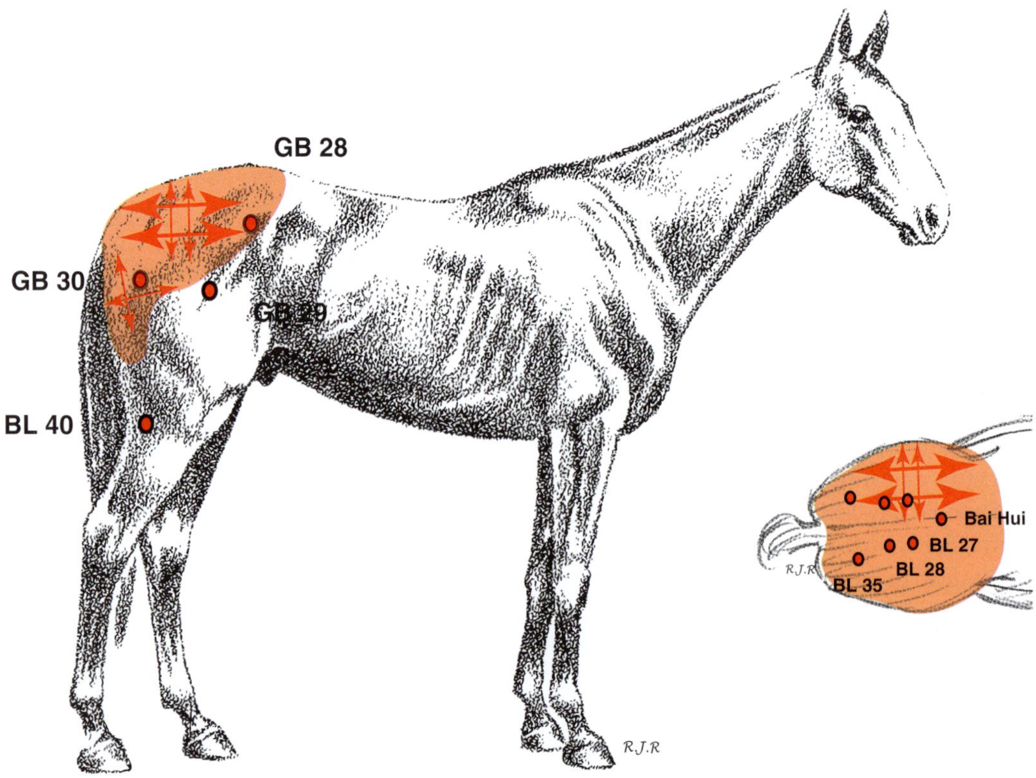

Figure 30.22 Oblique view of left stifle before the application of PBMT. Increased thermal gradients are visualized throughout the femoropatellar and femorotibial joints and surrounding tissues.

tested trial and error of daily practice, it is safe to say that administration of PBMT at least 7–10 days post-regenerative intraarticular administration is beneficial. There is some clinical evidence in the field that administering 24 hours post intra-articular injection has its benefits. This recommendation may change as more information becomes available.

Consistent clinical results are obtained when PBMT is applied to the primary and compensatory secondary areas. As in other anatomical areas, IRTI can help identify all affected areas (Figure 30.22). This thermographic image reveals increased thermal gradients (areas of hyperthermia) throughout the femoropatellar and femoraltibial joints and surrounding soft tissue structures of the left stifle (diffuse red areas and small focal white areas). PBMT was administered with a combination of an on-contact scanning technique and several point treatments over the areas identified on the image. The dosage ranged from 20 to 30 J/cm^2. All complementary acupuncture points were stimulated, as seen in Table 30.10 and Figure 30.23 (Fleming, 1998). The thermographic image in Figure 30.24 allows objective measurement and visualization of the reduction within the thermal gradients in 24 hours (red and white areas reduced). The patient also palpated less painful over most of the hyperthermic areas.

Table 30.10 Stifle pain.

Condition/ disorder	Corresponding acupuncture points
Stifle pain	Bai Hui, BL 20, BL 21, BL 27, BL 36, BL 37, BL 38, LV 8, SP 9, KI 10

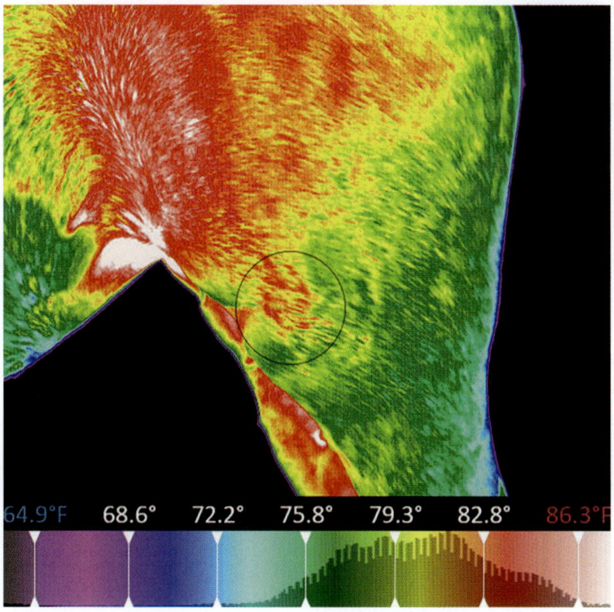

Figure 30.23 Acupuncture points and recommended area of treatment for the painful stifle disorders.

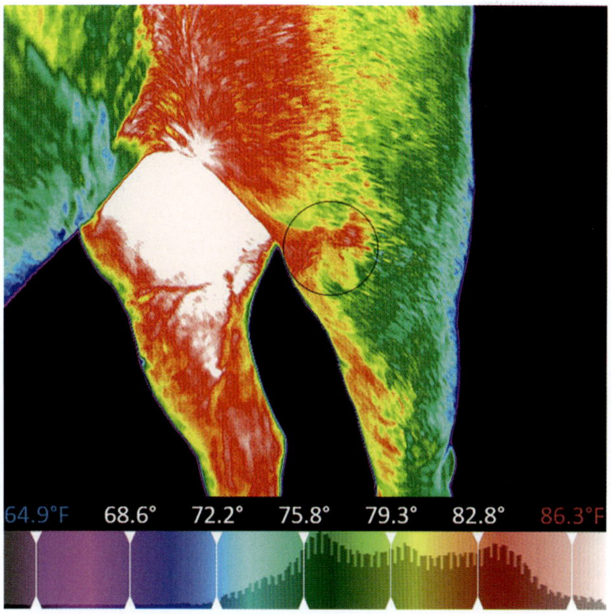

Figure 30.24 The same stifle 24 hours post PBMT treatment. The objective progress in reducing inflammation can be visualized by the reduction in the thermal gradients throughout.

Case Studies

Presentation

A 4-year-old standardbred gelding presented with a history of intermittent left rear leg lameness. Out of the previous five starts, this gelding had finished first and second twice, but in the last two races, it had tried to make a break. An intra-articular injection of HA and corticosteroid 3 weeks prior had resulted in no improvement.

Work-up

Digital palpation revealed swelling and soreness over both the medial and the lateral patellar ligaments and soreness over the medial patellar collateral ligament. The patient was 2/5 lame. Radiographs revealed only slight osseous change over the medial condyle of the femur. Ultrasound study revealed numerous areas of fluid and swelling within both the medial and the lateral patellar ligaments, with no evidence of tears. All other soft-tissue structures were within normal limits.

Diagnosis

Strain of both the medial and lateral patellar and the medial collateral patellar ligaments.

Treatment Plan

- Systemic non-steroidal anti-inflammatory administration for 10 days.
- On-contact administration of PBMT locally throughout both the medial and the lateral soft-tissue structures surrounding the left stifle joint at a dose of 25 J/cm^2 daily for 3 days, then every other day for six more treatments.
- Administration of PBMT to the left and right hip, the lumbosacral area, and the right stifle at appropriate dosages.
- Stimulation at the end of each session of the following acupuncture points with 50–150 J/point: Bai Hui, BL 20, BL 21, BL 27, BL 36, BL 37, BL 38, LIV 8, SP 9, and KI 10.
- Hand-walking for the first 3 days, then jogging for 2 mi on the regular training schedule. Training at speed and paddock turnout were restricted until a re-evaluation could be completed.

Resolution

Re-check revealed no pain or noticeable swelling upon digital palpation. The trainer stated that after the first week of therapy, the patient was sound at the jog. Then, 2 days prior to this follow-up exam, the trainer had difficulty restricting speed at the jog. The ultrasound exam revealed a resolution of the swelling and fluid previously present on both the medial and the lateral collateral patellar ligaments.

Recommendations

- Increase jogging distance and train normally in 1 week.
- Administer two more PBMT sessions, 1 in 2 days and 1 immediately after training.

Results

Training sessions went well, with no evidence of lameness. The patient was cleared to race after requalification due to time off. PBMT was administered after the qualifying race. He was trained again the following week, and PBMT was administered after he was cooled out. The patient was entered to race and had a PBMT session 2 days prior to the event. He raced at his previous level and finished third. PBMT was administered the day after the race, and the patient was hand-walked. The normal training scheduled was followed after the day off. Two more PBMT sessions were administered before a race the following week. The patient finished first and had a personal record of 3/10th of a second faster than its previous lifetime mark (the track was fast). This therapy regimen was followed for the next 5 weeks. The total purse money after initiating PBMT as part of a treatment and maintenance program was approximately $46 000. The total cost of PBMT sessions was $4,200. The horse was then sold to another owner for $80 000 and hauled to another track in another state. Over the next few weeks, the performance of the horse gradually declined after it won the first race for the new owner.

The Hock (Tarsus) and Metatarsus

The hock has three functions: it absorbs energy in the early stance phase, provides forward propulsion in the late stance phase, and raises and lowers the height of the hoof during the swing phase. Biomechanical studies, using radiopharmaceutical uptake with nuclear scintigraphy, have shown the greatest amount of compression occurs on the distal medial aspect of the tibia and the proximal lateral aspect of the third metatarsus. This suggests that the forces ascending the limb are transferred from medial to lateral through this structure (Badoux, 1987; Murray *et al.*, 2004). This area is subjected to a large amount of torque and a large compressive force. These biomechanical forces are the etiology for most of the lameness disorders that clinically transpire here.

The hock is composed of three rows of tarsal bones. The talus and calcaneus make up the proximal row. A central tarsal bone is the main component of the intermediate row, along with portions of the fused first and second tarsal bones. The third row comprises the third and fourth tarsal bones, in addition to the fused first and second tarsals. There are three metatarsal bones, and they have the same general anatomy as the corresponding metacarpal bones, with only a slight difference in angulation and length (Riegel & Hakola, 1996).

The hock joint comprises three areas of articulation: the tarsocrural, intertarsal, and tarsometatatarsal articulations. These contain four communicating synovial sacs for lubrication.

There are six common ligaments surrounding the hock joint: laterally, the long and short lateral ligaments; medially, the long and short medial ligaments; the plantar ligament on the plantar surface; and the dorsal ligament on the dorsal surface. Throughout these soft-tissue structures is a complex neurovascular supply which also supplies the remainder of the distal limb.

This complex anatomical structure, and the amount and direction of biomechanical forces ascending through it, is

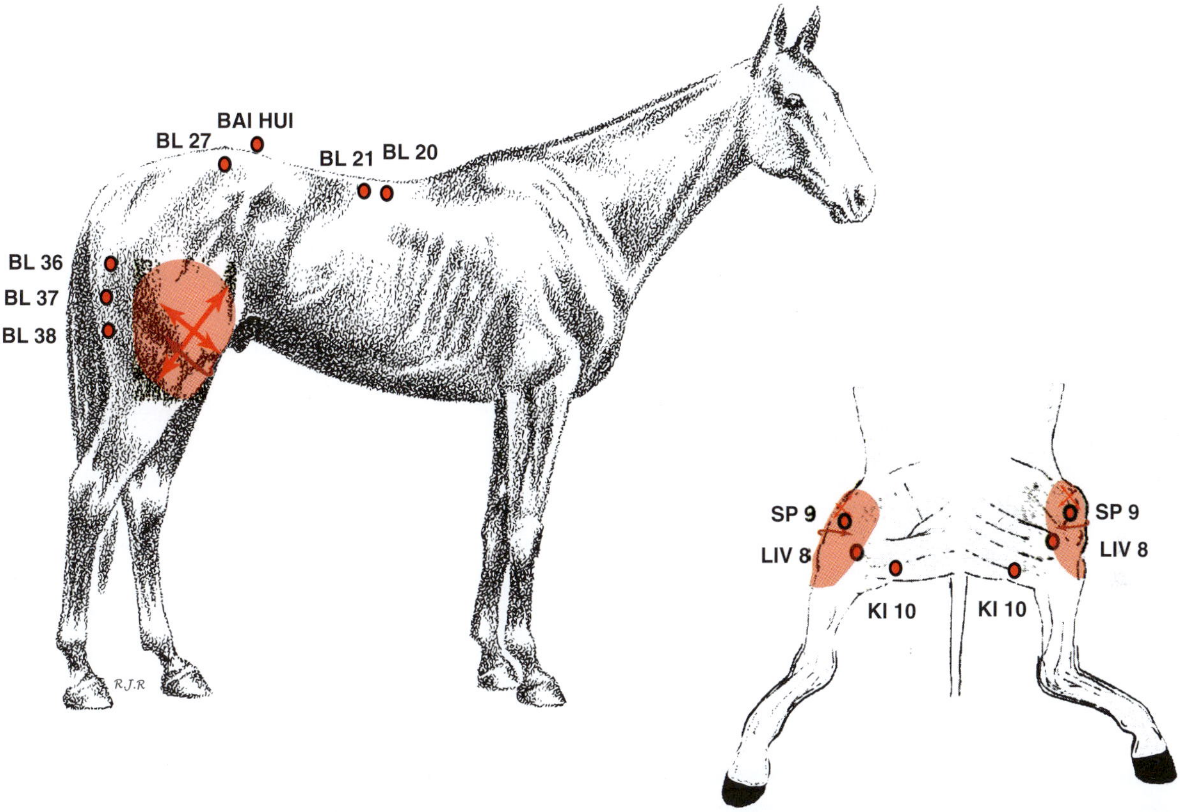

Figure 30.25 Infrared thermal image of the right tarsus. In this APMLO view, increased thermal gradients are present. These are areas of increased blood flow that correlate to inflammation and should receive further examination and special attention when applying PBMT.

often the primary source of hind-limb lameness. The structures are very superficial and are easily accessible to saturation of photonic energy (Figures 30.25 and 30.26).

Figures 30.26 and 30.27 are infrared thermal images of the tarsal and metatarsal areas. There are areas of increased thermal gradients, hyperthermia (areas of red and white) throughout both distal limbs on both images. These hyperthermic areas correlate with areas of inflammation. The identification of these areas necessitates further examination of these anatomical structures and further diagnostics. These IRTI also serve as a "roadmap" for the application of PBMT.

The disorders in this area that respond well to PBMT are synovitis, joint capsulitis, cunean bursitis, cunean tendonitis, fracture repair, bone spavin (osteoarthritis and osteitis), bog spavin (tarsocrural synovitis), and curbs (tarsal plantar desmitis), and in some cases osteochondrosis, stringhalt, and capped hocks (hygroma). These disorders can occur as a single manifestation, but normally a combination of several maladies occurs simultaneously.

Before initiating any PBMT treatment plan, establish an accurate diagnosis of the primary and all possible

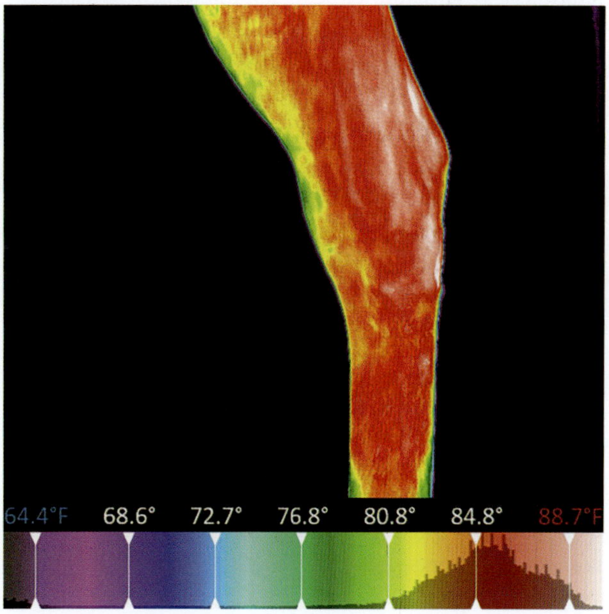

Figure 30.26 Infrared thermal image of the dorsal view of the right tarsus and an APMLO view of the left. All areas of increased thermal gradients should be examined thoroughly and receive PBMT.

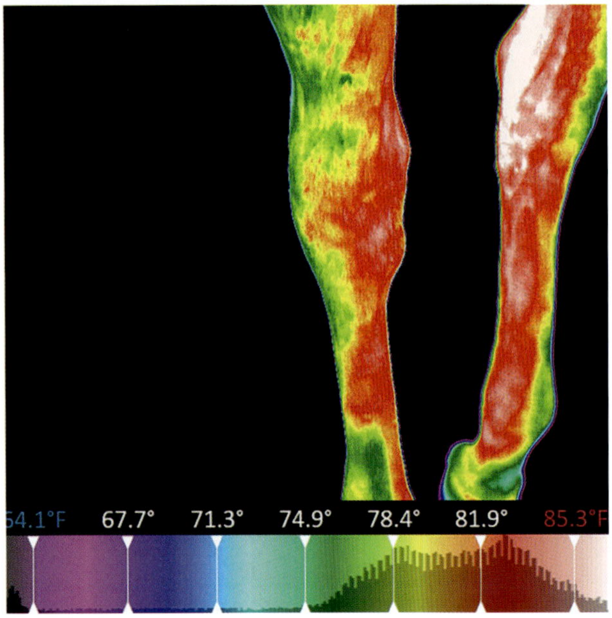

Figure 30.27 Acupuncture points and the recommended area of treatment for the painful disorders of the hock.

secondary disorders. Administer dosages in the range of 10–25 J/cm^2 on-contact utilizing either a scanning or point-to-point application technique. On-contact treatment may not be possible if the target area is too painful for the patient to tolerate even the slight contact pressure of the handpiece (e.g., acute cunean tendonitis). If this occurs, administer the therapy off-contact until the analgesic effect is initiated, which will eventually lead to an on-contact technique.

Treatment of this area is performed while the patient is weight-bearing. It is often necessary to pick up a forelimb to keep the hind limb stationary. Apply the therapy to the entire area circumferentially at all angles. It is often easier to administer therapy to the medial structures from the opposite side of the patient. Administer at least 60% of the total dose at all angles directly over the area of concern. Visualize the anatomy beneath the skin and ensure the primary area of concern and all surrounding soft tissues and joint spaces receive adequate amounts of energy.

The frequency of the therapy sessions will depend on the severity of the condition, whether it is acute or chronic, the compliance of the owner and trainer, and the schedule of competitive events. Acute cases should initially be treated very aggressively, daily or every other day, then tapered in frequency once a favorable clinical response is noted, until the therapeutic goal is reached and the issue is resolved. When managing chronic issues, the initial therapy sessions should not be as aggressive, but should be administered every other day until a therapeutic goal is reached, at which point a maintenance regime should be initiated to maintain the goal. The clinical success of the application of PBMT to any of the boney structures within this region relies on the ability of the photonic energy to reach the target. It is difficult to reach many of these structures, since it is difficult, if not impossible, to place this area through passive range of motion during administration.

Bone spavin is common in all breeds of horse, especially the Icelandic horse, where it is thought to be a heritable condition (Axelsson *et al.*, 2001). It is the most common cause of chronic hind-limb lameness. A very painful condition that is not just osteoarthritis, it also includes osteitis, synovitis, and joint capsulitis. The distal intertarsal, tarsometatarsal, and proximal intertrarsal joints can be individually involved, or the condition can occur throughout the entire joint. It often begins on the dorsolateral aspect of these joints, a region of high compression strain (Tranquille *et al.*, 2009). Therefore, even when there is no radiographic evidence of change, ensure that these areas receive a saturating dose of photonic energy from every angle.

Osteochondrosis is a condition in which the cartilage at the end of the long bones fails to develop normally. If this condition results in a fragment of the cartilage being displaced, it is defined as osteochondritis dissecans. Wittwer *et al.* (2006) published a study examining 167 South German coldbloods, with a mean age of 14 months. They found an incidence of 61.7% of osteochondrotic lesions in the fetlock or hock joints and 26.9% of osseus fragments. Lesions in racing thoroughbreds and standardbreds are usually seen by age 2, but in warmbloods (which are older when they begin training), clinical signs may not manifest until 5–6 years of age.

The success of treatment of osteochondrosis with PBMT is contingent upon the location of the lesion. When the lesion can be fully saturated with photonic energy, the clinical results of utilizing PBMT in conjunction with traditional care (both systemic and intra-articular) are very consistent. When the lesion is inaccessible to light energy, the clinical results will be the same as if the patient were solely on a traditional therapeutic regime. Even though these lesions seem very superficial, they are covered by the skin, fibrous soft-tissue structures, and synovial fluid. Therefore, administer dosages of 25–30 J/cm^2 on-contact, not only directly over the lesion but also over all surrounding tissues and joint spaces. Therapy should be administered as often as possible, with at least 12 treatments over 30 days, until a follow-up radiographic exam can determine the progress of the case. PBMT should be administered in combination with systemic and intra-articular therapy such as PRP. If intra-articular PRP is administered, the first therapy session should be at least several days post-injection.

Soft-tissue disorders, tendonitis, desmitis, and any inflammation within the associated bursa respond well to PBMT. These structures usually lie just beneath the dermis and are readily accessible to photonic stimulation. Administer dosages of 15–20 J/cm^2 on-contact from the origin to the insertion. Include the bursa sac beneath, the surrounding soft tissues, and the underlying joint. In all cases, the general rule is to treat the entire hock circumferentially, with a high percentage of the energy administered directly to the primary and any secondary structures that may also be involved.

Acute tendonitis/desmitis will often respond after the first PBMT session. After the first treatment, it is not unusual for the patient to appear unsound on the opposite hind limb. These conditions are often bilateral, with one limb being more painful than the other. This transformation is not as distinct as a nerve block to the area, but it is visible in most of the patients. With the hock being the primary cause of lameness, there will always be compensatory areas that would benefit from therapy. Ideally, treatment should be administered to both hocks, stifles, hips, and the lumbosacral areas. Treat as aggressively as possible, daily or every other day for three or four sessions, then less frequently once a clinical response is noted until the treatment goal is reached. These acute cases will often require a maintenance treatment plan to avoid reoccurrence. The maintenance plan will be unique to each patient, depending upon the disciple and the compliance of the client, owner, and trainer, and will be partially determined by the athlete's competition schedule.

The goal when treating a chronic case of tendonitis/desmitis is to maintain the soundness of the animal throughout the competitive season. These cases have a history of systemic and localized pharmaceutical treatment. PBMT sessions should be tailored to each athlete's schedule. Initially, treat aggressively, and then maintain performance at the highest level possible.

The literature states that PBMT plays a protective role in the degradation of cartilage and synovitis in rabbits with progressive osteoarthritis (Wang *et al.*, 2014b). Inflammation of the synovial membrane and joint capsule can be caused by direct injury to the joint, constant concussive force resulting from poor conformation, or most disorders within the hock (tarsocrural synovitis, commonly referred to as "bog spavin," is a good example). Treat these conditions early and aggressively with a dose of 10–15 J/cm^2 on-contact.

Table 30.11 Acupuncture points for hock pain.

Condition/disorder	Corresponding acupuncture points
Hock pain	BL 18, BL 19, BL 23, BL 35, BL 39, BL 60, BL 62, ST 45, LV 4

Stimulation of the complementary acupuncture points with PBMT should be accomplished after all localized therapy has been administered. Administer 120–150 J/point to the points listed in Table 30.11 and illustrated in Figure 30.27 (Fleming, 1998).

Conclusion

PBMT provides an excellent therapeutic option for a variety of equine disorders. The biochemical cascade of events that occurs upon stimulation, results in an alleviation of pain, a modulation of the inflammatory cycle, and an increase in circulation. When administered at the correct dosage, utilizing a good application technique, with a sufficient number of treatments, PBMT will accelerate the healing process, allowing a faster return to competition and improved quality of life. PBMT has become an integral part of our standard of care for equine patients and should be considered and included in most treatment plans.

References

Anders, J.J. *et al.* (2004). Phototherapy promotes regeneration and functional recovery of injured peripheral nerve. *Neurol Res.* 26(2):233–239.

Anon (1965). British Equine Veterinary Association survey of equine disease 1962–1963. *Vet Rec.* 77:528.

Assis, L. *et al.* (2016). Aerobic exercise training and low-level laser therapy modulate inflammatory response and degenerative process in an experimental model of knee osteoarthritis in rats. *Osteoarthr Cartil.* 24(1):169–177.

Axelsson, M. *et al.* (2001). Risk factors associated with hindlimb lameness and degenerative joint disease in the distal tarsus of Icelandic horses. *Equine Vet J.* 33(1):84–90.

Ayyildiz, S. *et al.* (2015). Evaluation of low-level laser therapy in TMD patients. *Case Rep Dent.* 2015:424213.

Badoux, D. (1987). Some biomechanical aspects of the structure of the equine tarsus. *Anat Anz.* 64(1):53–61.

Bathe, A.P. (1994). 245 fractures in thoroughbred racehorses: results of a 2-year prospective study. *Proc Am Assoc Equine Pract.* 40:175–178.

Bjordal, J.M. *et al.* (2006). Low-level laser therapy in acute pain: a systematic review of mechanisms of action and clinical effects in randomized placebo-controlled trials. *Photomed Laser Surg.* 24(2):158–168.

Budak, M.T. *et al.* (2009). Gene expression in the lamellar dermis-epidermis during the developmental phase of carbohydrate overload-induced laminitis in the horse. *Vet Immunol Immunopathol.* 131(1–2):86–96.

Burns, T.A. *et al.* (2015). Laminar inflammatory events in lean and obese ponies subjected to high carbohydrate feeding: implications for pasture-associated laminitis. *Equine Vet J.* 47(4):489–493.

Calisto, F.C. *et al.* (2015). Use of low-power laser to assist the healing of traumatic wounds. *Acta Cir Bras.* 30(3):204–208.

Chang, W. *et al.* (2014). Therapeutic outcomes of low-level laser therapy for closed bone fracture in the human wrist and hand. *Photomed Laser Surg.* 32(4):212–218.

Chow, R. *et al.* (2011). Inhibitory effects of laser irradiation on peripheral mammalian nerves and relevance to analgesic effects: a systematic review. *Photomed Laser Surg.* 29(6):365–381.

Coyne, M.J. *et al.* (2008). Cloning and expression of ADAM-related metalloproteases in equine laminitis. *Vet Immunol Immunopathol.* 129(3–4):231–241.

Dyce, K.M. *et al.* (2002). The neck, back, and vertebral column of the horse. In: *Textbook of Veterinary Anatomy*, 3 edn, pp. 598–624. Saunders, Philadelphia, PA.

Enwemeka, C.S. (2009). Intricacies of dose in laser phototherapy for tissue repair and pain relief. *Photomed Laser Surg.* 27(3):387–393.

Fekrazad, R. *et al.* (2016). Effects of photobiomodulationand mesenchymal stem cells on articular cartilage defects in a rabbit model. *Photomed Laser Surg.* 34(11):543–549.

Fleming, P. (1994). Acupuncture treatment for musculoskeletal and neurological conditions in horses. In: *Veterinary Acupuncture: Ancient Art to Modern Medicine*, pp. 183–194. Mosby, Maryland Heights, MO.

Fleming, P. (1998). Equine acupuncture. In: *Complementary and Alternative Veterinary Medicine*, 1 edn, p. 182. Mosby, Maryland Heights, MO.

Ginani, F. *et al.* (2015). Effect of low-level laser therapy on mesenchymal stem cell proliferation: a systemic review. *Lasers Med Sci.* 30(8):2189–2194.

Ip, D. and Fu, N.Y. (2015). Can combined use of low-level lasers and hyaluronic acid injections prolong the longevity of degenerative knee joints? *Clin Interv Aging.* 10:1255–1258.

Jang, H. and Lee, H. (2012). Meta-analysis of pain relief effects by laser irradiation on joint areas. *Photomed Laser Surg.* 30(8):405–417.

Jeffcoat, L.B. (1980a). Disorders of the thoracolumbar spine of the horse – a survey of 443 cases. *Equine Vet J.* 12(4):197–210.

Jeffcoat, L.B. (1980b). Guidelines for the diagnosis and treatment of back problems in horses. *Proceedings of the 26th Annual Conference of the American Association of Equine Practitioners.* November 30–December 3, 2016. Anaheim, CA.

de Jesus, J.F. *et al.* (2016). Low-level laser therapy (780nm) on VEGF modulation at partially injured Achilles tendon. *Photomed Laser Surg.* 34(8):331–335.

Kazem, S.S. *et al.* (2010). Effect of low-level laser therapy on the fracture healing process. *Lasers Med Sci.* 25(1):73–77.

Lemos, G.A. *et al.* (2016). Low-level laser stimulates tissue repair and reduces the extracellular matrix degradation in rats with induced arthritis in the temporomandibular joint. *Lasers Med Sci.* 31(6):1051–1059.

Levine, D. *et al.* (2015). Effects of laser on endurance of the rotator cuff muscles. *Lasers Surg Med.* 47(S26):44–45.

Loftus, J.P. *et al.* (2008). Leukocyte-derived and endogenous matrix metalloproteinases in the lamellae of horses with naturally acquired and experimentally induced laminitis. *Vet Immunol Immunopathol.* 129(3–4):221–230.

Machado, B.C. *et al.* (2016). Effects of oral motor exercises and laser therapy on chronic temporomandibular disorders: a randomized study with follow-up. *Lasers Med Sci.* 31(5):945–954.

Maegawa, Y. *et al.* (2000). Effects of near-infrared low-level laser irradiation on microcirculation. *Lasers Surg Med.* 27(5):427–437.

Murray, R.M. *et al.* (2004). Nuclear scintigraphic evaluation of the distal tarsal region in normal horses. *Vet Radiol Ultrasound.* 45(4):345–351.

Nakamura, T. *et al.* (2014). Low level laser therapy for chronic knee joint pain patients. *Laser Ther.* 23(4):273–277.

Poyton, R.O. and Ball, K.A. (2011). Therapeutic photobiomodulation: nitric oxide and a novel function of mitochondrial cytochrome c oxidase. *Discov Med.* 11(57):154–159.

Rathgeber, R. (2001). Chapter 4). *Understanding Equine Acupuncture*, 1 edn, pp. 36–37. The Blood-Horse, Inc., Lexington, KY.

Ridgway, K. (1999). Acupuncture as a treatment modality for back problems. *Vet Clin North Am Equine Pract.* 15(1):211–221.

Riegel, R.J. and Hakola, S. (1996). *Illustrated Atlas of Clinical Equine Anatomy and Common Disorders of the Horse*, 1 edn, pp. 26–40. Primedia Equine Network, Kennett Square, PA.

Rogers, P. (1999). Treatment of back pain in the horse and dog by acupuncture. 1st Spanish Inter-University Meeting of Acupuncture and 3rd European Meeting of Acupuncture. Zaragoza, Spain.

Stashak, T.S. (1976). *Adam's Lameness in Horses*, 3 edn, pp. 15–18. Lea and Febiger, Philadelphia, PA.

Sutherland, E. *et al.* (1994). Cross reference of equine acupuncture points. In: *Veterinary Acupuncture: Ancient Art to Modern Medicine*. Mosby, Maryland Heights, MO.

Tranquille, C. *et al.* (2009). Effect of exercise on thickness of mature hyaline cartilage, calcified cartilage and subchondral bone thickness of equine tarsi. *Am J Vet Res*. 70 (12):1477–1483.

Wang, C.Z. *et al.* (2014a). Low-level laser irradiation improves functional recovery and nerve regeneration in sciatic nerve crush rat injury model. *PLoS One*. 9(8):e103348.

Wang, P. *et al.* (2014b). Effects of low-level laser therapy on joint pain, synovitis, anabolic, and catabolic factors in a progressive osteoarthritis rabbit model. *Lasers Med Sci*. 29(6):1875–1885.

Wittwer, C. *et al.* (2006). Prevalence of osteochondrosis in the limb joints of south German coldblood horses. *J Vet Med A Physiol Pathol Clin Med*. 53(10):531–539.

Xie, H. and Preast, V. (2007). *Xie's Veterinary Acupuncture*, 1 edn, p. 254. Blackwell Publishing, Hoboken, NJ.

Xie, H. *et al.* (1997). Equine back pain: a traditional Chinese medical review. *Equine Pract*. 19:2–11.

31

Laserpuncture for the Equine Patient

Ronald J. Riegel

American Institute of Medical Laser Applications, Marysville, OH, USA

Introduction

The use of photonic energy to stimulate acupuncture points was first developed in China and Russia, and initially applied clinically by Plog in 1973 (Plog, 1980; Jang *et al.*, 2019). The use of lasers to stimulate acupuncture points is termed "laser acupuncture" or "laserpuncture" (Lorenzini *et al.*, 2010). It harnesses the therapeutic benefits of traditional needle acupuncture and photobiomodulation therapy (Litscher, 2018). One of the key advantages of laserpuncture is its ability to provide a needle-free, painless, noninvasive alternative to conventional acupuncture. This method is also free from complications and can be performed swiftly with minimal patient restraint, making it a preferred choice for many patients with needle phobia (Martin & Klide, 1987; Schoen & Wynn, 1998).

Traditionally, an acupuncturist inserts an ultrathin metal needle into a specific acupuncture point. The needle can then be manually stimulated by gently twisting or moving it up and down. Several theories have been proposed to explain the mechanism of action, including the gate-control theory of pain and the endorphin-and-neurotransmitter model (Chow & Lee, 2013). Chow and Lee suggested that the stimulation from the metal needle alters the transmission of pain signals and modulates the release of endogenous endorphins and neurotransmitters, leading to physiological changes.

Laserpuncture is a noninvasive procedure that does not physically pierce the skin. Instead of the mechanical stimulation provided by traditional needle therapy, laser acupuncture irradiates acupoints and triggers physiological responses at the cellular level (Law *et al.*, 2015). The exact mechanism through which nonthermal, low-intensity laser irradiation stimulates acupoints is yet to be fully understood. It is plausible that the process of laserpuncture operates differently compared to our current comprehension of acupuncture. The prevailing theories propose that laserpuncture operates by modulating inflammation, alleviating pain, and enhancing circulation. This is achieved when the appropriate irradiation parameters are employed (Chung *et al.*, 2012).

The physiological response to laserpuncture can vary significantly. This is due to the diverse anatomical structures of the skin, including its color, thickness, and the density of the underlying tissues. These factors present challenging optical properties that can affect the scattering and absorption of light as it penetrates the skin (Whittaker, 2004). Moreover, the power output of the laser, how the energy is emitted, and the dosage of energy also play a crucial role in determining the level of light penetration and scattering. For laserpuncture, visible red light and infrared radiation (625–1000 nm) are commonly used (Wan *et al.*, 1981; Anderson & Parrish, 1981).

Applying photonic energy for tissue stimulation at the average depth of a needle acupuncture point necessitates an energy dose of 80–200 J/point. Deeper points, those surrounded by substantial muscle masses and bone, mandate a higher energy dose of 125–225 J/point (Fuchtenbusch & Rosin, 2006). The administration of laser acupuncture should be carried out deliberately, employing a low power setting of 0.5 W or less, and utilizing either a pulsed or a combination of pulsed and super-pulsed emission modes. The selection of wavelengths within the therapeutic window is crucial to ensure efficacy.

Laser therapy software often comes equipped with preconfigured protocols. These protocols guide the application of photonic energy to stimulate specific acupuncture points. Each setting dictates the use of particular wavelengths, power output (wattage), and the duration of application (time) necessary to activate each acupoint individually. While these presets serve as a foundational starting point, they can be customized to cater to the unique needs of each patient. Moreover, the software may also feature preconfigured settings intended to either stimulate or sedate an acupoint, providing a tailored approach to treatment.

Laser Therapy in Veterinary Medicine: Photobiomodulation, Second Edition. Edited by Christopher J. Winkler and Lisa A. Miller.

Laser therapy equipment typically includes interchangeable photoprobes or handpieces designed to administer photonic energy to acupoints. These probes are crafted from nontoxic, polished optical glass, which ensures easy cleaning. The optical properties of either the handpiece or the photoprobe facilitate the delivery of a safe and optimal power density when they are applied directly on-contact to the acupuncture point.

Despite a substantial decrease in photonic energy as the laser beam traverses from superficial to deeper tissue, the stimulatory effect remains potent enough to irradiate even the most challenging acupuncture points. For optimal penetration, it is advisable to apply the laser treatment directly on the skin using the appropriate acupuncture handpiece or photoprobe. This can be done either by keeping the handpiece or probe stationary, or by gently massaging the skin with them in a circular motion while applying a light pressure.

Laser acupuncture is best utilized as a component of a comprehensive wholistic (treatment of the entire patient) laser treatment plan. Implementation of laserpuncture can significantly enhance rehabilitation protocols by offering pain relief and promoting increased circulation within the muscular tissues (Le Jeune *et al.,* 2016). If it is the only therapy, its frequency of application will depend on the severity of the disorder and the client's compliance to the treatment schedule. A recommended schedule is twice-weekly treatments until the therapeutic objective is achieved.

In a 2015 study, a meta-analysis of human research on laser acupuncture for treating musculoskeletal pain was conducted. Among the well-designed studies where appropriate doses were administered twice weekly, two-thirds reported consistent positive clinical outcomes after long-term follow-up, as opposed to immediately after treatment (Law *et al.,* 2015).

Anatomical Location of Equine Acupuncture Points Using Western Nomenclature

All acupuncture point location descriptions in this chapter are given according to the International Veterinary Acupuncture Society (IVAS) (www.ivas.org) unless otherwise indicated. For graphical diagrams of many of these points, refer to the tables and figures in Chapters 29 and 30. Additional information about equine acupuncture points is available in Riegel and Hakola (1996), Fleming (1998), Fuchtenbusch and Rosin (2006), Xie and Preast (2007), and Bessent (2011).

In the Western nomenclature system, each point receives a unique combination of letters and numbers to create its name. The prefix, composed of letters, is an abbreviation of the meridian on which the point lies. The numeric suffix represents the sequential position of the point on the meridian. For example, there are 67 points on the Bladder Meridian (BL). BL 1 would be the first point on this meridian, and BL 67 would be the last. The term "cun" describes a unit of measure relative or proportionate to an individual body. A distance of 1 cun equals the width of an individual horse's 18th (last) rib. Many practitioners often use their own fingers to gauge cun measurements: 1 cun is approximately equal to the width of the index and middle fingers, or about 3 cm (1.18 in.), while 2 cun is the width of four fingers (a hand), or about 6 cm.

Heart Meridian

HT 7

The superficial location is in the depression on the medial surface of the radius, just cranial to the cranial border of the flexor carpi ulnaris muscle, at the level of the dorsal aspect of the accessory carpal bone.

Deeper, there is a location between the flexor carpi ulnaris and the superficial digital flexor muscle.

HT 8

On the caudolateral aspect of the third metacarpal, half the distance from the carpus to the fetlock, just cranial to the deep digital flexor tendon.

HT 9

On the palmarolateral aspect of the front foot, in the depression just proximal to the coronary band, approximately two-thirds of the distance from the dorsal midline of the coronary band to the palmar border of the lateral bulb of the heel.

Pericardium Meridian

PC 7

In the depression, just cranial to the cranial border of the chestnut, midway between the proximal and distal ends of the chestnut.

PC 8

On the fore limb, half the distance from the carpus to the fetlock, on the caudal aspect of the superficial digital flexor tendon.

PC 9

On the palmar midline of the front foot, in the depression between the bulbs of the heel.

Lung Meridian

LU 1
In the depression in the middle of the pectoralis descendens muscle, 1.5 cun lateral to the pectoralis sulcus (in the first intercostal space).

LU 7
In the depression on the medial surface of the radius, 1.5 cun proximal to the most medial prominence of the styloid process, 0.5 cun distal to the level of PC 6.

LU 10
On the medial side of the fore limb, at the halfway junction of the third metacarpal, between the suspensory ligament and the palmar digital vein.

LU 11
On the palmaromedial aspect of the front foot, in the depression just proximal to the coronary band, approximately two-thirds of the distance from the dorsal midline of the coronary band to the palmar border of the medial bulb of the heel.

Stomach Meridian

ST 25
In the depression, 1.5 cun lateral to the umbilicus.

ST 34
Approximately 3 cun proximal to the proximal and lateral edge of the patella.

ST 35
In the large depression ventral to the ventral border of the patella, between the middle and lateral patellar ligaments.

ST 36
In the depression just lateral to the tibial crest, in the muscular groove between the tibialis cranialis and long digital extensor muscles, 2 cun distal to the proximal edge of the tibial crest.

ST 45
On the dorsal midline of the rear foot, in the depression just proximal to the coronary band.

Small-Intestine Meridian

SI 1
On the dorsolateral aspect of the front foot, in the depression just proximal to the coronary band, approximately one-third of the distance from the dorsal midline of the coronary band to the palmar border of the lateral bulb of the heel.

SI 3
On the lateral side of the fore limb, in the depression just distal to the end of the fourth metacarpal (lateral splint) bone and proximal to the fetlock, on the palmarolateral border of the third metacarpal bone.

SI 4
On the lateral surface of the fore limb, distal to the carpal joint, upper one-third of the distance from carpus to fetlock, cranial to the suspensory ligament.

SI 6
Distal to the tip of the ulna, over the lateral ulnar muscle.

SI 9
In the large depression caudal to the proximal humerus, along the caudal border of the deltoid muscle, and between the long and lateral heads of the triceps brachii muscle.

SI 10
At 2 cun craniodorsal to SI 9.

SI 16
On the dorsal border of the brachiocephalic muscle at the level of the second cervical vertebrae.

Large-Intestine Meridian

LI 1
On the dorsomedial aspect of the front foot, in the depression just proximal to the coronary band, approximately one-third of the distance from the dorsal midline of the coronary band to the palmar border of the medial bulb of the heel.

LI 4
On the medial side of the fore limb, in the depression just palmar to the second metacarpal (medial splint) bone and distal to its base. This would be at the level between the proximal and middle thirds of the third metacarpal (cannon) bone. There are three depressions on the palmar aspect of the second metacarpal bone, which is located on the level of the second depression.

LI 6
At 3 cun proximal to the lateral distal tuberositas radii, between the extensor carpi radialis and common digital extensor muscles.

LI 11
In the transverse cubital crease, in the depression, just cranial to the lateral epicondyle of the humerus between the extensor carpi radialis and common digital extensor muscles. This point is easily palpated when the elbow is flexed.

LI 15
Just cranial to the point of the shoulder (cranial part of the greater or lateral tuberosity of the humerus).

LI 16
Along the cranial border of the scapula, in a depression two-thirds of the distance from TH 15 to the point of the shoulder.

LI 17
At 2 cun craniodorsal to LI 16, on the brachiocephalic muscle.

LI 18
With the head extended, along the line of the ventral mandible to the depression just above the jugular groove.

Liver Meridian

LV 1
On the dorsomedial aspect of the rear foot, in the depression just proximal to the coronary band, approximately one-third of the distance from the dorsal midline of the coronary band to the plantar border of the medial bulb of the heel.

LV 3
On the medial side of the hind limb, in the depression just plantar to the second metatarsal (medial splint) bone and distal to its base. This would be at the level between the proximal and middle thirds of the third metatarsal (cannon) bone.

LV 4
In the cranial aspect of the hock, on the saphenous vein, medial to the cunean tendon.

LV 8
Posterior to the medial condyle of the femur, in the depression cranial to the insertion of the semitendinosus and semimembranosus muscles, and caudal to the saphenous vein.

Gall-Bladder Meridian

GB 20
In the large depression just caudal to the lateral canthus.

GB 21
In the depression, cranial to the cranial border of the subclavius muscle, dorsal to the dorsal border of the omotransversarius muscle, and dorsal to the seventh cervical vertebra. Some authors put it at the level of the midpoint of the cranial border of the scapula.

GB 27
At 0.5 cun craniodorsal to the cranial aspect of the iliac spine.

GB 28
In a depression midway between GB 27 and GB 29.

GB 29
In the depression located midway on a line from the ventral aspect of the tuber coxae (coxal tuber) to the palpable middle of the third trochanter of the femur.

GB 30
In the depression caudoventral to the dorsal border of the caudal portion of the greater trochanter, in the biceps femoris muscle.

GB 34
In the interosseous space between the tibia and fibula and between the long and lateral digital extensor muscles, craniodistal to the head of the fibula.

GB 39
In the depression, 3 cun proximal to the most lateral prominence of the lateral malleolus of the tibia, caudal to the tibial border, cranial to the deep digital flexor muscle.

GB 44
On the dorsolateral aspect of the rear foot, in the depression just proximal to the coronary band, approximately one-third of the distance from the dorsal midline of the coronary band to the plantar border of the lateral bulb of the heel.

Spleen Meridian

SP 1
On the plantaromedial aspect of the rear foot, in the depression just proximal to the coronary band, approximately two-thirds of the distance from the dorsal midline of the coronary band to the plantar border of the medial bulb of the heel.

SP 6
In the depression 3 cun proximal to the most medial prominence of the medial malleolus of the tibia, just caudal to

the caudal border of the tibia and dorsal to the combined heads of the deep digital flexor muscle, tibialis caudalis muscle, and lateral digital flexor muscle. This point is usually located just distal to where the saphenous vein crosses the caudal border of the tibia. Since the fibula does not exist in the horse, SP 6 is located opposite GB 39 on the lateral aspect of the leg.

SP 9
In the depression, just ventral to the medial condyle of the tibia, caudal to the caudal border of the tibia, over the popliteus muscle, and cranial to the saphenous vein.

SP 13
Directly ventral to the tuber coxae.

Kidney Meridian

KI 1
On the plantar midline of the rear foot, in the depression between the bulbs of the heel.

KI 3
On the medial aspect of the hock area, in the middle of the webbed area cranial to the calcaneal tendon, at the level of the tip of the tuber calcanei (calcanean tuber).

KI 10
On the medial side of the popliteal fossa at the level of BL 40, between the semitendinosus and semimembranosus muscles.

Bladder Meridian

BL 10
In a depression, just caudal to the wings of the atlas, 2 cun from the dorsal midline.

BL 11
In the depression, just cranial to the craniodorsal border of the scapular cartilage, 1.5 cun lateral to the dorsal midline, over the cervical portion of the trapezius muscle.

BL 13
At the caudal edge of the scapular cartilage (eighth intercostal space), 3 cun lateral to the dorsal midline.

BL 14
At the ninth intercostal space, 3 cun lateral to the dorsal midline within the intercostal muscle group.

BL 15
At the 10th intercostal space, 3 cun lateral to the dorsal midline (in the iliocostal muscle groove).

BL 17
In the depression 3 cun lateral to the dorsal midline, in the 12th intercostal space, in the muscular groove between the longissimus thoracis and iliocostalis thoracis muscles.

BL 18
In the depression, 3 cun lateral to the dorsal midline. This point has two locations: in the 13th and 14th intercostal spaces, in the muscular groove between the longissimus thoracis and iliocostalis thoracis muscles.

BL 19
In the depression 3 cun lateral to the dorsal midline, in the 15th intercostal space, in the muscular groove between the longissimus thoracis and iliocostalis thoracis muscles.

BL 20
In the depression 3 cun lateral to the dorsal midline, in the 17th (last) intercostal space, in the muscular groove between the longissimus thoracis and iliocostalis thoracis muscles.

BL 21
In the depression 3 cun lateral to the dorsal midline, in the depression caudal to the 18th (last) rib, between T18 and L1 (T–L junction), in the muscular groove between the longissimus lumborum and iliocostalis lumborum muscles.

BL 22
In the first lumbar intervertebral space (L1–L2), 3 cun lateral to the dorsal midline.

BL 23
In the depression 3 cun lateral to the dorsal midline, between the spinous processes of L2 and L3, in the muscular groove between the longissimus lumborum and the iliocostalis lumborum muscles.

BL 25
In the depression 3 cun lateral to the dorsal midline, between the spinous processes of the fifth and sixth lumbar vertebrae (L4 and L5, if L6 is missing). Usually on a line extending from the dorsal midline to the cranial edge of the tuber coxae (coxal tuber).

BL 26
In the depression 3 cun is lateral to the dorsal midline, between the spinous processes of the sixth (or fifth if the sixth is missing) lumbar and the first sacral vertebrae.

BL 27
In the depression 3 cun lateral to the dorsal midline and 1.5 cun lateral to the first sacral foramen.

BL 28
In the depression 3 cun lateral to the dorsal midline and 1.5 cun lateral to the second sacral foramen.

BL 32
In the second sacral intervertebral space, 1.5 cun lateral to the dorsal midline.

BL 35
At the dorsal end of the muscular groove between the biceps femoris and semitendinosus muscles.

BL 36
In the muscular groove between the biceps femoris and semitendinosus muscles, 2 cun distal to the tuber ischii (ischial tuber).

BL 37
In the muscular groove between the biceps femoris and semitendinosus muscles, 5 cun distal to the tuber ischii (ischial tuber).

BL 38
In the muscular groove between the biceps femoris and semitendinosus muscles, 8 cun distal to the tuber ischii (ischial tuber).

BL 39
In the depression just medial to the caudal division of the biceps femoris muscle, at the ventral end of the muscular groove between the biceps femoris and semitendinosus muscles; level with the stifle.

BL 40
In the depression, at the midpoint of the transverse crease of the popliteal fossa, between the caudal division of the biceps femoris and semitendinosus muscles. It is more easily found with the stifle flexed.

BL 54
In the depression at the intersection of two lines: one from the caudal portion of the greater trochanter to the lumbosacral space, the other from the dorsal aspect of the tuber coxae (coxal tuber) to the tuber ischii (ischial tuber).

BL 60
On the lateral aspect of the hock area, in the middle of the webbed area cranial to the calcaneal tendon, at the level of the tip of the tuber calcanei (calcanean tuber).

BL 62
In the depression, just plantardistal to the most lateral prominence of the lateral malleolus of the tibia.

BL 63
In the depression proximal to the base of the fourth metatarsal bone and dorsal to the long plantar ligament.

BL 67
On the plantarolateral aspect of the rear foot, in the depression just proximal to the coronary band, approximately two-thirds of the distance from the dorsal midline of the coronary band to the plantar border of the lateral bulb of the heel.

Triple-Heater Meridian

TH 1
On the dorsal midline of the front foot, in the depression just proximal to the coronary band.

TH 5
In the groove between the tendons of the lateral digital extensor and common digital extensor muscles, at the level of the midportion of the cranial border of the chestnut.

TH 7
On the radial side of the ulna, 3 cun proximal to the carpus.

TH 10
One cun superior to the olecranon process in a depression with elbow flexed (1 cun dorsocranial to SI 8).

TH 11
At 1 cun cranial to TH 10.

TH 13
Two-thirds of the distance from TH 11 to TH 14.

TH 14
In the caudal margin of shoulder joint, at the level of the point of the shoulder.

TH 16
At the caudal boarder of the brachiocephalic muscle, between the first and second cervical vertebral spaces, cranial and dorsal to SI 16.

TH 17
In the depression between the mandible and the mastoid process, caudoventral to the ear.

Conception-Vessel Meridian

CV 12
On the ventral midline, in the depression halfway between the xiphoid process and the umbilicus.

CV 24
On the ventral midline, 1 cun ventral to the border of the lower lip.

Governing-Vessel Meridian

Bai Hui (Hundred Meetings)
In the depression on the dorsal midline in the lumbosacral space.

GV 14
On the dorsal midline, in the depression between the spinous processes of the seventh cervical and the first thoracic vertebrae.

GV 24
On the dorsal midline at the rostral end of the mane.

GV 26
On the midline, between the ventral limits of the nostrils.

Other Points

Yin-Tang
In the depression at the junction of the frontal bones, on the dorsal midline of the face, at the level of the lateral canthi.

Tong-Tang (Communicating Hall)
At the dorsal midline, at the level of the medial canthus of the eye.

Chou-Jin (Pulling Tendon)
On the midline of the upper lip.

ER-Jian (Ear Tip)
At the tip of the ear, on its outer surface, at the junction of the medial, middle, and lateral branches of the auricular vein.

Ear Shen-Men
In the inter-ridge groove 0.5 cun above the distal end of the common cutaneous ridge.

References

Anderson, R.R. and Parrish, J.A. (1981). The optics of human skin. *J Invest Dermatol.* 77(1):13–19.

Bessent, C. (2011). *Equine Acupuncture Points and Meridians.* Herbsmith, Hartland, WI.

Chow, T.Y. and Lee, M.C. (2013). Acupuncture. *Mayo Clin Proc.* 88(10):1141–1146.

Chung, H. *et al.* (2012). The nuts and bolts of low-level laser light therapy. *Ann Biomed Eng.* 40(2):516–533.

Fleming, P. (1998). Equine acupuncture. In: *Complementary and Alternative Veterinary Medicine*, 1 edn. Mosby, Maryland Heights, MO.

Fuchtenbusch, A. and Rosin, P. (2006). *Laser Therapy and Acupuncture on Horses.* Self-published.

Jang, I. *et al.* (2019). Early history of laser acupuncture: who used it first? *Integr Med Res.* 8(2):129–130.

Law, D. *et al.* (2015). Laser acupuncture for treating musculoskeletal pain: a systematic review with meta-analysis. *J Acupunct Meridian Stud.* 8(1):2–16.

Le Jeune, S. *et al.* (2016). Acupuncture and equine rehabilitation. *Vet Clin North Am Equine Pract.* 32(1):73–85.

Litscher, G. (2018). *Definition of Laser Acupuncture and All Kinds of Photo Acupuncture. Multidisciplinary Digital Publishing Institute*, Basel.

Lorenzini, L. *et al.* (2010). Laser acupuncture for acute inflammatory, visceral, and neuropathic pain relief: an experimental study in the laboratory rat. *Res Vet Sci.* 88(1):159–165.

Martin, B.B. and Klide, A.M. (1987). Treatment of chronic back pain in horses. Stimulation of acupuncture points with a low-powered infrared laser. *Vet Surg.* 16(1): 106–110.

Plog, F.M.W. (1980). Biophysical application of the laser beam. In: *Lasers in Medicine.* (ed. H.K. Koebner), pp. 21–37. John Wiley, New York.

Riegel, R.J. and Hakola, S. (1996). *Illustrated Atlas of Clinical Equine Anatomy and Common Disorders of the Horse*, 1 edn. Primedia Equine Network, Kennett Square, PA.

Schoen, A.M. and Wynn, S.G. (1998). *Complementary and Alternative Veterinary Medicine Principles and Practice*, 1 edn, pp. 173–184. Mosby, Maryland Heights, MO.

Wan, S. *et al.* (1981). Transmittance of nonionizing radiation in human tissue. *Photochem Photobiol.* 34(6):679–681.

Whittaker, P. (2004). Laser acupuncture: past, present, and future. *Lasers Med Sci.* 19(2):69–80.

Xie, H. and Preast, V. (2007). *Xie's Veterinary Acupuncture*, 1 edn. Blackwell Publishing, Hoboken, NJ.

32

Laser Therapy for the Treatment of Equine Wounds

Ronald J. Riegel

American Institute of Medical Laser Applications, Marysville, OH, USA

Introduction

In the equine species, the innate flight response often leads to traumatic injuries. This instinctive behavior causes horses to flee without regard for their surroundings, resulting in lacerations, abrasions, contusions, penetrating, and contaminated wounds. It seems that all equines will eventually sustain some form of wound. Managing these injuries is a long-term, labor-intensive process to restore disrupted tissues to normal anatomic activity. This process can be frustrating, but it is crucial for minimizing the visible evidence of the initial injury. An effective approach to speeding up the healing process and restoring tissues is utilizing laser therapy, also known as photobiomodulation therapy (PBMT). This treatment is vital in managing equine injuries, making it an indispensable tool in equine veterinary practice.

The Scientific Evidence of PBMT on Wound Healing

Wound healing is the patient's natural, systemic response to any traumatic injury to the skin or other tissues, such as muscle or tendon. When any traumatic incident occurs, it initiates a biochemical cascade of events to repair the damage (Nguyen *et al.*, 2009). This process is divided into four overlapping phases: hemostasis (clotting), inflammation, tissue growth (proliferation), and maturation (Stadelmann *et al.*, 1998). PBMT has been shown to significantly stimulate the healing of chronic wounds (AlGhamdi *et al.*, 2012; Mester *et al.*, 1971; Peplow *et al.*, 2010a). Understanding the mechanisms by which PBMT affects each phase allows for tailored treatment modifications, resulting in consistent acceleration of the healing process.

PBMT is vital in every phase of wound healing, supporting and enhancing the natural progression of physiological events. The process begins when photonic energy reaches the electron transport chain within the mitochondria's inner membrane. This energy is absorbed by chromophores and photoacceptor molecules in fibroblasts and endothelial cells, resulting in an electronically excited molecular state.

This state changes fundamental molecular processes, resulting in biological effects at the cellular level due to secondary biochemical reactions and cellular signaling (Passarella & Karu, 2014). These reactions correct deficiencies in the respiratory chain, enhancing cellular metabolism (Karu, 1998).

As a result, the production of adenosine triphosphate (ATP) increases, along with the release of nitric oxide (NO) and reactive oxygen species (ROS). These events trigger various biochemical changes that stabilize cellular functions.

This biochemical cascade allows PBMT to activate fibroblasts and macrophages, release growth factors and neurotransmitter substances, induce vasodilation, and affect collagen synthesis. These processes are vital for wound healing (Karu, 1999; Karu & Kolyakov, 2005; Woodruff *et al.*, 2004). Additional details on the fundamental principles of photobiomodulation (PBM) can be found in earlier chapters.

Phases of Wound Healing

Hemostatis Phase

When a patient suffers a traumatic injury, their body rapidly responds to stop the bleeding within the first few minutes. Blood vessels constrict to reduce blood loss, and platelets aggregate to form a plug, filling the vessel's gap.

Laser Therapy in Veterinary Medicine: Photobiomodulation, Second Edition. Edited by Christopher J. Winkler and Lisa A. Miller.

But how do the platelets know where to go? Signaling molecules such as cytokines, chemokines, and hormones guide the platelets to the injury site, releasing fibrin, a non-globular protein that forms a net-like structure. This mesh acts as a "glue," helping the platelets stick together to form a clot. This clot seals the broken blood vessel and prevents further hemorrhage (Versteeg *et al.*, 2013). Once the clot has formed, the next step is to clean up the area and prepare it for healing. The chemokines released by platelet activation attract inflammatory cells and white blood cells to the injury site. These cells help fight infection and initiate the next phase of tissue repair.

PBMT should not be applied until hemostasis is achieved. Using PBMT during active hemorrhage can result in vasodilation (Plass *et al.*, 2012), potentially increasing bleeding and hindering clot formation. This concept is still under research, as some studies indicate that laser irradiation of whole blood can accelerate coagulation and enhance fibrinolysis by affecting the vessel wall and platelet-wall interaction (Savolainen, 1993). However, PBMT-induced vasoconstriction lasts only 5–10 minutes, after which the body experiences vasodilation, peaking around 20 minutes post-insult. This vasodilation, caused by factors released by platelets and other cells, especially histamine (Werner & Gross, 2003), also makes blood vessels more porous, complicating the clotting process. Therefore, while PBMT may benefit coagulation and fibrinolysis, it must be used cautiously and only after establishing hemostasis.

Laser-irradiated mast cells, such as those in the RBL-2H3 model, have been shown to release histamine (Wu *et al.*, 2010). This process begins with a photoacceptor called cytochrome C oxidase (CCO), which absorbs photons and initiates mitochondrial signaling. These signals are transmitted from the mitochondria to the cytosol, leading to cytosolic alkalization. This alkalization opens calcium (Ca^{2+}) channels on the cell membrane (transient receptor potential vanilloid channels), allowing calcium ions to enter the cell. This influx of calcium ions enhances histamine release (Wu *et al.*, 2010; Young *et al.*, 1990).

The increased porosity and chemokine release from platelet activation attract inflammatory cells (leukocytes) to the wound site, facilitating their entry and initiating the next phase of the healing process (Gutowska-Owsiak *et al.*, 2014).

Inflammatory Phase

The inflammatory phase is vital to the healing process as it readies the wound for repair. Foreign substances and dead tissue are removed during this phase, while vascular and cellular responses prepare the area for the following healing stages. The intensity of this inflammatory response, including these vascular and cellular actions, is directly related to the severity of the tissue trauma.

The vascular response begins with initial vasoconstriction, lasting only a few minutes, followed by sustained vasodilation mediated by histamine, prostaglandins, kinins, and leukotrienes. This process is crucial for increasing blood flow to the wound, delivering necessary inflammatory cells and factors to combat infection and remove devitalized tissue.

The transdermal application of PBMT can modify vascular endothelial function by enhancing its antioxidant and angiogenic potential (Michael *et al.*, 2012; Szymczyszyn *et al.*, 2016).

The cellular aspect of the inflammatory phase begins within hours of injury and involves the recruitment of leukocytes from the bloodstream via various vasoactive mediators, chemoattractants, platelets, and mast cells (Singer & Clark, 1999). Neutrophilic diapedesis, stimulated by these mediators and chemoattractants, starts within minutes and peaks several days after the injury. Neutrophils, the first line of defense, eliminate cellular debris and bacteria through phagocytosis. They are drawn to the site by fibronectin, growth factors, and substances such as kinins (proteins or polypeptides like bradykinin).

Neutrophils play a crucial role in wound healing by phagocytizing debris and killing bacteria through the release of free radicals in a process known as the "respiratory burst" (Greenhalgh, 1998). They also help cleanse the wound by secreting proteases that break down damaged tissue. With a lifespan of only around 2 days at the wound site, functional neutrophils undergo apoptosis after completing their tasks and are subsequently engulfed and degraded by macrophages (Martin & Leibovich, 2005). Neutrophilic migration halts once contaminating substances are cleared from the injury. These cells become trapped within the clot, which is sloughed off during the later phases of repair. Any remaining cells are phagocytosed by incoming tissue macrophages or modified wound fibroblasts (Leibovich & Ross, 1975; Simpson & Ross, 1972).

Macrophages are arguably the most essential cells in the early phases of wound healing. They phagocytose debris and bacteria and secrete collagenases and elastases, which break down injured tissue. Additionally, they release cytokines and platelet-derived growth factor (PDGF), a critical cytokine that stimulates the chemotaxis and proliferation of fibroblasts and smooth muscle cells. Macrophages also secrete substances that attract endothelial cells to the wound, promoting their proliferation and angiogenesis (Deodhar & Rana, 1997; Newton *et al.*, 2004).

Macrophage-derived growth factors are pivotal for new tissue formation. This is evidenced by the fact that wounds in macrophage-depleted animals exhibit defective repair.

Studies have shown that experimental wounds rendered monocytopenic demonstrate impaired fibroplasia and granulation tissue formation, leading to delayed wound healing (Godwin *et al.*, 2013).

T-lymphocytes migrate into the wound during the inflammatory phase, approximately 72 hours after injury. The cellular release of interleukin 1 (IL1) attracts them to the wound, which also helps regulate collagenase. Lymphocytes secrete lymphokines such as heparin-binding epidermal growth factor and basic fibroblast growth factor. Additionally, they play a role in cellular immunity and antibody production (de Loura Santana *et al.*, 2016).

The inflammatory phase is a complex sequence of biochemical and physiological events. If these events deviate, the result can be suppuration, chronic prolonged inflammation, and excessive fibrosis. PBMT modulates this phase primarily by increasing the production and release of nitric oxide (NO), a potent vasodilator (Chung *et al.*, 2012). This increases blood vessel permeability, facilitating the entry of leukocytes and macrophages into the wound site.

Mediators such as cytokines and chemokines regulate the immunological process of inflammation through complex signaling mechanisms (Viegas *et al.*, 2007). These inflammatory mediators are released when immune cells are irradiated with specific wavelengths of light (Chung *et al.*, 2012). PBMT further modulates the inflammatory process by regulating the inflammatory cytokine IL1β. In male Wistar rats with a cryoinjury, IL1β levels decreased in those receiving PBMT (660 nm, 20 mW, 5 J/cm^2) but remained unchanged in those not receiving PBMT (Fernandes *et al.*, 2013).

Proliferative Phase

Granulation tissue comprises inflammatory cells, fibroblasts, and neovasculature within a matrix of fibronectin, collagen, glycosaminoglycans, and proteoglycans (Falanga *et al.*, 1988). The formation of granulation tissue, which appears approximately 3–5 days after injury, signifies the onset of the proliferative phase of wound healing. This phase can be divided into angiogenesis, fibroplasia (collagen deposition and granulation tissue formation), re-epithelialization, and contraction (Clark, 1996). It overlaps with the latter part of the inflammatory phase rather than being a distinct stage.

Angiogenesis

Angiogenesis is the process by which microvascular endothelial cells create new capillary blood vessels from existing ones, essential for the survival of granulation tissue within a wound bed. This process is triggered by tissue damage and hypoxia, making it a complex and dynamic mechanism.

Angiogenesis (the formation of new blood vessels) is regulated by various soluble factors in the serum and surrounding extracellular matrix (ECM). These angiogenic inducers include growth factors, chemokines, angiogenic enzymes, endothelial-specific receptors, and adhesion molecules such as integrins. Many of these inducers are released during the inflammatory phase of tissue repair (Li *et al.*, 2003; Liekens *et al.*, 2001).

PBMT has been the focus of numerous studies in recent years, primarily for its role in promoting angiogenesis across various research models. Hamblin (2008) highlighted the beneficial effects of nitric oxide (NO), a key component of PBMT, including pain relief, edema resolution, improved lymphatic drainage, and enhanced wound healing through angiogenesis promotion. Tuby *et al.* (2006) demonstrated that PBMT, using an 804 nm wavelength laser, could promote cardioprotection and angiogenesis following heart attacks in mice. Dungel *et al.* (2014) explored PBMT's potential in promoting angiogenesis and improving ischemic wound healing using different wavelengths (470 and 629 nm) at 50 mW/cm^2. Larkin *et al.* (2012) used a Class 4 laser to determine a therapeutic dose range for increasing blood flow to the biceps brachii muscle of the forearm. Their study, using venous occlusion plethysmography, concluded that a setting of 3 W (360 J) was an effective treatment modality.

Fibroplasia

Fibroplasia, the process of fibroblast and mesenchymal cell proliferation and differentiation, is crucial in the body's response to injury. Starting 3–5 days after injury, it involves a series of complex processes mediated by various growth factors. Fibroblasts and mesenchymal cells migrate, proliferate, and differentiate in response to fibronectin, PDGF, fibroblast growth factor, and transforming growth factors. Fibronectin acts as an anchor for myofibroblasts as they migrate within the wound. These fibroblasts grow and create a new, provisional ECM by secreting collagen and fibronectin, forming new granulation tissue. This stroma, rich in fibronectin and hyaluronan, replaces the fibrin-containing clot, providing a physical barrier to infection and a surface for mesenchymal cell migration (Song *et al.*, 2010).

PBMT has shown a proliferative effect on various human and animal cell types, including fibroblasts, keratinocytes, endothelial cells, lymphocytes, muscle cells, and stem cells (Basso *et al.*, 2012; Hamblin & Demidova, 2006; Peplow *et al.*, 2010b). The exact mechanism of this proliferation is not completely understood, but irradiated cells release ROS, leading to the expression of transcription factors such as nuclear factor kappa B (NF-κB). This, in turn, activates a form of nitric oxide synthase (NOS), which promotes cell proliferation (Alexandratou *et al.*, 2002; Chen *et al.*, 2011; Lubart & Breitbart, 2000).

Mouse fibroblasts and endothelial cells were irradiated with various wavelengths: visible red light from 625 to 675 nm using a potassium titanyl phosphate (KTP)-pumped tunable dye laser and near-infrared light at 810 nm using a diode laser (power density 5 mW/cm^2; energy density 10 J/cm^2). Cellular proliferation was measured 72 hours post-irradiation using a colorimetric assay for viable cells. Compared to control cells, fibroblasts irradiated by the visible red wavelengths exhibited increased proliferation, while those irradiated with the near-infrared 810 nm wavelength light displayed growth inhibition (Moore, 2005).

PBMT improved the remodeling of the ECM during tendon healing by activating matrix metallopeptidase 2 (MMP2) and stimulating collagen synthesis (Guerra *et al.*, 2013). Additionally, light-emitting diode (LED) irradiation emitting wavelengths in the range of 625–635 nm maintained human fibroblast viability and increased collagen synthesis *in vitro* using human fibroblast (HS68) cultures (Huang *et al.*, 2007).

Re-epithelialization

Re-epithelialization, the process where skin cells migrate to cover a wound, often occurs simultaneously with fibroplasia, the formation of fibrous tissue. This process involves cells at the wound edges moving a short distance, typically less than 1 mm, from one side of the wound to the other. Re-epithelialization tends to be faster in partial-thickness wounds because migrating cells can originate from the remaining skin at the wound's edge and from residual epidermal appendages. With the basement membrane intact, the regeneration process is quicker. Incisional wounds usually epithelialize within 48–72 hours post-injury.

In equine practice, a significant percentage of wounds are full-thickness and require second-intention healing, where the wound heals from the bottom up by first forming a bed of granulation tissue. Once this tissue forms, the skin begins to re-epithelialize. The rate of re-epithelialization varies by wound location; for example, wounds in a horse's flank region epithelialize at about 0.2 mm per day, whereas those in the distal limb regions, like the hooves, heal at a slower rate of approximately 0.09 mm per day (Jacobs *et al.*, 1984).

PBMT has been shown to effectively stimulate epithelial cell proliferation, aiding the healing process. In one case study, a patient with thalassemia intermedia and a non-healing ankle ulcer was treated with PBMT, receiving 17.3 J/cm^2 daily for 2 weeks, followed by an average of 6.5 J/cm^2 for another 2 weeks. This treatment led to complete re-epithelialization with no recurrence during a 6-month follow-up (Dixit *et al.*, 2014).

Leite *et al.* (2015) studied rats with a 1.5 mm punched dorsum skin wound on a high-fat diet. The study showed that PBMT accelerated cutaneous wound healing by modulating oxidative stress in rats with a metabolic disorder under a high-fat diet.

Contraction

Wound contraction begins simultaneously with collagen synthesis and involves the inward movement of wound edges, helping to close the wound. This contraction is driven by the proliferation and activity of myofibroblasts, differentiated fibroblasts present in the granulation tissue. Myofibroblasts contain smooth-muscle actin filaments that connect with other fibroblasts and the ECM, contracting to pull the wound margins toward the center (Darby *et al.*, 1990). The rate of wound contraction affects the speed of second-intention healing and the esthetic quality of the resulting scar. Specific cytokines regulate wound contraction, but inflammation can inhibit it. Once myofibroblasts have completed their role, excess cells undergo apoptosis.

PBMT enhances the transformation and proliferation of fibroblasts into myofibroblasts, accelerating wound contraction. This effect was demonstrated in a study where wounds were irradiated with a helium-neon laser (Pourreau-Schneider *et al.*, 1990). Another study evaluated PBMT's effects on wound healing by examining ECM components and myofibroblast proliferation. In this study, cutaneous wounds were inflicted on Wistar rats, and PBMT was applied at dosages of 4 and 8 J/cm^2. Lesions were analyzed at various intervals using histology, immunohistochemistry, and electron microscopy. Results showed that PBMT-treated groups experienced reduced inflammatory reactions, increased collagen deposition, and greater myofibroblast proliferation (Medrado *et al.*, 2003). Applying PBMT immediately post-operatively enhances tissue repair in patients with diabetes by modulating inflammation, increasing myofibroblast synthesis, and improving collagen organization (de Loura Santana *et al.*, 2015).

Maturation Phase

When collagen production and degradation levels equalize, the maturation phase of tissue repair begins. During this phase, type III collagen, which predominates during proliferation, is replaced by type I collagen (Dealey, 2012). Disorganized collagen fibers are rearranged, crosslinked, and aligned along tension lines (Wood *et al.*, 2010).

The timing of the maturation phase can vary significantly, influenced by factors such as wound size and whether it was closed or left open (Lorenz & Longaker, 2008). Collagen deposition peaks within the first week of primary wound care and between 7 and 14 days in second-intention healing.

Collagen deposition provides tensile strength to the wound. Although this period corresponds to the fastest gain in strength, it accounts for only 20% of the wound's final strength. The majority of the wound's strength develops in the following weeks (Stashak & Theoret, 2008).

By the third week, the body balances collagen synthesis and lysis, preventing excessive collagen accumulation and avoiding scar tissue formation.

As wound healing progresses, the wound's tensile strength increases. Collagen, a critical structural component of the skin, gradually strengthens. By the third week, collagen achieves approximately 20% of its total tensile strength, continuing to increase until the 12th to 14th week, reaching about 80% of its full potential (Mercandetti & Cohen, 2015).

Research by Stadler *et al.* (2001) demonstrated that PBMT significantly enhances wound tensile strength in a murine diabetic mouse model using an 830 nm wavelength at a dosage of 5 J/cm^2. Similarly, Vasilenko *et al.* (2010) found that 635 and 670 nm wavelengths improved tensile strength in full-thickness skin incisions in rats, further supporting PBMT's effectiveness in wound healing. Kilik *et al.* (2014) evaluated PBMT with a 635 nm wavelength, administering equal daily doses of 5 J/cm^2 at power densities of 1, 5, and 15 mW/cm^2, three times a day. This study, involving both normal and diabetic rats with open skin wounds, confirmed that PBMT enhances wound tensile strength regardless of health status. Collectively, these studies highlight PBMT's potential in strengthening wounds during the healing phase.

Paraguassu *et al.* (2014) explored PBMT's effects on collagen expression during healing in normal and hypothyroid rats using a GaAlAs laser emitting a wavelength of 660 nm, 40 mW, and 1 W/cm^2. The researchers found that PBMT increased the immune expression of collagen type I during tissue repair, improving the quality of newly formed tissue in hypothyroid rats (Paraguassu *et al.*, 2014).

The content and arrangement of collagen fibers determine wound tensile strength. PBMT stimulates better alignment and normal distribution of type I and type III collagen during healing (Paraguassu *et al.*, 2014; Wood *et al.*, 2010). This results in stronger and less exuberant scars, which are crucial for the cosmetic resolution of wounds in horses (Oliveira *et al.*, 2009; Peplow *et al.*, 2010a). Redondo (2015) further noted that PBMT increases fibroblast multiplication, differentiation, motility, and collagen production, leading to earlier wound closure.

Equine PBMT Treatment Techniques

Dosing

Dosages are determined by several factors, including:

- The anatomical area of the wound
- Whether the wound is open or closed
- The stage of healing of the wound
- The anatomical tissues involved (e.g., tendons vs. muscle)
- The distance to the target tissues
- The presence or absence of infection and contamination

These factors must be considered for each individual patient, as there are no universal dosages. "Treat to effect" is crucial, meaning the dosage should be sufficient to achieve the desired therapeutic effect. While there is a wide margin of safety in dosage determination, dosages that are not administered frequently enough or at inhibitory wavelengths will affect the clinical outcome of the treatment.

The dosages detailed in Table 32.1 are guidelines that can be considered where applicable. For instance, treating an open wound in the lower extremity might require a different dosage than treating a closed wound in the upper extremity.

The goal of applying PBMT to any wound is to safely and effectively administer enough energy to saturate all target tissues, eliciting a biological and physiological response. To acclimate the patient to the procedure, starting with a lower power density treatment can be achieved in several ways:

- **Decrease the power output and increase the treatment time:** This method involves reducing the power output and extending the treatment duration.
- **Increase the spot size:** Increasing the spot size decreases the power density. This can be easily achieved by increasing the distance between the handpiece and the target tissue.

Table 32.1 Recommended dosages for equine wounds.

Wound type	Dosage (J/cm$^{2)}$
Abrasion	4 ± 2
Incisional	4–6
Wheal	2–4
Contusion	4–8
Laceration (sutured)	4–6
Laceration (open)	8–12
Laceration (muscle and tendon tissue involvement)	10–12
Laceration (tendon and hoof involvement)	10–12
Puncture (not infected and minimal muscle damage)	6–8
Puncture (not infected with muscle damage)	8–10
Puncture (not infected with muscle and tendon damage)	8–12
Puncture (infected)	10–12
Chronic	10–12
Chronic (profuse granulation tissue)	10–14

- **Use a pulsed/frequency emission:** These settings mean the laser alternates between emitting and not emitting. The average power output is a fraction of that in continuous wave mode. For example, a laser set to 10 W pulsed delivery at a 50% duty cycle will emit an average of only 5 W over a given period versus 10 W if emitting continuously.
- **Increase the scanning speed:** Moving the handpiece more quickly across the target tissue does not reduce the power density but helps minimize potential discomfort in sensitive tissues.

Therapy laser equipment may include software with preset protocols calculated for the wound area. These protocols need to be adapted to the individual case but serve as initial treatment guidelines. The total dose can also be manually calculated by measuring the area and multiplying by the desired dose.

Application Technique

The majority of equine wounds are initially treated using an off-contact method, which can be administered using either a scanning or a point-to-point technique. To treat the wound, maintain the handpiece perpendicular to the target tissue and distribute the calculated dosage at 90° angles in a grid-like pattern over the wound. It is crucial to include a sufficient margin of healthy tissue surrounding the wound, ideally around 6 cm. Ensure that all areas of epithelialization within the wound receive adequate therapy.

After a few initial treatments, transitioning to on-contact treatment may be possible. This method is particularly suitable for closed wounds and areas of epithelialization surrounding an open wound. However, treating on-contact over an open wound bed can be challenging due to patient sensitivity and concerns about handpiece contamination. Therefore, proceed cautiously and thoroughly clean and disinfect the wound bed before performing on-contact treatment.

Frequency of Treatment

Acute wounds, whether open or closed, should receive PBMT daily until a visible clinical response is noted. Once a clinical response is observed, therapy sessions can be spaced out, with a day or more between sessions, until the wound is completely resolved. PBMT response is cumulative, meaning each treatment contributes to the healing process. If there is no clinical response after the second treatment, despite a correct diagnosis and no hindering conditions, increase the dosage in small increments to ensure it reaches the target tissue.

Chronic wounds require a different approach. Initially, these wounds should receive two to three daily treatments, which can then be spaced according to clinical progress and medical management. Chronic wounds often undergo initial debridement, placing them in the acute wound classification. The goal for treating these injuries is complete resolution; however, some patients may require periodic maintenance doses of PBMT.

General Wound Management

PBMT is an adjunct to the standard of care in wound management. This noninvasive therapy provides pain relief, modulation of the inflammatory reaction, and increased circulation.

Following an initial physical examination and assessment, a treatment plan is determined. After lavage and debridement, a decision is made on whether to manage the wound as closed or open. PBMT is then integrated into the standard wound care protocol as follows:

- **Closed wounds:** If the wound is closed with sutures, staples, or glue after the initial exam, PBMT can be administered immediately post-closure, treating it as an incision.
- **Delayed closure:** If the wound is closed after several days of lavage to remove contamination or reduce infection, PBMT should be administered after each lavage and before bandaging. Initially, the wound is treated as open and then managed as closed.
- **Open wounds:** For wounds left to heal by second intention and managed as open wounds throughout the healing process, PBMT should be administered at each bandage change after cleaning, lavage, and debridement, but before applying any moist dressings or bandages.

Blue Light

In addition to red and infrared lights, blue light therapy (BLT) is another potent tool in equine wound management. With shorter wavelengths of 380 nm to 500 nm, blue light cannot penetrate deeply into the wound but has bactericidal properties that complement red and infrared light when administered simultaneously.

Research has shown that BLT applied to the skin has bactericidal (Halstead *et al.*, 2016), anti-contamination (Wang *et al.*, 2017), and anti-inflammatory (Shnitkind *et al.*, 2006) effects. It has also demonstrated a wide range of antimicrobial effects against Gram-positive and Gram-negative bacteria (Huang *et al.*, 2023). While the detailed mechanism of action is not entirely understood, it is believed to rely on photodynamic effects following the light excitation of endogenous microbial chromophores (Plavski *et al.*, 2018; Cieplik *et al.*, 2014). Additionally, BLT combined with silver nanoparticles has been found to be highly effective against a multidrug-resistant isolate of *Pseudomonas aeruginosa* both *in vitro* and *in vivo* (Nour El Din 2016).

Blue light is typically applied off-contact, using a slow-scanning technique. Emissions vary depending on the equipment, but it is generally administered in pulsed or super-pulsed mode. The entire wound bed should be saturated with blue light. Since BLT does not cause thermal buildup in tissues, more infected areas can safely receive a higher dose over a longer period.

Types of Wounds

Traumatic wounds can be categorized as either closed or open. Closed wounds are those where the skin is not broken through all layers, indicating tissue damage without loss of skin continuity. Examples include abrasions, contusions, hematomas, and wheals. Open wounds penetrate through the skin into the subcutaneous and other underlying tissues. These include incisions, lacerations, avulsions, and punctures.

Chronic wounds in horses require special treatment due to the risk of excessive granulation tissue. Additionally, burns, tendon lacerations, and trauma to the hoof necessitate individualized wound management protocols.

Closed Wounds

Abrasions

Abrasions are friction injuries, such as rope burns, affecting the superficial layers of the skin or mucous membranes. These injuries do not penetrate through all skin or mucous membrane layers and are characterized by oozing serum and minimal bleeding. A scab forms superficially, leading to second-intention healing.

Before treating friction injuries, ensure any bleeding has stopped. If a scab has formed, avoid disturbing it. Initially, treatment should be performed off-contact for patient comfort, transitioning to on-contact treatment during the first therapy session or shortly thereafter. The size of the injury determines the treatment dosage. For smaller injuries, start with a dosage of 2–6 J/cm^2. Larger injuries may require a higher dosage. Typically, resolution is achieved after two to four therapy sessions.

Contusions and Hematomas

Contusions result from trauma that ruptures subcutaneous blood vessels, causing localized bruising of underlying tissues beneath intact skin. The dorsal surface of the carpus is particularly susceptible to such injuries from striking a fence or stall door. Contusions are classified into three degrees:

- **First-degree contusions:** These display a small amount of hemorrhage beneath and into the skin, with minimal to no hematoma formation. PBMT should be applied at a dosage of 4–5 J/cm^2, on-contact if possible. Typically, these injuries require only one or two treatments to resolve.
- **Second-degree contusions:** These involve hematoma formation, often resulting from a kick or bite from another horse. Small hematomas will be absorbed, while large ones can lead to a seroma, scar tissue beneath the dermis, and potential blemishes (Garvican & Clegg, 2007). A hematoma over the carpal area may form a carpal hygroma. PBMT is noninvasive and aids in managing second-degree contusions. Treat these lesions aggressively to resolve the hematoma and minimize scar tissue formation. Apply PBMT initially off-contact at a dosage of 6–8 J/cm^2. Transition to on-contact treatment when the patient is comfortable with it. Treat daily for several consecutive days, then every other day until resolved.
- **Third-degree contusions:** These are severe, with underlying tissue damage beyond repair. Although the skin is not broken from the original blow, thrombosis of the vasculature occurs, eventually leading to the sloughing of the superficial tissues. Apply PBMT throughout all phases of the healing process, starting immediately after injury and continuing until both epithelialization and contraction are complete. An initial 6–8 J/cm^2 dosage is usually sufficient, but higher dosages may be needed as the dermal structure disintegrates.

Wheals

A wheal is a bulge or serous-filled blister in the skin; no hemorrhagic extravasation is present. Apply therapy at a dosage of 2–4 J/cm^2. If only slightly painful, treat off-contact, then attempt to transition to on-contact administration after administering a few 100 J. Wheals usually resolve after one or two treatments.

Open Wounds

Incisions

These are definitive wounds produced by surgical instruments or a surgical laser and are characterized by minimal tissue damage. They can be shallow or deep, hemorrhage profusely or not at all, elicit minimal pain, and may have only a modicum of tissue separation. Incised wounds are sutured or stapled. PBMT administered off-contact at a dosage of 4–6 J/cm^2 is an adjunct therapy to the standard post-surgical management. No contraindications exist for applying laser therapy over metal staples or any suture material. Three or four treatments generally lead to resolution.

Lacerations and Avulsions

Lacerations are types of wounds that result in rough, jagged skin edges. They often involve significant damage to the underlying tissues, such as tendons, their sheaths, joint capsules, ligaments, muscles, and neurovascular structures. Due to their nature, lacerations are more prone to contamination and infection compared to incisional wounds. Their treatment often begins with surgical debridement and suturing, but treatment approach may vary depending on the location and circumstances. Lacerations may sometimes be managed as second-intention healing or left as open wounds.

Avulsions, on the other hand, refer to the partial or complete tearing away of the skin and tissue. These are also treated as open wounds.

The severity of the injury determines the dosage and frequency of PBMT administration. For minor lacerations with minimal damage to the underlying tissues, a daily dosage of 4–6 J/cm^2 for several days is recommended. This is followed by further treatment as needed to speed up the healing process. However, when a laceration or avulsion involves tendon, muscle, ligament, or hoof involvement, higher dosages of PBMT are required.

Administration of PBMT to complex lacerations and avulsions involving multiple tissues should be aggressive. Due to the density of the underlying tendon and muscle tissues, dosages in the range of 10–12 J/cm^2 should be administered daily for 3–6 days and then every other day until resolution. Treatment of lacerations and avulsions deep into the muscle tissues may require even higher dosages to provide enough therapeutic energy to the target tissues.

Materials like bandages, cast materials, splints, and leg wraps can block emitted photonic energy. Laser therapy must, therefore, coincide with bandage changes so that it may be applied directly to the lesions. An alternative approach is to provide a treatment window within the bandage or cast material that allows direct access to the laceration. However, care must be taken when considering the placement and composition of a therapy window since immobilization must often be maintained to support the wound and prevent dehiscence.

Punctures

Puncture, or penetrating wounds, generally look minor at the skin's surface but can cause significant trauma to the underlying structures. Common causes are horn gores and sharp objects in the animal's stall, such as nails and steel pitchforks. Puncture wounds are commonly complicated by contamination. The skin can heal before the underlying tissues, resulting in abscessation. Punctures are not usually sutured but managed as an open, draining wound.

Apply only a small portion of the recommended dose to the opening in the skin. Treat all the surrounding structures circumferentially, directing the energy to the deep structures. Encourage healing from the inside of the wound out to the surface. Dose according to the anatomical area and consider the depth of the wound. A range of 6–12 J/cm^2 should be considered. If the wound is contaminated, account for the amount of energy absorbed by pus or exudate within the wound and administer appropriately.

Chronic Wounds

A primary objective in wound management is to prevent wounds from becoming chronic. However, various factors can hinder this goal, including a weakened immune system, advanced age, endocrine disorders such as Cushing's disease, patient noncompliance, and long-term steroid use. These factors can lead to chronic wounds, which are inherently challenging to manage. Infected wounds on the distal limbs pose an even more significant concern due to their increased risk of complications.

Exuberant granulation tissue, or proud flesh, is a common complication of chronic wounds, especially those below the carpus or tarsus. While granulation tissue production is part of normal healing and moves the skin toward the wound center, excessive granulation tissue can impede contraction and normal epithelialization, enlarging the wound by pushing the edges apart.

Treating proud flesh often requires surgical intervention to trim the excess tissue to just below the dermis. This highly vascularized tissue can cause significant bleeding and repeat trimming may be necessary to reduce the tissue gradually. Over time, the skin edges will start to pull across the wound. A helpful rule of thumb is that "skin cells do not climb mountains": if there is a protrusion of granulation tissue, the skin edges will not close properly.

Early administration of PBMT in the management of chronic wounds helps control the production of proud flesh. Increased epithelialization and the effect of laser therapy on fibroblasts promote contraction, encouraging the wound to close normally (Calisto *et al.*, 2015; Hawkins & Abrahamse, 2006; Kuffler, 2016; Reddy, 2004). Administer PBMT off-contact with dosages of 10–14 J/cm^2 daily for 3–5 days, then every other day until the therapeutic goal is reached. As with other wounds, treat to effect. Apply most of the dose along the epithelial border and the first few centimeters of the tissue margin. Continue application over granulation tissue until noticeable serum leakage or slight hemorrhage occurs. The owner or trainer must be forewarned of this possibility, and the therapist should administer PBMT with the handpiece in one hand and a gauze sponge in the other. This technique minimizes the need for surgical removal of granulation tissue.

Many chronic wounds require surgical intervention to encourage healing and create a more optimal environment for continued healing. Surgical intervention aims to convert a chronic wound into an acute state. Reasons for such intervention include the removal of devitalized tissues or foreign bodies, reducing excessive granulation tissue, thorough lavage of contaminated wounds, and establishing drainage.

Each chronic wound case will require a unique PBMT treatment plan. Aggressive treatment initiates and promotes the healing process. Frequent treatments at appropriate dosages can transform these challenging cases into positive clinical outcomes.

Wounds Requiring Special Consideration

Burns

Most equine burns are superficial and can be easily managed, often resulting from friction, such as rope burns, or the improper application of topical agents. Severe burns are less common and typically result from barn fires, which can lead to rapid burn shock or hypovolemia, causing cardiovascular complications. Further complications can arise from concurrent smoke inhalation and corneal ulceration (Fox, 1988; Fubini, 1987). Hanson (2005) provides a comprehensive management plan for burn injuries in horses.

PBMT is a scientific, evidence-based treatment for burns. While early studies showed inconsistent results (Al-Watban *et al.*, 2005; Cambier *et al.*, 1996; Schlager *et al.*, 2000), recent research has been more promising. For example, a study on diabetic rats found that third-degree burns healed faster when treated with 660 and 780 nm laser wavelengths at 35 mW, delivering a dose of 20 J/cm^2 with a laser beam diameter of 2 mm (Meireles *et al.*, 2008). Another study using a pulsed low-level laser with an 890 nm wavelength on third-degree burns in a rat model showed a significant increase in wound closure compared to the control group (Ezzati *et al.*, 2009).

PBMT is a valuable addition to the traditional standard-of-care management of burns. Some beneficial clinical physiological responses provided by PBMT to burn patients include:

- Pain management (Chow *et al.*, 2009; Takenori *et al.*, 2016)
- Increased cellular metabolism (Yadav *et al.*, 2016)
- Enhanced circulation and angiogenesis (Rhee *et al.*, 2016)
- Improved nerve regeneration and function (Takhtfooladi *et al.*, 2015)
- Increased tissue proliferation and regeneration (Macedo *et al.*, 2015)

PBMT should be gently administered to burns off-contact. Gentle administration can be achieved by setting the therapy laser's frequency (duty cycle) to deliver 50% of the energy over time compared to continuous wave (CW). Hold the handpiece perpendicular to the target tissue at a greater distance than normally used for the given anatomical area. In severe burns, nerve endings may be nonfunctional, so the patient might not move voluntarily if the therapy becomes uncomfortable.

A broad range of dosages can be used to treat these patients. For superficial burns, start therapy with 4–6 J/cm^2. For more severe burns (second or third-degree), begin with a low initial dose of 4–6 J/cm^2, applied off-contact in a gentle manner, then gradually increase the dosage according to the depth of the target tissue.

Tendon Lacerations

Lacerations of tendons are serious injuries due to the loss of biomechanical function, decreased tensile strength within the tissues, and the complication of inelastic scar tissue filling the area, which predisposes the patient to further injury. PBMT has been shown to positively impact tendon healing by stimulating the synthesis and organization of collagen I, MMP9, and MMP2 (Da Re Guerra *et al.*, 2016).

PBMT dosages in the 12–20 J/cm^2 range should be administered on contact with the tendon structures distal to the carpus and tarsus. As healing progresses, incorporate passive range-of-motion exercises while administering the therapy. Regularly monitor tissue healing with ultrasonic examinations and adjust the treatment frequency accordingly.

Trauma to the Hoof

The wavelengths and power of therapeutic lasers cannot penetrate the hoof wall. Depending on the laser's optics, any therapy laser emitting over a few 100 mW of power will cause a very small percentage of thermal buildup in the target tissues. Consider the consequences of even slight thermal energy buildup within the vasculature of the laminar corium and the stratum internum. However, PBMT can be safely administered to the coronary band and all the descending neurovascular supply to the foot.

The management of hoof trauma has been well described (DeBowes & Yovich, 1989; Stashak, 1989). Adding PBMT to these established techniques will increase circulation and provide some degree of pain relief. Initiate therapy at a dosage of 6–8 J/cm^2 in the fetlock area and follow all neurovascular pathways distal to the coronary band. Apply therapy to the entire coronary band, focusing on the area proximal to the injury. Treat all areas not directly involved with the injury on-contact if the patient allows it. Painful areas should be treated off-contact. Daily application is ideal, transitioning to every other day or three sessions per week.

Case Study: Treatment of an Open Distal Limb Wound

Presentation

A 19-year-old Paint mare was presented with a severe laceration of the left rear leg (Figure 32.1) after trying to jump a smooth-wire electric fence. There was involvement of the tendon sheaths, but the joint capsule and tendon integrity were not compromised. The tissues were contaminated, so the decision was made to treat it as an open wound.

Treatment

The wound was cleaned, lavaged with sterile saline, and wrapped with a commercial, semi-occlusive, multilayer hydrophilic-gel wound product. Sulfamethoxazole and trimethoprim were administered orally twice a day for 8 days. Phenylbutazone was administered for 2 days for pain management. Tetanus antitoxin was administered. The bandage was changed each day, and the wound was lavaged with saline before the leg was rewrapped with the hydrophilic-gel wound product beneath nonstick gauze pads incorporated into a stout three-layered support bandage.

PBMT was initiated 8 days after injury and applied during bandage changes (Figure 32.2). Dosing was 12 J/cm^2, administered off-contact utilizing a scanning technique throughout the wound and with a border of about 3 cm of skin around the epithelial margin. The wound was treated proximal to distal at 90° angles, with more energy administered to the epithelial margin and skin border than the wound bed. Several attempts were made to treat the epithelial margin and skin border on-contact, but the patient would not allow it. After each treatment, the wound bed (granulation tissue) oozed serum, and a small amount of hemorrhage was visible.

The above therapy protocol was repeated daily for two additional days and repeated on days 9 and 10. On day 12, the saline lavage was discontinued and replaced with garden-hose hydrotherapy, with PBMT applied after the therapy and prior to bandaging (Figure 32.3). Treatments were then repeated on days 14, 15, 17, 21, 24, 26, 31, 33, 38, and 43 (Figures 32.4–32.6).

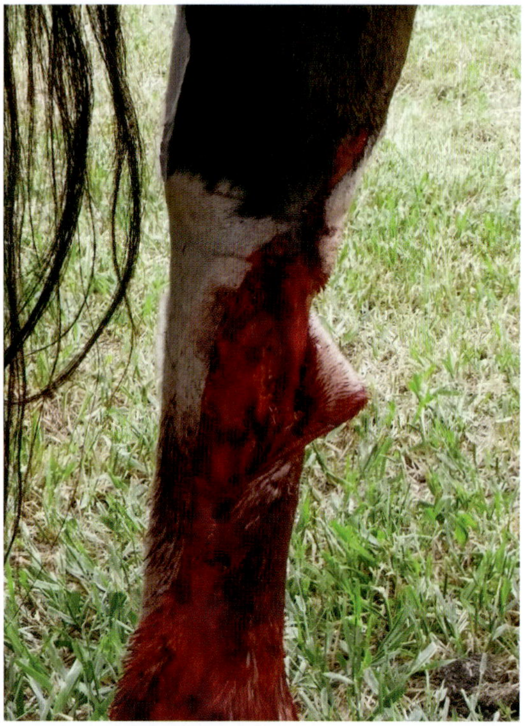

Figure 32.1 Initial presentation of a laceration of the left rear leg of a 19-year-old Paint mare, induced by trying to jump a smooth wire electric fence. Note the flap of skin, the abrasion extending dorsally through the hock, and the slight trauma to the underlying tendons. Courtesy of Courtenay Marshall, LVT.

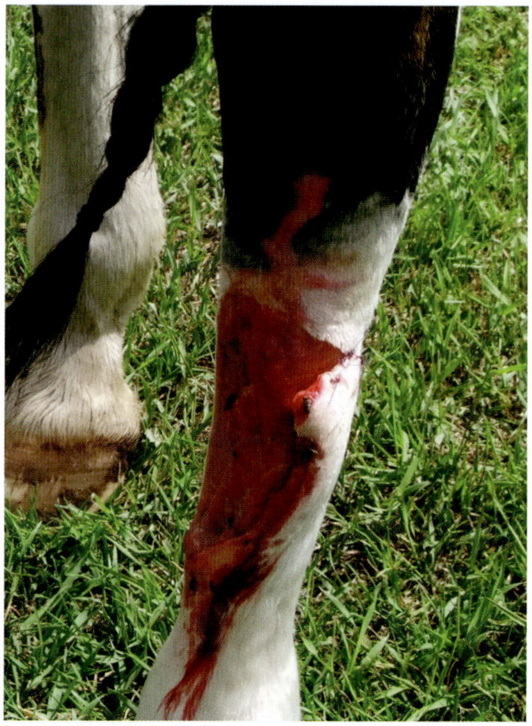

Figure 32.2 Day 8. Picture taken before the first application of PBMT. Courtesy of Courtenay Marshall, LVT.

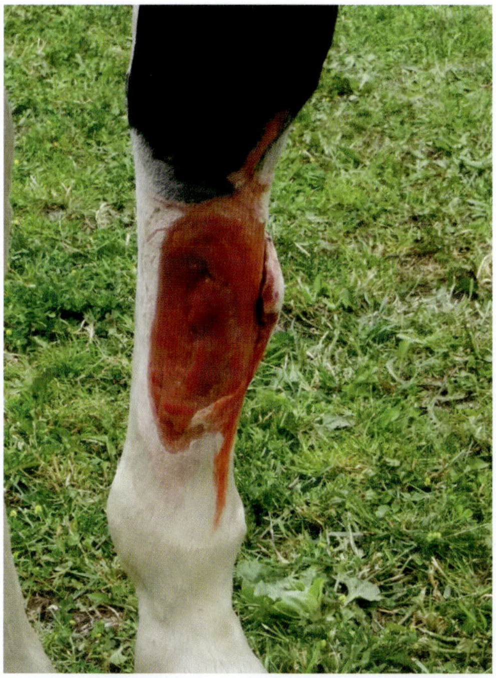

Figure 32.3 Day 12. The picture was taken after the first two laser therapy sessions on days 8 and 9. Note the early healing along the epithelial margin, the reduction in swelling and inflammation, and the early adherence of some areas of the skin flap. Courtesy of Courtenay Marshall, LVT.

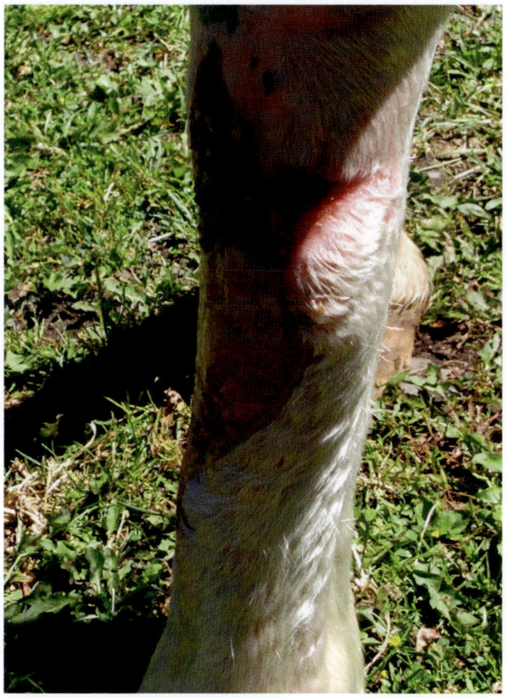

Figure 32.4 Day 18. Appearance of the wound 18 days after the injury and after six therapy laser sessions. This image was taken at a different angle to emphasize the general health of the wound bed, the adherence of the skin flap, the lack of production of exuberant granulation tissue, and the epithelialization of the wound margins. Courtesy of Courtenay Marshall, LVT.

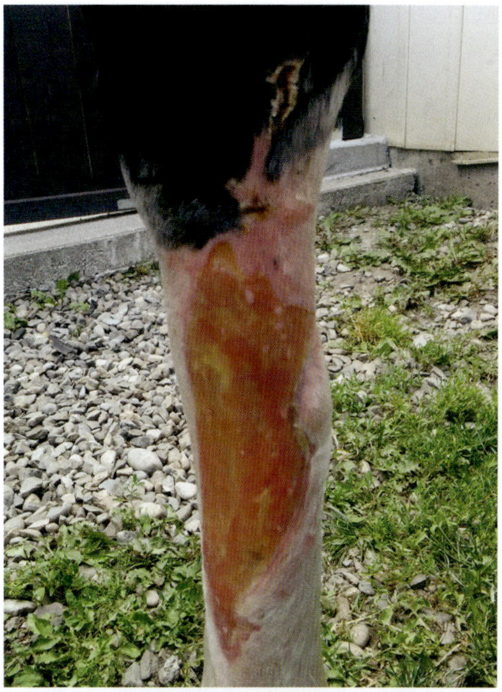

Figure 32.5 Day 26. Progress after eight laser therapy sessions. Note the lack of excessive granulation tissue, the total adherence and healing of the skin flap, and the advancement of the epithelial margins. Courtesy of Courtenay Marshall, LVT.

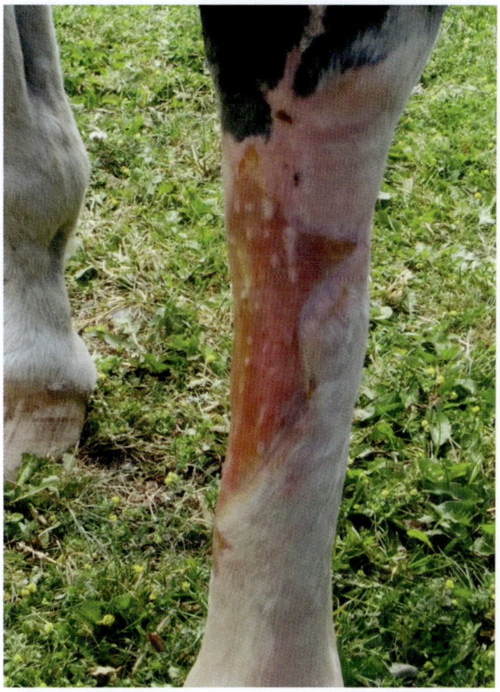

Figure 32.6 Day 32. Progress after 10 laser therapy sessions. Note the degree of contraction of the wound, the health of the wound bed, the almost total healing over the tarsus, and the epithelialization throughout all margins. Courtesy of Courtenay Marshall, LVT.

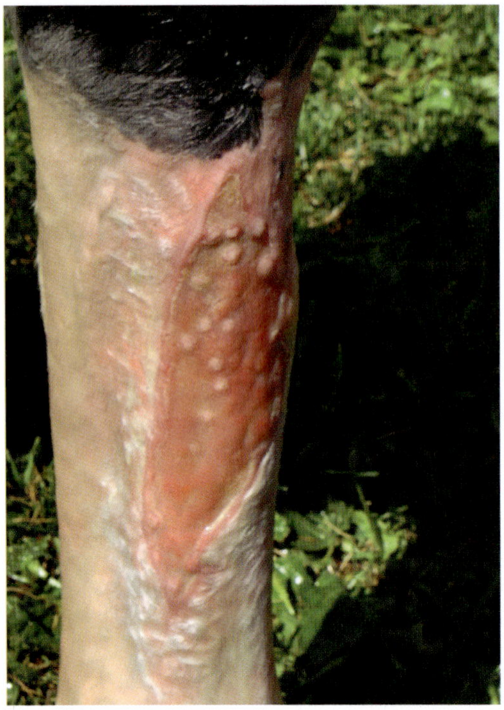

Figure 32.7 Day 44. Progress after 13 laser therapy sessions. Note the continuing progress of epithelialization, the lack of excessive granulation tissue, and the good contraction of the wound. The range of motion was normal, and there was no indication of adhesions. Courtesy of Courtenay Marshall, LVT.

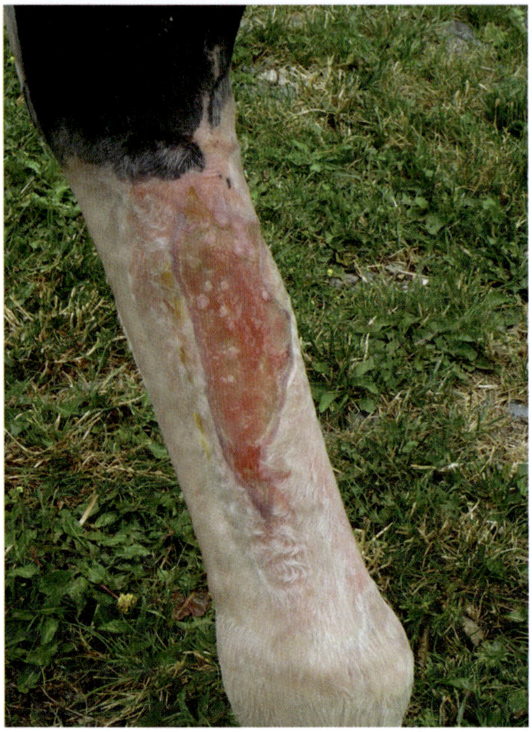

Figure 32.8 Day 46. Continued rapid healing of the wound. At this time, the patient was ridden for a short period of time with no sign of lameness. Courtesy of Courtenay Marshall, LVT.

The wound was never scrubbed after the initial cleaning. Moist wraps were applied after each laser therapy session. The wound never required debridement. PBMT was applied aggressively, which avoided the need for debridement of the granulation tissue. The wound contracted very well with the epithelial margin advancing across the wound bed very naturally. On day 43, the animal's range of motion was back to normal, and it was ridden with no sign of lameness. The prognosis remained very good for this 19-year-old to return to normal function and resume her career as a trail horse in the Rocky Mountains within a few months of the injury (Figures 32.7 and 32.8).

Conclusion

PBMT is a scientifically and clinically proven therapy for treating wounds. It offers pain relief, modulates the inflammatory reaction, and increases circulation. The physiological effects of PBMT accelerate the healing of all types of wounds. Incorporating this therapy into wound-management protocols will benefit all equine patients with wounds.

References

Alexandratou, E. *et al.* (2002). Human fibroblast alterations induced by low power laser irradiation at the single cell level using confocal microscopy. *Photochem Photobiol Sci.* 1(8):547–552.

AlGhamdi, K.M. *et al.* (2012). Low-level laser therapy: a useful technique for enhancing the proliferation of various cultured cells. *Lasers Med Sci.* 27(1):237–249.

Al-Watban, F.A. *et al.* (2005). Burn healing with a diode laser: 670 nm at different doses as compared to a placebo group. *Photomed Laser Surg.* 23(3):245–250.

Basso, F.G. *et al.* (2012). Biostimulatory effect of low-level laser therapy on keratinocytes in vitro. *Lasers Med Sci.* 28(2):367–374.

Calisto, F.C. *et al.* (2015). Use of low-power laser to assist the healing of traumatic wounds. *Acta Cir Bras.* 30(3):204–208.

Cambier, D.C. *et al.* (1996). Low-power laser and healing of burns: a preliminary assay. *Plast Reconstr Surg.* 97(3):555–558.

Chen, A.C. *et al.* (2011). Low-level laser therapy activates NF-kB via generation of reactive oxygen species in mouse embryonic fibroblasts. *PLoS One.* 6(7):e22453.

Chow, R.T. *et al.* (2009). Efficacy of low-level laser therapy in the management of neck pain: a systemic review and meta-analysis of randomized placebo or active treatment controlled trials. *Lancet.* 374(9705):1897–1908.

Chung, H. *et al.* (2012). The nuts and bolts of low-level laser (light) therapy. *Ann Biomed Eng.* 40(2):516–533.

Cieplik, F. *et al.* (2014). Blue light kills Aggregatibacter actinomycetemcomitans due to its endogenous photosensitizers. *Clin Oral Investig.* 18(7):1763–1769.

Clark, R.A.F. (1996). Overview and general considerations of wound repair. In: *The Molecular and Cellular Biology of Wound Repair*, 2nd edn, pp. 3–33. Plenum Press, New York.

Da Re Guerra, F. *et al.* (2016). Low-level PBMT modulates pro-inflammatory cytokines after partial tenotomy. *Lasers Med Sci.* 31(4):759–766.

Darby, I. *et al.* (1990). α-Smooth muscle actinis transiently expressed by myofibroblasts during experimental wound healing. *Lab Investig.* 63(1):21–29.

Dealey, C. (2012). The physiology of wound healing. In: *The Care of Wounds: A Guide for Nurses*, 4th edn, pp. 3–12. Wiley-Blackwell, Hoboken, NJ.

Debowes, R.M. and Yovich, J.V. (1989). Penetrating wounds, abscesses, gravel, and bruising of the equine foot. *Vet Clin North Am Eq Pract.* 5(1):179–194.

Deodhar, A.K. and Rana, R.E. (1997). Surgical physiology of wound healing: a review. *J Postgrad Med.* 43(2):52–56.

Dixit, S. *et al.* (2014). Closure of chronic non healing ankle ulcer with low level laser therapy in a patient presenting with thalassemia intermedia: case report. *Indian J Plast Surg.* 47(3):432–435.

Dungel, P. *et al.* (2014). Low level light therapy by LED of different wavelength induces angiogenesis and improves ischemic wound healing. *Lasers Surg Med.* 46(10):773–780.

Ezzati, A. *et al.* (2009). Low-level laser therapy with pulsed infrared laser accelerates third-degree burn healing process in rats. *J Rehabil Res Dev.* 46(4):543–554.

Falanga, V. *et al.* (1988). Wound healing. *J Am Acad Dermatol.* 19(3):559–563.

Fernandes, K.P. *et al.* (2013). Effect of photobiomodulation on expression of IL-1beta in skeletal muscle following acute injury. *Lasers Med Sci.* 28(3):1043–1046.

Fox, S.M. (1988). Management of a large thermal burn in a horse. *Compend Contin Educ Pract Vet.* 10:88–95.

Fubini, S.L. (1987). Burns. In: *Current Therapy in Equine Medicine*, 2nd edn, pp. 639–641. Saunders, Philadelphia, PA.

Garvican, E. and Clegg, P. (2007). Clinical aspects of equine carpal joints. *UK Vet Comp Anim.* 12(1):5–12.

Godwin, J.W. *et al.* (2013). Macrophages are required for adult salamander limb regeneration. *Proc Natl Acad Sci USA.* 110(23):9415–9420.

Greenhalgh, D.G. (1998). The role of apoptosis in wound healing. *Int J Biochem Cell Biol.* 30(9):1019–1030.

Guerra, F.R. *et al.* (2013). LLLT improves tendon healing through increase in MMP activity and collagen synthesis. *Lasers Med Sci.* 28(5):1281–1288.

Gutowska-Owsiak, D. *et al.* (2014). Histamine enhances keratinocyte-mediated resolution of inflammation by promoting wound healing and response to infection. *Clin Exp Dermatol.* 39(2):187–195.

Halstead, F.D. *et al.* (2016). Antibacterial Activity of Blue Light against Nosocomial Wound Pathogens Growing Planktonically and as Mature Biofilms. *Appl Environ Microbiol.* 82(13):4006–4016.

Hamblin, M.R. (2008). The role of nitric oxide in low level light therapy. *Proc of SPIE.* 6846(684602).

Hamblin, M.R. and Demidova, T.N. (2006). Mechanisms of low level light therapy. *Proc of SPIE.* 6140(612001):1–12.

Hanson, R.R. (2005). Management of burn injuries in the horse. *Vet Clin North Am Equine Pract.* 21(1):105–123.

Hawkins, D. and Abrahamse, H. (2006). The role of laser fluence in cell viability, proliferation, and membrane integrity of wounded human skin fibroblasts following helium-neon laser irradiation. *Lasers Surg Med.* 38(1):74–83.

Huang, P.J. *et al.* (2007). In vitro observations on the influence of copper peptide aids for the LED photoirradiation of fibroblast collagen synthesis. *Photomed Laser Surg.* 25(3):183–190.

Huang, S. *et al.* (2023). The parameters affecting antimicrobial efficacy of antimicrobial blue light therapy: a review and Prospect. *Biomed.* 11(4):1197.

Jacobs, K.A. *et al.* (1984). Comparative aspects of the healing of excisional wounds on the leg and body of horses. *Vet Surg.* 13(2):83–90.

Karu, T. (1998). Primary and secondary mechanisms of the action of monochromatic visible and near infrared radiation on cells. In: *The Science of Low Power Laser Therapy*, pp. 53–94. Gordon and Breach Science Publishers, London.

Karu, T. (1999). Primary and secondary mechanisms of action of visible to near-IR radiation on cells. *J Photochem Photobiol B.* 49(1):1–17.

Karu, T. and Kolyakov, S.F. (2005). Exact action spectra for cellular responses relevant to phototherapy. *Photomed Laser Surg.* 23(4):355–361.

Kilik, R. *et al.* (2014). Effect of equal doses achieved by different power densities of low-level laser therapy at 635 nm on open skin wound healing in normal and diabetic rats. *Biomed Res Int.* 2014:269253.

Kuffler, D.P. (2016). Photobiomodulation in promoting wound healing: a review. *Regen Med.* 11(1):107–122.

Larkin, K.A. *et al.* (2012). Limb blood flow after class 4 laser therapy. *J Athl Train.* 47(2):178–183.

Leibovich, S.J. and Ross, R. (1975). The role of macrophage in wound repair: a study with hydrocortisone and antimacrophage serum. *Am J Pathol.* 78(1):71–100.

Leite, S.N. *et al.* (2015). Phototherapy improves wound healing in rats subjected to high-fat diet. *Lasers Med Sci.* 30 (5):1481–1488.

Li, J. *et al.* (2003). Angiogenesis in wound repair: angiogenic growth factors and the extracellular matrix. *Microsc Res Tech.* 60(1):107–114.

Liekens, S. *et al.* (2001). Angiogenesis: regulators and clinical applications. *Biochem Pharmacol.* 61(3):253–270.

Lorenz, H.P. and Longaker, M.T. (2008). Wounds: biology, pathology, and management. In: *Surgery – Basic Science and Clinical Evidence*, pp. 191–208. Springer, New York.

de Loura Santana, C. *et al.* (2015). Tissue reponses to postoperative laser therapy in diabetic rats submitted to excisional wounds. *PLoS One.* 10(4):e0122042.

de Loura Santana, C. *et al.* (2016). Effect of laser therapy on immune cells infiltrate after excisional wounds in diabetic rats. *Lasers Surg Med.* 48(1):45–51.

Lubart, R. and Breitbart, H. (2000). Biostimulative effects of low-energy lasers and their implications for medicine. *Int J Drug Dev Res.* 50(3–4):471–475.

Macedo, A.B. *et al.* (2015). Low-level laser therapy (LLLT) in dystrophin-deficient muscle cells: effects on regeneration capacity, inflammation response and oxidative stress. *PLoS One.* 10(6):e0128567.

Martin, P. and Leibovich, S.J. (2005). Inflammatory cells during wound repair: the good, the bad and the ugly. *Trends Cell Biol.* 15(11):599–607.

Medrado, A.R. *et al.* (2003). Influence of low level laser therapy on wound healing and its biological action upon myofibroblasts. *Lasers Surg Med.* 32(3):239–244.

Meireles, G.C. *et al.* (2008). Effectiveness of laser photobiomodulation at 660 or 780 nm on the repair of third-degree burns in diabetic rats. *Photomed Laser Surg.* 26(1):47–54.

Mercandetti, M. and Cohen, A.J. (2015). Wound healing and repair. Medscape. Available from: http://emedicine.medscape.com/article/1298129-overview (accessed November 30, 2016).

Mester, E. *et al.* (1971). Effect of laser rays on wound healing. *Am J Surg.* 122(4):532–535.

Michael, C.H. *et al.* (2012). Immediate effects of monochromatic infrared energy on microcirculation in healthy subjects. *Photomed Laser Surg.* 30(4):193–199.

Moore, P. (2005). Effect of wavelength on low-intensity laser irradiation-stimulated cell proliferation in vitro. *Lasers Surg Med.* 36(1):8–12.

Mosca, R.C. *et al.* (2019). Photobiomodulation therapy for wound care: a potent, noninvasive, Photoceutical approach. *Adv Skin Wound Care.* 32(4):157–167.

Newton, P.M. *et al.* (2004). Macrophages restrain contraction of an in vitro wound healing model. *Inflammation.* 28(4):207–214.

Nguyen, D.T. *et al.* (2009). The pathophysiological basis for wound healing and cutaneous regeneration. In: *Biomaterials for Treating Skin Loss*, pp. 25–57. Elsevier, Philadelphia, PA.

Nour El Din, S. *et al* (2016). in vitro and in vivo antimicrobial activity of combined therapy of silver nanoparticles and visible blue light against Pseudomonas aeruginosa. *Int. J Nanomedicine* 11(17): 1749–1758.

Oliveira, F.S. *et al.* (2009). Effect of low-level laser therapy (830nm) with different therapy regimes on the process of tissue repair in partial lesion calcaneous tendon. *Lasers Surg Med.* 41(4):271–276.

Paraguassu, G. *et al.* (2014). Effect of laser phototherapy (660nm) on type I and III collagen expression during wound healing in hypothyroid rats: an immunohistochemical study in a rodent model. *Photomed Laser Surg.* 32(5):281–288.

Passarella, S. and Karu, T. (2014). Absorption of monochromatic and narrow band radiation in the visible and near IR by both mitochondrial and nonmitochondrial photoacceptors results in photobiomodulation. *J Photochem Photobiol B.* 140:344–358.

Peplow, P.V. *et al.* (2010a). Laser photobiomodulation of wound healing: a review of experimental studies in mouse and rat animal models. *Photomed Laser Surg.* 28(3):291–325.

Peplow, P.V. *et al.* (2010b). Laser photobiomodulation of proliferation of cells in culture: a review of human and animal studies. *Photomed Laser Surg.* 28(Suppl. 1):S3–S40.

Plass, C.A. *et al.* (2012). Light-induced vasodilation of coronary arteries and its possible clinical implication. *Ann Thorac Surg.* 93(4):1181–1186.

Plavskii, V.Y. *et al.* (2018). Porphyrins and flavins as endogenous acceptors of optical radiation of blue spectral region determining photoinactivation of microbial cells. *J Photochem Photobiol B.* 183:172–183.

Pourreau-Schneider, N. *et al.* (1990). Helium-neon laser treatment transforms fibroblasts into myofibroblasts. *Am J Pathol.* 137(1):171–178.

Reddy, G.K. (2004). Photobiological basis and clinical role of low-intensity lasers in biology and medicine. *J Clin Laser Med Surg.* 22(2):141–150.

Redondo, M.S. (2015). Laser therapy approach to wound healing in dogs. Vet Times. Available from: www.vettimes.co.uk/article/laser-therapy-approach-towound-healing-in-dogs/(accessed November 30, 2016).

Rhee, Y.H. *et al.* (2016). Low-level laser therapy promoted aggressive proliferation and angiogensis through decreasing of transforming growth factor-β1 and increasing of AKT/hypoxia inducible factor-1α in anaplastic thyroid cancer. *Photomed Laser Surg.* 34(6):229–235.

Savolainen, H.O. (1993). Effects of continuous wave and pulsed laser on blood coagulation. An in-vitro thromboelastographic study. *Ann Chir Gynaecol.* 82(1):37–41.

Schlager, A. *et al.* (2000). Low-power laser light in the healing of burns: a comparison between two different wavelengths (635 nm and 690 nm) and a placebo group. *Lasers Surg Med.* 27(1):39–42.

Shnitkind, E. *et al.* (2006). Anti-inflammatory properties of narrow-band blue light. *J Drugs Dermatol.* 5(7):605–610.

Simpson, D.M. and Ross, R. (1972). The neutrophilic leukocyte in wound repair-a study with antineutrophil serum. *J Clin Invest.* 51(8):2009–2023.

Singer, A.J. and Clark, R.A.F. (1999). Cutaneous wound healing. *N Engl J Med.* 341(10):738–746.

Song, G. *et al.* (2010). Use of the parabiotic model in studies of cutaneous wound healing to define the participation of circulating cells. *Wound Repair Regen.* 18(4):426–432.

Stadelmann, W.K. *et al.* (1998). Physiology and healing dynamics of chronic cutaneous wounds. *Am J Surg.* 176(2A Suppl):26S–38S.

Stadler, I. *et al.* (2001). 830-nm irradiation increases the wound tensile strength in a diabetic murine model. *Lasers Surg Med.* 28(3):220–226.

Stashak, T.S. (1989). Management of lacerations and avulsion injuries of the foot and pastern region and hoof wall cracks. *Vet Clin North Am Equine Pract.* 5(1):195–220.

Stashak, T.S. and Theoret, C.L. (2008). Physiology of wound healing. In: *Equine Wound Management*, pp. 5–29. Wiley-Blackwell, Ames, IA.

Szymczyszyn, A. *et al.* (2016). Effect of the transdermal low-level laser therapy on endothelial function. *Lasers Med Sci.* 31(7):1301–1307.

Takenori, A. *et al.* (2016). Immediate pain relief effect of low level laser therapy for sports injuries: randomized, double-blind placebo clinical trial. *J Sci Med Sport.* S1440 S2440 (16):30002–30010.

Takhtfooladi, M.A. *et al.* (2015). Effect of low-level laser therapy (685 nm, 3 J/cm^2) on functional recovery of the sciatic nerve in rats following crushing lesion. *Lasers Med Sci.* 30(3):1047–1052.

Tuby, H. *et al.* (2006). Modulations of VEGF and iNOS in the rat heart by low level laser therapy are associated with cardioprotection and enhanced angiogenesis. *Lasers Surg Med.* 38(7):682–688.

Vasilenko, T. *et al.* (2010). The effect of equal daily dose achieved by different power densities of low-level laser therapy at 635 and 670 nm on wound tensile strength in rats: a short report. *Photomed Laser Surg.* 28(2):281–283.

Versteeg, H.H. *et al.* (2013). New fundamentals in hemostasis. *Physiol Rev.* 93(1):327–358.

Viegas, V.N. *et al.* (2007). Effect of low-level laser therapy on inflammatory reactions during wound healing: comparison with meloxicam. *Photomed Laser Surg.* 25(6):467–473.

Wang, Y. *et al.* (2017). Antimicrobial blue light inactivation of pathogenic microbes: state of the art. *Drug Resist Updat.* 33–35:1–22.

Werner, S. and Grose, R. (2003). Regulation of wound healing by growth factors and cytokines. *Physiol Rev.* 83(3):835–870.

Wood, V.T. *et al.* (2010). Collagen changes and realignment induced by low-level laser therapy and low-intensity ultrasound in the calcaneal tendon. *Lasers Surg Med.* 42(6):559–565.

Woodruff, L.D. *et al.* (2004). The efficacy of laser therapy in wound repair: a meta-analysis of the literature. *Photomed Laser Surg.* 22(3):241–247.

Wu, Z.H. *et al.* (2010). Mitochondrial signaling for histamine release in laser-irradiated RBL-2H3 mast cells. *Lasers Surg Med.* 42(6):503–509.

Yadav, A. *et al.* (2016). Photobiomodulation effects of superpulsed 904 nm laser therapy on bioenergenetics status in burn would healing. *J Photochem Photobiol B.* 162:77–85.

Young, S.R. *et al.* (1990). Effect of light on calcium uptake by macrophages. *Laser Ther.* 5:53–57.

33

Laser Therapy in Equine Rehabilitation

Steve Adair

Department of Large Animal Clinical Science, University of Tennessee, College of Veterinary Medicine, Knoxville, TN, USA

Introduction

LASER is an acronym for light amplification by stimulated emission of radiation (Wikipedia, 2024a). A laser is a device that produces light that is coherent, collimated (parallel), and monochromatic (Wikipedia, 2024a). Lasers may be used in a wide range of applications, from bar code scanners to surgical lasers. Lasers use this light to stimulate various body processes such as waste removal, reduction of swelling, increased tissue repair processes, biostimulating effects, and stimulation of wound healing (Hamblin *et al.*, 2017). Currently, the most common term used to describe the use of lasers in tissue healing and regeneration is photobiomodulation (PBM) (Wikipedia, 2024b). Other terms that may be used colloquially are low-level laser therapy (LLLT) and high-intensity laser therapy (HILT). This chapter discusses the use of lasers in equine rehabilitation.

Lasers used in equine rehabilitation are classified based on their ability to cause ocular damage (Wikipedia, 2024a). The following are the most common classes of lasers used in equine rehabilitation:

Class 1M – safe under all conditions of normal use (Figure 33.1).
Class 3B – can cause immediate eye damage upon exposure (Figure 33.2).
Class 4 – can burn skin; in some cases, even scattered light from these lasers can cause eye and/or skin damage (Figure 33.3).

The wavelengths of light used for laser therapy fall between 600 and 1070 nm (Chung *et al.*, 2012). Wavelengths in the range of 600–700 nm are used to treat superficial tissue, and longer wavelengths in the range of 780–950 nm, which penetrate further, are used to treat deeper-seated tissues (Chung *et al.*, 2012). As a general rule, the higher the wavelength, the deeper the penetration of laser photons. However, it should be noted that there is a decrease in penetration depth in the range of 970–990 nm due to increased chromophore and water absorption (Hamblin and Demidova, 2006; Hamblin *et al.*, 2017). Duesterdieck-Zellmer *et al.* evaluated penetration of laser light using a Class 4 laser (800 & 970 nm wavelength) in an ex-vivo model (Duesterdieck-Zellmer *et al.*, 2016). They found that most of the laser energy was absorbed or scattered by the skin. Only 1–20% and 0.1–4% of energy were absorbed by SDFTs (superficial digital flexor tendons) and DDFTs (deep digital flexor tendons), respectively, depending on skin color, skin thickness, and applied wavelength. Ryan and Smith, using an 810 nm laser, found that when applying laser to a subcutaneous structure in the horse, the area should be clipped and cleaned beforehand (Ryan & Smith, 2007). They also found that laser light transmission was not affected by individual horse, coat color, or leg. However, it was associated with the condition of the leg (clipped). Limbs clipped dry and cleaned with alcohol were associated with greater transmission of light than the unprepared limbs. They recommended that the area to be treated should be clipped and cleaned beforehand. Luna *et al.* evaluated the penetration of a Class 1 and Class 4 laser in equine skin (Luna *et al.*, 2020). They found that the Class 1 device provided a greater penetration than a Class 4 laser in unclipped light and dark skin, suggesting that the former may produce a better therapeutic clinical effect (Luna *et al.*, 2020).

Laser therapy has also been subjectively divided into LLLT and HILT primarily based on the energy output (Ahmad *et al.*, 2022). Lasers with an energy output of <500 mW (Class 1, 2, 3) are considered low-level lasers while lasers with an energy output of >500 mW (Class 4) are considered high-intensity lasers. Both LLLT and HILT can use many of the same wavelengths, though HILT lasers

Laser Therapy in Veterinary Medicine: Photobiomodulation, Second Edition. Edited by Christopher J. Winkler and Lisa A. Miller.

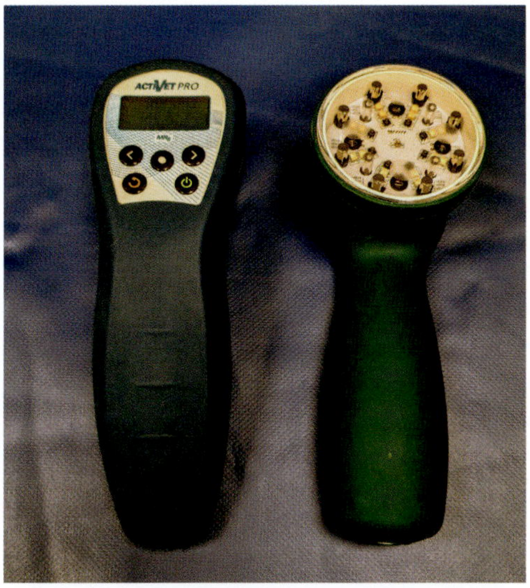

Figure 33.1 Class 1M laser (Steve Adair (Chapter Contributor)).

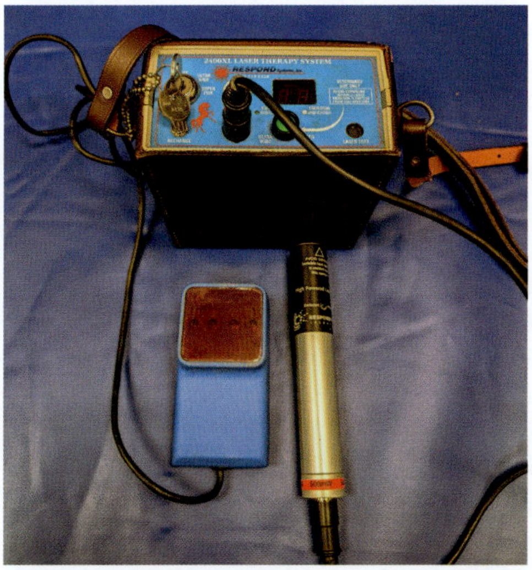

Figure 33.2 Class 3B laser (Steve Adair (Chapter Contributor)).

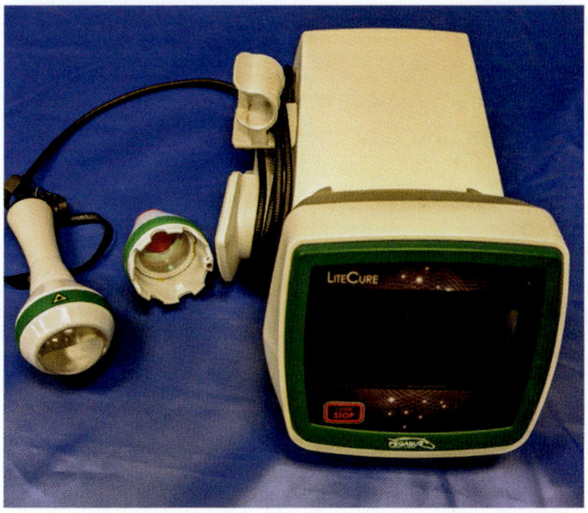

Figure 33.3 Class 4 laser (Steve Adair (Chapter Contributor)).

usually will have longer wavelengths. LLLT lasers generally do not have a thermal effect, while HILT does, meaning extra care must be taken not to damage tissue due to the photothermic effect. Most of the recent research on horses uses HILT.

PBM in Equine Literature

Much of the literature on laser usage in the horse pertains to surgical conditions. The literature pertaining to the use of therapeutic lasers in the horse is sparser and often has conflicting results. The efficacy of laser therapy in treating different conditions is unclear. Zielinska *et al.* using HILT found that an efficient photothermal effect can be achieved in skin with a nonclipped coat, but that clipping the treatment area increases photobiostimulation of the tissue, while reducing the photothermal effect (Zielińska *et al.*, 2020). These authors also found that while it reduces joint pain and lameness grade, it poorly limits joint discomfort after a flexion test is performed (Zielińska *et al.*, 2023b). Pluim *et al.* evaluated healing of experimentally induced suspensory branch lesions following HILT and showed improved healing compared to conservative therapy (Pluim *et al.*, 2020, 2022). However, Rushing reviewed the literature looking at the effects of HILT on suspensory ligaments and concluded that the two studies they evaluated provided only weak evidence to show that horses treated with both HILT and conservative management return to primary function sooner than horses treated with conservative management alone (Rushing, 2023). Pluim *et al.* using HILT reported a decrease in lameness and improvement in ultrasound scores within 2 weeks of starting therapy in 150 sports horses with either a tendinopathy or desmopathy (Pluim *et al.*, 2018). They also reported a decrease in re-injury rate. Ahmed *et al.* evaluated the effects of a Class 1M laser on equine longissimus and gluteal muscles and found that LLLT has a positive effect on horse muscles that showed a change in their firing frequency that is equal with changes seen with analgesia in subjects experiencing pain (Ahmed *et al.*, 2021). Zielinska *et al.* evaluated the effect of HILT on equine longissimus muscle and skin temperature and found it increased skin temperature and decreased longissimus muscle pain, as shown by decreased withdrawal from digital palpation (Zielińska *et al.*, 2023a). Haussler *et al.* found that LLLT produced significant reductions in back pain, epaxial muscle hypertonicity, and trunk stiffness (Haussler *et al.*, 2020). The effect of high-intensity lasers on tendon and ligaments injuries has shown that it promoted analgesic and anti-edema effects, with visual lameness reduction in horses with tendon and ligament injuries, and reduced lesion percentage, but did not influence change in lesion echogenicity (Zielińska *et al.*, 2020). Kidtiwong *et al.* found that HILT in superficial flexor tendonitis had the ability to reduce inflammation but had no effect on reducing the cross-sectional area of the treated tendon (Kidtiwong *et al.*, 2022). Michanek *et al.* found no effect of LLLT on experimentally created equine wounds (Michanek *et al.*, 2021). Freeman *et al.* conducted a literature review on factors that influenced equine wound healing and found there is currently insufficient evidence to figure out whether laser therapy provides benefits in wound healing in the horse (Freeman *et al.*, 2021). Peat *et al.* evaluated the effect of irradiating mesenchymal stem cells (MSC) with a 1064 nm laser; they found that 1064 nm irradiation shows promise in the photobiomodulation of MSCs to enhance their therapeutic properties (Peat *et al.*, 2018). In a 2023 review on laser therapy, Millis and Berg found conflicting results and unclear application for clinical use (Millis & Bergh, 2023). They concluded that although some beneficial effects were reported for light therapy, the studies also had limited scientific quality regarding these therapies, with a high or moderate risk of bias. Many of the aforementioned studies provide potential evidence that both LLLT and HILT may be beneficial in treating various conditions found in the equine. However, it is important to recognize the limitations of these studies and that well-designed clinical trials are necessary with correctly and consistently reported parameters. Many of the studies in current literature either fail to report the laser parameters adequately or do so incorrectly, making it difficult to evaluate the quality of the study.

Dosimetry

Laser therapy dosage is described as energy density at the tissue surface. This measurement is also known as the fluence and is expressed in Joules/cm^2 (J/cm^2). When determining dose, an area wider than the injured tissue should be treated. We treat 1–2 cm outside of the boundary of the affected structure. One should measure the area to be treated and then decide the fluence you will use. As an example, if you want to deliver 10 J/cm^2 to a 100 cm^2 area you would multiply 100 by 10 to arrive at a total dose of 1000 J that must be delivered. You should treat in a grid pattern and keep the laser perpendicular to the skin surface. Ideally, you should treat in on-contact fashion, as this will improve the depth of penetration. However, for some conditions (i.e., wounds), noncontact may be preferred. The dose needed for a particular condition is dependent on several factors, including the anatomical area, the laser used, and the wavelength.

We do not use set protocols based on specific clinical conditions. Instead, we base our dose and treatment frequency on depth of lesion, size of lesion, and whether the condition is acute or chronic. The more superficial a tissue, the less energy is needed. In our practice, we use 4–8 J/cm^2 for superficial lesions (i.e., wounds); 8–15 J/cm^2 for tendons and ligaments; and 15–35 J/cm^2 for deep muscles (Riegel, 2018). The frequency of treatment is case dependent. For postsurgical applications, we typically treat daily for 2–4 days. For acute conditions, we typically treat daily until a response is noted. Then we decrease to every-other-day treatment until resolution of signs. For chronic conditions, we follow a similar treatment frequency as for an acute condition, and then decrease to the minimum needed to maintain a positive clinical response. In our practice, the most common use of laser therapy is to decrease pain and inflammation associated with musculoskeletal injuries both before and during the rehabilitation process and for wound healing. We also use lasers in conjunction with injection of orthobiologics because of its biostimulatory effect. In this case, we follow a similar frequency to postsurgical applications.

When selecting proper dosages some guidance can be obtained from the literature. Chen *et al.*, using a GaAs laser (820 nm) and InGaAs, P laser (635 nm) with a power output of 40 mW and a pulsed frequency rate of 50 Hz found the best dose to stimulate porcine tenocytes in culture was 2 J/cm^2 (Chen *et al.*, 2009). Duesterdieck-Zellmer *et al.* found that 1–20% and 0.1–4% of energy was absorbed by SDFTs and DDFTs, respectively, depending on skin color, skin thickness, and applied wavelength (Duesterdieck-Zellmer *et al.*, 2016). By extrapolating these figures to clinical use we use 8–15 J/cm^2 for treating tendonitis of the SDFTs and DDFTs, using a multi-wavelength (810–980 nm) high-intensity laser. This dose is also used for treating desmitis. For tendonitis of the SDFT or suspensory branch lesion we would use 10 J/cm^2 and for a DDFT or mid-body suspensory ligament lesion we would go with 15 J/cm^2 (Figure 33.4). We would typically treat once daily until a response is noted and then every other day until resolution of signs. Following the injection of an orthobiologics we would use similar dosages but would treat immediately following the injection and then daily for an additional 3–4 days.

We typically use 20–30 J/cm^2 for treatment of muscle pain (Figure 33.5). This is supported by work from Zielinska *et al.*, who showed a reduction in longissimus muscle pain using 20 J/cm^2 (Zielińska *et al.*, 2023a). The thicker the muscle, the higher the total energy that is delivered (total joules). For acute pain we typically treat daily until a response is seen, then every other day until pain is gone.

The application of laser light to equine wounds is controversial. Michanek *et al.* found no effect on experimentally induced wounds when using 637 and 956 nm wavelength

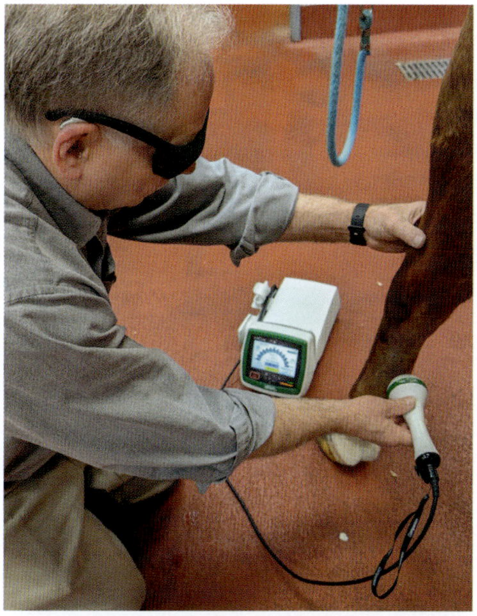

Figure 33.4 Class 4 laser being used to treat superficial digital flexor tendonitis (Steve Adair (Chapter Contributor)).

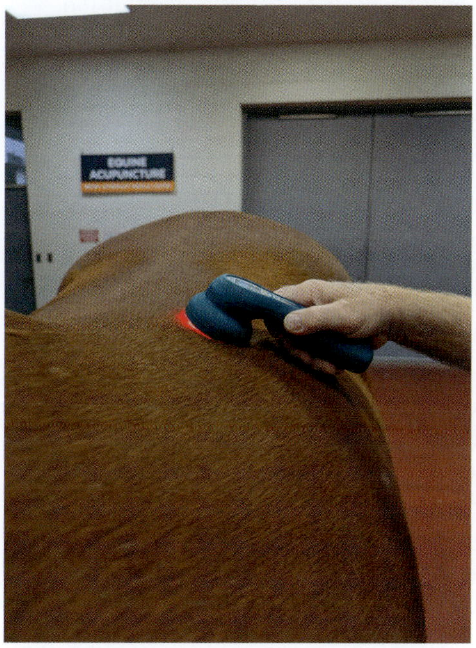

Figure 33.5 Class 1M laser being used to treat longissimus muscle pain (Steve Adair (Chapter Contributor)).

light emitting diodes (delivering 0.2 and 1.2 J/cm^2 for each wavelength, respectively) (Michanek *et al.*, 2021). However, Hoisang *et al.* showed a significant effect in treating chronic wounds in dogs using an 830 nm laser with a fluence of 4 J/cm^2 (Hoisang *et al.*, 2021). Lopez and Brundage reviewed the literature dealing with wound photobiomodulation and

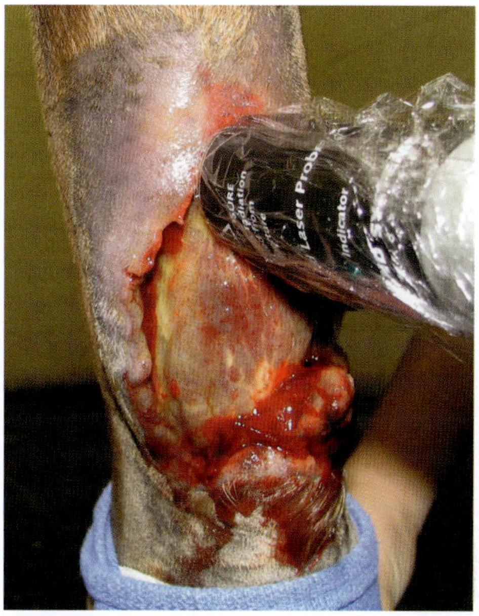

Figure 33.6 Class 3B laser being used to treat wound over flexor tendons. Note the sterile plastic wrap covering laser head for protection (Steve Adair (Chapter Contributor)).

also found conflicting results in the equine – one study that showed benefit used a fluence of 5.1 J/cm^2 and a wavelength of 635 nm, while another study that showed no effect used 2 J/cm^2 and a wavelength of 830 nm (Lopez & Brundage, 2019). Based on these studies, we typically use a higher fluence of 6 J/cm^2 and a multi-wavelength laser. We treat daily until we note evidence of epithelization, and then every other day until most of the wound is epithelized. We treat the entire surface of the wound, using sterile plastic wrap over the laser head to protect both the wound and the laser (Figure 33.6). Once the wound is epithelized, we stop treatment.

When performing laser therapy, adequate safety precautions must be observed. Proper signage and eye protection should be used, based on the class of the laser and its wavelength. Individuals using the laser should have appropriate laser safety training. This is mandatory at our facility, and if a person has not been trained, they are not allowed into the room where laser therapy is being performed. While signage and eye protection are unnecessary for Class 1M lasers, we have a blanket policy that they must be used regardless of the class of laser. Further information on safety is included in Chapter 5.

Conclusion

The use of photobiomodulation therapy in equine rehabilitation is becoming more common place. Alongside the application of cold, PBM is also valuable to treat inflammation that occurs not only in the acute condition but also any inflammation that may occur during the rehabilitation process. Additionally, because of its ability to stimulate growth factors and regenerative cells, it is beneficial during the healing process of different tissues and especially following the administration of biological products. The one thing that is lacking is appropriate dosage protocols. At this time, dosages are arbitrary or have been adapted from other animal models or human medicine. This approach often leads to dosage regimes that are often inadequate or in some cases excessive. There is a need to have well-designed clinical trials in the horse that establish a set dosage protocol based on the condition being treated, the laser wavelength and its fluence. Standard protocols must be instituted and all researchers need to report the protocols used in parameters accepted by the laser community. Researchers should also utilize quantifiable measurements when evaluating response. It is very important that the studies be designed such that they can be repeated by other researchers. Only by doing the aforementioned can we be assured that appropriate dosimetry is being used regardless of the laser.

References

Ahmad, M.A. *et al.* (2022). Effects of low-level and high-intensity laser therapy as adjunctive to rehabilitation exercise on pain, stiffness and function in knee osteoarthritis: a systematic review and meta-analysis. *Physiotherapy*. 114:85–95. doi:10.1016/j.physio.2021.03.011.

Ahmed, W. *et al.* (2021). An investigation into the short-term effects of photobiomodulation on the mechanical nociceptive thresholds of *M. longissimus* and *M. gluteus* medius, in relation to muscle firing rate in horses at three different gaits. *J Equine Vet*. 98:103363. doi:10/gmd6mn.

Chen, C.-H. *et al.* (2009). Low-level laser irradiation promotes cell proliferation and mRNA expression of type I collagen and decorin in porcine Achilles tendon fibroblasts *in vitro*. *J Orthop Res*. 27(5):646–650. doi:10.1002/jor.20800.

Chung, H. *et al.* (2012). The nuts and bolts of low-level laser (light) therapy. *Ann Biomed Eng*. 40(2):516–533. doi:10.1007/s10439-011-0454-7.

Duesterdieck-Zellmer, K.F. *et al.* (2016). Ex vivo penetration of low-level laser light through equine skin and flexor tendons. *Am J Vet Res*. 77:991–999. doi:10.2460/ajvr.77.9.991.

Freeman, S.L. *et al.* (2021). BEVA primary care clinical guidelines: wound management in the horse. *Equine Vet J*. 53(1):18–29. doi:10.1111/evj.13289.

Hamblin, M.R. and Demidova, T.N. (2006). Mechanisms of low level light therapy. *Proceedings SPIE* 6410 614001 http://proceedings.spiedigitallibrary.org/proceeding.aspx?articleid=1276129 (Accessed: 1 February 2013).

Hamblin, M.R. *et al.* (2017). *Handbook of Low-level Laser Therapy*. Pan Stanford publishing, Singapore.

Haussler, K.K. *et al.* (2020). Effects of low-level laser therapy and chiropractic care on back pain in quarter horses. *J Equine Vet*. 86:102891. doi:10.1016/j.jevs.2019.102891.

Hoisang, S. *et al.* (2021). Assessment of wound area reduction on chronic wounds in dogs with photobiomodulation therapy: a randomized controlled clinical trial. *Vet World*:2251–2259. doi:10/gmnqhn.

Kidtiwong, A. *et al.* (2022). Superficial digital flexor tendinitis treatment using high-intensity laser therapy and therapeutic ultrasound in polo ponies. *Vet Integr Sci*. 20(2):253–266. doi:10.12982/VIS.2022.020.

Lopez, A. and Brundage, C. (2019). Wound photobiomodulation treatment outcomes in animal models. *J Vet Med*. 2019:e6320515. doi:10.1155/2019/6320515.

Luna, S.P.L. *et al.* (2020). Penetration profiles of a class IV therapeutic laser and a photobiomodulation therapy device in equine skin. *J Equine Vet*. 85:102846. doi:10.1016/j.jevs.2019.102846.

Michanek, P. *et al.* (2021). Effect of infrared and red monochromatic light on equine wound healing. *Equine Vet J*. 53(1):143–148. doi:10.1111/evj.13266.

Millis, D.L. and Bergh, A. (2023). A systematic literature review of complementary and alternative veterinary medicine: laser therapy. *Animals*. 13(4):667. doi:10.3390/ani13040667.

Peat, F.J. *et al.* (2018). *In vitro* effects of high-intensity laser photobiomodulation on equine bone marrow-derived mesenchymal stem cell viability and cytokine expression. *Photomed Laser Surg*. 36(2):83–91. doi:10.1089/pho.2017.4344.

Pluim, M. *et al.* (2018). Short- and long term follow-up of 150 sports horses diagnosed with tendinopathy or desmopathy by ultrasonographic examination and treated with high-power laser therapy. *Res Vet Sci*. 119:232–238. doi:10.1016/j.rvsc.2018.06.003.

Pluim, M. *et al.* (2020). High-power laser therapy improves healing of the equine suspensory branch in a standardized lesion model. *Front Vet Sci*:7 Available at: https://www.frontiersin.org/article/10.3389/fvets.2020.00600 (Accessed: 3 June 2022).

Pluim, M. *et al.* (2022). Histological tissue healing following high-power laser treatment in a model of suspensory ligament branch injury. *Equine Vet J*. 54(6):1114–1122. doi:10.1111/evj.13556.

Riegel, R.J. (2018). *Laser Therapy in Veterinary Medicine: Photobiomodulation*. John Wiley & Sons Inc., Chichester, West Sussex; Hoboken, N.J.

Rushing, J. (2023). Does high-intensity laser therapy speed return to primary function in horses with suspensory ligament desmopathy? *Vet Evid.* 8(1). doi:10.18849/ve.v8i1.564.

Ryan, T. and Smith, R.K.W. (2007). An investigation into the depth of penetration of low level laser therapy through the equine tendon *in vivo*. *Ir Vet J.* 60(5):295–299.

Wikipedia. (2024a). "Laser." Available at: https://en.wikipedia.org/w/index.php?title=Laser&oldid=1207944925 (Accessed: 1 March 2024).

Wikipedia. (2024b). "Low-level laser therapy." Available at: https://en.wikipedia.org/w/index.php?title=Low-level_laser_therapy&oldid=1210691587 (Accessed: 1 March 2024).

Zielińska, P. *et al.* (2020). Effects of high intensity laser therapy in the treatment of tendon and ligament injuries in performance horses. *Animals.* 10(8):1327. doi:10/gmv8kq.

Zielińska, P. *et al.* (2023a). A preliminary study of the influence of high intensity laser therapy (HILT) on skin surface temperature and longissimus dorsi muscle tone changes in thoroughbred racehorses with back pain. *Animals.* 13(5):794. doi:10.3390/ani13050794.

Zielińska, P. *et al.* (2023b). A case series of 11 horses diagnosed with bone spavin treated with high intensity laser therapy (HILT). *J Equine Vet.* 120:104188. doi:10.1016/j.jevs.2022.104188.

34

Laser Therapy in Food-Animal Practice

Julie Gard Schnuelle

Department of Clinical Sciences, Auburn University College of Veterinary Medicine, Auburn, AL, USA

Introduction

In the past, food-animal medicine has relied heavily on antibiotics for therapeutic treatments and disease prevention (Patel *et al.*, 2020). Antibiotics have been utilized extensively to prevent and/or treat postoperative infections, infections following traumatic injuries, and systemic infections. Antibiotics kill the bacteria and/or prevent bacterial replication, resulting in a removal of the infection. Antibiotics can decrease wound healing times by preventing infection, inflammation, and pain. Not every antimicrobial utilized in animals is utilized in humans. However, it has been stated that widespread antibiotic usage in food-producing animals may contribute to antibiotic-resistant infections in humans (Patel *et al.*, 2020). Antibiotic-resistant infections are a global threat and were responsible for an estimated 1.27 million deaths in people worldwide and 35 000 deaths in the United States in 2019 (CDC, 2019). The US Food and Drug Administration's (FDA) Center for Veterinary Medicine (CVM) developed a multipronged, multiyear strategy designed to slow the emergence of resistance arising from the use of antibiotics in animals, while continuing to ensure the availability of safe and effective antibiotics for use in animals and humans (FDA, 2022a). The strategy seems to be working with the number of domestic sales of antimicrobials in food-producing animals decreasing by 36% from 2015 to 2022 (FDA, 2022b). Antimicrobial resistance is a serious issue, and even though strategies have made inroads, there is a tremendous need for investigation of alternative therapies to further reduce antibiotic usage.

Consumers are looking for food and products that do not have added drugs, hormones, or antibiotics. The increased market share of organically produced food has highlighted these consumer expectations. When utilizing antimicrobials or drugs in food-producing animals, a meat and/or milk withdrawal time will result; dairy cattle that are given a drug such as Banamine® (Flunixin meglumine) will result in the nonsaleable milk from that cow for 48 hours, while cattle will not be able to be slaughtered for meat for 8 days following administration of Banamine. This is an increased cost to the producer.

Alternative therapies in livestock and food-producing animals have thus grown in popularity, as they do not result in antimicrobial resistance or withdrawal times. Examples of popular alternative therapies include hyperbaric oxygen therapy (HPOT). HPOT causes an increase in the amount of oxygen flow to areas of the body to increase healing. The cost of HPOT causes a barrier for use in food-producing animals, except in the case of seed stock producers where the animals are worth considerably more than commercial stock. Photobiomodulation therapy (PBMT, or laser therapy) is a popular alternative therapy that can aid in healing and pain relief without consequential drug withdrawal or promotion of antibiotic resistance. PBMT has been utilized in human and companion animal medicine for years to aid in the reduction of pain caused by various conditions from traumatic injuries to chronic conditions such as arthritis. There have been multiple studies confirming its positive effects on the reduction and control of pain in humans and animals (Moore & Calderhead, 1991; Boerner *et al.*, 1996; Bjordal *et al.*, 2006; Sattayut & Bradley, 2012; Cotler *et al.*, 2015). Consumers are demanding changes in food-animal farming practices that focus on animal welfare, and therapies that promote healing, reduce pain, and promote animal well-being. PBMT is thus a practice that focuses on animal welfare.

Laser therapy has historically been well received by owners of companion animals, such as small animals and equines, but its use in food animals has not been utilized as widely. However, food animals that are of higher value genetically, organically produced, or bucking stock are more likely to receive PBMT. Utilization within the

Laser Therapy in Veterinary Medicine: Photobiomodulation, Second Edition. Edited by Christopher J. Winkler and Lisa A. Miller.

commercial animal sector has increased and will continue to increase as familiarity with the equipment grows and consistent clinical results are clearly shown. PBMT has not been utilized in food animals to the extent that it has been with companion animals, but it is starting to be seen, especially in cattle, swine, camelids, sheep, and goats.

General Applications of PBMT in Food-Animal Medicine

The general applications of PBMT are similar to what is utilized in other species. Since there is a similarity in most conditions, it is easy to extrapolate the multitude of benefits seen in the equine species to cattle, swine, camelids, sheep, goats, deer, and exotic ruminants. These applications include acute inflammatory conditions such as mastitis, postoperative edema, traumatic injuries, and chronic painful conditions such as osteoarthritis.

Traumatic injuries occur in all species and often necessitate cleansing, immediate surgical closure, or monitored second-intention healing. The standard of care includes antibiotic therapy, pain management, cleansing, debriding, and bandaging. Hydrotherapy, osmotic soaks, and poultices, along with systemic anti-inflammatory drug administration, are routinely instituted to manage edema within or surrounding a wound. PBMT has been shown in numerous case and clinical studies to decrease healing times by elevating blood flow to the injured site, increasing lymphatic drainage, and stimulating fibroblast migration into the site (Márquez Martínez *et al.*, 2008; Kuffler, 2016). Often, PBMT is utilized as an adjunctive therapy to promote healing of wounds. The blood supply to a wound is increased when PBMT is applied to an area (Maegawa *et al.*, 2000). Increasing the blood supply and oxygenation is imperative to increasing wound healing and preventing secondary bacterial growth from bacteria such as *Clostridia* spp. that proliferate in an anaerobic environment. Cattle, sheep, goats, and horses are very predisposed to *Clostridia* diseases, so improving the circulation and oxygenation to the traumatized tissue is preventative as well as therapeutic.

In cases of mastitis, such as with *Escherichia* coli (*E. coli*), endotoxins are released, causing severe inflammatory reactions and vasoconstriction. Mastitis is an extremely painful condition. Dairy cows and dairy sheep and goats are the most predisposed to *E. coli* mastitis. Utilization of PBMT is quite beneficial in cases of mastitis, especially early in the course of the disease, as it minimizes the inflammatory reaction and increases the blood supply. Wang *et al.* (2014) investigated the effects of laser therapy on a rat model of lipopolysaccharide-induced mastitis and its underlying molecular mechanisms. They demonstrated that the number of polymorphonuclear (PMN) cells in the mammary alveolus and the myeloperoxidase activity were decreased after laser therapy (Wang *et al.*, 2014). These results suggest that laser therapy is beneficial in decreasing somatic cell count (primarily made up of PMN cells) and improving milk nutritional quality in cows with an intramammary infection. PBMT has the added benefit, in food-animal patients, of having no withdrawal times.

Application Techniques Unique to Food-Animal Species

Food animals pose additional challenges beyond those encountered when treating companion animals with PBMT. Domesticated cattle, sheep, goats, and swine often do not mind human touch, and usually do not resist the contact of the therapy laser handpiece. However, food animals require different levels of restraint, even though they are domesticated. Beef cattle, especially bucking stock, are not as easy to handle as dairy cattle. Sedation may be necessary if an animal is extremely fractious, as is seen with bucking stock or in exotic animals and wildlife such as deer. Additional restraint and sedation may also be necessary if the animal is extremely sensitive around the area being treated, such as a postoperative area or an area such as the foot, which poses a hazard to the operator. Initiate laser therapy utilizing a noncontact technique to acclimate the patient to the sensation of the laser. Follow up with hand contact, and finally treat using an on-contact technique with the laser handpiece touching the skin.

Each food-animal species has unique considerations when applying PBMT. The presence of any organic debris, the thickness and color of the hair coat or wool, and the color and thickness of the skin and underlying tissues all need to be considered when determining the dosage to be administered, the power required for penetration, the administration technique, and the frequency of treatments. Cleaning of all organic debris within the area requiring treatment, even the lanolin in sheep's wool, is a stringent requirement before successful administration of PBMT.

The thickness of cattle hide can be problematic. Administration at a higher power level, utilizing longer treatment times, and treating more frequently is often necessary to achieve penetration to the target cells in cattle. The teat skin is an exception to this statement and is much thinner than the rest of the hide, so it will require a lower power setting and a shorter treatment time. In sheep, the wool is especially problematic and will have to be sheared unless the area does not have wool (such as the mammary gland). Goats may also have to be sheared as necessary. Objections may be raised from the client, such as with a show animal.

In short, there are unique conditions present in all species of food animals that require common sense and good judgment to ensure consistent clinical results.

Dosing

In the food-animal field, there are many body types, body conditions, body colors, hair coat lengths (e.g., sheep versus pigs), and hair coat colors. The goal of PBMT is to administer a safe dose to the skin, sufficient to penetrate through all the unique anatomical structures of the patient that cause a loss of irradiance, and produce a physiological response within the target tissues.

There is wide range of individual characteristics to consider. Examples are the umbilicus of the newborn lamb versus the lumbosacral spine of a 275 kg Duroc boar, post-umbilical herniation in a piglet versus spondylosis in a Holstein bull, and a laceration on the shoulder of an alpaca versus a laceration on the shoulder of an Angus bull. There are no scientific evidence-based research papers identifying specific dosages for any of the food-animal species. The mantra for the application of PBMT in any of the food animals is "dose to effect." The dosages recommended in Table 34.1 are based on a collection of anecdotal clinical cases and cross-species extrapolation. They are a general guide from which estimates of an appropriate dosage can be made on a case-by-case basis.

Table 34.1 Dosages for PBMT of food animals, by species.

					Dose (J/cm^2)	
Species	**Patient**	**Weight (lb)**	**Weight (kg)**	**Skin hair coat color**	**Superficial**	**Deep**
Bovine (beef)	Adult	1200–1500	545–680	Black	10–15	15–25
				Light	8–10	12–20
	Yearling	450–650	205–295	Black	8–12	12–20
				Light	8–10	10–15
	Calf	60–75	27–34	Black	6–8	8–12
				Light	4–8	6–10
Bovine (dairy)	Adult	1200–1650	545–748	Black	12–20	20–23
				Light	10–15	15–25
	Yearling	400–800	181–362	Black	8–15	20–25
				Light	8–12	12–20
	Calf	60–85	27–39	Black	6–10	10–15
				Light	6–8	8–12
Camelid (llama)	Adult	250–450	113–205	Black/dark	8–10	10–12
				Light	6–8	8–10
	Cria	20–30	9–14	Black/dark	4–6	6–8
				Light	2–4	4–6
Camelid (alpaca)	Adult	110–190	50–86	Black/dark	6–8	8–12
				Light	4–6	6–10
	Cria	18–20	8–9	All	2–4	4–8
Caprine	Adult doe	140–170	63–77	Black/dark	6–8	8–12
				Light	4–6	6–8
	Adult buck	170–190	77–86	Black/dark	8–10	10–12
				Light	6–8	8–10
	Kid	4–120	2–54	Black/dark	2–8	4–10
				Light	2–4	4–6
Ovine	Adult	160–220	73–100	All	8–10	10–15

(Continued)

Table 34.1 (Continued)

Species	Patient	Weight (lb)	Weight (kg)	Skin hair coat color	Dose (J/cm²) Superficial	Deep
	Lamb	90	90	All	6–8	8–10
	Birth lamb	5–80	2–36	All	2–4	4–6
Porcine	Adult	280–500	127–227	All	8–10	10–20
	Shoat	20–120	9–54	All	4–6	6–8
	Pig	1–20	0.5–9.0	All	2–4	4–6

These dosages are a general guide from which estimates of an appropriate dosage can be made on a case-by-case basis. Reevaluate before each therapy laser session and apply an appropriate dosage within the suggested ranges. If clinical improvement is not seen within three sessions, increase the dosage. Clipping of the hair coat greatly decreases the required dosage.

Some general dosing guidelines are applicable in almost all food-animal species.

When to Increase the Suggested Dosage

- The animal has black pigmented skin and the hair coat cannot be clipped (e.g., black Angus show stock).
- Treating any of the bovine breeds with very thick skin. Thicker skin requires more energy to be administered so that an effective amount can reach the target tissues and produce a clinical response.
- Applying laser therapy to any of the ovine species that are not shorn. There is a great deal of energy lost within the thick, dense layer of wool, even with a baby lamb. Lanolin is also present, which will absorb a portion of the administered photons.
- There is an excessive amount of edema and swelling, as with mastitis and postpartum edema.
- The target cells are beneath thick layers of either adipose or muscle tissues.
- Applying laser therapy to areas where excessive granulation tissue has already formed.

When to Decrease the Suggested Dosage

- Treatment is applied directly over the bed of an open wound.
- Treating very young stock.

Numerous therapy lasers on the market are preprogrammed with software containing preset protocols for many different maladies in different species. Often, similar anatomical areas and circumstances exist between the equine or companion-animal protocol and that of food animals.

Most wound protocols are based on the area of the wound, and their application is therefore almost universal across species. Postoperative application of PBMT to surgical incisions is similar regardless of species. The use of preprogrammed software protocols for wounds and postoperative treatment of incisions can provide an initial dosage recommendation; adjustments can then be made during each subsequent reevaluation.

Treatment of acute musculoskeletal injuries such as torn tendons and ligaments and of chronic conditions such as osteoarthritis and back pain in both bucking and breeding stock is highly beneficial. The equine or companion-animal software protocols for similar anatomical areas are a good place to start. Preset protocols for osteoarthritis in horses are very similar to those required for cattle, though an increase is usually warranted due to the thicker skin (increase the total dosage 25%). The equine preset protocols for the lumbosacral spine can be used for the treatment of both acute and chronic back pain in bucking stock and aged bovine breeding stock. Preset protocols for tendonitis and other soft-tissue injuries are comparable between species. Laminitis is not just a problem in the equine species, and since it is seen in the bovine, ovine, caprine, and porcine species, preset protocols for equine laminitis can be used here, too.

Conditions Responsive to PBMT in Food Animals

There are numerous acute conditions such as mastitis, udder edema, traumatic injuries, foot rot, lacerations, and postoperative edema, as well as chronic conditions, such as osteoarthritis in stifle and fetlock joints, that benefit from PBMT.

Foot Conditions

Acute and chronic laminitis occurs not only in horses but also in cattle, sheep, goats, and pigs. Laser therapy can be applied as an adjunctive treatment in all laminitis cases. The laser beam should be directed at the coronary band around the foot, at the bulbs of the heel, and at the medial portion of the coronary band in the interdigital space for cattle, sheep, goats, wild and exotic ruminants, and pigs.

A similar method is applied for the treatment of foot rot in cattle, except that the treatment area should include the entire pastern and the fetlock. The area to be treated should continue more proximally if swelling has progressed to that level. Utilizing PBMT for cases of soft soles or abscess on the solar surface of the foot can be beneficial. Abscesses can be treated off-contact with a similar technique to that used for a wound in the equine species (see Chapters 29–33).

Mastitis and Udder Edema

Mastitis and udder edema are two interrelated conditions for which PBMT has been demonstrated to be efficacious (Wang *et al.*, 2014). In food animals, PBMT is used to treat mastitis and udder edema most commonly in dairy cattle and dairy sheep and goats. In a recent study, the effect of laser treatment along with antibiotics on mastitis on dairy cows was evaluated. Cows with local and systemic signs of mastitis were treated with either intramuscular injections of approved antibiotics in label doses alone (controls) or with the same intramuscular treatment protocol and laser irradiation (STP-99 laser) of inflamed glands for 5 consecutive days (2 minutes a day). The laser head was kept at 10 cm under the treated area and the depth of penetration of the laser beam exceeded 70 cm. Pulse wave variable frequency and length was 1 second, and peak radiated power was a maximum of 1.5 W. Laser irradiation significantly ($p < 0.05\%$) increased the recovery rate by 31.2% and 16.6% above intramammary treatment alone and systemic antibiotic treatment alone, respectively (Malinowski *et al.*, 2019).

Beneduci *et al.* (2007) also found that the application of PBMT was an aid in the treatment of cows with mastitis. Beneduci *et al.* (2007) reported a significant decrease in milk somatic cell counts following use of PBMT on mastitic mammary glands with a STP-8 laser once a day for 30 seconds for 5 days. Somatic cell counts above 50.000 cells/mL are routinely utilized as an indicator of subclinical and/or clinical mastitis in lactating dairy cows. Somatic cells increase in mastitis due to an increase of white blood cells, especially neutrophils, within the mammary gland. The white blood cells are recruited to fight off the infection within the gland. However, with abrupt decreases in milk production, the dilution of the somatic cells decreases resulting in an increase in somatic cell count. Hence, increased somatic cell counts are not always an indicator of mastitis. Malinowski *et al.* (2019) reported an increase in milk somatic cell counts following application of PBMT. The increase in somatic cell counts in the study was attributed to a biostimulating effect of the laser by accelerating blood and lymph circulation. An increase in the margination of white blood cells, stage of mastitis, and/or concurrent decrease in the amount of milk produced could all contribute to these findings.

A study by Fenyő *et al.* (2008), found that the application of linearly polarized light to the mammary gland of cattle significantly increased milk production while decreasing the somatic cell counts of the milk. The positive effects of laser therapy on the mammary gland are highlighted in this study (Fenyő *et al.*, 2008).

Mastitis is an incredibly painful condition of the udder. The severity and frequency of mastitis in companion animals are quite low in comparison to those in dairy animals. Early detection and frequent milking or stripping of the udder is of utmost importance in the treatment of this condition. PBMT can be utilized to reduce pain, increase the blood supply and lymphatic drainage, and reduce edema. This allows a more complete, less painful milking and stripping of the udder.

Most veterinary-specific therapy lasers with software protocols have a setting for "edema and swelling" that can be used on an udder with mastitis and edema. However, the udder can be quite large, so often the quarters in cattle, or halves in sheep, goats, and camelids should be treated separately. Additionally, the udder needs to be treated frequently, at least twice daily until the mastitis resolves. The ideal approach is to administer a portion of the PBMT dose immediately before milking, to aid in milk let down and emptying of the quarter. Before it is extracted from the quarter, the liquid milk is yet another layer of density that is photo absorbing. When milk is present, it absorbs photons, and fewer reach the target tissue (mammary alveoli). Therefore, an additional dosage of PBMT following milking is indicated to effectively treat the affected tissue.

Administration of PBMT concurrently with massage is beneficial for the stimulation of milk let down, which is often inhibited by the pain associated with mastitis. Some laser therapy equipment emits its energy through optics contained within a rolling massage-ball handpiece. This is an ideal application handpiece for mastitis since it combines the delivery of photonic energy with massage. If there are areas where hard, turgid, edematous tissue is present, these need to be treated at a higher dosage, administered at a higher power, more frequently and for longer periods. PBMT administered to these tissues, using this massage technique, will stimulate a release of oxytocin, further improving milk let down.

Dosages administered to the udder are governed by the color of the skin (black versus white), the hair coat length (long versus short or clipped), and the mass and density of the tissue. An udder with both black skin and hair will require a higher dosage, since the pigment is an incidental absorber of photons and will prevent some of the energy from penetrating to the target tissue. Immediately postpartum, when the udder is usually very edematous, a higher dosage is needed. Dosages for patients with shorter hair, lighter skin and hair color, and less dense udders should start at 12 J/cm^2. Dosages for patients with longer hair, dark skin or hair, or dense mammary tissue can be as high as 20 J/cm^2.

One suggested protocol for dairy cattle with mastitis begins with 2 mL of oxytocin given IV immediately prior to milking out the udder. Then following milking, apply 7 minutes of treatment of a wavelength blend of 808 and 980 nm, at a fluence of 10 J/cm^2, an irradiance of 2.24 W/cm^2, at 12 W continuous wave (CW) power, for a total of 5040 total joules to each quarter affected by mastitis in an area (about 500 cm^2 in size, on all sides surrounding the udder). Treat as much of the area of teat cistern, annular ring, gland cistern, and milk ducts as possible utilizing an on-contact method with a large deep tissue applicator (large contact treatment head), in a continuously moving grid pattern at a speed of 1–3 in./second (2.5–7.5 cm/second). The teat of the infected quarters should be included in the treatment area but should be treated off-contact, with the applicator held 1–2 in. (2–5 cm) from the skin while using a scanning motion as the area is treated, so as not to contaminate the teat itself with any bacteria on the surface of the treatment head.

Reproductive Applications

The use of PBMT to increase fertility has not been thoroughly explored. However, anything that can be done to minimize lameness will increase fertility. It has been shown that lameness has a negative effect on conception rates (Bicalho *et al.*, 2007). Utilizing PBMT on the vulvar lips postpartum to decrease swelling, and on any lacerations of the vulvar lips, is beneficial. Vaginal or cervical prolapse, preputial lacerations, preputial edema, preputial abscesses, and post-castration edema are other conditions that benefit from PBMT. Additional case studies and clinical research need to be performed with food animals to scientifically evaluate the benefits of PBMT in this area.

Swelling and Edema

Cattle, like horses, develop a significant amount of ventral edema, especially following wounds or suture lines located on the ventrum of the body. Livestock spend a great deal of time standing, adding to the amount of edema. Preputial lacerations in bulls, stallions and geldings are good examples of wounds that result in a collection of severe ventral edema surrounding them. Traditionally, hydrotherapy and Epsom salt soaks are often employed twice daily with wrapping and elevation of the prepuce to help manage this swelling and edema in bulls. In addition to the hydrotherapy, PBMT accelerates the reduction of swelling and edema. Fresh wounds on the prepuce should be treated off-contact, administering a dosage of 5–10 J/cm^2 twice daily, if possible, followed by 10–12 J/cm^2 on-contact to the surrounding margins of the laceration, to prevent or help relieve the accumulation of ventral edema. When the patient can tolerate on-contact therapy directly over the laceration, this administration technique should be used throughout the entire area of the wound and surrounding tissues. The benefits of administering PBMT to these types of lesions are vasodilation and an increase in the blood supply, increased lymphatic drainage, and relief of pain. Administer therapy for this type of edema and swelling twice a day for 3–4 days, and then once a day until resolution.

Conclusion

PBMT is a primary or adjunctive therapy that can provide acceleration of wound healing and significant pain relief in cattle, small ruminants, camelids, pigs, and wild and exotic ruminants. Additionally, utilization of PBMT does not require withdrawal times, because there is no drug residue within the tissues. This is extremely beneficial in the organic food-production industry, where the use of any drugs is strictly prohibited.

Utilization of PBMT will continue to grow in the food-animal industry as veterinarians, producers, and owners realize the multiple benefits this modality can provide.

References

Beneduci, A. *et al.* (2007). Evaluation of the effects induced by near infrared low intensity laser radiation on bovine affected by subacute mastitis: a simple-quarter foremilk sampling study. *J Anim Vet Adv.* 6:761–767.

Bicalho, R.C. *et al.* (2007). Visual locomotion scoring in the first seventy days in milk: impact on pregnancy and survival. *J Dairy Sci.* 90(10):4586–4591.

Bjordal, J.M. *et al.* (2006). Low-level laser therapy in acute pain: a systematic review of mechanisms of action and clinical effects in randomized placebo-controlled trials. *Photomed Laser Surg.* 24(2):158–168.

Boerner, E. *et al.* (1996). Double-blind study on the efficacy of the laser therapy. *Proc SPIE.* 2929:75–79.

CDC (2019). *Antibiotic Resistance Threats in the United States*. U.S. Department of Health and Human Services, Atlanta, GA https://www.cdc.gov/drugresistance/national-estimates.html#:~:text=In%20the%20U.S.%2C%20more%20than,Resistance%20(AR)%20Threats%20Report. (Accessed 03/05/2024).

Cotler, H.B. *et al.* (2015). The use of low level laser therapy (LLLT) for musculoskeletal pain. *MOJ Orthop Rheumatol.* 2(5):00068.

Fenyő, M. *et al.* (2008). Effect of polarized light treatment on milk production and milk somatic cell count of cows. *Acta Vet Brno.* 77:225–229.

Food and Drug Administration (FDA) (2022a). FDA-TRACK: Progress on FDA's support of antimicrobial stewardship in veterinary settings. https://www.fda.gov/about-fda/fda-track-agency-wide-program-performance/fda-track-progress-fdas-support-antimicrobial-stewardship-veterinary-settings (Accessed 03/05/2024).

Food and Drug Administration (FDA) (2022b). *Summary Report on Antimicrobials Sold or Distributed for Use in Food-Producing Animals*. U.S. Department of Health and Human Services, Rockville, MD Available from URL: https://www.fda.gov/animal-veterinary/antimicrobial-resistance/2022-summary-report-antimicrobials-sold-or-distributed-use-food-producing-animals. Accessed 03/05/2024.

Kuffler, D.P. (2016). Photobiomodulation in promoting wound healing: a review. *Regen Med.* 11(1):107–122.

Maegawa, Y. *et al.* (2000). Effects of near-infrared low-level laser irradiation on microcirculation. *Lasers Surg Med.* 27(5):427–437.

Malinowski, E. *et al.* (2019). The effect of low intensity laser irradiation of inflamed udders on the efficacy of antibiotic treatment of clinical mastitis in dairy cows. *Vet Ital.* 55(3):253–260. doi:10.12834/VetIt.818.3989.2 PMID: 31599550.

Márquez Martínez, M.E. *et al.* (2008). Effect of IR laser photobiomodulation on the repair of bone defects grafted with organic bovine bone. *Lasers Med Sci.* 23(3):313–317.

Moore, K. and Calderhead, R.G. (1991). The clinical application of low incident power density 830 nm gallium aluminum arsenide diode laser radiation in the therapy of chronic intractable pain. *Int J Opto Electronics.* 6(5):503–520.

Patel, S.J. *et al.* (2020). Antibiotic stewardship in food-producing animals: challenges, progress, and opportunities. *Clin Therio.* 42:1649–1658.

Sattayut, S. and Bradley, P. (2012). A study of the influence of low intensity laser therapy on painful temporomandibular disorder patients. *Laser Ther.* 21(3):183–192.

Wang, Y. *et al.* (2014). Low-level laser therapy attenuates LPS-induced rats mastitis by inhibiting polymorphonuclear neutrophil adhesion. *J Vet Med Sci.* 76(11):1443–1450.

Part VIII

Laser Therapy and Alternative and Regenerative Therapies

35

Laser Acupuncture

Ronald B. Koh

UC Davis School of Veterinary Medicine, Davis, CA, USA

Introduction

Laser acupuncture (LA), a modern extension of the ancient Chinese medical practice, has been gaining attention in both human and veterinary medicine. It integrates the principles of traditional acupuncture with the technological advancements of photobiomodulation therapy (PBMT), and it has been defined as "photonic stimulation of acupuncture points and areas to initiate therapeutic effects similar to that of needle acupuncture and related therapies together with the benefits of photobiomodulation (PBM)" (Litscher, 2018). Its noninvasive, pain-free approach is increasingly being integrated into veterinary settings, offering an innovative modality particularly suitable for small and zoological companion animals, as well as for those averse to needles or have difficulty remaining still for acupuncture treatments. Additionally, LA is an advantageous option for treating patients with severe comorbidities or those with increased risks of complications such as bleeding and infection. In addition, the duration of LA treatment is generally shorter, allowing for the stimulation of more acupoints, potentially enhancing overall treatment efficacy. As LA is a specialized branch of acupuncture, practitioners must possess knowledge of both the anatomical locations and the clinical indications of acupuncture points (acupoints). This knowledge is critical for optimizing the effectiveness of LA treatments.

While traditional acupuncture has ancient roots, LA emerged much more recently, in the early 1970s, following the invention of the laser beam in the 1960s and its surgical application shortly thereafter (Litscher, 2020). Friedrich Plog, a German-Canadian physician, is recognized for pioneering LA around 1973, exploring its nonsurgical applications soon after lasers became available for medical use (Jang *et al.*, 2019). His published work extensively elaborates on the methodology and application of LA (Plog, 1980, pp. 21–37) Since its initial clinical use, LA has seen rapid development and global research interest. There is substantial evidence supporting its application in treating conditions of humans such as myofascial pain, postoperative nausea and vomiting, knee osteoarthritis, chronic low-back pain, musculoskeletal pain, and nocturnal enuresis (Baxter *et al.*, 2008; Law *et al.*, 2015; Glazov *et al.*, 2016; Chen *et al.*, 2019; Hung *et al.*, 2021; Peixoto *et al.*, 2023; da Silva Mira *et al.*, 2024; Di Francesco *et al.*, 2024). In veterinary medicine, several clinical studies have established the efficacy of LA as an adjunct therapy in managing postsurgical pain in dogs and cats, along with chronic back pain in horses (Tomacheuski *et al.*, 2020; Nascimento *et al.*, 2019, Klide & Martin Jr, 1989, pp. 1375–1379).

Background of Acupuncture

Acupuncture, a key component of Traditional Chinese Medicine (TCM) and Traditional Chinese Veterinary Medicine (TCVM), is a time-honored medical practice. It involves inserting thin needles into the skin at strategic points to treat various conditions, alleviate pain, and promote overall health (Xie & Preast, 2007, pp. 3–15; Xie & Chrisman, 2009, pp. 1–4). The earliest known documentation of acupuncture appears in "*Huangdi Neijing*" (The Yellow Emperor's Inner Classic of Medicine), dating from roughly 475 to 225 BCE (Xie & Chrisman, 2009, pp. 1–4). The practice also extends to animals, with "*Bo Le Zhen Jing*" (Bole's Canon of Veterinary Acupuncture), the oldest known veterinary acupuncture text, authored by Dr. *Bo Le* in the period between 659 and 621 BCE (Song & Xie, 2012, pp. 5–6). Acupuncture for animals now includes a broad range of species and has seen substantial growth in recent decades due to increased research into its mechanisms and benefits for various conditions such as pain,

Laser Therapy in Veterinary Medicine: Photobiomodulation, Second Edition. Edited by Christopher J. Winkler and Lisa A. Miller.

musculoskeletal diseases, intervertebral disc disease, nausea and vomiting, behavioral problems, and reproductive disorders (Roynard *et al.*, 2018; Wright, 2019; Holyoak & Ma, 2022; Huntingford & Petty, 2022; Repac *et al.*, 2022; Koh & Harrison, 2023). In recent years, veterinary medicine programs in academic institutions have created an integrative medicine curriculum that includes acupuncture as an integral part of patient care in disease management (Memon *et al.*, 2021).

There are several techniques for the stimulation of acupoints, such as dry needling (DN), electroacupuncture (EA), aquapuncture (AA), and LA, as well as through moxibustion and material implantation (Xie & Preast, 2007, pp. 332–336; Koh & Harrison, 2023). Each of these methods has a distinct therapeutic objective. DN is the most common technique. It is the practice of inserting fine, sterile needles of varying gauges (28–36) and lengths (0.25–1.5 in.) into specific acupoints, where they are retained for 10–30 minutes. EA enhances acupoint stimulation by delivering electrical currents through inserted needles, typically over 10–30 minutes, and is particularly noted for its extended analgesic properties. It is especially effective in treating neuralgia, nervous system injuries, and chronic pain. EA at lower frequencies (2–10 Hz) is more efficacious in reducing inflammatory pain and in mitigating allodynia/hyperalgesia caused by nerve injuries than higher frequencies (100 Hz). AA involves the injection of a small volume of sterile fluid into the acupoints, such as saline or vitamin B_{12}, and is often employed subsequent to DN or EA to extend the stimulation effects. LA utilizes laser therapy to emit light that penetrates tissue to stimulate acupoints. Moxibustion is a technique that uses the heat from burning mugwort herb to stimulate acupoints.

Mechanisms of Action

The mechanism of acupuncture is intricately linked to the concept of the neural acupuncture unit (NAU), which provides a modern understanding of this ancient practice (Zhang *et al.*, 2012). The NAU encompasses a network of critical components within the body's tissue matrix, including free nerve endings, mast cells, autonomic and somatic nerve fibers, encapsulated cutaneous receptors, and sensory receptors found in muscles and tendons, such as muscle spindles and tendon organs (Zhang *et al.*, 2012). This structure is further supported by microcirculatory elements that can be visualized using electron microscopy (Wright, 2019). When an acupuncture needle is inserted into an acupoint, it activates the NAU, triggering a cascade of biological responses. This activation leads to the release of various neurotransmitters and inflammatory mediators such as endorphins and enkephalins, which have potent analgesic effects, as well as corticosteroids that modulate the immune response. By stimulating these NAUs, acupuncture can influence the nervous system, thereby altering pain perception, reducing inflammation, and initiating the healing processes that address a range of physiological imbalances.

Growing evidence demonstrates that acupuncture provides pain relief in animal models by triggering several bioactive substances via mechanisms at the peripheral, spinal, and supraspinal levels (Zhang *et al.*, 2014). Peripherally, acupuncture induces analgesic effect locally, primarily due to the release of adenosine, which acts as an antinociceptive neuromodulator (Goldman *et al.*, 2010). This process involves adenosine's inhibition of pain signals at adenosine A1 receptors on nociceptive nerve endings. Additionally, acupuncture can enhance local analgesia through mechanisms such as the upregulation of CB2 receptors (CB2R), reduction of prostaglandin E2 (PGE2) synthesis, and downregulation of cyclooxygenase-2 (COX-2) in inflamed tissues (Lee *et al.*, 2006; Su *et al.*, 2011). Furthermore, at the needle insertion site, acupuncture induces a micro-traumatic environment that triggers immunobiological responses, leading to the reduction of proinflammatory cytokines (e.g., IL-1β, TNF-α, and IL-6) and recruiting mast cells and macrophages to release bioactive molecules (e.g., histamine, serotonin, etc.) (Cui *et al.*, 2021). These processes collectively contribute to reducing inflammation, alleviating pain, and promoting healing, with the immunobiological effects potentially lasting beyond the immediate period of needle retention.

At the spinal level, acupuncture stimulates the release of spinal neurotransmitters such as opioids, serotonin, norepinephrine, and acetylcholine, potentially reducing the excitability of nerve cells in the dorsal horn, which is responsible for processing pain signals. Simultaneously, acupuncture inhibits the spinal transmission of pain signals by suppressing the activity of cytokines, glutamate, glial cells, and substance P, along with downregulating N-methyl-D-aspartate (NMDA) receptors, known to be pivotal in the pain pathway (Zhang *et al.*, 2014; Tahir *et al.*, 2021). At the supraspinal level, the brain's role in acupuncture's pain mitigation is intricate due to the complex nature of pain regulation and perception within the neural network. However, existing research indicates that acupuncture contributes to pain relief in the brain by several mechanisms (Kong *et al.*, 2013; Zhang *et al.*, 2014; Dewey & Xie, 2021; Tahir *et al.*, 2021): (i) altering the somatosensory cortex, which affects the sensory dimension of pain; (ii) stimulating the hypothalamus to release β-endorphin into the cerebrospinal fluid and bloodstream; (iii) activating the brainstem's descending pain inhibitory pathways; and (iv) reducing activity within the limbic system, thereby providing analgesic and calming effects.

LA employs red or near-infrared light with wavelengths between 600 and 1000 nm and power levels ranging from 5 to 500 mW (Hu et al., 2013). Typically, LA deposits 0.1–0.5 J/cm^2 at each acupoint or 1–4 J/cm^2 at Ashi points, potentially stimulating therapeutic benefits (Hu et al., 2013). While LA shares similarities with traditional acupuncture, its precise mechanisms are not yet entirely clear. It is thought that the therapeutic effects of LA might be attributed to the phenomenon of PBM, which is potentially amplified at acupoints due to their specialized characteristics. These characteristics may include higher levels of neural components, skin nitric oxide (NO), and neuronal nitric oxide synthase (nNOS) at the acupoints in contrast to non-acupoint areas, suggesting that acupoints have a distinct bioactive profile that could influence the efficacy of PBM (Ma, 2017). PBM is known to increase the local release of NO, reduce inflammation, stimulate ATP production, and regulate neuro-immune interactions (Hamblin, 2017), which can be particularly impactful when applied to acupoints with their specialized neuro-immune connections (Jiang *et al.*, 2017a). These acupoints may have an increased capacity to influence the body's healing processes, thus amplifying the therapeutic effects of PBM through mechanisms that involve neuro-immune regulation, angiogenesis, and cellular respiration (Li *et al.*, 2021). A study observed that LA results in a dose-dependent increase in NO release at specific acupoints (PC4, PC5). The experiment utilized a 658 nm near-infrared laser with intensities of 12, 24, and 48 mW over durations of 20, 40, and 60 minutes. A slight increase in NO at non-acupoints after 40 minutes suggests a general PBM effect. In contrast, the acupoints showed more than a twofold increase in NO release with 24 and 48 mW applications compared to non-acupoints, with the most efficient NO release at 24 mW. This finding indicates that the LA-induced release of NO is specific to acupoints and is dose-dependent. (Jiang *et al.*, 2017b).

Clinical Evidence

In the medical field, LA is emerging as a promising noninvasive modality (Hu et al., 2013; Chon *et al.*, 2019). Specifically, moderate-quality evidence supports its use in managing musculoskeletal and myofascial pain with minimal side effects in humans (Baxter *et al.*, 2008; Law *et al.*, 2015). This method also extends to veterinary medicine, demonstrating a viable and safe option for managing pain and other conditions in animals. Current research, while indicative of positive outcomes and safety, points to the need for more extensive, randomized controlled clinical trials to verify the efficacy of LA in animals. Additionally, the development and implementation of standardized treatment protocols including LA parameters are essential. Such measures would ensure the optimal therapeutic impact of LA for our companion animals, maintaining consistency and quality of care across the veterinary setting.

Human Research

Clinical research has revealed the efficacy of LA in a range of treatments. A 2008 systematic review suggested that LA provides a moderate level of evidence to alleviate myofascial pain and reduce postoperative nausea when administered with specific parameters, including a power of at least 10 mW and dosage starting from 0.5 J per point for pain and 0.3 J per point for nausea (Baxter *et al.*, 2008). A 2019 study found LA beneficial for osteoarthritis knee pain, although the effects may wane over time; the review called for more detailed analysis of LA's technical parameters (Chen *et al.*, 2019). A 2021 meta-analysis reported LA's notable success in reducing musculoskeletal pain and improving overall physical function, with variable wavelengths from 632.8 to 980 nm and power from 4 to 200 mW delivering energy from 0.275 to 43.2 J per acupoint, significantly outperforming placebo treatments (Hung *et al.*, 2021).

Another review endorsed LA for temporomandibular disorders (TMD), emphasizing its safety and efficacy in reducing chronic pain and improving jaw function. Common acupoints targeted were LI4, ST6, and ST7, with wavelengths between 690 and 810 nm, power density ranging from 0.76 to 240 W/cm^2, energy dose ranging from 0.375 to 26.25 J/cm^2, and duration of irradiation ranging from 5 seconds to 15 minutes (da Silva Mira *et al.*, 2024). Despite variations in LA parameters, LA was shown to be a viable option for TMD, offering pain relief and increased mobility without adverse effects. Recent systematic reviews and meta-analyses have bolstered the evidence suggesting that both traditional acupuncture and LA are more effective than placebos in in reducing TMD-associated chronic pain and improving mouth opening range (Peixoto *et al.*, 2023; Di Francesco *et al.*, 2024). Overall, LA is increasingly recognized as a potentially superior alternative to placebos for managing TMD symptoms, suggesting its value as an adjunct therapy for TMD.

Equine Research

In a study by Martin and Klide in 1987, the effectiveness of low-powered infrared laser stimulation of acupoints was investigated as a noninvasive treatment for chronic back pain in horses. The study involved 14 horses that had been suffering from chronic back pain ranging from 4 to 48 months and had not seen significant improvements from other treatments. These horses underwent treatment involving the stimulation of nine specific acupoints (T2, T4, TLR, T10, and HLIO, with T2 being the only nonbilateral point), using a low-powered infrared laser, characterized by a gallium-aluminum arsenide semiconductor with a power output of 300 μW, wavelength of 904 nm, and frequency of 360 Hz, with each point treated for 2 minutes. The treatments were administered weekly. On average, after 11 sessions, 10 out of the 14 horses showed a reduction in clinical signs of back pain, three showed no change, and one was lost to follow-up. Remarkably, a year after the treatments ceased, 9 of the 10 improved horses continued to perform at levels deemed satisfactory by their owners (Martin Jr & Klide, 1987).

In 1989, the research team continued their investigations into chronic back pain in horses over durations ranging from 2 to 108 months. The study was conducted on three groups of horses, each treated with different acupuncture methods: needle acupuncture ($n = 15$), LA ($n = 15$), and injection (saline) acupuncture ($n = 15$). The treatment frequency was once per week, with an average of 8 sessions for needle acupuncture, 11 sessions for LA, and 9 sessions for injection acupuncture. LA was performed following the parameters established in previous studies (Martin Jr & Klide, 1987). Posttreatment observations revealed that 37 horses experienced relief from pain symptoms and could resume training and competition: 13 in the needle acupuncture group, 11 in the LA group, and 13 in the injection acupuncture group. The results suggested that all three acupuncture modalities were comparably effective in mitigating chronic back pain in horses (Klide & Martin Jr, 1989, pp. 1375–1379).

A 2021 study evaluated the effectiveness of LA versus therapeutic ultrasound (TU) for treating chronic lower back pain in sport horses. The horses, diagnosed with such pain, were divided into two groups: one received high-intensity LA, and the other received TU applied to the lower back (T-18 to sacroiliac joint). The selected acupoints for LA were BL21, BL23, BL25, BL26, and *Bai-hui*, with either 1 W for 12 seconds per point, or 2 W for 6 seconds per point, providing a total of 12 J per acupoint and an energy density of 12 J/cm^2. After eight treatments every other day, both LA and TU significantly reduce lower back pain in sport horses measured by acupoint sensitivity scan and pressure algometry (Mongkolrat *et al.*, 2021).

A 2011 case series provided potentials on the efficacy of combining local laser therapy with LA to address pain relief, lameness improvement, and wound healing in horses suffering from laminitis. The study involved 21 horses undergoing low-level laser therapy (LLLT) applied both directly to acupoints and topically to the hoof to promote microcirculation and aid in abscess demarcation. Utilizing two different laser units emitting the same wavelength of 904 nm, a 90 W impulse laser probe and a 40 W impulse laser pen were used to stimulate acupoints (TH1, PC9, LU9, BL40, LIV8, KID7, GB41, TH5, BL18, BL23, and LIV13) for 20 seconds each. Acute cases received treatments every 2–3 days until a significant reduction in pain was observed, then spaced out to weekly sessions. Additionally, the affected hooves were treated with wet dressings containing aluminum acetate and arnica tincture. The outcomes showed notable improvements, with the average pain score decreasing significantly from 3.52 pretreatment to 1.14 posttreatment, highlighting the potential benefits of the combined application of LLLT and LA on laminitis in horses, and suggesting a necessity for more comprehensive studies to investigate their therapeutic effects in greater depth (Petermann, 2011, pp. 13–25).

Further work by Dr. Petermann reinforced the beneficial effects of combining local laser therapy with LA for treating acute and chronic tendinitis in horses, without the need for additional therapies like antibiotics or anti-inflammatories. The treatment involved 29 horses of various ages with conditions such as tendonitis of the superficial digital flexor tendon and suspensory ligament. Using a 904 nm gallium arsenide laser with a 90 W peak pulse power, the laser was applied directly to the affected areas for 1 minute, totaling 6 J of energy. Key acupuncture points SP2, LIV8, GB34, and PC6 were targeted, along with PC9, HT9, LU11/9, GB23, BL18, BL23, and correlating pressure-sensitive points along the spine, each receiving 30 seconds of treatment at 0.5 J per point. This method led to a significant resolution of lameness and restoration of activity levels in 97% of the cases after 6 months, with a continued athletic performance success rate of 90% at one to several years follow-up. These findings support the combined approach of local laser therapy and LA as a potent treatment for tendinopathy in horses (Petermann, 2016, pp. 43–51).

In addition to pain and wound management, LA has also been shown to offer potential benefits for reducing anxiety in horses under stress. In a 2019 study, a randomized controlled crossover trial was performed to assess the anti-anxiety effects of LA on horses. Twenty-four horses were randomly divided into two groups (those receiving LA and those receiving sham acupuncture) and the assigned treatments were exchanged following a 7-day washout interval. LA was performed with a commercial class I laser with an average output of 133 mW delivering 25 W Superpulsed laser light at 905 nm, 875 nm, and 640 nm. Acupoints *An-shen*, GV-24, HT-7, PC-6, BL-14, and BL-15 were stimulated for 1 minute per point at 2 J/cm^2. Key findings included the significantly smaller heart rate increase in response to an acute startle test in horses that received LA compared to the sham group. Additionally, the LA-treated horses exhibited a significantly faster return to baseline heart rate post-stressor. These outcomes suggest that administering LA provides a noninvasive means to promote relaxation and well-being in horses, particularly useful in high-stress situations that are common in the equine sports world or during veterinary interventions (Ying *et al.*, 2019).

Small Animal Research

Marques *et al.*'s study in 2015 provided valuable insights into the effectiveness of LA as a supplemental treatment for postoperative pain management in cats. The study involved 20 cats undergoing an ovariohysterectomy. These cats were then divided into two groups. One group received LA at specific points (bilateral ST-36 and SP-6), while the other (control) group did not receive any LA treatment. Treatment was performed prior to induction of anesthesia. A laser with a 904 nm wavelength and a frequency of 124 Hz was used to deliver energy to the acupoints ST36 and SP6, at a dosage of 3 J/cm^2 for a duration of 9 seconds at each point. Postoperative pain was assessed using validated pain scales (dynamic interactive visual analogue scale, dynamic interactive visual analog scale (DIVAS) and multidimensional composite pain scale (MCPS). The results indicated that both pain scores did not significantly differ between the treatment groups at any time point. However, the LA group required less additional pain medication postsurgery compared with the control group, suggesting that LA could reduce the need for conventional analgesics after an operation in cats (Marques *et al.*, 2015).

The 2019 study by Nascimento *et al.* expanded on previous research by Marques *et al.* (2015) to evaluate the effectiveness of LA and EA for postoperative pain management in cats. This later study was also prospective, randomized, and blinded. Thirty cats undergoing ovariohysterectomy were equally divided into three groups to receive either LA, EA, or no treatment (control group). The acupoints, laser parameters, and pain assessment scores were consistent with those used in the Marques *et al.* study (2015). Pain assessments were conducted within the first 24 hours postsurgery. Results showed no significant differences in both pain scores between the groups at any assessed time point. However, there was a notably higher need for rescue analgesia in the control group compared to the LA and EA groups, indicating that both LA and EA effectively reduced the requirement for additional pain relief. The study concluded that LA in particular offers advantages over EA, being a noninvasive, painless, and simpler application method for pain management in cats postsurgery (Nascimento *et al.*, 2019)

Research on the efficacy of LA in dogs is not widely found, but a preliminary study by Tomacheuski *et al.* in 2020 did address this topic by examining its effectiveness for postoperative pain management in dogs. The study included 16 dogs scheduled for ovariohysterectomy and divided them into two groups. One group received an intramuscular injection of meloxicam at a dosage of 0.2 mg/kg ($n = 8$), while the other group was treated with LA ($n = 8$) on specific acupuncture points including LI4, LIV3, SP6, ST36, and GB34. The parameters for LA were set at a wavelength of 904 nm, frequency of 124 Hz, and energy of 10 J, applied for 100 seconds on each acupoint. Pain levels were assessed using the Glasgow composite measure pain scale (GCMPS) and DIVAS before and for 24 hours following the surgery. The findings indicated that dogs receiving LA had lower pain scores for the entire 24-hour period postsurgery compared to those in the meloxicam group. Additionally, none of the dogs in the LA group required additional rescue analgesia, while three dogs in the meloxicam group did (Tomacheuski *et al.*, 2020). The study highlighted that LA could be as effective as traditional analgesic medication (such as meloxicam) in treating postoperative pain following soft tissue surgeries in dogs. This provides an important insight into multimodal veterinary pain management techniques, especially for animals that may not tolerate traditional medications well, or for owners seeking nonpharmacological options for their pets' care.

A 2019 study assessed the efficacy of EA versus LA for treating dogs with coxofemoral osteoarthritis. Thirty-one dogs with this condition were randomly divided into two groups for the treatment. The LA group received therapy with a Class IV laser directed at the hip acupuncture points BL54, GB29, and GB30. The settings for the laser were 0.4 W power, delivering a total energy of 12 J at a frequency of 10 Hz, for 30 seconds over each point. The EA group was treated at the same points with EA. Both groups received these treatments weekly over an 8-week span. Eight weeks after treatment, both EA and LA treatments significantly improved canine brief pain inventory (CBPI) scores, quality of life assessment, and hip joint range of motion compared to baselines. The EA group exhibited a more pronounced reduction in pain scores than the LA group. This comparison suggests that while both modalities can decrease pain and enhance life quality for dogs with coxofemoral osteoarthritis, EA may offer superior pain relief. Nevertheless, for dogs intolerant to needles, LA may present a viable adjunct for pain management (Chomsiriwat & Ma, 2019, pp. 11–20).

Clinical Indications

LA is frequently utilized in veterinary medicine as a noninvasive, holistic approach primarily for pain management, addressing both acute and chronic pain arising from various conditions, such as postsurgery, musculoskeletal injuries, and neuropathic pain from spinal cord disorders (Martin Jr & Klide, 1987; Klide & Martin Jr, 1989, pp. 1375–1379; Hu et al., 2013; Nascimento *et al.*, 2019; Tomacheuski *et al.*, 2020). In the realm of orthopedic issues, LA is particularly beneficial for conditions such as osteoarthritis, cranial cruciate ligament disease, patellar luxation, and hip or elbow dysplasia. Its capacity to reduce inflammation and alleviate pain makes it a valuable therapeutic option. Moreover, for tendon and ligament injuries, LA's biostimulative effect on tissue regeneration can be crucial in enhancing recovery (Law *et al.*, 2015; Petermann, 2016, pp. 43–51). By promoting cellular repair and improving blood flow, LA aids in reducing recovery times and improving functional outcomes in animals, which is vital for their return to normal activity and quality of life.

Wound care, including injury recovery and postoperative healing, is another common condition treated by LA due to its biostimulative effect, which can expedite the healing process by enhancing cellular activity and improving blood circulation (Ishak *et al.*, 2022; Petermann, 2015, pp. 33–42). Furthermore, this modality is beneficial for the relief of myofascial pain syndrome and trigger points (localized areas of muscle tension that can cause pain and dysfunction) (Chang *et al.*, 2021; Sajedi *et al.*, 2022). By targeting these points, LA can alleviate muscle spasms and restore normal function. This is especially beneficial for performance or athletic animals, where optimal muscle function is essential.

LA is not just limited to pain and wound management; its applications encompass neurological conditions as well. LA may be beneficial in managing spinal cord disorders such as intervertebral disk disease (IVDD) and degenerative lumbosacral stenosis (DLSS), which can otherwise lead to significant pain and mobility issues. LA decreases inflammation, inhibits apoptosis, and mitigates oxidative stress within the spinal cord lesions (On-Ong-Arj *et al.*, 2018). These therapeutic actions contribute to neural repair and functional recuperation, offering a ray of hope for the management of these often debilitating conditions in animals. Furthermore, there is emerging evidence of effects such as reducing anxiety, alleviating symptoms of depression, and improving memory, indicating a promising role for LA in a range of neurological disorders (Quah-Smith *et al.*, 2013; Sutalangka *et al.*, 2013; Ying *et al.*, 2019; Rangel & Pinheiro, 2021).

Overall, LA presents a promising and valuable adjunct or alternative to traditional acupuncture for a variety of conditions affecting animals. It has the potential to not only improve clinical outcomes but also enhance the overall well-being of animals, especially when traditional therapies are not suitable or have proven ineffective. Table 35.1 outlines the wide range of clinical conditions amenable to LA treatment. Additionally, Tables 35.2 and 35.3 detail commonly used acupoints for LA stimulation, tailored for selected conditions in small animals and horses.

Table 35.1 Clinical indications for laser acupuncture (Xie & Preast, 2007, pp. 247–308).

Category/system	Condition/disease
Various types of pain	Acute, chronic, nociceptive, visceral, and neuropathic pain
Musculoskeletal issues	Osteoarthritis, myofascial trigger points, dysplasia, cranial cruciate disease, patellar luxation, iliopsoas strain, tendinopathy, desmopathy, laminitis, navicular diseases, etc.
Neurological disorders	Intervertebral disc diseases, wobbler disease, myelopathy, peripheral neuropathy, facial paralysis, seizures, etc.
Gastrointestinal disorders	Colic, nausea, vomiting, diarrhea, constipation, poor appetite or inappetence, inflammatory bowel disease, megacolon, megaesophagus, pancreatitis, etc.
Dermatological disorders	Otitis, pruritus, allergies, atopy, lick granuloma, chronic wound, pressure sores, etc.
Respiratory disorders	Rhinitis, sinusitis, bronchitis, pneumonia, asthma, laryngeal paralysis or hemiplegia, heaves, chronic obstructive pulmonary disease (COPD), etc.
Behavioral disorders	Fears and phobias, separation anxiety, abnormal repetitive behaviors, aggression, hyperactivity, stereotypic behaviors, cognitive dysfunction
Reproductive disorders	Infertility, impotence, anestrus, low libido, agalactia
Other conditions	Incontinence, anhidrosis, liver diseases, kidney diseases, hyperadrenocorticism, heart diseases, cancer, etc.

Clinical Applications

LA represents a distinctive, cutting-edge therapeutic approach that synergistically integrates the principles of PBM with the ancient art of acupuncture. This integration demands practitioners to possess not only a comprehensive understanding of acupuncture theory, acupoint locations, and their clinical relevance, but also a fundamental grasp of the underlying mechanisms and parameters of PBM. Mastery of these dual aspects is essential to maximize the therapeutic efficacy of LA, ensuring that each treatment is tailored to the patient's unique medical needs.

Table 35.2 Commonly used acupoints for various clinical conditions in small animals (Xie & Preast, 2007, pp. 247–308; Huntingford & Petty, 2022).

Conditions	Common acupoints
Calming effect	GV-20, GV-21, *An-shen, Bai-hui*
General pain and inflammation	LI-4, LI-11, LIV-3, ST-36, BL-60
Dental pain	ST-6, LI-4, LIV-3, ST-36
Bone and arthritic pain	BL-11, BL-23, KID-3; combined with local acupoints
Neck pain or stiffness	GB-20, GB-21, GV-14, SI-3, Jing-jia-ji
Back pain	ST-36, LIV-3, BL-40, *Bai-hui, Hua-tuo-jia-ji*
Shoulder pain	LI-15, LI-4, SI-9, BL-11
Elbow pain	LI-4, LI-10, LI-11, LU-5, SI-9
Carpus pain	LI-4, TH-5, LI-11, SI-9
Coxofemoral or hip pain	GB-29, GB-30, BL-54, BL-40, LIV-3
Stifle pain	ST-35a or 35b, ST-36, GB-34, BL-54, LIV-3
Tarsus pain	BL-60, LIV-3, ST-41, BL-54
General gastrointestinal disorders	BL-20, BL-21, ST-36, LI-10, SP-6; add acupoints for additional signs
Poor appetite or inappetence	*Shan-gen*
Nausea and/or vomiting	PC-6
Diarrhea or constipation	GV-1
Otitis and ear pain	SI-19, LI-11, *An-shen*
Pruritis	GB-20, BL-17, SP-10, *An-shen*
Lick granuloma or wound	Circle the dragon
Rhinitis or sinusitis	LL-4, LI-20, *An-shen*
Cough or asthma	LU-1, BL-13
Incontinence	BL-23, BL-39, CV-3
Seizure or epilepsy	GB-20, GV-20, GV-1, *An-Shen, Nao-shu*
Liver diseases	BL-18, BL-20, LIV-3
Kidney diseases	BL-23, KID-3, SP-6
Heart diseases	BL-15, HT-7
Aging and cognition	ST-36, GV-20, BL-21, GV-4, HT-7

Table 35.3 Commonly used acupoints for various clinical conditions in horses (Xie & Preast, 2007, pp. 247–308; Repac *et al.*, 2022).

Conditions	Common acupoints
Calming effect	GV-20, GV-21, *An-shen, Bai-hui*
Arthritis	KID-1, BL-40, B-60, ST-36, LI-4
Back pain	BL-40, KID-1, *Hua-tuo-jia-ji, Bai-hui, Shen-shu*
Bowed tendons or tendonitis	Front: BL-18, LI-4, PC-9, SI-3 Hind: BL-18, LIV-1, LIV3, GB-34
Laminitis	Front: TH-1, PC-9, LI-3, SI-3, *Qian-ti-men* Hind: KID-1, ST-45, GB-41, LIV-3, *Hou-ti-men*
Navicular disease	PC-9, BL-13, LI-4 SI-9, TH-15
Fetlock pain	SI-3, LI-1, LI-3, SI-9, LI-16
Hip pain	BL-40, *Bai-hui, Huan-tiao, Huan-zhong*
Stifle pain	ST-35, ST-36, BL-40, GB-34, LIV-3
Cervical pain or wobbler syndrome	SI-3, BL-10, KID-1, GB-21, *Jing-jia-ji*
Suprascapular neuropathy (sweeney)	LI-10, LI-15, SI-9, TH-14
General gastrointestinal disorders	BL-20, BL-21, ST-36, LI-10, SP-6; add acupoints for additional signs
Poor appetite or inappetence	*Mi-jiao-gan*
Diarrhea or constipation	GV-1, SP-1
Abdominal pain or colic	BL-20, BL-21, ST-36, *Jiang-ya*
Laryngeal hemiplegia	LI-10, LI-18, GB-21, CV-23, *Hou-shu*
Facial paralysis	ST-4, ST-6, ST-36, LI-4, SI-19
Anhidrosis	LU-11, HT-9, KID-7, LI-11, BL-22
Asthma or COPD	BL-23, BL-26, BL-13, ST-36, *Ding-chuang*
Infertility	CV-4, CV-6, KID-7, BL-26
Impotence or low libido	BL-26, BL-23, KID-3, CV-4
Agalactia	BL-20, SP-6, ST-36, BL-18, SP-10
Poor performance	BL-21, BL-54, *Yan-chi, Qi-hai-shu, Shen- shu*
Aging and senility	ST-36, LI-10, BL-21, GV-4, *Bai-hui*

Generally, acupoints are selected based on a comprehensive evaluation of the patient's specific health conditions, clinical signs, and overall well-being. This process often incorporates the methodologies of TCVM to make a pattern diagnosis or differentiation. The strategic selection of acupoints targets the regulation of *Qi* (vital energy flow) and seeks to harmonize the body's *Yin* and *Yang*, aiming to restore equilibrium and promote healing (Xie & Preast, 2013, pp. 332–336).

The choice of acupuncture points can vary greatly depending on the clinician's experience and the specific condition being treated. Some acupoints are chosen for their local effects on the area of pain or discomfort, while others are selected for their systemic influence on the body's energy pathways. This customized approach may involve a combination of acupoints designed to mitigate the clinical signs and address the underlying cause of the patient's condition. The principle is to offer a tailored treatment plan that caters to the unique needs of each patient, ensuring a holistic approach to restoration and well-being.

By judiciously applying laser technology to specific acupoints, practitioners can invoke photochemical changes within cells, thereby facilitating healing and pain relief with precision and control. The expertise required encompasses a sound knowledge of tissue optics, laser physics, dosimetry, and the biological effects of light, which are all pivotal to the successful delivery of LA treatments in a clinical setting. In the realm of LA, technical parameters are crucial to ensure the effective stimulation of acupoints and to facilitate the desired therapeutic effects. These parameters encompass (i) wavelength (nm), which determines the depth of laser penetration; (ii) output power (W), which influences the intensity of the treatment; (iii) power density or irradiance (W/cm^2), which affects the amount of energy applied per unit area; (iv) energy density or fluence (J/cm^2), dictating the total energy delivered to a given area; (v) dose range (J), which must be tailored to treated areas or conditions; and (vi) the modality of the laser emission, whether continuous or pulsed, each with specific indications. Comprehensive information on PBM parameters can be found in dedicated sections (Chapters 2 and 4).

Determining the ideal parameters for LA is an ongoing area of research. Despite the lack of a universal consensus on these parameters, it is acknowledged that a synergistic approach, carefully considering variables such as wavelength, dose, fluence, irradiance, and the mode of pulse, is vital. The careful adjustment of these factors is necessary to precipitate the most beneficial cellular and physiological reactions, which is essential for the effective application of PBM within the realm of patient care. Table 35.4 outlines the parameters for LA, serving both as an informational guide for practitioners and as a reference tool. These parameters are derived from a combination of empirical evidence from clinical trials, specifications from laser equipment manufacturers, and insights from the author's own clinical practice. This synthesis of data ensures that the parameters are grounded in both research and practical application, offering a framework for safe and effective LA treatment.

Table 35.4 Guidelines for laser acupuncture parameters.

Parameters		Note & author's comments
Wavelength (nm)	600–950	600–700 nm is ideal for shallow points, while 780–950 nm is better for deeper points (Zein *et al.*, 2018).
Output power (mW)	5–500	Minimal 10 mW is suggested (Baxter *et al.*, 2008); At 40 mW, LA yields effects comparable to needle acupuncture (Litscher & Opitz, 2012); High power risks tissue overheating.
Power density or irradiance (W/cm^2)	0.01–2	Minimal 1.3 W/cm^2 is suggested to activate physiological effects of acupuncture (Litscher & Opitz, 2012); High irradiance risks tissue overheating.
Energy density or fluence (J/cm^2)	0.5–4	0.1–0.5 J/cm^2 per acupoint, or 1–4 J/ cm^2 per Ashi point (Hu *et al.* 2013).
Dosage per acupoint (J)	0.5–12 per point	Minimal 0.5 J per point (Baxter *et al.*, 2008)

Safety Concerns

LA is generally considered a safe and pain-free alternative to traditional acupuncture, presenting minimal to no adverse effects, and offering greater versatility (Hu et al., 2013; Chon *et al.*, 2019). However, it is not entirely without risks. Specific safety concerns may arise due to the nature of laser devices, requiring strict adherence to safety protocols to avoid or reduce any significant risks associated with their use (Yang *et al.*, 2020). Proper training in laser safety for clinical applications is crucial to ensure that both patients and practitioners are not exposed to harmful laser emissions. While laser therapy has been widely used for pain and wound healing, practitioners should always review a patient's medical history for any contraindications prior to treatment. Additional details on laser therapy safety can be found in Chapter 5.

Precautions are necessary with LA, particularly concerning the duration of exposure and the part of the body being treated (Yang *et al.*, 2020). The eyes are especially vulnerable to laser damage, making protective eyewear mandatory for both the patient and practitioner. As such, acupoints near the eyes should be avoided, and facial treatments should be conducted with extreme caution. While traditional acupuncture may cause minor adverse effects like tiredness, increased water intake, soreness, muscle spasm, and minor bleeding, such effects are less common with LA due to its noninvasive nature (Xie & Preast, 2007, p. 245–247; Chon *et al.*, 2019).

Contraindications for LA also exist, mirroring some of those for traditional acupuncture. It is generally contraindicated over cancerous areas, hemorrhagic areas, gonads, secretary glands, the abdomen of pregnant animals, the heart region of patients with cardiac conditions, and in patients with implanted electronic devices (e.g., pacemaker) (Xie & Preast, 2007, p. 245–247; Chon *et al.*, 2019). Additionally, certain acupoints associated with inducing labor should be avoided in non-full-term pregnancies due to their potential to stimulate uterine contractions (i.e., ST-36, SP-6, BL-40, BL-60, BL-67) (Xie & Preast, 2007, p. 245–247).

Summary

With its expanding use in veterinary medicine, LA stands as a testament to the growing field of integrative animal health care, where the convergence of ancient wisdom and modern technology can lead to better health solutions for our animal companions. LA is noted for its safety, noninvasive nature, and minimal side effects, making it a favorable choice either as a stand-alone therapy or in conjunction with traditional acupuncture. With its growing use, further research is essential to fully elucidate LA's mechanisms, determine its optimal application parameters, and verify its overall efficacy in veterinary practices.

References

Baxter, G.D. *et al.* (2008). Clinical effectiveness of laser acupuncture: a systematic review. *J Acupunct Meridian Stud.* 1(2):65–82. doi:10.1016/s2005-2901(09)60026-1.

Chang, W.H. *et al.* (2021). Comparison of the effects between lasers applied to myofascial trigger points and to classical acupoints for patients with cervical myofascial pain syndrome. *Biom J.* 44(6):739–747. doi:10.1016/j.bj.2020.05.020.

Chen, Z. *et al.* (2019). Laser acupuncture for patients with knee osteoarthritis: a systematic review and meta-analysis of randomized placebo-controlled trials. *Evid Based Complement Alternat Med.* 2019:6703828. doi:10.1155/2019/6703828.

Chomsiriwat, P. and Ma, A. (2019). Comparison of the effects of electro-acupuncture and laser acupuncture on pain relief and joint range of motion in dogs with coxofemoral degenerative joint disease. *Am J Trad Chin Vet Med.* 14(1):11–20.

Chon, T.Y. *et al.* (2019). Laser acupuncture: a concise review. *Med Acupunct.* 31(3):164–168. doi:10.1089/acu.2019.1343.

Cui, J. *et al.* (2021). Research progress on the mechanism of the acupuncture regulating neuro-endocrine-immune network system. *Vet Sci.* 8(8):149. doi:10.3390/vetsci8080149.

Dewey, C.W. and Xie, H. (2021). The scientific basis of acupuncture for veterinary pain management: a review based on relevant literature from the last two decades. *Open Vet J.* 11(2):203–209. doi:10.5455/OVJ.2021.v11.i2.3.

Di Francesco, F. *et al.* (2024). Efficacy of acupuncture and laser acupuncture in temporomandibular disorders: a systematic review and meta-analysis of randomized controlled trials. *BMC Oral Health.* 24(1):174. doi:10.1186/s12903-023-03806-1.

Glazov, G. *et al.* (2016). Low-level laser therapy for chronic non-specific low back pain: a meta-analysis of randomised controlled trials. *Acupunct Med.* 34(5):328–341. doi:10.1136/acupmed-2015-011036.

Goldman, N. *et al.* (2010). Adenosine A1 receptors mediate local anti-nociceptive effects of acupuncture. *Nat Neurosci.* 13(7):883–888. doi:10.1038/nn.2562.

Hamblin, M.R. (2017). Mechanisms and applications of the anti-inflammatory effects of photobiomodulation. *AIMS Biophys.* 4(3):337–361. doi:10.3934/biophy.2017.3.337.

Holyoak, G.R. and Ma, A. (2022). Evidence-based application of acupuncture in theriogenology. *Vet Sci.* 9(2):53. doi:10.3390/vetsci9020053.

Hu, W.L. *et al.* (2013). Explore laser acupuncture's role. In: *Acupuncture in Modern Medicine.* InTech, Available at: http://dx.doi.org/10.5772/55092.

Hung, Y.C. *et al.* (2021). The effectiveness of laser acupuncture for treatment of musculoskeletal pain: a meta-analysis of randomized controlled studies. *J Pain Res.* 14:1707–1719. doi:10.2147/JPR.S308876.

Huntingford, J.L. and Petty, M.C. (2022). Evidence-based application of acupuncture for pain management in companion animal medicine. *Vet Sci.* 9(6):252. doi:10.3390/vetsci9060252.

Ishak, A. *et al.* (2022). Effect of manual acupuncture and laser acupuncture on wound closure in rat with deep partial thickness burn injury. *Med Acupunct.* 34(4):240–250. doi:10.1089/acu.2021.0083.

Jang, I. *et al.* (2019). Early history of laser acupuncture: who used it first? *Integrat Med Res.* 8(2):129–130. doi:10.1016/j.imr.2019.04.009.

Jiang, W.L. *et al.* (2017a). Changes in nitric oxide releases of the contralateral acupoint during and after laser acupuncture at bilateral same-name acupoints in human. *Evid Based Complement Alternat Med.* 2017:5763458. doi:10.1155/2017/5763458.

Jiang, W.L. *et al.* (2017b). Effects of different-intensity laser acupuncture at two adjacent same-meridian acupoints on nitric oxide and soluble guanylate cyclase releases in human. *Microcirculation.* 24(7). doi:10.1111/micc.12390.

Katsoulis, J. *et al.* (2010). Laser acupuncture for myofascial pain of the masticatory muscles. A controlled pilot study. *Schweiz Monatsschr Zahnmed.* 120(3):213–225.

Klide, A.M. and Martin, B.B. Jr. (1989). Methods of stimulating acupuncture points for treatment of chronic back pain in horses. *J Am Vet Med Assoc.* 195(10):1375–1379.

Koh, R.B. and Harrison, T.M. (2023). Acupuncture in zoological companion animals. *Vet Clin North Am Exot Anim Pract.* 26(1):257–280. doi:10.1016/j.cvex.2022.07.008.

Kong, J.T. *et al.* (2013). Understanding central mechanisms of acupuncture analgesia using dynamic quantitative sensory testing: a review. *Evid Based Complement Alternat Med.* 2013:187182. doi:10.1155/2013/187182.

Law, D. *et al.* (2015). Laser acupuncture for treating musculoskeletal pain: a systematic review with meta-analysis. *J Acupunct Meridian Stud.* 8(1):2–16. doi:10.1016/j.jams.2014.06.015.

Lee, J.H. *et al.* (2006). Electroacupuncture inhibits inflammatory edema and hyperalgesia through regulation of cyclooxygenase synthesis in both peripheral and central nociceptive sites. *Am J Chin Med.* 34(6):981–988. doi:10.1142/S0192415X06004454.

Li, N. *et al.* (2021). The anti-inflammatory actions and mechanisms of acupuncture from acupoint to target organs via neuro-immune regulation. *J Inflamm Res.* 14:7191–7224. doi:10.2147/JIR.S341581.

Litscher, G. (2018). Definition of laser acupuncture and all kinds of photo acupuncture. *Medicine.* 5(4):117. doi:10.3390/medicines5040117.

Litscher, G. (2020). History of laser acupuncture: a narrative review of scientific literature. *Med Acupunct.* 32(4):201–208. doi:10.1089/acu.2020.1438.

Litscher, G. and Opitz, G. (2012). Technical parameters for laser acupuncture to elicit peripheral and central effects: state-of-the-art and short guidelines based on results from the Medical University of Graz, the German Academy of Acupuncture, and the Scientific Literature. *Evid Based Complement Alternat Med.* 2012:697096. doi:10.1155/2012/697096.

Ma, S.X. (2017). Nitric oxide signaling molecules in acupoints: toward mechanisms of acupuncture. *Chin J Integr Med.* 23(11):812–815. doi:10.1007/s11655-017-2789-x.

Marques, V.I. *et al.* (2015). Laser acupuncture for postoperative pain management in cats. *Evid Based Complement Alternat Med.* 2015:653270. doi:10.1155/2015/653270.

Martin, B.B. Jr. and Klide, A.M. (1987). Treatment of chronic back pain in horses. Stimulation of acupuncture points with a low powered infrared laser. *Vet Surg.* 16(1):106–110. doi:10.1111/j.1532-950x.1987.tb00919.x.

Memon, M.A. *et al.* (2021). Survey of integrative veterinary medicine training in AVMA-accredited veterinary colleges. *J Vet Med Educ.* 48(3):289–294. doi:10.3138/jvme.2019-0067.

Mongkolrat, N. *et al.* (2021). Comparison of high intensity laser stimulation of acupuncture points and therapeutic ultrasound for relief of chronic lower back pain in horses. *Am J Trad Chin Vet Med.* 16(2):31–40. doi:10.59565/001c.84098.

Nascimento, F.F. *et al.* (2019). Analgesic efficacy of laser acupuncture and electroacupuncture in cats undergoing ovariohysterectomy. *J Vet Med Sci.* 81(5):764–770. doi:10.1292/jvms.18-0744.

On-Ong-Arj, P. *et al.* (2018). Yellow laser stimulation at GV2 acupoint mitigates apoptosis, oxidative stress, inflammation, and motor deficit in spinal cord injury rats. *Evid Based Complement Alternat Med.* 2018:5407052. doi:10.1155/2018/5407052.

Palizgir, R. *et al.* (2023). Comparison of therapeutic effects of 940 nm diode laser acupuncture with transcutaneous electrical nerve stimulation in the myofascial pain dysfunction syndrome: a comparative randomized clinical trial. *Lasers Med Sci.* 38(1):233. doi:10.1007/s10103-023-03900-4.

Peixoto, K.O. *et al.* (2023). Temporomandibular disorders and the use of traditional and laser acupuncture: a systematic review. *Cranio.* 41(6):501–507. doi:10.1080/08869634.2021.1873605.

Petermann, U. (2011). Comparison of pre- and post-treatment pain scores of twenty one horses with laminitis treated with acupoint and topical low level impulse laser therapy. *Am J Trad Chin Vet Met.* 6(1):13–25.

Petermann, U. (2015). Combination of laser acupuncture and low level laser therapy for treatment of non-healing and infected wounds. *Am J Trad Chin Vet Med.* 10(2):33–42.

Petermann, U. (2016). Treatment of 29 cases of acute and chronic equine tendonitis with local laser therapy and laser acupuncture. *Am J Trad Chin Vet Med.* 11(2):43–51.

Plog, F.M.W. (1980). Biophysical application of the laser beam. In: *Lasers in Medicine.* (ed. H.K. Koebner), pp. 21–37. John Wiley, New York.

Quah-Smith, I. *et al.* (2013). Laser acupuncture for depression: a randomised double blind controlled trial using low intensity laser intervention. *J Affect Disord.* 148(2–3):179–187. doi:10.1016/j.jad.2012.11.058.

Rangel, C.R.G. and Pinheiro, S.L. (2021). Laser acupuncture and intravascular laser irradiation of blood for management of pediatric dental anxiety. *J Oral Sci.* 63(4):355–357. doi:10.2334/josnusd.21-0025.

Repac, J. *et al.* (2022). Clinical application of acupuncture in equine practice. *Vet Clin North Am Equine Pract.* 38(3):525–539. doi:10.1016/j.cveq.2022.07.001.

Roynard, P. *et al.* (2018). Acupuncture for small animal neurologic disorders. *Vet Clin North Am Small Anim Pract.* 48(1):201–219. doi:10.1016/j.cvsm.2017.08.003.

Sajedi, S.M. *et al.* (2022). Comparative efficacy of low-level laser acupuncture and cupping for treatment of patients with myofascial pain dysfunction syndrome: a double-blinded, randomized clinical trial: comparison of the effects of LLL acupuncture and cupping. *Galen Med J.* 11:1–13. doi:10.31661/gmj.v11i.2305.

da Silva Mira, P.C. *et al.* (2024). Laser acupuncture to reduce temporomandibular disorder (TMD) symptoms: systematic review and meta-analysis. *Lasers Med Sci.* 39(1):66. doi:10.1007/s10103-024-03999-z.

Song, D. and Xie, H. (2012). *Annotated Yuan Heng's Classical Collection on the Treatment of Equine Diseases*, pp. 5–6. China Agriculture Press, Beijing.

Su, T.F. *et al.* (2011). Cannabinoid CB2 receptors contribute to upregulation of β-endorphin in inflamed skin tissues by electroacupuncture. *Mol Pain.* 7:98. doi:10.1186/1744-8069-7-98.

Sutalangka, C. *et al.* (2013). Laser acupuncture improves memory impairment in an animal model of Alzheimer's disease. *J Acupunct Meridian Stud.* 6(5):247–251. doi:10.1016/j.jams.2013.07.001.

Tahir, A.H. *et al.* (2021). Peripheral and spinal mechanisms involved in electro-acupuncture therapy for visceral hypersensitivity. *Front Neurosci.* 15:696843. doi:10.3389/fnins.2021.696843.

Tomacheuski, R.M. *et al.* (2020). Postoperative analgesic effects of laserpuncture and meloxicam in bitches submitted to ovariohysterectomy. *Vet Sci.* 7(3):94. doi:10.3390/vetsci7030094.

Wright, B.D. (2019). Acupuncture for the treatment of animal pain. *Vet Clin North Am Small Anim Pract.* 49(6):1029–1039. doi:10.1016/j.cvsm.2019.07.001.

Xie, H. and Chrisman, C. (2009). Equine acupuncture: from ancient art to modern validation. *Am J Trad Chin Vet Med.* 4(2):1–4.

Xie, H. and Preast, V. (2007). *Xie's Veterinary Acupuncture.* Blackwell Publishin, Ames,IA 3–15, 245–247, 247–308, 332–336.

Xie, H. and Preast, V. (2013). *Traditional Chinese Veterinary Medicine: Fundamental Principles*, Vol. 1–43, 2 edn, pp. 249–302. Jing Tang, Florida.

Yang, J. *et al.* (2020). The safety of laser acupuncture: a systematic review. *Med Acupunct.* 32(4):209–217. doi:10.1089/acu.2020.1419.

Ying, W. *et al.* (2019). Effect of laser acupuncture on mitigating anxiety in acute stressed horses: a randomized, controlled study. *Am J Trad Chin Vet Med.* 14(1):33–40.

Zein, R. *et al.* (2018). Review of light parameters and photobiomodulation efficacy: dive into complexity. *J Biomed Opt.* 23(12):1–17. doi:10.1117/1.JBO.23.12.120901.

Zhang, Z.J. *et al.* (2012). Neural acupuncture unit: a new concept for interpreting effects and mechanisms of acupuncture. *Evid Based Complement Alternat Med.* 2012:429412. doi:10.1155/2012/429412.

Zhang, R. *et al.* (2014). Mechanisms of acupuncture-electroacupuncture on persistent pain. *Anesthesiology.* 120(2):482–503. doi:10.1097/ALN.0000000000000101.

36

Laser Therapy in Veterinary Regenerative Medicine

João C. Alves

Clinica Veterinária de Cães, Guarda Nacional Republicana, Lisbon, Portugal

1st Edition Contributor:

Debra Canapp

Veterinary Orthopedic and Sports Medicine Group, Orthobiologic Innovations, Annapolis Junction, MD, USA

Laser Therapy in Veterinary Regenerative Medicine

Regenerative medicine refers to the methodology of stimulating, replacing, engineering, or regenerating a patient's cells, tissues, or organs, with the end goal of restoring or establishing normal function of the tissue treated. This relatively new field of translational medicine holds the potential to stimulate the body's own repair mechanisms to heal previously unrepairable tissues and organs. Regenerative medicine is on the forefront of newly developing technologies and treatments in veterinary medicine for multiple disease processes, especially in musculoskeletal and neurologic diseases and injuries (Bashir *et al.*, 2014). Once injured or affected by disease, some tissues are able to heal back to their original strength and resilience. Many of the current regenerative medicine applications are geared toward tissues that historically heal poorly or with scar tissue, such as tendons, ligaments, cartilage, and muscle.

Veterinary regenerative medicine currently focuses on harvesting the patient's naturally occurring reparative cells and molecules, concentrating them through either patient-side mechanisms or culture expansion, and then returning them to the precise location of injury. The most successful and popular regenerative medicine techniques are the use of platelet-rich plasma (PRP) and adult-derived stem cells, either alone or in combination.

Platelet-Rich Plasma Therapy

Platelets have been shown to recruit, stimulate, and provide a scaffold for stem cells (Dohan Ehrenfest *et al.*, 2008; Drengk *et al.*, 2009; Mishra *et al.*, 2009; Schnabel *et al.*, 2009; Cho *et al.*, 2011; Torricelli *et al.*, 2011; Braun *et al.*, 2014; Broeckx *et al.*, 2014). Thus, PRP has been classified and used as a regenerative medicine therapy to aid in tissue healing. PRP, a fluid concentrate composed primarily of platelets and growth factors, is prepared from the patient's own blood sample. It has been shown to assist in healing by supplying growth factors, cytokines, chemokines, and other bioactive compounds (Boswell *et al.*, 2012). Many of these growth factors act individually or synergistically to help regulate cellular migration and proliferation, promote angiogenesis, promote matrix deposition in order to enhance tendon and wound healing, aid in cartilage health, and protect and counteract against the cartilage breakdown that is associated with osteoarthritis (Mishra & Pavelko, 2006; McCarrel & Fortier, 2009; McCarrel *et al.*, 2012; Hsu *et al.*, 2013; Patel *et al.*, 2013). Thus, PRP is becoming widely used in both human and veterinary medicine to aid in healing a wide range of tissues.

Recent studies have compared key parameters of the PRP products of well-known and commonly used commercial canine PRP systems and found variations in their composition (Stief *et al.*, 2011; Carr *et al.*, 2014; Franklin *et al.*, 2015). Historically, there has been an inadequate reporting of

Laser Therapy in Veterinary Medicine: Photobiomodulation, Second Edition. Edited by Christopher J. Winkler and Lisa A. Miller.

scientific details critical to outcome in many studies. For that reason, minimum reporting requirements for clinical studies evaluating PRP and stem cells have been developed (Murray *et al.*, 2017). With that in mind, it is important for both patient and practitioner to closely examine the data, record product values, monitor treatment sites, and record all outcomes to interpret and identify applications and any changes that may need to be discussed.

For osteoarthritis, PRP products are injected directly into the joint, with or without sedation. While not mandatory for all administrations, as proper needle positioning can be confirmed through the collection of synovial fluid, advanced imaging (diagnostic ultrasound, digital radiography, or fluoroscopy) should be available for guidance, as in some cases joint access can be challenging. Diagnostic ultrasound guidance is mandatory for soft-tissue injuries, as PRP is most effective when administered directly into the injury or lesion and such imaging ensures the accuracy of the injection. Sedation is usually required for ultrasound-guided soft-tissue injections.

Stem-Cell Therapy

Stem cells are defined as the body's progenitor cells, from which all other cells are derived. Many studies have shown that mesenchymal stem cells, produced from adult stem cells, regenerate and heal injured tissue, decrease inflammation, and stimulate angiogenesis. They support healing, activate local tissue-resident stem cells, provide a scaffold for further healing, protect other tissue cells from death, and remodel and break down scar tissue (Grassel & Lorenz, 2014; Mazor *et al.*, 2014; Ham *et al.*, 2015; Sampson *et al.*, 2015; Wolfstadt *et al.*, 2015). Several studies recently published in veterinary medicine show the benefit of stem-cell therapy when applied to canines. These studies include stem-cell therapy as an adjunct to surgery in fragmented coronoid cases (Kiefer *et al.*, 2013), canine hip osteoarthritis (Cuervo *et al.*, 2014), partial tears of the cranial cruciate ligament (Canapp *et al.*, 2016), muscle and tendon strains (Gary Brown *et al.*, 2012; Case *et al.*, 2013; Gibson *et al.*, 2017), bone defects (Jang *et al.*, 2008; Song *et al.*, 2017), wounds (Kim *et al.*, 2013), or inflammatory bowel disease (Pérez-Merino *et al.*, 2015).

The most widely used stem-cell therapy, autologous adult-derived mesenchymal cells, may be obtained from various sources in a patient's body. The most common places, based on research and clinical use, are the patient's bone marrow and adipose tissue. Only recently did a xenogeneic, ready-to-use product become available (Punzón *et al.*, 2022). Stem cells from both sources have repeatedly shown the ability to differentiate into cartilage, bone, tendons, and ligaments. Previously, both bone marrow- and adipose-derived stem cells (ASCs) could be either processed on-site or shipped to an institution for processing, culture expansion, and banking for future use (Martinello *et al.*, 2011). Currently, in compliance with Food and Drug Administration (FDA) guidelines released in December 2015, universities and institutions in the United States are under regulations that restrict certain stem-cell manipulations, expansion, and banking for commercial use. For that reason, only certified institutions can provide this service.

Like PRP, stem-cell therapy is considered a minimally invasive procedure and is typically performed with or without the use of sedation, depending on the application and the location of the injection. A vast amount of energy is spent in exploring stem-cell engraphment and viability once cells have been embedded into a target tissue (Li *et al.*, 2016). Cell delivery techniques and biological vehicles are current areas of debate, and exploration is needed to find the best combination to ensure long-term stem cell survival in order to increase the probability of tissue regeneration within the injured tissue (Zarembinski *et al.*, 2011).

Combination regenerative medicine therapy (combining PRP products with stem cells regardless of their source) has become common among small-animal practitioners. Recent studies have shown that PRP recruits and stimulates stem cells, thereby supporting the notion that PRP should be combined with stem cells prior to injection (Figure 36.1). This method supports both activation and scaffold provision for the stem cells (Del Bue *et al.*, 2008; Chen *et al.*, 2012; Uysal *et al.*, 2012; Xie *et al.*, 2012; Carvalho *et al.*, 2013; Manning *et al.*, 2013; Tobita *et al.*, 2013; Yun *et al.*, 2014).

No matter the source or content of the product, ensuring that it is directly situated in the site of injury through either ultrasound guidance or another assurance method is one of the most important requirements for a successful outcome, followed by continued viability of the cell in its new environment.

Studies support regenerative medicine as an efficacious tool in managing numerous orthopedic conditions, including routinely occurring osteoarthritis and soft-tissue injuries. Soft-tissue injuries and osteoarthritis are extremely common conditions afflicting active, working, and sporting dogs, due to the repetitive forces placed on their joints. Micro-trauma to the tendons, ligaments, and articular surfaces of joints can occur, creating an environment favorable to osteoarthritic development. Once the degenerative cascade of osteoarthritis is initiated, its progression can be insidious. Therapies for this debilitating condition have focused on treating the symptoms or slowing the progression of the disease. Regenerative medicine therapy may

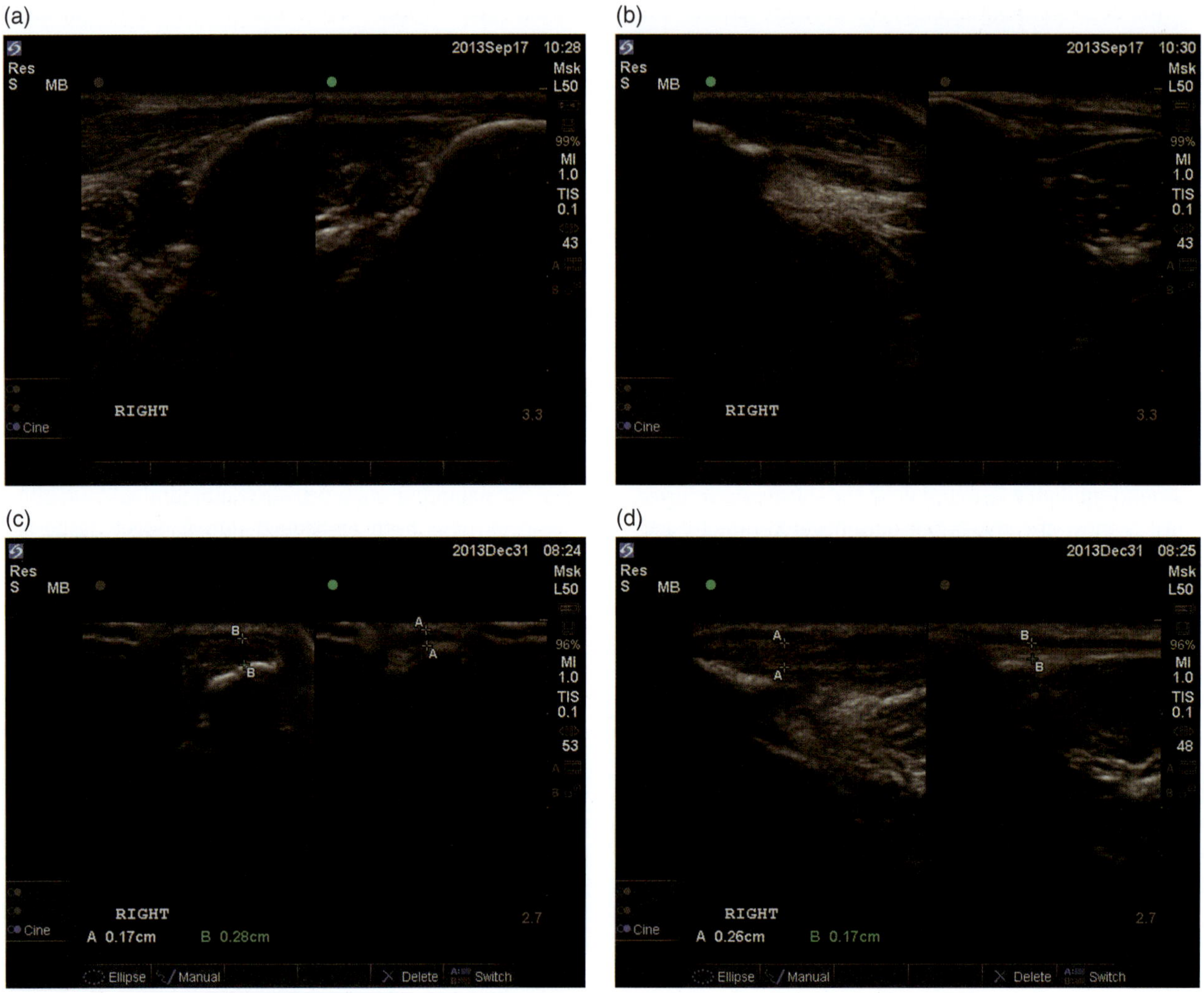

Figure 36.1 Initial ultrasound scans, (a) distal and (b) proximal, of a grade 2/3 patellar tendon strain, with normal comparison on the right. Scans of the same tendon, (c) cross-section and (d) longitudinal, 12 weeks post-injection of stem cells and PRP and initiation of weekly laser therapy. Note the decrease in inflammation, decreased thickness of the patellar tendon, and improved fiber pattern when compared to the normal side on the right.

not only treat symptoms and slow disease progression, but also help to induce repair of the underlying damage that initiated the cascade. Regenerative medicine technology gives new hope for extending the career and improving the quality of life of our canine companions.

Rehabilitation Therapy Following Regenerative Medicine Therapy

Rehabilitation therapy assists in tissue healing by decreasing inflammation, improving overall comfort, and eventually building muscle mass and increasing strength and range of motion. A well-structured, dedicated rehabilitation therapy program is recommended for at least 90 days following regenerative medicine therapy. Restricted activity and controlled exercise (focused on maintaining rather than strengthening muscle mass), is recommended for the first 8 weeks in order to minimize additional inflammation. This protocol also allows the regenerative medicine treatment to focus on tissue regeneration and not removal of inflammation. Studies have shown that implanted stem cells remain in the tissue for approximately 8–10 weeks, depending on the target tissue (Niemeyer *et al.*, 2008; Bai *et al.*, 2011).

Rehabilitation therapy sessions often include manual therapies, standard isometric exercises, and laser therapy. Laser therapy, correctly referred to as "photobiomodulation therapy" (PBMT), is recommended, as extensive literature supports the notion that light irradiation promotes stem-cell differentiation, proliferation, and viability. This will be explored extensively later in the chapter. Currently, all combination stem cell–PRP treatments performed at the author's veterinary practice are recommended to also receive laser therapy weekly to twice weekly at the site of injection. A power density (irradiance) of 0.25 W/cm^2 (250 mW/cm^2) and energy density (fluence) of 5 J/cm^2 is used, with either a single wavelength between 600 and 900 nm or, preferably, multiple wavelengths usually in the red to near-infrared range.

Underwater treadmill therapy is usually started 8 weeks after regenerative medicine treatment, due to its potential to aid inflammation to the target tissues via water's strengthening techniques. Therapeutic ultrasound, shockwave therapy, neuromuscular electrical stimulation or trans-electrical neuromuscular stimulation, and nonsteroidal anti-inflammatory drug (NSAID) usage are contraindicated within the first 8 weeks of regenerative medicine therapy, as their effects on stem cells and PRP have not been fully studied. Preliminary reports suggest detrimental effects on transplanted cells (Nicpon *et al.*, 2015). Rehabilitation therapy should be performed weekly in conjunction with a well-structured and explicit home-exercise program.

Once the targeted tissue has regenerated, as confirmed by diagnostic ultrasound or arthroscopy, the rehabilitation program can advance to focus on strengthening and conditioning. When appropriate muscle mass has been attained, the canine patient is then cleared for retraining and return to sport or normal daily activity.

Regenerative Medicine and Photobiomodulation

Ultimately, regenerative medicine's purpose is to assist the patient's body in regenerating injured tissue back to its original condition. Laser therapy has also been proven to stimulate many different cell lines via positive, restorative mechanisms. However, there is a scarcity of studies on the action of laser therapy on mesenchymal stem cells, and even less data on the actual mechanism of action of laser therapy on adult stem cells (Ginani *et al.*, 2015). Nevertheless, a 2015 landmark review article on photobiomodulation, looking precisely at its effects of proliferation and differentiation of both human- and animal-derived stem cells, helps define the importance of power density and energy density on the end stem-cell response (Emelyanov & Kiryanova, 2015). This article, which will be explored further throughout this chapter, finds that the influence of wavelength appears to be significant. Elevated values of proliferation or differentiation are primarily seen in studies using high power densities, low energy densities, and short exposure times. The greatest differentiation is attained using laser irradiation protocols different from those necessary to achieve maximal proliferation of the same cells. The article concludes that increased power density and reduced energy density are the essential parameters needed to increase the overall positive stem-cell response (Emelyanov & Kiryanova, 2015). In general, there is an overall agreement that power density and energy density (with less importance placed on specific light wavelength, as long as it is in the red or near-infrared range) are the most important parameters with regards to the effects of photobiomodulation (PBM) on stem cells and their use in regenerative medicine.

Unfortunately, all of these parameters are not always reported in every research article. When parameters are cited, they may differ greatly from study to study and often involve multiple different stem cell lines, species, and tissue origins. Using clinical research is important in determining when and how a tool can best be used to maximize its effectiveness. Researchers propose mechanisms involved in treating a broad spectrum of injuries or disease states, so that clinicians may decide whether the combination and synergism of regenerative medicine and laser therapy might be useful in each individual case.

This treatment-method approach of evaluating the literature as a practice guide is often referred to as "evidence-based medicine." Using research aids clinicians in determining when a therapy is anticipated to have a benefit for the patient in question. The veterinarian then takes this information and uses his or her judgment as to when and where to apply the therapy. At times, there may be little support for the use of a particular treatment in a particular species.

Research regarding the use of regenerative medicine (specifically in canine musculoskeletal injuries, canine neurological injuries, or canine wound healing) is becoming more frequently available, despite many protocols and indications being taken from human, alternate mammal, or animal model literature and applied to canine patients, making the parameters of the laser possibly confusing as they vary from trial to trial. Examples include hip osteoarthritis (Alves *et al.*, 2021), partial tears of cranial cruciate ligament (Canapp *et al.*, 2016), and muscle and tendon strains (Gary Brown *et al.*, 2012; Case *et al.*, 2013; Gibson *et al.*, 2017). Still, the use of these data across species has proven to be very successful clinically in the treatment of many musculoskeletal injuries seen in the canine. In spite of this experience, it is crucial for the veterinarian to be able to discern why a modality or treatment does or does not add benefit. This should be well-documented while developing the ongoing treatment plan.

Despite the current lack of species-specific data or consistency in reporting details, key opinion leaders, residing in a broad range of well-respected disciplines, believe that PBM of stem cells is a valuable tool for boosting stem cell viability and proliferation. Extraordinary therapies will become available as a result of this intellectual drive and the promising synergism between regenerative medicine and laser therapy.

In Vitro Laser Therapy and Stem Cells

Many years of dedicated research into a wide range of light applications, light wavelength ranges, power densities, and exposures across several species and cell lines have paved the way for the useful clinical application we see today. Early research in laser therapy and adult stem cells suggested that laser therapy escalates the proliferation of stem cells (Tuby *et al.*, 2007). Studies on human adipose mesenchymal stem cells suggest that this effect may derive from an enhanced mitochondrial membrane potential, reactive oxygen species, and vesicle transport phenomena, which have potential in cell proliferation, migration, and differentiation (Pan *et al.*, 2022). Additionally, as PBMT increases the production of nitric oxide, adenosine triphosphate, and cyclic adenosine monophosphate (cAMP), these can also initiate cell proliferation (Khorsandi *et al.*, 2020). It is also possible that PBMT may modulate the status of DNA methylation and the expression of tissue-specific genes during the differentiation procedure (Zamani *et al.*, 2020).

An investigation of the effect of a 635 nm diode laser with an output power of 60 mW at numerous dosages on rat bone marrow-derived mesenchymal stem cells (BMSCs) demonstrated 0.5 J/cm^2 to be an optimal energy density for the stimulation of cellular proliferation. At a higher dose of 5 J/cm^2, the stem cells secreted both vascular endothelial growth factor (VEGF) and nerve growth factor. This dosage also facilitated myogenic differentiation. The researchers concluded that laser therapy stimulates proliferation, facilitates myogenic differentiation, and increases growth factor secretion in BMSCs (Huo *et al.*, 2008). This study may provide data to support the preconditioning of BMSCs with laser light prior to implantation into the patient.

Irradiation of BMSCs cultured *in vitro* with a 632.8 nm laser with an output power of 10 mW and a power density of 0.5 mW/cm^2, using an increased exposure time of 10 minutes per day for 28 days, found that laser irradiation had a biostimulatory effect on the conversion of BMSCs into bone-forming cells and induced ossification (Abramovitch-Gottlib *et al.*, 2005).

Use of a 635 nm diode laser on an ASC stem cell line, with an output power of 50.2 mW and a power density of 5.5 mW/cm^2 at a one-time dose of 5 J/cm^2, showed no changes in cell morphology after 48 hours, although cell viability and proliferation were significantly increased (Mvula *et al.*, 2008).

Other studies looking at different cell populations, such as human dental pulp stem cells and cardiac stem cells, all show a positive effect of laser phototherapy with improved cell growth, supporting the overall synergistic effect of progenitor cells and laser light irradiation (Tuby *et al.*, 2007; Eduardo *et al.*, 2008). Similar *in vitro* results are seen in equine species. Equine peripheral blood mesenchymal stem cells incubated with growth factors and irradiated with laser light promoted differentiation into the tenocyte lineage (Gomiero *et al.*, 2016).

These cell-culture studies and prominent review articles support the notion that phototherapy can significantly "increase the initial number of stem cells before differentiation, thus increasing the number of differentiated cells for tissue engineering and regenerative and healing processes" (Ginani *et al.*, 2015). Yet, the issue remains that there is a deficiency in standardization of treatment parameters with regards to wavelength, power density, time, and polarization of light. The effect of PBMT can even extend to the point of inducing stem cell differentiation, with the differentiation of ASCs to osteoblasts, neurons, and adipocytes *in vitro* having been described recently (Muneekaew *et al.*, 2022; Tang *et al.*, 2022a, 2022b).

With reference to the wavelength used in these studies, the majority used the visible red spectrum in the 600–700 nm range. This is most likely due to historical support from studies looking at the positive effects of these wavelengths on *in vitro* biostimulation of cells in general. Though there have been significantly fewer studies looking at the infrared range, results have shown the positive proliferative and differentiation effects of an 810 nm wavelength on human bone-marrow cells (Tuby *et al.*, 2007; Soleimani *et al.*, 2012). A review of different parameters on mesenchymal stem cells showed that PBMT had a positive effect on cell proliferation when energy densities of 0.7–9 J/cm^2 and powers of 50–800 mW were considered (Fekrazad *et al.*, 2016).

One negative study showed that the application of laser therapy in the near-infrared range (808 nm, 800 mW, 4 J/cm^2) on murine bone-marrow stem cells resulted in a lower number of colony-forming units (CFUs) when compared to nontreated cells (Bouvet-Gerbettaz *et al.*, 2009). It has since been speculated that though it may have been the infrared spectrum that caused this result, the higher power could also have had an effect (Ginani *et al.*, 2015).

In Vivo Laser Therapy and Stem Cells

Regenerative medicine and PBMT are now also being looked at synergistically *in vivo*. Laser irradiation assisting in stem cell proliferation is a common area of research.

A study looking at human ASCs transplanted into rats and treated with laser therapy with an 830 nm wavelength showed a significant increase in the number of human stem cells in the irradiated group compared to the nonirradiated group (Min *et al.*, 2015). Other studies looking at the effect of stem cells treated with light irradiation include a number of different applications in injury repair that could be translated to canines. In reference to wound therapy, one group looked at cultured human adipose-derived mesenchymal stem cells treated with light from a light-emitting diode (LED) (660 nm, 10 mW/cm^2, 6 J/cm^2) prior to and following implantation into the wound beds of mice. The light-irradiated group appeared superior in many factors, including functional recovery (Park *et al.*, 2015a). In a rat model, PBMT plus ASCs significantly improved the healing of created femoral defects in osteoporotic female rats (Asgari *et al.*, 2022).

One of the few canine species-specific studies investigated the effect of canine ASCs on wound healing in athymic mice. When the ASCs were treated with laser therapy (632 nm, 17 mW, 1.2 J/cm^2 daily for 20 days), wound healing was enhanced through increased neovascularization and regeneration of skin appendages compared with the group receiving ASCs alone. In general, ASCs promoted skin regeneration through cell differentiation and secretion of necessary growth factors. In the ASC and laser-treated group, the survival of ASCs was increased through laser therapy decreasing cell apoptosis within the wound bed. In addition, the secretion of growth factors was increased in the ASC and laser-treated group compared with the ASC group alone (Kim *et al.*, 2012). In animal disease models, PBMT following mesenchymal stem cell (MSC) transplantation effectively increases cell differentiation, proliferation, migration, and activity, which contributes to the different diseases' treatment (Ahrabi *et al.*, 2019; Daigo *et al.*, 2020).

Vascularity within the area of stem cell injection or application, as seen in the previously cited studies, is often an important factor when looking at cell survivability. Stem cell survival inside the tissue needing treatment or repair is essential to their ability to aid in healing. In a recent study looking at human ASC implantation into ischemic mice limbs, the group that received both ASCs and LED light irradiation (660 nm, 50 mW/cm^2, 30 J/cm^2) showed an overall increase in ASCs due to decreased cell death. The secretion of growth factors was also triggered in this group compared with the group receiving ASCs alone. The ASC and LED light group demonstrated enhanced treatment efficacy, including neovascularization and tissue regeneration. Laser Doppler blood perfusion images showed that blood perfusion of the treatment site was significantly improved by ASC and LED light treatment. These data suggest that LED light irradiation is an effective biostimulator of ASCs with regard to vascular regeneration and growth factors, showing improvement in the survival of implanted stem cells in ischemic limbs (Park *et al.*, 2015b). The combination of PBMT and stem cell therapy has been shown to positively impact human patients following myocardial infarction. Interestingly, the effects are observed if the cells or the myocardium are targeted with the PBMT. This leads to significantly reduced scar tissue formation, increased angiogenesis, and increased cell survival, proliferation, and differentiation (El Gammal *et al.*, 2017). In managing temporomandibular joint disc disorders, the combination of PBMT and stem cells can also be used to modulate degenerative changes observed in the joint disc (Karic *et al.*, 2020).

Bone marrow-derived stem cells and laser therapies have also been explored. One study evaluated the effect of bone marrow aspirate (BMA), laser therapy, and their combination on bone healing in surgically created defects in rat calvaria. This study found the combination of BMA and laser therapy generated significantly greater bone formation compared to controls or either treatment alone (Nagata *et al.*, 2013; Fekrazad *et al.*, 2015).

The combination of laser therapy with regenerative medicine has also shown positive effects in neurologic injury. Once again, this is a necessary area for translational medicine to examine within the canine community. In a study involving induced peripheral nerve crush injuries in rats, laser therapy showed a synergistic effect when combined with transplantation of mesenchymal cells into the site of injury. This combined treatment provided greater functional recovery than either mesenchymal stem cell transplantation or laser therapy alone (Yang *et al.*, 2016). Another neurologic application demonstrated that applying laser light (660 nm, 50 mW, single exposure for 10 minutes) to adipose-derived rat stem cells elicited positive effects on stem cell differentiation, which in turn effectively treated ischemic stroke in rats, specifically improving motor function recovery when compared to controls and those receiving stem cells without laser irradiation (Shen *et al.*, 2015). Human studies have shown that the combined use of stem cells and PBMT can improve the symptoms of Parkinson's disease (Ahrabi *et al.*, 2022), which can open the door for future uses in a population of companion animals that is experiencing a growth in life expectancy.

The use of stem cells stimulated by PBMT is expanding to new applications. Exploring effects of PBMT on stem cells while they are still in situ within the host has developed ideas around preparing the body's resident stem cells to better react following injury. Mature mammalian cardiac tissue is known to have limited regenerative capabilities following acute injury. Early studies proposed that photobiostimulation of autologous BMSCs might stimulate these stem cells to migrate to a section of the heart suffering infarction and mitigate scarring. In one study, rats underwent myocardial infarction and had their exposed tibial bone marrow irradiated with laser light (804 nm, 10 mW/cm^2, 1 J/cm^2) for different time intervals. Infarct size and ventricular dilatation were significantly reduced in the rats receiving the laser treatment. The study concluded that laser irradiation applied in situ to the autologous bone marrow of rats following induction of myocardial infarction has promise in inducing BMSCs to move into the circulation to target and significantly reduce the scarring process post-myocardial infarction (Tuby *et al.*, 2011).

In a similar January 2016 research article (this involving irradiation of porcine long bones), targeting BMSCs showed a significant reduction in scarring, enhancement of angiogenesis, and functional improvement in both the acute and long-term phase following induction of myocardial infarction (Blatt *et al.*, 2016). Another study found that MSCs harvested from wild-type mice and stimulated with laser therapy showed an increased ability to maturate toward a monocyte lineage, which in turn increased phagocytosis activity toward soluble amyloid beta (Aβ), an unwanted substance found in the brain of Alzheimer's disease (AD) patients. Using these preliminary data, the same team then looked at weekly laser therapy application to the bone marrow of an AD mouse model for 2 months, starting at 4 months of age (progressive stage of AD). Their findings showed an improved cognitive capacity and spatial learning as compared to sham-treated AD mice. Furthermore, postmortem histology disclosed a significant reduction in Aβ brain burden (Farfara *et al.*, 2015). These data could be useful in cognitive disorders, which are now seen more commonly in our canine patients due to their increased lifespans.

In summary, these studies support the promise of synergism between PBMT and stem cells in a variety of applications, but they also show the diverse variability in treatment parameters. One review article nicely summarized the general effects of both power density and energy density in a graph pertaining to cell proliferation, illustrating the stages of change in cell response to laser stimulation. The data show a specific adaptation phase of the cells, or a prime treatment dosage. More importantly, they also defined a phase of photostress and photoshock, which illustrates there is a threshold of irradiation, which when exceeded can cause damage to stem cells (Emelyanov & Kiryanova, 2015).

Laser Therapy and PRP

Recent studies have also looked at the effect of laser therapy with PRP alone. Achilles tendon injuries are commonly seen in our canine companions, and even more frequently in our canine athletes. In a study on rat Achilles tendon injury, the relative amount of type I collagen was significantly greater in the PRP plus 830 nm laser irradiation group, while the quantity of type III collagen was significantly greater in the PRP-only group (both compared to the irradiation-only group). The study concluded that PRP treatment combined with irradiation at 830 nm produced a larger number of fibroblasts and increased the concentration of type I collagen, thereby accelerating the healing of the injured tendon (de Carvalho *et al.*, 2016).

Similar findings were also noted when PRP and laser therapy were applied to rabbit Achilles tendon injuries using a wavelength in the visible spectrum. This study compared untreated injured tendons to irradiated injured tendons (650 nm diode laser, 30 mW, 1.8 J/cm^2 for 15 consecutive days), and to irradiated injured tendons injected with PRP. Though laser treatment had advantages over no treatment, the combination of PRP and laser irradiation was even more efficient in decreasing tendon healing time (Allahverdi *et al.*, 2015).

Another study on treatment of Achilles tendon injury in rats combined PRP with 660 and 830 nm wavelengths at a dosage of 7 J/cm^2 applied to three points every other day for 13 days. Their results showed that the deposition of collagen type I was higher with combined PRP and laser treatment, suggesting a faster regeneration of the tendon (Barbosa *et al.*, 2013). These data are valuable for the canine world, since circumstances often create economic barriers to the use of stem cells in canine musculoskeletal injury. If these data can be translated, it would mean that canines could receive less expensive PRP treatment with the support of laser therapy, and thus reach a very healthy functional outcome for their tendon injury (Figure 36.2).

The effect on other musculoskeletal lesions, such as muscle injury, is not as well-researched. In a rat muscle injury model, the separate use of PRP and PBMT effectively repaired the damage caused by muscle injury. However, the combined use of the two treatment modalities reduced the area of injury, regenerating the cells and producing a healthier appearance. The muscle also demonstrated a better histological aspect (Ozaki *et al.*, 2016). In a rat model for rheumatoid arthritis, PBMT and PRP were evaluated alone and in combination. PBMT was performed using 808 nm wavelength, a power of 25 mW, and a fluence of 30 J/cm^2 for 33 seconds, delivering 0.825 J over a single point. The combined use of PBMT and

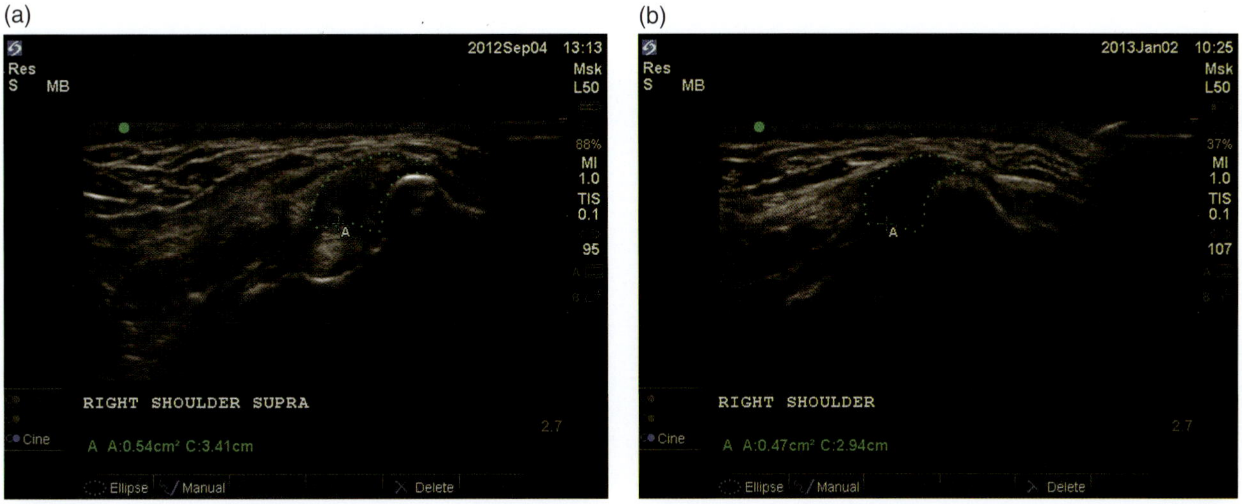

Figure 36.2 (a) Initial ultrasound scan, cross-section, of a supraspinatus tendon illustrating fibrous and calcified lesions within the outlined tendon. (b) Ultrasound scan, cross-section, 90 days post–stem cell and PRP injection. Note the improved fiber pattern, decrease in both inflammation and size of the tendon, and resolution of the fibrous and calcified lesions.

PRP led to a greater anti-inflammatory effect and increased joint preservation by morphological aspects (Gonçalves *et al.*, 2021). In bone lesions, the association of PRP and PBMT promises great results, improving bone healing and decreasing disease relapse (Fornaini *et al.*, 2017; Surmeli Baran *et al.*, 2021; Scribante *et al.*, 2023). Defined amounts of energy, with fluences of 5 J/cm^2 delivered in 2 minutes, or of 10 J/cm^2 delivered in 4 minutes, can lead to a significant increase in both proliferation and differentiation rates of *in vitro* osteoblasts (Ghidini *et al.*, 2021). A recent study looked at the combined use of PBMT and PRP compared to their isolated use in dogs. The authors concluded that PRP and photobiomodulation can improve objective outcomes and client-reported outcome measures in dogs with OA, but their combined use leads to greater, longer-lasting, clinically significant improvements. The PBMT treatment parameters included 980 nm wavelength, with a power of 6.5–8 W, an irradiance of 4.5–5.2 W/cm^2, and a fluence of 14.3–19.5 J/cm^2 over a 225cm^2 area (Alves *et al.*, 2023).

The adjunct use of PRP and PBMT can also extend to other fields than musculoskeletal conditions. Wavelengths in the 600–1200 nm range have been used to activate human platelets, enabling a sustained release of growth factors from PRP (Irmak *et al.*, 2020). The isolated use of PRP and PBMT is well-established for wound healing approaches. Their combined use is not as well documented, but there is evidence that they accelerate acute wound healing and decrease erythema (Picard *et al.*, 2015). There is also information from animal models showing that elastin and collagen deposition were fully restored in Methicillin-resistant *Staphylococcus aureus*-infected skin wounds treated with the combined approaches (Lee *et al.*, 2021).

Conclusion

Regenerative medicine and laser therapy have been used separately to stimulate healing and help the body regenerate injured tissues back to their original conditions. Leading areas of interest now involve looking at combining both regenerative medicine and PBMT in the hope of discovering a superior healing approach across species. Current applications of this therapy are expanding, using translational evidence-based medicine. Applications for sport-related conditions, neurologic injury, and wound healing in the canine include medial shoulder syndrome, shoulder tendinopathies, iliopsoas strain, Achilles tendon injury, early partial cranial cruciate ligament tear, carpal and tarsal ligament injuries, osteoarthritis, traumatic wound injury, intervertebral disk disease (IVDD), lumbosacral disease, and a wealth of other conditions seen routinely in canine patients. Continued emphasis on exploring this area of cutting-edge medicine, specifically for the canine patient, will be essential for our patients, veterinary medicine as a whole, and the world of translational medicine.

References

Abramovitch-Gottlib, L. *et al.* (2005). Low level laser irradiation stimulates osteogenic phenotype of mesenchymal stem cells seeded on a three-dimensional biomatrix. *Lasers Med Sci.* 20(3):138–146.

Ahrabi, B. *et al.* (2019). The effect of photobiomodulation therapy on the differentiation, proliferation, and migration of the mesenchymal stem cell: a review. *J Lasers Med Sci.* 10(5):S96–S103. doi:10.15171/jlms.2019.S17.

Ahrabi, B. *et al.* (2022). Photobiomodulation therapy and cell therapy improved Parkinson's diseases by neuro-regeneration and tremor inhibition. *J Lasers Med Sci.* 13(1): e28–e28. doi:10.34172/jlms.2022.28.

Allahverdi, A. *et al.* (2015). Evaluation of low-level laser therapy, platelet-rich plasma, and their combination on the healing of Achilles tendon in rabbits. *Lasers Med Sci.* 30(4):1305–1313.

Alves, J.C. *et al.* (2021). Platelet-rich plasma therapy in dogs with bilateral hip osteoarthritis. *BMC Vet Res.* 17(1):207. doi:10.1186/s12917-021-02913-x.

Alves, J.C. *et al.* (2023). A preliminary report on the combined effect of intra-articular platelet-rich plasma injections and photobiomodulation in canine osteoarthritis. *Animals.* 13:3247. doi:10.3390/ani13203247.

Asgari, M. *et al.* (2022). Photobiomodulation and stem cell on repair of osteoporotic bones. *Photobiomodulation Photomed Laser Surg.* 40(4):261–272. doi:10.1089/photob.2021.0127.

Bai, X. *et al.* (2011). Tracking long-term survival of intramyocardially delivered human adipose tissue- derived stem cells using bioluminescence imaging. *Mol Imaging Biol.* 13(4):633–645.

Barbosa, D. *et al.* (2013). Low-level laser therapy combined with platelet-rich plasma on the healing calcaneal tendon: a histological study in a rat model. *Lasers Med Sci.* 28 (6):1489–1494.

Bashir, J. *et al.* (2014). Mesenchymal stem cell therapies in the treatment of musculoskeletal diseases. *PM R.* 6(1):61–69.

Blatt, A. *et al.* (2016). Low-level laser therapy to the bone marrow reduces scarring and improves heart function post-acute myocardial infarction in the pig. *Photomed Laser Surg.* 34(11):516–524.

Boswell, S.G. *et al.* (2012). Platelet-rich plasma: a milieu of bioactive factors. *Arthroscopy.* 28(3):429–439.

Bouvet-Gerbettaz, S. *et al.* (2009). Effects of low-level laser therapy on proliferation and differentiation of murine bone marrow cells into osteoblasts and osteoclasts. *Lasers Surg Med.* 41(4):291–297.

Braun, H.J. *et al.* (2014). The effect of platelet-rich plasma formulations and blood products on human synoviocytes. *Am J Sports Med.* 42(5):1204–1210.

Broeckx, S. *et al.* (2014). Regenerative therapies for equine degenerative joint disease: a preliminary study. *PLoS One.* 9(1):e85917.

Canapp, S.O. *et al.* (2016). Partial cranial cruciate ligament tears treated with stem cell and platelet-rich plasma combination therapy in 36 dogs: a retrospective study. *Front Vet Sci.* 3. doi:10.3389/fvets.2016.00112.

Carr, B.J. *et al.*, (2014). Canine platelet rich plasma systems: a multicenter, prospective analysis. *Proceedings of the American College of Veterinary Surgeons Surgery Summit.* (October 15–18). San Diego, CA.

Carvalho, A.M. *et al.* (2013). Equine tendonitis therapy using mesenchymal stem cells and platelet concentrations: a randomized controlled trial. *Stem Cell Res Ther.* 4(4):85.

de Carvalho, P.K. *et al.* (2016). Analysis of experimental tendinitis in rats treated with laser and platelet-rich plasma therapies by Raman spectroscopy and histometry. *Lasers Med Sci.* 31(1):19–26.

Case, J.B. *et al.* (2013). Gastrocnemius tendon strain in a dog treated with autologous mesenchymal stem cells and a custom orthosis. *Vet Surg.* 42(4):355–360. doi:10.1111/j.1532-950X.2013.12007.x.

Chen, L. *et al.* (2012). Synergy of tendon stem cells and platelet-rich-plasma in tendon healing. *J Orthop Res.* 30(6):991–997.

Cho, H.S. *et al.* (2011). Individual variation in growth factor concentrations in platelet-rich plasma and its influence on human mesenchymal stem cells. *Korean J Lab Med.* 31(3):212–218.

Cuervo, B. *et al.* (2014). Hip osteoarthritis in dogs: a randomized study using mesenchymal stem cells from adipose tissue and plasma rich in growth factors. *Int J Mol Sci.* 15(8):13437–13460.

Daigo, Y. *et al.* (2020). Wound healing and cell dynamics including mesenchymal and dental pulp stem cells induced by photobiomodulation therapy: an example of socket-preserving effects after tooth extraction in rats and a literature review. *Int J Mol Sci.* 21(18):6850. doi:10.3390/ijms21186850.

Del Bue, M. *et al.* (2008). Equine adipose-tissue derived mesenchymal stem cells and platelet concentrations: their association in vitro and in vivo. *Vet Res Commun.* 32(1): S51–S55.

Dohan Ehrenfest, D.M. *et al.* (2008). Classification of platelet concentrates: from pure platelet-rich plasma (P-PRP) to leukocyte- and platelet-rich fibrin (L-PRF). *Trends Biotechnol.* 27(3):158–167.

Drengk, A. *et al.* (2009). Influence of platelet-rich plasma on chondrogenic differentiation and proliferation of chondrocytes and mesenchymal stem cells. *Cells Tissues Organs.* 189(5):317–326.

Eduardo, F.P. *et al.* (2008). Stem cell proliferation under low-intensity laser irradiation: a preliminary study. *Lasers Surg Med.* 40(6):433–438.

El Gammal, Z.H. *et al.* (2017). Effect of low-level laser-treated mesenchymal stem cells on myocardial infarction. *Lasers Med Sci.* 32(7):1637–1646. doi:10.1007/s10103-017-2271-1.

Emelyanov, A.N. and Kiryanova, V.V. (2015). Photomodulation of proliferation and differentiation of stem cells by the visible and infrared light. *Photomed Laser Surg.* 33(3):164–174.

Farfara, D. *et al.* (2015). Low-level laser therapy ameliorates disease progression in a mouse model of Alzheimer's disease. *J Mol Neurosci.* 55(2):430–436.

Fekrazad, R. *et al.* (2015). The effects of combined low level laser therapy and mesenchymal stem cells on bone regeneration in rabbit calvarial defects. *J Photochem Photobiol B.* 151:180–185.

Fekrazad, R. *et al.* (2016). Effect of photobiomodulation on mesenchymal stem cells. *Photomed Laser Surg.* 34 (11):533–542. doi:10.1089/pho.2015.4029.

Fornaini, C. *et al.* (2017). Laser and platelet-rich plasma to treat medication-related osteonecrosis of the jaws (MRONJ): a case report. *Laser Ther.* 26(3):223–227. doi:10.5978/islsm.17-CR-04.

Franklin, S.P. *et al.* (2015). Characteristics of canine platelet-rich plasma prepared with five commercially available systems. *Am J Vet Res.* 76(9):822–827.

Gary Brown, S. *et al.* (2012). Adipose-derived stem cell therapy for severe muscle tears in working German shepherds: two case reports. *Stem Cell Discov.* 02(02):41–44. doi:10.4236/scd.2012.22007.

Ghidini, G. *et al.* (2021). Photobiomodulation with a 645 nm diode laser of Saos-2 cells and platelet-rich plasma: the potential for a new mechanism of action. *Photobiomodulation Photomed Laser Surg.* 39(2):86–93. doi:10.1089/photob.2020.4839.

Gibson, M.A. *et al.* (2017). Semitendinosus myopathy and treatment with adipose-derived stem cells in working German shepherd police dogs. *Can Vet J.* 58(3):241–246.

Ginani, F. *et al.* (2015). Effect of low-level laser therapy on mesenchymal stem cell proliferation: a systemic review. *Lasers Med Sci.* 30(8):2189–2194.

Gomiero, C. *et al.* (2016). Tenogenic induction of equine mesenchymal stem cells by means of growth factors and low-level laser technology. *Vet Res Commun.* 40(1):39–48.

Gonçalves, A.B. *et al.* (2021). Photobiomodulation (λ=808nm) and platelet-rich plasma (PRP) for the treatment of acute rheumatoid arthritis in Wistar rats. *J Lasers Med Sci.* 12(1): e60–e60. doi:10.34172/jlms.2021.60.

Grassel, S. and Lorenz, J. (2014). Tissue engineering strategies to repair chondroal and osteochondral tissue in osteoarthritis: use of mesenchymal stem cells. *Curr Rheumatol Rep.* 16(10):452.

Ham, O. *et al.* (2015). Therapeutic potential of differentiated mesenchymal stem cells for treatment of osteoarthritis. *Int J Mol Sci.* 16(7):14961–14978.

Hsu, W.K. *et al.* (2013). Platelet-rich plasma in orthopaedic applications: evidence-based recommendations for treatment. *J Am Acad Orthop Surg.* 21(12):739–748.

Huo, J.F. *et al.* (2008). In vitro effects of low level laser irradiation for bone marrow mesenchymal stem cells: proliferation, growth factor secretion and myogenic differentiation. *Lasers Surg Med.* 40(10):726–733.

Irmak, G. *et al.* (2020). Sustained release of growth factors from photoactivated platelet rich plasma (PRP). *Eur J Pharm Biopharm.* 148:67–76. doi:10.1016/j.ejpb.2019.11.011.

Jang, B.-J. *et al.* (2008). Implantation of canine umbilical cord blood-derived mesenchymal stem cells mixed with beta-tricalcium phosphate enhances osteogenesis in bone defect model dogs. *J Vet Sci.* 9(4):387. doi:10.4142/jvs.2008.9.4.387.

Karic, V. *et al.* (2020). Photobiomodulation and stem cell therapy for temporomandibular joint disc disorders. *Photobiomodulation Photomed Laser Surg.* 38(7):398–408. doi:10.1089/photob.2019.4790.

Khorsandi, K. *et al.* (2020). Biological responses of stem cells to photobiomodulation therapy. *Curr Stem Cell Res Ther.* 15(5):400–413. doi:10.2174/1574888X15666200204123722.

Kiefer, K. *et al.*, (2013). Autologous and allogeneic stem cells as adjuvant therapy for osteoarthritis caused by spontaneous fragmented coronoid process in dogs. *VOS Proceedings 2013. 40th Annual Conference of the Veterinary Orthopedic Society. Veterinary Orthopedic Society* (March 9–13). Canyons Resort, UT.

Kim, H. *et al.* (2012). Enhanced wound healing effect of canine adipose-derived mesenchymal stem cells with low-level laser therapy in athymic mice. *J Dermatol Sci.* 68(3):149–156.

Kim, J. *et al.* (2013). The effects of topical mesenchymal stem cell transplantation in canine experimental cutaneous wounds. *Vet Dermatol.* 24(2):242. doi:10.1111/vde.12011.

Lee, W.-R. *et al.* (2021). Low-fluence laser-facilitated platelet-rich plasma permeation for treating MRSA-infected wound and photoaging of the skin. *Int J Pharm.* 595:120242. doi:10.1016/j.ijpharm.2021.120242.

Li, X. *et al.* (2016). Improving cell engraftment in cardiac stem cell therapy. *Stem Cells Int.* 2016:7168797.

Manning, C.N. *et al.* (2013). Controlled delivery of mesenchymal stem cells and growth factors using a nanofiber scaffold for tendon repair. *Acta Biomater.* 9(6):6905–6914.

Martinello, T. *et al.* (2011). Canine adipose-derived-mesenchymal stem cells do not lose stem features after a long-term cryopreservation. *Res Vet Sci.* 91(1):18–24.

Mazor, M. *et al.* (2014). Mesenchymal stem-cell potential in cartilage repair: an update. *J Cell Mol Med.* 18(12):2340–2350.

McCarrel, T. and Fortier, L. (2009). Temporal growth factor release from platelet- rich plasma, trehalose lyophilized platelets, and bone marrow aspirate and their effect on tendon and ligament gene expression. *J Orthop Res.* 27(8):1033–1042.

McCarrel, T.M. *et al.* (2012). Optimization of leukocyte concentration in platelet-rich plasma for the treatment of tendinopathy. *J Bone Joint Surg Am.* 4(19):e143 (1–8).

Min, K.H. *et al.* (2015). Effect of low-level laser therapy on human adipose-derived stem cells: in vitro and in vivo studies. *Aesth Plast Surg.* 39(5):778–782.

Mishra, A. and Pavelko, T. (2006). Treatment of chronic elbow tendinosis with buffered platelet-rich plasma. *Am J Sports Med.* 34(11):1774–1778.

Mishra, A. *et al.* (2009). Buffered platelet-rich plasma enhances mesenchymal stem cell proliferation and chondrogenic differentiation. *Tissue Eng Part C Methods.* 15(3):431–435.

Muneekaew, S. *et al.* (2022). Control of stem cell differentiation by using extrinsic photobiomodulation in conjunction with cell adhesion pattern. *Sci Rep.* 12(1):1812. doi:10.1038/s41598-022-05888-3.

Murray, I.R. *et al.* (2017). Minimum information for studies evaluating biologics in orthopaedics (MIBO). *J Bone Joint Surg.* 99(10):809–819. doi:10.2106/JBJS.16.00793.

Mvula, B. *et al.* (2008). The effect of low level laser irradiation on adult human adipose derived stem cells. *Lasers Med Sci.* 23(3):277–282.

Nagata, M.J. *et al.* (2013). Bone marrow aspirate combined with low-level laser therapy: a new therapeutic approach to enhance bone healing. *J Photochem Photobiol B.* 121:6–14.

Nicpon, J. *et al.* (2015). The effect of metamizole and tolfenamic acid on canine and equine adipose-derived mesenchymal stem cells (ASCs) an in vitro research. *Pol J Vet Sci.* 18(1):3–11.

Niemeyer, P. *et al.* (2008). Survival of human mesenchymal stromal cells from bone marrow and adipose tissue after xenogenic transplantation in immunocompetent mice. *Cytotherapy.* 10(8):784–795.

Ozaki, G.A.T. *et al.* (2016). Analysis of photobiomodulation associated or not with platelet-rich plasma on repair of muscle tissue by Raman spectroscopy. *Lasers Med Sci.* 31(9):1891–1898. doi:10.1007/s10103-016-2067-8.

Pan, L.-C. *et al.* (2022). Single cell effects of photobiomodulation on mitochondrial membrane potential and reactive oxygen species production in human adipose mesenchymal stem cells. *Cells.* 11(6):972. doi:10.3390/cells11060972.

Park, I.S. *et al.* (2015a). Vascular regeneration effect of adipose-derived stem cells with light-emitting diode phototherapy in ischemic tissue. *Lasers Med Sci.* 30(2):533–541.

Park, I.S. *et al.* (2015b). Enhancement of ischemic wound healing by spheroid grafting of human adipose-derived stem cells treated with low-level light irradiation. *PLoS One.* 10(6):e0122776.

Patel, S. *et al.* (2013). Treatment with platelet-rich plasma is more effective than placebo for knee osteoarthritis: a prospective, double-blinded, randomized trial. *Am J Sports Med.* 41(2):356–364.

Pérez-Merino, E.M. *et al.* (2015). Safety and efficacy of allogeneic adipose tissue-derived mesenchymal stem cells for treatment of dogs with inflammatory bowel disease: clinical and laboratory outcomes. *Vet J.* 206(3):385–390. doi:10.1016/j.tvjl.2015.08.003.

Picard, F. *et al.* (2015). Should we use platelet-rich plasma as an adjunct therapy to treat "acute wounds," "burns," and "laser therapies": a review and a proposal of a quality criteria checklist for further studies. *Wound Repair Regen.* 23(2):163–170. doi:10.1111/wrr.12266.

Punzón, E. *et al.* (2022). Equine umbilical cord mesenchymal stem cells demonstrate safety and efficacy in the treatment of canine osteoarthritis: a randomized placebo-controlled trial. *J Am Vet Med Assoc.* 260(15):1947–1955. doi:10.2460/javma.22.06.0237.

Sampson, S. *et al.* (2015). Stem cell therapies for treatment of cartilage and bone disorders: osteoarthritis, avascular necrosis, and non-union fractures. *PM R.* 7(4 Suppl):S26–S32.

Schnabel, L.V. *et al.* (2009). Mesenchymal stem cells and insulin-like growth factor-I gene- enhanced mesenchymal stem cells improve structural aspects of healing in equine flexor digitorum superficialis tendons. *J Orthop Res.* 27(10):1392–1398.

Scribante, A. *et al.* (2023). Laser devices and autologous platelet concentrates in prevention and treatment of medication-related osteonecrosis of the jaws: a systematic review. *Medicina.* 59(5):972. doi:10.3390/medicina59050972.

Shen, C.C. *et al.* (2015). Corrigendum to "low-level laser stimulation on adipose-tissue-derived stem cell treatments for focal cerebral ischemia in rats". *Evid Based Complement Alternat Med.* 2015:278951.

Soleimani, M. *et al.* (2012). The effects of low-level laser irradiation on differentiation and proliferation of human bone marrow mesenchymal stem cells into neurons and osteoblasts: an in vitro study. *Lasers Med Sci.* 27(2):423–430.

Song, J. *et al.* (2017). Use of stem-cell sheets expressing bone morphogenetic protein-7 in the management of a nonunion radial fracture in a Toy Poodle. *J Vet Sci.* 18(4):555. doi:10.4142/jvs.2017.18.4.555.

Stief, M. *et al.* (2011). Concentration of platelets and growth factors in canine autologous conditioned plasma. *Vet Comp Orthop Traumatol.* 24(2):122–125.

Surmeli Baran, S. *et al.* (2021). The effects of photobiomodulation on leukocyte and platelet-rich fibrin as barrier membrane on bone regeneration: an experimental animal study. *Photobiomodulation Photomed Laser Surg.* 39(4):245–253. doi:10.1089/photob.2020.4943.

Tang, W. *et al.* (2022a). Protocol to photoactivate adipose-derived stem cell differentiation using a tightly-focused femtosecond laser. *STAR Protocols.* 3(3):101574. doi:10.1016/j.xpro.2022.101574.

Tang, W. *et al.* (2022b). Stem cell differentiation with consistent lineage commitment induced by a flash of ultrafast-laser activation in vitro and in vivo. *Cell Rep.* 38(10):110486. doi:10.1016/j.celrep.2022.110486.

Tobita, M. *et al.* (2013). Periodontal tissue regeneration by combined implantation of adipose tissue-derived stem cells and platelet-rich plasma in a canine model. *Cryotherapy.* 15(12):1517–1526.

Torricelli, P. *et al.* (2011). Regenerative medicine for the treatment of musculoskeletal overuse injuries in competition horses. *Int Orthop.* 35(10):1569–1576.

Tuby, H. *et al.* (2007). Low level laser irradiation promotes proliferation of mesenchymal and cardiac stem cells in culture. *Lasers Surg Med.* 39(4):373–378.

Tuby, H. *et al.* (2011). Induction of autologous mesenchymal stem cells in the bone marrow by low- level laser therapy has profound beneficial effects on the infarcted rat heart. *Lasers Surg Med.* 43(5):401–409.

Uysal, C.A. *et al.* (2012). Adipose-derived stem cells enhance primary tendon repair: biomechanical and immunohistochemical evaluation. *J Plast Reconstr Aesthet Surg.* 65(12):1712–1719.

Wolfstadt, J.I. *et al.* (2015). Current concepts: the role of mesenchymal stem cells in the management of knee osteoarthritis. *Sports Health.* 7(1):38–44.

Xie, X. *et al.* (2012). Comparative evaluation of MSCs from bone marrow and adipose tissue seeded in PRP-derived scaffold for cartilage regeneration. *Biomaterials.* 33(29):7008–7018.

Yang, C.C. *et al.* (2016). Synergistic effects of low-level laser and mesenchymal stem cells on functional recovery in rats with crushed sciatic nerves. *J Tissue Eng Regen Med.* 10(2):120–131.

Yun, J.H. *et al.* (2014). Effects of bone marrow-derived mesenchymal stem cells and platelet-rich plasma on bone regeneration for osseointegration of dental implants: preliminary study in canine three-wall intrabony defects. *J Biomed Mater Res B Appl Biomater.* 102(5):1021–1030.

Zamani, A.R.N. *et al.* (2020). Modulatory effect of photobiomodulation on stem cell epigenetic memory: a highlight on differentiation capacity. *Lasers Med Sci.* 35(2):299–306. doi:10.1007/s10103-019-02873-7.

Zarembinski, T.I. *et al.*, (2011). The use of a hydrogel matrix as a cellular delivery vehicle in future cell-based therapies: biological and non-biological considerations. Available from: http://www.intechopen.com/booksregenerative-medicine-and-tissue-engineering-cells-and-biomaterials/the-use-of-a-hydrogel-matrix-as-a-cellular-delivery-vehicle-in-future-cell-based-therapies-biologica (accessed November 30, 2016).

Part IX

Integrating Laser Therapy into Veterinary Medicine and Complementary Technologies

37

Successful Implementation and Marketing of Laser Therapy

Diane J. Miller

The Animal Athlete, Newark, DE, USA

Introduction

You now have a therapy laser – or are considering purchasing one. This noninvasive modality can have a huge impact on the way you practice medicine. However, simply introducing a laser will not automatically grow your business. Like anything in your practice, laser therapy is a business segment that needs to be nurtured in order to grow and flourish. Can it be done? Absolutely! Can you realize a significant revenue stream within a year? Absolutely! However, it will depend on how well you integrate laser therapy into your practice and build an infrastructure to support it. Numerous articles have appeared in veterinary trade publications and journals recently, detailing the implementation, integration, and economics of laser therapy (Andersen, 2014; Arp, 2009a,b; Reeder, 2015; Tremayne, 2012; Zimlich, 2015). Despite the success stories featured in these articles, expecting your laser therapy business to grow without any planning or effort is unrealistic and sets you up for failure.

The business model for laser therapy is quite different from other traditional veterinary practice business models. We usually price an item based on a percentage markup or a flat dollar increase. That model makes sense for us. It is easy to handle in our practice-management software, it is something that we are familiar with, and it relates to most aspects of the practice. Laser therapy does not fit this model. Laser therapy, through the process of photobiomodulation (PBM), provides potential benefits in a vast array of disorders and conditions. The previous chapters have detailed the science, the mechanisms, and the many applications of PBMT. All patients presenting with pain, inflammation, or a process requiring healing may be candidates for laser. These attributes indicate that laser therapy will become part of multiple treatment protocols, and this can be rather intimidating when you are trying to integrate this modality into your practice.

When I lecture about how to "Maximize Patient Care and Grow Your Bottom Line with Laser Therapy," I stress that thinking in terms of traditional marketing is a mistake. The world of direct mail, newspaper advertising, and yellow page ads is gone. These media are a waste of marketing dollars. The return on these methods is so low that the time to a breakeven point is measured in months, not days – if it ever comes.

If you look at laser therapy with a myopic view of traditional marketing techniques, you will have a difficult time implementing and maintaining a solid laser therapy foundation. Instead, look beyond your everyday experiences, and learn from other business models that are disconnected from the veterinary industry. Look at other unique businesses and see how they set up their infrastructure and pricing, how they handle customer service, and other related business aspects. Their ideas may require some modification to fit the veterinary practice environment, but it will be well worth the effort.

In this chapter, you will see examples of different business strategies that will give you a better understanding of the elements you need to consider. There are many paths up the mountain, and these are in no way the only options. These concepts have been used by thousands of laser therapy practices, including companion, specialty, mixed, feline-only, equine-only, and mobile. Each has implemented these ideas and achieved results.

Pricing

One of the first questions to cross everyone's mind is, "How should I charge for laser therapy?" There is not a single answer that will satisfy the needs of all practices. Keep in mind that there are many options. However, if you follow the guidelines in this section, you will be able to develop a model that will work in almost any practice.

Laser Therapy in Veterinary Medicine: Photobiomodulation, Second Edition. Edited by Christopher J. Winkler and Lisa A. Miller.

Pricing Guidelines

Avoid using subjective descriptions as pricing classifications (e.g., acute versus chronic). This is the first mistake most practices make. Using subjective descriptions guarantees that at some time there will be an error in estimating. "My dog has a reoccurring problem with otitis. Is this acute or chronic?" Unless there are absolute definitions established, you are setting yourself up for confusion.

All staff must be able to give the same estimate every time; therefore, pricing components and parameters must be consistent. The worst-case scenario is that clients come in for the same condition on different occasions, find the condition interpreted differently by staff, and are invoiced for different amounts for the same therapy. If a client is provided two different prices depending on who gave the estimate, there is a problem with your pricing model, not the staff.

Clients must be able to follow your pricing structure. Every time a client comes in for a laser therapy session, they need to understand what they are being billed for and how the fee was determined. Since photobiomodulation therapy (PBMT) can be included in multiple treatment protocols, a client may see a laser therapy fee for different species, different conditions, and different treatment durations.

Do not micromanage your pricing model. It is easy to get carried away and develop models that consider the condition, the length of treatment, and the species being treated. This can get out of hand very quickly. If the pricing model is confusing enough for your own staff to make errors, then you can imagine what it looks like to your client.

One of the biggest problems is pricing by species. Since they are smaller patients, the application of laser therapy to feline, avian, and exotic species takes less time. However, you will need an additional technician in the room to restrain such patients. Thus, therapy time is short, but the expenses associated with that time are high. When applying laser therapy to a canine, the treatment time will be greater but the dog will likely be more cooperative, and the owner will be able to hold the leash while the dog lies or stands for the treatment. Therefore, the treatment time is longer but the expenses for that time are lower. These two scenarios thus even out in terms of revenue and expenses. As you devise a pricing structure, delve deeper into the process, and consider the total expense associated with a treatment before assigning a fee.

Select a model that allows for the least number of practice management software codes. It should not take your staff an exorbitant amount of time to locate the appropriate code and charge a client the correct amount. You should be able to develop a pricing structure with approximately 15 codes that will cover the majority of scenarios.

Core Pricing Structure

Notice in the following two examples how the fees are calculated by numbers rather than words ("acute versus chronic"). This means the fee determination is a numeric calculation and not a subjective interpretation.

1) **Core pricing by treatment site:** This model is based on the number of sites, body parts, or areas to be treated. The "Initial Site" charge is always billed. This is a higher fee, since it will cover the expenses associated with the services. Pricing for this is US$25–40 depending on the practice and the demographics. In addition, there are associated charges for "Additional Sites." This is a quantity field that depends on the number of sites treated. The fee is usually 50% of the "Initial Site" fee. By adding the "Additional Sites" to the "Initial Site," you calculate the total fee.
2) **Core pricing by block of time:** For some practices, mimicking their appointment schedule enables them to manage, book, and coordinate their laser therapy business. If the practice operates on 20-minute appointments, it is helpful to know that you can roughly treat two sites in a 20-minute block of time. The fee or charge for the first 20 minutes is approximately US$40, which covers the therapy of up to two sites. If the prescribed treatment protocol is more than two sites then the client will be charged for additional 20-minute blocks of time. As with the "by site" example, the additional slots of time will be at a reduced rate, usually about 50% of the initial fee.

The other pricing categories that will need to be taken into consideration are postsurgical applications, dental applications, prepaid bundles of 3, 6, 9, and 12, and redeemed prepaid sessions. The pricing for these will vary depending on your core pricing strategy.

The most significant takeaway is that it is imperative to minimize the chance of different estimate interpretations. Clients should not be confused about what they are being billed for each time their animal undergoes laser therapy, regardless of the species or condition.

Internet, Website, and Social Media Marketing

Internet and Websites

Traditional marketing venues are no longer valid. The standard marketing tools for the promotion of our businesses, products, and services used to be newspaper advertising, yellow pages, and direct mail. Over the last 10 years, the internet and social media have replaced these outdated tools. The continued investment of advertising dollars in older venues must be evaluated carefully, with hard-core returns established and monitored.

Your website is a critical extension of you and your practice. Free, cookie-cutter sites are not sufficient in the long term. Be cautious and look critically at the layout and photos being used on your site. If stock photos are supplied by the web designer, then you stand the risk of them appearing on other sites.

One of the best marketing tools is photos of patients in laser-safe goggles. These are fun to see, eye-catching, and an excellent way to promote your laser therapy business. When clients see these cute pet photos, their immediate reactions are, "Why are they wearing them?" and, "I want a photo with my pet!" When using photos of pets receiving laser therapy in goggles at your practice, clients see familiar "landmarks." This makes the photos personal and unique to your practice, while showcasing this innovative treatment modality.

Search the internet and look at a variety of websites (not just veterinary) to see what looks good and what does not from the perspective of the reader. Then, design your website with those thoughts in mind. It takes time and effort to build this important marketing tool.

Consider the audience when creating your website. For example, there needs to be different content for new versus existing clients. New clients need a lot more information about the practice itself. They have little or no experience or relationship with you. Therefore, you need to provide them with detailed information about your practice: who, what, when, and where. You should critically evaluate this information and ask yourself, "Why should they come to you?" That your practice is "nice" or "close" is not enough. Looking at your practice from this myopic perspective is not going to assist you in gaining or retaining clients. Your website will often provide a potential new client's first impression of your practice. It must be a fair and accurate representation.

The flip side is that website information also needs to appeal to existing clients. It is frustrating to view webpages that give line-item lists of services, with no additional information: Laser Therapy, Geriatrics, Wellness, Diagnostics, Laboratory, Surgery, Boarding, and Grooming often appear as a list of services. This type of information does not provide any significant medical or technical knowledge to your client. A line item like "Laser Therapy" requires additional information and clarification. You should link "Laser Therapy" to a whole page of technical information and subpages with testimonials, photos, and success stories. If it is important enough to mention, then it is important enough to provide technical and substantive information on. If sufficient information is not given, a client may perceive your practice as being lazy, lacking sufficient knowledge, or providing only a minimal version of the service. Remember, a client's perception is your reality.

Another byproduct of inadequate web design is that it forces clients to look elsewhere to obtain technical medical information. This leads clients to other sites: veterinary competition, blogs loaded with personal opinions wrapped up as authority, and self-professed experts with a beautiful webpage. When browsing is encouraged, clients may receive information that is inaccurate, medically dangerous, or contrary to your practice's philosophy regarding quality of care. Do not open the door to clients leaving your website to obtain additional information.

Social Media

Your website is used to display information that is relatively static, whereas Facebook and other social media are primarily used to disseminate information that is rapidly changing. Social media, in some form, is a marketing necessity for today's practice. To use social media effectively, you will need to make regular updates and posts. Pictures, testimonials, and new videos of patients receiving treatments keep people involved.

Appeal to your clients' egos. Having their pet posted on your Facebook page wearing laser-safe goggles and getting their laser therapy treatment will generate a buzz. It will become a contest to see which pet's picture receives the most "likes." Client ego is good for your business if executed correctly and you adhere to a regular posting schedule. Interspersing those postings with links to YouTube channels and technical and medical information about laser therapy and its benefits will not only keep clients engaged but also educate them before they even walk through your door.

Many laser therapy equipment manufacturers have YouTube channels and other sources of information to which you can create links on Facebook and your website. By linking to appropriate information, you encourage clients to become self-educated, informed, and updated. Guiding them to accurate information regarding PBMT and its applications can help emphasize your own practice philosophies about the technology.

Regardless of which social media channels you decide to use, there are some guidelines you will need to follow for your social media efforts to be affective and create goodwill rather than confusion.

Social Media Guideline

1) **Commit to a forum.** Unless you have a full-time staff member dedicated to social media, you will need to

prioritize which forum makes the best business sense for your practice. Select the one forum that will enable you to expand and grow your social presence while being manageable with the practice medical and operational needs. If you are finding this one forum to be expanding and becoming a valuable tool to the practice, consider hiring a person dedicated to social media management.

2) **Respond to positive as well as negative comments.** There is a tendency to ignore or minimally address positive comments. Effective use of social media (acknowledging and thanking posters, answering questions, and posting operational updates in a timely fashion) requires that same amount of time and attention to detail as negative interactions. In some respects, it is more important. If a client goes to the trouble of posting or communicating to you through social media, acknowledging this interaction requires the same consideration as if they had called and left a message on the answering machine. Delaying or ignoring their communication, just because it is positive, allows for it to possibly become a negative comment.
3) **Standardize your answers to negative comments.** Then disengage online. It is understood that you built this practice and it is very important to you on a personal level. But this is business, and you cannot be loved by everyone. Use negative comments to look at processes and operations with a critical eye to make improvements, but do not take them personally! Create a standardized response to address negative comments that acknowledges the issue but take the entire discussion offline, such as:

   "We appreciate your comment(s). If you have any questions regarding your pet's personal care, services received, or any issues at our practice; please reach out directly to the (designated individual – use their title, NEVER their full name) and we will schedule a time where we can discuss them."

   End the conversation there; do not respond further. You have given the individual the opportunity to connect to resolve their issue, and the onus is now on them to contact you to talk. Should a diatribe on the thread continue, delete the thread. If this has taken on a life of its own, then block individuals, especially when people are anonymous and may never have had services with you at all. If they do reach out, then take it seriously. The matter should be handled within days, not weeks.

   You are responding to a phantom until you have all the facts in front of you. If you plan on deleting the exchange, print a copy first and place it in a folder until you have it associated with anyone. Once you have identified the client, place the exchange in their records. You never know when you might need to refer to it.
4) **Monitor twice daily and review all comments and postings on your site.** The use of social media is very similar to voice mail. These must be reviewed and responded to daily at the very least, especially if you have enabled messaging through them. What you do not want is someone to have reached out with a question and then be ignored, or have a negative comment posted and then become viral on a whole new level before you have had a chance to see it. This is an absolute commitment. The minimum you should be reviewing social media is on your arrival to the practice and before you leave at the end of the day.
5) **Train your team to respond to social media.** As with anything in the practice, training of the team is essential. Depending on hours of operation, staff scheduling, and how active your social media is, you may need to have multiple team members reviewing and responding to this account. They are not to treat this as their own account. Some basic tenants are:
   1) Standardized statements (positives and negatives) are just that. They are to be used as written for the designated situation or comment. You will find that these responses will address 50–80% of the posts that you receive.
   2) The monitoring schedule MUST be adhered to – no excuses.
   3) Protect your staff. No personal information is to be given out for any team member under any circumstance. You should avoid last names of the team, family information, home locations, and links to their personal social media pages.
   4) Names for any submissions should always be per attorney-designated format
   5) If you do not know how to respond, ask.
6) **Act as an *educational* forum for products and services.** One of the biggest complaints from the veterinary community is that clients resort to "Dr. Google" for their educational needs regarding products, services, and medical conditions. That's no surprise, given that new technologies and treatment options are developed all the time. Social media fills a gap by linking to approved and accurate sources that reflect the medical philosophies of the practice. Inquisitive clients are a good thing and, if managed appropriately, can be very helpful. And let us face it, it is easier to get on the internet and do the research verses talking to the practice and getting answers. This is not to disparage or imply deficiency in the practice in any way; practice time is at a premium and resources are stretched thin just to address daily operational needs. Social media is a great tool to educate your clients with factual information. Use the educational resources you have available if you do not have

sufficient time to draft articles yourself. Provide an introductory paragraph and then include a link to vetted products and services and enable those to provide the "work" for you. This can be critical if you are incorporating a new technology or treatment protocol into your medicine. Training your clients to look to you first for educational information will reduce the time in the appointment explaining why your protocols differ from the internet.

7) **Obtain approval of the use of client and pet photos.** Secure releases and approval to post them online, especially if they also include children. Just because a client has shared a picture of their pet with you does not mean that they want it shared on the internet, and under no circumstance should any client's personal information be shared. There should be a signed release or acknowledgment before it gets posted (including posting Christmas cards). You may want to consult with an attorney and have a legal release approved for your state.

Some practices have had clients send the photo with a description sent to a designated email account like pictures@animalhospital.com that sends an automated response (also reviewed by an attorney) such as: "Thank you for your picture and description. We may use this for our social media, website, or other marketing materials. If you DO NOT want the picture or comments used in this manner, please respond to this email in 72 hours. A reason is not necessary." This gives them time to come to decision while letting them know the "why" does not matter. Sharing something with the practice does not automatically mean sharing with the world.

You may also want to discuss with your attorney how names should be listed (i.e.: Pet's Name: Muffin Jones, Muffin, Muffin J. People Names: Susan J., Susan). Or use another safe format.

Social media can be an asset within the practice, but like anything else, it will take time and effort to develop an infrastructure to support it. Should you decide to launch a program, it is imperative to have structure and consistency. Take your time, plan it out, identify staff involvement, and have a guide before you start. The prep work may take some time on the front end, but in the long run it will save you time and resources later.

The internet is the communication tool of the future and is critical to promoting your laser therapy business. Create laser therapy content on your website and social media platform that encourages visitors to submit emails, pet information, and questions, all of which can increase identification of laser therapy candidates. Making the most of the internet by creating these tools and incentives will identify patients that can benefit from laser therapy and will increase the success of your marketing tactics.

Daily Communication Opportunities

If laser therapy is a new business segment for your practice, you must spend the time and effort to develop, cultivate, and integrate it into your day-to-day activities. When you're busy practicing, it is easy to remain within your comfort zone and avoid that which is new. Therefore, you will need to develop specific actions that effectively nurture, cultivate, and integrate this new treatment modality into your practice. These actions can be anything from tagging appointments as laser opportunities to developing base protocols integrating laser therapy into the standard treatment of common conditions.

We can become so busy in the day-to-day operation of our practices that we become accustomed to operating in a basic stimulus–response mode. Whatever situation presents itself to us in the moment is what we address. Rarely do we look past this and take an "aerial view" of what our day and our interactions look like. Unfortunately, when busy, we miss dozens of opportunities to integrate laser therapy into our treatment protocols and to educate our clients about this technology. Every interaction with a client can be a laser opportunity to communicate who you are, how laser therapy differentiates you from other practices, how laser therapy impacts the quality of medicine you provide, and how laser therapy can benefit pets.

The 3Ps of Communication

When a client comes in for an appointment, there are multiple opportunities to start the communication and education process. Effective communication requires that we Prepare for it, Provide it, and Personalize it.

Prepare

In veterinary practice, there is never enough time to educate clients about services and products, especially when dealing with laser therapy. The education curve is significant, since this is a relatively new treatment modality. Staffing is stretched, and we often fall behind on appointments rather than get ahead of the schedule, so having time to discuss the features and benefits of laser therapy with each client is not always possible.

Preparing clients with rudimentary information about laser therapy before they come to the practice can help in effectively communicating with them during the visit. Some of the most effective tools for this process are the internet and other electronic information channels.

Websites and social media, email "blasts," and on-hold messaging are examples.

Collecting email addresses is a vital component of preparing your clients and should be a priority. Email is a free communication tool that allows you to share a whole new dimension of information. Email gives you the ability to embed links to videos, send targeted and market-specific information, and link recipients to your website. You can communicate with substantive information and allow recipients to review the material at their convenience, while reducing advertising expenditures drastically.

Provide

Provide clients with quality information during their visit to the practice. Use this time to educate them with detailed information, photos, videos, testimonials, and presentations. Information displays should not only include what is on the walls, but also the materials present throughout the lobby and exam rooms.

A practice is not a repository of expired magazines. These publications have no positive impact on your business. If it seems there is neither the staff nor the time to educate your client base about medical and technical issues, then do not encourage clients to read materials that provide no medical or business benefit. All publications, materials, and displays should have some value to the business and practice itself.

Develop laser therapy literature with a list of conditions that PBMT can be used for on one side, and text about your laser therapy services on the other. Laminate this resource and place it on chairs throughout the lobby. Usually, when a client picks something up from a chair before sitting, they will look at it. They should first see the list with their pet's condition included, then flip the document over to read about laser therapy and how it can help. You have thus prepared them with laser therapy information prior to getting them into the exam room, creating an opportunity to impact your business in a way outdated, unrelated magazines will not.

Personalize

Personalize the information you provide: "What does laser therapy mean for my pet?" Translate materials and communications into impact statements for the client.

Achieve client compliance by taking pictures and videos of pet treatments. This can be a huge asset on multiple levels. In essence, you are making the intangible tangible in the client's mind. Developing an infrastructure that incorporates photos and videos into laser therapy treatment protocols will be a substantial business asset and will make the laser therapy experience very personal. Re-creating a client experience via photos or videos is invaluable. For example, videos are essential when getting new clients to accept laser therapy for osteoarthritis, and when documenting improvement of a pet's quality of life through laser therapy follow-up maintenance sessions.

Appointment Process Touch Points

The entire appointment process and patient visit offers multiple opportunities to Prepare, Provide, and Personalize communications (Figure 37.1).

Published Practice Information (Prepare)

Regularly updating information on social media and ensuring that your website is informative provides the first touchpoint of the appointment process. By using internet communication tools, you can highlight technical products and services like laser therapy. This allows clients to learn and experience technical aspects before coming to the practice.

Email is a free marketing tool that becomes available when a concerted effort is made to collect and continually update email addresses. Sending email blasts that link clients directly to online portals can help educate them at their convenience. Many therapy laser manufacturers have technical information posted on their websites and YouTube channels, often showing unique case studies with wonderful results that can encourage your clients to consider PBMT as a treatment option for their pet. Linking to such information within your emails requires minimal effort and will help fill information gaps, creating an entirely new quality communication tool.

Making the Appointment (Prepare)

Analyze how an appointment is processed and how a patient visit is routed through your practice. Take into consideration what materials and steps are used from the moment the client enters the building through to their exit. Create reminders along that pathway for staff, and the tools they can use, to encourage clients to accept laser therapy as an option.

Tagging appointments when they are made allows your staff to be prepared for a laser opportunity before the client walks through the door. Tagging can involve noting the appointment in the practice software, highlighting travel sheets, placing notices on examination room doors, and distributing brochures to clients when they check in. Each of these actions is designed to remind the staff and the client of laser therapy as a treatment option during the appointment.

Figure 37.1 Appointment process touch points.

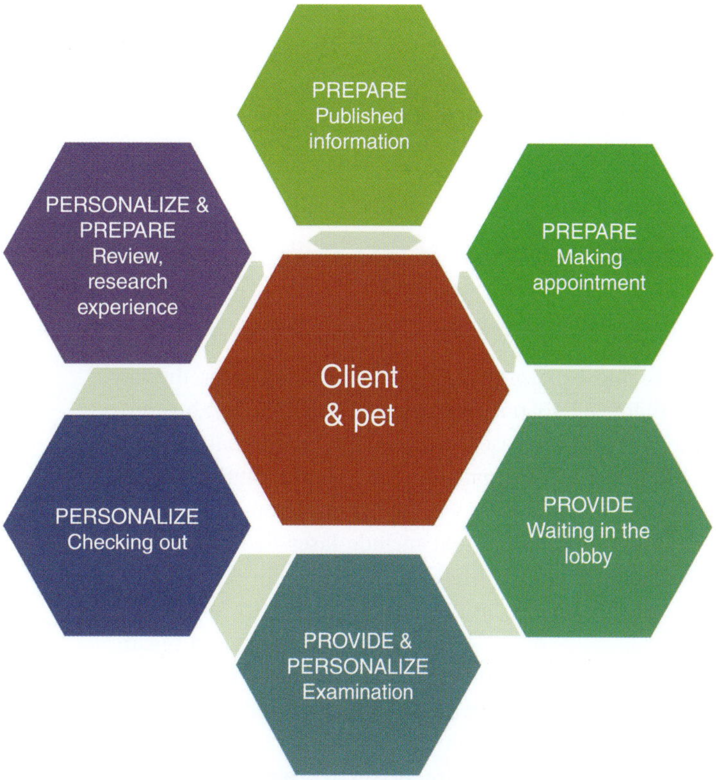

Lobby (Provide)

Examine all your materials critically for how they can increase your business. There is nothing wrong with warm and fuzzy, but there should be a practice pay-off as well. Many practices keep Christmas pictures and cards posted all year round. Yes, this can give a warm, fuzzy feeling, but these displays do not create income to pay staff salaries, monthly bills, or the lease. Limit this season-specific display to the month of December. During the remaining months, a more appropriate use of the space is to display pictures of laser therapy patients with their goggles on. This will create excitement and initiate questions and can have a positive impact on your practice revenue. Do not sacrifice warm and fuzzy: complement it with your practice's services.

Exam Room (Provide and Personalize)

Videos are a critical component of successful laser therapy client acceptance. They do not have to be lengthy, nor do they have to win any Academy Awards, to remain a valuable resource to you and your practice.

For example, videos documenting osteoarthritis need to present the animal in multiple motion states and be consistent in format. Videos should be taken in the same location within the practice and should consist of the same motion exercises. Record patients as they walk up and down a hallway in a frontal and posterior view, then while they are sitting, lying down, and getting up.

Without videos, you are asking clients to remember what a pet looked like several weeks ago. They will likely not remember all the subtle progress that has been made. By recording videos, comparisons can be drawn as treatment progresses. Seeing the first video prior to commencing laser therapy and comparing it to the latest session will present a dramatic benefit picture for the client. These views will enable a client to see their pet's progress in multiple motion states during multiple therapy sessions. This successful progression creates client compliance to continue with additional laser therapy treatments.

An additional benefit is that the video becomes a sales tool for others considering laser therapy. When you describe laser therapy to them and present videos of other pets with similar circumstances, they can visualize what you are trying to accomplish, and you stand a better chance of persuading them to accept laser therapy as part of their treatment program.

Checking Out (Personalize)

Invoices are the one communication tool that every client walks out of the practice with, and they should be considered one more valuable means of communication rather than a business byproduct. Placing a label on the bottom of the invoice with information about laser therapy, or a special offer, can promote the technology and turn an unread or unacknowledged document into a marketing opportunity. Staff should point out this additional information to the client to maximize invoices as a new revenue-generating tool.

Developing a Medical Infrastructure

Creating Base Protocols

Developing base protocols and integrating laser therapy into them will not only increase your laser therapy business but will also increase revenue from additional services. Make a habit of integrating laser therapy into three new protocols every quarter, so that an increasing number of protocols are in place that include laser therapy and are consistent for your entire team.

As an example, consider how your practice manages a feline abscess. Your practice already has a standard-of-care base protocol for treating this presentation. It may include clipping and cleaning of the wound, and application of systemic and topical antibiotics.

Your use of language is important in explaining your base protocol with the intention to add laser therapy. Never apologize or attempt to explain away what you wish to do. What should be conveyed to the pet owner is this: "We are going to clip and clean the wound we are going to apply PBMT to it (which will help to reduce pain, inflammation, and speed healing), and we will provide you an antibiotic to help combat the infection." The client hears a coherent treatment plan, presented with conviction and authority, that makes sense.

When you develop protocols in this fashion, the client understands all the components necessary to improve their pet's health and speed their healing. The more confident the practice is in providing a medical treatment protocol, the more likely the pet owner will comply.

Though we would like for clients to act solely in their pet's best interest, we know that sometimes they take actions based on their own convenience or needs. Include comments that emphasize the impact of your protocol on their time and convenience. This will personalize the plan and get a more positive response to your treatment suggestions. If you use a long-acting antibiotic injection on a difficult animal, saying, "This is because after day 2, I know you cannot pull the cat out from underneath the couch without getting sliced and diced," creates a picture of the impact it will have on them. Money becomes less of a deciding factor and convenience has a greater value. The resulting benefit is that the cat gets the antibiotic you ultimately wish to prescribe.

Creating base protocols using this approach will increase overall service revenue, while providing pets with quality medical care that meets your standards.

One Voice and One Message

Veterinarians as individuals have different preferences for drugs, treatment protocols, and other medical techniques. In general, this diversity has minimal impact on the day-to-day operations of a practice. When introducing laser therapy into the business model, however, there must be a united consensus between all those within the business who prescribe and apply this technology, on when and where it should be applied. Failure to achieve such a consensus can result in client distrust of medical recommendations and erode confidence in the practice as a whole.

For example: Mrs. Smith is a client of Dr. A. Her pets have been seeing him for years, and he has recommended laser therapy for a variety of conditions, such as wounds, otitis, and hotspots, in conjunction with cytology, cleaning, and topical medication. While Dr. A is on vacation, Mrs. Smith takes her pet to see Dr. B at the same practice for an otitis issue. She does not expect any changes in treatment methods. However, the end of the appointment is reached without any mention of laser therapy. When Mrs. Smith asks Dr. B about this, Dr. B responds, "It's not necessary; you should be all right without it." As a client, Mrs. Smith comes to one of two conclusions, and neither of them is good. The first is that Dr. A has been padding the bill and Mrs. Smith's pets have been receiving laser therapy when it is unwarranted. The second is that Dr. B is not practicing quality medicine. Neither of these messages is acceptable.

When you are introducing a new treatment protocol that includes laser therapy, it is imperative that the practice team is united and provides the same message. By developing these treatment protocols, you will provide clients with a uniform message and quality of care.

Advise with Conviction

Clients look to us as experts with all the answers, who can provide a course of action that is guaranteed to be a success. This is far from the case. Diagnosis and treatment can be a complicated puzzle, one in which the pieces do not always fit without close and sometimes extended investigation.

Qualifying words in our everyday language such as "try," "could," "would like to," and "maybe", can lead our clients to hear, "The treatment may or may not work," "This is unnecessary," or "I want you to pay for something unnecessary." This applies not only to laser therapy, but to every treatment protocol and client interaction. By using these words, we set ourselves up for client refusal, as they do not support the quality of medicine to which our clients and their pets are entitled.

As when changing any longstanding habits, there must be a concerted effort to remove these words from our everyday business vocabulary. We do our clients and their pets a disservice if we do not medically advise with conviction.

Everybody on Board

Describing laser therapy to a client can be an overwhelming task. Defining and explaining PBMT can be daunting. Nonetheless, clients do need some explanation of what laser therapy is, why it is referred to as "PBMT," how it works, and what its benefits are for their pet. Developing a standardized message about laser therapy for the entire practice is very important in getting clients to accept it, and it need not be nearly as intimidating as it sounds.

One of the basic analogies to use when explaining PBMT is comparing it to photosynthesis. Regardless of the educational background of your client, they are likely to be familiar with photosynthesis. Using photosynthesis as an analogy is helpful for the layperson: "Sunlight hits a plant and through the process of photosynthesis the plant creates its food and grows." We can take this a step further and use the same idea in describing laser therapy: "We have found that when certain wavelengths of light come in to contact with human or animal cells, their activity is stimulated to reduce inflammation, reduce pain, and speed healing." Though this definition is simplistic, it does help the client have a basic understanding of what is happening to their pet. More technical and scientific information can be given if the client requests it. Brochures from your laser therapy equipment manufacturer, links to your webpage (containing additional links to technical and scientific information), case studies, or and a simple one-page handout with detailed information can all be provided.

Regardless of how you approach laser therapy education with your client, it is critical that the entire team has a fundamental grasp of the core message and its impact. Each member will have a unique method of talking about laser therapy, but the core medical and technical information must be consistent.

Communication Tools

There are many existing communication tools currently in use in practices that we underutilize as marketing tools. These are often free, or through the economies of scale have minimal costs associated with them. They provide additional marketing exposure for products and services such as laser therapy. Some of these tools do require additional infrastructure design and support to incorporate them into laser therapy marketing, but such modifications should become part of your business practices. These existing communication tools include invoices, vaccine reminders, email notifications, on-hold messaging, social media, and activities within the practice.

To successfully use communication tools, there are specific considerations that should be addressed with every marketing effort. The days of "just placing an ad" or "donating to a club" are outdated. Calculated evaluations should take place for each and every marketing endeavor, in order to decide whether to retain it.

Know the Goal

You must have a goal to evaluate success. If you are investing resources, you should know what you hope to gain. Is it clients sending you laser therapy success stories? More photos of patients in goggles? More commitments for laser therapy bundles? Greater acceptance of laser therapy as an exam-room treatment option? There may be instances where the goal is not monetary but rather increased awareness. Regardless, the goal should be determined before initiating marketing using a communication tool.

Monitor Success

Any laser therapy marketing endeavor requires a quantitative measure of success. At minimum, one should know the breakeven point and be able to calculate the return on investment. Data should be tracked, monitored, and regularly evaluated.

Make Information Audience-Appropriate

Communications cannot be everything to everyone. The type of information used to communicate laser therapy to your clients can be based on specific conditions. Marketing to clients with senior pets with osteoarthritis-related conditions should be different from marketing to clients whose patients have hot spots. The audience determines the marketing message.

Include a Call to Action

Marketing messages need to provide a reason or incentive for a client to act on the service. This incentive could be in the form of discounts, information, opportunities, or something else entirely. A call to action should require a client to partake of a product or service within a specified time frame. Examples are encouraging clients to schedule an appointment for a free laser therapy assessment or purchasing six laser therapy sessions and getting one free.

Establish a Reasonable Time Frame

Ensure that the client has a reasonable time frame within which to act and avail themselves of a marketing offer. In most cases, the time frame should be no less than 30 days and no more than 90. Fewer than 30 days may not allow enough people to become aware of and act on your laser therapy offer. More than 90 days allows too much time to elapse before clients must decide to act, contributing to a lack of urgency.

Targeting Elite Markets

Do not limit your target market. There are many different market segments that can appreciate and utilize laser therapy. Some will require added investigation to identify, but most special-interest groups and clubs can easily be located via the Internet. The examples in this section should assist you to look at your clients and community differently.

Pet Insurance

Clients with pet insurance are often more willing to try an innovative treatment, as long as it is covered by their plan. On surveying the 11 known pet insurance companies in the United States in 2017, 10 reimbursed for laser therapy (with some requiring a supplemental "rehabilitation" or "premium" policy). Thus, your practice should recommend pet insurance programs that reimburses for laser therapy and should have some method of identifying clients with insurance in the practice management software. Ensuring that clients know their insurance covers laser therapy is beneficial for both the practice and the pet. The pet insurance industry has changed, and the reimbursement process usually no longer affects billing and payment for the practice. Money does not become a limiting factor for the acceptance of recommended treatments, and pets can receive the care and services that the veterinarian recommends.

Performance Animals

Performance animals are animal athletes. Some of the more common canine performance activities are agility, field trial, flyball, and Schutzhund. Dogs performing these very strenuous, endurance-oriented programs can receive a tremendous benefit from the regular administration of laser therapy. Pre- and post-event laser therapy sessions can provide a warm-up prior to the event and assist with recuperation afterwards (Borsa *et al.*, 2013). Since dogs participating in these sports are often costly, and owners have invested considerable time and money in them, keeping them physically fit and injury-free is a priority. The importance of laser therapy in the care of canine athletes is detailed in Chapter 21.

Figure 37.2 depicts a performance dog competing in Schutzhund. In this depiction of the obedience work shown, one can envision and appreciate the speed of the dog as it approaches the helper, its momentum as it takes the grip, and the follow-through. Note the body positioning, especially the curve of the dog's spine and the location of its rear quarters in relation to its shoulders. PBMT is truly a benefit to these animals, as it allows them to maintain this level of performance. The same is true of the physical demands and needs of military and police dogs.

Laser therapy is equally important to equine athletes. The physical stress on performance horses and their propensity for injury are significant. Incorporating laser therapy into an equine practice is easy, since portable, battery-powered devices are readily available. The new higher-power lasers allow deep penetration into tissues and reasonable treatment times even in large horses.

Service Dogs

Service dogs work across a diverse list of fields, including military and police, detection disciplines (explosives, cadavers, and drugs), handicap assistance, and search and rescue efforts. Creating a laser therapy program for service dogs helps them minimize injuries, facilitates their recuperation, and keeps them on the job. It is a benefit to the animal and to the community to keep these dogs working. If you do not have a program or plan to offer laser therapy for service dogs, make it a priority to develop one.

Integration Conclusion

Effective integration of laser therapy into the veterinary practice requires a business plan. Most successful practices have looked at the individual marketing components and outlined steps to ensure that key elements are addressed. The goal is to have a laser therapy program that is self-sustaining, meshes with existing protocols, and elevates the quality of patient care. Be realistic and self-critical in your marketing efforts, recognizing that traditional marketing channels are no longer effective. Continuing to invest time and money with minimal results is not a sound business strategy, and constant vigilance is needed to weed out ineffective marketing programs.

To successfully integrate laser therapy, you will need to step outside the box and be daring, looking at other successful professions and adapting their marketing techniques to fit veterinary medicine. With focused efforts, much can be

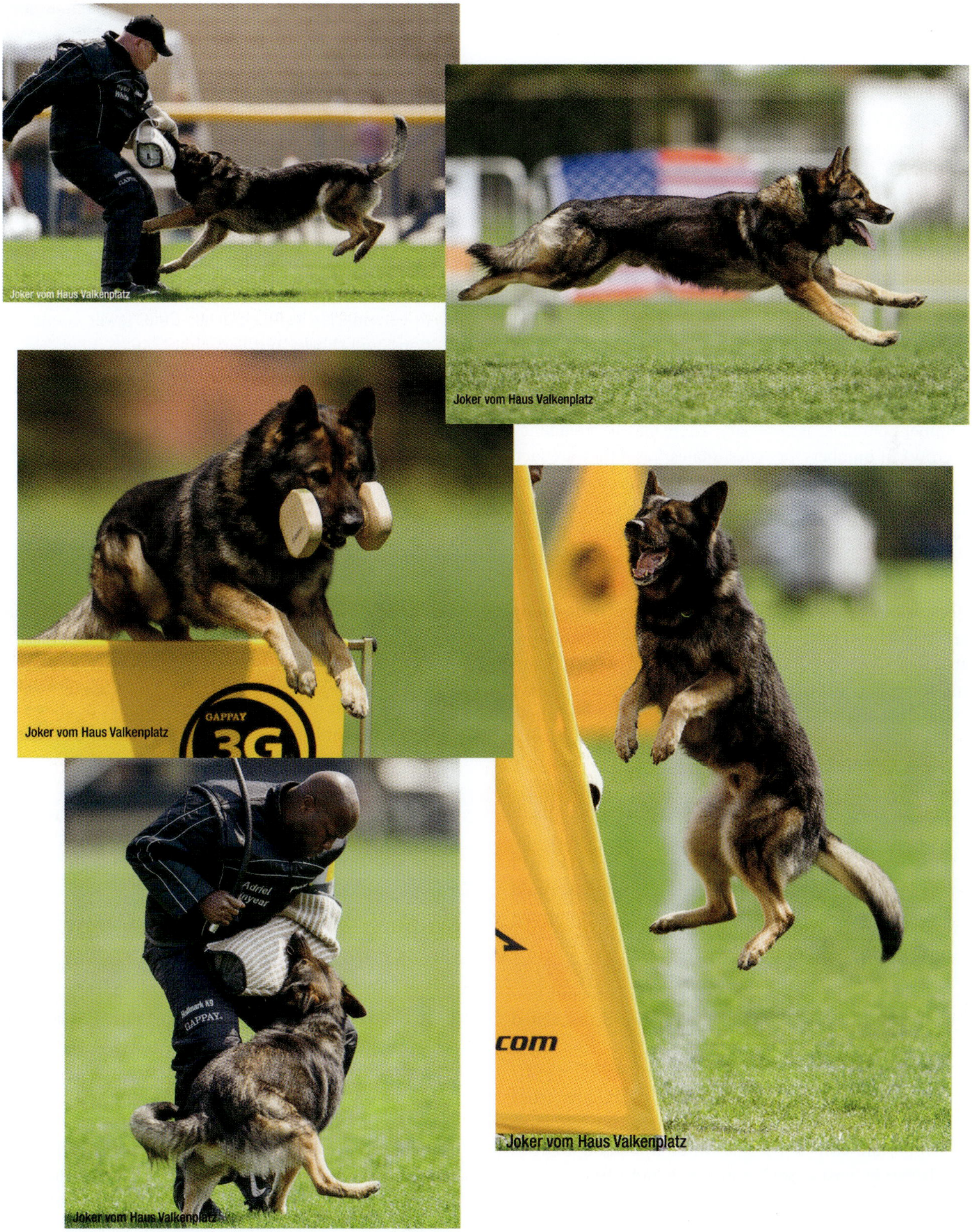

Figure 37.2 A performance dog competing in Schutzhund.

accomplished that will not only improve your laser therapy business but also provide patients with increased quality of care.

Return on Investment (ROI)

As a veterinarian you have recognized the medical value of laser therapy and its value in being a non-invasive, fear-free treatment modality for a variety of conditions. The final hurdle is the hardest: developing an infrastructure to support it within the practice that does not require excessive time and resources. Earlier in this chapter we discussed how to create that infrastructure, but one component was omitted, which we will discuss now: return on investment (ROI).

Using data to measure success or failure of a capital equipment purchase is necessary. There may be a tendency to throw out numbers, or "guestimates," as if they are fact. When businesses are evaluated by guestimates rather than actual data, very rarely are the two comparable. Such differences could translate into significant losses that directly affect resources for business improvements (i.e. a new technician, business renovations, and/or bonuses, etc.).

Determining the ROI for laser therapy involves assessing the financial and nonfinancial benefits of the therapy compared to its costs. It is very easy to get mired in deep financial gymnastics to determine ROI. However, for our use, we will provide enough information to understand the whole picture and enable you to develop a simplistic formula that can work in your practice.

1) **Define the objectives.** Bringing in a new treatment modality requires an identification of the goals and objectives. What are you trying to achieve and how will you integrate it into your medicine? Examples could include knowing what conditions you can treat improving patient outcomes, offering a fear-free treatment option, or developing a totally new revenue stream or business (such as starting a rehabilitation program).
2) **Identify the costs.** Determine all the costs associated with implementing laser therapy:
   - **Direct costs.** Technician time, room use/office visit/tech visit, equipment costs, supplies, and any other associated materials. The first three are the most important costs to consider when evaluating ROI.
   - **Indirect costs.** Staff training, administrative overhead, and facility expenses.
   - **Opportunity costs.** Consider any resources that could have been allocated to alternative treatments. Examples include prescriptions and other therapies such as acupuncture, massage, and other holistic services.
3) **Measure benefits.** Assess both the financial and nonfinancial benefits of laser therapy on a regular basis. A quarterly or year-end review will not allow you to be responsive to your laser therapy business unless and until it is established and successful. Delays in evaluating ROI could mean lost revenue if this is a new service for your practice. Such benefits may include:
   - **Health outcomes.** Evaluate how the laser has impacted your patient outcomes, shortened your treatment times, and affected your use of pain management.
   - **Cost savings.** Calculate potential cost savings related to veterinarian vs. technician time, fewer complications, and shorter recovery times.
   - **Increased revenue.** Determine if the inclusion of laser therapy can lead to higher patient volume or increased ancillary services.
   - **Patient/client satisfaction.** Include PBMT in your surveys to measure satisfaction with the therapy and its benefits to clients' pets.
4) **Calculate ROI:**

   The basic ROI formula is ROI = (Net benefit / Cost of investment) × 100, where
   - **Net benefit** is the total benefit minus the total cost.
   - **Cost of investment** includes all direct and indirect costs associated with the therapy. Cost can be a little more complicated. For example, staff time and overhead are part of the costs, but may already be allocated to your technician or office visit. If you have a dedicated laser therapy technician, you may need to incorporate their salary as part of costs. Be aware that there are relationships to other expenses in your practice, and if an expense starts to show significant changes as you grow your laser therapy business, you may have to make adjustments.
5) **Consider the time frame.** Decide on the time frame over which you want to measure ROI. Short-term and long-term impacts may vary, so consider both when calculating ROI. Take into consideration the structure of your finance agreement to map your financial strategy appropriately.
6) **Document and communicate.** Clearly document data and communicate it to the team during office meetings. Success is dependent on the entire team's understanding of PBMT's medical applications and being proficient in that understanding to feel comfortable in educating clients on laser therapy and its value to the pet.
7) **Continuous monitoring.** Continuously monitor laser therapy's utilization over time to assess whether initial ROI calculations are accurate or need adjustments. Have a doctor complete a Laser Therapy Scorecard

(see below) to assist in determining those who are embracing the modality and those who are not. Having a one-on-one discussion with the practice's veterinarians can assist in determining any reluctance and lack of adoption of laser therapy as a treatment option. If the reason is medical, reach out to your manufacturer or other resources for a peer-to-peer discussion or consider a continuing education opportunity. If the reason is "out of sight, out of mind," look to the information presented earlier in this chapter for suggestions on how to integrate laser therapy more firmly into your established infrastructure.

Calculating ROI for laser therapy can be complex, but even managing it on a simplistic level will enable you to evaluate its profitability within the practice. Equipment should never be purchased to "just break even." The goal is to make a profit and increase the practice's overall revenue year over year. To do this requires data monitoring so you can ensure that everyone has embraced the technology and you are sync to the fullest. When done right, pets benefit medically while the practice benefits financially: a perfect relationship.

Having reviewed the theories, definitions, and actions to take above; let us look at some numbers and how you can apply them to your laser therapy business from a financial perspective, following purchase of the laser (this example does not take into consideration any finance fees or interest).

- Laser purchase = $20 000
- The number of years in which you would want the laser paid off. (e.g. 3 years).
- $20 000 / 3 years = $6666 per year
- $6666 per year / 12 months = $556 per month
- $556 per month / 4 weeks = $139 per week
- $139 per week / 5 days in a week = $28 per day cost.
- Using the laser 4 times a day is $7 cost each time the laser is turned on.

What this example shows is that, every day, your laser costs a minimum of $28 per day. Using the laser will reduce your cost of the laser itself. Not using it will result in this amount rolling over to the remaining days of the week, increasing the financial obligation on the other days and extending the time required to recoup your initial capital equipment cost.

Direct costs, as noted above, include technician time, using the exam room, and the cost of the laser itself. This amount will vary based on how you schedule your office visits and laser therapy appointments in your practice. For this example, we will assume that your laser therapy appointment time matches your office visit time.

- Office/Therapy appointments = 20-minute blocks of time.
- Additional tech or office visit fee (e.g. $50).
- The technician is paid at a rate of $18 / hour or $6 every 20 minutes.
- $50 (Tech/Office visit) + $6 (Tech time) + $7 (Laser cost) = Total direct cost $63.

What this example shows is that if you use your laser a minimum of 4 times a day, for a 20-minute appointment, your direct cost is $63. Understanding how these numbers relate to your laser therapy business will enable you to accurately assess its health and will provide actual data from which you can make informed decisions about the business.

ROI RECAP

1) **Review data** monthly to determine if there are cyclical considerations. You can always make adjustments as you learn about your laser therapy business. Using the Laser Therapy Practice Scorecard (below) will assist you in creating an accurate picture of your own laser business and identify areas that need requiring improvement for success.
2) **Monitor data** monthly, quarterly, and yearly to effectively manage the business during its growth phase.
3) **Compare data** against any marketing or event plan to gauge effectiveness and reproducibility. Learn what marketing efforts are profitable and repeat them. Discontinue those that are not so that resources are focused on new efforts.
4) Look for **improvement** by taking a percentage of missed opportunities per condition for use as a goal during the following period. You can even tie compensations, bonuses, and rewards to meeting these numbers.
5) **Celebrate** your successes throughout the year with your team!

LASER THERAPY PRACTICE SCORECARD

Practice Scorecard : Staff Scorecard: ______________________

Date Period: __________ to __________ Total Clients Seen: ______________

EVALUATION	Comparison Period			Date	to	Date
	Total # of Conditions Seen (A)	Without Laser Treatment (B)	With Laser Treatment ©	Laser Fee Per Procedure (D)	Laser Revenue Per Period (E)	Missed Laser Opportunity (F)
Routine & Elective Surgeries	0	0	0	$0.00	$0.00	$0.00
Dental Cleanings & Extractions					$0.00	$0.00
Common Conditions:						
Otitis					$0.00	$0.00
Hot Spots					$0.00	$0.00
Lick Granulomas					$0.00	$0.00
Wounds					$0.00	$0.00
Edema					$0.00	$0.00
Other: ____________					$0.00	$0.00
					$0.00	$0.00
Osteo Conditions:						
Arthritis					$0.00	$0.00
Hip Dysplasia					$0.00	$0.00
Elbow Dysplasia					$0.00	$0.00
Degenerative Myelopathy					$0.00	$0.00
Other: ____________	0	0	0	$0.00	$0.00	$0.00
	0	0	0	$0.00	$0.00	$0.00
TOTAL REVENUE					**$0.00**	**$0.00**

Column A = data extracted from practice management software

Column B = data extracted from practice management software

Column C = data extracted from practice management software

Column D = Fees for laser therapy assigned for each condition (may vary by condition, site, time)

Column E = Column G * Column F for each row

Column F = Column G * Column E for each row

References

Andersen, D. (2014). Vets say why they use laser therapy. *Vet Pract News*. (August 20).

Arp, D. (2009a). Lasers financially therapeutic, too. *Vet Pract News*. (April 17).

Arp, D. (2009b). Spreading the warmth. *Vet Pract News*. (August 31).

Borsa, P.A. *et al.* (2013). Does phototherapy enhance skeletal muscle contractile function and postexercise recovery? A Systematic Review. *J Asthl Training*. 48 (1):57–67.

Reeder, J. (2015) Fired up about lasers. *Trends*. December.

Tremayne, J. (2012). Lasers offer a therapeutic plan for pain. *Vet Pract News*. (August 6).

Zimlich, R. (2015). Two practices shine light on laser therapy in the veterinary business model. *Vet Econ*. (June 1).

38

The Role of the Veterinary Technician in Photobiomodulation Therapy

Renaud "Ren" Houyoux

Heartland Veterinary Partners, Chicago, IL, USA

Introduction: Veterinary Technicians, the Primary Drivers of PBMT

At the time of writing of this textbook's first edition, photobiomodulation therapy (PBMT) was in its turbulent adolescent years: an emerging modality experiencing pushback from those skeptical about its efficacy or still adhering to the "we've always done it this way" mindset. While such hesitation was understandable, this is not the case today. We are now in PBMT's early professional adult years, and with a solid clinical base for validation, we can now focus on dynamically improving this AVMA-recognized treatment.

Our current understanding and application of PBMT is dictated by its level of evolution, and this momentum of improvement will continue as PBMT becomes more integrated in veterinary medicine. This is why it is imperative and the responsibility of all practitioners utilizing PBMT to take an active role in this continuing process. Just as we should not allow pain and debilitation to establish itself in any case for which we are responsible, we simply should not stand by and hope someone else will evolve this modality for us. Inaction is not an option, and it could indeed be argued that it goes against our primary tenet, *Primum Non Nocere* (Do No Harm).

Veterinary technicians, the drivers of PBMT, must shoulder the responsibility commensurate to the potential evolution of the laser therapy platform. Although credentials, schooling, and areas of interest will vary, all veterinary technicians use laser therapy to achieve the same goal: enable their patients to live the best quality of life they can. The patients are at the core of who we as technicians serve. As a wise colleague said, "To all my patients: Regardless of the direction, the journey has always been about you."

The veterinary technician has always held a crucial role in all aspects of PBMT in veterinary medicine, and this is well understood by the practices that utilize this modality on large numbers of patients daily. With the integration of PBMT into the care and knowledge of our community (notably in its inclusion within the 2015 AAHA Pain Management Guidelines), educating clients, administering and documenting treatments, adjusting treatment protocols and time frames, and keeping the attending veterinarian appraised of a patient's progression are all important tasks the technician must undertake and oversee to provide optimal care for their patients. With a firm understanding of the science and delivery platforms with appropriate power, veterinary-specific treatment protocols, and wavelength parameters, we can look forward to new and extended developments of applying PBMT in our field of veterinary medicine.

Aids and Avenues

1) A written document should be provided to each operator. It should include an organigram of the in-clinic photobiomodulation (PBM) team for immediate internal support and contact information for the laser manufacturer's customer support and local representative.
2) Maintain the laser therapy unit under warranty coverage. The laser fiber is the part of the unit most susceptible to wear and tear from regular use. It is suggested to have a spare fiber, as well as a spare set of any ancillary parts such as the various treatment heads.
3) Implement an ongoing training program for new team members. Nonclinical personnel should focus on their basic understanding and public core message to provide appropriate client support. Clinical personnel should understand the principles and applications of a targeted medical laser prescription. This includes approaches to anatomy when targeting specific areas, such as the cervical spine, iliopsoas muscle group, or stifle structures.

Laser Therapy in Veterinary Medicine: Photobiomodulation, Second Edition. Edited by Christopher J. Winkler and Lisa A. Miller.

4) Allow staff members to begin their training by treating their own or their coworkers' pets. Being more familiar with their own pets and their particular behaviors and responses, this assists laser operators to rapidly become confident in their treatment design and delivery technique and quickly develop proficiency in operating the platform.
5) When adding PBMT, or upgrading from one current laser therapy platform to another, clinics may receive client interest by hosting an "open house" to showcase their new service. This is a good opportunity to initiate treatments for new patients, as well as to offer a discount for initial laser prescriptions.
6) Consider presenting a "Laser Case of the Month" both on an in-clinic board and on social media, as methods to spark interest and begin conversations with clients. This concept should also be considered for inclusion in regularly scheduled staff meetings, keeping PBMT at the forefront of the clinic team's thoughts and repertoire.
7) Provide a laser incentive program for staff members to be rewarded when laser therapy is utilized.
8) Encourage the laser point person and PBMT team to attend continuing education events to deliver the best care and stay current with how laser therapy is developing and evolving. A cornucopia of events and materials are available, and new ones continue to be developed and published.
9) Participate in professional groups and organizations who are familiar with PBM and promote its use in the veterinary field. Targeted networking can be a very efficient resource in keeping a finger on the pulse of laser therapy and its future developments.

The Technician's Role in PBMT Training

When a practice decides to invest in a therapy laser, the technician takes a role to ensure this new modality is understood by all, that laser safety education is undertaken, that safety practices become muscle memory, and that the client base and local community are made aware of this new service addition available through the clinic. Since they are most familiar with treating specific conditions, technicians are best placed to shoulder the responsibility of PBMT training for the practice staff, enabling the creation of comprehensive training programs for their teams, including sessions discussing scheduling and fee ranges.

Typically, initial training is carried out by the manufacturer's representative. Prior to initial training, prepare the team by having them make a list of questions they have for the representative about PBM, and be sure to acquire written materials from the manufacturer for both in-house training and client education. The entire team must truly believe in the modality as a medical prescription and be eager to start offering it to their client base. Any lack of buy-in needs to be addressed during this initial training and implementation so that a simple core message and perception of value is adopted by the entire team at once prior to the introduction of this new service line. Regardless of which area of the clinic and to what capacity they contribute to its operations, all team members must have a solid core of training, understanding, and validation for PBMT.

It is imperative for any practice to establish a key technician who will oversee the use of the practice's laser unit(s), and nurture the training of other team members who may not have as much expertise, to make certain the therapy laser is used to its fullest potential. This technician often has a dual role serving as the practice's Veterinary Medical Laser Safety Officer (VMLSO), a title making them responsible for the safe use of the therapy laser, seeing to it that federal and state laser mandates are followed by the practice, and ensuring that all persons handling the laser are properly trained (Barat, 2006; Oleson, 2016). The successful integration and application of PBMT in clinical practice best occurs with the oversight provided by a VMLSO, who understands the importance of frequent cross-training to not only provide for an in-clinic cohesion among team members, but also enable the practice to optimize the potential use of the therapy laser every day.

Once laser therapy is implemented within the practice, ensure all its teams are motivated to promote and utilize this new tool in the veterinary arsenal. From this point, it will primarily be in-clinic technicians, led by the VMLSO, who will oversee and implement training sessions, remain the primary points of contact to the manufacturer for customer support and case consultations, maintain its use daily by the entire medical staff, and see that it is supported by the rest of the team. Like all services offered by the practice, the entire veterinary team must have a unified core message for the client regarding PBMT, a message established across all teams within the clinic.

Front and Center: The Technician Leads the Way in Client Communication and Preparation

After the clinical team has had their questions answered, they must be prepared for some typical client questions which may arise:

- How does the laser work to help with my pet's condition?
- What other types of lasers are there?

- Does the laser hurt? How does it feel?
- Is the laser safe? Why do we have to wear eye protection?
- Is this used in human medicine? Can you use it on me?
- How long does the treatment session take?
- Who can administer laser treatments? Why can't you give me one to use at home? Why shouldn't I just buy a laser online?
- What results should I expect? When? To what level?
- Do I need to restrict certain activities or encourage others?
- Why are lasers not used in every animal hospital?

As when explaining the benefits of good dental care, it is usually the responsibility of the veterinary technician to convey to clients the basics of PBMT. The veterinary technician often introduces the term "photobiomodulation therapy" to the client (Anders *et al.*, 2015) and clearly explains how this noninvasive, nonpharmacological modality will benefit a patient experiencing pain, inflammation, or any tissue damage indicating a need for tissue healing and normalization to enable a quicker and more comfortable return to function (Chung *et al.*, 2012). The canny laser operator can handle client questions, gauge patient response, and advise with an ongoing plan to deliver an optimal client and patient experience during PBMT sessions. These sessions are noninvasive and do not elicit pain, a perfect tool for a Fear-Free Certified Practice to utilize.

When a client hears the word "laser," most will more than likely think of those used now more than ever in human and veterinary medicine: the more invasive surgical lasers (or, thanks to television and Hollywood, things such as photon torpedoes and laser blasters). Like surgical lasers, therapy lasers produce a coherent, cohesive, and collimated beam of light, but this is where their likeness ends. Surgical and therapeutic lasers often operate with differing wavelengths, power densities, and delivery methods. The different combinations of these parameters (as well as duty cycle and pulse rate of emission) determine the effect laser light has on organic tissues. With CO_2 surgical lasers, the energy is absorbed by the target tissue's intracellular water, which is vaporized through a photothermal effect. With therapy lasers, the energy is absorbed by a different target site, the mitochondria. This initiates a cascade of effects that results in photobiomodulation. Laser therapy is a photoceutical modality. There are other similar applications depending on wavelength selection, but not all use a laser beam as opposed to incoherent multichromatic beams of photons (e.g., ultraviolet for disinfection, neoplasia analysis, heat diffusion imaging, and allied technologies such as thermography, digital thermal imaging, or fluorescence-assisted tissue healing).

In my experience, very few clients are interested in learning about the physics of laser therapy. It is usually counterproductive to share details of population inversions of electrons, their metastable states, and how photons share properties of both waves and particles, with clients who simply seek a noninvasive approach to healing their precious companion who is in pain or physically debilitated. For those clients with a scientific background, the technician could consider making the correlation between PBMT and vitamin-D synthesis. A brief explanation of PBMT coupled with an enthusiasm for the efficacy of the treatment will often be enough to spark interest in laser therapy for many clients.

I find my own preferred approach an easy way to explain to clients the concept of PBM: making it analogous to other processes of light interaction with tissues that are commonly known and understood by the lay person, such as photosynthesis in plants and vitamin D synthesis in humans. These are similar enough that a correlation can be made, allowing the client to grasp the concept of PBM and thus feel much more comfortable to comply as they proceed with the treatment. To put it plainly, structures within cells absorb specific wavelengths of light and convert that photonic energy into cellular repair and functioning. Energy is neither created nor destroyed, it only changes form. I have found the above approach best received by most of our client base so they can understand the concept of photobiomodulation.

It can sometimes be challenging to convey to a client how PBMT is a scientifically accepted and evidence-based modality. If the technician can explain how it works in layman's terms, the client will perceive the value of the therapy and be much more likely to accept the prescribed course of treatments.

The practice's client and patient base should also be examined to identify potential candidates for PBMT. Patient pools such as geriatrics, those on recurring scripts for pain management medications such as NSAIDs, those who have undergone an orthopedic procedure (especially those with surgical implants), those with organ debilitation, EOL/hospice care patients, and those patients diagnosed with chronic and incurable disease such as osteoarthritis, degenerative myelopathy, DJD, and spondylosis. The technician is beholden to ensure that all patients with conditions responsive to PBM are given the opportunity to benefit from it. Laser therapy offers large and impactful new opportunities to veterinary practices when the equipment is properly implemented and used (Reeder, 2015). If it is painful, inflamed, or displays any amount of tissue damage or dysfunction, it is likely a candidate for laser therapy (Karu, 1999; Fulop *et al.*, 2010; Farivar *et al.*, 2014; Pryor & Millis, 2015). The dedicated technician will listen for any of the categories mentioned above, and any word with the suffix "-itis."

Setting the Clock: Laser Therapy Scheduling

Just as with any other modality in the practice, PBMT sessions should be allotted scheduled appointments, with the understanding that any outpatient appointment may also become a candidate for laser therapy. Superficial and acute conditions typically require little time and can be accommodated quickly. Those pets suffering from chronic conditions involving deep tissues and multiple sites of treatment will inevitably require more time. The laser operator must be very clear in establishing to the client a frequency of treatment to ensure a maximum clinical response. To ensure client compliance to that schedule, it is helpful to prescribe a set or bundle of treatments and collect the appropriate fee in advance. This helps provide a speedy transition from patient to patient when the day is fully booked and prevents a bottleneck from occurring. It is also important to provide the client with a written plan for them to follow. This will help to set initial expectations on both ends as well as providing a vision of the pet's progress moving forward.

With such a wide range for potential patients, a successful clinic can establish a robust PBMT program with ample staff support, and implement a scheduling system involving multiple lasers and laser operators, which all see use daily. One laser, typically a larger unit with greater power output, may be operated by a technician with a set schedule for the entire day, usually on long-term patients with chronic conditions. A second laser can be focused on perianesthetic procedures (surgeries, dental procedures) at the same time, while a third laser is on hand for hospitalized patients or for veterinarians seeing ICU and outpatient appointments. These latter two units may be on more portable platforms (such as a rolling cart) for transfer between surgical and dental suites and to various multiple ICU and treatment areas as needed.

The reception team provides crucial assistance to a successful PBMT program, by flagging select appointments on the books for the day to give a "heads-up" to the technical and clinical teams, introducing clients to the potential need for PBMT and providing them brochures to peruse prior to the attending veterinarian completing their physical exam. The exam room technician can quickly reiterate a potential need for PBMT. In this manner, the client receives a consistent core message and indication for use of the laser from multiple members of the veterinary team.

Providing the Laser "Spa Day" Zen Experience

Whether some facilities see shorter unscheduled laser treatments performed in any outpatient exam room while maintaining a dedicated laser treatment area for ongoing scheduled treatments, the veterinary technician should see to it that the delivery venue is equally comfortable for all those concerned. PBMT treatments should be as relaxing for the patient and client as they are for the operator, giving them time to slow down and focus on a patient in a calm setting. It is not uncommon or unusual for some of our patients to start to become sedate or even doze off.

Design a setting that is as therapeutic psychologically as the laser's physiological effect on the tissues. Whenever possible, dedicate a room specifically designed and reserved for therapy laser treatments. Manage the environment to create a quiet, relaxed, comfortable experience for all involved. Other devices enhance a therapeutic environment, such as low music, pheromone dispensers, low natural light, and white noise units. Soft, natural lighting will provide a calming sensation during the treatment. Aromatics may be calming but be cautious with their use since some patients (or even clients) may respond negatively to certain odors. Natural, soothing sounds (such as birds chirping or a babbling brook) can be played at a low level. Have hypoallergenic treats on hand, as patients are easily and eagerly bribed this way to cooperate with the treatment. Treats provide an extra touch of care and empathy to patients and clients. The perception of the client will go a long way to ensuring their willingness to comply with ongoing treatment recommendations.

Small patients can be treated on a table, bringing them up to an ergonomically comfortable level for the technician. Treatments for larger patients can be done either on the floor or on a raised platform large enough for the patient, technician, and client. Regardless of where the patient is treated, it should be able to stand or lie on a very comfortable surface with good footing, especially important for patients suffering from a debilitating disease such as osteoarthritis or degenerative myelopathy. We can do so with nonslip surfaces and a good-quality padded fleece to place under the patient (Figure 38.1). Thick fleece liners can be cut to any shape and provide good traction and enhanced comfort for all involved. They can also greatly help with patients suffering from fecal or urinary incontinence by their wicking property. Disposable absorbent padding may also be on hand for incontinent patients. It is not uncommon to see a patient being treated after an anesthetic procedure within their metallic kennel during the recovery period, and the operator must account for possible reflection of the laser beam from such surfaces. A yoga mat or car windshield sun shield, over which a towel is draped, will minimize this potential for primary laser beam reflection within the kennel and the surrounding area.

Just as with the many other modalities, tools, and equipment we utilize in practice, the potential for adverse laser therapy events exists. Class IV lasers can present adverse

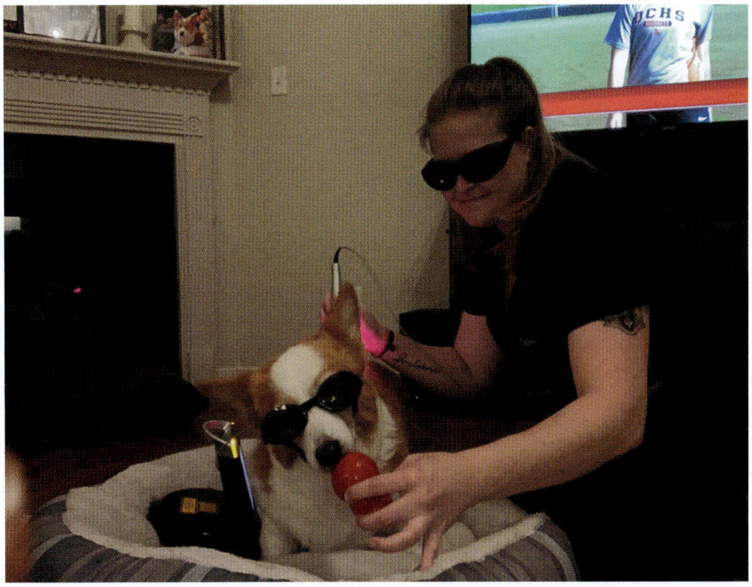

Figure 38.1 A relaxed patient being provided positive distraction by a therapist during a laser session.

conditions such as singed fur or a slight skin burn. These are more likely due to an inappropriate treatment design and delivery through operator error, and not the laser platform itself. This reinforces the fact that we must use the tool the way in which it is intended to operate, and maintain safety parameters while providing for an optimal clinical response. Pursuing laser safety education is essential for all operators within the practice. Delivered correctly, the treatment should be comfortable and not cause any pain to the patient. Treatments are noninvasive, require no sedation, and can be done on an outpatient basis in a relatively short amount of time. The client can be present and take an active role in reassuring patients new to these experiences that such sessions are safe and comfortable. It is very commonplace for clients to refer to outpatient treatments as a "spa day" for their beloved. Administering laser therapy treatments is an art when you consider the intricacies involved. The laser operator should adapt and individualize their technique for each patient. Even though treatments are usually of short duration and do not hurt, we cannot take away the pet's memory of years of veterinary visits, including rectal temperature checks, blood draws, and other uncomfortable procedures. The savvy technician will assume a nonthreatening body language and tone of voice, helping the patient to relax during the treatment and therefore become more amenable to future sessions via habituation.

As laser operators, technicians have the one-on-one interaction with both client and patient, and in turn have a positive impact on the lives of both (Jergler, 2013). The client is often present during the treatment. This enables the operator to be more time efficient as they can get an update of the client's observations of the patient's response to therapy at home. The savvy laser operator practices basic communication skills with clients. This is now also the best point for the laser operator to ensure the client understands the validation for application in this case, the plan moving forward, and any expectations and goals from the veterinarian prescribing these treatment sessions (Andersen, 2014). Polite conversation, appropriate body language, and active listening techniques will prove very useful for everyone involved in maintaining the patient's calm state, assessing its progress, and maintaining client compliance with future visits. It is better to be able to make small talk than to endure an uncomfortable silence during a PBMT session. Small talk can include part of the core message from the clinic to the client, the operator's observations in the modality and their part in the clinic's PBMT program. Other simple ways to engage with the client include seeking hints of the client's interests, such as a polo shirt with an NFL team logo or a baseball cap with a fly-fishing resort. In a well-developed program, the entire veterinary technician team will be cross trained and the client should become comfortable with multiple operators acting in like fashion.

The establishment of a therapeutic and safe setting for laser sessions can become an important source of relief and emotional benefit for the client. I recall a long-term client whose beloved pet was being successfully treated. This gentleman, a war veteran, would begin recalling instances of being in tough situations and explaining how he handled these to ensure his own and his team's safety. As I would start the laser, he would tell stories, such as, "So we had been in the bush on patrol for a few days. I am sure glad it had rained, otherwise I would not have seen the drops of water on the trip wire across the bush trail..." Not once did I initiate conversation in this area, preferring to keep it to the pet's medical treatment plan and assessment of the patient's response to laser therapy, but I always listened and validated his communication. I believe these laser sessions became a sort of "therapy" session for himself as he was dealing with the emotions of situations and experiences only a combat veteran could understand. Laser operators may find that many clients are prone to divulging personal details via such small talks during PBMT sessions and should be prepared to encounter such conversations with PBMT clients, which may strengthen the vet-client-patient relationship.

Going the Distance: Short-Term Versus Chronic Treatment in Phases

Assess each laser therapy patient as an individual, making sure to consider breed, age, predispositions, preexisting conditions, lifestyle, and current medical treatments, especially any pharmaceuticals the patient is receiving. No two patients or conditions are alike, and neither is their own individual response to therapy. The treatment plan, just like the administration of the treatment, needs to be tailored accordingly. Some patients with extreme pain or advanced chronic disease are more likely to require an extended habituation to treatment. They may be too sensitive in early sessions to allow direct contact of the handpiece to the treatment site, movement of joints through range of motion, or a massage technique. If the patient is improving, it is acceptable to allow them to respond as an individual, and to give them the time they need to reach their peak of response.

I find veterinary patients to be very adaptive and resilient. While humans tend to dwell on things and overrationalize, pets live in the moment and take everything as is, without wasting any time feeling sorry for themselves or questioning why things are the way they are. The astute laser technician keeps this in mind whenever performing a treatment. A young and otherwise healthy patient will be able to respond more rapidly and effectively than a geriatric patient, which may have preexisting conditions already taxing its body's energy, immune system, and overall ability to function and repair itself. Patients will quickly habituate to laser therapy treatments, rapidly learning that these sessions are not painful, noninvasive, and relatively short (Figure 38.2). It is not uncommon for a client to report that their dog is eager to come in for a treatment. Patients quickly associate a palliative response with therapy. They often visibly relax during treatment, offer access to the treatment site (even turning over on their own when appropriate) or lean into the therapy laser handpiece as the treatment is administered with an on-contact delivery technique (Figure 38.3). Successive treatment sessions become more relaxed as the patient's pain is reduced and the client comes to appreciate how his or her companion can resume past behaviors that became lost due to injury or the progression of osteoarthritis and degenerative joint disease.

The specific condition being treated, as well as return to function, will determine the frequency and duration of ongoing treatments. Laser therapy treatments have a cumulative effect; they build on one another. For acute conditions (e.g., otitis externa or trauma such as a snakebite wound), a series of treatments should be administered until complete resolution is achieved. A different approach is usually taken when treating a chronic condition such as

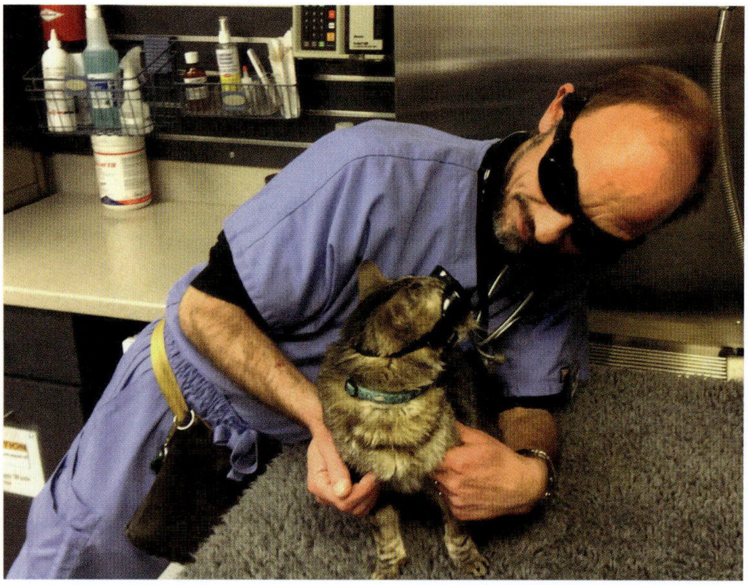

Figure 38.2 A patient and laser operator prior to a laser session.

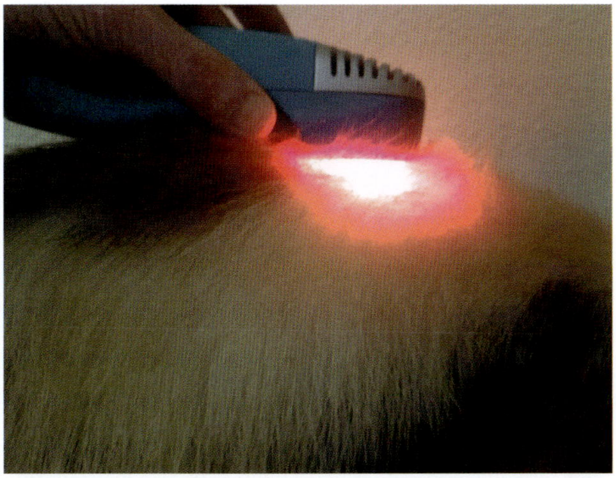

Figure 38.3 On-contact treatment technique.

osteoarthritis or chronic stomatitis. Chronic conditions can yet be managed and maintained, and their degenerative nature can be altered to be less aggressive and progressive. Since we cannot completely cure most chronic conditions, the goal is to promote comfort and mobility while preventing an active decline by adopting a proactive approach in our delivery of care, realizing that each patient will have an individual peak plateau response.

There are multiple ways to design a treatment plan for patients presenting with either an acute or chronic condition. Let us also not overlook the possibility of an acute-on-chronic situation for multiple conditions being addressed. While it is possible to underdose a patient with an inadequate total target dose (J/cm^2) or carry out treatment inappropriately, it is difficult, if not impossible, to overdose a patient. Damaged cells repairing themselves via PBM will only respond when the metabolic rate is less than normal. Healthy tissue cannot become "super tissue" through PBM. The best way to treat a patient is to reevaluate at each presentation and adjust the treatment plan accordingly. Flexibility must always be shown in treatment design, delivery, and frequency of therapy.

The technician's ability to think creatively and be adaptive to different situations remains a crucial requirement of the effective laser operator. An example of the "adapt and overcome" mantra might be where a patient is sensitive to the use of needles in acupuncture. Photonic energy could instead be administered to the acupuncture points, often with similar results to needling, such as in the treatment of point P6 to prevent nausea in a patient undergoing chemotherapy treatments (Lorenzini *et al.*, 2010; de Oliveira & de Freitas, 2016). Cats with pathological rib fractures secondary to asthma may also benefit from a timely application of PBM. Many "contraindications" hold over from a continuation of early lack of understanding carried out decades ago. For example, while it is not typically recommended that serial treatments be performed on active growth plates (de Oliveira *et al.*, 2013), it is not contraindicated to administer a single or a short series of palliative treatments to an acute epiphysitis case (Oliveira *et al.*, 2012; Son *et al.*, 2012), or to treat a puppy with active epiphyses for parvoviral enteritis abdominal pain. The current laser operator is encouraged to educate themselves on the physics and physiological effects of PBM and considerations for its safe use in the previous chapters of this text.

We must be aware that current dosing recommendations continue to evolve as this modality does. Overall, we can appreciate an increase in recommended dosages from what has been previously recommended in the past few decades:

- Superficial conditions: 3–5 J/cm^2 (pyotraumatic dermatitis, postop incision)
- Deep tissue conditions: 15–20 J/cm^2 (OA, ALG, pancreatitis, masticatory myositis)
- Refractory conditions: 30–40 J/cm^2 (degenerative myelopathy, gingivostomatitis, CRF)

It is typically recommended to use a conservative irradiance (W/cm^2) for superficial treatments to ensure patient comfort. Initially, technicians should set expectations for conditions to which PBMT will be recommended as an allied technology. Such conditions' treatment recommendations will continue to evolve as the team implements the daily use of PBM, and is thus expected to be an ongoing process.

If there is any level of pain, it needs to be addressed. An appropriate palliative plan is paramount to expect clinical success since, when left unabated, pain will quickly trump other basic needs for life such as nutrition and hydration. When a patient presents with pain, it is appropriate to treat daily until a clinical response is noted. If the patient is in intractable pain, it is advantageous to treat more often, such as twice (or three to four times) daily. Once a clinical response is noted and the pain level has been reduced to a tolerable level, an every-other-day treatment frequency is recommended until resolution, or until a peak plateau response is achieved, at which point a phasic tapering technique can be applied while moving forward in the course of treatment. With chronic conditions, the frequency of treatment should be tapered once the patient has reached the initial therapeutic goal; the cumulative effect of multiple treatments enable a tapering in treatment frequency to maintain the peak plateau response. Ongoing treatment phases are designed with increased times between treatments. If the patient does not have any relapses, this tapering can continue.

Prevention of such setbacks while maintaining a clinical effect is the key to effective tapering. Regardless of the planned treatment time frame, the client must understand that the patient needs to return immediately if there are any relapses. The plan should remain flexible, each patient treated as an individual. This is where each patient's unique physical status, daily routine and lifestyle, and potential secondary diseases especially come into play. No two patients are alike; treat the individual appropriately as for the individual they are. If poor response to therapy continues, consider reassessing the initial diagnosis.

Fortunately, only a small percentage of patients are truly beyond the reach of PBM therapy. It is a victory for medical professionals and the patients entrusted to our care if we can make a moment minimally painful and potentiate the body's ability to heal more quickly and effectively. With an appropriate treatment plan tailored for the individual, a clinical response and improvement are usually noted in the majority of our patient pool.

Due Diligence: Treatment Documentation by the Technician

Like all medical treatments, each laser therapy treatment needs to be included in the patient's medical record. The most efficient way of doing this is to design a form that is incorporated into the patient's daily record. This form should include specifics such as the date of the treatment, the name of the laser operator, the attending veterinarian, and the treatment's specifics: the sites being treated, their approximate size (cm^2), the power (W), length of time, and the total energy and target dose delivered to each site (joules and joules/cm^2 respectively). It is also important for this form to include the technician's notes about the patient's progress and response to treatments. These notes are crucial since they allow all the practice's technicians to have current information going forward, regardless of who is administering the treatment. Thankfully, most practice management software platforms easily integrate this information, even when a specific "Laser Treatment Form" has been created and integrated (Figure 38.4). Documenting the patient's progress helps determine the need for further treatments and at what time intervals they should be applied. The attending veterinarian can use the record to determine a course of future laser therapy treatments, declare resolution of a condition for their records, or be delivered to a referring veterinarian if the case was provided as a referral service.

AAHA American Animal Hospital Association

8 years and 7 months old

Laser Therapy

Date: 5/12/14
Operator: Ren

Initiating DVM: Dr.

Feline ☐ Coat ☐ Light ☐ Medium ☑ Dark
Canine: ☑ Skin Color ☐ Light ☐ Medium ☑ Dark
Weight ☐ 0-20 ☐ 20-40 ☑ 40-60 ☐ 60-80 ☐ 80-100 ☐ >100
Power: 7 Watts Time: 4:10
Energy: 1400 Joules

Probe:
☐ Small Ball (Contact Only!!)
☐ Large Ball (Contact/Non-Contact
☐ Small Cone (Non-Contact less than 6 watts)
☑ Large Cone (Non-Contact greater than 6 watts)

☐ Arthritis
☑ Pain Trauma
☐ Edema Swelling
☐ Acute pain
☐ Sprain Strain

☐ Head
☐ Neck
☐ Shoulder
☑ Elbow
☐ Carpus
☐ Back
☐ Hip
☐ Stifle
☐ Tarsus

Notes and Protocol Adjustments

Hx. STS Sx. 4/26, Tx. # 2 (single charge - Level 2).
Pt. QAR, standing during Tx, no RXN noted.

Site healing nicely, healthy granulation bed.
Active contraction @ wound edges.
Inflammation / edema greatly decreased since last Tx.
Pt. walking normally, appears comfortable.

Focused 75% of Tx. @ wound edges, 25% @ granulation bed.

Soft tissue bandage replaced P-Tx.

Very encouraging glidepath after initial Tx.

Plan: O will D/O Friday, may poss. call to set up an appointment on Wednesday as well.
Focus on wound healing for now, poss. consider chemotherapy after wound closure. RH

Figure 38.4 Sample laser treatment form.

Gold Nuggets: Technician Treatment Tips and Techniques

Occasionally, a client will report that a patient suffering from a chronic condition seemed a little stiffer the afternoon or evening after the first few treatments. This is a positive sign of response, indicating that the patient's tissues are being affected in a positive and reparative fashion by PBM. Typically, these symptoms are low-grade and transient, do not cause severe pain, and do not last more than 24 hours. If they are noted early in the treatment phase, it is encouraging, since it points to the patient's physical ability to respond, and actual tissue remodeling is occurring.

When given the option, it is always more efficient to make light and steady contact with the tissues to maximize photon transmission into them. However, there will be times when a contact technique will not be possible, such as the intraoperative treatment of a closed cystotomy incision or intestinal anastomosis site (Kirkby *et al.*, 2012). When not in contact with the tissue, the laser technician may elect to increase the total target dose by 20–40% to account for surface scatter of photons that occurs with a noncontact delivery technique.

The nearby healthy tissue margins surrounding the target treatment site should be treated as well. Proper illumination of both target tissue and nearby healthy tissues will ensure an optimal clinical response from the patient. To do so, the laser beam needs to make a full excursion over the affected area as well as approximately 2 in. of adjacent healthy peripheral tissue margins. The handpiece should be held perpendicular to the target tissues to ensure a uniform beam spot on all tissues being treated.

When treating any part of an extremity, treatment should be administered in a circumferential manner to ensure complete photonic penetration and saturation of the tissues. If the patient will allow, their joints should be moved through a passive range of motion while treating. With severely affected and painful patients, this may not always be possible during initial treatments. Most patients will habituate to treatments and reach a comfort level where they will allow some degree of limb motion and manipulation. Putting a joint through a passive range of motion during laser therapy administration ensures that the photonic energy reaches all target tissues and intraarticular surfaces. Monitoring of these sites by taking goniometric measurements at presentation and during ensuing treatments can be an effective tool in documenting the patient's progress. Thermography (digital thermal imaging) can also be utilized to establish baseline variance in thermal emission of contralateral sites and the ensuing change in said variance as the patient courses through treatment phases (Figure 38.5).

When treating an extremity, it is also recommended to perform a separate treatment to the spinal nerve root segments innervating that limb. This optimizes the treatment on the extremity by reducing the transmission of painful stimuli at the site of photobiomodulation in the pain pathway and thus decreasing the patient's perception of pain (Chow *et al.*, 2007).

Laser therapy should always be applied to any secondary, tertiary, and compensatory sites. For example, when treating the hip joint, it is useful to palpate the pectineus muscle (originating on the pubic crest and inserting on the medial shaft of the femur) to assess how tight, sensitive, or reactive

(a) (b)

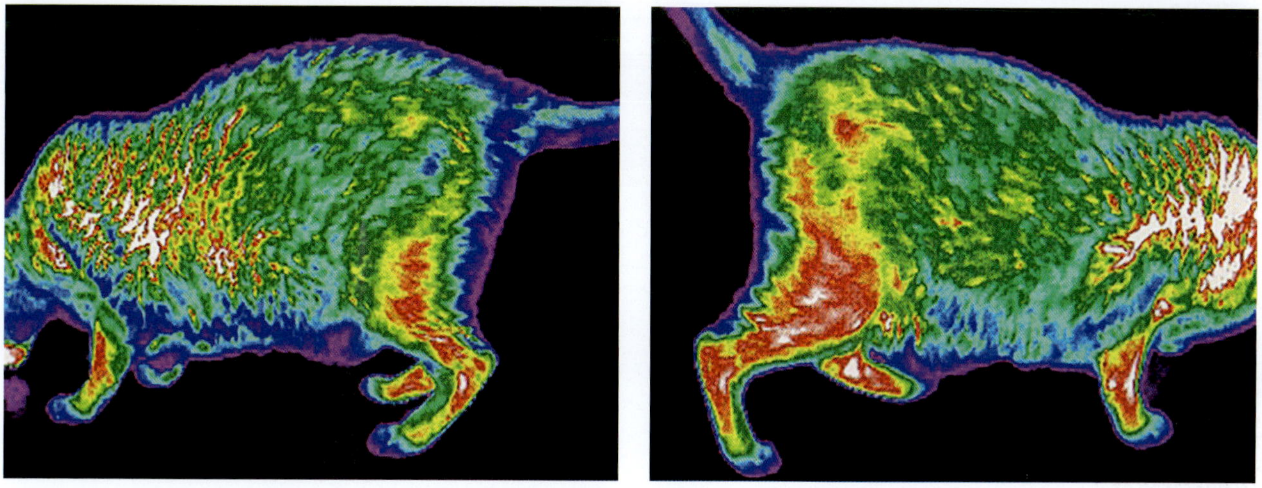

Figure 38.5 Left lateral (a) and right lateral (b) digital thermal imaging screening of a feline patient.

the muscle is. Often, a patient having hip discomfort will have compensatory pain in the pectineus muscle, exhibiting as very tight and reactive even to the lightest palpation or strumming. Continuing to palpate this muscle as further treatments are carried out can be a helpful tool by which to assess the patient's progress.

Another example of a compensatory site that should be treated in any hind-limb musculoskeletal disorder is the iliopsoas muscle group, originating from the ventral aspect of lumbar vertebrae L2–L7 and inserting on the lesser trochanters. These are frequent sites of compensatory pain, and can typically be evaluated for sensitivity via hip extension and external rotation of the pelvic limb.

With all treatments, the laser operator should be mindful of the need to monitor the patient for any reactivity or sensitivity to specific trigger points in the tissues being treated. If the patient does exhibit a focal sensitivity, special attention should be paid to that area. Monitoring decreased reactivity to previously sensitive trigger points is another good way to measure the patient's progression in response to laser therapy treatments.

Conclusion: Reaching New Horizons of Laser Therapy

Veterinary technicians continue to play an essential role in laser therapy. They should be involved in every aspect of this modality, including planning for and implementing laser therapy in the practice. They can oversee the training of other staff members and become a vital communication resource for clients. It is their responsibility to be adept in not just administering treatments but guiding the patient and client through their scheduled therapeutic regimen as well. With proper training, technicians can help ensure that laser therapy is administered utilizing a proper and consistent technique, individualized protocols, and effective client communication, for the welfare and benefit of their patients.

Although the experiences we accrue as we work through the years belong to us as individuals, the knowledge that we gain does not. This knowledge must be shared for the benefit of the patients entrusted to our care and the medical community. The experienced technician should responsibly pass on knowledge about laser therapy to newcomers in our ranks and help ignite the spark of motivation and innovation integral in furthering this technology as it continues to develop. Technicians should also monitor continuing technological developments that facilitate patient evaluation while undergoing laser therapy.

While there remains much to learn about laser therapy, what was proven to be valid, safe, and effective when used appropriately at the time of the first edition (Mandel & Hamblin, 2012), has now evolved into an established treatment modality that is widely accepted and utilized in the veterinary field. Now more than ever, this is a unique and exciting time to be a veterinary technician. With PBM platforms, we are enabling pain reduction and tissue healing at the speed of light. Semper Ad Lucem.

References

Anders, J. *et al.* (2015). Low-level light/laser therapy versus photobiomodulation therapy. *Photomed Laser Surg.* 33(4):183–184.

Andersen, D. (2014). Vets say why they use laser therapy. Vet Pract News. August 20.

Barat, K. (2006). Laser safety officer or advisor. In: *Laser Safety Management*, p. 9. Taylor & Francis, Boca Raton, FL.

Chow, R.T. *et al.* (2007). 830 nm laser irradiation induces varicosity formation, reduces mitochondrial membrane potential and blocks fast axonal flow in small and medium diameter rat dorsal root ganglion neurons: implications for the analgesic effects of 830 nm laser. *J Peripher Nerv Syst.* 12(1):28–39.

Chung, H. *et al.* (2012). The nuts and bolts of low-level laser (light) therapy. *Ann Biomed Eng.* 40(2):516–533.

Farivar, S. *et al.* (2014). Biological effects of low-level laser therapy. *J Lasers Med Sci.* 5(2):58–62.

Fulop, A. *et al.* (2010). A meta-analysis of the efficacy of laser phototherapy on pain relief. *Clin J Pain.* 26(8):729–736.

Jergler, D. (2013). Staffs embrace laser therapy. Vet Pract News. November 14.

Karu, T. (1999). Primary and secondary mechanisms of action of visible to near-IR radiation on cells. *J Photochem Photobiol B.* 49(1):1–17.

Kirkby, K. *et al.* (2012). The effects of low-level laser therapy in a rat model of intestinal ischemia-reperfusion injury. *Lasers Surg Med.* 44(7):580–587.

Lorenzini, L. *et al.* (2010). Laser acupuncture for acute inflammatory, visceral and neuropathic pain relief: an experimental study in the laboratory rat. *Res Vet Sci.* 88(1):159–165.

Mandel, A. and Hamblin, M. (2012). A renaissance in low-level laser (light) therapy – LLLT. *Photonics Lasers Med.* 1(4):231–235.

Oleson, S. (2016). Laser Safety Officer Information. Available from: https://www.lia.org/subscriptions/safety_bulletin/laser_safety_info/#The Laser Safety Officer (accessed November 30, 2016).

de Oliveira, R.F. and de Freitas, P.M. (2016). Laser therapy on points of acupuncture on nerve repair. *Neural Regen Res*. 11 (4):557–558.

Oliveira, S. *et al.* (2012). Low-level laser on femoral growth plate in rats. *Acta Cir Bras*. 27(2):117–122.

de Oliveira, F. *et al.* (2013). Helium-neon laser therapy interferes with epiphyseal plate growth in the femur and tibia of rabbits. *Photonics Lasers Med*. 2(4):349–354.

Pryor, B. and Millis, D.L. (2015). Therapeutic laser in veterinary medicine. *Vet Clin North Am Small Anim Pract*. 45(1):45–56.

Reeder, J. (2015). Fired up about lasers. *Trends*. December.

Son, J. *et al.* (2012). Bone healing effects of diode laser (808 nm) on a rat tibial fracture model. *In Vivo*. 26(4):703–709.

39

Infrared Thermal Imaging and Laser Therapy

Ronald J. Riegel

American Institute of Medical Laser Applications, Marysville, OH, USA

Introduction

Infrared thermal imaging first appeared in veterinary literature in 1964 (Smith, 1964) when it was used as a screening tool on performance horses. This early thermography equipment was rudimentary, cumbersome, and expensive. There was little understanding of how to image patients, much less the knowledge needed for interpretation. In the 1980s, courts in the United States accepted thermography as evidence of the patient experiencing pain (Archer & Zinn, 1983; Goodman & Zak, 1986; Lamb *et al.*, 1988). This evidentiary determination allowed the use of thermology to expand in human medicine to include cancer screening, identification of work-related injuries, and monitoring functional physiology.

In the 1960s and through the mid-1970s, several studies investigated the effectiveness and benefits of infrared thermography in veterinary medicine (Delahanty & Georgi, 1965; Clark & Cena, 1977). In 1975, Nelson and Osheim used infrared thermography in a regulatory capacity when they documented the abnormal characteristic infrared emission pattern on the area of the limb when a chemical substance was administered to the horse's digit. In 1977, Purohit *et al.* established a protocol for obtaining normal thermographic patterns of the horses' limbs and other anatomical areas. At the Olympic Games in Atlanta in 1996, infrared thermography was the most requested service by the equestrian teams.

Since its inception, infrared thermography has evolved technologically, developed established techniques and protocols, and now relies on standardized interpretation to become an invaluable screening tool in both human and veterinary fields. These functional physiological images provide an anatomical guide for administering PBMT, objectively monitoring the patient's response to therapy, and serving as a visualization to the client.

Introduction to Veterinary Infrared Thermal Imaging

Dramatic veterinary infrared thermal imaging improvements have occurred in the last 10 years. Technologically, there have been refinements in the mid-infrared range detector chips, faster microprocessors that convert thermal energy into an electrical signal, improvements in the display systems, and advances in analytical software to even include artificial intelligence-based interpretation.

Infrared thermal imaging is a noninvasive measurement, compilation, and analysis of the radiated electromagnetic thermal energy emitted by the patient. The process involves using an infrared camera system that captures the emitted radiation. A thermal microprocessor transforms this radiation into electrical signals, which can be displayed in colors or shades to represent different temperature values (Figure 39.1).

The system's software plays a crucial role in this process. It converts each quantum of infrared energy into a corrected temperature reading and assigns each temperature a specific color or shade. This results in a dynamic, two-dimensional representation of the temperature data emitted by the patient, known as a thermogram. These thermographic images are then used to visualize and assess the patient's functional physiology dependent on the circulation. Think vascular visualization! The skin is an accurate projector of heat from the underlying structures and their vascular supply. This heat energy travels from the deeper tissues to the skin's surface through a process called conduction (Flesch *et al.,* 1985). For example, muscles with a rich blood supply emit thermal energy due to the constant cellular metabolic activity. However, tendons, ligaments, bones, and areas with compromised sympathetic nerve supply radiate less thermal energy because of a lesser

Laser Therapy in Veterinary Medicine: Photobiomodulation, Second Edition. Edited by Christopher J. Winkler and Lisa A. Miller.

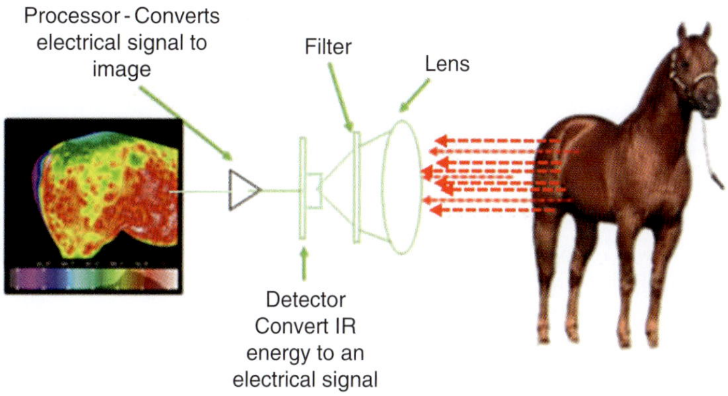

Figure 39.1 Thermal energy radiates from the patient, passes through the lens, and is converted into an electrical signal by the detector (microbolometer). This signal is then converted into a color or shade palette image that represents a graphical temperature distribution map of the examined body surface called a thermogram.

vascularization within the structures, or that vascularization is in a vasoconstrictive state.

In summary, an infrared image (a thermogram) is a visual map of the emitted skin surface temperatures. These recorded skin temperatures represent heat transferred from internal structures through various tissue layers via conduction. To interpret thermographic images, a basic understanding of the physiological mechanisms of skin blood flow and the factors within the patient that influence heat conduction to the skin must be considered to evaluate this dynamic process (Otsuka *et al.*, 2002).

Current Analytical and Diagnostic Techniques

Ideally, we would like to determine a definitive diagnosis for each patient. For anatomical diagnostics, we rely on images obtained via digital radiography, CT scanning, MRIs, and ultrasonography (Figure 39.2). Each imaging technology has one distinction: The images they produce tell us what has already happened. Infrared thermal imaging provides us with information on what is happening to the patient in real time. These images visualize the functional physiology of the patient at that moment.

The American Academy of Thermology (Veterinary Guidelines)

The American Academy of Thermology (AAT) has published internationally peer-reviewed guidelines on veterinary thermography (American Academy of Thermology, 2019). The first veterinary guidelines were written by a committee formed of veterinary and medical members of AAT in 2013, revised in 2016, and revised again in 2019. The mission and bylaws of the AAT support the incorporation of thermal imaging into veterinary clinical medicine. The AAT recognizes the need to promulgate continuing education in the science and methods of thermal imaging and the clinical application of heat asymmetry patterns obtained from thermal imaging among veterinarians and thermal technologists.

The following information is abbreviated, condensed, and paraphrased versions of the content within the 2019 revised version of the veterinary guidelines.

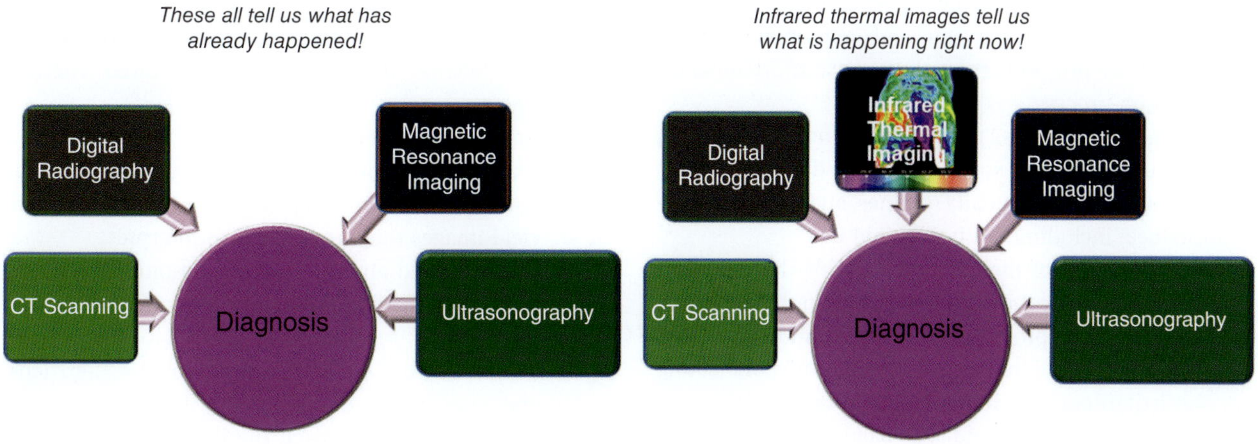

Figure 39.2 Digital radiography, CE scanning, MRIs, and ultrasound images all provide us with information about our patients that has already happened. Infrared thermal imaging provides us with information about the patient's physiology in real time.

Common Uses

The AAT guidelines list four common uses for infrared imaging in veterinary medicine:

1) As an adjunct to obtaining a diagnosis, changes in the thermal patterns of the scanned areas suggest a thermographic finding, which is further investigated through physical examination and using anatomical diagnostic imaging modalities.
2) As a method to enhance clinical assessment of the veterinary patient, include:
    - Evaluation and assessment of the patient's functional physiology:
        - Pre-physical exam screening tool to identify areas that would benefit from further evaluation.
            - A visualization of the patient's muscle and peripheral circulation.
            - Qualitative and quantitative assessment of the vasculature and blood flow to the tissues.
            - An evaluation of peripheral neuropathies.
            - Pre-procedure assessment to aid in the planning of interventional therapeutics or diagnostics.
            - Evaluation of an anatomical area of inflammation.
    - Objective patient monitoring:
        - Follow-up on baseline images of patients with known or suspected vasomotor instability.
        - Follow-up to detect a disease's improvement, progression, or spread, all of which could be visualized in numerous areas.
        - Evaluation of postsurgical swelling and wound healing.
        - Evaluation of unexpected postoperative complications.
        - To determine if areas of palpable soreness are associated with changes in circulation.
        - Monitoring of testicular temperature.
        - Monitoring of extremities post-cast application.
        - Monitoring progression and appropriateness of exercise protocols through the post-injury rehabilitation process.
3) As a method to assess thermal, functional, ergonomic, and musculoskeletal stress in animals during and after training, competition, daily routines, and travel and performance, including but not limited to:
    - Identification of the presence of hyperthermia indicating subclinical inflammation within that structure to allow for appropriate early intervention.
    - Identification of the onset of hypothermia, indicating an irritation of the nerve supply to the area.
    - Assessment of hoof and shoe balance in horses.
    - Assessment of the effects of the rider on a horse's back.
    - Evaluation of the ergonomic fitness of harnesses, thermal control/equipment vests, and foot protection booties in performance and working animals.
4) For regulatory medicine to determine welfare compliance within all equestrian and canine athletic disciplines, but not limited to:
    - Assessment of limb temperature changes for limb sensitivity in jumping events.
    - Identification of abnormal cold areas on the distal limbs suggestive of foreign substance application.
    - Assessment of thermal patterns on the palmar pastern areas on the equine suggestive of abnormal scar formation.
    - Assessment of thermal patterns of the equine distal limbs, indicating the application of a "soring" agent or the possibility of a nerve block.

Contraindications and Limitations

1) Infrared imaging is sensitive to environmental factors, and understanding these factors is imperative for its success.
2) Infrared imaging is contraindicated if utilized by untrained individuals who do not understand infrared radiation physics.
3) The value of the images is compromised if bilateral symmetrical images cannot be compared for evaluation.
4) Imaging is contraindicated if environmental factors cannot be controlled, including sunshine, ambient temperature, drafts, haircoat, topical moisture, topical liniments, and the presence of bandages, blankets, or articles of harness.

The 10 Guidelines

1) Establishment of communication with the owner (person responsible) and the patient is properly prepared for the examination.
2) Patient assessment, which includes a comprehensive exam, before the initiation of infrared thermal imaging.
3) Examination guidelines:
    - Use infrared camera imaging systems that meet the AAT's specifications. Industrial infrared systems will yield images that are difficult to interpret.
    - The preferred absolute detector resolution is 640 × 480 coupled with a suitable microbolometer and lens. When systems with 320 × 240 sensors are coupled with a high-quality microbolometer, lens, and compensatory software or firmware innovations, they can approach the image quality, spatial resolution, and spot measurement requirements in the 640 × 480 systems.

- Thermal sensitivity of <50 mK NETD (noise equivalent temperature difference) @30 °C.
  - Ability to perform accurate quantitative differential temperature analysis with a precision of $\leq \pm 0.05$ °C (50 mK).
- Ability to render images in hi-resolution color and grayscale.
- High-resolution image visual display for interpretation.
- **Temperature range** set to cover temperatures within the range of emissions (20–45 °C).
- Ability to archive images for future reference and comparison using the same patient positioning and distance from the camera.
- Software manipulation of the images should be maintained within strict parameters to ensure that the images' original quantitative temperature data is not compromised.
- Imaging software that can identify areas of temperature calculations and locations for reporting should be utilized. Appropriate infrared sympathetic skin response (SSR) instrumentation includes real-time display, electronic static image capture, storage, post-capture annotation, and hardcopy documentation capabilities.
- All studies should be performed in an environment where the ambient temperature is controlled, free from drafts, and where no exposure to infrared rays (such as incandescent lights or sunlight) may result in heating or reflective artifacts.

4) Review of the infrared thermography examination:
   - The temperature data and all images acquired during the exam of the entire patient should be reviewed to ensure that a complete and comprehensive evaluation has been performed and documented. Any exceptions to the routine examination protocol (i.e., study omissions or revisions) should be noted, and reasons should be given.
5) Presentation of exam finding:
   - The examiner must provide preliminary results as provided for by internal policy based on examination findings.
   - The examiner must present the record of the thermal images and, when applicable, explanations for suboptimal examination findings to the interpreting veterinarian for use in diagnosis and archival purposes.
6) Preparation and storage of exam findings:
   - Images should be presented to the interpreting veterinarian for use in analysis and archival purposes. Radiometric images in either radiometric image format or radiometric image convertible format such as JPEG or DICOM are acceptable. A color-to-temperature thermal scale must accompany each image.
   - The imaging clinic should adhere to all established federal and state regulations. Image data and the analysis/report will be archived for at least 7 years.
7) Exam time recommendations:
   - High-quality and accurate results are fundamental elements of the infrared study. The exam should take approximately 30–60 minutes.
8) Reporting:
   - A veterinary medical record report should be prepared within 24 hours of the study.
   - *Thermographic findings* should be documented, and any abnormalities should be noted. Findings include thermal asymmetry of >1 °C in >25% of the surface area of any individual region of interest and localized areas of hyperthermia or hypothermia.
   - *Thermographic impressions* include classification according to an accepted naming system or summarization of the thermographic findings. When recognized patterns (thermal signatures) are seen, the thermographic impressions may include the description of that pattern (e.g., a thermographic pattern of the animal's back consistent with overriding vertebral spinous processes); however, care should be taken not to make any statements about clinical diagnosis in this section of the report. These patterns have been associated with the disease, but do not prove it.
   - *Clinical impressions* are not to be included in the *thermographic findings* paragraph but rather in a separately identifiable paragraph that speaks to the generator or etiology of those findings. Any discussion that is clinically relevant should be reserved for this paragraph.
9) Continuing professional education:
   - Certification is considered the standard of practice for infrared technology.
10) Emerging technologies:
    - Technology is constantly being introduced that can challenge existing guidelines or that do not necessarily conform to currently accepted practices.
    - General industrial or personal thermal imaging cameras that do not meet the specification guidelines contained herein are not intended for use in veterinary medical thermology.
    - Technologies not otherwise covered in these guidelines that employ methodologies, hardware, or protocols that have gained federal regulatory approval for medical thermology may become available over time.

Important Veterinary Medical Thermography Parameters

As stipulated in the AAT guidelines, resolution, sensitivity, accuracy, and temperature range are essential when imaging veterinary patients with hair coats, scales, or feathers.

Resolution

Image resolution refers to the level of detail in an image. In the context of veterinary infrared camera equipment, this is quantified by the number of pixels in the image. Each pixel represents a single point of temperature measurement. Consequently, a higher resolution indicates a greater number of temperature points measured in each image. This enhanced resolution enables more accurate and detailed temperature analysis, which can be crucial in veterinary applications.

An infrared camera with a resolution of 640 × 480 measures 307,200 points of temperature in each image, while an infrared system with a resolution of 320 × 240 only measures 76,800 points of temperature. The AAT recommends a resolution of 640 × 480 for medical and veterinary thermography.

Sensitivity

The sensitivity of a thermal camera is its ability to detect minimal differences in temperature. The lower this value, the more sensitive the camera is. The AAT veterinary guidelines require a sensitivity of ±0.05 °C. The AAT medical guidelines require a sensitivity of ±0.02 ° C. When the thermal energy radiates from the patient, it must radiate through hair and air. Therefore, the higher the sensitivity, the more detailed the thermograms will be.

Temperature Range

The veterinary infrared camera system must be able to measure the temperature range emitted from a cold-blooded reptile covered in scales, an exotic bird covered in feathers, and those emitted through hair and air. This temperature range is 60° to 112 ° F (15.5–45 °C).

Many industrial cameras measure the temperature range from a negative value to several hundred degrees Fahrenheit without exploring all the scientific reasons for adhering to the range recommended by the AAT of 50°–112 °F.

Interpretation of Infrared Thermal Images Is Intuitive

Imaging Techniques

Two fundamental imaging techniques are used to assess a patient's functional physiology. The first technique involves a study that showcases thermal imagery of all anatomical regions of the patient at the time of the exam. The second technique employs serial imaging, facilitating a physiological comparison of the same anatomical area at different time intervals.

Each patient is its own control. Normal patients are sagittally symmetrical, both qualitatively and quantitatively. Thermal symmetry evaluation is based on comparisons between contralateral anatomical areas. Healthy patients are thermally symmetrical (Figure 39.3), whereas unhealthy patients are asymmetrical (Figure 39.4) due to inflammatory, neurological, and vascular conditions (Chudecka *et al.*, 2015).

The second approach to thermographic interpretation entails comparing the temperature data of a series of images over time. The images from each anatomical area considered for comparison must be framed the same and have the same temperature range (Figure 39.5).

Qualitative and Quantitative Analysis in Thermography

Optimal interpretation of infrared thermal images combines qualitative and quantitative analysis. Qualitative analysis visually represents the thermally detected temperature data and determines the location of the quantitative measurement sites. Quantitative analysis compares the numerical temperature data between specific regions of interest on the same image or between two serial images of the same region of interest of the same patient. This is the temperature data used to calculate the temperature difference (ΔT) between two anatomically demarcated areas.

Qualitative thermography analysis involves properly adjusting the palette over the temperature data within the region of interest to maximize the visual illustration of the thermal information. Qualitative analysis comparison of two images is only possible when both images are framed the same and have the same range of temperature data (Figure 39.6).

Quantitative analysis is the measurement of the detected temperature data. This step utilizes the analysis software to display and compare the minimum, average, and maximum temperatures within a defined area. The focal and

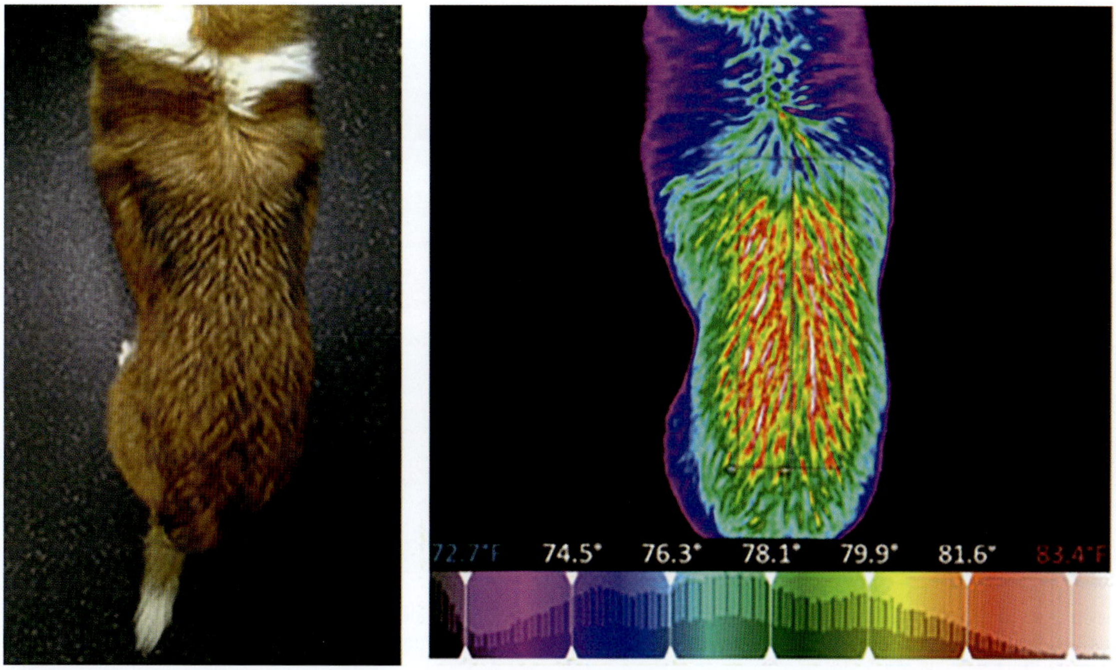

Figure 39.3 Normal patients are thermally symmetrical. Normal blood flow results in symmetrical surface temperatures within contralateral anatomical areas. Note the even blood flow bilaterally throughout the paravertebral musculature on this dorsal view.

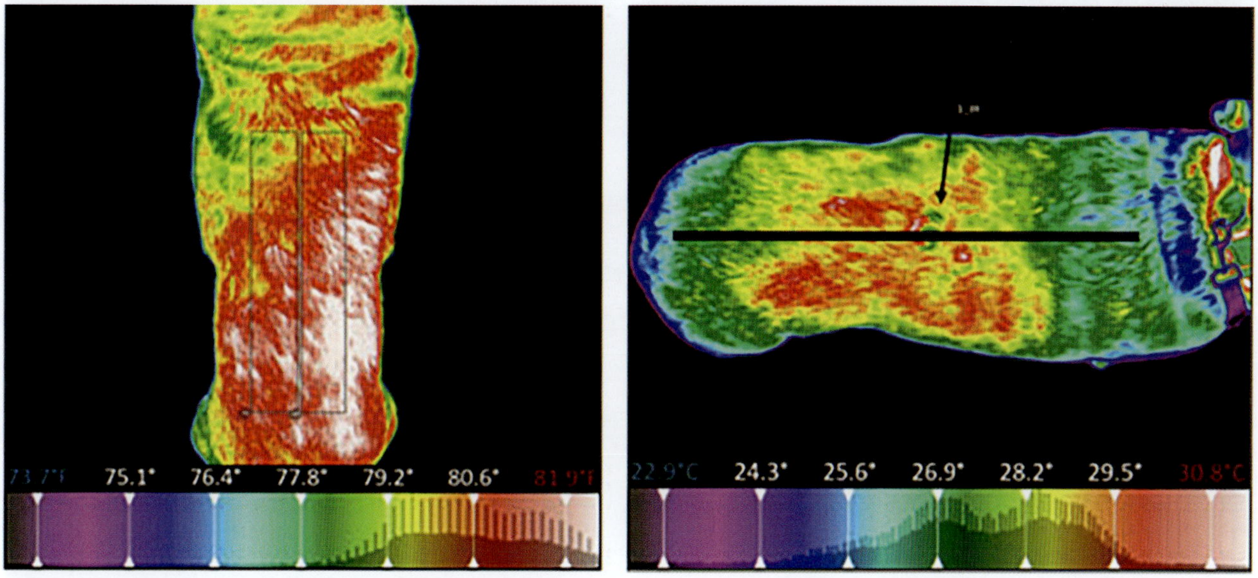

Figure 39.4 Unhealthy patients become thermally asymmetrical, resulting from abnormal blood flow through the contralateral anatomical areas. There is an asymmetrical circulatory pattern when comparing the right and left paravertebral muscles on both these dorsal images.

diffuse hyperthermic area defined by Zone 1 has minimum temperature readings of 84.8 °F, average temperature readings of 92.86 ° F, and maximum temperature readings of 96.4 °F.

In the image of Figure 39.7, the recorded temperature data from Zone 1, on the patient's right lateral image, can then be compared to the exact same area on the left contralateral anatomical area. The difference between the

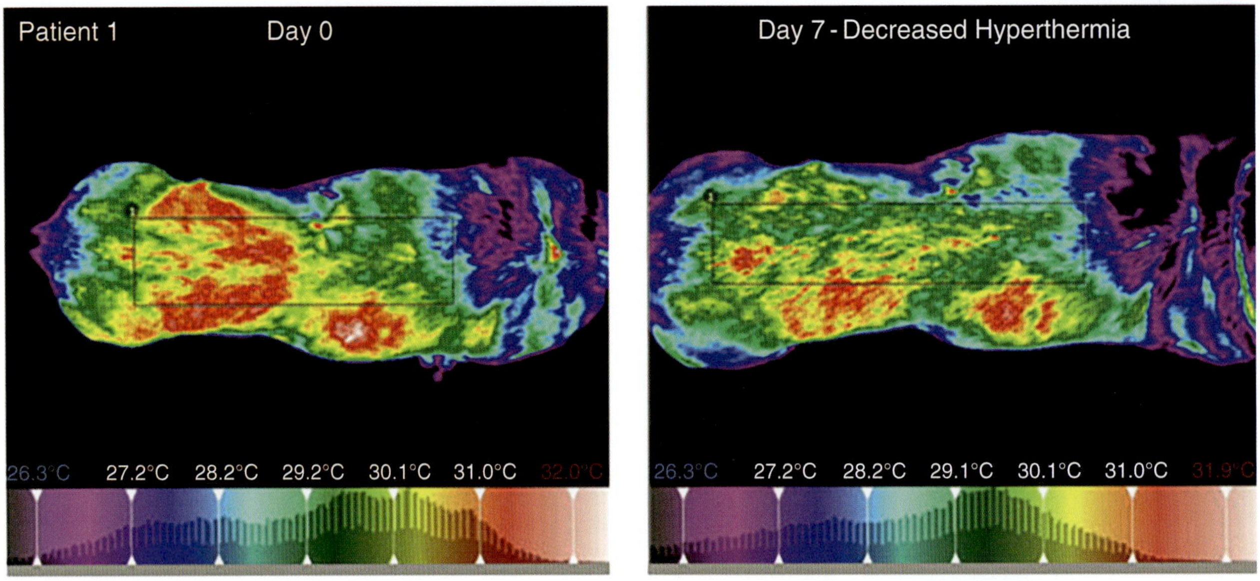

Figure 39.5 The interpretation of serial images requires the images to be framed the same and have the same temperature range. These two images were taken 7 days apart, and you can see a decrease in the areas of hyperthermia indicating a normalization of the circulation.

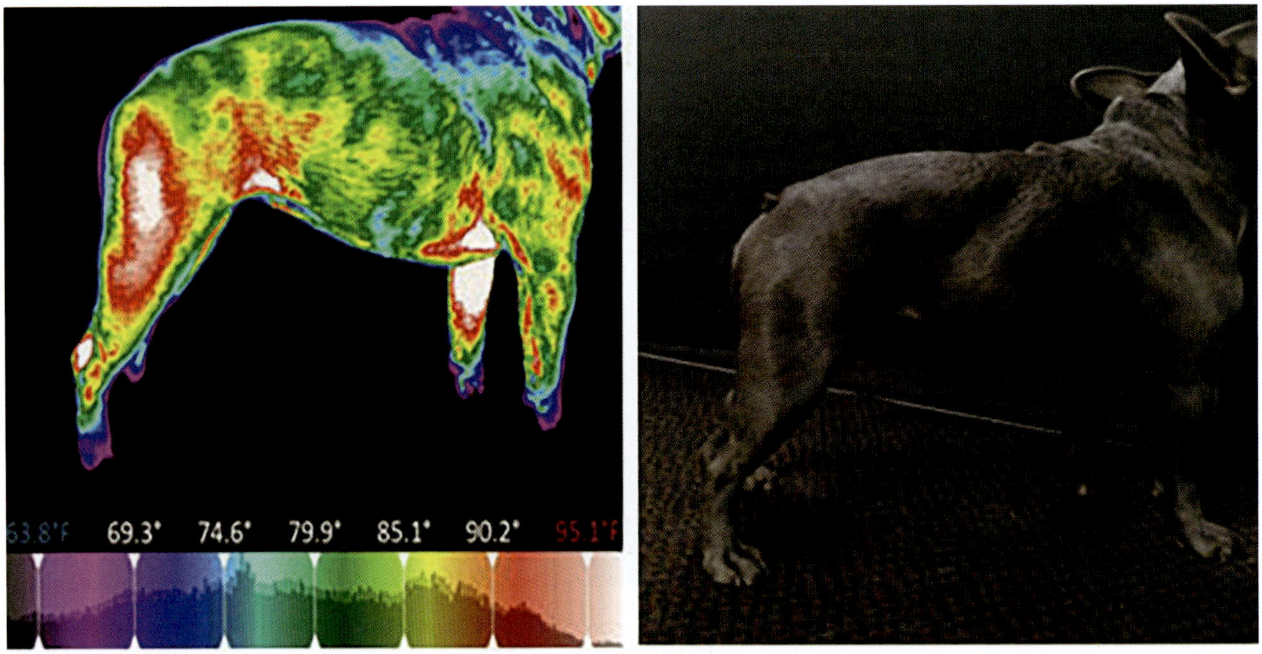

Figure 39.6 The qualitative analysis of this lateral (Region of Interest [ROI]) image contains only the temperature data emitted from the patient. There is a large focal area surrounded by a diffuse area of hyperthermic activity over the biceps femoris, portions of the fascia lata covering the vastus muscle, and the distal portion of the semitendinosus muscle. Images provided by Lauren Bueter BS, RVT, CCRP of Michiana Animal Rehab Services.

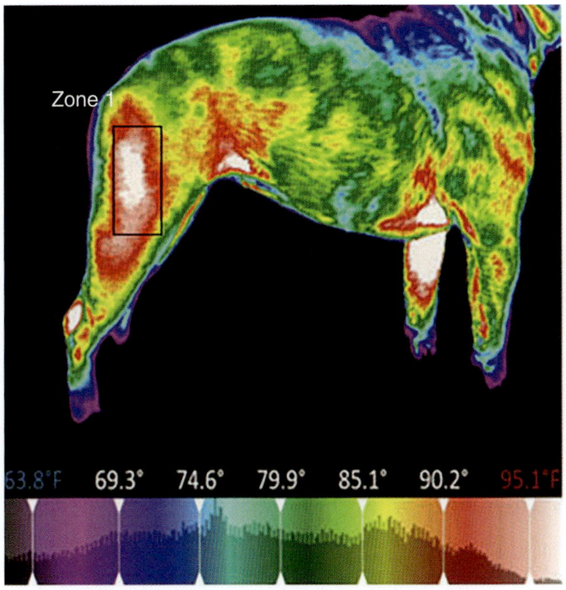

Zone 1	
Minimum	84.8°
Average	92.86°
Maximum	96.4°

Figure 39.7 The quantitative analysis of this lateral image contains an ROI defined by Zone 1. The software recognizes this zone's temperature data and displays the minimum, average, and maximum temperatures. Images provided by Lauren Bueter BS, RVT, CCRP of Michiana Animal Rehab Services.

temperature data from each of these zones is then used to calculate ΔT. Any difference >1 °C between these identical zones is significant.

Clinical Implications

Anatomical areas of hyperthermic activity (whether bilaterally symmetrical, asymmetrical, or localized) correlate to increased vascularization. The majority of these hyperthermic areas result from inflammation. Other causes include increased circulation from a strained or sprained tendon or ligamentous structure, an infection, or a neoplastic growth. Most patients will have numerous areas of hyperthermia as they age (Figure 39.8).

Patients may present thermally asymmetrical (bilaterally or locally) with decreased blood flow. These areas are referred to as hypothermic, or areas of hypothermia. The etiology of most of this reduced vascularization is neurological irritation, resulting in a vasoconstrictive state (Figure 39.9). Areas of muscle atrophy, infarction, or a scar will also manifest as areas of hypothermia.

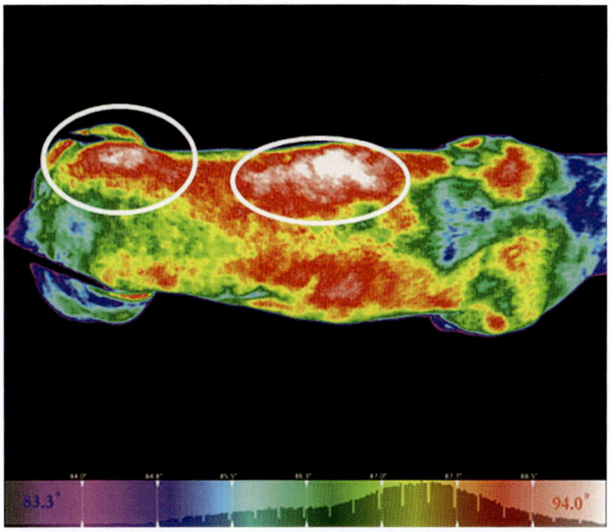

Figure 39.8 Asymmetrical bilateral hyperthermia from the level of T_{9-10}–L_{3-4}. Hyperthermia is more diffuse on the right than on the left. Still, both involve areas of the longissimus and latissimus dorsi, starting along the spinous processes and then distally over the thoracic and lumbar cavities. The hyperthermia on the left contains both focal and diffuse areas of radiated energy. There is a second focal and diffuse area of hyperthermia over the left gluteal region.

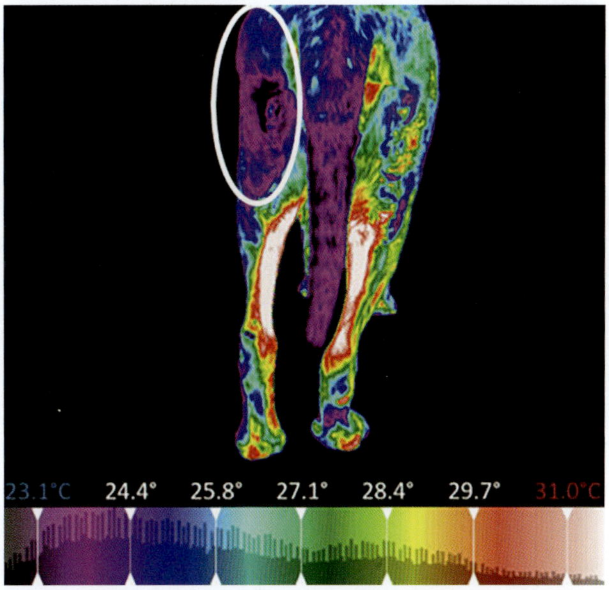

Figure 39.9 There is generalized hypothermia throughout the proximal portion of the entire left hind limb and qualitative evidence of small areas of hypothermia present on the proximal portion of the right hind limb. This seven-year-old patient was diagnosed with congenital hip dysplasia at 11 months of age. Bony changes along the spinal cord from L_{4-5}–S_{1-2} resulted in nerve irritation at the emergence of the spinal nerves.

Utilizing Infrared Thermal Imaging in Practice

Each practice employs a unique approach when incorporating infrared thermal imaging into their individual protocols and procedures. In all types of practices, infrared thermal imaging brings:

- **A way to identify all anatomical areas that would benefit from further evaluation and diagnostic procedures.** IRTI is a screening tool that provides real-time functional physiological information on each patient. This allows a proactive approach to detecting issues before they manifest clinically.
- **A visual guide, or "roadmap," for administering PBMT or any other therapeutic modality.** All anatomical structures that would benefit from PBMT will be identified. Therefore, treatment will be applied to the primary and any compensatory areas. This "wholistic" approach to the administration of any modality-based therapy makes treatment and/or recovery more effective and efficient.
- **A way to objectively monitor therapeutic/rehabilitation treatment protocols or regimens.** Serial images are taken over time, and each is quantitatively measured to compare ΔT.
- **A visual client education tool.** IRTI provides visual support to your clinical evaluation and provides a visualization of the patient's functional physiological state. An educated and understanding client will be more compliant with your diagnostic and therapeutic recommendations.

Photobiomodulation Therapy

The administration of PBMT is a key to unlocking the body's natural healing mechanisms. Photonic energy stimulates the photoreceptors inside our cells' mitochondria (Smith, 1991). This triggers a biochemical cascade of events that work to alleviate pain, modulate the inflammatory response, and increase microcirculation. Applying this photonic energy to the target cells of our patients induces an acceleration of their own healing processes (Passarella & Karu, 2014).

The chart in Figure 39.10 illustrates several scientifically proven clinical responses to PBMT (Viegas *et al.*, 2007; Samoilova *et al.*, 2008; Chung *et al.*, 2012; Mitchell and Mack, 2013; Cidral-Filho *et al.*, 2014).

Searching the http://www.pubmed.ncbi.nlm.nih.gov and www.researchgate.net websites for veterinary laser therapy or veterinary PBMT yields well over 1200 published papers.

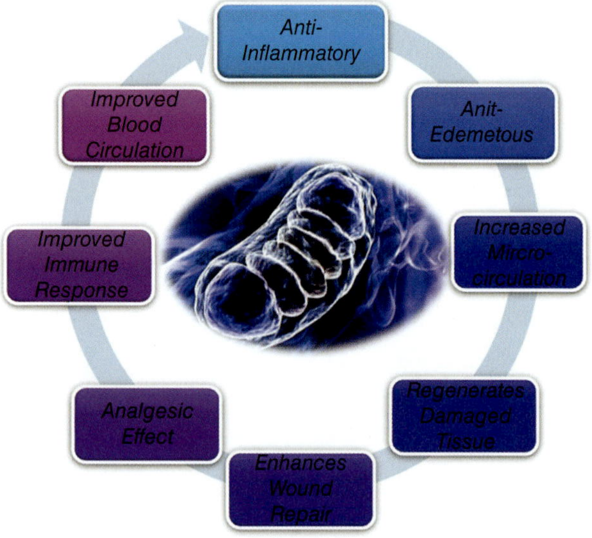

Figure 39.10 When photonic energy is absorbed by the photoreceptors within the mitochondria, a biochemical cascade of events results in these clinical responses within the patient.

Within the last 15 years, the majority of these appeared in peer-reviewed journals. It is no longer a question of the efficacy of PBMT but of what other conditions would also benefit from this therapy.

The literature does not tell us where to administer the therapy or how much or how often it should be administered to each of our patient's conditions. It does not matter what model therapy laser is being used, what wavelengths it is emitting, the power being using, or the technique of on-contact or off-contact, either scanning or in a point-to-point administration. If the therapy is not being administered where it is needed most, or to all areas that would benefit from the therapy, the efficacy is diminished. The patient may not respond to the therapy or have a prolonged period to reach the therapeutic goal.

All therapeutic modalities are more effective when administered exactly where needed and to all compensatory areas that would also benefit.

The Synergy Between PBMT and IRTI

What if you had a device to assist you, so that:

- when prescribing or administering PBMT, you knew exactly where to administer it?
- you could identify all the anatomical areas of the patient that would also benefit from PBMT?
- you could objectively monitor the patient's progress throughout the treatment plan?

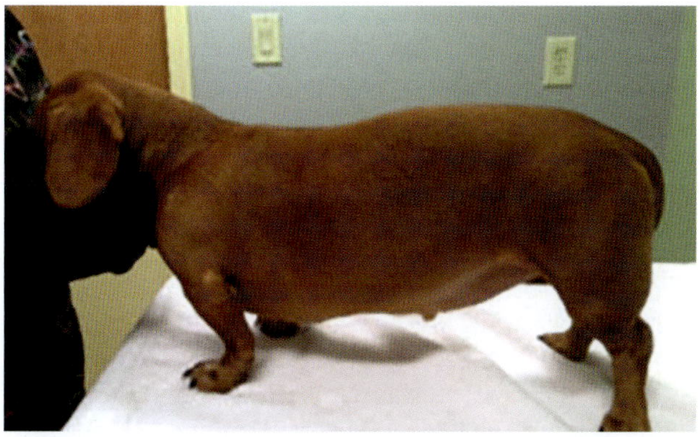

Figure 39.11 Presentation: Unable to place neck through PROM in any direction without a painful response. Pain palpable from T_{11}-L_3.

- you know when the patient has completely recovered?
- your client can visualize the patient's progress; would they then comply more with your recommendations?

Infrared thermal imaging provides accurate and concise answers to all these questions. Identifying all the areas of the patient that would benefit from further evaluation and anatomical diagnostics will enable you to ascertain each area that would also benefit from PBMT. The treatment times will be more efficient and beneficial, allowing a faster recovery. The patient in Figure 39.11 benefited from this approach.

Presentation: A 6-year-old SF Dachshund. A physical exam revealed that the patient is unable to place his neck through passive range of motion (PROM) in any direction without a painful response. Pain is palpable within the paravertebral musculature bilaterally from T_{11}-L_3.

The infrared thermal imaging, six screening views, revealed many areas of hyperthermia over the entire patient and an area of hypothermia over the cervical region.

Without the IRTIs, PBMT would have been prescribed for the cervical and painful thoracolumbar region (white ellipses). After reviewing the IRTIs with the owner, the treatment plan now includes administering PBMT to the areas of both the white ellipses and those areas demarcated by the black ellipses (Figure 39.12). The hypothermia within the cervical region indicates an area of vasoconstriction caused by nerve irritation, which suggests that placing the cervical area through PROM during the administration of PBMT may allow more saturation of the target tissues.

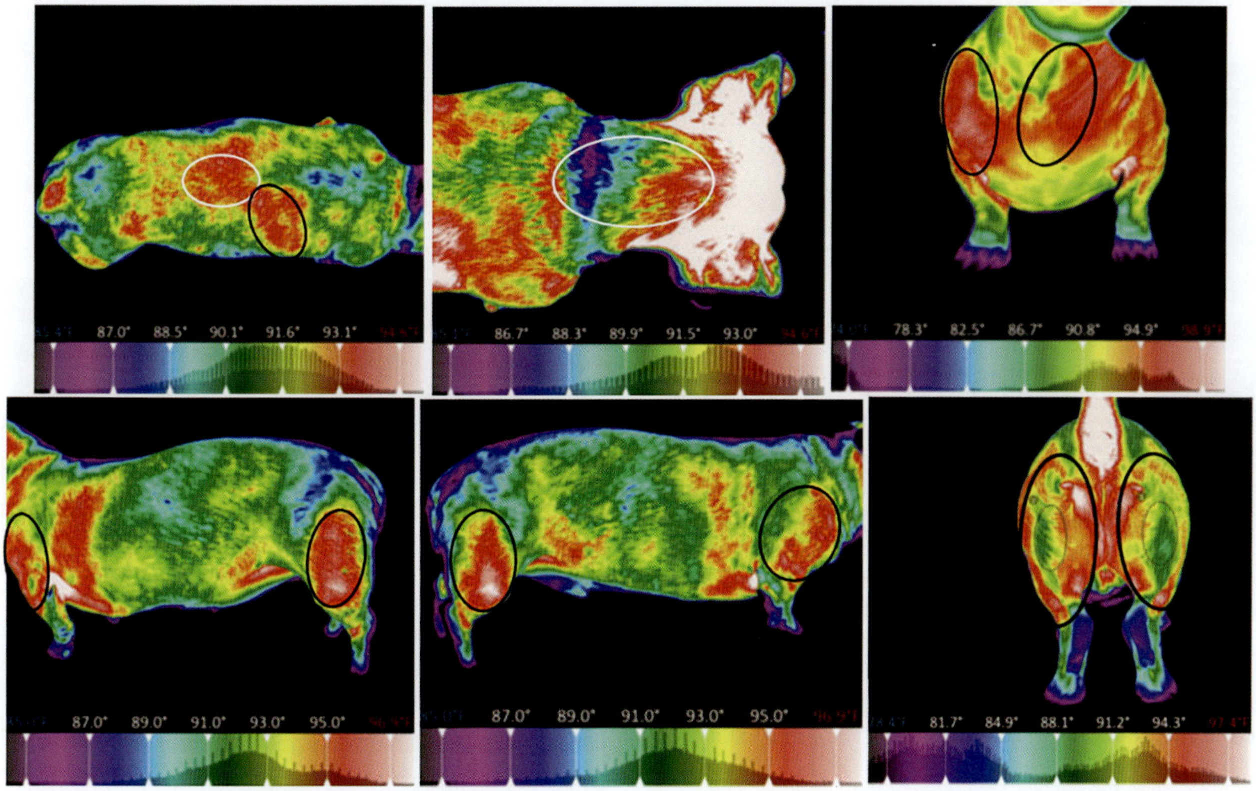

Figure 39.12 Without the IRTI screening, PBMT would have been applied to those areas demarcated by the white ellipses. IRTI revealed many areas of hyperthermia and the area of hypothermia over the cervical region. The treatment plan now includes the administration PBMT to all the black ellipses with consideration of placing the cervical area through PROM during administration.

PBMT was only a part of the treatment plan. Concurrently with PBMT, acupuncture, core strengthening and stability exercises, and proprioception training were all performed. This patient recovered without surgery in 3 weeks.

Objectively Monitoring PBMT

Infrared thermal imaging provides objective patient monitoring throughout pharmaceutical and/or multi-modality-based treatment protocols. The software allows the demarcation of specific bilateral anatomical areas, and a temperature measurement is made of all the temperature points within. Objective evaluations are made when a series of images of the same anatomical area with the same temperature range are measured. The temperature data collected will result in the ability to calculate a temperature change (ΔT) within that specific area. A lowering of the temperature data correlates to a decrease in the inflammatory processes. If the ΔT is increased within an initial area of hypothermia, this indicates a normalization, a reestablishment of the circulation. Both objective measurements indicate a response to therapy and an improvement in the patient.

Figure 39.13 is a case example of the objective ability of IRTI to monitor a patient's progress. This is an 11-year-old neutered Shepherd mix who presented with chronic back pain. A complete set of screening images was taken, but the dorsal view best exemplifies the objective ability of infrared thermal imaging to monitor the patient.

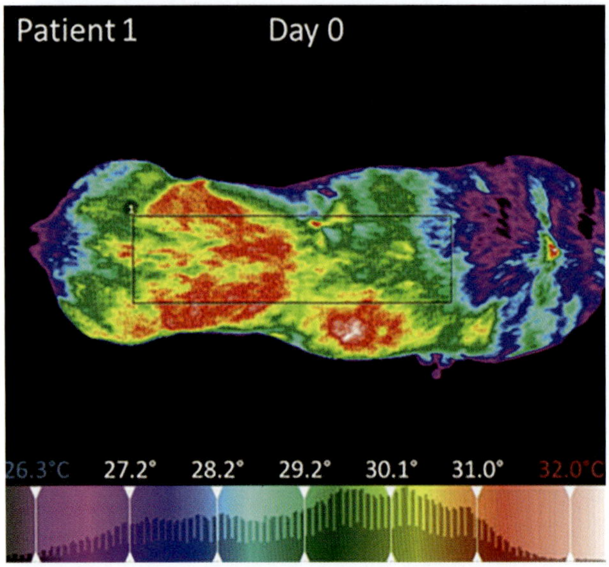

Figure 39.13 This dorsal image was taken before any administration of PBMT. Bilateral areas of hyperthermia are evident from L_1-S_1. These areas qualitatively appear red in color, begin at L_1, and expand bilaterally caudally and distally to the area of both hips. Additional diffuse hyperthermia (yellow) areas extend from L_1 along the paravertebral epaxial muscles to S_1. The software delineated a zone (1) that started at T_8 to the lumbosacral joint and laterally included all paravertebral musculature. All the temperature data within this zone was measured and had a minimum of 27.8 ° C (82.04 °F), an average of 30.7 °C (87.26 ° F), and a maximum of 31.8 °C (89.24 °F).

PBMT was administered on-contact in the areas demarcated by the four ellipses, utilizing a scanning technique, at a dose of 10 J/cm^2 (Figure 39.14). The goal was to relieve pain and modulate the inflammation within the targeted structures. This was repeated every 24 hours for 4 consecutive days.

On day 7, the patient was reimaged 36 hours after the last PBMT session. The temperature data emitted from the delineated zones was significantly reduced. ΔT was calculated between the average temperatures within the zones as 2.5 °C (4.5 °F) (Figure 39.15). This reduction in hyperthermia was greater than 1 °C, which is stated in the literature as significant (Purohit & McCoy, 1980; Soroko *et al.,* 2017).

A 4-year-old Quarter Horse was presented with a 1/5 lameness in the left stifle. Twenty-four IRTIs were taken on an IRTI screening exam. There was a pronounced thermal asymmetry between the stifles, with the left stifle exhibiting hyperthermia within the joint and surrounding soft tissues. Moderate pressure during palpation of the stifle and surrounding structures elicited a slightly painful response. The patient was on an off-day between performance competitions; hence, the treatment plan was to administer PBMT and then recheck the next day to monitor the recovery, ensuring the patient was safe to compete.

The initial image of the horse's left stifle (Figure 39.16, left) was used as a guide for administering PBMT. A handheld unit with a spot size of 4 cm^2, emissions

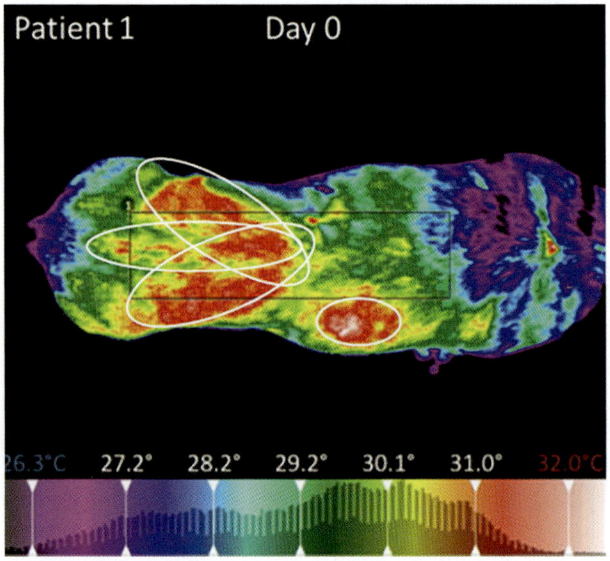

Figure 39.14 PBMT was administered on-contact within the three elongated ellipses using a scanning technique at a dose of 10 J/cm^2.

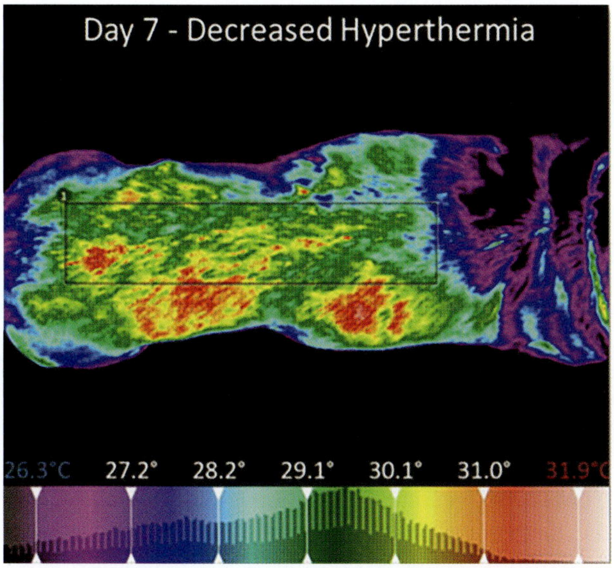

Figure 39.15 This dorsal image was taken 72 hours after the last PBMT session. All the thermal gradients are normalizing with a marked reduction in the area and intensity of hyperthermia. Zone (1) temperatures: minimum of 27.6 °C (81.68 °F), average of 28.2 °C (82.76 °F), and a maximum of 30.8 °C (87.44 °F). Delta T (ΔT) = 2.5 °C (4.5 °F).

utilizing a combination of continuous wave, pulsed, and superpulsed wavelengths of 660 nm, 860 nm, and 905 nm, were administered using a point-to-point technique applied at all angles to the joint and along all of the soft tissue structures surrounding the joint at an average dosage of 15 J/cm^2.

The second image of the horse's left stifle (Figure 39.16, right) was taken 22 hours after the PBMT session. Within the ellipse, the hyperthermia present prior to therapy has almost resolved. The temperature data emitted from the stifle decreased by 2.4 °F. Strong digital palpation revealed no painful response in the joint or surrounding structures. The patient competed that day and placed second in the event.

Objective Assessment of Recovery

When managing a horse's leg injury, there is always the question of, "How soon can the horse return to training?" The visualization provided by infrared thermal imaging has not only provided a PBMT administration guide but also reinforced recommendations to continue therapy until it is safe to return to training.

This 4-year-old performance horse exhibited tenderness throughout the flexor tendons on both front limbs. Ultrasonic exams revealed no significant lesions. PBMT was administered daily for 4 days. The trainer wanted to immediately put the horse back into training since the tenderness and swelling within these structures appeared resolved. The oblique image of both forelimbs in Figure 39.17 revealed focal areas of hyperthermia still present in these structures. Visualization of this image by the trainer convinced the trainer to continue PBMT for another 3 days and then reimage.

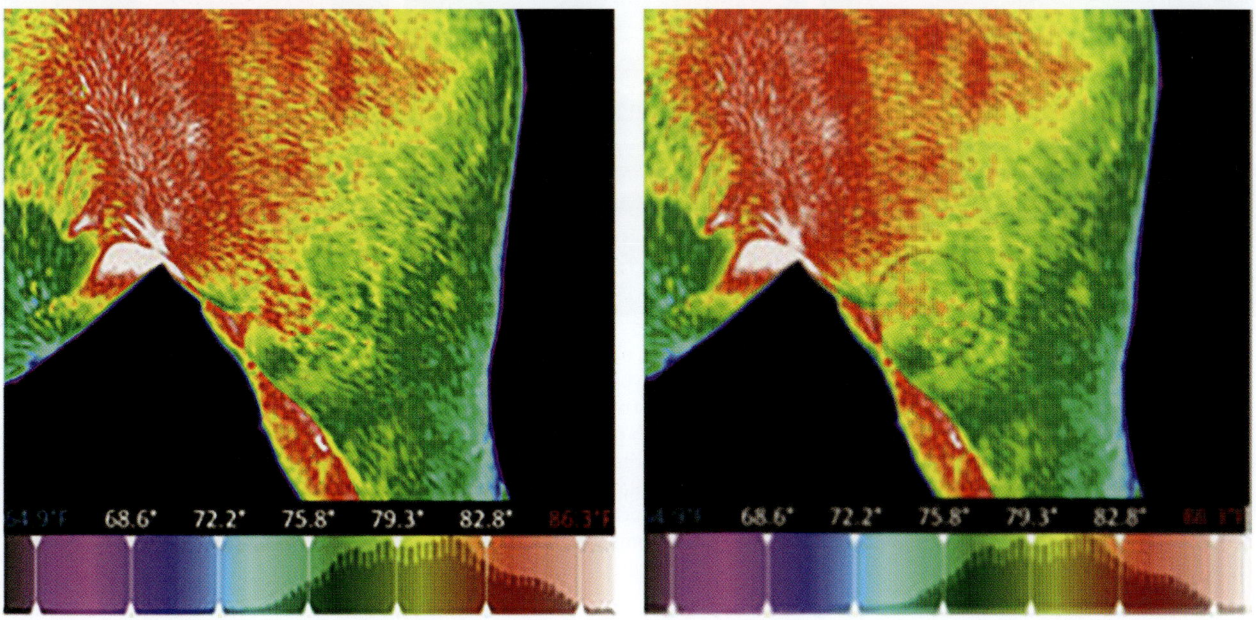

Figure 39.16 The IRTI on the left was taken before the administration of PBMT. PBMT was administered on contact, using a point-to-point method, at a dose of 15 J/cm^2. The right image was taken 22 hours after PBMT. Within the ellipse, the temperature decreased by 2.4 °F. The areas and intensity of hyperthermia present initially have all been reduced.

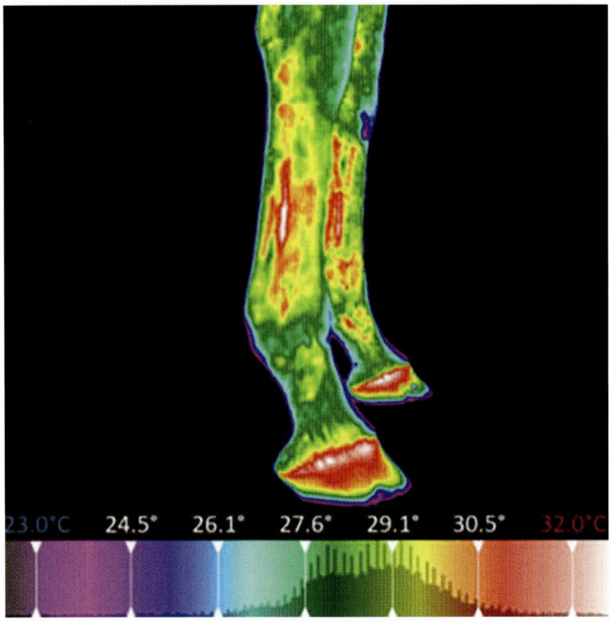

Figure 39.17 This oblique view of the distal forelimbs revealed focal and diffuse areas of hyperthermia. These correlate with inflammation within the deep digital flexor, the inferior check ligament, and suspensory tendons. This visualization prevented this horse from returning to training before the strains on these structures were resolved.

Case Examples

Objectively Monitor Patient Response to Treatment

Case shared by Lauren Bueter BS, RVT, CCRP, Michiana Animal Rehabilitation Services

A 2-year-old FS French Bull Dog presented with a complaint of lethargy and difficulty moving around. These three screening views were taken on October 21, 2019 (Figure 39.18).

Upon physical exam, the patient showed pain upon palpation over the musculature of the left shoulder and throughout the hyperthermic areas on the right hindlimb. There was a slight sensitivity to digital palpation along the paravertebral musculature from the midcervical region to the lumbosacral joint. There was a reluctance to allow PROM to be performed on the neck. There was a slight lameness in the left hindlimb.

The owner visualized these thermographic findings and complied with the recommendation of a radiographic study of the cervical and thoracic spine. Hemivertebrae were present throughout the thoracic spine, but no obvious cervical lesions were found except a possible narrowing at the axis/C_3 space. Fourteen pairs of ribs were noted.

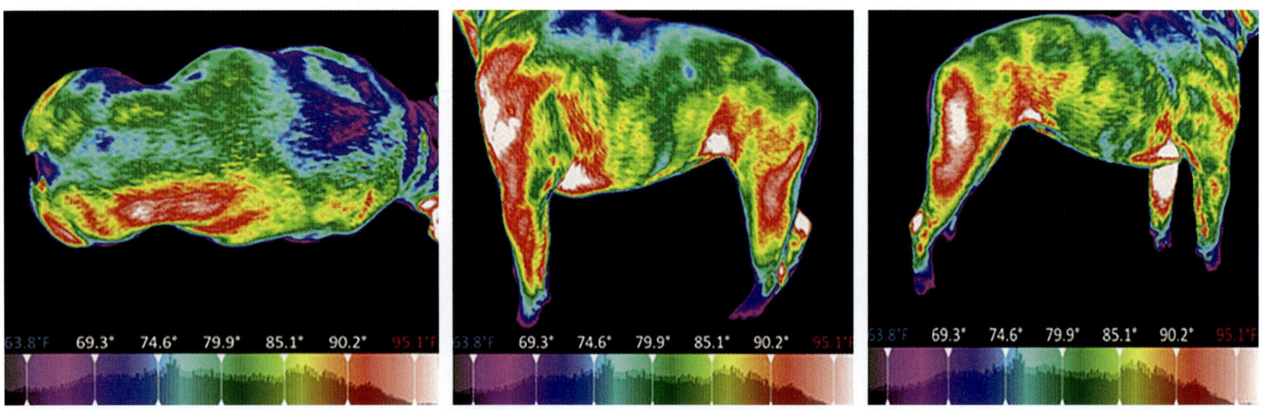

Figure 39.18 (Oct 21, 2019) Asymmetrical thermographic findings of hyperthermia and hypothermia bilaterally within the contralateral anatomical areas throughout all three images. Focal and diffuse hypothermic gradients originate over the spinous processes and the adjacent musculature from the last two cervical vertebrae to the area of the first few lumbar areas. These thermographic findings repeat on all three images. There is hypothermic asymmetry throughout both gluteal areas. The left gluteal area exhibits a larger area of vasoconstriction than the right. The left shoulder has a large focal area of hyperthermia centered over the scapulohumeral joint. This area extends proximally to include the cranial musculature of the scapula and distally through the triceps brachii and the extensor group of muscles. This focal area radiates into more diffuse areas. A more focal and diffuse area of hyperthermia exists over the biceps femoris, semitendinosus, semimembranosus muscles, and the tarsus when compared contralaterally to the hyperthermic areas on the left hindlimb. Hypothermia is present throughout all four distal limbs from the carpus to the phalanges.

The treatment plan included PBMT along the cervical, thoracic, and lumbar spine three times per week and over both shoulders and hips. Therapeutic exercises were done upon each PBMT therapy visit, prioritizing increasing the core strength and proprioception. Acupuncture treatments were performed once per week (Figure 39.19).

The PBMT administration was changed each week based on information from the IRTI. More energy was administered to the areas of hypothermia over the spine with the goal of reestablishing circulation. The left gluteal area responded to PBMT, and it was applied bilaterally with a slightly higher dosage on the left. Quantitative temperature data was recorded weekly.

Thermal asymmetry is determined by the difference in the temperature data emitted between contralateral anatomical areas. Figure 39.20 recorded the average temperature data from the right and left thorax, the right and left lumbar, and the right and left shoulder. The difference in the average temperature from one area compared to its contralateral area is the calculation of ΔT on that day at that exact time. Analysis and calculations of ΔT were made from the different anatomical areas over time. These are the numerical values within the red ellipses. Normalization is defined as a progression toward thermal symmetry. The patient is thermally symmetrical when the average temperatures from contralateral anatomical areas are the same. This same principle is true when a series of images is analyzed. If there is little or no difference between the average temperature of the images, the area is emitting the same temperature data that it did on the previous date. Example: on February 2, 2020, ΔT between the right and left thorax was only 0.6 °F. Therefore, measuring the same area on this date at that time, the right and left thorax are thermally symmetrical.

Thermal asymmetry in each anatomical area has normalized, resulting in a state where the blood circulation is the same. This correlates to a decrease in inflammation within the areas of hyperthermia, or a restoration of the innervation to that area in the case of the areas of hypothermia. There is still hypothermia evident over the gluteal area of the left rear leg, even though the degree of lameness has lessened. This correlates with the possibility of permanent

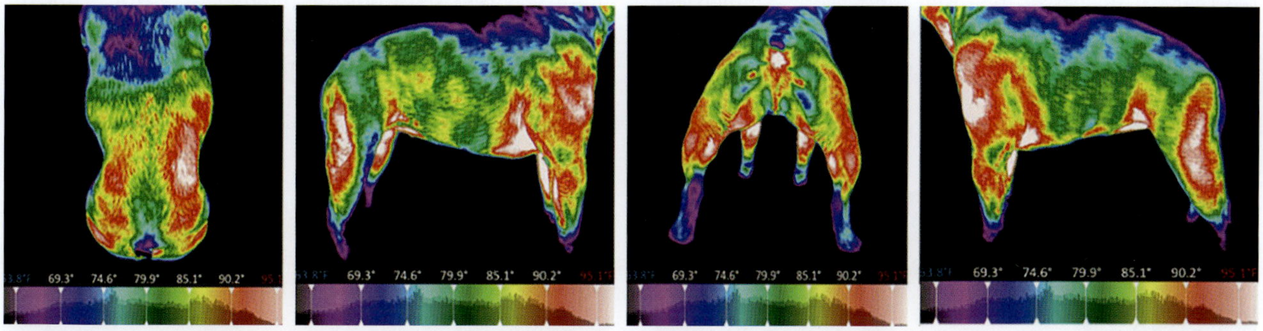

Figure 39.19 (Dec 6, 2019) The asymmetrical hypothermic and hyperthermic thermographic findings were still present throughout the contralateral anatomical areas in all four images. Overall, the temperature data from each region was reduced. Circulation is being reestablished in the hypothermia areas present over the left gluteal musculature. Quantitatively, the temperature data over the left shoulder has decreased, and qualitatively, the hyperthermia has reduced in area. The hypothermia along the thoracic spine has remained unchanged.

ROI (F°)	10/21/2019	ΔT	12/06/2019	ΔT	2/02/2020	ΔT
Right Thorax	86.3		84.3		86.1	
Left Thorax	83.8	1.5	82.8	2.0	85.5	0.6
Right Lumbar	88		88.1		89.7	
Left Lumbar	85.9	2.1	86.9	1.2	88.4	1.3
Right Shoulder	88.8		92.3			
Left Shoulder	90.8	2.0	92.5	0.2		

Figure 39.20 Average temperature data from each anatomical region compared to the contralateral anatomical area. This is expressed as ΔT (change in temperature). This determines thermal asymmetry. A comparison can be made from the contralateral anatomical area at that time and then as a series of images comparing the change of temperature between two dates.

irritation to the innervating spinal nerves. The prognosis of this patient needing perpetual therapy to maintain the current quality of life can be quantitatively and qualitatively realized through the visualization of these images by the owner.

IRTI as a Guide to PBMT Administration

Presentation: 8-year-old Gran Prix Warmblood. Performance declining; behavior issues.

A comprehensive set of infrared thermal images was taken before the physical and lameness evaluation. Figure 39.21 is an oblique infrared thermal image of the spine. Infrared thermal imaging of the back revealed focal and diffuse areas of hyperthermia throughout the epaxial musculature and directly over the spinous processes of the thoracic and lumbar vertebrae. Several asymmetrical areas of hyperthermia are qualitatively seen as focal and diffuse white and shades of red. This hyperthermia extends bilaterally throughout the longissimus dorsi and into the gluteal area before descending distally to the coxofemoral joint. Uncharacteristically, there is no focal area of increased circulation over the lumbosacral joint. All infrared thermal images of the distal limbs were symmetrical and typical of a horse in training.

The entire horse was examined, including observation while in motion. It was concluded that this is one of the rare cases with a primary back problem. Digital palpation, extension, and flexion tests revealed no significant issues in any of the distal limbs. In motion, both rear limbs were short in stride.

Digital palpation detected soreness, rigidity, and areas of spasticity throughout the epaxial musculature. The areas of soreness were more prevalent in the left paravertebral musculature than in the right. Soreness was also detected bilaterally within both superficial gluteus muscles. The areas of soreness correlated with the image in Figure 39.21.

The differential diagnosis included overriding dorsal spinous processes, dorsal spinous ligament injuries, and muscle strain and pain due to the rigorous training schedule.

PBMT and massage were prescribed as the only therapy for this patient. A pharmaceutical approach was not considered due to the withdrawal times during competition. PBMT was administered on-contact to all the areas highlighted in Figure 39.22, with special emphasis on administration to the area within the white ellipse till the muscle spasticity is resolved. Manual massage techniques, tender digital and palm pressure stroking, and kneading with cross-frictional fiber work were performed while applying the PBMT. After the therapy session, the horse was walked for at least an hour and at no point was released from the handler's control. After the walk, stretching exercises focused on the back muscles. This therapy protocol was applied twice daily for 4 days, then once daily, increasing the controlled walking exercise time with each session.

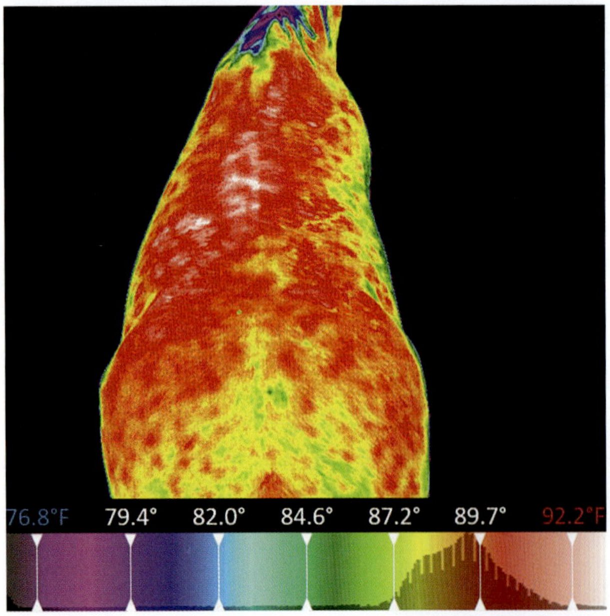

Figure 39.21 An oblique infrared thermal image of the spine of an 8-year-old Gran Prix Warmblood with asymmetrical hyperthermia visible dorsally.

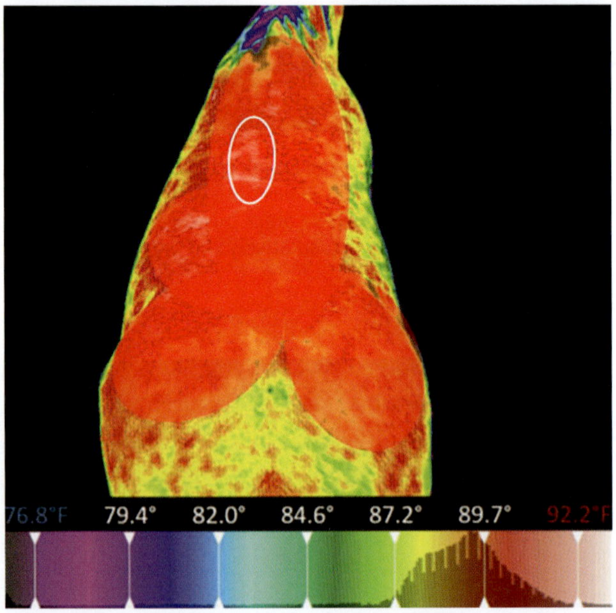

Figure 39.22 DTI of the same 8-year-old Gran Prix Warmblood detailing the focus for PBMT and massage therapy.

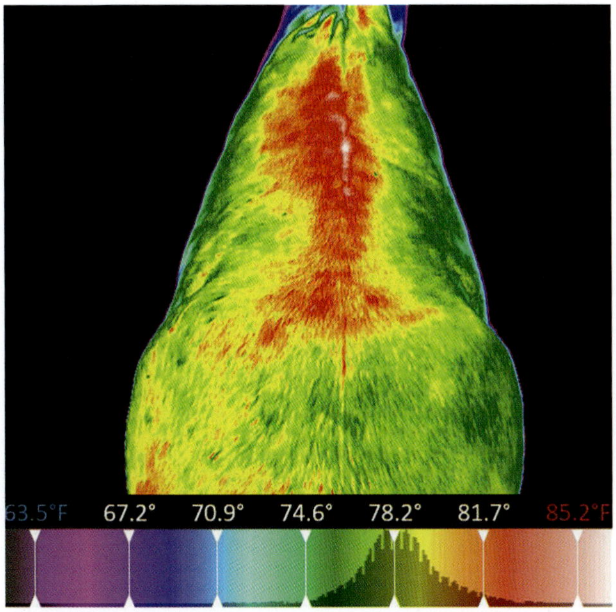

Figure 39.23 Dorsal oblique DTI of the same 8-year-old Gran Prix Warmblood following PMBT, massage therapy, and stretching exercises twice daily for 4 days, then once daily for 10 days.

After 10 days of utilizing this treatment protocol, the patient was rechecked. Figure 39.23 is the dorsal oblique image of this patient's back. Qualitatively, the asymmetrical bilateral hyperthermia is 85% resolved. Four focal areas of hyperthermia are still present over the spinous process of the vertebrae, which provides visualization for the client to consider further diagnostics of this area to obtain a definitive diagnosis.

Conclusion

There is a synergy between infrared thermal imaging and PBMT. IRTI provides a functional physiological exam of the entire patient. All anatomical areas that would benefit from PBMT are easily identified, providing a precise treatment guide and an application roadmap. Applying any modality is more beneficial when applied to all the areas that would respond to treatment. By continuously capturing infrared thermal images, you can monitor the patient's progress in real-time throughout the treatment process. Client visualization reinforces your recommendations, provides them with proof of efficacy, and determines when an issue is totally resolved. Combining the technology of IRTI and the benefits of PBMT allows better care and a higher quality of life for our patients.

References

American Academy of Thermology: 2019. Guidelines: Neuromusculoskeletal thermography. https://aathermology.org/organization-2/guidelines/. Accessed 17 March 2024.

Archer, S.D. & Zinn, J.A. (1983). Thermograms: Persuasive Tools in Soft-Tissue Injury Cases. *Trial* 19: Feb.

Chudecka, M. *et al.* (2015). The use of thermal imaging in the evaluation of the symmetry of muscle activity in various types of exercises (symmetrical and asymmetrical). *J Hum Kinet.* 49:141–147.

Chung, H. *et al.* (2012). The nuts and bolts of low-level laser (light) therapy. *Ann Biomed Eng.* 40(2):516–533.

Cidral-Filho, F.J. *et al.* (2014). Light emitting diode therapy induces analgesia in a mouse model of postoperative pain through activation of peripheral opioid receptors and the L-arginine/nitric oxide pathway. *Lasers Med Sci.* 29 (2):695–702.

Clark, J.A. and Cena, K. (1977). The potential of infrared thermography in veterinary diagnosis. *Vet Rec.* 100:404.

Delahanty, D.D. and Georgi, J.R. (1965). Thermography in equine medicine. *J Am Vet Med Assoc.* 147:235–238.

Flesch, U. *et al.* (1985). Physics of skin surface temperatures. *Thermol Methods*:21–37.

Goodman, A.R. and Zak, P.A. (1986). The heat is on: thermograms as evidence under the Frye standard. *West New England Law Rev.* 8(1).

Lamb, C.R. *et al.* (1988). The first twenty-one years of veterinary diagnostic ultrasound: a bibliography. *Vet Radiol Ultrasound.* 29:37–45.

Mitchell, U.H. and Mack, G.L. (2013). Low-level laser treatment with near-infrared light increases venous nitric oxide levels acutely; a single-blind, randomized clinical trial of efficacy. *Am J Phys Med Rehab.* 92(2):151–156.

Otsuka, K. *et al.* (2002). Imaging of skin thermal properties with estimation of ambient radiation temperatures. *IEEE Eng Med Biol.* 21:65–71.

Passarella, S. and Karu, T. (2014). Absorption of monochromatic and narrow band radiation in the visible and near IR by both mitochondrial and non-mitochondrial photoacceptors results in photobiomodulation. *J Photochem Photobiol B.* 140:344–358.

Purohit, R.C. and McCoy, M.D. (1980). Thermography in the diagnosis of inflammatory process in the horse. *Am J Vet Res.* 41(8):1167–1174.

Purohit, R.C. *et al.* (1977). Value of clinical thermography in veterinary medicine. *Auburn Vet.* 33:104–108.

Samoilova, K.A. *et al.* (2008). Role of nitric oxide in the visible light-induced rapid increase of human skin microcirculation at the local and systemic levels: II: healthy volunteers. *Photomed Laser Surg.* 26(5):443–449.

Smith, K.C. (1991). The photobiological basis of low laser radiation therapy. *Laser Ther.* 3(1):19–24.

Smith, W.M. (1964). Applications of thermography in veterinary medicine. *Am NY Acad Sci.* 121:248–254.

Soroko, M. *et al.* (2017). The influence of breed, age, gender, training level and ambient temperature on forelimb and back temperature in racehorses. *Anim Sci J.* 88(2):347–355.

Viegas, V.N. *et al.* (2007). Effect of low-level laser therapy on inflammatory reactions during wound healing: comparison with meloxicam. *Photomed. Laser Surg.* 25(6):467–473.

Appendix A

Glossary

Ablation The process of removal of tissue by cutting or vaporization.

Absorption The conversion of light to other forms of energy when coming into contact with a chromophore within material media.

Active medium A material selected for containment within a given optical cavity to undergo stimulated emission for the production of radiant energy (photons). The specific medium used within the optical cavity of a laser resonator determines the specific wavelength of laser light produced by that resonator.

Articulated arm A delivery system consisting of an apparatus of tubes and seven 360°-swiveling elbow joints, each joint containing a mirror of high reflectance.

Atom The smallest unit having all the unique physical and chemical properties of any one of the elements, of which there are 108 varieties presently known. An atom consists of a nucleus containing neutrons (uncharged particles) and protons (positively charged particles), around which smaller, negatively charged particles known as electron rotate in orbits that can be elliptic or circular and are constrained to have only certain sizes and distances from the nucleus. In a normal (neutral) atom, the number of electrons is equal to the number of protons.

Attenuation The progressive weakening of a light ray as it penetrates deeper into a material medium. In general, it is caused by both absorption and scattering. In homogeneous, isotropic materials, it is exponential in nature: the ray loses a constant fraction of its intensity in every unit distance of forward travel.

Average power An expression (in Watts) of the total amount of laser energy delivered divided by the duration of the laser exposure. For a pulsed laser, the product of the energy per pulse (Joule) and the pulse frequency (Hertz).

Beam of light A bundle of rays of light traveling in the same general direction with an included solid angle that is less than 90°. May be divergent, convergent, or collimated.

Chromophore A substance, molecule, or tissue type exhibiting selective light-absorbing qualities (often to specific wavelengths), facilitating its conversion to other forms of energy. Also known as a *photoacceptor*.

Coherence A unique characteristic of laser radiation, manifested in two ways: spatial and temporal. Spatial coherence is the coincidence of the crests and valleys of the electrical waves of light rays in a beam, along surfaces that are everywhere perpendicular to the rays. Temporal coherence is the constancy of speed of propagation, frequency, and wavelength of the light waves.

Collimation The property of a beam of light in which all the rays are parallel to one another; the beam has no divergence, and its included solid angle is zero degrees. A characteristic of laser radiation.

Contact mode A laser technique in which the delivery system of the laser comes into direct contact with the skin. Synonymous with "on-contact."

Continuous wave A type of exposure where laser light is continuously emitted as long as the activation switch is depressed. By definition, a continuous wave always possesses a duty cycle of 100%.

Delivery system A means of delivery of laser light from resonator to patient. Its distal end is typically fitted with either a handpiece or other piece of equipment (a microscope or endoscope) for the refinement of laser light delivery to the patient.

Drug-to-light interval The period of time between the administration of a photosensitizer and its activation by light.

Duty cycle The percentage of a given single cyclical period of time in which laser light is being emitted, or "on." For example, in a period of 1 second, if the laser were on for 0.8 seconds and off for 0.2 seconds, the laser's duty cycle would be 80%.

Laser Therapy in Veterinary Medicine: Photobiomodulation, Second Edition. Edited by Christopher J. Winkler and Lisa A. Miller.

Electron The small, negatively charged particle which orbits the nucleus of an atom.

Energy The ability to do work, such as lifting a mass against the force of gravity. The product of power (Watts) and duration (seconds). $1\,J = 1\,W \times 1$ second.

Energy density A synonymous term with fluence (see Fluence).

Excimer A diatomic molecule consisting of a halogen atom (Cl or F) and an atom of noble gas (argon, dkrypton, or xenon), which exists only in the excited state of one or both atoms, and dissociates after emitting radiation in the ultraviolet portion of the spectrum.

Excitation The process by which an atom or molecule or ion increases its energy above the normal, or ground, level. It requires absorption of a quantum of energy from outside having exactly the value corresponding to the difference between the ground level and some permitted higher level.

Exposure The synonymous term used in this textbook for a temporal mode.

Fluence The energy delivered by a laser beam to a target, divided by the irradiated area of that target. The basic unit is $1\,J/cm^2$.

Frequency The number of cycles per second of a sinusoidal wave of light passing a fixed point in space; or the number of pulses per second in the output power of a pulsed laser.

Gaussian The name given to a laser beam that has the most fundamental transverse electromagnetic mode (TEM_{00}), or bell-shaped distribution of power density across the beam.

Handpiece That part of a laser's delivery system held in the hand of a surgeon for delivery of laser light to the patient. Handpieces come in a variety of designs, some with the means to adjust spot size in order to further manipulate control of fluence and power density during a surgical procedure. They are typically made of autoclavable materials to facilitate sterility.

Hertz The basic unit of frequency in the International System (SI) of units, measured in cycles per second.

Hollow waveguide A delivery system consisting of a flexible hollow metal tube, the inner surface of which carries high reflectance.

Index of refraction The ratio of the speed of light in free space to its speed in a material medium. The refractive index of every material medium is greater than unity, except near wavelengths where the medium exhibits significant absorption.

Intensity Synonymous with Irradiance and Power Density of a ray or beam of light (see power density).

Ion An atom in which the number of orbiting electrons is not equal to the number of protons on the nucleus. It has a net electric charge that is either positive or negative, but not zero.

Irradiance Synonymous with intensity and power density of a ray or beam of light (see power density).

Joule (J) The basic unit of energy or work in the International System (SI) of units, equal to an exposure of 1 W of power for 1 second.

Kilogram (Kg) The basic unit of mass in the International System (SI) of units, equal to 1000 g.

Laser An apparatus for the purpose of generating coherent, collimated, monochromatic electromagnetic radiation. The acronym *LASER* stands for ***L**ight **A**mplification by **S**timulated **E**mission of **R**adiation.*

Laser light The spectrum of electromagnetic radiation producible by a laser apparatus, ranging from 100 to 20 000 nm, and consisting of sinusoidal waves of orthogonal electric and magnetic fields that are both perpendicular to its axis of propagation. Characteristics particular to laser light include coherence, collimation, and monochromaticity.

Longitudinal modes Those discrete wavelengths of standing waves of light reflected back and forth between the mirrors of an optical cavity in such a way that the forward and backward waves reinforce each other.

Mass The essential property of matter. Mass is convertible into energy according to the eq. $E = Mc^2$, where E is energy, M is mass, and c is the velocity of light in free space.

Matter The fundamental substance of which all materials in the universe are composed. Its most important property is mass. Its basic unit is the atom.

Meter The basic unit of length in the International System (SI) of units.

Molecule A collection of atoms bound together by forces associated with the outermost electrons. Inorganic molecules are usually smaller than organic, the most complex of which can contain thousands of atoms.

Monochromaticity The property of having just one wavelength. A characteristic of laser radiation.

Micrometer (μm) One millionth (10^{-6}) of a meter. Also known as a *micron*.

Microsecond (μsec) One millionth (10^{-6}) of a second.

Mie scattering A type of scattering caused by particles greater than or equal to the wavelength of the laser light being scattered, predominantly occurring in a forward direction of propagation.

Millisecond (msec) One thousandth (10^{-3}) of a second.

Mode For the purpose of this textbook, the state in which the laser is operating with Superpulse either on or off.

Nanometer (nm) One billionth (10^{-9}) of a meter. In this textbook, the basic unit of a wavelength of laser light.

Nanosecond One billionth (10^{-9}) of a second.

Non-contact mode A laser technique in which the photobiomodulation delivery system does not come into contact with the skin. Light radiation may be focused or defocused depending on operator's technique and procedure.

Optical cavity A chamber or volume of space coaxial with and located between two mirrors whose geometry is such that a paraxial ray of light traveling back and forth between the mirrors will always remain within the cavity.

Optical fiber A delivery system consisting of a solid slender filament of optically transparent material (quartz, glass, or polymethylmethacrylate) having a diameter between 0.1 and 1.0 mm and an index of refraction significantly greater than unity. It is usually clad with a thin coating of another material having a lower index of refraction. It transmits light by total internal reflection, even around bends of short radius.

Peak power The highest power in a laser pulse.

Photobiomodulation (PBM) In medicine, the utilization of light energy to achieve physiological and biochemical changes within tissues in order to obtain a beneficial therapeutic outcome.

Photobiomodulation therapy (PBMT) A noninvasive application of low-level light energy to stimulate cells within tissues to reduce pain and inflammation, promote wound healing, and aid in improving diverse mental and physical health issues.

Photochemolysis Breakdown of living tissue or inorganic polymers by rupture of interatomic bonds caused by energetic photons at wavelengths shorter than 319 nm. This process occurs at average power densities below $1\ \text{W/cm}^2$.

Photodynamic therapy The selective removal of unwanted cells and tissues through the release of reactive (singlet) oxygen by a chemical substance (photosensitizer) following that substance's activation by light.

Photon A massless quantum of radiant energy, transmitted through free space and material media in straight lines at the speed of light. It is equivalent to a wavelet, and its energy is proportional to the frequency of this equivalent wavelet.

Photosensitizer A chemical substance applied topically or systemically with selective uptake by cells that, when activated by light, releases reactive (singlet) oxygen to cause local cell death.

Picosecond One trillionth (10^{-12}) of a second.

Planck's constant The proportionality factor (h) in the equation relating photonic energy to the frequency of the equivalent wavelet:

$$E_p = hf$$

This factor is named after Max Planck and its value is 6.626×10^{-34} J-sec.

Plume The smoke produced from aerosolization of by-products due to laser-tissue interaction. It is composed primarily of water vapor, with cellular debris, particulate matter, carbonaceous and inorganic materials, and potentially biohazardous products.

Population inversion A condition of having more atoms or molecules of a medium in an excited state within a laser resonator than in unexcited or less-excited states.

Power The amount of work performed in a unit of time, such as the time-rate of transfer of energy from one place to another, or transformation of energy from one form to another. The basic unit of power is the watt (W). 1 W = 1 J/1 second.

Power density The power transmitted by a laser beam per unit area of cross-section of that beam, or the power falling upon the target of a laser beam per unit area of the irradiated surface of that target. Also known as intensity and irradiance. The basic unit of power density in laser surgery is $1\ \text{W/cm}^2$.

Pulse duration A measurement of the total amount of time that a pulse is emitted; also known as pulse width.

Pumping The process of adding energy to a laser medium in such a way that its atoms or molecules are excited, creating a population inversion.

Radiation The transport of energy through space from one point to another, with or without the need for an intervening material medium. It occurs in straight lines and at constant speed in a homogeneous, isotropic medium.

Radical A group of connected atoms or ions that passes unchanged through a chemical reaction, and may form an important constituent of a molecule.

Randomly diffused radiant flux Light within tissue having such strong scattering that the probability of photon travel is equal in all possible directions. The exact opposite of collimated, coherent radiation such as laser light. When dealing with randomly diffused radiant flux, power density is the number of photons per unit time passing through a small sphere, divided by the equatorial cross-section of that sphere.

Ray of light The axis of a light wave.

Rayleigh scattering A type of scattering caused by particles less than the wavelength of the laser light being scattered. Unlike Mie scattering, Rayleigh scattering is strongly dependent on the wavelength of laser light and may occur in any direction.

Reflection The redirection of a ray of light from its impact point on the boundary surface between two different media back into the hemisphere of space, centered at the impact point, from which that ray originated, in such a way that the angle of incidence is equal to the angle of reflection (both measured from the perpendicular to the reflecting surface in the plane defined by the incident and reflected rays). In general, some of the intensity of the ray will be lost by penetration into the reflecting medium, so that the reflected ray is relatively weaker than the incident ray.

Refraction The change in direction of a ray of light upon striking the interface between two media of different refractive indices, in such a way that the angle of incidence is always less in the medium of higher index. In general, refraction is accompanied by reflection of some of the intensity of the incident ray, except where the angle of incidence is greater than the critical angle for total reflection in dense-to-rare crossing of the interface.

Repeat pulse A type of exposure where the laser light is emitted intermittently in short bursts as long as the trigger is depressed.

Repetition rate Number of pulses per second, also known as the pulse rate, usually expressed in Hertz.

Resonator That part of a laser apparatus consisting of the optical cavity and the active medium contained therein.

Scattering The change in direction of a ray of light in a material medium or living tissue without a change of wavelength; the result is the dispersal of the ray of light throughout tissue.

Second (sec) The basic unit of time in the International System (SI) of units.

Single pulse A type of exposure where laser light is emitted in only a single timed burst with depression of the trigger.

Singlet oxygen The lowest excited state of the O_2 molecule. Highly cytotoxic in its reaction with surrounding organic compounds.

Spectrum A continuous range of wavelengths or frequencies of electromagnetic radiation. The whole electromagnetic spectrum spans more than 20 orders of magnitude, from long radio waves to ultra-short cosmic rays.

Speed of propagation The distance traveled per unit time by a light wave or photon, without regard to direction. In free space, it is 2.998×10^8 m/sec.

Spontaneous emission The emission of a photon of light by an excited atom or molecule as it returns to a lower level of energy without an external influence. The source of all light in nature.

Spot size In focused laser beam systems, the diameter (in millimeters) of the circular pattern that laser light produces on its target tissue that contains 86% of the total power of the laser beam, or the diameter of the aperture of a handpiece to create just such a circular pattern when held at optimal focal distance from the target tissue. Spot size is inversely proportional to power density.

Stimulated emission The triggering of an excited atom or molecule by an incident photon to emit an identical photon, parallel to and synchronized with the incident photon, but without absorption of the incident photon.

Superpulse A mode of laser light delivery characterized by extremely short pulses of high peak power, in which the pulse durations are shorter than thermal relaxation time, while the spacing between pulses is greater than the thermal relaxation time. Such intense pulses of high power exceed the power of a continuous wave exposure and help to facilitate efficient ablation, while the interval between pulses minimizes collateral thermal trauma. Superpulse may be available in different forms of exposure.

Temporal mode The pattern of time-variation of output power from a laser apparatus. In this textbook, temporal mode is synonymous with *exposure*. Usually available in three pre-programmed forms: continuous wave, repeat pulse, or single pulse.

Thermal relaxation time The rate at which an irradiated tissue diffuses heat; it is dependent on a particular tissue's wavelength-dependent absorption coefficient.

Transmission The passage of laser light directly through tissue without any tissue effects, due to lack of an appropriate absorptive or scattering medium relative to the laser's wavelength.

Transverse electromagnetic mode The distribution of power density across a laser beam as a function of angular position and radial distance from the axis. It is usually abbreviated as TEM_{mn}, where **m** and **n** are integers equal to the number of troughs of power density in the *x*-direction and *y*-direction, respectively, of a three-dimensional (3-D) plot of the intensity profile of the beam in which the *z*-direction is the beam axis of propagation.

Vaporization The conversion of liquid water into vapor.

Velocity (of a photon or wave) The vector whose direction is the direction of travel at the point or moment in question, and whose magnitude is the speed of the wave or photon at that point and moment.

Watt (W) The basic unit of power in the International System (SI) of units. 1 W equals 1 J/sec.

Wavelength The distance between any two successive crests of the electric wave of a ray of light. In this book, measured in nanometers.

Appendix B

Certifying and Academic Laser Organizations

American Board of Laser Surgery (ABLS)
Administrative Office
55 Corporate Drive, 3rd Floor
Trumbull, CT 06611
Phone: 203-332-2507
www.americanboardoflasersurgery.org
lasers1060@gmail.com

American Institute of Medical Laser Applications (AIMLA)
18070 Raymond Rd
Marysville, Ohio 43040
Phone: 937-642-9813
www.aimla.org
aimladvm@aol.com

American Laser Medicine College and Board (ALMCB)
(Advanced-level training and certification in laser surgery and laser dentistry)
Peter Vitruk, PhD
Peter@americanlaserstudyclub.org

American Laser Study Club (ALSC)
www.americanlaserstudyclub.org
ALSC@americanlaserstudyclub.org

American Society for Laser Medicine and Surgery (ASLMS)
2100 Stewart Avenue, Suite 240
Wausau, WI 54401
Phone: 715-845-9283/877-258-6028
www.aslms.org
information@aslms.org

Laser Institute of America (LIA)
13501 Ingenuity Drive, Suite 128
Orlando, FL 32826
Phone: 1-800-345-2737
www.lia.org
https://www.lia.org/contact

International Academy for Laser Medicine and Surgery (IALMS)
Borgo Pinti 57
50121 Florence IT
(+39) 055.234.2330
http://ialms.international/
secretary@ialms.international

North American Association for PhotobiomoduLation Therapy (NAALT)
Terrance L. Baker, MD, MS
3700 Koppers Street, Suite 100
Baltimore, MD 21227
Phone: 410-592-9889
www.naalt.org
www.naalt.org/contact/

World Association for Photobiomodulation Therapy (WALT)
3435 Main Street
B36A, Foster Hall
Buffalo, NY, 14214
https://waltpbm.org/
INFO@WALTPBM.ORG

Laser Therapy in Veterinary Medicine: Photobiomodulation, Second Edition. Edited by Christopher J. Winkler and Lisa A. Miller.

Index

Note: *Italic* page numbers refer to *figure* and **Bold** page numbers reference to **tables**.

a

Laser Therapy in Veterinary Medicine: Photobiomodulation, Second Edition. Edited by Christopher J. Winkler and Lisa A. Miller.